the calorie carb and fat bible 2006

Juliette Kellow BSc RD and Rebecca Walton

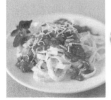   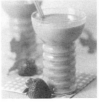 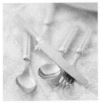

The UK's Most Comprehensive Calorie Counter

The Calorie, Carb & Fat Bible 2006

© Weight Loss Resources 2006

Published by:
Weight Loss Resources
Remus House
Peterborough
PE2 9JX

Tel: 01733 345592
www.weightlossresources.co.uk

Companies and other organisations wishing to make bulk purchases of the Calorie, Carb and Fat Bible should contact their local bookstore or Weight Loss Resources direct.

Whilst every effort has been made to ensure accuracy, the publishers cannot be held responsible for any errors or omissions.

ISBN 1 904512 03 8

Authors: Juliette Kellow BSc RD
          Rebecca Walton

Design & Layout: Joanne Readshaw / Jonathan Slater

Printed and bound in Finland by:
WS Bookwell Oy

Contents

Losing weight – the easy way

CHINESE TAKEAWAYS, curries, chocolate, chips and a glass of wine! Imagine being told the best diet to help you lose weight includes all these foods and more. It sounds too good to be true, doesn't it? But the truth is, these are exactly the types of foods you can still enjoy if you opt to lose weight by counting calories.

But you'd be forgiven for not knowing you can still eat all your favourite foods – and lose weight. In recent years, endless trendy diets that cut carbs, boost protein intakes or skip entire groups of foods, have helped to make dieting a complicated business. Added to this, an increasing number of celebrities and so-called nutrition experts have helped mislead us into thinking that dieting is all about restriction and denial. Is it any wonder then that most of us have been left feeling downright confused and miserable about what we should and shouldn't be eating to shift those pounds?

But dieting doesn't have to be complicated or an unhappy experience. In fact, there's really only one word you need to remember if you want to shift those pounds healthily and still eat all your favourite foods. And that's the CALORIE!

It's calories that count

When it comes to losing weight, there's no getting away from the fact that it's calories that count. Ask any qualified nutrition expert or dietitian for advice on how to fight the flab and you'll receive the same reply: quite simply you need to create a calorie deficit or shortfall. In other words, you need to take in fewer calories than you use up so that your body has to draw on its fat stores to provide it with the energy it needs to function properly. The result: you start losing fat and the pounds start to drop off!

Fortunately, it couldn't be easier to create this calorie deficit. Regardless of your age, weight, sex, genetic make up, lifestyle or eating habits, losing weight is as simple as reducing your daily calorie intake slightly by modifying your diet and using up a few more calories by being slightly more active each day.

Better still, it's a complete myth that you need to change your eating and exercise habits dramatically. You'll notice I've said you need to reduce your calorie intake 'slightly' and be 'slightly' more active. It really is just LITTLE differences between the amount of calories we take in and the amount we use up that make BIG differences to our waistline over time. For example, you only need to consume one can of cola more than you need each day to gain a stone in a year. It's no wonder then that people say excess weight tends to 'creep up on them'.

10 simple food swaps you can make every day (*and won't even notice!*)

Make these simple swaps every day and in just 4 weeks you'll lose 7lb!

SWAP THIS...	FOR THIS...	SAVE...
300ml full-fat milk *(195 calories)*	300ml skimmed milk *(100 calories)*	95 calories
1tsp butter *(35 calories)*	1tsp low-fat spread *(20 calories)*	15 calories
1tbsp vegetable oil *(100 calories)*	10 sprays of a spray oil *(10 calories)*	90 calories
1tsp sugar *(16 calories)*	Artificial sweetener *(0 calories)*	16 calories
1tbsp mayonnaise *(105 calories)*	1tbsp fat-free dressing *(10 calories)*	95 calories
Regular sandwich *(600 calories)*	Low-fat sandwich *(350 calories)*	250 calories
Can of cola *(135 calories)*	Can of diet cola *(0 calories)*	135 calories
Large (50g) packet of crisps *(250 calories)*	Small (25g) packet of crisps *(135 calories)*	115 calories
1 chocolate digestive *(85 calories)*	1 small chocolate chip cookie *(55 calories)*	30 calories
1 slice thick-cut wholemeal bread *(95 calories)*	1 slice medium-cut wholemeal bread *(75 calories)*	20 calories
	TOTAL CALORIE SAVING:	*861 calories*

The good news is the reverse is also true. You only need to swap that daily can of cola for the diet version or a glass of sparking water and you'll lose a stone in a year – it really is as easy as that!

Of course, most people don't want to wait a year to shift a stone. But there's more good news. To lose 1lb of fat each week you need to create a calorie deficit of just 500 calories a day. That might sound like a lot, but you can achieve this by simply swapping a croissant for a wholemeal fruit scone, a regular sandwich for a low-fat variety, a glass of dry white wine for a gin and slimline tonic and using low-fat spread on two slices of toast instead of butter. And losing 1lb a week, amounts to a stone in 14 weeks, or just under 4 stone in a year!

Taking control of calories

By now you've seen it really is calories that count when it comes to shifting those pounds. So it should be no surprise that a calorie-controlled diet is the only guaranteed way to help you shift those pounds – and that's a science fact! But better still, a calorie-controlled diet is one of the few that allows you to eat just about anything, whether it's pizza, wine or chocolate. Providing you count the calories – and stick to your daily allowance – you can eat whatever you want, whenever you want!

And that's where this book can really help. Gone are the days when it was virtually impossible to obtain information about the calorie contents of foods. This book provides calorie information for more than 21,000 different branded and unbranded foods so that counting calories has never been easier.

The benefits of counting calories
✔ *It's guaranteed to help you lose weight providing you stick to your daily calorie allowance*
✔ *You can eat all your favourite foods*
✔ *No foods are banned or restricted*
✔ *It's a great way to lose weight slowly and steadily*
✔ *Nutrition experts agree that it's a proven way to lose weight*

Calorie counting made easy

Forget weird and wacky science, complicated diet rules and endless lists of foods to fill up on or avoid every day! Counting calories to lose weight couldn't be easier. Quite simply, you set yourself a daily calorie allowance to help you lose between ½-2lb a week and then add up the calories of everything you eat and drink each day, making sure you don't go over your limit.

To prevent hunger from kicking in, it's best to spread your daily calorie allowance evenly throughout the day, allowing a certain amount of calories for breakfast, lunch, dinner and one or two snacks. For example, if you are allowed 1,500 calories a day, you could have 300 calories for breakfast, 400 calories for lunch, 500 calories for dinner and two snacks or treats of 150 calories each. You'll find more detailed information on p16-20 (Your step-by-step guide to using this book and shifting those pounds).

QUESTION
What affects the calorie content of a food?

ANSWER:
Fat, protein, carbohydrate and alcohol all provide the body with calories, but in varying amounts:

- *1g fat provides 9 calories*

- *1g alcohol provides 7 calories*

- *1g protein provides 4 calories*

- *1g carbohydrate provides 3.75 calories*

The calorie content of a food depends on the amount of fat, protein and carbohydrate it contains. Because fat provides more than twice as many calories as an equal quantity of protein or carbohydrate, in general, foods that are high in fat tend to contain more calories. This explains why 100g of chips (189 calories) contains more than twice as many calories as 100g of boiled potato (72 calories).

DIET MYTH:
Food eaten late at night stops you losing weight

DIET FACT:

It's not eating in the evening that stops you losing weight. It's consuming too many calories throughout the day that will be your dieting downfall! Providing you stick to your daily calorie allowance you'll lose weight, regardless of when you consume those calories. Nevertheless, it's a good idea to spread your calorie allowance throughout the day to prevent hunger from kicking in, which leaves you reaching for high-calorie snack foods.

Eat for good health

While calories might be the buzz word when it comes to shifting those pounds, it's nevertheless important to make sure your diet is healthy, balanced and contains all the nutrients you need for good health. Yes, you can still lose weight by eating nothing but, for example, chocolate, crisps and biscuits providing you stick to your calorie allowance. But you'll never find a nutrition expert or dietitian recommending this. And there are plenty of good reasons why.

To start with, an unbalanced diet is likely to be lacking in essential nutrients such as protein, vitamins, minerals and fibre, in the long term putting you at risk of nutritional deficiencies. Secondly, research proves that filling up on foods that are high in fat and/or salt and sugar can lead to many different health problems. But most importantly, when it comes to losing weight, it's almost impossible to stick to a daily calorie allowance if you're only eating high-calorie foods.

Filling up on lower-calorie foods also means you'll be able to eat far more with the result that you're not constantly left feeling unsatisfied. For example, six chocolates from a selection box contain around 300 calories, a lot of fat and sugar, few nutrients – and are eaten in just six mouthfuls! For 300 calories, you could have a grilled skinless chicken breast (packed with protein and zinc), a large salad with fat-free dressing (a great source of fibre, vitamins and minerals), a slice of wholemeal bread with low-fat spread (rich in fibre and B vitamins) and a satsuma (an excellent source of vitamin C). That's a lot more food that will take you a lot more time to eat! Not convinced? Then put six chocolates on one plate, and the chicken, salad, bread and fruit on another!

Bottom line: while slightly reducing your calorie intake is the key to losing weight, you'll be healthier and far more likely to keep those pounds off if you do it by eating a healthy diet. You'll find more information about healthy eating on p21-24.

Eight steps to a healthy diet
1 *Enjoy your food*
2 *Eat a variety of different foods*
3 *Eat the right amount to be a healthy weight*
4 *Eat plenty of foods rich in starch and fibre*
5 *Don't eat too much fat*
6 *Don't eat sugary foods too often*
7 *Look after the vitamins and minerals in your food*
8 *If you drink alcohol, keep within sensible limits.*

Fat facts

Generally speaking, opting for foods that are low in fat can help slash your calorie intake considerably, for example, swapping full-fat milk for skimmed, switching from butter to a low-fat spread, not frying food in oil and chopping the fat off meat and poultry. But don't be fooled into believing that all foods described as 'low-fat' or 'fat-free' are automatically low in calories or calorie-free. In fact, some low-fat products may actually be higher in calories than standard products, thanks to them containing extra sugars and thickeners to boost the flavour and texture. The solution: always check the calorie content of low-fat foods, especially for things like cakes, biscuits, crisps, ice creams and ready meals. You might be surprised to find there's little difference in the calorie content when compared to the standard product.

Uncovering fat claims on food labels

Many products may lure you into believing they're a great choice if you're trying to cut fat, but you need to read between the lines on the labels if you want to be sure you're making the best choice. Here's the lowdown on what to look for:

LOW FAT	by law the food must contain less than 3g of fat per 100g. These foods are generally a good choice if you're trying to lose weight.
REDUCED FAT	by law the food must contain 25 percent less fat than a similar standard product. This doesn't mean the product is low-fat (or low-calorie) though! For example, reduced-fat cheese may still contain 14g fat per 100g.
FAT FREE	the food must contain less than 0.15g fat per 100g. Foods labelled as Virtually Fat Free must contain less than 0.3g fat per 100g. These foods are generally a good choice if you're trying to lose weight.
LESS THAN 8% FAT	this means the product contains less than 8g fat per 100g. It's only foods labelled 'less than 3% fat' that are a true low-fat choice.
X% FAT FREE	the Food Standards Agency believe terms such as 90% and 95% fat free are misleading and so shouldn't be used. Another way of describing a food that claims to be 90% fat free is to say that it contains 10% fat (10g fat per 100g) – and that's a fair amount!
LIGHT OR LITE	there are no rules for the use of these terms and so manufacturers often use them as they wish, for example, to imply a product has less fat or fewer calories. The Food Standards Agency recommends manufacturers explain exactly what the claim means on the label.

10 easy ways to slash fat (and calories)

1   Eat fewer fried foods – grill, boil, bake, poach, steam, roast without added fat or microwave instead.

2   Don't add butter, lard, margarine or oil to food during preparation or cooking.

3   Use spreads sparingly. Butter and margarine contain the same amount of calories and fat – only low fat spreads contain less.

4   Choose boiled or jacket potatoes instead of chips or roast potatoes.

5   Cut off all visible fat from meat and remove the skin from chicken before cooking.

6   Don't eat too many fatty meat products such as sausages, burgers, pies and pastry products.

7   Use semi-skimmed or skimmed milk instead of full-fat milk.

8   Try low-fat or reduced-fat varieties of cheese such as reduced-fat Cheddar, low-fat soft cheese or cottage cheese.

9   Eat fewer high-fat foods such as crisps, chocolates, cakes, pastries and biscuits.

10   Don't add cream to puddings, sauces or coffee.

Getting started

Hopefully by now, you're excited about getting started. But before rushing into things, it's worth taking time to prepare yourself mentally for the weeks ahead. Here are some top tips to put you on the road to success.

1. Put previous failures behind you

Don't dwell on dieting successes and failures you've had in the past. The chances are if you need to lose weight now, they weren't right for you. Instead, make a promise to yourself that this will be the last time you'll ever need to lose weight.

2. Use your head

Add up all the hours you've wasted in the last month worrying about your weight and what you eat. Then compare them with the number of hours you've spent feeling great about your size, shape and diet! Hold on to the fact that before too long, you'll be changing those negative thoughts for positive ones.

3. Visualise the new slim you

Spend some time visualising your new life as a slimmer, fitter and healthier you. Find somewhere quiet where you won't be disturbed, sit in a comfortable chair and close your eyes. In your mind's eye see yourself as the slimmer you. How does it feel? How much more confident are you? How do you look? What are you wearing? What are you doing in your new life? What ambitions do you have? What changes have you made? Hold onto this image of the new you and as you continue on the road to losing weight, take time to revisit it at regular intervals. Holding onto this image will help you to stay focussed and boost your determination if things get tough.

4. Prepare to fit food around your lifestyle

Forget about trying to change the way you live to accommodate a new way of eating – it's guaranteed to result in failure. Trying to turn yourself into a Domestic Goddess when you work incredibly long hours or only buying foods from a health food shop when you have a family of four to feed will quickly result in you ditching your new way of eating. Instead, fit your diet around your lifestyle and you'll be far more likely to shift those pounds.

5. Identify bad habits

More often than not, we eat out of habit rather than because we are hungry – and this can easily sabotage good intentions. Spend some time identifying those occasions when you eat out of habit. For example, do you always go straight to the fridge when you get home? Do you always have a biscuit with your morning coffee? Do you always buy a cake when you walk past the bakery? Then look at ways to swap these old habits for new, healthier ones. For example, go straight to the fruit bowl when you get in; swap your coffee and biscuit for sparkling water and fruit; or take a different route home that avoids the bakery.

6. Avoid 'all or nothing' thinking

Prepare yourself for the fact that you will probably overindulge from time to time. But also prepare for how you will deal with this. Remember, one small over-indulgence doesn't mean you've 'blown your diet' or give you free licence to go on a food fest! Simply put the indulgence behind you and move on. Tomorrow is another day.

7. Think positively about food

Dieting shouldn't be about denial and deprivation. Instead of thinking about all the foods you should be eating less of, focus on all the foods you will be able to eat more of. And don't picture them in a negative light. Think of words to describe them that makes them sound delicious, for example, a juicy, crunchy apple, a mouth-watering bowl of strawberries or a satisfying, filling slice of wholegrain bread.

8. Healthy eating is for life

Ban the word 'diet' from your vocabulary and instead focus on the fact you'll be changing your eating habits for life. 'Going on a diet' infers you start on a particular day, finish on a particular day and only change what you eat in between, so that once your 'diet' is finished you return to the eating habits that made you pile on the pounds in the first place! Instead, use this time to kickstart a long-term healthy eating plan you can sustain for life.

What you'll need

One of the advantages of calorie counting is that you don't need to spend a fortune on expensive equipment or food. However, it's worth arming yourself with a few essential tools:

✔ *A notepad and pen – use this to keep track of everything you eat and drink*

✔ *A calculator – to tot up all those calories.*

✔ *A set of food scales – they don't need to cost a fortune. A simple set of scales is all you need to weigh portions of food.*

✔ *A tape measure – to measure your vital statistics.*

✔ *The Calorie, Carb & Fat Bible – it contains all the information you need to succeed!*

Your step-by-step guide to using this book and shifting those pounds

1. Find your perfect weight

Use the weight charts, body mass index table and information on pages 25-27 to determine the right weight for you. Then set yourself a weight to aim for. If you have a lot of weight to lose, you may find it helpful to break your total weight loss down into smaller chunks of, for example, a stone or half a stone. This will make dieting seem less daunting and will give your motivation and confidence a boost as you reach each target.

2. Set a realistic time scale

With today's hectic lifestyles, everything tends to happen at breakneck speed, so it's no wonder that when it comes to losing weight, most of us want to shift those pounds in an instant. But it's probably taken years to accumulate that extra weight, with the result that it's unrealistic to expect to lose the excess in just a few weeks! Instead, prepare yourself to lose weight slowly and steadily. It's far healthier to lose weight like this. But better still, research shows you'll be far more likely to maintain your new, lower weight.

If you only have a small amount of weight to lose, aim for a weight loss of around 1lb a week. But if you have more than 2 stone to lose, you may prefer to aim for 2lb each week. Remember though, it's better to keep going at 1lb a week than to give up because trying to lose 2lb a week is making you miserable! The following words may help you to keep your goal in perspective:

'Never give up on a goal because of the time it will take to achieve it – the time will pass anyway.'

3. Calculate your calorie allowance

Use the calorie tables on pages 28-29 to find out how many calories you need each day to maintain your current weight. Then use the table below to discover the amount of calories you need to subtract from this amount every day to lose weight at your chosen rate. For example, a 35 year-old woman who is moderately active and weighs 12 stone needs 2,188 calories a day to keep her weight steady. If she wants to lose 1/2lb a week, she needs 250 calories less each day, giving her a daily calorie allowance of 1,938 calories. If she wants to lose 1lb a week, she needs 500 calories less each day, giving her a daily calorie allowance of 1,688 calories, and so on.

TO LOSE...	Cut your daily calorie intake by	In three months you could lose...	In six months you could lose...	In one year you could lose...
½lb a week	250	6.5lb	13lb	1st 12lb
1lb a week	500	13lb	1st 12lb	3st 10lb
1½lb a week	750	1st 5.5lb	2st 11lb	5st 8lb
2lb a week	1,000	1st 12lb	3st 10lb	7st 6lb

Danger Zone

Although you may lose a little more than 2lb each week when you first start dieting, in the long term you should never try to lose more than this. Severely restricting restrict your calorie intake in an effort to lose weight quickly means you'll lose protein (in the form of muscle) as well as fat. This is bad news as muscle burns calories and helps to set your metabolism. Ultimately, if you lose muscle, you'll also lose its calorie-burning capacity, making it even more difficult to shift those pounds – and keep them off.

If you find you are regularly losing more than 2lb a week, increase your calorie intake slightly. Generally, most people should avoid having less than 1,100 calories a day.

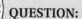

QUESTION:
Do I need to stick to exactly the same number of calories each day or is it OK to have a lower calorie intake during the week and slightly more at the weekend?

ANSWER:
The key to losing weight is to take in fewer calories than you need for as long as it takes to reach your target, aiming for a loss of no more than 2lb a week. In general, most nutrition experts recommend a daily calorie allowance. However, it's just as valid to use other periods of time such as weeks. If you prefer, simply multiply your daily allowance by seven to work out a weekly calorie allowance and then allocate more calories to some days than others. For example, a daily allowance of 1,500 calories is equivalent to 10,500 calories a week. This means you could have 1,300 calories a day during the week and 2,000 calories a day on Saturday and Sunday.

QUESTION:
Why are heavier people allowed more calories than those who have smaller amounts of weight to lose?

ANSWER:
This confuses a lot of people but is easily explained. Someone who is 3 stone overweight, for example, is carrying the equivalent of 42 small packets of butter with them everywhere they go – up and down the stairs, to the local shops, into the kitchen. Obviously, it takes a lot more energy simply to move around when you're carrying that extra weight. As a consequence, the heavier you are, the more calories you need just to keep your weight steady. In turn, this means you'll lose weight on a higher calorie allowance. However, as you lose weight, you'll need to lower your calorie allowance slightly as you have less weight to carry around.

4. Keep a food diary

Keeping a food diary before you even start to change your eating habits will help you identify opportunities for cutting calories by substituting one food for another, cutting portion sizes of high-calorie foods or eating certain foods less often. Simply write down every single item you eat or drink during the day and use this book to calculate the calories of each item. Then after a few days of eating normally, introduce some changes to your diet to achieve your daily calorie allowance. Remember to spread your daily calorie allowance evenly throughout the day to prevent hunger.

You'll find a template for a daily food diary on page 31. Remember to include every single item that passes your lips, including drinks, and be accurate about portion sizes.

Top Tip

If you only fill in your main food diary once a day, keep a pen and notepad with you to write down all those little extras you eat or drink during the day – that chocolate you ate in the office, the slither of cheese you had while cooking dinner and the few chips you pinched from your husband's plate, for example! It's easy to forget the little things if they're not written down, but they can make the difference between success and failure.

5. Control your portions

As well as making some smart food swaps to cut calories, it's likely you'll also need to reduce your serving sizes for some foods to help shift those pounds. Even 'healthy' foods such as brown rice, wholemeal bread, chicken, fish and low-fat dairy products contain calories so you may need to limit the amount you eat. When you first start out, weigh portions of foods like rice, pasta, cereal, cheese, butter, oil, meat, fish, and chicken rather than completing your food diary with a 'guesstimated' weight! That way you can calculate the calorie content accurately. Don't forget that drinks contain calories too, alcohol, milk, juices and sugary drinks all count.

6. Measure your success

It's important to keep a record of how well you're doing, but this doesn't mean jumping on the scales several times a day! Most people's weight fluctuates dramatically throughout the day – often making it look as though you've gained 4lb between 8am and 8pm! This will do little to keep you motivated, so weigh yourself just once a week, at the same time of day – most people prefer first thing in the morning – and wearing the same clothing. Don't just focus on what the bathroom scales say either – keep a record of your vital statistics, too. Many people find it doubly encouraging to see the inches dropping off, as well as the pounds!

Top Tip

If you can't stay off the scales, ask a friend to store them for you and weigh yourself just once a week when you're out shopping.

7. Stay motivated

Each time you lose half a stone – celebrate! Treat yourself to a little luxury – something new to wear, a little pampering or some other (non-food!) treat. Digging out some old pictures of yourself when you were bigger or trying on an item of clothing that used to be tight can also help to keep you feeling motivated. Once you've reviewed how well you've done, you should then use this book to set yourself a new daily calorie allowance based on your new weight to help you lose the next half stone (see point 3 - Calculate your calorie allowance, above).

8. Keep it off

What you do to stay slim is just as important as what you did to get slim. Quite simply, if you return to your old ways, you can expect to return to your old weight! The great thing about calorie counting is that you will learn so much about what you eat, and make so many important changes to your eating and drinking habits, that you'll probably find it difficult to go back to your old ways – and won't want to anyway. It's still a good idea to weigh yourself once a week to keep a check on your weight. The key is to deal with any extra pounds immediately, rather than waiting until you have a stone to lose. Simply go back to counting calories for as long as it takes to shift those pounds and enjoy the new slim you!

Healthy eating made easy

GONE ARE THE DAYS when a healthy diet meant surviving on bird seed, rabbit food and carrot juice! The new approach to eating healthily means we're positively encouraged to eat a wide range of foods, including some of our favourites – it's just a question of making sure we don't eat high fat, high sugar or highly processed foods too often.

Eating a healthy diet, together with taking regular exercise and not smoking, has huge benefits to our health, both in the short and long term. As well as helping us to lose or maintain our weight, a healthy diet can boost energy levels, keep our immune system strong and give us healthy skin, nails and hair. Meanwhile, eating well throughout life also means we're far less likely to suffer from health problems such as constipation, anaemia and tooth decay or set ourselves up for serious conditions in later life such as obesity, heart disease, stroke, diabetes, cancer or osteoporosis.

Fortunately, it couldn't be easier to eat a balanced diet. To start with, no single food provides all the calories and nutrients we need to stay healthy, so it's important to eat a variety of foods. Meanwhile, most nutrition experts also agree that mealtimes should be a pleasure rather than a penance. This means it's fine to eat small amounts of our favourite treats from time to time.

To help people eat healthily, the Food Standards Agency recommends eating plenty of different foods from four main groups of foods and limiting the amount we eat from a smaller fifth group. Ultimately, we should eat more fruit, vegetables, starchy, fibre-rich foods and fresh products, and fewer fatty, sugary, salty and processed foods.

The following guidelines are all based on the healthy eating guidelines recommended by the Food Standards Agency.

Bread, other cereals and potatoes

Eat these foods at each meal. They also make good snacks.

Foods in this group include bread, breakfast cereals, potatoes, rice, pasta, noodles, yams, oats and grains. Go for high-fibre varieties where available, such as wholegrain cereals, wholemeal bread and brown rice. These foods should fill roughly a third of your plate at mealtimes.

TYPICAL SERVING SIZES

- *2 slices bread in a sandwich or with a meal*

- *a tennis ball sized serving of pasta, potato, rice, noodles or couscous*

- *a bowl of porridge*

- *around 40g of breakfast cereal*

Fruit and vegetables

Eat five different servings every day

Foods in this group include all fruits and vegetables, including fresh, frozen, canned and dried products, and unsweetened fruit juice. Choose canned fruit in juice rather than syrup and go for veg canned in water without added salt or sugar. These foods should fill roughly a third of your plate at mealtimes.

TYPICAL SERVING SIZES

- *a piece of fruit eg apple, banana, pear*

- *2 small fruits eg satsumas, plums, apricots*

- *a bowl of fruit salad, canned or stewed fruit*

- *a small glass of unsweetened fruit juice*

- *a cereal bowl of salad*

- *3tbsp vegetables*

Milk and dairy foods

Eat two or three servings a day.

Foods in this group include milk, cheese, yogurt and fromage frais. Choose low-fat varieties where available such as skimmed milk, reduced-fat cheese and fat-free yoghurt. These foods should fill no more than a sixth of your plate at mealtimes.

TYPICAL SERVING SIZES

- *200ml milk*

- *a small pot of yoghurt or fromage frais*

- *a small matchbox-sized piece of cheese*

Meat, fish and alternatives

Eat two servings a day

Foods in this group include meat, poultry, fish, eggs, beans, nuts and seeds. Choose low-fat varieties where available such as extra-lean minced beef and skinless chicken and don't add extra fat or salt. These foods should fill no more than a sixth of your plate at mealtimes.

TYPICAL SERVING SIZES

- *a piece of meat, chicken or fish the size of a deck of cards*

- *1-2 eggs*

- *3 heaped tablespoons of beans*

- *a small handful of nuts or seeds*

Fatty and sugary foods

Eat only small amounts of these foods

Foods in this group include oils, spreading fats, cream, mayonnaise, oily salad dressings, cakes, biscuits, puddings, crisps, savoury snacks, sugar, preserves, confectionery and sugary soft drinks.

TYPICAL SERVING SIZES:

- *a small packet of sweets or a small bar of chocolate*
- *a small slice of cake*
- *a couple of small biscuits*
- *1 level tbsp mayo, salad dressing or olive oil*
- *a small packet of crisps*

How to make your plate a slimming plate

It's really easy. Stick to the same proportions of the different foods on your plate but choose lower-calorie foods from each section. If you want to be really strict, you could also replace any fatty and sugary foods on your plate for extra fruit and veggies.

Body Mass Index

Body Mass Index is a number calculated from an individual's weight and height, that is used to determine whether a person is within, or outside of, a normal weight range. Use the Body Mass Index Chart to look up your BMI, and use the table below to see what range you fall into.

BMI	
Less than 20	*Under Weight*
20-25	*Normal Weight*
25-30	*Over Weight*
30-40	*Obese*
Over 40	*Severely Obese*

The spread from 20-25 shows that what is normal covers quite a big range. This is because 'normal' weight for height covers both men and women, and people of different shapes and body composition. A man would normally be expected to have a higher BMI than a woman of the same height, because men tend to have more muscle than women (women naturally have more fat) and muscle weighs more per square inch than fat. For the same reason a slim, muscular woman will have a higher BMI (i.e. weigh more) than a slim, not very muscular woman of the same height.

What's the Right Weight for You?

As a general rule women, unless they are very strong and muscular, will tend to look at their best at the lower end of the normal range, men around the middle to top of the range. 'Ideal weight' is a very individual thing, probably the best thing to do is set a goal within the normal range as described above and, as you get closer to it, adjust to a level at which you feel at your best.

Body Mass Index Table

HEIGHT IN FEET / INCHES

	4'6	4'8	4'10	5'0	5'2	5'4	5'6	5'8	5'10	6'0	6'2	6'4	6'6	6'8	6'10
6st 7	22.0	20.5	19.1	17.8	16.7	15.7	14.7	13.9	13.1	12.4	11.7	11.1	10.6	10.0	9.5
7st 0	23.7	22.1	20.6	19.2	18.0	16.9	15.9	15.0	14.1	13.3	12.6	12.0	11.4	10.8	10.3
7st 7	25.4	23.6	22.0	20.6	19.3	18.1	17.0	16.0	15.1	14.3	13.5	12.8	12.2	11.6	11.0
8st 0	27.1	25.2	23.5	22.0	20.6	19.3	18.1	17.1	16.1	15.2	14.4	13.7	13.0	12.3	11.8
8st 7	28.8	26.8	25.0	23.3	21.8	20.5	19.3	18.2	17.1	16.2	15.3	14.5	13.8	13.1	12.5
9st 0	30.5	28.4	26.4	24.7	23.1	21.7	20.4	19.2	18.1	17.2	16.2	15.4	14.6	13.9	13.2
9st 7	32.2	29.9	27.9	26.1	24.4	22.9	21.5	20.3	19.2	18.1	17.1	16.2	15.4	14.7	14.0
10st 0	33.9	31.5	29.4	27.4	25.7	24.1	22.7	21.4	20.2	19.1	18.0	17.1	16.2	15.4	14.7
10st 7	35.6	33.1	30.8	28.8	27.0	25.3	23.8	22.4	21.2	20.0	18.9	18.0	17.0	16.2	15.4
11st 0	37.3	34.7	32.3	30.2	28.3	26.5	24.9	23.5	22.2	21.0	19.8	18.8	17.9	17.0	16.2
11st 7	39.0	36.2	33.8	31.6	29.6	27.7	26.1	24.6	23.2	21.9	20.7	19.7	18.7	17.8	16.9
12st 0	40.7	37.8	35.2	32.9	30.8	28.9	27.2	25.6	24.2	22.9	21.6	20.5	19.5	18.5	17.6
12st 7	42.3	39.4	36.7	34.3	32.1	30.1	28.3	26.7	25.2	23.8	22.5	21.4	20.3	19.3	18.4
13st 0	44.0	41.0	38.2	35.7	33.4	31.4	29.5	27.8	26.2	24.8	23.5	22.2	21.1	20.1	19.1
13st 7	45.7	42.5	39.6	37.0	34.7	32.6	30.6	28.8	27.2	25.7	24.4	23.1	21.9	20.8	19.8
14st 0	47.4	44.1	41.1	38.4	36.0	33.8	31.7	29.9	28.2	26.7	25.3	23.9	22.7	21.6	20.6
14st 7	49.1	45.7	42.6	39.8	37.3	35.0	32.9	31.0	29.2	27.6	26.2	24.8	23.5	22.4	21.3
15st 0	50.8	47.3	44.0	41.2	38.5	36.2	34.0	32.0	30.2	28.6	27.1	25.7	24.4	23.2	22.0
15st 7	52.5	48.8	45.5	42.5	39.8	37.4	35.2	33.1	31.2	29.5	28.0	26.5	25.2	23.9	22.8
16st 0	54.2	50.4	47.0	43.9	41.1	38.6	36.3	34.2	32.3	30.5	28.9	27.4	26.0	24.7	23.5
16st 7	55.9	52.0	48.5	45.3	42.4	39.8	37.4	35.2	33.3	31.4	29.8	28.2	26.8	25.5	24.2
17st 0	57.6	53.6	49.9	46.6	43.7	41.0	38.6	36.3	34.3	32.4	30.7	29.1	27.6	26.2	25.0
17st 7	59.3	55.1	51.4	48.0	45.0	42.2	39.7	37.4	35.3	33.3	31.6	29.9	28.4	27.0	25.7
18st 0	61.0	56.7	52.9	49.4	46.3	43.4	40.8	38.5	36.3	34.3	32.5	30.8	29.2	27.8	26.4
18st 7	62.7	58.3	54.3	50.8	47.5	44.6	42.0	39.5	37.3	35.3	33.4	31.6	30.0	28.6	27.2
19st 0	64.4	59.9	55.8	52.1	48.8	45.8	43.1	40.6	38.3	36.2	34.3	32.5	30.8	29.3	27.9
19st 7	66.1	61.4	57.3	53.5	50.1	47.0	44.2	41.7	39.3	37.2	35.2	33.3	31.7	30.1	28.6
20st 0	67.8	63.0	58.7	54.9	51.4	48.2	45.4	42.7	40.3	38.1	36.1	34.2	32.5	30.9	29.4
20st 7	69.4	64.6	60.2	56.3	52.7	49.4	46.5	43.8	41.3	39.1	37.0	35.1	33.3	31.6	30.1
21st 0	71.1	66.2	61.7	57.6	54.0	50.6	47.6	44.9	42.3	40.0	37.9	35.9	34.1	32.4	30.9
21st 7	72.8	67.7	63.1	59.0	55.3	51.9	48.8	45.9	43.3	41.0	38.8	36.8	34.9	33.2	31.6
22st 0	74.5	69.3	64.6	60.4	56.5	53.1	49.9	47.0	44.4	41.9	39.7	37.6	35.7	34.0	32.3
22st 7	76.2	70.9	66.1	61.7	57.8	54.3	51.0	48.1	45.4	42.9	40.6	38.5	36.5	34.7	33.1
23st 0	77.9	72.5	67.5	63.1	59.1	55.5	52.2	49.1	46.4	43.8	41.5	39.3	37.3	35.5	33.8
23st 7	79.6	74.0	69.0	64.5	60.4	56.7	53.3	50.2	47.4	44.8	42.4	40.2	38.2	36.3	34.5
24st 0	81.3	75.6	70.5	65.9	61.7	57.9	54.4	51.3	48.4	45.7	43.3	41.0	39.0	37.0	35.3
24st 7	83.0	77.2	71.9	67.2	63.0	59.1	55.6	52.3	49.4	46.7	44.2	41.9	39.8	37.8	36.0
25st 0	84.7	78.8	73.4	68.6	64.2	60.3	56.7	53.4	50.4	47.6	45.1	42.8	40.6	38.6	36.7
25st 7	86.4	80.3	74.9	70.0	65.5	61.5	57.8	54.5	51.4	48.6	46.0	43.6	41.4	39.4	37.5
26st 0	88.1	81.9	76.3	71.3	66.8	62.7	59.0	55.5	52.4	49.5	46.9	44.5	42.2	40.1	38.2
26st 7	89.8	83.5	77.8	72.7	68.1	63.9	60.1	56.6	53.4	50.5	47.8	45.3	43.0	40.9	38.9
27st 0	91.5	85.1	79.3	74.1	69.4	65.1	61.2	57.7	54.4	51.5	48.7	46.2	43.8	41.7	39.7
27st 7	93.2	86.6	80.8	75.5	70.7	66.3	62.4	58.7	55.4	52.4	49.6	47.0	44.7	42.4	40.4
28st 0	94.9	88.2	82.2	76.8	72.0	67.5	63.5	59.8	56.4	53.4	50.5	47.9	45.5	43.2	41.1
28st 7	96.5	89.8	83.7	78.2	73.2	68.7	64.6	60.9	57.5	54.3	51.4	48.7	46.3	44.0	41.9
29st 0	98.2	91.4	85.2	79.6	74.5	69.9	65.8	62.0	58.5	55.3	52.3	49.6	47.1	44.8	42.6
29st 7	99.9	92.9	86.6	80.9	75.8	71.1	66.9	63.0	59.5	56.2	53.2	50.5	47.9	45.5	43.3

WEIGHT IN STONES / LBS

Weight Chart

BMI categories shown:
- Very Underweight BMI 10-15
- Underweight BMI 15-20
- IDEAL WEIGHT BMI 20-25
- Overweight BMI 25-30
- Obese BMI 30-35
- Very Obese BMI 35-40
- Morbidly Obese BMI 35-40

Height axis: 6ft 6" / 197.5cm, 6ft 5" / 195cm, 6ft 4" / 192.5cm, 6ft 3" / 190cm, 6ft 2" / 187.5cm, 6ft 1" / 185cm, 6ft 0" / 182.5cm, 5ft 11" / 180cm, 5ft 10" / 177.5cm, 5ft 9" / 175cm, 5ft 8" / 172.5cm, 5ft 7" / 170cm, 5ft 6" / 167.5cm, 5ft 5" / 165cm, 5ft 4" / 162.5cm, 5ft 3" / 160cm, 5ft 2" / 157.5cm, 5ft 1" / 155cm, 5ft 0" / 152.5cm, 4ft 11" / 150cm, 4ft 10" / 147.5cm, 4ft 9" / 145cm, 4ft 8" / 142.5cm, 4ft 7" / 140cm, 4ft 6" / 137.5cm

Weight axis: 4st 7lb / 29kg, 5st 0lb / 32kg, 5st 7lb / 35kg, 6st 0lb / 38kg, 6st 7lb / 41kg, 7st 0lb / 45kg, 7st 7lb / 48kg, 8st 0lb / 51kg, 8st 7lb / 54kg, 9st 0lb / 57kg, 9st 7lb / 60kg, 10st 0lb / 64kg, 10st 7lb / 67kg, 11st 0lb / 70kg, 11st 7lb / 73kg, 12st 0lb / 76kg, 12st 7lb / 79kg, 13st 0lb / 83kg, 13st 7lb / 86kg, 14st 0lb / 89kg, 14st 7lb / 92kg, 15st 0lb / 95kg, 15st 7lb / 98kg, 16st 0lb / 102kg, 16st 7lb / 105kg, 17st 0lb / 108kg, 17st 7lb / 111kg, 18st 0lb / 114kg, 18st 7lb / 118kg, 19st 0lb / 121kg, 19st 7lb / 124kg, 20st 0lb / 127kg, 20st 7lb / 130kg, 21st 0lb / 133kg, 21st 7lb / 137kg, 22st 0lb / 140kg, 22st 7lb / 143kg, 23st 0lb / 146kg, 23st 7lb / 149kg

BMI axis: 10, 11, 12, 13, 14, 15, 16, 17, 18, 19, 20, 21, 22, 23, 24, 25, 26, 27, 28, 29, 30, 31, 32, 33, 34, 35, 36, 37, 38

Calories Required to Maintain Weight
Adult Males

AGE / ACTIVITY LEVEL

WEIGHT IN STONES / LBS	VERY SEDENTARY			MODERATELY SEDENTARY			MODERATELY ACTIVE			VERY ACTIVE		
	<30	30-60	60+	<30	30-60	60+	<30	30-60	60+	<30	30-60	60+
9st 0	1856	1827	1502	2010	1979	1627	2320	2284	1878	2784	2741	2254
9st 7	1913	1871	1547	2072	2026	1676	2391	2338	1933	2870	2806	2320
10st 0	1970	1914	1591	2134	2074	1724	2463	2393	1989	2955	2871	2387
10st 7	2027	1958	1636	2196	2121	1772	2534	2447	2045	3041	2937	2454
11st 0	2084	2001	1680	2258	2168	1820	2605	2502	2100	3127	3002	2520
11st 7	2141	2045	1724	2320	2215	1868	2677	2556	2156	3212	3067	2587
12st 0	2199	2088	1769	2382	2262	1916	2748	2611	2211	3298	3133	2654
12st 7	2256	2132	1813	2444	2310	1965	2820	2665	2267	3384	3198	2720
13st 0	2313	2175	1858	2506	2357	2013	2891	2719	2322	3470	3263	2787
13st 7	2370	2219	1902	2568	2404	2061	2963	2774	2378	3555	3329	2854
14st 0	2427	2262	1947	2630	2451	2109	3034	2828	2434	3641	3394	2920
14st 7	2484	2306	1991	2691	2498	2157	3106	2883	2489	3727	3459	2987
15st 0	2542	2350	2036	2753	2545	2205	3177	2937	2545	3813	3525	3054
15st 7	2599	2393	2080	2815	2593	2253	3248	2992	2600	3898	3590	3120
16st 0	2656	2437	2125	2877	2640	2302	3320	3046	2656	3984	3655	3187
16st 7	2713	2480	2169	2939	2687	2350	3391	3100	2711	4070	3721	3254
17st 0	2770	2524	2213	3001	2734	2398	3463	3155	2767	4155	3786	3320
17st 7	2827	2567	2258	3063	2781	2446	3534	3209	2823	4241	3851	3387
18st 0	2884	2611	2302	3125	2828	2494	3606	3264	2878	4327	3917	3454
18st 7	2942	2654	2347	3187	2876	2542	3677	3318	2934	4413	3982	3520
19st 0	2999	2698	2391	3249	2923	2591	3749	3373	2989	4498	4047	3587
19st 7	3056	2741	2436	3311	2970	2639	3820	3427	3045	4584	4112	3654
20st 0	3113	2785	2480	3373	3017	2687	3891	3481	3100	4670	4178	3721
20st 7	3170	2829	2525	3434	3064	2735	3963	3536	3156	4756	4243	3787
21st 0	3227	2872	2569	3496	3112	2783	4034	3590	3211	4841	4308	3854
21st 7	3285	2916	2614	3558	3159	2831	4106	3645	3267	4927	4374	3921
22st 0	3342	2959	2658	3620	3206	2880	4177	3699	3323	5013	4439	3987
22st 7	3399	3003	2702	3682	3253	2928	4249	3754	3378	5098	4504	4054
23st 0	3456	3046	2747	3744	3300	2976	4320	3808	3434	5184	4570	4121
23st 7	3513	3090	2791	3806	3347	3024	4392	3862	3489	5270	4635	4187
24st 0	3570	3133	2836	3868	3395	3072	4463	3917	3545	5356	4700	4254
24st 7	3627	3177	2880	3930	3442	3120	4534	3971	3600	5441	4766	4321
25st 0	3685	3220	2925	3992	3489	3168	4606	4026	3656	5527	4831	4387
25st 7	3742	3264	2969	4054	3536	3217	4677	4080	3712	5613	4896	4454
26st 0	3799	3308	3014	4116	3583	3265	4749	4135	3767	5699	4962	4521
26st 7	3856	3351	3058	4177	3630	3313	4820	4189	3823	5784	5027	4587
27st 0	3913	3395	3103	4239	3678	3361	4892	4243	3878	5870	5092	4654
27st 7	3970	3438	3147	4301	3725	3409	4963	4298	3934	5956	5158	4721
28st 0	4028	3482	3191	4363	3772	3457	5035	4352	3989	6042	5223	4787
28st 7	4085	3525	3236	4425	3819	3506	5106	4407	4045	6127	5288	4854
29st 0	4142	3569	3280	4487	3866	3554	5177	4461	4101	6213	5354	4921
29st 7	4199	3612	3325	4549	3913	3602	5249	4516	4156	6299	5419	4987
30st 0	4256	3656	3369	4611	3961	3650	5320	4570	4212	6384	5484	5054

Calories Required to Maintain Weight
Adult Females

AGE / ACTIVITY LEVEL

WEIGHT IN STONES / LBS	VERY SEDENTARY			MODERATELY SEDENTARY			MODERATELY ACTIVE			VERY ACTIVE		
	<30	30-60	60+	<30	30-60	60+	<30	30-60	60+	<30	30-60	60+
7st 7	1425	1473	1304	1544	1596	1412	1781	1841	1630	2138	2210	1956
8st 0	1481	1504	1338	1605	1629	1450	1852	1880	1673	2222	2256	2008
8st 7	1537	1535	1373	1666	1663	1487	1922	1919	1716	2306	2302	2059
9st 0	1594	1566	1407	1726	1696	1524	1992	1957	1759	2391	2349	2111
9st 7	1650	1596	1442	1787	1729	1562	2062	1996	1802	2475	2395	2163
10st 0	1706	1627	1476	1848	1763	1599	2133	2034	1845	2559	2441	2214
10st 7	1762	1658	1511	1909	1796	1637	2203	2073	1888	2644	2487	2266
11st 0	1819	1689	1545	1970	1830	1674	2273	2111	1931	2728	2534	2318
11st 7	1875	1720	1580	2031	1863	1711	2344	2150	1975	2813	2580	2370
12st 0	1931	1751	1614	2092	1897	1749	2414	2188	2018	2897	2626	2421
12st 7	1987	1781	1648	2153	1930	1786	2484	2227	2061	2981	2672	2473
13st 0	2044	1812	1683	2214	1963	1823	2555	2266	2104	3066	2719	2525
13st 7	2100	1843	1717	2275	1997	1861	2625	2304	2147	3150	2765	2576
14st 0	2156	1874	1752	2336	2030	1898	2695	2343	2190	3234	2811	2628
14st 7	2212	1905	1786	2397	2064	1935	2766	2381	2233	3319	2858	2680
15st 0	2269	1936	1821	2458	2097	1973	2836	2420	2276	3403	2904	2732
15st 7	2325	1967	1855	2519	2130	2010	2906	2458	2319	3488	2950	2783
16st 0	2381	1997	1890	2580	2164	2047	2976	2497	2362	3572	2996	2835
16st 7	2437	2028	1924	2640	2197	2085	3047	2535	2405	3656	3043	2887
17st 0	2494	2059	1959	2701	2231	2122	3117	2574	2449	3741	3089	2938
17st 7	2550	2090	1993	2762	2264	2159	3187	2613	2492	3825	3135	2990
18st 0	2606	2121	2028	2823	2298	2197	3258	2651	2535	3909	3181	3042
18st 7	2662	2152	2062	2884	2331	2234	3328	2690	2578	3994	3228	3093
19st 0	2719	2182	2097	2945	2364	2271	3398	2728	2621	4078	3274	3145
19st 7	2775	2213	2131	3006	2398	2309	3469	2767	2664	4162	3320	3197
20st 0	2831	2244	2166	3067	2431	2346	3539	2805	2707	4247	3366	3249
20st 7	2887	2275	2200	3128	2465	2383	3609	2844	2750	4331	3413	3300
21st 0	2944	2306	2235	3189	2498	2421	3680	2882	2793	4416	3459	3352
21st 7	3000	2337	2269	3250	2531	2458	3750	2921	2836	4500	3505	3404
22st 0	3056	2368	2303	3311	2565	2495	3820	2960	2879	4584	3552	3455
22st 7	3112	2398	2338	3372	2598	2533	3890	2998	2923	4669	3598	3507
23st 0	3169	2429	2372	3433	2632	2570	3961	3037	2966	4753	3644	3559
23st 7	3225	2460	2407	3494	2665	2608	4031	3075	3009	4837	3690	3611
24st 0	3281	2491	2441	3554	2699	2645	4101	3114	3052	4922	3737	3662
24st 7	3337	2522	2476	3615	2732	2682	4172	3152	3095	5006	3783	3714
25st 0	3394	2553	2510	3676	2765	2720	4242	3191	3138	5091	3829	3766
25st 7	3450	2583	2545	3737	2799	2757	4312	3229	3181	5175	3875	3817
26st 0	3506	2614	2579	3798	2832	2794	4383	3268	3224	5259	3922	3869
26st 7	3562	2645	2614	3859	2866	2832	4453	3307	3267	5344	3968	3921
27st 0	3618	2676	2648	3920	2899	2869	4523	3345	3310	5428	4014	3973
27st 7	3675	2707	2683	3981	2932	2906	4594	3384	3353	5512	4060	4024
28st 0	3731	2738	2717	4042	2966	2944	4664	3422	3397	5597	4107	4076
28st 7	3787	2768	2752	4103	2999	2981	4734	3461	3440	5681	4153	4128

Calories Burned in Exercise

This table shows the approximate number of extra* calories that would be burned in a five minute period of exercise activity.

ACTIVITY	CALORIES BURNED IN 5 MINUTES	ACTIVITY	CALORIES BURNED IN 5 MINUTES
Aerobics, Low Impact	25	Situps, Continuous	17
Badminton, Recreational	17	Skiing, Moderate	30
Cross Trainer	30	Skipping, Moderate	30
Cycling, Recreational, 5mph	17	Squash Playing	39
Dancing, Modern, Moderate	13	Tennis Playing, Recreational	26
Fencing	24	Toning Exercises	17
Gardening, Weeding	19	Trampolining	17
Hill Walking, Up and Down, Recreational	22	Volleyball, Recreational	10
Jogging	30	Walking, Uphill, 15% Gradient, Moderate	43
Kick Boxing	30	Walking Up and Down Stairs, Moderate	34
Netball Playing	23	Walking, 4mph	24
Rebounding	18	Weight Training, Moderate	12
Roller Skating	30	Yoga	13
Rowing Machine, Moderate	30		
Running, 7.5mph	48		

*Extra calories are those in addition to your normal daily calorie needs.

Food and Exercise Diary

DATE: ___ / ___ / ___

DAILY CALORIE ALLOWANCE [ ] **A**

FOOD/DRINK CONSUMED	SERVING SIZE	CALORIES
_____	_____	_____
_____	_____	_____
_____	_____	_____
_____	_____	_____
_____	_____	_____
_____	_____	_____
_____	_____	_____
_____	_____	_____
_____	_____	_____
_____	_____	_____
_____	_____	_____
_____	_____	_____
_____	_____	_____
_____	_____	_____
_____	_____	_____
_____	_____	_____
_____	_____	_____

TOTAL CALORIES CONSUMED [ ] **B**

EXERCISE/ACTIVITY	NO. MINS	CALORIES
_____	_____	_____
_____	_____	_____
_____	_____	_____
_____	_____	_____

CALORIES USED IN EXERCISE [ ] **C**

CALORIE BALANCE [ ] **D**

You are aiming for your Calorie Balance (Box D) to be as close to zero as possible - ie. you consume the number of calories you need.

Your Daily Calorie Allowance (Box A) should be set to lose 1-2lb a week, or maintain weight, depending on your goals.

Daily Calorie Allowance (A) *plus* Extra Calories used in Exercise (C) *minus* Total Calories Consumed (B) *equals* Calorie Balance (D)

$$A + C - B = D$$

Food Information

Nutritional Information

CALORIE VALUES are given per serving, plus calorie and nutrition values per 100g of product. This makes it easy to compare the proportions of fat, protein, carbohydrate and fibre in each food.

The values given are for uncooked, unprepared foods unless otherwise stated. Values are also for only the edible portion of the food unless otherwise stated. ie - weighed with bone.

Finding Foods

The Calorie, Carb & Fat Bible has a new Eating Out section which is arranged alphabetically by brand. In the General Foods and Drinks A-Z most foods are grouped together by type, and then put in to alphabetical order. This makes it easy to compare different brands, and will help you to find lower calorie and/or fat alternatives where they are available.

This format also makes it easier to locate foods. Foods are categorised by their main characteristics so, for example, if it is bread, ciabatta or white sliced, you'll find it under "Bread".

There are, however, some foods which are not so easy to categorise, especially combination foods like ready meals. The following pointers will help you to find your way around the book until you get to know it a little better.

FILLED ROLLS AND SANDWICHES - Bagels, baguettes, etc which are filled are listed as "Bagels (filled)" etc. Sandwiches are under "Sandwiches".

CURRIES - Popular types of curry, like Balti or Jalfrezi, are listed under their individual types. Unspecified or lesser known types are listed under their main ingredient.

BURGERS - All burgers, including chicken-type sandwiches from fast-food outlets, are listed under "Burgers".

CHIPS & FRIES - Are listed seperately, depending on the name of the particular brand. All other types of potato are listed under "Potatoes".

SWEETS & CHOCOLATES - Well-known brands, eg. Aero, Mars Bar, are listed under their brand names. Others are listed under "Chocolate" (for bars) and "Chocolates" (for individual sweets).

READY MEALS - Popular types of dishes are listed under their type, eg. "Chow Mein", "Casserole", "Hot Pot", etc. Others are listed by their main ingredient, eg. "Chicken With", "Chicken In", etc.

EATING OUT & FAST FOODS - By popular demand this edition has the major eating out and fast food brands listed separately, at the back of the book. They are alphabetised first by brand, then follow using the same format as the rest of the book.

Serving Sizes

Many ready-meal type foods are given with calories for the full pack size, so that an individual serving can be worked out by estimating the proportion of the pack that has been consumed. For example, if you have eaten a quarter of a packaged pasta dish, divide the calorie value given for the whole pack by 4 to determine the number of calories you have consumed. Where serving sizes are not appropriate, or unknown, values are given per 1oz/28g. Serving sizes vary greatly from person to person and, if you are trying to lose weight, it's very important to be accurate – especially with foods that are very high in calories such as those that contain a fair amount of fat, sugar, cream, cheese, alcohol etc.

Food Data

Nutrition information for basic average foods has been compiled by the Weight Loss Resources food data team using many sources of information to calculate the most accurate values possible. Some nutrition information for non-branded food records is from The Composition of Foods 5th Edition (1991). Reproduced under licence from The Controller of Her Majesty's Stationary Office. Where basic data is present for ordinary foodstuffs such as 'raw carrots'; branded records are not included.

Nutrition information for branded goods is from details supplied by retailers and manufacturers, and researched by Weight Loss Resources staff. The Calorie Carb & Fat Bible contains data for over 900 UK brands, including major supermarkets and fast food outlets.

The publishers gratefully acknowledge all the manufacturers and retailers who have provided information on their products. All product names, trademarks or registered trademarks belong to their respective owners and are used only for the purpose of identifying products.

Calorie & nutrition data for all food and drink items are typical values.

Caution

The information in The Calorie, Carb and Fat Bible is intended as an aid to weight loss and weight maintenance, and is not medical advice. If you suffer from, or think you may suffer from a medical condition you should consult your doctor before starting a weight loss and/or exercise regime, If you start exercising after a period of relative inactivity, you should start slowly and consult your doctor if you experience pain, distress or other symptons.

Weights, Measures and Abbreviations

ABBREVIATIONS	
kcal	*kilocalories / calories*
prot	*protein*
carb	*carbohydrate*
sm	*small*
med	*medium*
lge	*large*
tsp	*teaspoon*
tbsp	*tablespoon*
dtsp	*desertspoon*

BRAND ABBREVIATIONS USED

ASDA

Good for You	*GFY*

JD WETHERSPOON

JD Wetherspoon	*JDW*

MARKS & SPENCER   M&S

Count on Us	*COU*

MORRISONS

Better For You	*BFY*

SAINSBURY'S

Be Good to Yourself	*BGTY*
Way to Five	*WTF*
Taste the Difference	*TTD*

	Measure INFO/WEIGHT	per Measure KCAL	Nutrition Values per 100g / 100ml				
			KCAL	PROT	CARB	FAT	FIBRE
ACKEE							
Canned, Drained	1oz/28g	42	151	2.9	0.8	15.2	0.0
ADVOCAAT							
Average	1 Shot/25ml	65	260	4.7	28.4	6.3	0.0
AERO							
Creamy White Centre, Nestle*	1 Bar/46g	244	530	7.6	57.4	30.0	0.0
Honeycomb, Nestle*	1 Serving/40g	199	497	5.9	62.2	25.0	0.0
Minis, Nestle*	1 Bar/11g	57	518	6.8	58.1	28.7	0.8
Mint, Nestle*	1 Bar/48g	249	518	6.8	58.1	28.7	0.8
Mint, Snack Size, Nestle*	1 Bar/21.6g	116	529	5.4	61.6	29.0	0.0
Nestle*	1 Bar/46g	238	518	6.8	58.1	28.7	0.8
ALFALFA SPROUTS							
Raw	1oz/28g	7	24	4.0	0.4	0.7	1.7
ALMOND DRINK							
Ecomil, Holland & Barratt*	1 Serving/250g	128	51	1.0	6.6	2.3	0.3
ALMONDS							
Blanched, Average	1oz/28g	171	610	25.0	7.2	53.5	8.5
Chopped, Sainsbury's*	1 Serving/10g	61	614	25.4	6.5	55.8	7.4
Flaked, Tesco*	1 Tbsp/7g	43	614	21.1	6.9	55.8	7.4
Ground, Average	1 Serving/10g	62	625	24.0	6.6	55.8	7.4
Smoked, Sainsbury's*	1 Serving/40g	264	660	26.0	9.0	57.8	7.5
Sugared, Co-Op*	1 Almond/5.5g	27	455	7.0	74.0	14.0	2.0
Toasted, Average	1oz/28g	178	634	25.0	6.6	56.5	6.6
Whole, Average	1 Portion/20g	122	612	23.4	8.1	54.8	8.4
Yoghurt Coated, Holland & Barratt*	1 Pack/100g	536	536	10.9	45.3	37.0	2.8
ALOO TIKKI							
Budgens*	1 Serving/25.2g	51	202	5.9	27.8	7.5	4.1
Mini, Indian Selection, Somerfield*	1 Serving/25g	49	199	4.5	30.3	6.6	0.2
Mini, Indian Snack Selection, Occasions, Sainsbury's*	1 Tikki/17.9g	34	190	4.4	27.6	6.9	3.2
ANCHOVIES							
Fillets, Flat, John West*	1 Can/50g	113	226	25.0	0.1	14.0	0.0
Fillets, Marinated, Waitrose*	1 Serving/5g	9	177	22.0	2.0	9.0	0.0
In Oil, Canned, Drained, Average	1 Serving/30g	58	194	22.9	0.0	11.3	0.0
Salted, Finest, Tesco*	1 Serving/10g	9	93	18.2	0.0	2.2	0.0
With Olives, Marinated, H Forman & Son*	1 Pack/200g	320	160	20.2	0.2	8.7	0.0
ANGEL DELIGHT							
Banana Flavour, Kraft*	1 Sachet/59g	289	490	2.5	72.0	21.0	0.0
Banana Toffee Flavour, No Added Sugar, Kraft*	1 Sachet/59g	292	495	4.8	58.5	26.5	0.0
Butterscotch Flavour, Kraft*	1 Sachet/59g	280	475	2.4	73.5	19.0	0.0
Butterscotch Flavour, No Added Sugar, Kraft*	1 Sachet/47g	226	480	4.5	61.0	24.0	0.0
Chocolate Flavour With Topples, Kraft*	1 Sachet/59g	274	465	5.0	67.0	20.0	0.5
Chocolate Flavour, Kraft*	1 Sachet/67g	305	455	3.7	69.5	18.0	0.4
Chocolate Flavour, No Added Sugar, Kraft*	1 Sachet/59g	266	450	6.3	56.5	22.0	0.6
Forest Fruit Flavour, Kraft*	1 Sachet/59g	289	490	2.5	71.5	21.5	0.0
Raspberry Flavour, Kraft*	1 Sachet/59g	289	490	2.5	72.0	21.0	0.0
Raspberry Flavour, No Added Sugar, Kraft*	1 Sachet/59g	292	495	4.8	59.5	26.0	0.0
Strawberry Flavour With Topples, Kraft*	1 Sachet/59g	266	450	2.8	74.5	14.0	0.0
Strawberry Flavour, Kraft*	1 Sachet/59g	286	485	2.5	71.0	21.0	0.0
Strawberry Flavour, No Added Sugar, Kraft*	1 Sachet/47g	230	490	4.8	59.0	26.5	0.0
Tangerine Flavour, No Added Sugar, Kraft*	1 Sachet/59g	292	495	4.8	58.0	27.0	0.9
Toffee Flavour, Kraft*	1 Sachet/59g	283	480	2.6	70.0	21.0	0.0
Vanilla Ice Cream Flavour, Kraft*	1 Sachet/59g	289	490	2.5	71.5	21.5	0.0
Vanilla Ice Cream Flavour, No Added Sugar, Kraft*	1 Sachet/59g	295	500	4.8	59.5	27.0	0.0

A

	Measure INFO/WEIGHT	per Measure KCAL	Nutrition Values per 100g / 100ml				
			KCAL	PROT	CARB	FAT	FIBRE
ANGEL HAIR							
Pasta, Sainsbury's*	1 Serving/100g	357	357	12.3	73.1	1.7	2.5
ANTIPASTO							
Artichoke, Sainsbury's*	1 Serving/50g	68	135	2.0	3.6	12.5	2.3
Misto Cotto, Arrosto Erbe, Waitrose*	1 Slice/9g	11	129	22.2	0.0	4.4	0.0
Mixed Mushroom, Sainsbury's*	1/4 Jar/72g	70	97	2.7	1.4	9.0	3.7
Mixed Pepper, Sainsbury's*	1/4 Jar/68g	23	34	1.3	4.2	1.3	3.5
Seafood, Drained, Sainsbury's*	1/2 Jar/84g	150	178	14.3	4.1	11.6	1.4
Sun Dried Tomato, Sainsbury's*	1 Tomato/5g	12	232	4.7	15.5	16.8	6.6
Wild Mushroom, Sainsbury's*	1 Serving/100g	97	97	2.7	1.4	9.0	3.7
APPLES							
Bites, Average	1 Pack/118g	58	49	0.3	11.7	0.1	2.2
Braeburn, Average	1 Apple/165g	79	48	0.4	11.3	0.1	1.8
Cape, Tesco*	1 Apple/100g	50	50	0.4	11.8	0.1	1.8
Cooking, Baked With Sugar, Flesh Only	1 Serving/140g	109	78	0.5	20.1	0.1	1.7
Cooking, Raw, Peeled	1oz/28g	10	35	0.3	8.9	0.1	1.6
Cooking, Stewed With Sugar	1 Serving/140g	104	74	0.3	19.1	0.1	1.2
Cooking, Stewed Without Sugar	1 Serving/140g	46	33	0.3	8.1	0.1	1.5
Dried, Average	1 Pack/250g	554	222	1.1	57.3	0.3	6.7
Empire, Tesco*	1 Apple/100g	50	50	0.4	11.8	0.1	1.8
English Cox, Average	1 Apple/108g	53	49	0.4	11.6	0.1	2.2
Fuji, Organic, Sainsbury's*	1 Apple/167g	82	49	0.4	11.6	0.1	1.8
Gala, Average	1 Apple/152g	74	49	0.4	11.5	0.1	1.4
Golden Delicious, Average	1 Med Apple/102g	49	48	0.4	11.5	0.1	1.7
Granny Smith, Average	1 Sm Apple/125g	62	50	0.4	11.9	0.1	2.0
Pink Lady, Average	1 Apple/125g	62	50	0.4	11.7	0.1	1.8
Sliced, Average	1oz/28g	14	49	0.4	11.6	0.1	1.8
Slices, Canned, Average	1oz/28g	8	27	0.2	6.4	0.1	1.5
Stewed, Sainsbury's*	1/4 Can/100g	71	71	0.2	17.4	0.0	1.2
APPLETISE							
Schweppes*	1 Glass/200ml	98	49	0.0	11.8	0.0	0.0
APRICOTS							
& Prunes, In Fruit Juice, Breakfast, Sainsbury's*	1 Pot/150g	134	89	1.1	21.2	0.1	0.7
Canned, In Syrup	1oz/28g	18	63	0.4	16.1	0.1	0.9
Dried, Sainsbury's*	1 Pack/150g	219	146	0.6	34.8	0.6	6.3
Dried, Tropical Wholefoods*	1 Serving/20g	240	240	2.4	55.2	1.1	7.8
Halves, In Fruit Juice, Average	1 Sm Can/221g	87	40	0.5	9.2	0.1	1.0
Raw, Average	1 Apricot/40g	13	34	1.0	7.5	0.1	1.5
ARCHERS*							
Aqua, Peach	1 Bottle/275ml	206	75	0.3	5.1	0.0	0.0
Peach Schnapps, (Calculated Estimate)	1 Shot/35ml	91	260	0.0	0.0	0.0	0.0
ARTICHOKE							
Hearts, Canned, Drained, Average	1/2 Can/117g	35	30	1.9	5.5	0.1	2.2
Hearts, Chargrilled in Olive Oil, TTD, Sainsbury's*	1/4 Jar/73g	150	205	1.0	3.4	20.8	0.0
Hearts, Marinated & Grilled, Waitrose*	1 Serving/50g	57	114	3.0	3.0	10.0	3.0
Raw, Fresh	1oz/28g	13	47	3.3	10.5	0.2	5.4
ASPARAGUS							
Boiled in Salted Water	5 Spears/125g	33	26	3.4	1.4	0.8	1.4
Canned, Average	1 Can/250g	48	19	2.3	2.0	0.2	1.6
Raw, Average	1oz/28g	7	25	3.1	1.8	0.7	1.8
AUBERGINE							
Baked Topped, Marks & Spencer*	1 Serving/150g	165	110	2.4	7.4	7.7	0.9
Fried, Average	1oz/28g	85	302	1.2	2.8	31.9	2.3
In Hot Sauce, Yarden*	1 Serving/35g	96	273	1.5	8.8	25.8	0.0

	Measure INFO/WEIGHT	per Measure KCAL	Nutrition Values per 100g / 100ml				
			KCAL	PROT	CARB	FAT	FIBRE
AUBERGINE							
Marinated & Grilled, Waitrose*	1/2 Pack/100g	106	106	1.0	3.0	10.0	2.0
Parmigiana, Marks & Spencer*	1 Pack/350g	333	95	4.6	7.6	5.3	1.1
Raw, Fresh	1 Sm/120g	18	15	0.9	2.2	0.4	2.0
AUTHENTIC MIX							
Bacon & Mushroom Taglietelle, Schwartz*	1 Pack/33g	112	340	9.9	73.8	0.6	0.5
Bombay Potatoes, Schwartz*	1 Pack/33g	110	332	15.3	61.7	2.7	0.2
Cajun Chicken, Schwartz*	1 Pack/38g	112	294	6.6	61.5	2.4	0.0
Chargrilled Chicken Pasta, Schwartz*	1/4 Packet/9g	28	316	9.1	59.7	4.5	0.5
Chicken & White Wine, Schwartz*	1/2 Pack/35g	113	322	10.3	65.2	2.2	0.3
Chicken Balti, Schwartz*	1oz/28g	91	324	13.5	54.4	5.8	0.0
Chilli Con Carne, Schwartz*	1 Pack/40.9g	126	308	8.2	64.6	1.9	0.5
Creamy Pork & Mushroom, Schwartz*	1/4 Pack/10g	30	302	9.9	63.3	1.0	1.0
Creamy Tikka Masala, Schwartz*	1oz/28g	97	346	13.7	63.6	4.1	0.2
For Chicken Fajitas, Schwartz*	1 Pack/35g	114	325	10.4	63.3	3.3	0.5
For Spagetti Bolognese, Schwartz*	1 Pack/40g	120	300	10.4	61.2	1.5	0.4
For Spaghetti Carbonara, Schwartz*	1/2 Pack/16g	70	436	9.5	56.0	19.3	0.3
Hot Chilli Con Carne, Schwartz*	1 Pack/41g	126	308	10.6	61.8	0.8	0.2
Lamb Casserole, Schwartz*	1 Pack/35g	116	332	7.7	68.0	3.3	1.3
Lasagne, Schwartz*	1 Pack/36g	113	313	6.6	70.1	0.7	0.3
Mexican Chilli Chicken, Schwartz*	1 Pack/35g	113	322	8.8	64.2	3.3	0.4
Thai Green Curry, Schwartz*	1 Serving/41g	141	344	11.2	67.6	3.2	0.2
Thai Lemon Chicken, Schwartz*	1 Serving/10g	37	365	3.6	78.3	4.2	0.0
Thai Red Curry, Schwartz*	1 Serving/20g	70	349	5.7	70.2	5.0	0.7
Thai Yellow Curry, Schwartz*	1 Packet/35g	126	360	7.3	64.2	8.2	0.8
Tuna Napolitana, Schwartz*	1 Serving/30g	107	357	10.3	49.7	13.0	0.3
AVOCADO							
Average	1 Med/145g	276	190	1.9	1.9	19.5	3.4

	Measure INFO/WEIGHT	per Measure KCAL	Nutrition Values per 100g / 100ml				
			KCAL	PROT	CARB	FAT	FIBRE
BACARDI*							
& Diet Coke	1 Serving/275ml	85	31	0.0	1.0	0.0	0.0
37.5% Volume	1 Shot/25ml	52	207	0.0	0.0	0.0	0.0
40% Volume	1 Shot/25ml	56	222	0.0	0.0	0.0	0.0
Breezer, Apple, Half Sugar, Crisp	1 Serving/275ml	121	44	0.0	3.7	0.0	0.0
Breezer, Cranberry	1 Serving/275ml	154	56	0.0	7.1	0.0	0.0
Breezer, Lemon, Diet	1 Bottle/275ml	96	35	0.0	1.2	0.0	0.0
Breezer, Lime	1 Serving/275ml	182	66	0.0	9.1	0.0	0.0
Breezer, Orange	1 Serving/275ml	179	65	0.0	8.2	0.0	0.0
Breezer, Orange & Vanilla, Diet	1 Bottle/275ml	96	35	0.0	1.2	0.0	0.0
Breezer, Orange, Diet	1 Serving/275ml	80	29	0.0	0.0	0.0	0.0
Breezer, Pineapple	1 Serving/275ml	171	62	0.0	8.6	0.0	0.0
Breezer, Raspberry, Half Sugar, Refreshing	1 Serving/275ml	122	44	0.0	3.7	0.0	0.0
Breezer, Watermelon	1 Serving/275ml	151	55	0.0	6.8	0.0	0.0
BACON							
Average	1 Rasher/25g	74	295	15.0	22.9	16.1	0.9
Back, Dry Cured, Average	1 Rasher/31g	77	250	28.1	0.3	15.1	0.3
Back, Dry Fried Or Grilled, Average	1 Rasher/25g	76	304	26.5	0.1	21.9	0.0
Back, Lean, Average	1 Rasher/33g	57	174	16.3	0.1	12.0	0.5
Back, Smoked, Average	1 Rasher/25g	66	265	20.9	0.0	19.9	0.0
Back, Smoked, Lean, Average	1 Rasher/25g	41	163	28.2	1.1	5.0	0.2
Back, Smoked, Rindless, Average	1 Rasher/25g	60	241	21.0	0.1	17.4	0.0
Back, Tendersweet, Average	1 Rasher/25g	63	251	29.8	0.5	14.4	0.1
Back, Unsmoked, Average	1 Rasher/32g	78	243	21.3	0.4	17.3	0.0
Back, Unsmoked, Rindless, Average	1 Rasher/23g	56	241	22.5	0.0	16.9	0.0
Chops, Average	1oz/28g	62	222	22.3	0.0	14.8	0.0
Chops, Coated In American Style BBQ Glaze, Tesco*	1 Serving/200g	330	165	18.6	3.8	8.4	1.3
Chops, In Cheese Sauce, Tesco*	1 Serving/185g	405	219	12.6	10.0	14.3	1.1
Collar Joint, Lean & Fat, Boiled	1oz/28g	91	325	20.4	0.0	27.0	0.0
Collar Joint, Lean & Fat, Raw	1oz/28g	89	319	14.6	0.0	28.9	0.0
Collar Joint, Lean Only, Boiled	1oz/28g	53	191	26.0	0.0	9.7	0.0
Fat Only, Cooked, Average	1oz/28g	194	692	9.3	0.0	72.8	0.0
Fat Only, Raw, Average	1oz/28g	209	747	4.8	0.0	80.9	0.0
Gammon Rasher, Lean Only, Grilled	1oz/28g	48	172	31.4	0.0	5.2	0.0
Joint, British, Sainsbury's*	1 Serving/100g	253	253	20.6	1.3	18.5	0.0
Lean Only, Fried, Average	1 Rasher/25g	83	332	32.8	0.0	22.3	0.0
Lean Only, Grilled, Average	1 Rasher/25g	73	292	30.5	0.0	18.9	0.0
Lean, Average	1oz/28g	40	142	19.6	0.9	6.7	0.2
Loin Steaks, Grilled	1 Serving/120g	229	191	25.9	0.0	9.7	0.0
Medallions, Average	1 Rasher/18g	27	151	29.4	0.9	3.3	0.1
Middle, Fried	1 Rasher/40g	140	350	23.4	0.0	28.5	0.0
Middle, Grilled	1 Rasher/40g	123	307	24.8	0.0	23.1	0.0
Middle, Raw	1 Rasher/43g	104	241	15.2	0.0	20.0	0.0
Rindless, Average	1 Rasher/20g	30	151	18.5	0.0	8.5	0.0
Smoked, Average	1 Rasher/28g	46	166	24.8	0.3	7.4	0.0
Smoked, Crispy, Cooked, Average	1 Serving/10g	46	460	53.0	2.1	26.9	0.0
Smoked, Rindless, Average	1 Rasher/20g	21	106	19.8	0.0	3.0	0.0
Streaky, Cooked, Average	1 Rasher/20g	68	342	22.4	0.3	27.8	0.0
BACON BITS							
Average	1oz/28g	66	235	19.6	0.0	17.4	0.0
BACON VEGETARIAN							
Rashers, Morningstar Farms*	2 Rashers/16.5g	59	345	11.5	13.4	27.6	3.9
Rashers, Redwood Foods*	1 Serving/18g	33	185	23.8	12.4	4.4	0.0
Rashers, Tesco*	1 Rasher/20g	46	230	23.3	6.0	12.8	7.5

INFO/WEIGHT	Measure	per Measure KCAL	Nutrition Values per 100g / 100ml				
			KCAL	PROT	CARB	FAT	FIBRE
BACON VEGETARIAN							
Realeat*	2 Rashers/35.7g	99	275	28.0	26.6	6.2	1.7
BAGEL							
Bacon, & Soft Cheese, Boots*	1 Serving/148g	481	325	12.0	31.0	17.0	2.2
Chicken, Lemon & Watercress, Safeway*	1 Pack/153g	329	215	12.8	28.2	4.1	0.0
Cream Cheese, & Salmon, Smoked, Marks & Spencer*	1 Bagel/23g	64	280	10.9	31.7	12.2	2.9
Cream Cheese, Marks & Spencer*	1 Bagel/22.5g	81	352	7.8	31.0	21.8	1.8
Ham, & Pesto, COU, Marks & Spencer*	1 Pack/173g	260	150	11.1	23.5	1.4	1.7
Pastrami, & Swiss Cheese, Bagelmania*	1 Pack/173.8g	339	195	12.3	25.7	6.6	4.2
Soft Cheese, & Salmon, Smoked, American, Sainsbury's*	1 Bagel/130.9g	356	272	8.3	31.8	12.4	1.7
Soft Cheese, & Salmon, Smoked, Finest, Tesco*	1 Pack/173g	396	229	13.1	31.2	5.8	1.7
Soft Cheese, & Salmon, Smoked, Shapers, Boots*	1 Pack/158g	344	218	12.0	29.0	6.0	0.9
Tuna, & Salad, BGTY, Sainsbury's*	1 Bagel/170g	325	191	10.4	26.0	4.2	1.0
Tuna, & Sweetcorn Relish, Safeway*	1 Bagel/162g	284	175	11.5	26.2	2.7	0.0
Turkey, & Cranberry, Bagelmania*	1 Pack/198.2g	325	164	9.0	24.5	3.7	1.1
Turkey, Pastrami & American Mustard, Shapers, Boots*	1 Bagel/146g	296	203	11.0	32.0	3.4	1.4
BAGUETTE							
All Day Breakfast, Darwins Deli*	1 Serving/184g	498	271	13.4	31.9	11.7	0.0
Cheese & Chive, Safeway*	1/4 Baguette/65g	216	333	7.9	37.1	14.7	1.4
Cheese & Ham, French, Shell*	1oz/28g	82	292	8.9	37.2	12.0	0.0
Cheese & Onion, Asda*	1oz/28g	102	366	12.0	39.8	17.6	1.3
Cheese & Pickle, Fullfillers*	1 Baguette/280g	767	274	11.9	35.5	11.1	0.0
Cheese, Mixed, & Spring Onion, Asda*	1 Pack/190g	629	331	9.5	32.1	18.3	1.3
Cheese, Tomato & Basil, Asda*	1/4 Bread/42g	138	329	10.0	40.8	14.0	1.3
Chicken & Mayonnaise, Asda*	1 Pack/190g	407	214	9.7	30.5	8.7	1.3
Chicken & Spicy Tomato, Snack, Sainsbury's*	1 Baguette/160g	344	215	14.1	31.2	3.7	2.2
Chicken & Stuffing, Hot, Sainsbury's*	1 Baguette/227g	543	239	13.7	29.6	7.2	0.0
Chicken Salad, Asda*	1 Serving/158.3g	325	206	9.0	29.0	6.0	2.1
Chicken Salad, Shapers, Boots*	1 Serving/133g	230	173	9.4	26.0	3.6	2.2
Chicken Tikka, Asda*	1 Pack/190g	439	231	10.4	32.8	9.4	1.3
Chicken Tikka, Hot, Sainsbury's*	1 Pack/190g	386	203	8.5	28.4	6.1	0.0
Chicken, Honey & Mustard, BGTY, Sainsbury's*	1 Pack/186.8g	340	182	11.0	30.0	2.0	0.0
Egg & Tomato, Oldfields*	1 Pack/198g	416	210	8.7	27.0	7.6	0.0
Egg Mayonnaise & Cress, Cafe, Sainsbury's*	1 Pack/100g	480	480	13.8	60.2	20.4	0.0
Ham & Cheese, French, Marks & Spencer*	1 Serving/100g	495	495	23.7	56.4	19.5	1.9
Ham & Cheese, Snack 'n' Go, Sainsbury's*	1 Baguette/178g	381	215	12.6	29.6	5.1	1.9
Ham Salad, With Mustard Mayonnaise, Sainsbury's*	1 Baguette/100g	412	412	17.6	49.6	15.9	0.1
Mozarella, Tomato, & Pesto, Darwins Deli*	1 Serving/210g	531	253	11.7	29.7	9.7	0.0
Prawn Mayonnaise, Asda*	1 Pack/190g	399	210	9.1	32.5	4.9	1.3
Prawn, French, Shell*	1 Baguette/63g	171	272	9.7	32.4	11.5	0.0
Steak & Onion, Snack 'n' Go, Sainsbury's*	1 Baguette/177g	396	225	14.3	30.6	5.0	2.2
Tuna Melt, Sainsbury's*	1 Serving/204g	373	183	11.3	25.8	3.9	0.0
Turkey & Ham, Asda*	1 Baguette/360g	774	215	11.6	30.7	5.1	1.3
BAILEYS*							
Glide	1 Serving/200ml	212	106	0.0	18.0	1.2	0.0
Irish Cream, Original	1 Glass/37g	130	350	3.2	20.0	15.7	0.0
BAKE							
Aubergine & Spinach, BGTY, Sainsbury's*	1 Pack/360g	148	41	2.2	4.0	1.8	1.3
Bean & Pasta, Asda*	1 Pack/450g	599	133	5.0	17.0	5.0	1.7
Broccoli & Three Cheese, Marks & Spencer*	1 Serving/225g	315	140	6.3	6.3	9.7	1.8
Cauliflower & Broccoli Bake, Tesco*	1/2 Pack/250g	178	71	2.8	5.8	4.1	1.0
Cheese & Spinach, Tesco*	1 Serving/140g	258	184	4.8	22.4	8.3	1.6
Chicken & Mushroom, COU, Marks & Spencer*	1 Serving/360g	324	90	7.3	10.3	2.3	1.1
Chicken Arrabbbiata, Marks & Spencer*	1 Pack/450g	540	120	7.6	16.0	3.0	2.0

B

	Measure INFO/WEIGHT	per Measure KCAL	Nutrition Values per 100g / 100ml				
			KCAL	PROT	CARB	FAT	FIBRE
BAKE							
Chicken Spiralli, Marks & Spencer*	1 Serving/400g	400	100	7.9	9.1	3.8	1.1
Chicken, Bacon & Potato, British Classics, Tesco*	1/2 Pack/375g	435	116	7.0	12.2	4.4	1.4
Chicken, Broccoli & Mushroom, Safeway*	1 Serving/175g	425	243	8.9	22.4	13.1	3.0
Chicken, Tomato, & Mascarpone, Healthy Living, Tesco*	1 Serving/400g	468	117	7.6	15.5	2.7	0.8
Cod & Prawn, COU, Marks & Spencer*	1 Pack/400g	320	80	6.5	8.8	2.0	1.0
Creamy Peppercorn, Vegetarian, Tesco*	1 Serving/140g	322	230	3.6	27.0	12.0	1.2
Fish & Vegetable, Young's*	1 Serving/374.8g	446	119	5.6	10.0	6.3	1.3
Garlic Mushroom, Waitrose*	1/2 Pack/200g	420	210	4.1	20.3	12.7	0.8
Mushroom, Leek & Spinach, Cumberland, Sainsbury's*	1 Pack/450g	518	115	3.6	12.9	5.4	1.2
Paprika, Eat Smart, Safeway*	1 Serving/25g	90	360	6.6	76.9	2.5	4.6
Potato & Brie, Finest, Tesco*	1/2 Pack/200g	284	142	4.3	8.6	10.0	1.1
Potato & Vegetable, Co-Op*	1 Bake/340g	425	125	4.0	11.0	8.0	1.0
Potato, Cheese, & Bacon, Homepride*	1 Serving/210g	277	132	1.6	3.2	12.5	0.0
Potato, Cheese, & Onion, Tesco*	1 Pack/400g	376	94	2.4	10.0	4.9	1.0
Potato, Mushroom & Leek, Marks & Spencer*	1 Serving/225g	225	100	3.5	10.0	5.9	2.0
Potato, Tomato & Mozzarella, Marks & Spencer*	1 Bake/450g	585	130	5.2	9.8	7.6	1.8
Roast Onion & Potato, COU, Marks & Spencer*	1 Pack/450g	338	75	1.9	13.6	1.3	1.5
Roast Potato, Cheese & Onion, Asda*	1/2 Pack/200g	288	144	4.2	14.0	8.0	1.1
Salmon & Broccoli, Weight Watchers*	1 Serving/330g	311	94	5.1	10.2	3.6	0.8
Salmon & Broccoli, Young's*	1 Bake/375g	409	109	6.3	9.6	5.1	1.3
Salmon & Prawn, Marks & Spencer*	1 Bake/328.6g	461	140	7.4	6.6	9.5	0.7
Smoked Haddock & Prawn, BGTY, Sainsbury's*	1 Pack/350g	319	91	7.5	13.6	0.7	1.1
Spicy Bean & Potato, Safeway*	1 Pack/385.7g	405	105	3.9	14.2	3.2	2.1
Spicy Chickpea & Apricot, Safeway*	1 Pack/400g	340	85	2.2	12.5	2.9	3.2
Tomato & Mascarpone, Sainsbury's*	1 Pack/400g	608	152	3.9	17.6	7.3	2.1
Tuna & Pasta, Healthy Living, Tesco*	1 Pack/400g	360	90	8.3	10.7	1.5	0.9
Tuna Conchiglie, Marks & Spencer*	1 Serving/400g	500	125	8.6	10.2	5.4	0.9
Vegetable & Lentil, Somerfield*	1 Pack/350g	319	91	4.9	13.8	1.8	2.5
Vegetable, Marks & Spencer*	1 Serving/300g	255	85	1.8	9.8	4.3	3.2
BAKE MIX							
Potato, Creamy Cheddar Cheese, Colman's*	1 Pack/45g	189	420	11.5	34.8	26.0	9.6
Potato, Ham & Leek, Colman's*	1 Pack/44g	181	412	9.9	40.4	24.0	2.1
Quick Quisine, Atkins*	1 Serving/100g	286	286	44.0	16.0	2.7	19.8
BAKING POWDER							
Average	1 Tsp/2g	3	163	5.2	37.8	0.0	0.0
BALTI							
Chicken & Mushroom, Tesco*	1 Serving/350g	326	93	12.3	4.2	3.0	0.7
Chicken & Naan Bread, Somerfield*	1 Pack/335g	489	146	10.0	16.0	5.0	0.0
Chicken & Potato Wedges, Healthy Living, Tesco*	1 Pack/450g	387	86	6.0	10.8	2.1	1.1
Chicken & Rice, COU, Marks & Spencer*	1 Serving/400g	360	90	7.3	13.2	0.9	2.5
Chicken & Rice, Good Choice, Iceland*	1 Pack/400g	440	110	5.2	18.1	1.9	0.7
Chicken & Rice, Patak's*	1 Pack/370g	440	119	6.1	16.7	3.5	1.7
Chicken Ceylon, Finest, Tesco*	1 Pack/400g	588	147	14.4	0.9	9.5	5.0
Chicken Tikka & Wedges, Healthy Living, Tesco*	1 Pack/450g	428	95	6.2	11.8	2.5	1.3
Chicken Tikka, Finest, Tesco*	1/2 Pack/200g	280	140	15.8	1.1	8.6	3.2
Chicken Tikka, Indian, Tesco*	1 Serving/350g	427	122	11.2	5.6	6.1	0.6
Chicken Tikka, Tesco*	1 Pack/350g	466	133	11.1	6.4	7.0	0.7
Chicken Tikka, Weight Watchers*	1 Pack/320g	224	70	4.8	10.2	1.1	0.6
Chicken With Naan Bread, Perfectly Balanced, Waitrose*	1 Pack/375g	450	120	12.1	9.7	3.6	2.8
Chicken With Naan Bread, Sharwood's*	1 Pack/375g	540	144	6.5	15.4	6.3	2.2
Chicken With Rice & Naan, Iceland*	1 Serving/148g	589	398	15.0	66.4	8.0	3.1
Chicken With Rice, Curry Break, Patak's*	1 Pack/220g	198	90	4.7	11.6	2.8	0.0
Chicken With Rice, Weight Watchers*	1 Pack/329g	253	77	4.8	10.7	1.7	0.5

	Measure INFO/WEIGHT	per Measure KCAL	Nutrition Values per 100g / 100ml				
			KCAL	PROT	CARB	FAT	FIBRE
BALTI							
Chicken, BGTY, Sainsbury's*	1 Pack/400g	356	89	5.1	15.8	0.6	0.7
Chicken, Blue Parrot Cafe, Sainsbury's*	1 Can/400g	308	77	8.9	4.6	2.5	0.8
Chicken, From Indian Meal For One, Sainsbury's*	1 Pack/300g	384	128	12.9	3.7	6.8	2.1
Chicken, Iceland*	1 Pack/544g	740	136	12.0	5.7	7.2	1.6
Chicken, Indian Takeaway, Iceland*	1 Pack/402.2g	362	90	7.8	4.0	4.8	0.7
Chicken, Marks & Spencer*	1 Pack/350g	350	100	10.8	3.9	4.3	1.5
Chicken, Morrisons*	1 Pack/350g	441	126	12.1	2.3	7.6	1.5
Chicken, Ready Meals, Marks & Spencer*	1oz/28g	34	120	10.2	4.7	6.5	1.6
Chicken, Safeway*	1 Pack/350g	485	139	9.5	5.4	8.7	2.1
Chicken, Sainsbury's*	1 Serving/200g	230	115	12.8	4.2	5.2	3.5
Chicken, Takeaway, Sainsbury's*	1 Pack/400g	404	101	10.4	4.8	4.5	1.4
Chicken, Tesco*	1 Pack/460g	662	144	6.1	17.4	5.6	1.6
Chicken, Tin, Sainsbury's*	1 Serving/200g	168	84	9.4	4.0	3.4	1.0
Chicken, With Garlic & Coriander Naan, Frozen, Patak's*	1 Pack/375g	431	115	6.3	11.1	5.0	1.1
Chicken, With Pilau Rice, Asda*	1 Pack/504g	625	124	5.0	15.0	4.9	1.2
Chunky Vegetable, Aldi*	1 Can/400g	404	101	1.5	9.3	6.4	1.4
Prawn, Budgens*	1 Pack/350g	375	107	5.6	5.2	7.1	1.3
Vegetable & Rice, Tesco*	1 Pack/450g	378	84	2.0	15.6	1.6	1.3
Vegetable With Naan Bread & Raita, Eat Smart, Safeway*	1 Pack/371g	315	85	3.8	12.5	1.9	3.1
Vegetable, Asda*	1/2 Can/200g	206	103	2.2	10.0	6.0	2.5
Vegetable, GFY, Asda*	1 Pack/450g	324	72	1.9	14.0	0.9	1.5
Vegetable, Indian Meal for 2, Finest, Tesco*	1/2 Pack/150g	144	96	1.6	6.1	7.2	2.9
BAMBOO SHOOTS							
Canned, Average	1 Sm Can/120g	11	9	1.1	0.9	0.1	0.9
BANANA							
Chips	1oz/28g	143	511	1.0	59.9	31.4	1.7
Raw, Average	1 Med/118g	116	98	1.7	23.2	0.3	0.9
BANANA SPLIT							
Fresh Cream, Tesco*	1 Serving/240g	463	193	1.7	17.2	13.0	0.3
BANGERS & MASH							
& Beans, Blue Parrot Cafe, Sainsbury's*	1 Pack/300g	354	118	5.3	14.8	4.2	2.1
Balance, Spar*	1 Pack/400g	324	81	3.4	10.8	2.7	1.8
Co-Op*	1 Pack/300g	375	125	4.0	13.0	6.0	0.8
Eat Smart, Morrisons*	1 Serving/405g	340	84	5.9	10.7	2.0	1.7
Good Intentions, Somerfield*	1 Pack/447.7g	394	88	5.3	12.1	2.0	0.7
Meal for One, Marks & Spencer*	1 Pack/370g	481	130	4.7	9.5	7.9	1.1
Morrisons*	1 Pack/300g	306	102	3.0	12.3	4.9	0.8
Sausage, & Cabbage Mash, Eat Smart, Safeway*	1 Pack/400g	340	85	6.4	9.0	2.5	1.3
BARS							
AM, Breakfast Muffin, Apple & Sultana, McVitie's*	1 Bar/45g	168	373	4.4	54.9	16.7	1.6
AM, Cereal, Apple, McVitie's*	1 Bar/40g	160	400	4.3	65.4	13.5	3.1
AM, Cereal, Apricot, McVitie's*	1 Bar/30g	146	486	6.5	68.8	20.5	0.5
AM, Cereal, Berry, McVitie's*	1 Bar/30g	146	486	6.5	68.8	20.5	0.5
AM, Cereal, Fruit & Nut, McVitie's*	1 Bar/35g	167	477	6.6	64.9	21.4	3.4
AM, Cereal, Grapefruit, McVitie's*	1 Bar/35g	136	389	5.1	70.9	9.4	3.1
AM, Cereal, Orange Marmalade, McVitie's*	1 Bar/40g	151	378	4.5	53.3	18.0	1.8
AM, Cereal, Raisin & Nut, McVitie's*	1 Bar/35.1g	148	422	6.4	62.1	16.4	2.4
AM, Cereal, Strawberry, McVitie's*	1 Bar/35g	138	395	5.7	70.5	10.1	2.7
AM, Granola, Almond, Raisin & Cranberry, McVitie's*	1 Bar/35g	133	380	7.1	62.9	11.4	4.0
AM, Muesli Fingers, McVitie's*	1 Bar/35g	154	440	6.0	59.8	19.6	3.1
All Day Breakfast, Weight Watchers*	1 Bar/50g	179	358	6.8	72.2	4.6	3.2
All Fruit, Apple & Passionfruit, Jordans*	1 Bar/30g	89	295	1.2	71.0	0.7	5.2
All Fruit, Apple & Strawberry, Jordans*	1 Bar/30g	89	297	1.3	72.1	0.4	4.9

B

BARS

INFO/WEIGHT	Measure	per Measure KCAL	KCAL	PROT	CARB	FAT	FIBRE
Almond, Apricot & Mango, Marks & Spencer*	1 Bar/50g	205	410	8.9	60.2	14.9	5.0
Alpen*, Apple & Blackberry With Yoghurt	1 Bar/29g	117	404	5.4	71.8	10.6	0.0
Alpen*, Fruit & Nut	1 Bar/28g	110	394	6.5	71.2	9.2	0.0
Alpen*, Fruit & Nut With Milk Chocolate	1 Bar/29g	125	431	7.0	68.0	14.5	0.0
Alpen*, Strawberry With Yoghurt	1 Bar/29g	119	409	5.7	72.6	10.6	0.0
Alpini, Continental Chocolate, Thorntons*	1 Bar/35.6g	194	539	7.0	55.1	32.2	2.1
Apple & Cinnamon, Breakfast Snack, Tesco*	1 Bar/37.5g	139	365	4.3	58.8	12.5	2.0
Apple & Cinnamon, Chewy, GFY, Asda*	1 Bar/27g	95	351	6.0	76.0	2.6	3.5
Apple & Custard, Danish, Tesco*	1 Serving/125g	335	268	3.6	29.5	15.1	5.6
Apple & Raisin, Snack, Geobar, Traidcraft*	1 Bar/35g	127	362	3.3	76.4	4.8	2.3
Apple & Raspberry, Chewy & Crisp, Tesco*	1 Bar/27.0g	123	456	3.4	66.8	19.5	2.8
Apple, All Bran, Kellogg's*	1 Bar/40g	158	395	8.0	48.0	19.0	5.0
Apple, Geobar, Traidcraft*	1 Bar/35.1g	132	376	5.3	69.0	8.8	3.5
Apple, Granola, McVitie's*	1 Bar/35g	128	366	6.6	63.1	9.7	4.3
Apple, Pear & Berry, Shapers, Boots*	1 Bar/30g	78	261	1.2	64.0	0.1	10.0
Apricot & Almond, Chewy & Crisp, Tesco*	1 Bar/27g	122	452	6.2	60.0	20.8	2.6
Apricot & Almond, Eat Natural*	1 Serving/50g	202	403	11.2	53.3	16.1	0.0
Apricot & Almond, Yoghurt Coated, Eat Natural*	1 bar/50g	236	471	8.3	52.0	25.5	4.3
Apricot & Almond, Yoghurt Coated, Mini, Eat Natural*	1 Mini Bar/15g	71	471	8.3	52.0	25.5	4.3
Apricot & Coconut, Chewy & Crisp, Sainsbury's*	1 Bar/27g	123	457	5.2	58.8	22.3	4.0
Apricot & Raisin, Thorntons*	1 Bar/40g	185	462	8.0	46.0	27.3	3.5
Apricot, Dried Fruit, Sunsweet*	1 Bar/33g	96	292	3.6	72.5	0.1	0.0
Apricot, Fruity Grain, Tesco*	1 Bar/37g	50	134	1.3	25.3	3.0	0.9
Apricot, Oat Snack, Waitrose*	1 Bar/27g	121	447	4.9	65.2	18.5	2.4
Banana Break, Breakfast in a Bar, Jordans*	1 Bar/40g	152	381	5.7	69.1	9.1	5.0
Banana, Fruit Break, Lyme Regis Foods*	1 Bar/42g	162	385	9.0	51.9	15.7	3.9
Biscuit & Raisin, Reduced Fat, Tesco*	1 Bar/21g	85	406	4.9	68.5	12.5	1.8
Blue Riband, Double Choc, Nestle*	1 Bar/22g	113	513	4.8	66.4	25.3	1.1
Blue Riband, Nestle*	1 Bar/21.1g	104	495	4.5	64.5	24.5	1.0
Blueberrry, Fruit & Grain, Asda*	1 Bar/37g	124	335	4.1	64.0	7.0	3.9
Boohbah, Milk & White Chocolate, Marks & Spencer*	1 Bar/75g	405	540	7.9	54.7	32.3	1.2
Breakaway, Nestle*	1oz/28g	139	496	6.8	59.7	25.5	0.0
Breakfast, Apple Crisp, Morning Start, Atkins*	1 Bar/37g	145	392	29.2	25.4	21.4	13.8
Breakfast, Blueberry, Free From, Sainsbury's*	1 Bar/35g	163	467	3.8	62.6	22.4	0.2
Breakfast, Chocolate Chip Crisp, Morning Start, Atkins*	1 Bar/37g	137	370	31.8	22.5	18.8	15.0
Breakfast, Muesli, Country Garden*	1 Bar/25g	94	376	5.6	67.6	9.2	3.6
Breakfast, Vitality, Fruit & Fibre, Asda*	1 Bar/29g	113	390	6.0	69.0	10.0	4.1
Breakfast, Vitality, Tropical Fruit, Asda*	1 Bar/28g	101	361	6.0	75.0	4.1	4.4
Breakfast, Vitality, With Cranberries, Asda*	1 Bar/27g	103	381	6.3	77.8	4.8	3.0
Breakfast, With Cranberries, Asda*	1 Bar/28g	105	376	6.0	77.0	4.9	3.0
Brunch, Cranberry & Orange, Cadbury*	1 Bar/35g	154	440	5.9	67.7	15.9	0.0
Brunch, Hazelnut, Cadbury*	1 Bar/35g	163	465	7.1	61.0	21.6	0.0
Brunch, Raisin, Cadbury*	1 Bar/35g	151	430	5.7	66.7	15.8	0.0
Cappuccino Coll, Marks & Spencer*	1 Bar/35g	185	529	6.0	50.0	35.0	1.0
Caramel Crisp, Go Ahead, McVitie's*	1 Bar/33g	141	428	4.8	75.1	12.0	0.8
Caramel Crunch, Go Ahead, McVitie's*	1 Bar/24g	106	440	4.7	76.6	13.8	0.8
Caramel Mighty, Asda*	1 Serving/40g	186	464	5.0	66.0	20.0	1.5
Caramel Nougat, Soft, Shapers, Boots*	1 Bar/25g	86	343	2.9	60.4	10.0	0.6
Caramel Shortcake, Jive, Aldi*	1 Bar/29g	135	467	4.6	56.0	25.0	1.4
Caramel, Endulge, Atkins*	1 Bar/24g	89	369	7.8	54.4	12.6	8.6
Caramel, Snack, SlimFast*	1 Bar/26g	94	360	3.1	66.3	11.2	0.0
Caramelised Nut & Raisin Crunch, TTD, Sainsbury's*	1 Bar/50g	206	412	8.3	64.4	13.5	5.3
Cereal & Milk, Rice Krispies, Kellogg's*	1 Bar/20g	84	421	7.0	70.0	13.0	0.3

BARS

INFO/WEIGHT	Measure	per Measure KCAL	KCAL	PROT	CARB	FAT	FIBRE
Cereal & More, Marks & Spencer*	1 Bar/40g	154	385	20.0	58.2	7.8	2.9
Cereal, Almond, Orco*	1 Bar/21g	90	430	7.8	60.0	17.7	2.0
Cereal, Apple & Blackberry, With Yoghurt, Alpen*	1 Bar/29g	122	419	5.5	73.8	11.1	0.0
Cereal, Apple & Cinnamon, Tesco*	1 Serving/38g	137	365	4.3	58.9	12.5	2.1
Cereal, Apple & Cinnamonr, Fruit 'n' Grain, Asda*	1 Bar/37g	131	353	4.5	68.0	7.0	2.9
Cereal, Apple & Raisin, Harvest, Quaker*	1 Bar/22g	87	396	5.0	70.0	11.5	4.0
Cereal, Apple & Raspberry, Chewy & Crisp, Tesco*	1 Bar/27g	123	456	3.3	66.7	19.6	3.0
Cereal, Apple & Raspberry, Waitrose*	1 Bar/25g	90	359	5.0	77.1	3.4	4.6
Cereal, Apple & Sultana, Go Ahead, McVitie's*	1 Bar/35g	137	391	6.3	74.0	8.4	3.5
Cereal, Apple, Chewy, BGTY, Sainsbury's*	1 Bar/25g	85	340	4.8	76.0	2.0	2.0
Cereal, Apricot & Yoghurt, COU, Marks & Spencer*	1 Bar/20g	74	370	4.8	82.3	2.2	3.1
Cereal, Apricot & Yoghurt, Shapers, Boots*	1 Bar/27g	99	366	3.7	75.0	5.7	3.3
Cereal, Apricot Fruit & Cereal, Organic, Organix*	1 Bar/30g	122	408	7.2	55.3	20.4	6.2
Cereal, Apricot, Lyme Regis Foods*	1 Bar/35.1g	131	373	6.5	61.1	11.4	6.8
Cereal, Apricot, Organic, Evernat*	1oz/28g	101	360	5.6	64.9	8.7	7.2
Cereal, Apricot, Perfectly Balanced, Waitrose*	1 Bar/25g	89	356	4.9	76.9	3.2	3.8
Cereal, Balance With Fruit, Sainsbury's*	1 Bar/25g	100	401	5.8	75.2	8.6	1.9
Cereal, Balance, Orco*	1 Bar/21g	81	388	5.3	78.2	6.0	0.0
Cereal, Banana, Value, Tesco*	1 Bar/21g	80	387	6.0	73.9	7.5	3.7
Cereal, Banoffee, COU, Marks & Spencer*	1 Bar/20g	75	375	4.5	82.5	2.0	1.9
Cereal, Benefit With Fruit, Harvest Morn*	1 Bar/27g	108	401	5.8	75.2	8.6	1.9
Cereal, Berry & Cream, COU, Marks & Spencer*	1 Bar/20g	72	360	5.3	79.7	2.3	3.1
Cereal, Blueberry Flavour, Breakfast, Sweet Mornings*	1 Bar/38g	152	399	4.5	66.0	13.0	2.5
Cereal, Brownie, COU, Marks & Spencer*	1 Bar/20g	73	365	5.5	79.7	2.6	4.6
Cereal, Cheerios & Milk Bar, Nestle*	1 Bar/24g	98	407	7.6	64.5	13.2	0.0
Cereal, Chewy & Crisp With Choc Chips, Tesco*	1 Bar/27g	125	463	9.2	54.0	23.4	3.8
Cereal, Chewy & Crisp With Roasted Nuts, Tesco*	1 Bar/27g	127	471	9.3	57.0	22.9	2.5
Cereal, Chewy Apple, Fruitus*	1 Bar/34.9g	132	378	5.4	64.8	10.8	5.4
Cereal, Chewy, BGTY, Sainsbury's*	1 Serving/25g	85	342	4.9	75.8	2.1	1.9
Cereal, Choc Chip & Nut, Chewy & Crisp, Sainsbury's*	1 Bar/27g	129	476	8.8	51.8	26.0	4.4
Cereal, Chocolate & Orange, Healthy Living, Tesco*	1 Bar/25g	96	384	4.0	77.7	6.3	1.9
Cereal, Chocolate & Orange, Tesco*	1 Bar/25g	96	384	4.0	77.7	6.3	1.9
Cereal, Chocolate & Raisin, Seeds Of Change*	1 Bar/29g	112	385	5.5	69.3	9.5	0.0
Cereal, Chocolate Milk, Kellogg's*	1 Bar/26.7g	122	450	9.0	67.0	16.0	1.5
Cereal, Cinnamon Grahams, Nestle*	1 Bar/25g	107	426	7.2	66.2	14.7	1.9
Cereal, Coco Pops & Milk Bar, Kellogg's*	1 Bar/20g	84	420	7.0	67.0	14.0	1.0
Cereal, Coconut Muesli, Kellogg's*	1 Bar/25g	108	430	5.0	65.0	17.0	5.0
Cereal, Cranberrry & Blackcurrant, Healthy Living, Tesco*	1 Bar/25g	79	316	5.5	68.2	2.3	8.6
Cereal, Cranberry & Orange, BGTY, Sainsbury's*	1 Bar/26g	93	358	2.7	75.8	4.9	2.3
Cereal, Cranberry & Orange, Weight Watchers*	1 Bar/28g	102	365	4.5	77.6	4.1	2.3
Cereal, Cranberry, Benefit, Aldi*	1 bar/27g	101	375	6.2	76.5	4.9	3.0
Cereal, Cranberry, Chewy, Safeway*	1 Bar/25g	86	345	4.7	75.7	2.3	3.9
Cereal, Cranberry, Eat Smart, Safeway*	1 Bar/25g	86	345	4.7	75.7	2.3	3.9
Cereal, Cranberry, Waitrose*	1 Bar/25g	91	363	4.5	78.3	3.5	2.9
Cereal, Crunchy Nut, Kellogg's*	1 Bar/25g	112	446	6.0	70.0	16.0	1.5
Cereal, Dark Chocolate, Le Noir, Orco*	1 Bar/21g	95	451	7.3	69.9	15.8	0.0
Cereal, Frosties & Milk, Kellogg's*	1 Bar/24.9g	103	413	6.0	71.0	12.0	1.5
Cereal, Frosties, Chocolate, Kellogg's*	1 Bar/25g	103	412	6.0	72.0	12.0	1.6
Cereal, Frosties, Kellogg's*	1 Bar/25g	103	411	7.0	72.0	11.0	1.0
Cereal, Fruit & Fibre, Harvest Morn*	1 Bar/29g	114	392	6.5	69.1	10.0	4.1
Cereal, Fruit & Fibre, Sainsbury's*	1 Bar/28g	111	397	5.7	70.9	10.1	3.8
Cereal, Fruit & Nut Break, Jordans*	1 Bar/37g	135	374	7.0	63.2	10.4	8.1
Cereal, Fruit & Nut, Alpen*	1 Bar/28g	111	396	6.4	71.1	9.3	0.0

BARS

	INFO/WEIGHT	KCAL	KCAL	PROT	CARB	FAT	FIBRE
Cereal, Fruit N Fibre, Kellogg's*	1 Serving/25g	96	384	4.0	72.0	10.0	4.0
Cereal, Fruit, Nut, & Milk Chocolate, Alpen*	1 Serving/29g	122	421	6.6	68.3	13.4	0.0
Cereal, Ginger & Raisin, BGTY, Sainsbury's*	1 Bar/40g	91	228	2.0	48.5	2.8	0.0
Cereal, Ginger, Waitrose*	1 Bar/25g	92	367	4.9	79.3	3.3	3.3
Cereal, Golden Grahams, Nestle*	1 Bar/25g	106	425	6.5	68.8	13.7	0.0
Cereal, Hazelnut & Pistachio, Go Ahead, McVitie's*	1 Bar/35g	147	420	5.6	67.8	14.1	2.4
Cereal, Hazelnut & Sultana, Organic, Seeds Of Change*	1 Bar/29g	118	407	6.3	65.9	13.1	0.0
Cereal, Hazelnuts & Raisins, Organic, Tesco*	1 Bar/30g	144	481	7.2	50.3	27.9	3.8
Cereal, Lemon & Sultana, Eat Smart, Safeway*	1 Bar/25g	89	355	4.2	78.4	2.2	2.6
Cereal, Lemon, Holly Mill*	1 Bar/40g	172	430	5.7	51.0	22.6	4.4
Cereal, Lemon, Marks & Spencer*	1 Bar/25g	90	360	4.1	79.0	2.8	2.8
Cereal, Maple, Healthy Living, Tesco*	1 Bar/25g	93	372	5.5	76.6	4.9	2.0
Cereal, Milk Chocolate, Weetos, Weetabix*	1 Bar/20g	88	440	6.0	71.0	14.5	0.0
Cereal, Mixed Berry, Fruitus*	1 Bar/35g	132	376	5.7	63.8	13.8	6.6
Cereal, Mixed Berry, Go Ahead, McVitie's*	1 Bar/35g	134	383	4.6	77.1	6.3	3.1
Cereal, Muesli Break, Breakfast in a Bar, Jordans*	1 Bar/46g	178	387	5.9	66.6	10.8	4.3
Cereal, Muncho Chocolate & Coconut, Orco*	1 Bar/21g	93	441	5.0	71.4	15.0	0.0
Cereal, Nesquik, Nestle*	1 Bar/25g	108	433	6.2	68.7	14.9	0.0
Cereal, Nut & Chocolate, Chewy, Safeway*	1 Bar/27g	127	471	8.7	57.9	22.7	4.1
Cereal, Nuts & Raisins, Organic, Evernat*	1oz/28g	108	385	6.5	62.2	12.3	6.8
Cereal, Nutty, Free From, Sainsbury's*	1 Bar/25g	114	454	6.8	61.8	20.0	2.3
Cereal, Orange & Grapefruit, Healthy Eating, Tesco*	1 Bar/24.9g	90	361	4.1	79.9	2.8	2.2
Cereal, Orange, Lyme Regis Foods*	1 Bar/35g	132	377	4.6	73.4	9.5	5.2
Cereal, Peach Melba, Tesco*	1 Serving/25g	103	413	4.4	63.7	13.0	2.5
Cereal, Pink Grapefruit, Chewy, BGTY, Sainsbury's*	1 Bar/25g	86	345	5.0	76.5	2.1	2.4
Cereal, Pure Points, Weight Watchers*	1 Bar/50g	179	358	6.8	72.2	4.6	3.2
Cereal, Raisin & Apricot, Weight Watchers*	1 Bar/28g	100	358	6.8	72.2	4.6	3.2
Cereal, Raisin & Coconut, Value, Tesco*	1 Serving/21g	84	400	5.5	67.2	11.6	5.0
Cereal, Raisin & Nut Snack Bar, Benecol*	1 Bar/25g	98	390	3.9	68.5	11.1	2.0
Cereal, Redberry & Chocolate Sveltesse, Nestle*	1 Bar/25g	97	389	5.4	69.2	9.9	6.8
Cereal, Roast Hazelnut, Organic, Jordans*	1 Bar/33g	150	455	8.0	56.7	21.8	7.8
Cereal, Roasted Peanut, Weight Watchers*	1 Bar/26g	104	400	9.5	66.1	10.8	2.8
Cereal, Strawberry, BGTY, Sainsbury's*	1 Bar/26g	100	385	3.8	82.0	4.6	5.2
Cereal, Strawberry, Fruit 'n' Grain, Asda*	1 Bar/37g	126	340	4.2	65.0	7.0	4.5
Cereal, Strawberry, Value, Tesco*	1 Serving/21g	80	382	5.5	77.8	5.4	3.3
Cereal, Sultana & Honey, Jordans*	1 Bar/36g	130	361	6.0	65.9	8.2	9.2
Cereal, Toffee Apple, Chewy, Eat Smart, Safeway*	1 Bar/25g	89	355	4.0	78.3	2.8	2.9
Cereal, White Choc Chip, Harvest*	1 Bar/22g	94	425	6.0	67.0	15.5	3.5
Cereal, White Chocolate Muesli, Kellogg's*	1 Bar/25g	110	440	5.0	70.0	16.0	2.0
Cereal, With Fig, Fitness, Nestle*	1 Bar/23.5g	88	366	4.3	71.5	6.8	5.5
Cereal, With Pink Grapefruit, Chewy, Sainsbury's*	1 Bar/25g	86	345	5.0	76.5	2.1	2.4
Choc Chip & Nut, Chewy & Crisp, Sainsbury's*	1 Bar/27.1g	129	476	8.8	51.8	26.0	4.4
Chocolate & Hazelnut, Meal Replacement, Tesco*	1 Bar/65g	250	385	24.2	41.0	11.0	6.3
Chocolate & Orange, Crispy, Free From, Sainsbury's*	1 Bar/30g	132	440	4.8	68.2	16.2	1.2
Chocolate & Orange, Shapers, Boots*	1 Bar/26g	98	378	4.2	73.0	13.0	1.5
Chocolate & Raisin Oat Snack, Waitrose*	1 Bar/27g	112	416	5.4	67.2	14.0	2.1
Chocolate & Raisin, Shapers, Boots*	1 Bar/27g	95	353	4.7	76.0	9.1	2.7
Chocolate & Raspberry, COU, Marks & Spencer*	1 Bar/25g	90	360	5.4	78.2	2.7	3.2
Chocolate & Toffee, Free From, Sainsbury's*	1 Bar/29.9g	140	465	4.8	71.0	18.0	0.8
Chocolate Brownie, Big Softies, To Go, Fox's*	1 Bar/25g	87	348	5.5	74.9	2.9	0.0
Chocolate Caramel, SlimFast*	1 Bar/26g	99	382	3.0	72.0	12.0	1.2
Chocolate Chip, SlimFast*	1 Bar/26g	98	378	4.9	70.4	11.4	1.8
Chocolate Chip, Snack, SlimFast*	1 Bar/26g	99	382	4.9	70.4	11.4	1.8

BARS	Measure INFO/WEIGHT	per Measure KCAL	Nutrition Values per 100g / 100ml				
			KCAL	PROT	CARB	FAT	FIBRE
Chocolate Cookie Dough, Meal, SlimFast*	1 Bar/56g	220	393	14.3	64.3	8.9	3.6
Chocolate Creme, Endulge, Atkins*	2 Fingers/28g	141	504	12.5	38.6	34.3	2.5
Chocolate Crunch, SlimFast*	1 Bar/60g	215	359	23.4	47.8	10.3	6.7
Chocolate Decadence, Atkins*	1 Bar/60g	227	378	27.1	30.7	20.4	11.6
Chocolate Flavour Almond, Carbolite*	1 Bar/28g	124	438	8.7	52.0	36.0	3.8
Chocolate Hazelnut, Advantage, Atkins*	1 Bar/60g	236	393	32.3	29.0	20.3	8.3
Chocolate Heaven, Ainsley Harriott*	1 Bar/27.1g	147	543	7.0	56.0	32.0	2.5
Chocolate Muesli, SlimFast*	1 Bar/26g	97	373	4.6	53.8	14.2	6.5
Chocolate Muesli, Snack, SlimFast*	1 Bar/26g	99	379	4.7	64.5	13.3	6.5
Chocolate Peanut, SlimFast*	1 Bar/26g	99	381	5.4	66.5	13.1	1.2
Chocolate Truffle, Marks & Spencer*	1 Bar/35g	168	480	5.9	41.7	32.5	8.3
Chocolate, Caramel, & Biscuit, Asda*	1 Bar/29.5g	152	508	8.0	56.0	28.0	2.5
Chocolate, Crisp, Weight Watchers*	1 Bar/25g	92	369	5.4	75.1	10.2	0.8
Chocolate, Crispy, Blue Parrot Cafe, Sainsbury's*	1 Bar/24g	107	446	3.6	68.8	17.4	0.8
Chocolate, Digestive, Farmfoods*	1 Bar/21g	104	495	6.7	63.6	23.8	2.3
Chocolate, Double Cream, Nestle*	1 Bar/47g	250	531	8.5	54.8	30.9	0.0
Chocolate, Geobar, Traidcraft*	1 Bar/35g	126	360	5.2	72.6	5.4	4.8
Chocolate, Meal Replacement, SlimFast*	1 Bar/39g	122	314	19.9	46.2	9.4	5.5
Chocolate, Milk, Diabetic, Thorntons*	1/2 Bar/37g	174	470	7.3	43.0	33.1	2.2
Chocolate, Milk, Fimbles, Kinnerton*	1 Bar/12.1g	65	539	5.8	57.0	31.8	1.9
Chocolate, Polar, Sainsbury's*	1 Bar/25g	133	533	5.5	63.0	28.6	1.2
Chocolate, SlimFast*	1 Bar/39g	107	274	20.6	35.3	9.0	5.5
Chocolate, Soya, Dairy Free, Free From, Sainsbury's*	1 Bar/50g	274	548	10.8	47.5	35.0	4.3
Chocolate, Toffee Pecan, Marks & Spencer*	1 Bar/36g	179	498	4.9	58.3	27.3	0.7
Chocolate, Viennese, Continental, Thorntons*	1 Bar/38g	206	542	4.2	53.9	34.2	0.8
Chocolate, White, Creamy, Dairyfine, Aldi*	1 Bar/40g	220	551	5.5	58.0	33.0	0.0
Cinnamon, Danish Pastry, Cafe Creations, Health Valley*	1 Bar/40g	130	325	5.0	67.5	6.3	5.0
Club, Fruit, Jacobs*	1 Biscuit/25g	124	496	5.6	62.2	25.0	2.3
Club, Milk Chocolate, Jacobs*	1 Biscuit/24g	123	511	5.8	62.6	26.4	2.0
Club, Mint, Jacobs*	1 Biscuit/24g	124	517	5.6	62.5	27.2	1.7
Club, Orange, Jacobs*	1 Biscuit/24g	125	519	5.6	62.2	27.6	1.7
Coconut Chocolate Crisp, Weight Watchers*	1 Bar/25g	89	356	3.6	71.2	10.4	3.2
Coconut, Cool, Tesco*	1 Bar/25g	121	484	3.9	60.4	25.2	2.8
Coconut, Mueslix, Kellogg's*	1 Bar/25g	105	420	5.0	67.0	16.0	5.0
Cookie, Apple Crumble, COU, Marks & Spencer*	1 Bar/27g	90	335	5.8	72.6	2.6	2.3
Cookie, Maryland*	1 Bar/24.1g	120	498	7.6	60.0	22.5	0.0
Cookie, Oreo, Nabisco*	1 Bar/35g	180	514	2.0	66.0	29.0	0.0
Cookies & Cream, Myoplex*	1 Bar/100g	250	250	29.0	20.0	6.0	2.0
Corn Flakes & Chocolate Milk, Kellogg's*	1 Bar/40g	176	440	9.0	66.0	16.0	2.0
Cranberry & Boysenberry, Altu*	1 Serving/40g	155	387	10.6	63.9	9.9	3.4
Cranberry & Honey, Soft & Chewy, Sunny Crunch*	1 Bar/30g	115	382	6.0	73.1	8.3	3.1
Cranberry & Raisin, Geobar, Traidcraft*	1 Bar/35g	131	374	3.7	72.6	8.0	2.3
Cranberry, Perfectly Balanced, Waitrose*	1 Bar/25g	91	363	4.5	78.3	3.5	2.9
Crazy Caramel, Tesco*	1 Treat Bar/20g	94	469	4.1	66.0	21.0	1.1
Creme Brulee Chocolate, Marks & Spencer*	1 Bar/36g	178	495	4.4	54.0	29.2	0.4
Crispy Chocolate Peanut, Carb Minders*	1 Bar/60g	240	400	35.0	38.3	16.7	0.0
Crispy Lemon Yoghurt, Carb Minders*	1 Bar/60g	240	400	33.3	38.3	15.0	3.3
Crispy Orange, Reduced Fat, Tesco*	1 Bar/22g	95	431	3.6	75.5	12.7	0.6
Crispy Raspberry, Carb Minders*	1 Bar/60g	240	400	35.0	40.0	15.0	1.7
Crunchy Caramel, Tesco*	1 Bar/21g	98	467	4.6	56.0	25.0	1.4
Crunchy Crispy Treat, Kids, Tesco*	1 Bar/24g	109	453	3.6	62.5	20.9	1.5
Dairy Milk, Crispies, Cadbury*	1 Bar/49g	250	510	7.6	58.6	27.4	0.0
Dark Chocolate, Diabetic, Thorntons*	1 Bar/75g	345	460	5.4	28.5	35.8	8.1

B

BARS

INFO/WEIGHT	Measure	per Measure KCAL	Nutrition Values per 100g / 100ml				
			KCAL	PROT	CARB	FAT	FIBRE
Date & Fig, Lyme Regis Foods*	1 Bar/42g	169	402	7.3	58.2	15.5	8.9
Date & Fruit, Lyme Regis Foods*	1 Bar/42g	169	402	7.3	58.2	15.5	8.9
Date & Walnut, Eat Natural*	1 Bar/50g	221	441	8.0	57.1	20.1	3.3
Digestive, Milk Chocolate, Marks & Spencer*	1 Bar/23g	117	510	6.6	64.6	25.1	1.9
Digestive, Milk Chocolate, McVitie's*	1 Bar/23g	118	511	6.6	64.6	25.1	1.9
Digestive, Milk Chocolate, Tesco*	1 Bar/19g	96	506	6.8	61.6	25.8	2.4
Digestive, Milk Chocolate, Value, Tesco*	1 Bar/24g	119	495	6.7	63.6	23.8	0.0
Double Caramel, Go Ahead, McVitie's*	1 Cake/32g	97	302	4.0	65.3	4.4	0.7
Double Chocolate Treat, Shapers, Boots*	1 Bar/23g	92	400	3.6	74.0	9.9	0.7
Double Chocolate, Breakfast Snack, Tesco*	1 Bar/37.4g	142	385	5.3	52.7	17.0	3.3
Echo, Mint, Fox's*	1 Bar/25g	130	518	7.9	60.7	26.6	1.6
Echo, White Chocolate & Biscuit, Fox's*	1 Bar/26g	132	510	7.8	59.5	26.7	1.2
Fruit & Fibre, Whole Grain, Sainsbury's*	1 Bar/27g	109	405	6.2	70.1	11.1	3.8
Fruit & Nut Crisp, Go Ahead, McVitie's*	1 Bar/23.0g	99	430	5.3	71.3	13.7	1.7
Fruit & Nut, Coconut, Shepherdboy*	1 Bar/38g	167	439	11.6	42.3	24.8	5.8
Fruit & Nut, Eat Natural*	1 Bar/50g	223	446	11.6	49.8	22.3	5.3
Fruit & Nut, Organic, Eat Natural*	1 Bar/50g	244	488	10.2	42.9	30.6	0.0
Fruit & Nut, With Sunflower Seeds, Shepherdboy*	1 Bar/50g	216	431	17.1	40.4	22.3	5.1
Fruit 'n Fibre, Kellogg's*	1 Bar/25g	95	380	5.0	71.0	16.0	5.0
Fruit, Apple, Hellema*	1 Bar/33.1g	127	384	4.5	74.0	7.5	2.0
Fruit, Kidz Organic, Lyme Regis Foods*	1 Bar/20g	73	364	9.5	67.3	7.4	1.4
Fruit, Nut & Seed Bars, The Village Bakery*	1 Bar/25g	93	373	5.7	73.7	6.2	0.1
Fruit, Organic, The Village Bakery*	1 Bar/42.6g	150	348	4.9	67.0	6.6	5.5
Fruits Of The Forest, Advantage, Atkins*	1 Bar/60g	224	374	31.0	32.9	17.4	7.7
Fruits Of The Forest, Meal, SlimFast*	1 Bar/60g	225	375	24.0	48.3	9.8	6.7
Fruitsome, Citrus, Rowntree's*	1 Bar/35g	140	400	4.1	65.1	13.7	2.3
Fruity Cereal Bar, Free From, Sainsbury's*	1 Bar/25.1g	100	399	4.4	72.3	10.2	2.6
Fruity Cereal, Banoffee, Go, Soreen*	1 Serving/40g	143	358	6.0	72.8	4.8	0.0
Fruity Cereal, Go, Soreen*	1 Bar/40g	133	332	5.5	68.1	4.2	0.0
Frusli, Absolutely Apricot, Jordans*	1 Bar/33g	120	365	5.0	63.8	10.0	6.3
Frusli, Blueberry Burst, Jordans*	1 Bar/33g	126	381	5.5	68.3	9.5	4.6
Frusli, Cranberry & Apple, Jordans*	1 Bar/33.3g	131	385	5.1	68.9	9.9	5.8
Frusli, Raisin & Hazelnut, Jordans*	1 Bar/34g	129	379	5.7	66.0	10.3	2.1
Frusli, Tangy Citrus, Jordans*	1 Bar/33g	124	376	4.4	67.7	9.8	4.8
Fudge Mallow Delight, Whipple Scrumptious, Wonka*	1 Bar/38g	205	537	4.6	59.2	31.3	0.6
Ginger Oat, Snack, Waitrose*	1 Bar/27.0g	119	441	4.8	63.5	18.6	2.2
Ginger, Perfectly Balanced, Waitrose*	1 Bar/25g	92	367	4.9	79.3	3.3	3.3
Gold Bar, McVitie's*	1 Bar/23g	121	524	6.0	64.6	26.8	0.6
Granola, Almond & Raisin, McVitie's*	1 Serving/35g	133	380	7.0	62.9	11.3	4.1
Granola, Alpen*	1 Serving/29g	119	410	5.9	72.4	10.7	0.0
Granola, Nature Valley*	1 Bar/42g	180	429	9.5	69.0	14.3	4.8
Granola, Peanut Butter, Quaker*	1 Bar/28g	110	393	7.1	64.3	12.5	3.6
Harvest Cheweee, Apple & Raisin, Quaker*	1 Bar/22g	89	405	5.5	68.0	12.0	3.0
Harvest Cheweee, Choc Chip, Quaker*	1 Bar/22g	95	430	5.5	68.0	16.0	3.5
Harvest Cheweee, Toffee, Quaker*	1 Bar/22g	94	427	5.0	68.2	15.0	3.2
Harvest Cheweee, White Chocolate Chip, Quaker*	1 Bar/22g	94	425	6.0	67.0	15.5	3.5
Honey & Almond, Crunchy, Jordans*	1 Bar/33g	153	465	8.8	56.1	22.8	5.8
Honey, Natural, Trail Mix, Kallo*	1 Bar/40g	196	490	15.7	40.9	33.2	5.7
Italian Tiramisu, Marks & Spencer*	1 Bar/35g	184	527	6.3	49.1	34.0	0.8
K-Time, Honey Nut Crunch, Kellogg's*	1 Bar/33.4g	126	382	5.0	82.7	2.5	1.8
K-Time, Mixed Berry, Kellogg's*	1 Bar/28g	104	372	4.9	80.1	2.2	3.8
Lemon, Sicilian, Continental, Thorntons*	1 Bar/40g	201	502	4.1	55.4	29.3	0.4
Macadamia & Fruit, Eat Natural*	1 Bar/50g	243	485	7.3	44.6	30.8	0.0

BARS

INFO/WEIGHT	Measure per Measure KCAL	KCAL	PROT	CARB	FAT	FIBRE
Mango & Brazil, Tropical Wholefoods*	1 Bar/40g	172	429	4.7	61.4	19.1	4.2
Maple & Pecan, Crunchy, Jordans*	1 Bar/33g	153	464	7.7	56.8	22.9	6.5
Mighty, Asda*	1 Bar/40.9g	189	462	4.8	57.1	23.8	1.4
Mighty, Caramel, Treatsize bar, Asda*	1 bar/20.0g	96	479	3.9	64.0	23.0	1.0
Milk Chocolate Chip & Hazelnut, Snack, Benecol*	1 Bar/25g	99	395	4.7	64.5	13.1	2.5
Milk Chocolate Coated Orange Flavour, Energy, Boots*	1 Bar/70g	274	391	5.2	70.0	10.0	2.8
Milk Chocolate Whirls, Asda*	1 Bar/26g	116	447	3.7	72.0	16.0	0.8
Milk Chocolate, Mueslix, Kellogg's*	1 Bar/25g	110	440	6.0	63.0	18.0	2.0
Milk Chocolate, Wafer, Somerfield*	1oz/28g	148	529	7.0	60.0	29.0	0.0
Mint, Double Take, Sainsbury's*	1 Bar/20g	107	534	7.2	56.9	30.8	1.3
Mixed Nut Feast, Eat Natural*	1 Bar/50g	278	555	18.8	27.9	40.9	5.5
Muesli, Cookie Coach Co*	1 Bar/75g	289	385	6.8	65.1	11.1	0.0
Muffin, Cadbury*	1 Bar/68g	270	403	5.6	38.0	25.4	0.0
Nuts & Choc Chip, Asda*	1 Bar/27g	127	471	8.0	58.0	23.0	2.8
Nutty Crunch Surprise, Wonka*	1 Bar/37g	202	543	4.9	58.7	32.1	0.9
Nutty Nougat Caramel, Tesco*	1 Bar/20g	99	493	8.5	54.0	27.0	2.4
Oat Crunchy, Blueberry & Cranberry, Waitrose*	1 Bar/60g	262	437	8.0	67.0	15.2	7.4
Oats, Raisins, Honet & Apricots, Geobar, Traidcraft*	1 Bar/35g	132	376	5.3	69.0	8.8	3.5
Orange Crunch, Go Ahead, McVitie's*	1 Bar/23g	99	430	4.1	78.0	12.8	0.8
Orange Flavour, Crispy, Tesco*	1 Bar/22g	89	403	3.6	68.5	12.7	0.6
Orange Truffle, Marks & Spencer*	1 Bar/33g	177	535	6.6	55.6	31.9	1.4
Orchard Fruits & Yoghurt, Fruit & Fibre, Sainsbury's*	1 Bar/27g	102	379	5.9	75.3	6.0	4.1
Peach, Apricot & Almond, Altu*	1 Bar/40g	158	395	7.9	65.2	11.4	4.3
Peanut Butter, Chewy, Granola, SlimFast*	1 Bar/56g	123	220	8.0	35.0	6.0	0.0
Peanut, Cashew & Thai Sweet Chilli, Altu*	1 Bar/40g	172	430	14.7	47.0	20.3	3.1
Pear & Ginger, Fruit Break, Lyme Regis Foods*	1 Bar/42g	160	381	2.7	45.4	20.9	9.9
Pecan Apricot & Peach, Marks & Spencer*	1 Bar/50g	255	510	9.3	38.2	35.5	4.9
Penguin, Chukka, McVitie's*	1 Bar/28g	135	481	6.1	65.1	21.8	0.0
Penguin, McVitie's*	1 Bar/25g	133	531	5.4	65.4	27.5	1.5
Penguin, Mint, McVitie's*	1 Bar/25g	133	531	5.4	65.0	27.7	1.5
Penguin, Orange, McVitie's*	1 Bar/25g	133	531	5.4	65.0	27.7	1.5
Penguin, Snack, McVitie's*	1 Bar/24g	121	504	5.2	54.6	29.5	0.0
Raisin & Apricot, Geobar, Traidcraft*	1 Bar/35g	132	376	5.3	69.0	8.8	3.5
Raisin & Chocolate, Traidcraft*	1 Bar/35.1g	127	362	4.2	75.0	5.0	1.8
Raisin & Hazelnut, Weight Watchers*	1 Bar/24g	95	396	5.0	71.3	10.0	2.9
Raisin & Oatmeal, Breakfast Snack, Tesco*	1 Bar/37.5g	135	355	5.6	56.8	11.7	2.8
Rice Crisp, Cranberry & Orange, Go Ahead, McVitie's*	1 Bar/22.1g	92	417	3.9	77.0	10.4	1.0
Rice Crisp, With Honey, Go Ahead, McVitie's*	1 Bar/21.9g	91	415	4.1	76.1	10.5	0.8
Rice Krispies, Kellogg's*	1 Bar/20g	86	430	3.0	79.0	11.0	1.5
Rice, Chocolate & Toffee, Ultra Slim, Tesco*	1 Bar/26g	99	381	5.0	67.3	11.9	5.4
Roasted Nut, Chewy & Crisp, Sainsbury's*	1 Bar/27g	120	446	10.1	46.6	24.3	3.9
Roasted Nut, Chewy, Safeway*	1 Bar/26.9g	130	483	10.3	54.4	24.9	3.6
Rocky, Caramel, Fox's*	1 Bar/24g	115	480	6.1	60.7	23.8	0.8
Rocky, Fox's*	1 Bar/25g	126	505	7.2	59.0	26.6	1.8
Rocky, Funki Fudge, Fox's*	1 Biscuit/24.0g	125	520	6.9	60.3	27.7	1.1
Sandwich, Chocolate Viennese, Fox's*	1 Biscuit/14g	76	542	6.9	57.4	31.6	1.6
Sandwich, Chocolate, Rik & Rok*	1 biscuit/22g	105	477	6.5	70.0	19.0	0.0
Sandwich, Milk Chocolate Orange, Farmfoods*	1 Biscuit/26g	131	503	6.1	65.7	24.1	1.4
Sandwich, Milk Chocolate Orange, Tesco*	1 Biscuit/25.3g	136	536	6.2	62.2	29.1	1.8
Sandwich, Milk Chocolate, Orange, Somerfield*	1oz/28g	141	504	6.0	66.0	24.0	0.0
Sandwich, Milk Chocolate, SmartPrice, Asda*	1 Bar/25g	132	528	6.0	63.0	28.0	0.0
Sandwich, Milk Chocolate, Somerfield*	1oz/28g	142	507	6.0	66.0	25.0	0.0
Sandwich, Milk Chocolate, Value, Tesco*	1 Biscuit/25.1g	132	529	4.8	64.5	28.0	1.3

BARS

INFO/WEIGHT	Measure	per Measure KCAL	KCAL	PROT	CARB	FAT	FIBRE
School, Apricot, & Peach, Fruit Bowl*	1 Bar/20g	72	361	0.5	83.0	3.0	2.0
School, Blackcurrant, Apple, & Pear, Fruit Bowl*	1 Bar/20g	72	361	0.5	83.0	3.0	2.0
School, Cherry, Fruit Bowl*	1 Serving/20g	72	361	0.5	83.0	3.0	0.0
School, Strawberry, Fruit Bowl*	1 Bar/20g	72	361	0.5	83.0	3.0	2.0
Smarties, Nestle*	1 Bar/45g	238	528	6.2	58.2	30.0	0.9
Snack, Chocolate & Hazelnut, Benecol*	1 Bar/25g	99	397	4.7	64.5	13.1	2.5
Special K, Apple & Pear, Kellogg's*	1 Bar/23g	92	400	8.0	73.0	8.0	2.0
Special K, Peach & Apricot, Kellogg's*	1 Bar/23g	90	391	8.0	73.0	9.0	2.5
Special K, Red Fruits, Kellogg's*	1 Bar/21.5g	86	390	8.0	78.0	5.0	1.5
Strawberry, Breakfast, Carb Control, Tesco*	1 Bar/37g	144	389	7.0	40.5	23.2	4.1
Strawberry, Morning Shine, Atkins*	1 Bar/37g	145	392	28.9	24.9	21.6	14.1
Strawberry, Organic, Seeds Of Change*	1 Bar/26.2g	101	390	5.4	75.7	7.3	0.0
Strawberry, Shapers, Boots*	1 Bar/22g	75	343	2.5	77.0	11.0	0.9
Sultana, Apple & Yoghurt, Balance, Sainsbury's*	1 Bar/27g	104	387	6.1	77.4	5.9	2.3
Three Musketeer, Candy, Mars*	1 Bar/60.4g	258	430	3.3	76.2	13.2	1.7
Titan, Aldi*	1 Bar/55g	255	466	5.5	66.0	20.0	0.0
Toffee & Banana, Weight Watchers*	1 Bar/18g	67	372	6.1	77.2	3.9	1.7
Toffee Brazil Nut, Diabetic, Thorntons*	1 Serving/20g	93	467	3.2	49.0	35.1	0.5
Toffee Crisp, Nestle*	1 Bar/48g	245	511	4.3	60.6	27.9	0.0
Toffee Crunch, Simply Lite, Perfect Days*	1 Bar/51g	200	392	23.5	49.0	17.7	9.8
Toffee Delight Meal Replacement, SlimFast*	1 Bar/78g	248	318	20.6	45.3	9.6	5.9
Toffee, SlimFast*	1 Bar/39g	122	314	19.7	47.1	8.5	5.6
Tracker, Breakfast, Banana, Mars*	1 Bar/37g	176	476	4.7	63.3	22.6	9.4
Tracker, Breakfast, Lemon, Mars*	1 Bar/26g	124	477	4.6	64.3	22.4	0.0
Tracker, Chocolate Chip, Mars*	1 Bar/37g	174	470	7.0	61.0	22.0	0.0
Tracker, Forest Fruits, Mars*	1 Bar/26g	123	474	4.6	64.1	22.2	0.0
Tracker, Roasted Nut, Mars*	1 Bar/27g	139	515	9.8	53.5	29.1	0.0
Tracker, Strawberry, Mars*	1 Bar/27g	129	479	4.7	63.6	22.8	0.0
Tracker, Yoghurt, Mars*	1 Bar/27g	133	491	6.3	64.2	23.2	0.0
Triple Dazzle, Wonka*	1 Bar/39g	195	504	5.9	61.9	25.9	0.0
Trophy, Organic Four Fruits, Village Bakery*	1 Bar/42.5g	150	348	5.0	67.0	6.6	5.3
Trophy, Organic, Four Seeds, Village Bakery*	1 Bar/42.6g	175	410	9.6	58.5	15.3	5.6
Vanilla Fudge, Diabetic, Thorntons*	1 Bar/34g	156	460	3.3	69.2	18.8	0.6
Very Berry, Cookie, Big Softies, Fox's*	1 Bar/26.2g	85	325	5.7	69.7	2.5	2.5
Wafer Biscuit, Break, Two Finger, Morrisons*	1 Pack/22g	113	527	8.2	57.4	29.4	1.2
Wafer Biscuit, Milk Chocolate Coated, Value, Tesco*	1 Bar/24g	126	526	6.9	61.4	28.1	1.7
Wafer, Chocolate Flavour Crisp, Carbolite*	1 Bar/25g	120	482	8.5	52.3	34.8	2.0
Wafer, Florida Orange, Tunnock's*	1 Biscuit/20g	104	519	5.1	64.0	29.0	0.0
White Chocolate, Mueslix, Kellogg's*	1 Bar/25g	110	440	6.0	64.0	18.0	3.0
Wild & Whippy, Tesco*	1 Treat Bar/17.5g	80	447	3.7	72.0	16.0	0.8
Wild Fruit, GranoVita*	1oz/28g	99	353	6.4	53.9	12.4	0.0
Yoghurt & Muesli, Meal, SlimFast*	1 Bar/60g	221	368	24.0	46.2	11.7	6.7

BASIL

INFO/WEIGHT	Measure	per Measure KCAL	KCAL	PROT	CARB	FAT	FIBRE
Dried, Ground	1 Tsp/1.4g	3	251	14.4	43.2	4.0	0.0
Fresh	1 Tbsp/5.3g	2	40	3.1	5.1	0.8	0.0

BASS

INFO/WEIGHT	Measure	per Measure KCAL	KCAL	PROT	CARB	FAT	FIBRE
Sea, Raw, Average	1oz/28g	32	113	20.3	0.0	3.5	0.1

BATTER MIX

INFO/WEIGHT	Measure	per Measure KCAL	KCAL	PROT	CARB	FAT	FIBRE
For Pancakes & Yorkshire Puddings, McDougalls*	1 Pancake/38g	83	218	6.3	24.8	10.4	1.9
For Yorkshire Puddings & Pancakes, Morrisons*	1 Pudding/30g	43	143	6.4	23.1	2.8	4.1
For Yorkshire Puddings & Pancakes, Tesco*	1 Serving/17g	61	359	12.3	74.4	1.4	7.7
Greens*	1 Bag/125g	296	237	8.7	34.3	7.2	0.0
Made Up With Water & Egg, Safeway*	1 Serving/100g	143	143	6.4	23.1	2.8	4.1

	Measure INFO/WEIGHT	per Measure KCAL	Nutrition Values per 100g / 100ml				
			KCAL	PROT	CARB	FAT	FIBRE
BATTER MIX							
Pancakes, Sainsbury's*	1 Pancake/63g	96	152	6.5	27.4	1.8	3.1
SmartPrice, Asda*	1 Pack/128g	421	329	11.0	69.0	1.0	3.3
Tesco*	1 Pack/130g	467	359	12.3	74.4	1.4	7.7
BAY LEAVES							
Dried	1oz/28g	88	313	7.6	48.6	8.4	0.0
BEAN SPROUTS							
Average	1/2 Pack/100g	27	27	2.3	3.2	0.6	1.2
Mung, Canned, Drained	1 Serving/90g	9	10	1.6	0.8	0.1	0.7
Mung, Raw	1oz/28g	9	31	2.9	4.0	0.5	1.5
Mung, Stir-Fried in Blended Oil	1 Serving/90g	65	72	1.9	2.5	6.1	0.9
BEANFEAST							
Bolognese, Batchelors*	1 Serving/65g	196	302	23.9	39.0	5.6	13.5
Mexican Chilli, Batchelors*	1 Serving/65g	203	312	24.3	42.7	4.9	13.6
Savoury Mince, Batchelors*	1 Serving/65g	205	316	24.7	39.5	6.6	12.7
BEANS							
& Meatballs, In Tomato Sauce, Sainsbury's*	1/2 Can/200g	216	108	5.5	13.3	3.6	2.6
& Peas, Marks & Spencer*	1oz/28g	13	48	4.2	6.5	0.5	6.1
Aduki, Dried, Boiled in Unsalted Water	1 Tbsp/30g	37	123	9.3	22.5	0.2	5.5
Aduki, Dried, Raw	1 Tbsp/30g	82	272	19.9	50.1	0.5	11.1
Baked, & Jumbo Sausages, Asda*	1 Serving/210g	317	151	7.0	15.0	7.0	2.6
Baked, & Pork Sausages, Co-Op*	1/2 Can/210g	189	90	4.0	12.0	3.0	4.0
Baked, & Pork Sausages, Sainsbury's*	1 Serving/210g	248	118	5.7	13.9	4.4	3.4
Baked, & Sausage In Tomato Sauce, SmartPrice, Asda*	1/2 Can/203g	256	126	5.0	13.0	6.0	0.0
Baked, & Sausage, Asda*	1/2 Can/205g	252	123	6.0	16.0	3.9	3.0
Baked, & Sausage, GFY, Asda*	1 Serving/217g	178	82	4.7	10.0	2.6	1.8
Baked, & Sausages, Value, Tesco*	1 Can/140g	119	85	4.8	13.1	1.5	2.6
Baked, Barbecue, Heinz*	1/2 Can/100g	82	82	4.9	14.9	0.3	4.0
Baked, Cheezy, Heinz*	1oz/28g	53	189	11.6	24.5	4.9	6.2
Baked, Curried, Average	1/2 Can/210g	203	97	4.9	17.2	0.9	3.6
Baked, In Tomato Sauce, Average	1 Can/400g	346	86	4.8	16.0	0.5	3.3
Baked, In Tomato Sauce, Healthy Range, Average	1/2 Can/210g	143	68	3.9	12.8	0.2	2.8
Baked, In Tomato Sauce, Reduced Sugar & Salt, Average	1/2 Can/210g	159	76	4.6	13.7	0.3	3.8
Baked, Jalfrezi, Meanz Beanz, Heinz*	1 Serving/195g	135	69	4.5	9.8	1.3	3.6
Baked, Mexican, Mean Beanz, Heinz*	1 Serving/195g	137	70	4.5	12.3	0.3	3.6
Baked, Sweet Chilli, Mean Beanz, Heinz*	1 Serving/195g	142	73	4.5	13.0	0.3	3.6
Baked, Tikka, Mean Beanz, Heinz*	1 Serving/195g	172	88	4.8	10.6	3.0	3.5
Baked, With Chicken Nuggets, Heinz*	1 Can/200g	210	105	6.8	12.5	3.2	3.2
Baked, With Pork Sausages, In Tomato Sauce, Heinz*	1/2 Can/207g	193	93	5.3	10.7	3.3	2.7
Baked, With Vegetable Sausages, Heinz*	1 Can/200g	212	106	6.1	12.2	3.6	2.9
Blackeye, Canned, Average	1 Can/172g	206	120	8.5	19.8	0.8	3.3
Blackeye, Dried, Raw	1oz/28g	87	311	23.5	54.1	1.6	8.2
Borlotti, Canned, Average	1oz/28g	29	103	7.6	16.9	0.5	4.7
Broad, Canned, Average	1oz/28g	25	91	8.4	13.1	0.8	4.4
Broad, Canned, Drained, Average	1 Can /195g	134	69	6.8	8.9	0.8	6.2
Broad, Dried, Raw	1oz/28g	69	245	26.1	32.5	2.1	27.6
Butter, Canned, Average	1oz/28g	22	79	5.9	12.9	0.5	4.1
Butter, Dried, Boiled, Average	1oz/28g	30	106	7.2	18.7	0.6	5.2
Butter, Dried, Raw	1oz/28g	81	290	19.1	52.9	1.7	16.0
Cannellini, Canned, Average	1oz/28g	26	94	7.2	15.0	0.5	5.7
Chilli, Canned, Average	1 Can/420g	381	91	5.2	15.9	0.7	4.4
Curried, Mixed, Morrisons*	1 Tin/420g	420	100	4.2	12.1	3.9	5.6
Dwarf, Sainsbury's*	1oz/28g	7	25	1.9	3.1	0.5	2.2
Edamame, Sainsbury's*	1 Serving/150g	212	141	12.3	6.8	6.4	4.2

	Measure INFO/WEIGHT	per Measure KCAL	Nutrition Values per 100g / 100ml KCAL	PROT	CARB	FAT	FIBRE
BEANS							
Flageolet, Canned, Average	1 Can/265g	235	89	6.8	14.1	0.6	3.5
French, Canned, Average	1oz/28g	6	22	1.7	3.5	0.3	2.5
French, Raw	1oz/28g	7	24	1.9	3.2	0.5	2.2
Green, Cut, Average	1oz/28g	6	22	1.7	3.7	0.2	2.1
Green, Fine, Average	1 Serving/75g	18	25	1.8	3.4	0.4	2.6
Green, Sliced, Average	1oz/28g	6	23	1.9	3.5	0.2	2.1
Green, Sliced, Frozen, Average	1 Serving/50g	13	26	1.8	4.4	0.1	4.1
Green, Whole, Average	1oz/28g	6	22	1.6	3.0	0.4	1.7
Haricot, Canned, In Salted Water, Safeway*	1 Can/265g	257	97	6.6	16.6	0.5	4.9
Haricot, Dried, Boiled in Unsalted Water	1oz/28g	27	95	6.6	17.2	0.5	6.1
Haricot, Dried, Raw	1oz/28g	80	286	21.4	49.7	1.6	17.0
Kidney, Red, Canned, Average	1/2 Can/90g	92	102	7.8	16.7	0.6	5.6
Kidney, Red, Dried, Boiled in Unsalted Water	1oz/28g	29	103	8.4	17.4	0.5	6.7
Kidney, Red, Dried, Raw	1oz/28g	74	266	22.1	44.1	1.4	15.7
Kidney, Red, In Chilli Sauce, Sainsbury's*	1 Can/420g	340	81	5.1	14.3	0.4	4.3
Kidney, White, Dry, Raw, Unico*	1/2 Cup Dry/80g	270	338	22.5	61.3	1.1	21.3
Mixed, Canned, Average	1 Can/300g	300	100	6.8	15.7	1.2	4.1
Mixed, Spicy, Average	1 Serving/140g	109	78	4.9	13.4	0.5	3.9
Mixed, With Lentils, Waitrose*	1 Pack/300g	399	133	5.1	11.6	7.3	3.1
Mixed, With Passata, Tesco*	1 Can/300g	237	79	6.0	12.1	0.7	3.9
Mung, Whole, Dried, Boiled in Unsalted Water	1oz/28g	25	91	7.6	15.3	0.4	3.0
Mung, Whole, Dried, Raw	1oz/28g	78	279	23.9	46.3	1.1	10.0
Pinto, Dried, Boiled in Unsalted Water	1oz/28g	38	137	8.9	23.9	0.7	0.0
Pinto, Dried, Raw	1oz/28g	92	327	21.1	57.1	1.6	0.0
Refried, Average	1 Serving/215g	162	76	4.6	12.7	0.7	1.8
Runner & Carrots, Marks & Spencer*	1 Serving/240g	60	25	1.0	4.8	0.1	2.1
Runner, Average	1oz/28g	6	20	1.4	2.8	0.4	2.2
Soya, In Water, Salt Added, Sainsbury's*	1 Serving/100g	102	102	4.0	5.1	7.3	6.1
Soya, Dried, Average	1oz/28g	104	370	34.2	15.4	18.3	19.6
Soya, Dried, Boiled in Unsalted Water	1oz/28g	39	141	14.0	5.1	7.3	6.1
BEEF							
Brisket, Raw, Lean	1oz/28g	39	139	21.1	0.0	6.1	0.0
Brisket, Raw, Lean & Fat	1oz/28g	61	218	18.4	0.0	16.0	0.0
Cooked, Sliced, From Supermarket, Average	1 Slice/35g	35	101	17.4	2.6	2.4	0.4
Escalope, Healthy Range, Average	1 Serving/170g	233	137	24.2	1.2	4.0	0.4
Flank, Pot-Roasted, Lean	1oz/28g	71	253	31.8	0.0	14.0	0.0
Flank, Pot-Roasted, Lean & Fat	1oz/28g	87	309	27.1	0.0	22.3	0.0
Flank, Raw, Lean	1oz/28g	49	175	22.7	0.0	9.3	0.0
Flank, Raw, Lean & Fat	1oz/28g	74	266	19.7	0.0	20.8	0.0
For Casserole, Lean, Diced, Average	1oz/28g	35	126	23.0	0.0	3.8	0.0
Fore Rib, Lean & Fat, Average	1oz/28g	40	144	21.7	0.1	6.3	0.2
Fore-Rib, Raw, Lean	1oz/28g	41	145	21.5	0.0	6.5	0.0
Fore-Rib, Roasted, Lean	1oz/28g	66	236	33.3	0.0	11.4	0.0
Fore-Rib, Roasted, Lean & Fat	1oz/28g	84	300	29.1	0.0	20.4	0.0
Grill Steak, Average	1 Steak/170g	501	295	19.3	2.1	23.2	0.1
Grill Steak, Peppered, Average	1 Serving/172g	419	244	23.7	5.3	14.2	0.3
Joint, For Roasting, Average	1oz/28g	38	134	24.5	1.4	3.5	0.0
Joint, Sirloin, Roasted, Lean	1oz/28g	53	188	32.4	0.0	6.5	0.0
Joint, Sirloin, Roasted, Lean & Fat	1oz/28g	65	233	29.8	0.0	12.6	0.0
Mince, Cooked, Average	1 Serving/75g	214	286	24.0	0.0	20.3	0.0
Mince, Extra Lean, Stewed	1oz/28g	50	177	24.7	0.0	8.7	0.0
Mince, Lean, Raw, Average	1 Serving/100g	131	131	21.0	0.0	5.3	0.0
Mince, Raw, Average	1oz/28g	67	239	18.7	0.3	18.0	0.1

	Measure INFO/WEIGHT	per Measure KCAL	KCAL	PROT	CARB	FAT	FIBRE
BEEF							
Mince, Steak, Extra Lean, Average	1oz/28g	37	131	20.5	0.4	5.6	0.0
Mince, Steak, Raw, Average	1 Serving/125g	195	156	21.6	0.0	7.7	0.0
Mince, Stewed	1oz/28g	59	209	21.8	0.0	13.5	0.0
Peppered, Sliced, Average	1 Slice/20g	26	129	18.2	1.3	5.6	1.0
Roast, Sliced, Average	1 Slice/35g	48	136	26.1	0.4	3.6	0.2
Salt, Average	1 Serving/70g	80	114	21.7	1.0	2.5	0.1
Salted, Dried, Raw	1oz/28g	70	250	55.4	0.0	1.5	0.0
Silverside, Pot Roasted, Lean	1oz/28g	54	193	34.0	0.0	6.3	0.0
Silverside, Pot-Roasted, Lean & Fat	1oz/28g	69	247	31.0	0.0	13.7	0.0
Silverside, Raw, Lean	1oz/28g	38	134	23.8	0.0	4.3	0.0
Silverside, Raw, Lean & Fat	1oz/28g	60	215	20.4	0.0	14.8	0.0
Silverside, Salted, Boiled, Lean	1oz/28g	52	184	30.4	0.0	6.9	0.0
Silverside, Salted, Boiled, Lean & Fat	1oz/28g	63	224	27.9	0.0	12.5	0.0
Silverside, Salted, Raw, Lean	1oz/28g	39	140	19.2	0.0	7.0	0.0
Silverside, Salted, Raw, Lean & Fat	1oz/28g	64	227	16.3	0.0	18.0	0.0
Steak, Braising, Braised, Lean	1oz/28g	63	225	34.4	0.0	9.7	0.0
Steak, Braising, Braised, Lean & Fat	1oz/28g	69	246	32.9	0.0	12.7	0.0
Steak, Braising, Lean, Raw, Average	1oz/28g	40	145	24.8	0.0	5.0	0.0
Steak, Braising, Raw, Lean & Fat	1oz/28g	45	160	20.7	0.0	8.6	0.0
Steak, Economy, Average	1oz/28g	53	190	26.9	1.2	8.7	0.4
Steak, Fillet, Cooked, Average	1oz/28g	54	191	28.6	0.0	8.5	0.0
Steak, Fillet, Lean, Average	1oz/28g	42	150	21.0	0.0	7.3	0.0
Steak, Fillet, Lean, Cooked, Average	1oz/28g	52	186	28.7	0.0	8.0	0.0
Steak, Frying, Average	1 Steak/110g	128	116	23.7	0.0	2.5	0.0
Steak, Rump, Cooked, Average	1oz/28g	69	246	29.1	0.5	14.1	0.0
Steak, Rump, Lean, Cooked, Average	1oz/28g	50	179	31.0	0.0	6.1	0.0
Steak, Rump, Marinated Strips, Asda*	1oz/28g	66	235	17.6	0.1	18.3	0.1
Steak, Rump, Raw, Lean	1oz/28g	35	125	22.0	0.0	4.1	0.0
Steak, Rump, Raw, Lean & Fat	1oz/28g	49	174	20.7	0.0	10.1	0.0
Steak, Sirloin, Fried, Lean	1oz/28g	53	189	28.8	0.0	8.2	0.0
Steak, Sirloin, Fried, Lean & Fat	1oz/28g	65	233	26.8	0.0	14.0	0.0
Steak, Sirloin, Grilled, Medium-Rare, Lean	1oz/28g	49	176	26.6	0.0	7.7	0.0
Steak, Sirloin, Grilled, Medium-Rare, Lean & Fat	1oz/28g	60	213	24.8	0.0	12.6	0.0
Steak, Sirloin, Grilled, Rare, Lean	1oz/28g	46	166	26.4	0.0	6.7	0.0
Steak, Sirloin, Grilled, Rare, Lean & Fat	1oz/28g	60	216	25.1	0.0	12.8	0.0
Steak, Sirloin, Grilled, Well-Done, Lean	1oz/28g	63	225	33.9	0.0	9.9	0.0
Steak, Sirloin, Grilled, Well-Done, Lean & Fat	1oz/28g	72	257	31.8	0.0	14.4	0.0
Steak, Sirloin, Raw, Lean	1oz/28g	38	135	23.5	0.0	4.5	0.0
Steak, Sirloin, Raw, Lean & Fat	1oz/28g	56	201	21.6	0.0	12.7	0.0
Steak, Tender, Quick Cook, Average	1oz/28g	36	127	21.2	2.3	3.7	0.3
Stewed Steak, Average	1 Serving/220g	258	117	15.8	3.3	4.6	0.0
Stewing Steak, Lean & Fat, Raw, Average	1oz/28g	41	146	22.1	0.1	6.4	0.1
Stewing Steak, Raw, Lean	1oz/28g	34	122	22.6	0.0	3.5	0.0
Stewing Steak, Stewed, Lean	1oz/28g	52	185	32.0	0.0	6.3	0.0
Stewing Steak, Stewed, Lean & Fat	1oz/28g	57	203	29.2	0.0	9.6	0.0
Strips, For Stir Fry, Raw, Average	1 Serving/125g	146	117	23.6	0.0	2.5	0.3
Topside, Lean & Fat, Average	1oz/28g	61	220	27.5	0.0	12.2	0.0
Topside, Raw, Lean	1oz/28g	32	116	23.0	0.0	2.7	0.0
Wafer Thin Sliced, Cooked, Average	1 Slice/10g	13	129	24.5	0.5	3.2	0.2
BEEF &							
Beer, Princes*	1/2 Can/205g	215	105	14.0	5.5	3.0	0.0
Chips, Steak, Healthy Eating, Tesco*	1 Pack/450g	473	105	6.3	13.8	2.7	0.5
Onions, Minced, Asda*	1/2 Can/196g	314	160	13.0	4.6	10.0	0.1

	Measure INFO/WEIGHT	per Measure KCAL	Nutrition Values per 100g / 100ml				
			KCAL	PROT	CARB	FAT	FIBRE
BEEF &							
Onions, With Gravy, Minced, Lean, Sainsbury's*	1 Sm Tin/198g	285	144	17.0	3.1	7.0	0.2
Yorkshire Pudding, Minced, Sainsbury's*	1 Pack/350g	375	107	8.4	10.7	3.4	1.1
BEEF BORDELAISE							
Sainsbury's*	1 Pack/400.8g	525	131	8.7	9.7	6.4	1.0
BEEF BOURGUIGNON							
Extra Special, Asda*	1 Serving/300g	279	93	9.3	5.7	3.7	0.7
Finest, Tesco*	1 Serving/300g	351	117	15.5	3.5	4.5	1.2
BEEF BRAISED							
& Mashed Potato, Sainsbury's*	1 Pack/450g	473	105	7.7	10.3	3.9	0.8
& Veg With Mashed Potato, Sainsbury's*	1 Pack/453g	331	73	6.5	8.9	1.3	1.2
& Vegetables With Mashed Potato, BGTY, Sainsbury's*	1 Pack/453g	331	73	6.5	8.9	1.3	1.2
& Vegetables, With Mash, Eat Smart, Morrisons*	1 Serving/400g	272	68	5.6	8.7	1.2	1.7
Steak, & Cabbage, COU, Marks & Spencer*	1 Pack/380g	323	85	8.3	6.7	2.6	1.9
Steak, & Carrots, Mini Favourites, Marks & Spencer*	1 Serving/200g	140	70	8.0	4.2	2.5	1.3
Steak, & Mash, GFY, Asda*	1 Pack/400g	260	65	3.4	11.0	0.8	0.7
Steak, & Mash, Good Intentions, Somerfield*	1 Pack/450g	284	63	5.7	7.4	1.2	0.6
Steak, & Mash, Healthy Living, Tesco*	1 Pack/450g	419	93	7.0	10.2	2.7	0.7
Steak, & Mustard Mash, Healthy Eating, Tesco*	1 Pack/450g	392	87	7.4	9.5	2.1	0.7
Steak, COU, Marks & Spencer*	1/2 Pack/225g	180	80	11.9	3.6	2.2	0.7
Steak, With Colcannon Mash, Tesco*	1 Pack/450g	477	106	9.5	9.0	3.5	0.9
With Mashed Potato, Aberdeen Angus, Waitrose*	1 Serving/400g	432	108	4.6	10.1	5.5	1.1
With Parsnip Mash, Eat Smart, Safeway*	1 Pack/400g	300	75	6.8	8.2	1.2	1.1
BEEF CANTONESE							
Sainsbury's*	1/2 Pack/175g	200	114	5.5	20.1	1.3	0.5
BEEF CHASSEUR							
& Potato Mash, BGTY, Sainsbury's*	1 Pack/450g	387	86	7.8	8.4	2.4	1.3
Somerfield*	1 Serving/275g	287	104	14.8	5.2	2.7	2.1
BEEF CRISPY							
Chilli, Tesco*	1 Pack/250g	473	189	10.8	21.0	6.9	0.5
BEEF DINNER							
Roast, Birds Eye*	1 Dinner/340g	385	113	9.1	12.9	2.7	1.5
Roast, Iceland*	1 Serving/340g	354	104	8.5	9.1	3.7	1.6
Sliced, Farmfoods*	1 Serving/300g	195	65	4.0	10.6	0.7	1.7
Tesco*	1 Pack/400g	340	85	6.7	9.2	2.4	2.9
BEEF ESCALOPE							
BGTY, Sainsbury's*	1 Serving/300g	321	107	22.1	0.1	2.1	0.1
BEEF HOT & SOUR							
Chef's Selection, Marks & Spencer*	1 Pack/329g	395	120	9.2	8.4	5.3	1.3
With Garlic Rice, BGTY, Sainsbury's*	1 Pack/400g	428	107	5.9	17.0	1.7	0.6
BEEF IN							
Ale Gravy, Chunky, Birds Eye*	1 Pack/340g	272	80	7.4	8.3	2.0	1.5
Ale With Mushrooms, BGTY, Sainsbury's*	1 Pack/250.6g	193	77	10.2	5.6	1.5	0.4
Black Bean Sauce, Chinese, Tesco*	1 Pack/400g	396	99	9.1	8.7	3.1	0.5
Black Bean Sauce, Marks & Spencer*	1 Pack/350g	333	95	6.0	12.8	2.2	1.8
Burgundy Red Wine, GFY, Asda*	1 Pack/405g	348	86	8.0	9.0	2.0	1.1
Creamy Peppercorn Sauce, Steak, Tesco*	1 Steak/150g	189	126	16.5	2.6	5.5	0.1
Gravy, Roast, Birds Eye*	1 Portion/114g	117	103	13.5	3.2	4.0	0.1
Gravy, Sliced, Sainsbury's*	1 Serving/125g	100	80	13.5	2.6	1.8	0.2
Gravy, Sliced, Tesco*	1 Serving/200g	152	76	11.3	3.1	2.1	0.2
Madeira & Mushroom Gravy, Sliced, Finest, Tesco*	1 Pack/400g	536	134	15.2	4.3	6.2	1.0
Madras Sauce, BGTY, Sainsbury's*	1 Can/400g	344	86	9.5	4.0	3.6	0.9
Oriental Sauce, Lean Cuisine, Findus*	1 Pack/350g	420	120	4.5	20.0	2.5	1.5
Oyster Sauce, Asda*	1 Serving/100g	82	82	7.0	4.4	4.0	1.7

	Measure INFO/WEIGHT	per Measure KCAL	Nutrition Values per 100g / 100ml				
			KCAL	PROT	CARB	FAT	FIBRE
BEEF IN							
Red Wine Sauce, Marks & Spencer*	1oz/28g	34	120	13.2	3.6	5.9	0.3
Red Wine With Mashed Potato, Eat Smart, Safeway*	1 Serving/400g	340	85	4.6	12.6	1.4	0.7
Red Wine With Mashed Potato, Healthy Living, Tesco*	1 Pack/400g	288	72	3.4	10.2	1.9	1.7
Red Wine With Parsley Rice, Healthy Living, Tesco*	1 Serving/440g	374	85	5.2	12.2	1.7	0.6
Red Wine With Spinach Mash, Waitrose*	1 Pack/400g	380	95	7.4	10.1	2.6	0.8
Red Wine, Balanced Lifestyle, Aldi*	1 Pack/600g	426	71	10.5	2.4	2.1	1.8
BEEF MEAL							
Roast, Mini Favourite, Marks & Spencer*	1 Pack/200g	140	70	9.1	6.0	1.3	0.7
BEEF PLATTER							
Hillcrest, Aldi*	1 Pack/400g	312	78	7.7	7.2	2.0	2.4
BEEF SZECHUAN							
Sizzling Hot Spicy, Oriental Express*	1 Pack/400g	380	95	6.4	13.2	1.9	2.0
BEEF TERIYAKI							
With Noodles, BGTY, Sainsbury's*	1 Pack/400g	320	80	7.7	10.1	1.0	1.0
BEEF WELLINGTON							
Extra Special, Asda*	1 Serving/218.4g	604	277	11.0	20.0	17.0	0.9
Finest, Tesco*	1/3 Pack/216g	525	243	13.0	12.3	15.7	1.5
Marks & Spencer*	1oz/28g	76	270	10.7	17.5	18.3	1.4
Sainsbury's*	1 Wellington/175g	473	270	14.7	18.0	15.5	0.4
BEEF WITH							
Black Bean Sauce, Chilli, Sainsbury's*	1 Pack/300g	336	112	8.7	8.6	4.8	1.0
Honey & Black Pepper, Waitrose*	1 Pack/350g	326	93	9.1	9.4	2.1	1.8
Onion & Gravy, Minced, Princes*	1 Serving/200g	342	171	9.9	5.5	12.2	0.0
Onions & Gravy, Minced, Tesco*	1 Can/198g	224	113	14.0	2.8	5.1	0.8
Onions, Minced, Co-Op*	1/2 Can/196g	274	140	12.0	4.0	8.0	0.9
Oyster Sauce, Ooodles Of Noodles, Oriental Express*	1 Pack/425g	378	89	4.9	14.2	1.3	1.5
Peppercorn Sauce, Rib Eye Joint, Sainsbury's*	1 Serving/181.8g	300	165	22.2	3.4	7.0	0.1
Peppercorn Sauce, Steak, Just Cook, Sainsbury's*	1/2 Pack/128g	174	136	17.7	3.4	5.7	1.2
Red Wine Sauce, Rump Steak, Tesco*	1 Serving/150g	180	120	17.2	0.1	5.7	3.3
Shiraz Wine Sauce, Pot Roast, Finest, Tesco*	1 Pack/350g	350	100	14.1	5.1	2.6	0.9
Vegetable Rice, Hot & Sour, COU, Marks & Spencer*	1 Pack/400g	360	90	5.5	14.4	1.4	0.6
Vegetables & Gravy, Minced, Birds Eye*	1 Pack/178g	155	87	9.1	5.1	3.4	0.6
Whisky, Collops, Sainsbury's*	1 Pack/450g	513	114	8.0	4.1	7.3	1.2
BEER							
Bitter, Canned	1 Can/440ml	141	32	0.3	2.3	0.0	0.0
Bitter, Draught	1 Pint/568ml	182	32	0.3	2.3	0.0	0.0
Bitter, Keg	1 Pint/568ml	176	31	0.3	2.3	0.0	0.0
Bitter, Low Alcohol	1 Pint/568ml	74	13	0.2	2.1	0.0	0.0
Brown Ale, Bottled	1 Bottle/330ml	99	30	0.3	3.0	0.0	0.0
Extra Light, Sleeman Breweries*	1 Bottle/341ml	90	26	0.0	0.7	0.0	0.0
Ginger, Classic, Schweppes*	1 Can/330ml	115	35	0.0	8.4	0.0	0.0
Ginger, Light, Waitrose*	1 Glass/250ml	3	1	0.0	0.0	0.1	0.1
Ginger, Sainsbury's*	1 Can/330ml	178	54	0.0	13.0	0.0	0.0
Ginger, Tesco*	1 Serving/200ml	70	35	0.1	8.2	0.1	0.0
Ginger, Traditional Style, Tesco*	1 Can/330ml	218	66	0.0	16.1	0.0	0.0
Guinness*, Draught	1 Pint/568ml	210	37	0.3	3.2	0.1	0.0
Guinness*, Stout	1 Pint/568ml	170	30	0.4	3.0	0.0	0.0
Mackeson, Stout	1 Pint/568ml	205	36	0.4	4.6	0.0	0.0
Mild, Draught	1 Pint/568ml	136	24	0.2	1.6	0.0	0.0
Ultra, Michelob*	1 Bottle/275ml	88	32	0.0	0.9	0.0	0.0
Weissbier, Alcohol Free, Erdinger*	1 Bottle/500ml	125	25	0.4	5.3	0.0	0.0
Wheat, Tesco*	1 Bottle/500ml	155	31	0.5	0.4	0.0	0.0

B

	Measure INFO/WEIGHT	per Measure KCAL	Nutrition Values per 100g / 100ml				
			KCAL	PROT	CARB	FAT	FIBRE
BEETROOT							
& Roasted Red Onion, Marks & Spencer*	1 Serving/125g	94	75	1.5	12.6	2.1	2.5
Baby, Pickled, Average	1oz/28g	10	37	1.7	7.3	0.1	1.2
Pickled, In Sweet Vinegar, Average	1oz/28g	16	57	1.2	12.8	0.1	1.5
Pickled, In Vinegar, Average	1 Serving/50g	19	37	1.6	7.5	0.1	1.2
Raw, Average	1oz/28g	9	32	1.6	6.0	0.1	1.9
BHAJI							
Aubergine & Potato	1oz/28g	36	130	2.0	12.0	8.8	1.7
Bhajia Selection, Occasions, Sainsbury's*	1 Serving/15g	32	211	4.8	19.7	12.6	3.2
Cabbage & Pea With Vegetable Oil	1oz/28g	50	178	3.3	9.2	14.7	3.4
Cauliflower	1oz/28g	60	214	4.0	4.0	20.5	2.0
Mushroom	1oz/28g	46	166	1.7	4.4	16.1	1.3
Mushroom, Marks & Spencer*	1 Pack/225g	293	130	3.6	5.1	10.4	3.9
Okra, Bangladeshi With Butter Ghee	1oz/28g	27	95	2.5	7.6	6.4	3.2
Onion, Asda*	1 Mini Bhaji/49g	96	196	6.0	20.0	10.0	2.0
Onion, Delicately Spiced, Sainsbury's*	1 Bhaji/35g	96	275	7.3	22.2	15.4	4.1
Onion, Indian Meal For One, Tesco*	1 Bhaji/100g	204	204	5.5	29.2	7.3	1.3
Onion, Indian Starter Selection, Marks & Spencer*	1 Bhaji/22g	65	295	5.7	15.8	23.3	2.8
Onion, Indian Style Selection, Co-Op*	1 Bhaji/18.2g	40	220	8.0	29.0	8.0	6.0
Onion, Marks & Spencer*	1 Serving/80g	164	205	5.2	25.8	9.1	1.6
Onion, Marks & Spencer*	1 Serving/115g	219	190	4.8	24.0	8.5	1.5
Onion, Mini Indian Selection, Tesco*	1 Bhaji/23g	40	172	6.1	15.4	9.5	4.6
Onion, Mini, Asda*	1 Bhaji/19.2g	56	297	9.0	36.0	13.0	4.5
Onion, Mini, Morrisons*	1 Bhaji/18g	58	320	5.7	36.3	16.8	3.2
Onion, Mini, Sainsbury's*	1 Serving/22g	43	196	5.9	18.7	10.8	3.4
Onion, Mini, Snack Selection, Sainsbury's*	1 Serving/22g	57	257	7.3	22.2	15.4	4.1
Onion, Mini, Tesco*	1 Serving/23g	48	210	7.3	26.7	8.2	1.3
Onion, Mini, Waitrose*	1 Bhaji/21g	51	243	5.0	13.9	18.6	4.2
Onion, Morrisons*	1 Bhaji/50g	111	222	5.7	20.3	13.1	3.5
Onion, Safeway*	1 Bhaji/23g	40	175	5.7	20.3	7.5	3.5
Onion, Sainsbury's*	1 Bhaji/35g	90	257	7.3	22.2	15.4	4.3
Onion, Somerfield*	1 Bhaji/15g	39	262	5.0	15.0	20.0	0.0
Onion, Tesco*	1 Serving/18g	45	246	6.0	18.0	16.9	3.3
Onion, Waitrose*	1 Bhaji/45g	100	223	5.6	17.7	14.4	4.3
Onion, With Tomato & Chilli Dip, Marks & Spencer*	2 Bhajis/107.5g	205	190	4.8	24.0	8.5	1.5
Potato & Onion	1oz/28g	45	160	2.1	16.6	10.1	1.6
Potato, Onion & Mushroom	1oz/28g	58	208	2.0	12.0	17.5	1.5
Potato, Spinach & Cauliflower	1oz/28g	47	169	2.2	7.1	15.1	1.4
Spinach	1oz/28g	23	83	3.3	2.6	6.8	2.4
Spinach & Potato	1oz/28g	53	191	3.7	13.4	14.1	2.3
Turnip & Onion	1oz/28g	36	128	1.3	7.1	10.9	2.2
Vegetable With Vegetable Oil	1oz/28g	59	212	2.1	10.1	18.5	2.4
BHUNA							
Chicken & Rice, Sainsbury's*	1 Pack/500.7g	696	139	7.3	13.3	6.3	1.5
Chicken Tikka, Tesco*	1 Pack/350g	438	125	11.3	5.0	6.7	0.9
Chicken, Curry, Tesco*	1 Serving/300g	396	132	11.4	4.5	7.6	0.5
Chicken, Hyderabadi, Sainsbury's*	1 Pack/400g	472	118	12.6	5.2	5.2	1.3
Chicken, Indian Takeaway, Tesco*	1 Serving/350g	410	117	6.4	10.0	5.7	2.0
King Prawn, Sainsbury's*	1 Pack/400g	352	88	7.7	4.8	4.2	1.2
Lamb, & Rice, Sainsbury's*	1 Serving/124g	168	135	7.3	15.6	4.8	1.4
Prawn, Co-Op*	1 Pack/400g	300	75	3.0	6.0	4.0	1.0
BIERWURST							
Average	1 Slice/10g	25	253	14.5	1.0	21.2	0.1

	Measure INFO/WEIGHT	per Measure KCAL	Nutrition Values per 100g / 100ml				
			KCAL	PROT	CARB	FAT	FIBRE
BILBERRIES							
Fresh, Raw	1oz/28g	8	30	0.6	6.9	0.2	1.8
BILTONG							
Average	1 Serving/25g	64	256	50.0	0.0	4.0	0.0
BIRIYANI							
Seafood, Keralan*	1 Pack/450g	619	138	7.1	14.4	5.7	1.7
BIRYANI							
Chicken Tikka With Basmati Rice, Sharwood's*	1 Pack/373g	481	129	6.3	16.2	4.3	0.9
Chicken Tikka With Pilau Rice, Iceland*	1 Pack/500g	520	104	4.3	15.8	2.6	1.4
Chicken Tikka, BGTY, Sainsbury's*	1 Pack/450g	491	109	9.7	13.2	1.9	1.3
Chicken Tikka, Healthy Eating, Tesco*	1 Pack/450g	482	107	6.4	18.6	0.8	1.0
Chicken Tikka, Healthy Living, Tesco*	1 Pack/450g	482	107	6.4	18.6	0.8	1.0
Chicken Tikka, Northern Indian, Sainsbury's*	1 Pack/450g	698	155	9.4	16.5	5.7	1.2
Chicken With Rice, Tesco*	1 Pack/475g	518	109	7.2	12.1	3.5	1.0
Chicken, Easy Steam, Healthy Living, Tesco*	1 Pack/400g	424	106	7.0	15.5	1.8	0.6
Chicken, Healthy Choice, Nisa Heritage*	1 Pack/400g	380	95	6.6	12.0	2.3	1.0
Chicken, Healthy Eating, Tesco*	1 Pack/370g	289	78	8.5	10.0	0.5	0.4
Chicken, Indian, Asda*	1 Pack/450g	779	173	9.0	23.0	5.0	0.7
Chicken, Marks & Spencer*	1 Pack/400g	800	200	7.8	19.8	10.1	1.2
Chicken, Rice Bowl, Eat Smart, Safeway*	1 Pack/300g	255	85	5.5	11.3	1.6	2.4
Chicken, Tesco*	1 Pack/500g	640	128	6.0	15.0	4.9	0.6
Chicken, Waitrose*	1 Pack/450g	657	146	10.1	15.4	4.9	1.6
Chicken, Weight Watchers*	1 Pack/330g	308	93	6.2	14.6	1.1	0.6
Vegetable & Rice, Patak's*	1 Pack/370g	481	130	2.5	18.8	5.5	0.7
Vegetable & Rice, Sainsbury's*	1/2 Pack/125.0g	229	183	4.4	32.4	4.0	0.7
Vegetable With Curry, Budgens*	1 Serving/250g	378	151	3.4	22.9	5.1	1.5
Vegetable, Healthy Living, Tesco*	1 Pack/450g	455	101	2.7	17.9	2.1	1.6
Vegetable, Perfectly Balanced, Waitrose*	1 Serving/350g	238	68	2.6	14.0	0.2	2.7
Vegetable, Sainsbury's*	1 Serving/225g	329	146	2.4	16.3	7.9	1.1
Vegetable, Waitrose*	1 Pack/450g	486	108	2.8	15.2	4.0	2.2
BISCUITS							
Abbey Crunch, McVitie's*	1 Biscuit/9g	43	477	6.0	72.8	17.9	2.5
Abernethy, Simmers*	1 Biscuit/12.4g	61	490	5.7	69.2	21.9	0.0
Ace Milk Chocolate, McVitie's*	1 Biscuit/24g	122	510	6.1	66.2	24.5	1.6
After Eight, Nestle*	1 Biscuit/5g	26	525	6.5	62.6	27.7	1.5
All Butter Viennese, Marks & Spencer*	1 Biscuit/7g	40	571	7.1	71.4	31.4	1.4
All Butter, Asda*	1 Biscuit/9g	44	487	6.0	64.0	23.0	1.9
All Butter, Tesco*	1 Biscuit/9g	44	486	6.3	63.5	23.0	1.9
Almond Butter Thins, Extra Special, Asda*	1 Biscuit/4g	15	375	5.0	60.0	12.5	2.5
Almond Fingers, Co-Op*	1oz/28g	109	390	4.0	59.0	15.0	2.0
Almond Fingers, Tesco*	1 Finger/46g	180	391	6.2	58.4	14.7	1.0
Almond Thins, All Butter, Occasions, Sainsbury's*	1 Biscuit/3.1g	14	450	6.7	72.8	14.7	3.1
Almond Thins, All Butter, TTD, Sainsbury's*	1 Biscuit/3.5g	18	450	6.7	72.8	14.7	3.1
Almond Thins, Continental, Tesco*	1 Biscuit/3g	15	450	6.7	72.8	14.7	3.1
Almond Thins, Sainsbury's*	1 Biscuit/3g	13	430	7.0	80.3	9.0	1.0
Almond, Cantuccini*	1 Biscuit/8g	39	483	10.0	70.0	17.0	0.0
Almond, Marks & Spencer*	1oz/28g	140	500	7.3	62.7	24.4	2.2
Amaretti, Doria*	1 Biscuit/4g	17	433	6.0	84.8	7.8	0.0
Amaretti, Marks & Spencer*	1 Biscuit/6g	30	480	9.6	71.3	17.2	3.8
Amaretti, Sainsbury's*	1 Biscuit/6g	27	450	6.5	80.5	11.3	1.1
Animal Bites, Cadbury*	1 Pack/25g	120	480	7.1	69.8	19.0	0.0
Animals, Milk Chocolate, Cadbury*	1 Biscuit/19g	94	493	6.6	69.8	20.9	0.0
Animals, Mini Packs, Cadbury*	1 Pack/25g	123	491	6.7	70.7	20.2	0.0
Anirnals, Minis, Cadbury*	1 Biscuit/2.1g	10	480	6.5	68.5	20.1	0.0

BISCUITS

INFO/WEIGHT	Measure	per Measure KCAL	KCAL	PROT	CARB	FAT	FIBRE
Apple & Sultana, Go Ahead, McVitie's*	1 Biscuit/15g	56	386	6.0	72.7	7.9	3.3
Apple Crumble, Officially Low Fat, Fox's*	1 Biscuit/23.3g	84	365	5.4	80.4	2.4	2.5
Apple Strudel, Big Softies, Fox's*	1 Biscuit/23g	80	348	5.3	77.0	1.6	2.8
Apricot, Low Fat, Marks & Spencer*	1 Biscuit/23g	79	343	6.1	69.6	4.4	7.8
Arrowroot, Thin, Crawfords*	1 Biscuit/7.4g	33	473	7.4	76.7	15.2	2.2
BN, Chocolate Flavour, McVitie's*	1 Biscuit/18g	83	460	6.6	71.0	16.7	2.6
BN, Strawberry Flavour, McVitie's*	1 Biscuit/18g	71	395	5.6	78.0	6.8	0.0
BN, Vanilla Flavour, McVitie's*	1 Biscuit/18g	85	470	5.9	74.0	16.6	1.2
Banana Milk Shake, Creams, Safeway*	1 Biscuit/13.0g	60	460	5.6	70.9	16.8	1.8
Belgian Chocolate, Selection, Finest, Tesco*	1 Biscuit/10g	52	515	6.0	62.0	27.0	3.0
Belgian, Marks & Spencer*	1oz/28g	143	510	5.0	67.0	25.0	2.0
Bisc & Bounty, Masterfoods*	1 Bar/25g	132	526	4.8	52.3	33.0	0.0
Bisc & M&M's, Masterfoods*	1 Biscuit/17g	90	527	5.8	59.2	29.6	0.0
Bisc & Mars, Masterfoods*	1 Bar/27g	141	523	5.3	61.4	28.5	0.0
Bisc & Twix, Masterfoods*	1 Bar/27g	140	520	5.2	61.1	28.3	0.0
Biscotti, Almond, Pan Ducale*	1 Serving/30g	130	433	10.0	60.0	16.7	3.3
Biscotti, Cantuccini*	1 Biscotti/7g	31	444	10.0	65.0	16.0	0.0
Blackcurrant With Wheat Bran, Bisca*	4 Biscuits/30g	126	420	6.0	72.0	12.0	5.5
Boasters, Hazelnut & Choc Chip, McVitie's*	1 Biscuit/16g	88	549	7.0	55.5	33.3	2.4
Bourbon Creams, Asda*	1 Biscuit/14g	70	485	6.0	68.0	21.0	2.2
Bourbon Creams, Sainsbury's*	1 Biscuit/13g	60	476	5.7	70.4	19.1	1.7
Bourbon Creams, Tesco*	1 Biscuit/14g	68	485	5.6	67.8	21.3	2.2
Bourbon Creams, Value, Multipack, Tesco*	1 Biscuit/13g	62	494	5.9	68.0	22.8	1.7
Bourbon, Belmont, Aldi*	1 Biscuit/14g	68	490	5.6	68.8	21.4	1.9
Brandy Snaps	1oz/28g	122	437	2.5	64.0	20.3	0.8
Brandy Snaps, All Butter, Fox's*	1 Biscuit/12g	54	452	2.7	79.5	13.9	0.9
Breakfast, Aldi*	4 Biscuits/60g	213	355	13.7	69.5	2.5	7.5
Butter Crinkle Crunch, Fox's*	1 Biscuit/11g	52	470	5.7	70.2	18.2	1.9
Butter Puffs, Marks & Spencer*	1 Biscuit/10.5g	53	525	10.5	60.9	26.6	2.5
Butter Puffs, McVitie's*	1 Biscuit/10g	52	523	10.4	60.7	26.5	2.5
Butter Thins, Belgian Chocolate, The Best, Safeway*	1 Biscuit/10.1g	49	487	6.4	64.0	22.8	0.8
Butter, Dark Chocolate, Green & Black's*	1 Biscuit/8.3g	41	511	6.5	60.6	24.4	0.0
Cantuccini, Sainsbury's*	1 Biscuit/8g	35	440	10.4	63.1	16.2	4.4
Caramel Crunch, Go Ahead, McVitie's*	1 Bar/24g	106	440	4.7	76.6	13.8	0.8
Caramel Log, Tunnock's*	1 Biscuit/25g	118	472	4.2	64.3	24.0	0.0
Caramel Rocky Rounds, Fox's*	1 Biscuit/15g	72	480	6.2	62.3	22.9	1.1
Caramel Shortbread, Millionaires, Fox's*	1 Serving/16g	75	483	6.1	57.9	25.3	0.1
Caramel Shortcake, Boots*	1 Piece/70g	317	453	4.8	59.0	22.0	1.0
Caramel Shortcake, Mr Kipling*	1 Shortcake/36g	177	506	4.2	57.6	28.8	1.3
Caramel Shortcake, Squares, Marks & Spencer*	1 Serving/40g	190	475	5.5	59.7	23.9	1.0
Caramel Shortcake, Squares, Tesco*	1 Square/54g	274	507	4.6	54.1	30.4	0.4
Caramel Shortcake, Tesco*	1 Shortcake/45g	217	482	4.6	57.8	25.8	0.5
Caramelised, Lotus*	1 Biscuit/9g	44	488	5.0	72.0	20.0	0.8
Caramels, Milk Chocolate, McVitie's*	1 Serving/17g	81	478	5.6	65.8	21.4	1.8
Cheese Savouries, Sainsbury's*	1 Serving/50g	268	536	11.6	53.3	30.6	2.5
Cherry Bakewell, Big Softies, Fox's*	1oz/28g	98	350	5.8	72.3	2.6	2.3
Cherry Bakewell, Handfinished, Marks & Spencer*	1 Biscuit/40g	200	495	5.9	62.1	24.0	0.5
Choc Chip, Patersons*	1 Biscuit/16.67g	79	474	5.6	64.0	21.6	3.1
Chocahoops, Cadbury*	1 Biscuit/12.7g	66	510	5.8	62.7	26.4	0.0
Choco Leibniz, Dark Chocolate, Bahlsen*	1 Biscuit/14g	72	514	7.0	64.0	26.0	0.0
Choco Leibniz, Orange Flavour, Bahlsen*	1 Biscuit/14g	70	504	7.9	58.5	26.4	0.0
Chocolate & Coconut, Duchy Originals*	1 Biscuit/12.5g	71	543	6.3	52.1	34.4	2.6
Chocolate Fingers, Caramel, Cadbury*	1 Finger/8g	39	490	5.8	63.2	23.8	0.0

BISCUITS

	INFO/WEIGHT	KCAL	KCAL	PROT	CARB	FAT	FIBRE
Chocolate Fingers, Milk, Cadbury*	1 Biscuit/6g	31	520	6.8	62.9	26.9	0.0
Chocolate Fingers, Milk, Extra Crunchy, Cadbury*	1 Biscuit/5g	25	505	6.6	66.2	23.6	0.0
Chocolate Fingers, Milk, Mini, Marks & Spencer*	1 Finger/2.9g	15	515	7.1	59.5	27.9	3.4
Chocolate Fingers, Plain, Cadbury*	1 Biscuit/6g	30	508	6.2	60.6	26.8	0.0
Chocolate Fingers, White, Cadbury*	1 Biscuit/6g	32	530	6.7	62.4	28.2	0.0
Chocolate Flavour, Taillefine*	1 Biscuit/8g	33	408	5.8	70.8	10.8	5.8
Chocolate Ginger, Organic, Duchy Originals*	1 Biscuit/12.4g	62	518	4.6	59.7	29.0	2.1
Chocolate Ginger, Thorntons*	1 Biscuit/18.8g	97	512	5.9	58.2	28.4	0.0
Chocolate Kimberley, Jacobs*	1 Biscuit/20g	86	428	3.9	64.4	17.2	1.1
Chocolate Mousse Meringue, Occasions, Sainsbury's*	1 Biscuit/47g	245	522	5.6	55.7	30.7	3.2
Chocolate Orange, Thick Milk, Marks & Spencer*	1 Biscuit/13g	68	520	7.1	59.7	28.1	1.1
Chocolate Seville, Thorntons*	1 Biscuit/19g	97	512	5.7	59.0	28.1	0.0
Chocolate Teddy, Arnotts*	1 Biscuit/16.7g	81	478	6.6	69.3	19.2	2.0
Chocolate, Milk, Digestive, Homeblest*	I Biscuit/12g	60	481	7.0	64.1	21.8	2.9
Chocolate, Plain, Break, Tesco*	1 Biscuit/21g	110	524	6.3	60.4	28.6	1.9
Chocolinis, Milk Chocolate, Go Ahead, McVitie's*	1 Biscuit/12g	56	466	7.7	77.2	14.0	2.0
Chocolinis, Plain Chocolate, McVitie's*	1 Biscuit/12g	56	468	6.9	77.0	14.7	2.6
Christmas Shapes, Assorted, Sainsbury's*	1 Biscuit/14.60g	77	525	5.2	59.0	29.8	1.7
Classic, Creams, Fox's*	1 Biscuit/14g	72	516	4.4	65.2	25.8	1.7
Classic, Fox's*	1 Biscuit/9g	43	480	4.6	68.6	20.8	2.2
Classic, Milk Chocolate, Fox's*	1 Biscuit/13g	67	517	6.1	64.9	24.0	1.6
Coconut Crinkle, Sainsbury's*	1 Biscuit/11g	54	500	6.4	59.6	26.2	3.7
Coconut Macaroon, Tesco*	1 Macaroon/30g	134	448	5.5	63.7	19.0	1.6
Coconut Ring, Asda*	1 Biscuit/7.6g	39	486	6.0	66.0	22.0	2.6
Coconut Rings, Happy Shopper*	1 Biscuit/8g	42	500	6.2	70.0	21.7	2.6
Coconut Rings, Tesco*	1 Biscuit/9g	44	485	6.2	66.1	21.7	2.6
Continental Chocolate, Parkwood, Aldi*	1 Biscuit/13g	65	499	7.5	62.5	24.3	2.6
Cool Coconut, Tesco*	1 Biscuit/25g	121	484	3.9	60.4	25.2	2.9
Cranberry With Hip & Honey, Bisca*	4 Biscuits/30g	123	410	6.5	69.0	12.0	6.5
Crunchy Caramel, Tesco*	1 Bar/21g	98	467	4.8	56.2	25.2	1.4
Curls, Marks & Spencer*	1 Curl/8g	43	540	5.0	63.8	30.0	1.3
Custard Creams, 25% Less Fat, Sainsbury's*	1 Biscuit/13g	59	469	5.8	72.7	17.3	1.3
Custard Creams, 25% Less Fat, Tesco*	1 Biscuit/12.5g	61	473	5.8	72.2	17.9	1.2
Custard Creams, BGTY, Sainsbury's*	1 Biscuit/12g	57	473	5.8	72.2	17.9	1.2
Custard Creams, Jacobs*	1 Biscuit/16g	77	481	5.3	68.0	20.9	1.6
Custard Creams, Sainsbury's*	1 Cream/13g	67	514	5.5	70.4	23.4	1.6
Custard Creams, SmartPrice, Asda*	1 Biscuit/12.6g	63	486	6.0	69.0	21.0	1.6
Custard Creams, Tesco*	1 Biscuit/12g	61	509	6.1	65.0	25.0	1.5
Custard Creams, Value, Multipack, Tesco*	1 Biscuit/13g	62	496	6.0	67.3	22.6	1.6
Custard Creams, Waitrose*	1 Biscuit/11.9g	62	514	5.5	70.4	23.4	1.6
Dark Chocolate All Butter, Marks & Spencer*	1 Biscuit/15g	72	480	6.9	52.4	27.2	11.4
Dark Chocolate Ginger, Marks & Spencer*	1 Biscuit/13.1g	64	495	5.6	68.2	22.3	1.6
Digestive, 25% Less Fat, Tesco*	1 Biscuit/14g	65	462	7.3	71.0	16.5	3.8
Digestive, BGTY, Sainsbury's*	1 Biscuit/15g	70	468	7.4	71.0	17.2	3.8
Digestive, Caramels, Milk Chocolate, McVitie's*	1 Biscuit/16g	76	477	5.6	65.7	21.4	1.8
Digestive, Caramels, Plain Chocolate, McVitie's*	1 Biscuit/17g	82	481	5.7	65.5	22.1	2.1
Digestive, Chocolate	1 Biscuit/ 17g	84	493	6.8	66.5	24.1	2.2
Digestive, Chocolate Chip, Asda*	1 Biscuit/13.8g	69	491	6.0	65.0	23.0	2.9
Digestive, Chocolate Chip, Waitrose*	1 Biscuit/15g	71	473	5.6	62.9	22.1	2.3
Digestive, Cracker Selection, Tesco*	1 Biscuit/12g	56	464	7.1	65.2	19.4	4.3
Digestive, Creams, McVitie's*	1 Biscuit/12g	60	502	5.6	68.2	23.0	2.1
Digestive, Economy, Sainsbury's*	1 Biscuit/13g	65	498	6.8	66.3	22.8	3.3
Digestive, Finger, Reduced Fat, Sainsbury's*	1 Finger/8g	39	482	6.8	63.6	22.2	3.2

B

BISCUITS

	Measure INFO/WEIGHT	per Measure KCAL	Nutrition Values per 100g / 100ml				
			KCAL	PROT	CARB	FAT	FIBRE
Digestive, Fingers, Morrisons*	1 Biscuit/8g	39	482	6.8	63.6	22.2	3.2
Digestive, GFY, Asda*	1 Biscuit/14g	65	461	6.0	71.0	17.0	3.6
Digestive, Good Intentions, Somerfield*	1 Biscuit/15.3g	64	426	7.3	71.0	16.5	3.8
Digestive, Hovis, Jacobs*	1 Biscuit/12g	56	469	7.8	66.0	19.3	2.9
Digestive, Jacobs*	1 Biscuit/14g	67	479	6.6	65.7	21.1	3.4
Digestive, Lemon & Ginger, McVitie's*	1 Biscuit/15g	72	480	6.7	66.7	20.7	2.7
Digestive, Light, McVitie's*	1 Biscuit/15g	67	445	7.1	67.9	16.1	3.5
Digestive, Marks & Spencer*	1oz/28g	143	510	6.5	67.2	23.9	2.8
Digestive, McVitie's*	1 Biscuit/15g	74	495	7.0	67.6	21.9	2.8
Digestive, Milk Chocolate Homewheat, McVitie's*	1 Biscuit/17g	86	505	6.8	65.8	23.9	2.3
Digestive, Milk Chocolate, 25% Less Fat, Tesco*	1 Biscuit/17g	79	466	7.4	69.0	17.8	2.6
Digestive, Milk Chocolate, BGTY, Sainsbury's*	1 Biscuit/17g	77	480	7.4	72.5	17.8	2.6
Digestive, Milk Chocolate, Budgens*	1 Biscuit/12.7g	66	511	6.8	66.4	24.2	2.4
Digestive, Milk Chocolate, GFY, Asda*	1 Biscuit/17g	78	457	7.0	69.0	17.0	3.2
Digestive, Milk Chocolate, Marks & Spencer*	1 Biscuit/17g	89	522	6.4	65.3	26.1	2.1
Digestive, Milk Chocolate, Mini, McVitie's*	1 Bag/40g	198	496	6.6	61.9	24.7	2.9
Digestive, Milk Chocolate, Mini, Tesco*	1 Pack/30g	153	510	6.6	59.8	27.1	1.8
Digestive, Milk Chocolate, Safeway*	1 Biscuit/17g	86	504	7.0	61.5	25.5	2.2
Digestive, Milk Chocolate, Sainsbury's*	1 Biscuit/17g	87	509	6.8	66.4	24.0	2.4
Digestive, Milk Chocolate, Somerfield*	1 Biscuit/17g	87	513	7.0	67.0	24.0	0.0
Digestive, Milk Chocolate, Tesco*	1 Biscuit/17g	85	499	6.9	63.7	24.1	2.4
Digestive, Munch Bites, McVitie's*	1 Pack/40g	205	513	6.5	64.5	25.5	2.0
Digestive, Organic, Sainsbury's*	1 Biscuit/12.4g	58	483	6.6	60.9	23.7	5.8
Digestive, Organic, Tesco*	1 Biscuit/13g	60	464	7.7	66.3	20.8	4.6
Digestive, Parkside, Lidl*	1 Biscuit/13g	64	498	6.8	66.3	22.8	3.3
Digestive, Plain	1 Biscuit/14g	66	471	6.3	68.6	20.9	2.2
Digestive, Plain Chocolate Homewheat, McVitie's*	1 Biscuit/17g	83	486	6.0	61.5	24.0	4.0
Digestive, Plain Chocolate, BGTY, Sainsbury's*	1 Biscuit/17g	81	478	6.8	72.6	17.8	3.1
Digestive, Plain Chocolate, Tesco*	1 Biscuit/17g	85	499	6.2	63.5	24.4	2.8
Digestive, Plain Chocolate, Value, Tesco*	1 Biscuit/14g	71	497	6.5	62.2	24.7	3.1
Digestive, Reduced Fat, Marks & Spencer*	1 Biscuit/15.6g	77	480	7.2	73.3	17.5	3.4
Digestive, Reduced Fat, McVitie's*	1 Biscuit/15g	70	467	7.1	72.8	16.3	3.4
Digestive, SmartPrice, Asda*	1 Biscuit/15g	71	474	7.0	62.0	22.0	5.0
Digestive, Sweetmeal, Sainsbury's*	1 Biscuit/14g	72	498	6.0	66.4	23.1	3.3
Digestive, Sweetmeal, Tesco	1 Biscuit/18g	80	444	8.4	70.0	14.5	3.1
Digestive, Value, Tesco*	1 Biscuit/15g	73	487	6.9	62.8	23.1	3.2
Digestive, Waitrose*	1 Biscuit/14g	67	469	6.5	73.4	16.6	0.0
Echo, Fox's*	1 Bar/25g	128	510	7.8	59.5	26.7	1.2
Festive Box, Cadbury*	1oz/28g	139	495	6.8	65.2	23.2	0.0
First Class, Bahlsen*	1 Serving/125g	711	569	7.5	53.4	36.2	0.0
Florentines, Sainsbury's*	1 Florentine/8g	40	506	10.0	47.2	30.8	7.0
For Cheese, Bran Cracker, Christmas, Tesco*	1oz/28g	127	454	9.7	62.8	18.2	3.2
For Cheese, Chive Cracker, Christmas, Tesco*	1oz/28g	125	448	9.3	66.6	16.0	2.4
For Cheese, Cornish Wafer, Christmas, Tesco*	1oz/28g	148	530	8.0	56.8	31.2	2.4
For Cheese, Cream Cracker, Christmas, Tesco*	1oz/28g	118	421	9.9	71.9	12.7	5.1
For Cheese, Digestive, Hovis, Christmas, Tesco*	1oz/28g	127	453	4.2	74.6	18.2	7.0
For Cheese, Hovis Cracker, Christmas, Tesco*	1oz/28g	125	447	10.2	60.0	18.5	4.4
For Cheese, Poppy Snack, Christmas, Tesco*	1oz/28g	129	461	10.0	64.4	18.2	3.1
For Cheese, Sesame Carlton, Christmas, Tesco*	1oz/28g	133	476	9.1	61.5	21.5	2.7
For Cheese, Small High Bake Water, Christmas, Tesco*	1oz/28g	116	414	10.5	76.4	7.4	3.0
For Cheese, Whole Grain, Christmas, Tesco*	1oz/28g	128	458	9.0	63.9	18.5	4.1
Fruit Jambos, Rowntree's*	1 Biscuit/10.7g	47	435	4.7	73.6	13.4	1.7
Fruit Shewsbury, Mini Pack, Patersons*	1 Biscuit/16.67g	81	484	4.9	64.9	22.7	1.9

BISCUITS

	Measure INFO/WEIGHT	per Measure KCAL	Nutrition Values per 100g / 100ml				
			KCAL	PROT	CARB	FAT	FIBRE
Fruit Shortcake, McVitie's*	1 Biscuit/8g	39	483	5.9	69.6	20.1	2.1
Fruit Shortcake, Sainsbury's*	1 Biscuit/8g	39	483	5.9	69.6	20.1	2.1
Fruit Shortcake, Tesco*	1 Biscuit/9g	43	473	5.8	70.1	18.8	1.9
Fruit Shorties, Parkside, Aldi*	1 Biscuit/26g	120	461	6.4	69.1	17.7	2.1
Fruit, All Butter, Sainsbury's*	1 Biscuit/9g	45	477	5.6	66.0	21.2	1.9
Fruity Iced, Blue Parrot Cafe, Sainsbury's*	1 Pack/20g	83	415	6.0	82.0	7.0	1.1
Fruity Oat, Doves Farm*	1 Biscuit/16.7g	80	471	7.6	62.7	21.1	4.0
Fudge Flavour Choc Chip, Go Eat*	1 Biscuit/14.9g	77	510	6.5	59.2	27.4	1.7
Garibaldi, Asda*	1 Biscuit/10g	39	394	5.0	71.0	10.0	2.6
Garibaldi, Sainsbury's*	1 Biscuit/9g	35	389	5.7	67.1	10.9	3.3
Garibaldi, Tesco*	1 Section/10g	40	397	5.1	70.8	10.4	2.6
Ginger Crinkle Crunch, Fox's*	1oz/28g	124	442	4.6	77.0	12.8	1.5
Ginger Crinkle, Sainsbury's*	1 Biscuit/11g	53	486	6.2	63.8	22.9	2.9
Ginger Crunch Creams, Fox's*	1 Biscuit/14g	73	518	4.6	64.8	26.7	0.0
Ginger Nuts, Asda*	1 Biscuit/10g	45	447	5.0	73.0	15.0	0.0
Ginger Nuts, McVitie's*	1 Biscuit/12g	57	473	5.6	75.3	16.6	1.7
Ginger Nuts, Milk Chocolate, McVitie's*	1 Biscuit/14g	68	489	5.8	71.8	19.9	1.5
Ginger Nuts, Tesco*	1 Biscuit/8g	37	460	5.5	72.9	16.2	1.8
Ginger Snap, BGTY, Sainsbury's*	1 Biscuit/12g	51	427	6.5	78.2	9.8	1.8
Ginger Snap, Fox's*	1 Biscuit/8g	35	443	4.6	77.1	12.8	1.5
Ginger Snap, Less Than 10% Fat, Sainsbury's*	1 Biscuit/12.0g	51	424	6.5	78.9	9.1	1.9
Ginger Snap, Marks & Spencer*	1 Biscuit/8g	36	445	5.4	76.7	12.9	1.5
Ginger Snap, Sainsbury's*	1 Biscuit/10g	46	461	5.5	76.9	14.6	1.7
Ginger Thins, Asda*	1 Biscuit/5g	23	462	6.0	73.0	16.0	1.9
Ginger, Safeway*	1 Biscuit/12g	55	456	5.9	73.9	15.3	1.7
Ginger, Traditional, Fox's*	1 Biscuit/8.2g	32	404	4.4	70.1	11.7	1.4
Gingered, Duchy Originals*	1 Biscuit/15.7g	76	472	6.0	64.8	21.0	2.5
Gingernut	1 Biscuit/11g	50	456	5.6	79.1	15.2	1.4
Golden Crunch Creams, Fox's*	1 Biscuit/13g	66	511	4.3	65.6	25.7	1.2
Golden Crunch, Go Ahead, McVitie's*	1 Biscuit/9g	38	419	7.7	75.2	9.7	2.1
Golden Crunch, Patersons*	1 Biscuit/15g	69	474	5.1	62.5	22.6	4.8
Golden Shortie, Jacobs*	1 Biscuit/11g	54	492	6.0	64.9	23.2	0.0
Golden Syrup, McVitie's*	1 Biscuit/12.4g	61	508	5.1	67.3	24.2	2.2
Happy Faces, Jacobs*	1 Biscuit/16g	78	485	4.8	66.1	22.3	1.6
Happy Hippos, Kinder, Nestle*	1 Hippo/22g	126	573	9.5	47.0	38.5	0.0
Hazelnut Crispies, Occasions, Sainsbury's*	1 Biscuit/6.9g	36	518	6.0	64.3	26.3	0.0
Hazelnut Meringue, Sainsbury's*	1 Biscuit/6g	24	404	5.0	43.0	23.5	1.1
Hob Nobs Munch Bites, McVitie's*	1 Pack/40g	203	508	6.8	63.4	25.2	2.8
Hob Nobs, Chocolate Creams, McVitie's*	1 Biscuit/12g	60	503	6.7	60.3	26.1	4.0
Hob Nobs, McVitie's*	1 Biscuit/14g	67	476	7.7	62.2	21.7	5.6
Hob Nobs, Milk Chocolate, McVitie's*	1 Biscuit/16g	79	493	7.3	63.7	23.2	3.7
Hob Nobs, Minis, McVitie's*	1 Bag/30g	150	499	6.8	64.0	23.9	3.8
Hob Nobs, Plain Chocolate, McVitie's*	1 Biscuit/16.2g	80	498	6.7	63.3	24.3	4.2
Hob Nobs, Vanilla Creams, McVitie's*	1 Biscuit/12g	60	501	6.1	62.3	25.2	3.6
Honey & Oatmeal, Walkers*	1 Biscuit/34g	158	465	6.7	64.1	22.4	3.8
Iced Gems, Jacobs*	1 Portion/30g	116	388	5.0	85.5	2.9	1.5
Jaffa Cakes, Continental, Bahlsen*	1oz/28g	117	419	4.0	55.9	25.5	0.0
Jaffa Cakes, Dark Chocolate, Marks & Spencer*	1 Cake/11g	43	395	4.0	62.4	14.1	3.1
Jaffa Cakes, Lunch Box, McVitie's*	1 Cake/6.6g	28	395	4.2	74.3	9.0	1.4
Jaffa Cakes, McVitie's*	1 Biscuit/12g	45	375	4.1	70.0	8.5	2.0
Jaffa Cakes, Mini Roll XL, McVitie's*	1 Cake/44g	169	384	3.5	66.9	11.4	0.0
Jaffa Cakes, Mini, Asda*	1 Cake/5g	21	412	3.9	63.0	16.0	1.9
Jaffa Cakes, Mini, Co-Op*	1 Biscuit/5g	19	385	4.0	65.0	12.0	3.0

BISCUITS

	Measure INFO/WEIGHT	per Measure KCAL	Nutrition Values per 100g / 100ml				
			KCAL	PROT	CARB	FAT	FIBRE
Jaffa Cakes, Mini, McVitie's*	1 Cake/5.9g	26	441	5.1	83.1	10.2	1.7
Jaffa Cakes, Mini, Tesco*	1 Serving/5g	19	380	4.0	64.0	12.0	2.0
Jaffa Cakes, Morrisons*	1 Cake/13g	50	384	4.4	73.2	8.1	0.0
Jaffa Cakes, Plain Chocolate, Sainsbury's*	1 Cake/13g	46	384	4.4	73.3	8.1	1.3
Jaffa Cakes, Sainsbury's*	1 Serving/11g	41	373	4.3	69.3	8.8	2.0
Jaffa Cakes, SmartPrice, Asda*	1 Cake/11g	43	379	4.4	70.0	9.0	1.4
Jaffa Cakes, Tesco*	1 Cake/12g	45	378	4.2	70.4	8.8	1.4
Jaffa Cakes, Value, Tesco*	1 Cake/11g	41	377	4.4	70.3	8.7	1.4
Jaffa Viennese, Marks & Spencer*	1 Biscuit/17.2g	79	465	5.9	61.1	21.7	0.9
Jam Rings, Crawfords*	1 Biscuit/12g	56	470	5.5	73.0	17.2	1.9
Jam Sandwich Creams, Marks & Spencer*	1 Serving/15g	70	465	4.8	61.3	22.3	1.1
Jam Sandwich Creams, Sainsbury's*	1 Biscuit/16g	77	486	5.0	67.0	21.8	1.6
Jammie Dodgers, Bite Size, Burton's*	1 Pack/30g	134	448	5.1	74.1	14.2	0.0
Jammie Dodgers, Burton's*	1 Biscuit/19g	85	448	4.8	68.8	16.7	1.7
Jammie Dodgers, Mini, Burton's	1 Biscuit/29g	123	424	6.5	74.3	13.2	0.0
Jestives, Fruit & Nut, Cadbury*	1 Biscuit/17g	85	500	6.7	60.7	25.6	0.0
Jestives, Milk Chocolate, Cadbury*	1 Biscuit/17g	86	506	6.4	64.4	24.8	0.0
Lebkuchen, Sainsbury's*	1 Biscuit/10g	39	400	5.7	76.1	8.0	1.3
Lemon Butter, Thins, Sainsbury's*	1 Biscuit/13g	65	515	5.3	60.7	27.9	2.2
Lemon Curd Sandwich, Fox's*	1 Biscuit/14g	69	494	4.7	66.2	23.4	1.3
Lemon Puff, Jacobs*	1 Biscuit/13g	69	533	4.3	58.8	31.2	2.8
Lemon Thins, Sainsbury's*	1 Biscuit/10g	47	468	5.6	72.3	17.3	1.7
Lemon, All Butter, Half Coated, Finest, Tesco*	1 Biscuit/17g	84	505	5.6	60.4	26.9	3.6
Lincoln, McVitie's*	1 Biscuit/8g	41	514	6.3	69.0	23.6	2.0
Lincoln, Sainsbury's*	1 Biscuit/8g	40	479	7.2	66.1	20.6	2.1
Malt, Basics*	1 Biscuit/8g	36	470	7.1	73.6	15.7	0.0
Malted Milk, Asda*	1 Biscuit/8g	39	490	7.0	66.0	22.0	2.0
Malted Milk, Chocolate, Tesco*	1 Biscuit/10g	52	500	6.7	64.4	24.0	1.9
Malted Milk, Milk Chocolate, Asda*	1 Biscuit/11g	56	509	7.0	64.0	25.0	1.7
Malted Milk, Sainsbury's*	1 Biscuit/8g	40	488	7.1	65.5	21.9	2.0
Malted Milk, Tesco*	1 Biscuit/8g	39	488	7.2	65.6	21.9	2.0
Marie, Crawfords*	1 Biscuit/7g	33	475	7.5	76.3	15.5	2.3
Milk Chocolate, All Butter, Marks & Spencer*	1 Biscuit/14g	70	500	7.5	58.3	26.4	4.6
Milk Chocolate, Marks & Spencer*	1oz/28g	143	510	6.7	62.0	26.2	1.0
Milk Chocolate, Tesco*	1 Biscuit/25.3g	134	535	6.4	62.1	29.0	1.8
Mini Assortment, Marks & Spencer*	4 Biscuits/10g	48	480	6.1	63.9	22.5	2.8
Mint, Plain Chocolate, Tesco*	1 Biscuit/25.3g	135	538	5.1	63.0	29.5	1.7
Mixed Berries, Wheat Free, Nairn's*	1 Biscuit/10g	43	433	8.0	75.6	13.9	6.7
Morning Coffee, Asda*	1 Biscuit/4.8g	23	455	8.0	72.0	15.0	2.4
Morning Coffee, Somerfield*	1oz/28g	132	471	8.0	78.0	15.0	0.0
Morning Coffee, Tesco*	1 Biscuit/4.8g	23	450	7.6	72.3	14.5	2.4
Nice, Asda*	1 Biscuit/8g	38	480	6.0	68.0	21.0	2.4
Nice, Cream, Tesco*	1 Serving/10g	50	503	5.3	66.2	24.1	1.9
Nice, Family Selection, Elkes*	1 Biscuit/8g	38	485	6.5	68.0	20.8	2.4
Nice, Fox's*	1 Biscuit/8g	38	474	5.9	65.9	20.4	3.8
Nice, Jacobs*	1 Biscuit/7g	33	471	6.1	68.5	19.2	1.8
Nice, Sainsbury's*	1 Biscuit/8g	34	485	6.5	68.0	20.8	2.4
Nice, Value, Multipack, Tesco*	1 Biscuit/8g	39	485	6.5	68.0	20.8	2.4
Nice, Value, Tesco*	1 Biscuit/5g	24	489	6.9	64.6	22.6	2.4
Oat & Raisin, Organic, Ashbourne*	1oz/28g	129	460	5.6	62.2	22.8	2.8
Oat & Wholemeal, Crawfords*	1 Biscuit/14g	67	482	7.7	64.2	21.6	4.8
Oat Crunch, Weight Watchers*	1 Biscuit/23g	103	449	7.2	65.3	17.7	6.1
Oat, Santiveri*	1 Biscuit/5.4g	21	428	10.0	58.8	17.0	7.0

BISCUITS

	Measure	per Measure KCAL	KCAL	PROT	CARB	FAT	FIBRE
Oaten, Organic, Duchy Originals*	1 Biscuit/16g	71	441	9.8	62.3	16.9	5.3
Oatmeal Crunch, Jacobs*	1 Biscuit/8g	37	458	6.8	65.9	18.6	3.6
Orange Chocolate, Organic, Duchy Originals*	1 Biscuit/12.6g	66	509	5.5	60.0	28.0	3.0
Orange Munchy Bites, Blue Riband, Nestle*	1 Box/125g	653	522	5.2	61.4	27.9	2.0
Parmesan Cheese, Sainsbury's*	3 Biscuits/10g	53	553	14.7	56.4	29.9	1.8
Party Rings, Fox's*	1 Biscuit/6g	27	453	4.3	77.8	13.8	1.3
Party Rings, Iced, Fox's*	1 Biscuit/6g	29	459	5.1	75.8	15.0	0.0
Peanut Butter Cups, Mini, Reese's*	5 Pieces/39g	220	564	10.3	56.4	30.8	2.6
Peanut Butter, American Style, Sainsbury's*	1 Biscuit/12.5g	66	504	5.2	68.7	23.1	2.2
Petit Beurre, Stella*	1 Biscuit/6g	26	440	9.0	73.0	15.0	0.0
Pink Wafers, Crawfords*	1 Biscuit/7g	36	521	2.5	68.6	26.5	1.1
Pink Wafers, Sainsbury's*	1 Biscuit/8g	36	486	4.6	64.2	23.4	1.7
Puffin, Chocolate, Asda*	1 Biscuit/25g	133	533	5.0	63.0	29.0	1.2
Puffin, Orange, Asda*	1 Biscuit/25g	133	529	5.0	62.0	29.0	2.2
Raisin & Honey, Doves Farm*	1 Biscuit/16.6g	85	501	4.7	59.5	27.1	4.2
Ratafias, Sainsbury's*	1 Biscuit/1.9g	9	450	6.5	80.5	11.3	1.1
Rich Shorties, Asda*	1 Biscuit/10.3g	49	486	6.0	66.0	22.0	2.0
Rich Shorties, Crawfords*	1 Biscuit/10g	50	501	6.4	69.8	21.8	0.0
Rich Tea Creams, Fox's*	1 Biscuit/11.4g	50	456	5.3	62.7	20.4	1.4
Rich Tea Finger, Marks & Spencer*	1 Biscuit/5g	24	471	7.4	77.9	14.4	0.4
Rich Tea Finger, Tesco*	1 Biscuit/5g	23	451	7.4	72.9	14.4	2.3
Rich Tea, 25% Less Fat, Tesco*	1 Biscuit/10g	44	435	7.1	77.0	11.0	1.3
Rich Tea, Asda*	1 Biscuit/10g	45	447	7.0	71.0	15.0	2.3
Rich Tea, BGTY, Sainsbury's*	1 Biscuit/10g	39	430	7.8	75.9	10.6	2.4
Rich Tea, Balanced Lifestyle, Parkwood, Aldi*	1 Biscuit/10g	42	421	7.3	75.5	10.0	2.1
Rich Tea, Belmont, Aldi*	1 Biscuit/10g	44	454	7.4	71.5	15.4	2.3
Rich Tea, Economy, Sainsbury's*	1 Biscuit/8g	33	470	7.8	77.5	14.3	2.4
Rich Tea, Marks & Spencer*	1 Biscuit/10g	46	460	6.9	71.6	15.7	2.4
Rich Tea, McVitie's*	1 Biscuit/8g	39	475	7.5	76.3	15.5	2.3
Rich Tea, Milk Chocolate, Sainsbury's*	1 Biscuit/13.1g	66	504	6.3	68.5	22.7	2.1
Rich Tea, Plain Chocolate, Sainsbury's*	1 Biscuit/13g	65	497	6.6	66.0	23.0	2.6
Rich Tea, Reduced Fat, Marks & Spencer*	1 Biscuit/10g	43	430	7.8	75.9	10.6	2.4
Rich Tea, Reduced Fat, Somerfield*	1 Biscuit/10g	42	430	7.8	75.9	10.6	2.4
Rich Tea, Sainsbury's*	1 Biscuit/10g	45	454	7.5	71.4	15.4	2.3
Rich Tea, Somerfield*	1 Biscuit/8g	36	472	7.5	76.2	15.2	2.3
Rich Tea, Tesco*	1 Biscuit/10g	45	454	7.4	71.5	15.4	2.3
Rich Tea, Value, Tesco*	1 Biscuit/7.8g	36	453	7.2	72.4	15.0	2.3
Riva Milk, McVitie's*	1 Biscuit/25.2g	135	540	6.4	57.7	31.5	1.6
Rolo, Nestle*	1 Biscuit/22g	110	498	5.4	62.0	25.4	0.6
Rosemary & Raisin, Marks & Spencer*	1 Biscuit/7.1g	34	490	5.1	62.5	24.1	1.8
Sandwich, Viennese, Marks & Spencer*	1 Biscuit/15g	80	535	7.2	58.0	30.6	1.7
Savoury, Gluten, Wheat & Dairy Free, Sainsbury's*	1 Biscuit/16.5g	75	467	11.7	65.1	17.7	2.4
Savoury, Organic, Marks & Spencer*	1 Biscuit/7g	28	395	7.0	58.4	14.6	8.7
Shortbread, Chocolate Chip, Tesco*	1 Serving/20g	105	525	7.5	55.0	30.6	3.0
Shortbread, Organic, Waitrose*	1 Biscuit/12.5g	64	495	5.8	63.0	24.4	1.8
Shortcake Ring, Creations, Fox's*	1 Biscuit/20g	105	515	7.8	59.1	27.4	1.0
Shortcake, Asda*	1 Biscuit/14g	73	518	5.0	66.0	26.0	1.0
Shortcake, Caramel, Mini, Finest, Tesco*	1 Serving/15g	74	493	4.3	56.3	27.8	1.0
Shortcake, Caramel, Mini, Thorntons*	1 Piece/20.1g	98	492	4.8	46.3	31.6	0.6
Shortcake, Chocolate Caramel, TTD, Sainsbury's*	1 Shortcake/41g	211	515	4.6	50.3	32.8	1.4
Shortcake, Cranberry & Caramel, TTD, Sainsbury's*	1 Serving/40g	192	480	4.0	55.4	26.9	1.3
Shortcake, Crawfords*	1 Biscuit/10.3g	52	518	6.4	68.1	24.4	2.0
Shortcake, Dairy Milk Chocolate, Cadbury*	1 Bar/49g	252	515	7.5	59.2	27.5	0.0

BISCUITS

Measure INFO/WEIGHT	per Measure KCAL	Nutrition Values per 100g / 100ml				
		KCAL	PROT	CARB	FAT	FIBRE
Shortcake, Dutch, Marks & Spencer* 1 Biscuit/17g	90	530	5.7	58.2	30.6	0.9
Shortcake, Extremely Chocolatey, Marks & Spencer* 1 Biscuit/23g	120	522	7.8	60.0	28.7	0.9
Shortcake, Jacobs* 1 Biscuit/10g	49	485	6.7	65.6	21.8	2.0
Shortcake, Marbled Nutty Caramel, Tesco* 1 Serving/44g	220	506	5.3	53.8	29.9	1.4
Shortcake, Mini Pack, Patersons* 1 Biscuit/16.69g	82	490	5.5	60.8	25.0	3.2
Shortcake, Organic, Waitrose* 1 Biscuit/13g	64	495	5.8	63.0	24.4	1.8
Shortcake, Sainsbury's* 1 Biscuit/11g	53	484	7.2	66.6	21.0	2.0
Shortcake, Snack, Cadbury* 1 Biscuit/8g	42	525	7.0	64.2	26.6	0.0
Shortcake, Value, Tesco* 1 Biscuit/10g	49	486	7.1	66.5	21.2	2.1
Shortcake, Waitrose* 1 Biscuit/13g	67	512	6.0	68.1	24.0	1.9
Shortcake, With Real Milk Chocolate, Cadbury* 1 Biscuit/15g	75	500	6.3	65.8	23.5	0.0
Shorties, Cadbury* 1 Biscuit/15g	77	511	6.5	67.3	24.0	0.0
Shorties, Fruit, Value, Tesco* 1 Serving/10g	46	457	5.7	69.3	17.4	3.0
Shorties, Rich, Tesco* 1 Biscuit/10g	48	484	6.4	65.6	21.8	2.0
Shorties, Sainsbury's* 1 Biscuit/10g	50	500	6.4	69.8	21.8	2.0
Signature Collection, Cadbury* 1 Biscuit/15g	80	530	6.2	60.1	29.5	0.0
Spiced, Whole Wheat, Prodia* 1 Biscuit/5g	17	339	7.1	41.4	19.4	8.5
Sports, Fox's* 1 Biscuit/7.1g	30	434	6.1	61.5	18.8	1.8
St Clements Big Softies, Fox's* 1 Biscuit/14g	50	355	6.0	75.2	2.1	3.3
Stem Ginger, Brakes* 2 Biscuits/25g	124	495	5.6	62.6	24.7	0.0
Strawberry Mallows, Go Ahead, McVitie's* 1 Biscuit/18g	69	385	4.3	70.6	9.5	0.9
Strawberry, Cream Tease, McVitie's* 1 Biscuit/19g	97	510	4.8	65.9	25.2	1.2
Sultana & Cinnamon, Weight Watchers* 2 Cookies/23g	101	441	4.3	72.3	15.0	3.0
Summer Fruits, Big Softies, Fox's 1 Bar/25g	89	356	5.9	77.8	2.6	0.0
Tangy Jaffa Viennese, Creations, Fox's* 1 Biscuit/17g	76	447	5.0	63.5	19.2	0.9
Taxi, McVitie's* 1 Biscuit/26.5g	131	504	4.2	63.3	26.0	0.7
Toffee Apple Flavoured, Officially Low Fat, Fox's* 1 Bar/25.7g	91	350	5.6	75.9	2.6	2.4
Toffee Chip Crinkle Crunch, Fox's* 1 Biscuit/11g	51	460	4.6	69.6	18.2	0.0
Toffee, Choc Dips, KP 1 Pot/32g	171	534	4.4	62.2	29.7	1.2
Treacle Crunch Creams, Fox's* 1 Biscuit/13g	65	502	4.5	65.3	24.8	1.4
Triple Chocolate, Fox's* 1 Biscuits/20.9g	100	478	5.7	57.3	25.1	2.5
Viennese Creams, Raspberry, Marks & Spencer* 1 Biscuit/17.3g	88	520	4.6	60.4	28.6	1.3
Viennese Creams, Strawberry, Marks & Spencer* 1 Biscuit/16.5g	78	485	6.4	63.0	22.2	1.7
Viennese Finger, Mr Kipling* 1 Finger/32g	167	523	4.3	54.9	31.8	0.0
Viennese Whirl, Fox's* 1 Biscuit/25g	130	518	6.7	60.1	27.8	0.0
Viennese, Bronte* 2 Biscuits/50g	212	424	4.4	45.6	24.8	0.0
Viennese, Mini Pack, Patersons* 1 Biscuit/20.07g	106	527	5.4	67.1	30.8	1.6
Viscount* Mint 1 Biscuit/16g	83	521	4.8	62.7	27.9	1.3
Water 1oz/28g	123	440	10.8	75.8	12.5	3.1
Water, Asda* 1 Biscuit/5.8g	24	395	10.0	73.0	7.0	6.0
Water, Carr's* 1 Biscuit/8g	35	434	10.3	79.1	7.6	3.2
Water, High Bake, Jacobs* 1 Biscuit/5.3g	21	414	10.5	76.4	7.4	3.0
Water, High Bake, Sainsbury's* 1 Biscuit/5g	21	412	9.8	76.3	7.5	3.2
Water, High Bake, Tesco* 3 Biscuits/16g	64	401	10.5	73.1	7.4	3.0
Water, High Bake, Waitrose* 1 Cracker/6g	24	408	10.3	75.0	7.4	2.6
Water, Table, Large, Carr's* 1 Biscuit/8g	35	434	10.3	79.1	7.6	3.2
Water, Table, Small, Carr's* 1 Biscuit/3.4g	13	438	10.4	80.0	7.7	3.3
Wheat, Healthy Living, Tesco* 2 Biscuits/38g	126	336	11.8	68.0	1.9	10.1
White Chocolate, Marks & Spencer* 1oz/28g	150	535	6.8	60.8	29.3	0.7
Wholemeal Brans, Fox's* 1 Biscuit/20g	90	451	8.5	58.8	20.2	7.5
Yorkie, Nestle* 1 Biscuit/25g	128	510	6.7	60.4	26.8	1.3

BITES

Apple & Cinnamon, All Butter, Marks & Spencer* 1 Biscuit/10g	50	510	5.5	64.6	25.2	2.1

	Measure INFO/WEIGHT	per Measure KCAL	Nutrition Values per 100g / 100ml				
			KCAL	PROT	CARB	FAT	FIBRE
BITES							
Bacon, Crispy, Shapers, Boots*	1 Bag/23g	99	431	8.0	66.0	15.0	3.0
Bagel, Smokey Ham Flavour, COU, Marks & Spencer*	1 Pack/25g	91	365	10.5	75.6	2.5	5.2
Cheese & Ham, Sainsbury's*	1 Pack/21g	65	309	9.7	14.4	23.6	1.0
Ciabatta, Fried Onion, Occasions, Sainsbury's*	1 Bite/12g	44	368	10.9	37.6	19.3	1.0
Ciabatta, Garlic & Herb, Occasions, Sainsbury's*	1 Bite/12g	48	398	8.9	42.2	21.5	3.2
Egg & Bacon, Mini, Savoury, Tesco*	1 Bite/18g	55	305	8.8	20.2	21.0	2.7
Mini Apricot & Orange, COU, Marks & Spencer*	1 Bag/25g	86	345	3.4	76.9	2.5	4.1
Mini, Raspberry, COU, Marks & Spencer*	1 Pack/27g	90	340	3.8	74.9	2.7	4.5
Oat & Cranberry, Yoghurt Coated, Marks & Spencer*	1 Bite/12.5g	62	480	5.6	69.6	19.2	3.2
BITTER LEMON							
Low Calorie, Tesco*	1 Glass/200ml	6	3	0.0	0.8	0.0	0.0
Sainsbury's*	1 Glass/250ml	45	18	0.1	4.4	0.1	0.1
BLACK GRAM							
Urad Gram, Dried, Raw	1oz/28g	77	275	24.9	40.8	1.4	0.0
BLACK PUDDING							
Average	1 Pudding/40g	101	252	10.2	19.0	14.9	0.6
BLACKBERRIES							
In Fruit Juice, Average	1/2 Can/145g	52	36	0.6	7.9	0.2	1.3
Raw, Average	1oz/28g	8	30	0.8	6.0	0.3	1.6
BLACKCURRANTS							
Fresh, Raw	1oz/28g	8	28	0.9	6.6	0.0	3.6
In Fruit Juice, Average	1 Serving/30g	11	38	0.7	8.6	0.2	2.5
Stewed With Sugar	1oz/28g	16	58	0.7	15.0	0.0	2.8
Stewed Without Sugar	1oz/28g	7	24	0.8	5.6	0.0	3.1
BLISS*							
Berries, Bliss*	1 Bottle/275ml	170	62	0.0	7.8	0.0	0.0
BLUEBERRIES							
Chocolate Covered, Waitrose*	1 Serving/25g	120	481	4.0	65.6	22.4	3.0
Dried, Whitworths*	1 Pack/75g	226	301	0.9	74.2	0.1	11.4
Sainsbury's*	1 Punnet/150g	66	44	0.9	10.2	0.1	3.2
BOILED SWEETS							
Average	1oz/28g	92	327	0.0	87.1	0.0	0.0
Blackcurrant & Liquorice, Co-Op*	1 Sweet/8g	32	405	0.9	91.0	5.0	0.0
Cherry Drops, Bassett's*	1 Roll/47g	183	390	0.0	98.1	0.0	0.0
Clear Fruits, Sainsbury's*	1 Sweet/7g	26	372	0.1	92.9	0.0	0.0
Cough Sweets, Fundays, Bassett's*	1oz/28g	107	383	0.0	94.9	0.0	0.0
Fruit Drops, Co-Op*	1 Sweet/6g	24	395	0.2	98.0	0.0	0.0
Fruit Rocks, Assorted, Marks & Spencer*	1oz/28g	107	381	0.0	95.2	0.0	0.0
Fruit Sherbets, Assorted, Marks & Spencer*	1 Sweet/8g	34	425	0.0	89.7	7.3	0.0
Lockets, Mars*	1 Pack/43g	165	383	0.0	95.8	0.0	0.0
Pear Drops, Marks & Spencer*	1oz/28g	109	390	0.0	96.9	0.0	0.0
BOK CHOY							
Tesco*	1 Serving/100g	11	11	1.0	1.4	0.2	1.2
BOLOGNESE							
Beef, Asda*	1 Pack/392g	412	105	8.0	7.0	5.0	0.0
Extra Meaty, Marks & Spencer*	1oz/28g	31	110	9.0	4.8	6.1	0.3
Fusilli, Ready Meals, Marks & Spencer*	1oz/28g	38	135	7.0	13.1	6.2	1.0
Meat Free, Asda*	1 Serving/229g	179	78	6.0	11.0	1.1	0.6
Meatless, Granose*	1 Pack/400g	400	100	8.0	8.0	4.0	0.0
Medaglione, Rich Red Wine, Waitrose*	1 Serving/125g	253	202	11.6	29.6	4.1	3.1
Pasta, Minced Beef, Italian Express*	1 Pack/320g	317	99	5.7	17.5	0.7	1.9
Penne, BGTY, Sainsbury's*	1 Pack/400g	410	103	6.9	16.9	1.5	0.9
Penne, Heinz*	1 Pack/300g	213	71	3.8	11.8	0.9	0.6

B

	Measure INFO/WEIGHT	per Measure KCAL	Nutrition Values per 100g / 100ml				
			KCAL	PROT	CARB	FAT	FIBRE
BOLOGNESE							
Ravioli, Beef, Asda*	1 Serving/125g	206	165	7.0	28.0	2.8	1.2
Shells, BGTY, Sainsbury's*	1 Can/400g	340	85	5.0	11.8	2.0	0.7
Shells, Italiana, Weight Watchers*	1 Can/395g	280	71	5.2	9.6	1.3	0.7
Shells, Ready Meals, Marks & Spencer*	1 Pack/390g	585	150	7.8	11.4	8.3	0.9
Vegetarian, Marks & Spencer*	1 Pack/360g	360	100	4.5	12.5	3.5	2.1
BOMBAY ALOO							
Marks & Spencer*	1oz/28g	20	70	1.8	9.5	2.7	2.0
BOMBAY MIX							
Average	1oz/28g	141	503	18.8	35.1	32.9	6.2
BON BONS							
Apple, Lemon & Strawberry, Co-Op*	1/4 Bag/50g	203	405	1.0	88.0	5.0	0.0
Bassett's*	5 Bonbons/200g	834	417	1.1	85.4	7.5	0.0
Fruit, Bassett's*	1 Serving/6.6g	27	380	0.1	94.2	0.0	0.0
BOOST							
Cadbury*	1 Bar/55g	297	540	5.9	62.3	29.3	0.0
Treat Size, Cadbury*	1 Bar/24.3g	128	535	5.3	59.6	30.5	0.0
With Glucose & Guarana, Cadbury*	1 Bar/61g	323	530	5.8	60.3	29.6	0.0
With Glucose, Cadbury*	1 Bar/61g	326	535	5.3	59.6	30.5	0.0
BOUILLON							
Beef, Benedicta*	1floz/30ml	22	73	7.5	9.5	0.5	0.0
Beef, Touch of Taste*	1 Serving/15ml	11	73	7.5	9.5	0.5	0.0
Chicken, Benedicta*	1fl oz/30ml	23	75	4.0	8.0	3.0	5.6
Fish, Benedicta*	1fl oz/30ml	21	69	7.5	9.0	0.3	0.0
Vegetable, Benedicta*	1fl oz/30ml	30	101	7.5	17.0	0.3	0.0
Vegetable, Herbamare Concentre*	1 Serving/5g	15	298	4.6	13.5	25.4	0.3
BOUNTY							
Calapuno, Mars*	1 Pack/175g	919	525	6.3	54.3	31.4	0.0
Dark, Mars*	1 Funsize/29g	137	471	3.2	54.1	26.8	0.0
Milk, Mars*	1 Funsize/29g	137	471	3.7	56.4	25.6	0.0
BOURNVITA							
Powder, Made Up With Semi-Skimmed Milk	1 Mug/227ml	132	58	3.5	7.8	1.6	0.0
Powder, Made Up With Whole Milk	1 Mug/227ml	173	76	3.4	7.6	3.8	0.0
BOVRIL							
Beef Extract, Bovril*	1 Tsp/5g	10	197	10.8	29.3	4.1	0.0
Chicken Savoury Drink, Bovril*	1 Serving/12.5g	15	129	9.7	19.4	1.4	2.1
BOYSENBERRIES							
Canned, In Syrup	1oz/28g	25	88	1.0	20.4	0.1	1.6
BRAN							
Wheat	1 Tbsp/7g	14	206	14.1	26.8	5.5	36.4
BRANDY							
37.5% Volume	1 Shot/25ml	52	207	0.0	0.0	0.0	0.0
40% Volume	1 Shot/25ml	56	222	0.0	0.0	0.0	0.0
Cherry	1 Shot/25ml	64	255	0.0	32.6	0.0	0.0
BRANDY SNAP							
Baskets, Askeys*	1 Basket/20g	98	490	1.9	72.7	21.3	0.0
BRATWURST							
Frozen, Lidl*	1 Sausage/80g	235	294	12.8	0.5	26.8	0.0
BRAZIL NUTS							
Average	6 Whole/20g	137	687	15.5	2.9	68.3	4.9
Milk Chocolate, Tesco*	1 Nut/8g	47	585	9.9	38.0	43.7	1.9
BREAD							
10 Seed, Organic, The Village Bakery*	1 Slice/25g	66	263	9.0	43.8	5.7	3.8
Amazing Grain, Nimble*	1 Slice/22g	49	224	10.7	41.3	1.8	7.0

BREAD

INFO/WEIGHT	Measure per Measure KCAL	Nutrition Values per 100g / 100ml KCAL	PROT	CARB	FAT	FIBRE
Apricot & Sesame Seed, LifeFibre*	1 Slice/43g	148	344	8.1	55.0	10.3	6.2
Bagel, 4 Everything, Finest, Tesco*	1 Bagel/100g	268	268	11.1	51.9	1.8	2.5
Bagel, Caramelised Onion & Poppyseed, Waitrose*	1 Bagel/86g	222	258	9.7	49.2	2.5	2.4
Bagel, Cinnamon & Raisin, New York Bagel Co*	1 Bagel/85g	226	266	10.7	51.3	2.0	2.7
Bagel, Cinnamon & Raisin, Tesco*	1 Bagel/85g	207	243	9.3	47.5	1.7	2.3
Bagel, Fruit & Spice, Sainsbury's*	1 Bagel/85.1g	234	275	9.7	54.3	2.1	3.8
Bagel, Multigrain, Sainsbury's*	1 Bagel/113g	293	259	10.0	49.6	3.1	2.0
Bagel, Onion & Poppy Seed, Tesco*	1 Bagel/85g	217	255	10.0	46.7	3.1	3.6
Bagel, Onion, Tesco*	1 Bagel/85g	233	274	10.5	52.4	2.4	1.9
Bagel, Original, New York Bagel Co*	1 Bagel/85g	230	271	11.2	53.2	1.5	2.2
Bagel, Original, Organic, New York Bagel Co*	1 Bagel/85g	220	259	9.3	52.2	1.4	4.1
Bagel, Plain, GFY, Asda*	1 Bagel/84.2g	218	259	10.0	50.0	2.1	1.8
Bagel, Plain, New York Bagel Co*	1 Bagel/85g	216	254	10.6	49.2	1.7	3.6
Bagel, Plain, Organic, Waitrose*	1 Serving/86g	228	265	9.0	52.1	2.3	2.2
Bagel, Plain, Tesco*	1 Bagel/85g	220	259	9.8	50.2	2.1	1.8
Bagel, Plain, Waitrose*	1 Bagel/85g	226	266	10.4	50.7	2.4	1.5
Bagel, Poppy Seed, New York Bagel Co*	1 Bagel/85g	233	274	11.4	50.8	2.8	3.2
Bagel, Sesame Seed, GFY, Asda*	1 Bagel/83.8g	228	271	11.0	51.0	2.5	2.6
Bagel, Sesame, New York Bagel Co*	1 Bagel/84g	228	272	11.4	52.7	1.8	2.2
Bagel, Simply Plain, Marks & Spencer*	1 Bagel/85g	230	270	10.4	51.7	2.1	1.3
Bagel, White, Asda*	1 Bagel/86g	227	264	10.0	49.0	3.1	0.0
Baguette, French, Tesco*	1 Serving/60g	144	240	7.8	49.5	1.2	3.4
Baguette, Harvester, French Style, Somerfield*	1 Serving/110g	276	251	10.6	47.9	1.9	3.7
Baguette, Homebake, Half, Tesco*	1 Serving/60g	141	235	7.8	49.1	0.8	1.2
Baguette, Marks & Spencer*	1/4 Baguette/64.8g	187	287	9.8	58.6	1.4	3.2
Baguette, Mediterranean Herb, Sainsbury's*	1 Serving/60g	203	339	8.5	40.8	15.7	2.3
Baguette, Part Baked, Half, Tesco*	1/2 Baguette/150g	360	240	7.8	49.5	1.2	3.4
Baguette, Part Baked, Happy Shopper*	1/2 Baguette/55g	142	258	8.2	53.9	1.0	2.2
Baguette, Ready To Bake, Safeway*	1/4 Baguette/56.3g	147	263	8.4	54.8	1.2	2.3
Baguette, Ready To Bake, Sainsbury's*	1/2 Baguette/62g	150	242	7.8	49.7	1.3	2.8
Baguette, Ready To Bake, Waitrose*	1/2 Baguette/65g	170	262	8.9	53.8	1.2	2.5
Baguette, Soft Bake, Somerfield*	1 Serving/60g	170	284	10.3	57.3	1.5	1.9
Baguette, Take & Bake, Budgens*	1 Serving/60g	154	256	8.1	53.6	1.0	2.2
Baguette, White, Ready To Bake, Asda*	1 Serving/60g	168	280	10.0	56.0	1.8	2.6
Baguette, White, Sainsbury's*	1 Serving/50g	132	263	9.3	53.1	1.5	2.7
Baguette, White, Sandwich, Somerfield*	1 Serving/60g	155	259	9.4	52.1	1.4	1.7
Baltic Rye, Organic, The Village Bakery*	1oz/28g	68	243	8.0	50.3	1.4	2.9
Baps, Brown, Large, Asda*	1 Bap/58g	140	242	10.0	47.0	1.6	0.0
Baps, Brown, Malted Grain, Large, Tesco*	1 Bap/100g	238	238	8.5	44.0	3.1	1.9
Baps, Cheese Top, Sainsbury's*	1 Bap/75g	218	291	12.1	41.6	8.5	2.0
Baps, Cheese Topped, White, Tesco*	1oz/28g	86	307	12.2	48.0	7.0	0.7
Baps, Floured, Marks & Spencer*	1 Bap/60g	168	280	11.5	46.8	6.2	2.0
Baps, For Burger, Somerfield*	1oz/28g	77	276	10.0	48.0	4.0	0.0
Baps, Giant Malted, Sainsbury's*	1 Bap/108.5g	281	260	8.6	45.7	4.8	5.7
Baps, Malted Grain, Large, Tesco*	1 Serving/93g	231	248	8.7	46.2	3.2	1.9
Baps, Multigrain, Tesco*	1 Serving/97.5g	239	244	8.7	45.1	3.2	1.9
Baps, White Sandwich, Kingsmill*	1 Bap/80g	209	261	10.1	46.2	4.0	2.2
Baps, White Soft, Giant, Somerfield*	1 Bap/105.2g	261	249	9.1	44.7	3.8	2.3
Baps, White Soft, Somerfield*	1oz/28g	69	248	11.0	44.0	3.0	0.0
Baps, White, Floured, Waitrose*	1 Bap/60g	147	244	8.0	48.6	2.0	1.1
Baps, White, Giant, Sainsbury's*	1 Bap/103g	267	259	9.0	49.9	2.6	2.7
Baps, White, Giant, Waitrose*	1 Bap/104g	261	251	8.8	45.3	3.8	2.1
Baps, White, Large, Budgens*	1 Bap/50g	146	291	10.2	54.0	3.8	1.6

B

BREAD

	Measure INFO/WEIGHT	per Measure KCAL	KCAL	PROT	CARB	FAT	FIBRE
Baps, White, Large, Tesco*	1 Bap/86g	210	244	9.0	47.7	1.9	2.9
Baps, White, Medium, Morrisons*	1 Bap/62g	152	245	8.6	48.5	2.0	2.4
Baps, White, Sliced, Large, Asda*	1 Bap/58g	148	255	10.0	50.0	1.7	0.0
Baps, White, Soft, Floured, Marks & Spencer*	1 Bap/63g	176	280	11.5	46.8	6.2	2.0
Baps, White, Warburtons*	1 Bap/57g	144	252	9.8	43.4	4.3	2.7
Baps, Wholemeal, Diet Choice, Waitrose*	1 Bap/68g	171	252	9.6	41.4	5.3	5.6
Baps, Wholemeal, Giant, Sainsbury's*	1 Bap/110g	275	250	11.7	43.5	3.2	6.1
Baps, Wholemeal, Large, Tesco*	1 Bap/95g	223	235	10.5	39.1	4.1	7.6
Baps, Wholemeal, Sainsbury's*	1 Bap/60g	151	252	9.6	41.4	5.3	5.6
Baps, Wholemeal, Tesco*	1 Bap/46g	104	227	9.6	41.4	5.3	5.6
Batch, Multiseed, Organic, Tesco*	1 Slice/54g	138	256	13.6	33.9	7.3	8.2
Batch, Oatmeal, Finest, Tesco*	1 Slice/50g	120	240	9.3	42.7	3.5	5.4
Batch, Seeded, Finest, Tesco*	1 Slice/65g	168	259	9.3	41.8	6.1	6.1
Batch, Seeded, Warburtons*	1 Thick Slice/46g	127	277	11.0	38.7	8.3	3.0
Batch, White, Warburtons*	1 Thick Slice/42g	98	233	9.8	43.6	2.1	2.7
Best Of Both, Medium Sliced, Hovis*	1 Slice/40g	86	214	9.2	39.6	2.2	5.6
Best With Less, Hovis*	1oz/28g	55	195	11.3	33.4	1.9	7.5
Black Olive, Finest, Tesco*	1 Serving/72g	184	255	9.7	39.7	6.4	2.9
Bloomer, Multi Seed, Organic, Sainsbury's*	1 Serving/60g	160	266	10.9	40.3	6.8	8.8
Bloomer, Multiseed, Sliced, Marks & Spencer*	1 Slice/53.6g	151	280	10.5	43.6	7.2	3.1
Bloomer, Soft Grain, Marks & Spencer*	1 Slice/34g	80	235	9.5	45.5	1.5	3.6
Bloomer, Vienna, Marks & Spencer*	1oz/28g	79	281	9.6	55.8	2.1	2.7
Bloomer, White, Bake Off, Somerfield*	1oz/28g	69	246	9.0	47.0	3.0	0.0
Bloomer, White, Seeded, Bake Off, Somerfield*	1oz/28g	68	243	9.0	46.0	3.0	0.0
Bloomer, Wholemeal, Organic, Marks & Spencer*	1 Slice/50g	120	240	8.7	35.5	8.0	5.2
Breadcakes, Big Brown, Morrisons*	1 Breadcake/63g	154	245	9.0	44.6	3.4	4.3
Brioche, Finest, Tesco*	1 Bun/52g	207	398	10.8	38.3	22.4	2.0
Brioche, Loaf, Butter, Sainsbury's*	1/8 Loaf/50g	174	347	8.0	55.0	10.5	2.2
Brioche, Marks & Spencer*	1 Brioche/50g	182	363	7.8	40.2	20.5	1.5
Brioche, Rolls, Tesco*	1 Roll/26g	92	349	8.5	54.0	11.0	0.0
Brown	1 Med Slice/34g	74	218	8.5	44.3	2.0	3.5
Brown, Brace's*	1 Serving/26.5g	57	219	10.1	38.0	3.0	3.7
Brown, Crusty Golden, Hovis*	1 Slice/44g	102	231	8.7	43.0	2.7	3.3
Brown, Danish, Sliced, Weight Watchers*	1 Slice/19g	41	215	11.0	38.8	2.0	7.3
Brown, Danish, Warburtons*	1 Slice/19g	38	200	8.6	37.7	1.6	9.6
Brown, Farmhouse, Linwoods*	1 Slice/25g	56	225	7.3	44.4	1.7	5.8
Brown, Fibre Rich, Allinson*	1 Slice/24g	51	212	13.2	33.6	2.8	8.0
Brown, Free From, Sliced, Tesco*	1 Slice/45g	121	268	5.4	43.2	8.2	3.6
Brown, Gluten & Wheat Free, Sliced, Dietary Specials*	1 Slice/25g	56	224	3.4	41.0	5.2	9.4
Brown, Good Health, Warburtons*	1 Slice/34.8g	79	226	10.3	39.6	2.9	7.2
Brown, Harvest, Marks & Spencer*	1oz/28g	67	240	8.8	44.5	2.7	3.7
Brown, High Fibre, Ormo*	1 Slice/24g	57	239	9.2	42.9	2.6	7.5
Brown, Honey & Oat Bran, Vogel*	1 Serving/100g	220	220	7.9	39.2	4.5	5.7
Brown, Malted, Farmhouse Gold, Morrisons*	1 Slice/38g	94	248	8.2	49.6	1.4	3.0
Brown, Medium Sliced, Best Of Health, Hovis*	2 Slices/76g	158	208	10.1	36.4	2.4	6.9
Brown, Medium Sliced, Sainsbury's*	1 Slice/36g	81	225	8.2	43.8	1.9	3.9
Brown, Medium Sliced, Tesco*	2 Slices/72g	157	218	8.0	41.6	2.2	4.5
Brown, Medium, Irwin's*	2 Slices/67g	143	213	9.7	42.9	0.3	4.4
Brown, Mixed Grain, Vogel*	1 Serving/45g	102	227	9.8	47.1	1.3	6.4
Brown, New Look, Weight Watchers*	1 Slice/12.2g	28	235	14.1	39.9	2.6	5.1
Brown, Original Wheatgerm, Medium Sliced, Hovis*	1 Slice/33g	77	233	10.8	40.1	3.3	3.7
Brown, Premium Gold Malted, TTD, Sainsbury's*	1 Slice/43g	93	217	8.5	40.3	2.4	2.4
Brown, Premium, Warburtons*	1 Slice/23.7g	60	249	10.6	43.2	3.7	5.1

BREAD

INFO/WEIGHT	Measure	per Measure KCAL	KCAL	PROT	CARB	FAT	FIBRE
Brown, Sainsbury's*	1 Slice/34g	81	239	8.4	46.8	2.1	4.2
Brown, Seeded Batch, Warburtons*	1 Slice/28.1g	78	279	11.3	39.4	8.5	3.2
Brown, Sliced, Medium, Asda*	1 Slice/36g	80	223	8.0	44.0	1.7	4.6
Brown, Soda, Marks & Spencer*	1 Slice/40g	92	229	9.2	43.6	3.6	4.9
Brown, Soy & Linseed, Vogel*	1 Slice/50g	116	232	11.2	33.3	4.9	0.0
Brown, Thick, Country Baked, Lidl*	1 Slice/38g	82	217	8.1	42.6	1.6	4.5
Brown, Thick, Warburtons*	1 Slice/37.9g	80	211	9.4	39.2	1.8	6.2
Brown, Thin Sliced, Sainsbury's*	1 Slice/28.9g	65	225	8.2	43.8	1.9	3.9
Brown, Toasted	1 Med Slice/24g	65	272	10.4	56.5	2.1	4.5
Brown, Toastie, Kingsmill*	1 Thick Slice/43.9g	101	230	9.5	40.5	3.3	4.7
Brown, Weight Watchers*	1 Slice/12g	25	209	11.9	36.5	1.8	6.3
Buns, Burger, Farmfoods*	1 Bun/53g	131	248	8.0	47.5	2.9	2.2
Buns, White, Burger, Waitrose*	1 Serving/64g	169	264	10.0	47.2	3.9	2.7
Carbs So Low, Nimble*	1 Slice/22g	45	204	11.6	34.4	2.2	5.9
Cheese & Onion, Somerfield*	1oz/28g	67	241	8.0	44.0	4.0	0.0
Cheese & Onion, Tear & Share, Sainsbury's*	1/4 Bread/71g	202	285	9.8	40.6	9.3	1.9
Cheese & Tomato, Tear & Share, Sainsbury's*	1/4 Bread/72g	211	293	8.0	35.7	13.2	1.5
Cheese Onion & Garlic, Sainsbury's*	1 Baguette/190g	688	362	7.8	36.8	20.4	2.0
Cheese, Morrisons*	1 Serving/96g	297	311	9.9	35.9	14.2	3.0
Cheese, Onion & Garlic, Tear & Share, Waitrose*	1/4 Bread/112g	326	290	9.4	33.9	13.0	2.1
Cheese, Onion Mustard Seed, Cluster, Sainsbury's*	1 Cluster/100g	276	276	10.0	40.6	8.1	3.1
Cholla, Average	1/10 Loaf/154g	421	274	6.9	40.9	9.3	1.0
Cholla, Marks & Spencer*	1 Serving/67.9g	190	280	10.2	46.6	6.1	2.3
Ciabatta Stick, Organic, Marks & Spencer*	1 Stick/140g	315	225	8.9	48.5	1.4	4.2
Ciabatta, Black Olive, Part Baked, Sainsbury's*	1/4 Ciabatta/67g	172	257	8.8	46.8	3.8	2.4
Ciabatta, Black Olive, Ready To Bake, Sainsbury's*	1/4 Ciabatta/66g	170	257	8.8	46.8	3.8	2.4
Ciabatta, Extra Special, Asda*	1 Slice/19g	49	260	10.0	44.0	4.9	4.8
Ciabatta, Finest, Tesco*	1/4 Ciabatta/70g	185	264	9.3	42.5	6.3	2.3
Ciabatta, Green Olive, Tesco*	1/4 Loaf/70g	155	222	7.4	38.2	4.4	1.9
Ciabatta, Half, Heat & Serve, TTD, Sainsbury's*	1/2 Ciabatta/67g	182	274	10.4	44.8	5.9	2.7
Ciabatta, Half, Marks & Spencer*	1 Loaf/135g	354	262	10.3	48.1	4.1	2.1
Ciabatta, Half, Organic, Sainsbury's*	1/2 Roll/63g	152	241	9.1	48.7	1.0	2.3
Ciabatta, Italian Style, Flutes, The Best, Safeway*	1 Flute/125g	319	255	8.8	47.2	3.5	2.2
Ciabatta, Italian Style, Safeway*	1/4 Loaf/75g	194	258	8.9	47.7	3.5	2.2
Ciabatta, Marks & Spencer*	1 Ciabatta/130g	341	262	10.3	48.1	4.1	2.1
Ciabatta, Olive, Safeway*	1 Serving/25g	60	238	8.2	43.7	3.4	2.3
Ciabatta, Oregano & Feta, TTD, Sainsbury's*	1/2 Loaf/200g	574	287	10.4	36.5	11.0	2.4
Ciabatta, Organic, Marks & Spencer*	1oz/28g	59	209	7.8	42.5	0.9	1.9
Ciabatta, Organic, Tesco*	1/3 Loaf/100g	240	240	8.7	43.2	3.6	2.4
Ciabatta, Part Baked, Half, Sainsbury's*	1/2 Ciabbatta/67g	174	260	8.9	47.7	3.7	2.2
Ciabatta, Plain, Tesco*	1/4 Loaf/73g	174	240	9.8	41.5	3.9	2.4
Ciabatta, Ready To Bake, Marks & Spencer*	1 Serving/150g	393	262	10.3	48.1	4.1	2.1
Ciabatta, Ready To Bake, Sainsbury's*	1/2 Ciabatta/66g	172	260	8.9	47.7	3.7	2.2
Ciabatta, Spicy Topped, Finest, Tesco*	1 Serving/73g	163	223	9.2	34.0	5.5	1.7
Ciabatta, Sun Dried Tomato & Basil, Tesco*	1/4 Loaf/75g	193	257	8.9	42.4	5.7	2.4
Ciabatta, Sun Dried Tomato & Olive, TTD, Sainsbury's*	1 Serving/62g	161	260	10.0	39.7	6.8	2.5
Ciabatta, Sun Dried Tomato, Safeway*	1 Serving/127g	375	295	8.8	46.6	8.3	2.8
Ciabatta, Sweet Pepper, Healthy Eating, Tesco*	1 Serving/50g	135	270	11.8	49.5	2.7	2.8
Ciabatta, Tomato & Basil, GFY, Asda*	1 Serving/55g	143	260	9.0	51.0	2.2	0.0
Ciabatta, Tomato & Mozzarella, Iceland*	1 Ciabatta/150g	374	249	10.0	29.6	10.1	3.3
Cinnamon Swirl, Asda*	1 Serving/25g	87	349	6.0	52.0	13.0	1.6
Cottage Loaf, Stonebaked, Asda*	1 Serving/67g	155	232	10.0	45.0	1.3	3.2
Country Grain, COU, Marks & Spencer*	1 Slice/25g	58	233	11.0	42.8	2.0	5.6

BREAD

	Measure INFO/WEIGHT	per Measure KCAL	Nutrition Values per 100g / 100ml				
			KCAL	PROT	CARB	FAT	FIBRE
Crusty Loaf, Harvest Blend, Warburtons*	1 Slice/28.6g	64	220	11.3	37.4	2.8	4.3
Danish, Medium Sliced, Tesco*	1 Slice/20g	47	234	9.4	45.4	1.7	3.3
Danish, White, Medium Sliced, BFY, Morrisons*	1 Slice/17g	42	245	10.2	49.1	1.8	2.2
Farmhouse Loaf, Hovis*	1 Slice/44g	100	228	9.0	44.6	1.5	2.3
Fiery Green Pepper & Cheese, The Best, Safeway*	1/4 Loaf/75g	180	240	12.3	38.4	4.1	3.4
Fig & Almond, Bröderna Cartwright*	4 Slices/100g	267	267	9.2	39.7	7.5	0.0
Focaccia, Mini, Sun Dried Tomato & Basil, Sainsbury's*	1oz/28g	90	321	8.0	41.8	13.6	0.0
Focaccia, Onion & Herb, Tesco*	1/2 Pack/190g	547	288	8.7	35.2	12.5	3.7
Focaccia, Oregano, The Best, Safeway*	1 Serving/55.6g	151	270	9.1	45.0	5.7	1.8
Focaccia, Roast Cherry Tomato & Olive, GFY, Asda*	1/2 Pack/148g	350	237	9.0	41.0	4.1	2.8
Focaccia, Roasted Onion & Cheese, Marks & Spencer*	1 Serving/88.9g	240	270	10.4	45.7	4.6	2.8
Focaccia, Rolls, Rosemary & Rock Salt, TTD, Sainsbury's*	1 Roll/120g	344	287	10.5	42.7	8.2	3.3
Focaccia, Safeway*	1/6 Slice/47g	131	279	9.5	46.9	5.9	3.4
Foccacia, Mixed Herb, TTD, Sainsbury's*	1 Serving/67g	179	269	9.7	38.0	8.7	3.8
Foccacia, Tomato & Cheese, TTD, Sainsbury's*	1 Serving/67g	167	251	10.4	35.5	7.5	3.8
Fougasse, Caramelised Onion & Cheese, Tesco*	1oz/28g	80	284	11.1	43.1	6.3	3.5
French Stick	1 Serving/60g	162	270	9.6	55.4	2.7	1.5
French Stick, Part Baked For Home Baking, Budgens*	1 Stick/200g	526	263	8.4	54.8	1.2	2.3
French's*	1 Serving/23g	57	247	11.0	46.0	3.0	6.0
French, Safeway*	1/5 Slice/41g	110	268	9.8	58.5	0.5	2.4
French, Sliced, Parisian*	2 Slices/39g	100	256	5.1	48.7	2.6	0.0
Fruit & Cinnamon Loaf, Finest, Tesco*	1 Slice/37g	134	363	6.4	54.6	13.2	1.5
Fruit Loaf, Apple & Cinnamon, Soreen*	1 Serving/10g	31	307	6.9	60.5	4.2	0.0
Fruit Loaf, Apple, Marks & Spencer*	1 Slice/39.2g	99	255	8.5	51.9	1.5	3.3
Fruit Loaf, Asda*	1 Slice/16g	45	280	8.0	54.0	3.5	2.1
Fruit Loaf, Banana, Soreen*	1 Slice/25g	78	313	6.8	60.9	4.7	0.0
Fruit Loaf, Luxury, Christmas, Soreen*	1 Serving/28g	85	303	4.5	66.6	2.1	0.0
Fruit Loaf, Mothers Pride*	1 Slice/36g	92	256	8.2	49.3	2.9	2.6
Fruit Loaf, Rich, Soreen*	1/10 Loaf/30g	93	310	7.4	60.7	4.1	0.0
Fruit Loaf, Sliced, Tesco*	1 Slice/36g	100	278	6.9	51.2	5.1	3.7
Fruit Loaf, With Orange, Warburtons*	1 Slice/33.3g	88	268	7.7	51.5	3.4	3.0
Fruit Loaf, With Strawberry, Summer, Warburtons*	1 Slice/35g	92	262	7.7	50.3	3.3	3.0
Fruit, Continental, Schneider Brot*	1 Slice/65g	198	305	5.4	57.0	5.4	0.0
Fruit, Raisin Swirl, Sun-Maid*	1 Slice/33.1g	95	287	8.3	50.4	5.8	2.6
Fruited, Richly, Waitrose*	1 Serving/34g	95	279	10.4	49.3	4.5	3.1
Garlic, & Herb, Giant Feast, Sainsbury's*	1 Serving/50g	159	317	8.0	42.1	12.9	2.6
Garlic, & Herb, Tear & Share, Tesco*	1 Serving/73g	218	300	6.3	40.0	12.7	1.7
Garlic, & Parsley, Tesco*	1 Loaf/230g	699	304	9.0	41.0	11.6	2.7
Garlic, & Red Onion, Somerfield*	1 Serving/60g	177	295	9.6	38.9	11.1	2.1
Garlic, 25% Less Fat, Sainsbury's*	1/2 Baguette/85g	268	315	7.8	39.4	14.0	3.1
Garlic, 30% Less Fat, Morrisons*	1 Serving/80g	226	283	5.9	41.1	10.8	1.9
Garlic, Asda*	1/2 Baguette/85g	302	355	7.6	39.4	18.6	2.0
Garlic, BGTY, Sainsbury's*	1 Serving/40g	126	315	7.8	39.4	14.0	3.1
Garlic, Baguette, 25% Less Fat, Tesco*	1 Serving/100g	292	292	7.0	40.7	11.3	1.8
Garlic, Baguette, 50% Less Fat, Asda*	1/4 Baguette/43g	123	287	10.0	46.0	7.0	2.5
Garlic, Baguette, 50% Less Fat, BGTY, Sainsbury's*	1/2 Baguette/80g	222	277	7.9	43.6	7.9	1.9
Garlic, Baguette, Asda*	1/4 Baguette/42g	148	352	8.0	44.0	16.0	1.2
Garlic, Baguette, BGTY, Sainsbury's*	1 Serving/60g	166	277	7.9	43.6	7.9	1.9
Garlic, Baguette, Co-Op*	1/2 Baguette/80g	308	385	9.0	47.0	18.0	2.0
Garlic, Baguette, Extra Strong, Sainsbury's*	1/2 Baguette/85g	278	327	8.4	40.0	14.8	3.4
Garlic, Baguette, GFY, Asda*	1/4 Baguette/42.5g	106	246	8.0	40.0	6.0	2.1
Garlic, Baguette, Good Intentions, Somerfield*	1/2 Baguette/85g	209	246	7.0	37.8	7.4	1.6
Garlic, Baguette, Healthy Living, Tesco*	1/3 Baguette/66g	172	260	8.9	41.3	6.6	2.9

BREAD

INFO/WEIGHT	Measure per Measure KCAL	KCAL	PROT	CARB	FAT	FIBRE
Garlic, Baguette, Italian, Asda*	1/4 Baguette/48g 173	364	7.0	39.0	20.0	3.4
Garlic, Baguette, Italiano, Tesco*	1 Serving/60g 196	326	7.8	39.8	15.1	2.5
Garlic, Baguette, Morrisons*	1/2 Baguette/95g 295	311	6.3	37.8	15.0	1.5
Garlic, Baguette, Organic, Tesco*	1 Serving/60g 192	320	8.5	41.1	13.5	2.5
Garlic, Baguette, Reduced Fat, Waitrose*	1/2 Baguette/85g 230	270	8.1	41.5	8.0	2.7
Garlic, Baguette, Sainsbury's*	1/2 Baguette/85g 332	391	8.9	48.6	19.2	2.3
Garlic, Baguette, Slices, Tesco*	1 Serving/60g 187	312	9.8	33.8	15.3	1.7
Garlic, Baguette, Tesco*	1 Serving/60g 213	355	7.6	39.4	18.6	2.0
Garlic, Baguette, Value, Tesco*	1/2 Baguette/85g 279	328	8.1	41.1	14.6	2.8
Garlic, Baguette, Waitrose*	1/2 Baguette/85g 290	341	7.1	37.8	17.9	0.0
Garlic, Baguette, White, Homebake, Tesco*	3rd Baguette/55g 160	290	7.0	43.1	10.0	1.9
Garlic, Baguette, With Cheese, Healthy Living, Tesco*	1 Serving/50g 115	229	9.4	43.0	2.2	2.1
Garlic, Caramelised, TTD, Sainsbury's*	1/4 Bread/75g 218	290	9.8	41.5	9.4	3.0
Garlic, Ciabatta, & Herb Butter, Sainsbury's*	1/2 Loaf/105g 345	329	8.5	38.8	15.5	0.0
Garlic, Ciabatta, BGTY, Sainsbury's*	1/2 Ciabatta/105g 306	291	8.7	36.2	12.4	2.7
Garlic, Ciabatta, Finest, Tesco*	1 Serving/65g 205	316	8.1	40.1	13.7	2.4
Garlic, Ciabatta, Hand Stretched, Sainsbury's*	1/4 Pack/75g 244	325	8.4	41.0	14.1	2.9
Garlic, Ciabatta, Healthy Living, Tesco*	1/4 Bread/60g 151	251	8.6	44.6	4.2	2.6
Garlic, Ciabatta, Italian, Sainsbury's*	1 Serving/145g 454	313	10.0	41.6	11.8	2.9
Garlic, Ciabatta, Italiano, Tesco*	1 Serving/65g 211	324	7.7	40.9	14.4	2.2
Garlic, Ciabatta, Safeway*	1/4 Ciabatta/52.9g 180	340	8.7	41.0	15.6	2.6
Garlic, Finest, Tesco*	1/4 Loaf/60g 187	311	7.7	40.3	13.2	1.8
Garlic, Flatbread, BGTY, Sainsbury's*	1/4 Bread/56g 177	316	9.6	46.6	10.1	2.7
Garlic, Flatbread, Tesco*	1 Serving/82.5g 251	302	6.7	45.3	10.4	3.0
Garlic, Focaccia, & Herb, Safeway*	1/6 Focaccia /50g 154	308	9.1	42.9	11.1	2.1
Garlic, Focaccia, & Onion, GFY, Asda*	1/4 Focaccia/55g 150	272	12.0	47.0	4.0	0.0
Garlic, Focaccia, & Rosemary, Sainsbury's*	1/4 Focaccia/75g 219	292	8.0	43.0	9.8	2.8
Garlic, Foccacia, & Herb, Italian Style, Morrisons*	1/6 Focaccia/76g 259	341	8.5	44.7	14.3	2.5
Garlic, Foccacia, & Rosemary, Tesco*	1/4 loaf/73g 193	266	9.0	42.1	6.8	3.7
Garlic, GFY, Asda*	1 Slice/31g 104	337	11.0	53.0	9.0	1.1
Garlic, Good Choice, Iceland*	1 Slice/40g 156	389	7.7	43.9	22.8	0.0
Garlic, Herb, With Garlic & Herb Butter, Tesco*	1 Serving/73g 218	300	6.3	40.0	12.7	1.7
Garlic, Homebake, Tesco*	1 Serving/60g 209	348	7.1	33.7	20.5	1.5
Garlic, Italian Style Stone Baked, Morrisons*	1/2 Pack/115g 420	365	7.9	40.4	19.1	1.9
Garlic, Marks & Spencer*	1 Slice/20g 76	380	7.5	39.5	21.6	1.0
Garlic, Micro, McCain*	1/2 Bread/54g 202	374	7.8	45.1	18.0	0.0
Garlic, Organic, Waitrose*	1 Baguette/170g 536	315	8.7	39.1	13.7	1.8
Garlic, Pizza Bread, Co-Op*	1 Pizza/240g 756	315	8.0	41.0	13.0	2.0
Garlic, Reduced Fat, Waitrose*	1 Pack/170g 551	324	6.9	49.4	11.0	0.9
Garlic, Safeway*	1/4 Baguette/72g 242	336	8.2	45.9	13.3	2.7
Garlic, Slices, BGTY, Sainsbury's*	1 Slice/27g 82	305	9.4	48.9	8.0	2.9
Garlic, Slices, Frozen, Sainsbury's*	1 Slice/26g 105	405	8.3	42.2	22.6	3.9
Garlic, Slices, GFY, Asda*	1 Slice/31g 80	259	8.9	48.1	3.3	3.0
Garlic, Slices, Healthy Living, Tesco*	1 Slice/52g 131	251	8.6	44.6	4.2	2.6
Garlic, Slices, Italiano, Tesco*	1 Slice/27g 83	312	9.1	45.1	10.6	2.4
Garlic, Slices, Sainsbury's*	1 Slice/25g 93	372	9.1	47.3	16.3	3.2
Garlic, Slices, Savoury, Tesco*	1 Slice/26g 96	371	7.0	48.7	16.5	2.7
Garlic, Stonebake, Marks & Spencer*	1 Loaf/85g 264	310	9.3	41.4	11.9	3.1
Garlic, Stonebaked, With Cheese, Morrisons*	1/2 Pack/128g 413	323	10.2	38.4	14.3	1.8
Garlic, Tear & Share, Sainsbury's*	1/3 Bread/95g 285	300	9.7	37.8	12.2	2.7
Garlic, To Share, Marks & Spencer*	1/4 Loaf/82.1g 230	280	6.5	33.2	13.0	1.3
Garlic, With Cheese Slices, Asda*	1 Serving/32g 121	378	10.0	44.0	18.0	1.6
Garlic, With Cheese, Asda*	1 Slice/34g 130	382	11.0	44.0	18.0	0.0

BREAD

INFO/WEIGHT	Measure	per Measure KCAL	Nutrition Values per 100g / 100ml KCAL	PROT	CARB	FAT	FIBRE
Garlic, With Cheese, Italian Style, Morrisons*	1/2 Pack/135g	431	319	10.8	45.1	10.6	2.1
Granary	1 Slice/25g	59	235	9.3	46.3	2.7	4.3
Granary, COU, Marks & Spencer*	1 Slice/25g	62	246	11.7	45.1	2.1	5.7
Granary, Crusty, Farmhouse, Marks & Spencer*	1 Slice/50g	120	240	9.4	43.4	3.0	2.6
Granary, Hovis*	1 Serving/35g	83	238	10.1	42.3	3.1	5.3
Granary, Malted, Medium Brown, Asda*	1 Slice/35g	81	231	9.0	43.0	2.6	3.3
Granary, Medium Sliced, Hovis*	1 Slice/32.9g	81	246	9.6	45.8	2.7	5.3
Granary, Thick Sliced, COU, Marks & Spencer*	1 Slice/26g	65	250	11.7	45.1	2.1	5.7
Granary, Thick Sliced, Hovis*	1 Slice/42.2g	103	245	9.0	47.8	1.9	4.1
Granary, Waitrose*	1 Slice/40g	88	220	9.4	39.9	2.5	4.3
Hi Bran, Burgen*	1 Slice/43.9g	94	214	13.2	33.5	3.0	7.9
Hi Bran, Marks & Spencer*	1 Slice/26.2g	55	210	12.6	32.5	3.0	6.3
Hi Bran, Medium Sliced, Allinson*	1 Slice/44g	93	212	13.2	33.6	2.8	8.0
Hi Fibre, Seed, LifeFibre Company*	1 Slice/35g	109	313	12.5	43.6	10.1	2.7
Hovis, Marks & Spencer*	1 Slice/21g	47	222	10.1	38.5	3.0	4.6
Irish Barm Brack, Tesco*	1 Serving/75g	233	310	16.0	47.6	6.9	3.0
Irish Brown Soda, Tesco*	1 Serving/50g	110	219	9.2	36.2	3.8	6.4
Irish Brown, Ormo*	1 Serving/100g	229	229	9.2	43.6	3.6	4.9
Irish Brown, Soda, Sainsbury's*	1 Serving/100g	208	208	8.8	36.4	3.0	5.3
Irish Cottage Wheaten, Tesco*	1 Serving/40g	79	198	9.1	35.4	1.9	6.1
Italian Style Pesto, TTD, Sainsbury's*	1/4 Bread/99g	247	249	9.1	39.4	6.1	4.4
Italian Style Red Pepper, Safeway*	1 Serving/80g	184	230	9.1	42.2	2.3	2.1
Juvela*	1 Slice/25g	60	240	3.3	50.0	3.0	1.7
Light Grain, Eat Smart, Safeway*	1 Slice/26.5g	66	245	9.7	45.5	2.5	3.5
Loaf, Crusty, Farmhouse, Poppy Seed, Marks & Spencer*	1 Slice/40g	104	260	9.4	47.6	3.3	2.3
Malt Loaf, Family, Asda*	1 Serving/20g	54	270	8.0	56.0	1.5	5.0
Malt Loaf, Fruit, Sainsbury's*	1oz/28g	86	308	7.9	63.8	2.4	2.4
Malt Loaf, Fruity, Sliced, 97% Fat Free, Soreen*	1 Slice/33g	103	312	7.7	65.9	2.0	0.0
Malt Loaf, Fruity, Soreen*	1 Serving/42g	130	310	7.4	65.6	2.0	0.0
Malt Loaf, Organic, Tesco*	1 Slice/28g	82	292	7.2	61.2	2.0	2.3
Malt Loaf, Ready Spread Snack, Soreen*	2 Slices/64g	220	344	6.4	57.0	10.0	3.0
Malt Loaf, Sticky, Marks & Spencer*	3 Slices/47.5g	139	295	6.9	64.9	2.3	3.1
Malt Loaf, Tesco*	1 Slice/50g	146	291	8.6	58.0	2.7	4.8
Malt Loaf, Value, Tesco*	1 Slice/25g	72	289	8.9	60.2	1.4	3.3
Malted Brown, Granary, Hovis*	1 Med Slice/35g	79	225	9.1	42.7	2.0	3.3
Malted Brown, Kingsmill*	1 slice/44g	103	234	9.4	43.4	2.5	2.7
Malted Brown, Slice, BGTY, Sainsbury's*	1 Slice/22g	53	239	12.1	41.4	2.8	5.8
Malted Brown, TTD, Sainsbury's*	1 Slice/44g	103	234	8.8	42.9	3.0	3.1
Malted Brown, Thick Sliced, Organic, Tesco*	1 Slice/44g	116	264	7.8	53.8	2.0	3.3
Malted Danish, Nimble*	1 Slice/22g	49	222	8.3	43.7	1.6	5.3
Malted Grain, Co-Op*	1 Slice/43g	99	230	8.0	46.0	2.0	3.0
Malted Oat, Duchy Originals*	1 Serving/80g	195	244	8.8	43.6	3.8	3.7
Malted Wheat Country, Gold, Kingsmill*	1 Slice/41g	96	234	9.4	43.4	2.5	2.7
Malted Wheat Loaf, Thick Sliced, Village Green, Aldi*	1 Slice/38g	96	253	10.3	49.9	1.4	3.1
Malted Wheat, Eat Smart, Safeway*	1 Slice/26g	60	230	10.0	42.8	1.8	5.3
Malted Wheat, Gold, Kingsmill*	1 Slice/45g	108	240	9.8	43.8	2.9	3.6
Malted Wheat, The Best, Safeway*	1 Slice/44g	103	235	9.1	45.6	1.8	4.7
Malted, & Seeded, Batch, Organic, Waitrose*	1 Slice/50g	118	236	10.9	39.5	3.9	6.2
Malted, Crusty, Sainsbury's*	1 Slice/42.1g	109	259	8.6	48.6	3.3	4.4
Malted, Danish, Sliced, Warburtons*	1 Slice/19g	41	218	10.2	41.3	1.4	6.9
Malted, Danish, Weight Watchers*	1 Slice/19g	41	218	10.2	41.3	1.4	6.9
Malted, Floury Batch, Sainsbury's*	1 Roll/68g	190	280	8.7	51.6	4.3	4.2
Malted, Sunblest*	1 Serving/45g	115	256	9.9	49.1	2.2	3.8

BREAD	INFO/WEIGHT	KCAL	KCAL	PROT	CARB	FAT	FIBRE
Malted, Wheat Loaf, Crusty, Finest, Tesco*	1 Slice/50g	115	230	9.8	44.2	1.5	4.4
Mediterranean Olive, Waitrose*	1 Slice/30g	82	273	7.4	40.1	9.2	4.9
Mediterranean Style Seed, Safeway*	1 Slice/25g	65	259	11.4	37.2	7.2	9.1
Mediterranean Style, Marks & Spencer*	1/6 Loaf/47.6g	151	315	10.9	42.5	11.1	1.2
Milk Roll, Warburtons*	1 Slice/18g	46	253	11.0	45.1	2.7	2.7
Mixed Grain From Powder, Sainsbury's*	1 Serving/100g	228	228	7.7	46.0	1.5	4.4
Mixed Seed Loaf, Organic, Marks & Spencer*	1oz/28g	73	261	9.3	37.5	8.7	5.1
Mixed Seed, Organic, Duchy Originals*	2 Slices/85g	229	269	10.9	39.1	8.1	5.3
Multigrain, Bakers Choice, Marks & Spencer*	1 Slice/25g	61	242	13.4	33.7	6.0	6.4
Multigrain, Batch, Finest, Tesco*	1 Slice/50g	127	254	9.8	47.7	2.7	4.2
Multigrain, Crusty, Finest, Tesco*	1 Slice/40g	98	245	9.0	44.7	3.4	5.0
Multigrain, Farmhouse Baker's, Marks & Spencer*	1 Slice/51.1g	115	225	13.0	31.2	5.4	5.1
Multigrain, Gluten Free, Sainsbury's*	1 Slice/17g	39	229	5.1	40.8	5.0	5.6
Multigrain, Sliced Loaf, Gluten-Free, Dietary Specials*	2 Slices/66.4g	151	229	5.1	40.8	5.1	5.6
Multigrain, Soft Batch, Sainsbury's*	1 Slice/44g	106	242	11.3	34.5	6.5	5.6
Multigrain, Sunblest*	1 Slice/30g	76	254	9.0	47.0	2.5	4.5
Multigrain, Sunflower, Allinson*	1 Slice/47g	113	240	9.8	36.9	4.7	3.9
Multigrain, TTD, Sainsbury's*	1 Slice/44g	106	242	10.2	35.9	6.4	5.3
Multigrain, Tesco*	1 Slice/31g	66	214	11.1	36.8	3.2	8.9
Multigrain, Thick Sliced, Tesco*	1 Slice/50g	113	225	8.4	42.2	2.5	3.9
Naan	1 Naan/160g	538	336	8.9	50.1	12.5	1.9
Naan, Bombay Brasserie, Sainsbury's*	1 Naan/140g	372	266	9.8	49.6	3.1	2.9
Naan, Co-Op*	1oz/28g	60	216	7.7	36.9	4.2	1.3
Naan, Fresh, BGTY, Sainsbury's*	1 Serving/150g	368	245	9.4	44.9	3.1	2.2
Naan, Fresh, Sharwood's*	1oz/28g	70	251	7.3	48.0	3.3	2.0
Naan, Garlic & Coriander, Fresh, Sharwood's*	1oz/28g	71	252	7.7	47.8	3.3	2.2
Naan, Garlic & Coriander, Large, Sainsbury's*	1/2 Naan/75g	209	279	7.1	46.3	7.3	2.9
Naan, Garlic & Coriander, Mini, Long Life, Sharwood's*	1oz/28g	76	272	6.5	42.9	7.4	2.4
Naan, Garlic & Coriander, Mini, Sainsbury's*	1 Naan/50g	148	295	8.6	44.2	9.3	3.7
Naan, Garlic & Coriander, Mini, Sharwood's*	1 Naan/59g	144	244	7.1	46.2	3.4	2.0
Naan, Garlic & Coriander, Mini, Tesco*	1 Naan/60g	157	261	8.2	44.1	5.7	1.5
Naan, Garlic & Coriander, TTD, Sainsbury's*	1/2 Naan/70g	185	265	8.7	44.8	5.7	3.0
Naan, Garlic & Coriander, Tesco*	1 Naan/150g	374	249	7.1	36.5	8.3	2.1
Naan, Garlic, Sainsbury's*	1 Mini Naan/50g	131	262	7.7	46.7	4.9	3.9
Naan, Healthy Eating, Tesco*	1 Naan/70g	165	236	8.0	46.1	2.1	2.6
Naan, Indian Meal For One, BGTY, Sainsbury's*	1 Serving/45g	115	257	10.3	44.2	4.3	2.1
Naan, Indian Meal For One, Sainsbury's*	1 Serving/50g	145	289	9.7	47.6	6.6	2.1
Naan, Indian Meal For Two, Sainsbury's*	1 Naan//125g	357	285	8.7	45.9	7.4	1.9
Naan, Indian Style, Lidl*	1 Naan/140g	332	237	8.7	44.2	2.5	0.0
Naan, Indian Style, Mini, Asda*	1 Naan/50g	152	304	8.0	50.0	8.0	2.8
Naan, Keema Filled, Mini, Indian Takeaway, Safeway*	1 Naan/23g	58	253	10.1	38.3	6.6	2.1
Naan, King Prawn, Marks & Spencer*	1 Serving/185g	360	195	9.1	25.3	6.3	2.5
Naan, Long Life, Sharwood's*	1oz/28g	72	258	7.3	45.8	5.1	2.0
Naan, Marks & Spencer*	1 Bread/84g	260	310	12.0	43.8	9.8	2.1
Naan, Mini, Asda*	1 Serving/100g	304	304	8.0	50.0	8.0	2.8
Naan, Mini, Healthy Living, Tesco*	1 Naan/60g	128	213	7.8	44.1	1.9	2.9
Naan, Mini, Plain, Tesco*	1 Naan/60g	175	292	9.3	47.6	7.2	2.5
Naan, Mini, Sainsbury's*	1 Serving/50g	157	314	8.7	41.5	12.4	4.3
Naan, Northern Indian, Sainsbury's*	1 Serving/125g	356	285	8.7	45.9	7.4	1.9
Naan, Onion & Mint, Marks & Spencer*	1/2 Naan/135g	351	260	8.9	35.8	8.7	2.5
Naan, Onion Bhaji, Sharwood's*	1 Pack/130g	378	291	7.3	48.4	7.6	2.2
Naan, Onion Bhajia, Marks & Spencer*	1 Naan/140.4g	399	285	9.5	34.2	12.1	2.0
Naan, Peshwari, Fresh, Sharwood's*	1oz/28g	67	240	6.8	41.9	5.0	2.5

B

BREAD

	Measure INFO/WEIGHT	per Measure KCAL	Nutrition Values per 100g / 100ml				
			KCAL	PROT	CARB	FAT	FIBRE
Naan, Peshwari, Long Life, Sharwood's*	1oz/28g	71	252	6.2	42.0	6.6	2.6
Naan, Peshwari, Marks & Spencer*	1 Serving/127g	394	310	9.2	45.8	10.1	1.9
Naan, Peshwari, Northern Indian, Sainsbury's*	1 Bread/160g	458	286	6.3	49.7	6.9	2.8
Naan, Peshwari, Sharwood's*	1 Naan/130g	334	257	7.2	45.1	5.3	2.5
Naan, Peshwari, Tesco*	1 Naan/215.0g	684	318	7.5	48.9	12.4	4.8
Naan, Plain, Finest, Tesco*	1/2 Naan/85g	308	362	9.2	48.2	14.7	2.3
Naan, Plain, Mini, Asda*	1 Naan/58g	156	269	8.0	49.0	4.6	2.3
Naan, Plain, Mini, Fresh, Sharwood's*	1oz/28g	70	251	7.3	48.0	3.3	2.0
Naan, Plain, Mini, Tesco*	1 Serving/60g	158	263	7.5	43.9	6.4	2.1
Naan, Plain, Nisa Heritage*	1 Naan/150g	401	267	9.0	44.2	6.2	1.9
Naan, Plain, Original, Mild, Patak's*	1 Serving/130g	399	307	9.5	48.0	8.6	0.0
Naan, Plain, Sainsbury's*	1/2 Naan/74.9g	209	279	7.3	46.7	7.0	2.7
Naan, Plain, Sharwood's*	1 Bread/120g	326	272	8.5	42.9	7.4	2.4
Naan, Plain, TTD, Sainsbury's*	1 Naan/140g	352	251	8.2	43.1	5.1	2.9
Naan, Plain, Tesco*	1 Naan/150g	429	286	7.8	47.6	7.2	2.5
Naan, Plain, Value, Tesco*	1 Naan/135g	363	269	8.1	42.9	7.2	1.6
Naan, Plain, Waitrose*	1 Naan/130g	403	310	6.8	49.3	9.5	1.4
Naan, Tandoor Baked, Waitrose*	1 Naan/139.8g	372	266	9.8	49.6	3.1	2.9
Naan, Tandoori, Sharwood's*	1 Bread/130g	330	254	7.3	45.0	5.0	2.0
Oat, Waitrose*	1oz/28g	71	253	8.5	44.9	4.4	3.6
Oatmeal, Batch, Tesco*	1 Slice/50g	135	269	9.3	50.1	3.5	4.0
Oatmeal, Farmhouse, Soft, Marks & Spencer*	1 Slice/45g	110	245	11.1	39.5	4.4	5.2
Oatmeal, Farmhouse, Waitrose*	1 Slice/40g	110	276	9.4	47.9	5.2	4.6
Oatmeal, Sliced Loaf, Tesco*	1 Slice/50g	111	222	7.4	40.5	3.4	2.8
Olive, Waitrose*	1 Slice/28g	86	306	9.0	43.6	10.6	2.0
Panettone, Marks & Spencer*	1/8 Loaf/51g	184	360	6.5	53.4	13.2	2.0
Panini, Tesco*	1 Serving/75g	207	276	10.1	45.2	6.1	2.7
Paratha, Lachha, Waitrose*	1 Paratha/75g	322	429	7.8	46.0	23.8	1.8
Pave, Mixed Olive, Waitrose*	1oz/28g	59	209	6.3	41.6	1.9	2.6
Pave, Sundried Tomato, Waitrose*	1oz/28g	76	271	10.8	53.4	1.6	3.3
Petit Pain, Harvester, Somerfield*	1 Serving/70g	188	269	10.6	52.2	2.0	3.2
Petit Pain, Homebake, Mini, Tesco*	1 Roll/50g	120	240	7.8	48.5	1.2	3.4
Petit Pain, Organic, Tesco*	1 Roll/100g	235	235	7.8	49.1	0.8	1.2
Petit Pain, Ready To Bake, Sainsbury's*	1 Petit Pain/44g	117	265	12.1	49.4	1.9	3.0
Petit Pain, Ready to Bake, Co-Op*	1 Petit Pain/33g	73	220	7.0	46.0	1.0	3.0
Petit Pain, Waitrose*	1 Roll/69g	190	275	9.3	55.9	1.6	3.1
Petit Pain, White, Part Baked, Asda*	1 Roll/128g	330	258	8.0	53.0	1.6	2.0
Petit Pain, White, Soft Bake, Somerfield*	1 Roll/70g	174	248	9.2	49.9	1.3	1.8
Pitta, Brown, Organic, Waitrose*	1 Pitta/61g	138	226	6.4	47.5	1.4	6.6
Pitta, Cypriana Supreme*	1oz/28g	67	239	8.5	48.6	1.2	0.0
Pitta, Feta, Sun Dried Tomato, TTD, Sainsbury's*	1 Pitta/71g	208	293	9.5	43.1	9.2	2.9
Pitta, Garlic & Coriander, Asda*	1 Bread/57g	149	261	8.0	53.0	1.9	0.0
Pitta, Garlic & Herb, Tesco*	1 Pitta/60g	134	223	9.6	44.6	2.0	3.0
Pitta, Garlic, Morrisons*	1 Pitta/60g	149	249	9.7	51.1	1.8	0.0
Pitta, Garlic, Pride Valley*	1 Pitta/63g	157	249	9.7	51.1	1.8	2.7
Pitta, Garlic, Sainsbury's*	1 Pitta/60g	153	255	9.5	52.0	1.0	2.5
Pitta, Iceland*	1 Pitta/50g	126	251	8.6	50.0	1.8	2.3
Pitta, Lower Carb, Mini, Tesco*	1 Serving/100g	204	204	17.7	24.2	4.0	9.9
Pitta, Mexican, Santa Maria*	1 Pitta/66g	165	250	7.5	52.0	1.0	0.0
Pitta, Mini, Marks & Spencer*	1 Pitta/13g	34	260	9.2	52.1	2.4	1.8
Pitta, Mini, Safeway*	1 Pitta/25g	53	212	7.6	47.6	1.2	2.0
Pitta, Organic, Tesco*	1 Pitta/60g	124	206	8.3	40.2	1.4	5.7
Pitta, Pockets, Sainsbury's*	1 Serving/75g	188	250	8.5	52.0	1.0	3.5

BREAD

INFO/WEIGHT	Measure	per Measure KCAL	Nutrition Values per 100g / 100ml KCAL	PROT	CARB	FAT	FIBRE
Pitta, Sesame, Sainsbury's*	1 Pitta/59g	156	264	9.8	50.8	2.4	3.1
Pitta, Somerfield*	1 Pitta/56g	141	251	8.6	50.0	1.8	2.3
Pitta, Tex Mex Style, Mini, Morrisons*	1 Pitta/18g	43	240	9.2	48.7	0.9	3.3
Pitta, Value, Tesco*	1 Pitta/53g	138	263	10.1	51.2	1.9	2.7
Pitta, White	1 Pitta/75g	199	265	9.2	57.9	1.2	2.2
Pitta, White Picnic, Waitrose*	1 Pitta/30g	75	249	10.3	49.3	1.2	3.5
Pitta, White, Co-Op*	1 Pitta/63g	151	240	10.0	47.0	1.0	3.0
Pitta, White, Greek Style, Asda*	1 Pitta/50g	127	253	8.0	51.0	1.9	0.0
Pitta, White, Marks & Spencer*	1 Pitta/61g	156	255	8.9	51.6	2.4	0.0
Pitta, White, Mini, Safeway*	1 Pitta/54g	119	220	8.0	49.4	1.2	1.9
Pitta, White, Mini, Sainsbury's*	1 Pitta/30g	75	249	10.3	49.3	1.2	3.5
Pitta, White, Mini, Tesco*	1 Pitta/18g	47	262	10.1	51.2	1.9	2.6
Pitta, White, Morrisons*	1 Pitta/60g	157	262	10.1	51.2	1.9	0.0
Pitta, White, Organic, Sainsbury's*	1 Pitta/59g	150	254	10.3	50.7	1.1	2.5
Pitta, White, Sainsbury's*	1 Pittta/59g	147	249	10.3	49.3	1.2	3.5
Pitta, White, Tesco*	1 Pitta/56g	148	265	9.8	55.1	2.1	3.4
Pitta, White, Waitrose*	1 Pitta/60g	149	249	10.3	49.3	1.2	3.5
Pitta, Wholemeal, Asda*	1oz/28g	72	257	10.7	50.0	1.6	0.0
Pitta, Wholemeal, Healthy Eating, Co-Op*	1 Pitta/63g	135	215	12.0	37.0	2.0	9.0
Pitta, Wholemeal, Lemon, TTD, Sainsbury's*	1 Pitaa/80g	199	249	10.0	38.0	6.3	6.8
Pitta, Wholemeal, Marks & Spencer*	1 Pitta/60.9g	140	230	10.7	40.6	2.8	7.2
Pitta, Wholemeal, Morrisons*	1 Pitta/60g	135	225	11.9	46.4	2.0	0.0
Pitta, Wholemeal, Safeway*	1 Pitta/54g	125	232	9.7	44.2	1.9	6.5
Pitta, Wholemeal, Sainsbury's*	1 Pitta/59g	146	247	12.5	45.9	1.5	5.3
Pitta, Wholemeal, Somerfield*	1 Pitta/55.9g	127	227	10.6	41.0	2.3	6.2
Pitta, Wholemeal, Tesco*	1 Av Pitta/60g	145	241	11.0	51.5	2.3	7.4
Plum Loaf, Lincolnshire, Soreen*	1/10 Loaf/29.1g	88	302	8.1	57.8	4.3	0.0
Potato & Rosemary, Marks & Spencer*	1 Serving/40g	108	270	9.4	42.2	6.8	2.3
Potato & Rosemary, Tesco*	1oz/28g	67	241	8.2	42.0	4.5	2.2
Pumpernickel Rye, Kelderman*	1 Slice/50g	93	185	6.0	38.0	1.0	0.0
Pumpkin Seed, Raisin & Sunflower Seed, Sainsbury's*	1 Slice/30g	77	255	11.6	45.9	2.8	3.4
Raisin & Pumpkin Seed, Organic, Tesco*	1 Slice/30g	76	253	9.7	40.6	5.8	3.8
Raisin Loaf With Cinnamon, Warburtons*	1 Slice/33g	91	276	7.5	52.9	3.8	4.2
Roasted Onion, Marks & Spencer*	1 Slice/50g	125	250	9.0	46.7	3.3	2.1
Roasted Shallot & Gruyere, Safeway*	1/4 Loaf/52.6g	151	285	11.2	43.1	7.3	9.1
Rolls, American Style Deli, Tesco*	1 Roll/65g	162	249	7.8	46.8	3.4	1.6
Rolls, Batch, Seeded, Marks & Spencer*	1 Roll/76g	220	290	10.7	39.7	9.6	4.0
Rolls, Batched Sandwich, Warburtons*	1 Roll/60g	148	246	9.6	42.7	4.1	0.0
Rolls, Best Of Both, Square, Hovis*	1 Roll/52g	120	231	10.8	35.7	5.0	4.6
Rolls, Best of Both, Hovis*	1 Roll/29g	68	235	9.8	39.5	4.2	4.2
Rolls, Blackpool Milk, Warburtons*	1 Slice/18g	45	251	10.8	45.3	3.0	2.8
Rolls, Brioche, Plain Chocolate Chip, Sainsbury's*	1 Roll/35g	131	374	8.5	49.0	16.0	5.9
Rolls, Brioche, Sainsbury's*	1 Roll/32g	116	362	8.5	56.0	11.5	3.6
Rolls, Brown, Carb Control, Tesco*	1 Roll/45g	98	218	20.5	20.7	5.9	10.7
Rolls, Brown, Crusty	1 Roll/50g	128	255	10.3	50.4	2.8	3.5
Rolls, Brown, Free From, Tesco*	1 Roll/65g	174	268	5.4	43.2	8.2	3.6
Rolls, Brown, Large, Asda*	1 Roll/57g	138	242	10.0	47.0	1.6	0.0
Rolls, Brown, Malted Grain, Somerfield*	1 Roll/60g	147	245	8.7	45.2	3.2	3.0
Rolls, Brown, Malted Grain, Tesco*	1 Roll/58g	144	248	8.7	46.2	3.2	1.9
Rolls, Brown, Marks & Spencer*	1 Roll/105g	242	230	9.2	37.3	6.1	4.4
Rolls, Brown, Mini, Marks & Spencer*	1 Serving/32.7g	81	245	9.8	35.5	7.6	3.8
Rolls, Brown, Old Fashioned, Waitrose*	1 Roll/63g	152	241	9.6	41.3	4.1	4.7
Rolls, Brown, Seeded, Organic, Sainsbury's*	1 Roll/70g	166	237	9.9	39.1	4.6	6.5

BREAD

	Measure INFO/WEIGHT	per Measure KCAL	Nutrition Values per 100g / 100ml				
			KCAL	PROT	CARB	FAT	FIBRE
Rolls, Brown, Soft	1 Roll/50g	134	268	10.0	51.8	3.8	3.5
Rolls, Brown, Soft, Marks & Spencer*	1 Roll/45.7g	106	230	8.7	44.0	2.2	5.2
Rolls, Brown, Soft, Organic, Sainsbury's*	1 Serving/70g	166	237	9.9	39.1	4.6	6.6
Rolls, Brown, Soft, Somerfield*	1oz/28g	68	243	9.0	42.0	3.0	0.0
Rolls, Brown, Soft, Tesco*	1 Roll/50g	118	235	9.0	41.6	3.6	4.5
Rolls, Brown, Square, Marks & Spencer*	1 Roll/105g	242	230	9.2	37.3	6.1	4.4
Rolls, COU, Marks & Spencer*	1 Serving/51.1g	120	235	9.8	44.0	2.3	3.4
Rolls, Cheese Topped, Sandwich Rolls, Warburtons*	1 Roll/62g	168	270	12.1	40.7	6.5	2.6
Rolls, Cheese Topped, Village Green*	1 Roll/56g	159	284	13.1	41.2	7.4	4.8
Rolls, Ciabatta, Best, Safeway*	1 Serving/100g	211	211	7.3	39.1	2.9	1.8
Rolls, Ciabatta, Cheese Topped, Mini, Finest, Tesco*	1 Roll/30g	85	282	11.5	40.9	8.1	3.8
Rolls, Ciabatta, Finest, Tesco*	1 Roll/45g	93	206	7.7	33.5	4.6	2.3
Rolls, Ciabatta, Marks & Spencer*	1 Roll/80g	210	262	10.3	48.1	4.1	2.1
Rolls, Ciabatta, Mini, Finest, Tesco*	1 Roll/30g	89	297	9.9	49.1	6.8	4.1
Rolls, Ciabatta, Mixed Olive, TTD, Sainsbury's*	1 Roll/73g	216	296	10.3	39.6	10.7	3.3
Rolls, Ciabatta, Ready To Bake, Sainsbury's*	1 Roll/75g	198	264	9.1	48.9	3.6	2.3
Rolls, Ciabatta, Ready to Bake, TTD, Sainsbury's*	1 Roll/72g	197	274	10.4	44.8	5.9	2.7
Rolls, Ciabatta, Sun Dried Tomato, Mini, Finest, Tesco*	1 Roll/30g	79	262	8.7	42.3	6.4	2.6
Rolls, Ciabatta, Tesco*	1 Serving/80g	194	242	9.8	41.8	3.9	2.4
Rolls, Country Grain, Mini, Marks & Spencer*	1 Serving/30.9g	85	275	10.2	38.9	9.7	3.8
Rolls, Crisp, Original, Organic, Kallo*	1 Roll/8.7g	35	390	11.0	74.0	5.6	3.0
Rolls, Crusty, French, Marks & Spencer*	1 Roll/65g	159	245	8.1	50.5	1.2	3.3
Rolls, Crusty, Part-Baked, Budgens*	1 Roll/50g	148	296	9.4	61.4	1.4	2.5
Rolls, Finger, Morrisons*	1 Roll/46g	119	259	10.7	50.0	1.8	2.3
Rolls, Finger, Sainsbury's*	1 Roll/40g	102	256	10.3	47.9	2.6	2.4
Rolls, Focaccia, Tesco*	1 Serving/75g	227	302	8.7	45.6	9.4	3.8
Rolls, For Hamburgers	1 Roll/50g	132	264	9.1	48.8	5.0	1.5
Rolls, Granary Malted Wheatgrain, Soft, Marks & Spencer*	1 Roll/80g	208	260	9.3	47.2	3.9	2.3
Rolls, Granary, Bakers Premium, Tesco*	1 Roll/65g	158	243	9.9	47.8	1.3	2.3
Rolls, Granary, Mini, Tesco*	1 Roll/34g	92	271	10.0	43.5	6.5	3.8
Rolls, Granary, Waitrose*	1 Roll/59g	160	271	10.0	47.2	6.4	3.8
Rolls, Green Olive, Marks & Spencer*	1 Roll/75g	210	280	11.2	44.0	6.0	1.8
Rolls, Hot Dog, Sliced, Asda*	1 Roll/84g	197	234	7.0	44.0	3.3	0.0
Rolls, Hot Dog, Tesco*	1 Roll/85g	200	235	7.3	44.0	3.3	1.9
Rolls, Malted Grain Submarine, Marks & Spencer*	1 Serving/109.1g	300	275	8.9	53.6	4.3	3.0
Rolls, Malted Grain, Soft, Weight Watchers*	1 Roll/42g	95	226	9.8	42.2	2.0	4.5
Rolls, Malted Wheat & Poppy Seed, Safeway*	1 Roll/54g	140	260	10.6	48.7	2.8	3.4
Rolls, Malted, Sainsbury's*	1 Roll/68g	190	280	8.7	51.6	4.3	4.2
Rolls, Mediterranean Style, TTD, Sainsbury's*	1 Roll/75g	192	256	8.5	41.9	6.0	5.8
Rolls, Mini Submarine, Marks & Spencer*	1 Roll/23g	63	275	11.4	47.7	4.9	1.1
Rolls, Morning Breakfast, Marks & Spencer*	1 Roll/55g	160	290	10.3	53.8	4.3	0.6
Rolls, Morning, Tesco*	1 Roll/48g	117	243	10.4	44.8	2.5	4.7
Rolls, Multigrain, Torpedo, Sainsbury's*	1 Roll/111.9g	328	293	10.5	47.7	6.7	6.3
Rolls, Oatmeal, Soft, Marks & Spencer*	1 Roll/80g	224	280	12.3	43.4	6.4	2.7
Rolls, Pain Raisin, Mini, Marks & Spencer*	1oz/28g	87	310	5.3	42.3	13.6	1.3
Rolls, Panini, Marks & Spencer*	1 Roll/86g	211	245	8.3	39.3	6.2	1.6
Rolls, Panini, Sainsbury's*	1 Roll/90g	249	276	11.0	44.1	6.2	3.0
Rolls, Part Baked, Mini, Tesco*	1 Serving/50g	120	240	7.8	49.5	1.2	3.4
Rolls, Poppy Seeded Knot, Waitrose*	1 Roll/60g	169	282	10.3	48.3	5.3	2.2
Rolls, Rye, Toasting, Good & Hot*	1 Roll/65g	143	220	7.3	44.6	1.1	7.1
Rolls, Sandwich, Warburtons*	1 Roll/40g	98	245	9.3	42.4	4.3	2.4
Rolls, Scottish, White, Tesco*	1 Roll/48g	117	243	10.4	44.8	2.5	4.7
Rolls, Seeded, Sandwich, Warburtons*	1 Roll/77g	240	312	13.3	41.2	10.4	0.0

BREAD

INFO/WEIGHT	KCAL	KCAL	PROT	CARB	FAT	FIBRE
Rolls, Snack, Mini, Tesco*	1 Roll/35g	95	271	19.0	43.0	6.0	4.0
Rolls, Soft, Sandwich, Warburtons*	1 Roll/80g	210	264	11.0	45.0	4.4	0.0
Rolls, Square, Hovis*	1 Roll/47g	116	247	8.4	44.8	3.8	2.0
Rolls, Submarine, Malted Wheat, Organic, Tesco*	1 Serving/108g	279	258	10.1	45.2	4.1	4.8
Rolls, Submarine, Sainsbury's*	1 Roll/117g	305	261	9.1	47.4	3.9	2.4
Rolls, Submarine, Tesco*	1 Roll/100g	272	272	8.1	50.6	4.2	1.9
Rolls, Sun Dried Tomato, Homebake, Tesco*	1 Roll/50g	123	246	11.3	44.0	3.0	0.0
Rolls, Sunflower Seed, Toasting, Good & Hot*	1 Roll/65g	163	250	8.5	41.0	5.0	8.0
Rolls, Tomato & Basil, Sub, COU, Marks & Spencer*	1 Roll/32.5g	87	265	11.0	48.7	2.7	2.4
Rolls, White, BGTY, Sainsbury's*	1 Roll/50g	114	227	9.1	45.3	1.0	3.0
Rolls, White, Basics, Somerfield*	1 Roll/44g	107	243	8.9	48.2	1.6	2.1
Rolls, White, Big Square, Hovis*	1 Roll/73g	183	250	8.4	45.2	3.9	2.1
Rolls, White, Cheese Topped, Asda*	1 Roll/46g	121	264	10.0	46.0	4.4	2.0
Rolls, White, Cheese Topped, Sainsbury's*	1 Roll/75g	218	291	12.1	41.6	8.5	2.0
Rolls, White, Co-Op*	1 Roll/55g	138	250	9.0	46.0	3.0	2.0
Rolls, White, Crusty	1 Roll/50g	140	280	10.9	57.6	2.3	1.5
Rolls, White, Crusty, Bake At Home, Morrisons*	1 Roll/100g	254	254	11.4	47.9	1.9	2.6
Rolls, White, Deli, Tesco*	1 Roll/65g	180	277	8.7	52.0	3.8	2.7
Rolls, White, Finger, SmartPrice, Asda*	1 Roll/50g	121	242	9.0	48.0	1.6	2.1
Rolls, White, Finger, Tesco*	1 Roll/50g	125	251	9.7	55.5	0.4	1.5
Rolls, White, Finger, Waitrose*	1 Roll/49g	121	247	9.4	45.6	3.0	2.7
Rolls, White, Floured, Batch, Tesco*	1 Roll/76g	193	254	8.8	47.3	3.3	2.2
Rolls, White, Floured, Warburtons*	1 Roll/50g	124	247	9.8	43.3	3.8	2.7
Rolls, White, Floury Batch, Sainsbury's*	1 Roll/65g	167	257	8.7	46.6	4.0	3.1
Rolls, White, Floury, Roberts*	1 Roll/63.0g	160	254	8.4	49.5	2.5	2.0
Rolls, White, Golden Sun, Lidl*	1 Roll/36g	89	248	8.3	48.6	2.3	0.0
Rolls, White, Good Health, Warburtons*	1 Roll/54g	122	226	9.6	42.0	2.0	4.1
Rolls, White, Hot Dog, Safeway*	1 Roll/52.8g	131	248	8.6	46.1	3.2	2.5
Rolls, White, Hot Dog, Sainsbury's*	1 Roll/85g	235	277	7.3	48.8	5.8	2.4
Rolls, White, Hot Dog, Tesco*	1 Roll/85g	200	235	7.3	44.0	3.3	1.9
Rolls, White, Kingsmill*	1 Roll/60g	151	252	9.3	44.5	4.1	2.4
Rolls, White, Large, Sliced, Warburtons*	1 Serving/89g	230	258	10.1	44.4	4.5	2.7
Rolls, White, Low Price, Sainsbury's*	1 Roll/44g	107	243	8.9	48.2	1.6	2.1
Rolls, White, Milk, Warburtons*	1 Serving/18.3g	45	251	10.8	45.3	3.0	2.8
Rolls, White, Morning, Co-Op*	1 Roll/47g	134	285	12.0	53.0	3.0	2.0
Rolls, White, Morning, Marks & Spencer*	1 Roll/50g	136	272	8.8	53.8	1.5	2.7
Rolls, White, Old Fashioned, Waitrose*	1 Roll/57g	157	275	8.8	49.8	4.5	2.8
Rolls, White, Organic, Sainsbury's*	1 Roll/65g	170	262	8.7	49.9	3.0	1.0
Rolls, White, Part Baked, Morrisons*	1 Roll/75g	227	303	9.6	63.0	1.4	2.6
Rolls, White, Ploughman's, Sainsbury's*	1 Roll/65g	185	285	8.6	54.1	3.8	2.3
Rolls, White, Premium Soft, Rathbones*	1 Roll/65g	190	293	9.3	50.3	6.0	2.7
Rolls, White, Savers, Safeway*	1 Roll/40g	113	283	10.4	54.6	1.8	20.0
Rolls, White, Scottish, Morning, Safeway*	1 Roll/40g	113	283	10.4	56.4	1.8	1.6
Rolls, White, Seeded, Sainsbury's*	1 Roll/80g	217	271	10.9	43.4	5.9	4.8
Rolls, White, Seeded, Soft, Marks & Spencer*	1 Roll/72g	205	285	11.7	46.2	5.7	1.8
Rolls, White, SmartPrice, Asda*	1 Roll/44g	106	242	9.0	48.0	1.6	2.1
Rolls, White, Snack, Sainsbury's*	1 Roll/67g	159	237	7.9	49.2	1.0	2.3
Rolls, White, Soft	1 Roll/45g	121	268	9.2	51.6	4.2	1.5
Rolls, White, Soft, Boulders, Hovis*	1 Roll/74g	206	279	11.0	51.5	3.0	2.3
Rolls, White, Soft, COU, Marks & Spencer*	1 Roll/37g	94	255	10.7	47.1	2.7	1.5
Rolls, White, Soft, Farmhouse, Warburtons*	1 Roll/59g	148	250	9.7	43.0	4.4	2.5
Rolls, White, Soft, Finger, Marks & Spencer*	1 Roll/64g	189	295	10.1	47.5	7.2	2.2
Rolls, White, Soft, Marks & Spencer*	1 Roll/49g	120	245	9.7	45.8	2.8	2.0

B

BREAD

INFO/WEIGHT	Measure per Measure	KCAL	Nutrition Values per 100g / 100ml			
			KCAL	PROT	CARB	FAT	FIBRE

	Measure INFO/WEIGHT	per Measure KCAL	KCAL	PROT	CARB	FAT	FIBRE
Rolls, White, Soft, Premium, Village Green, Aldi*	1 Roll/65g	168	259	8.3	47.5	4.0	1.9
Rolls, White, Soft, Sandwich, Warburtons*	1 Roll/79g	209	264	11.0	45.0	4.4	0.0
Rolls, White, Soft, Tesco*	1 Serving/63g	154	245	8.8	48.9	1.6	2.4
Rolls, White, Softgrain, GFY, Asda*	1 Roll/54.0g	128	237	9.0	46.0	1.9	2.9
Rolls, White, Spar*	1 Roll/45g	113	251	8.6	46.6	3.4	2.4
Rolls, White, Split, Asda*	1 Roll/45g	113	251	10.0	45.0	3.4	2.8
Rolls, White, Submarine, Marks & Spencer*	1 Serving/109g	300	275	11.0	47.0	5.0	1.0
Rolls, White, Value, Tesco*	1 Roll/35g	81	231	8.0	45.7	1.8	2.3
Rolls, White, Warburtons*	1 Roll/57g	141	248	9.7	42.8	4.2	0.0
Rolls, White, Weight Watchers*	1 Roll/54g	135	251	11.7	47.1	1.8	4.2
Rolls, Wholemeal	1 Roll 45g	108	241	9.0	48.3	2.9	5.9
Rolls, Wholemeal With Cracked Wheat, Allinson*	1 Roll/58g	134	231	11.0	38.0	3.9	7.0
Rolls, Wholemeal, Asda*	1 Roll/58g	131	225	11.0	39.0	2.8	6.0
Rolls, Wholemeal, Budgens*	1 Roll/55.2g	147	268	11.7	48.1	3.2	4.0
Rolls, Wholemeal, COU, Marks & Spencer*	1 Roll/110g	226	205	11.3	33.4	2.8	7.1
Rolls, Wholemeal, Deli, Tesco*	1 Serving/65g	156	240	9.0	40.2	4.8	5.7
Rolls, Wholemeal, Deli, With Cracked Wheat, Tesco*	1 Roll/65g	156	240	9.0	40.2	4.8	5.7
Rolls, Wholemeal, Finger, Soft, Marks & Spencer*	1 Roll/69g	179	260	11.9	37.4	6.8	4.4
Rolls, Wholemeal, Floury Batch, Sainsbury's*	1 Roll/68g	150	220	10.7	36.0	3.7	6.6
Rolls, Wholemeal, Food Explorers, Waitrose*	1 Roll/32.0g	74	231	10.6	40.2	3.1	5.7
Rolls, Wholemeal, Healthy Living, Tesco*	1 Roll/68g	134	198	10.7	34.4	2.0	10.1
Rolls, Wholemeal, Kingsmill*	1 Roll/68g	167	245	10.7	41.5	4.0	5.1
Rolls, Wholemeal, Milk, Warburtons*	1 Roll/22g	51	231	12.5	38.1	3.2	7.0
Rolls, Wholemeal, Mini, Assorted, Waitrose*	1 Roll/35.6g	85	236	9.0	38.1	5.3	5.2
Rolls, Wholemeal, Mini, Tesco*	1 Roll/34g	82	240	10.9	36.4	5.6	5.8
Rolls, Wholemeal, Old Fashioned, Waitrose*	1 Roll/57g	135	236	11.1	37.2	4.8	6.6
Rolls, Wholemeal, Organic, Sainsbury's*	1 Roll/66g	152	230	10.7	41.0	2.7	6.6
Rolls, Wholemeal, Organic, Tesco*	1 Roll/65g	177	273	10.3	44.1	6.2	5.5
Rolls, Wholemeal, Ploughman's, Sainsbury's*	1 Roll/67g	153	229	10.7	39.3	3.2	8.6
Rolls, Wholemeal, Sainsbury's*	1 Serving/64.8g	153	236	10.7	40.8	3.3	7.4
Rolls, Wholemeal, Sandwich, Warburtons*	1 Roll/58g	124	214	10.2	35.1	3.7	6.6
Rolls, Wholemeal, Soft, Marks & Spencer*	1 Roll/55g	134	244	12.4	37.9	4.7	6.3
Rolls, Wholemeal, Soft, Sainsbury's*	1 Roll/60g	133	221	9.9	37.8	3.4	6.5
Rolls, Wholemeal, Square, Hovis*	1 Roll/52g	118	227	11.1	36.3	4.2	6.1
Rolls, Wholemeal, Submarine, Warburtons*	1 Serving/94g	231	246	10.9	40.6	4.4	6.3
Rolls, Wholemeal, Sunflower & Honey, Sainsbury's*	1 Roll/85g	225	265	9.2	45.4	5.1	4.5
Rolls, Wholemeal, Tasty, Kingsmill*	1 Roll/53g	125	236	10.7	39.2	4.0	7.4
Rolls, Wholemeal, Tesco*	1 Roll/58g	137	235	10.5	39.1	4.1	7.6
Rolls, Wholewhite, Kingsmill*	1 Roll/63g	158	251	9.5	43.7	4.2	3.5
Rolls, Wholmeal, Deli, Tesco*	1 Roll/65g	156	240	9.0	40.2	4.8	5.7
Roti, Tesco*	1 Bread/95g	256	269	8.4	46.4	5.5	3.2
Rye	1 Slice/25g	55	219	8.3	45.8	1.7	4.4
Rye With Sesame Seeds, Ryvita*	1 Slice/9g	31	339	10.5	58.5	7.0	16.0
Rye With Sunflower Seeds, Organic, Sunnyvale*	1 Slice/25g	50	198	5.1	30.3	6.3	0.0
Rye, Dark, Sliced, Trianon*	1 Slice/41g	74	180	6.5	35.0	1.5	0.0
Rye, German Style, Kelderman*	1 Slice/62g	96	155	5.6	30.2	1.4	7.7
Rye, Light, Finest, Tesco*	1 Slice/20g	47	237	10.4	44.3	2.0	3.7
Rye, Organic, Waitrose*	1 Serving/100g	207	207	6.4	42.7	1.2	5.1
Rye, Swedish Style, Kelderman*	1 Slice/50g	93	185	7.2	31.5	3.2	4.3
Rye, Wholemeal, Organic, Mestemacher*	1 Serving/71g	127	179	5.7	33.5	2.5	8.1
Rye, Wholemeal, With Sunflower Seeds, Organic, Biona*	1 Slice/72g	144	202	7.1	35.0	3.7	0.0
Rye, With Sunflower Seeds, Mestemacher*	1 Slice/80g	146	182	6.1	32.3	3.1	0.0
Scottish Plain, Mothers Pride*	1oz/28g	64	227	8.7	44.6	1.5	3.0

BREAD

INFO/WEIGHT	Measure	per Measure KCAL	Nutrition Values per 100g / 100ml KCAL	PROT	CARB	FAT	FIBRE
Sfilatino, Ready to Bake, TTD, Sainsbury's*	1 Sfilatino/125.9g	327	260	8.9	47.7	3.7	2.2
Soda	1oz/28g	72	258	7.7	54.6	2.5	2.1
Soda Farls, Tesco*	1 Farl/142g	325	229	7.1	42.2	3.2	2.6
Soda, Fruit, Marks & Spencer*	1 Slice/40.4g	104	260	5.9	51.3	4.6	2.5
Soda, Marks & Spencer*	1 Slice/40g	82	205	8.7	39.2	1.6	4.2
Softgrain, Farmhouse, Marks & Spencer*	1 Slice/25g	60	238	8.4	42.8	3.7	3.2
Softgrain, Medium Sliced, GFY, Asda*	1 Slice/35g	79	226	7.0	46.0	1.5	3.7
Softgrain, Mighty White*	1 Slice/36g	81	224	7.2	45.5	1.5	3.7
Soya & Linseed, Burgen*	1 Slice/36g	102	285	17.9	29.2	10.5	6.2
Stoneground, Small Loaf, Organic, Sainsbury's*	1 Slice/24g	50	208	10.0	37.9	2.1	7.9
Submarine, Malted Grain, Marks & Spencer*	1 Roll/109g	300	275	8.9	53.8	4.3	3.0
Sunflower & Honey, Marks & Spencer*	1 Serving/67g	206	308	12.9	34.0	13.4	5.6
Sunflower & Pumpin Seed, Batched, Organic, Tesco*	1 Slice/30g	73	243	11.0	33.1	7.4	5.2
Sunflower Seed, Bolletje, Delhaize*	1 Slice/44g	106	240	7.5	35.0	7.0	6.0
Sunny, Hovis*	1 Slice/44g	110	250	8.2	41.5	5.7	2.0
Three Grain, Organic, Schneider Brot*	1 Slice/71.5g	119	165	5.8	30.4	2.2	0.0
Toaster, White, Rathbones*	2 Slices/76g	185	243	9.1	48.6	1.3	2.3
Tomato & Chilli, BGTY, Sainsbury's*	1/4 Bread/65g	155	238	11.9	36.9	4.7	2.8
Tomato & Garlic, Morrisons*	1 Serving/125g	271	217	5.9	31.4	7.6	2.5
Tomato & Herb, Tear & Share, Tesco*	1/4 Pack/73g	164	226	6.3	40.2	4.4	2.1
Veda Malt, St Michael*	1 Serving/45g	99	219	7.1	45.3	1.1	2.2
Walnut, Waitrose*	1 Slice/33g	104	315	10.8	43.2	11.0	4.3
Wheat Free, Organic, The Stamp Collection*	1 Slice/35g	66	188	6.5	39.5	0.4	0.4
Wheat, Tasty, Kingsmill*	1 Serving/38g	84	221	10.1	37.6	3.4	6.8
Wheaten, Marks & Spencer*	1 Slice/33g	74	225	9.3	42.9	3.5	3.9
Wheatgerm, Original, Medium, Hovis*	1 Slice/33g	66	199	11.5	32.7	2.5	3.7
Wheatgerm, Thin Sliced, Hovis*	1 Slice/21g	47	222	10.1	38.5	3.0	4.6
Wheatgrain, Robertson*	1 Slice/30g	90	300	9.3	57.3	4.0	4.0
White	1 Slice/25g	59	235	8.4	49.3	1.9	1.5
White, Batch Loaf, Extra Special, Asda*	1 Slice/47g	109	233	9.0	45.0	1.9	2.2
White, Big & Bouncy, Hovis*	1 Slice/50g	117	233	8.3	46.3	1.6	2.2
White, COU, Marks & Spencer*	1 Slice/26g	60	231	10.6	41.9	2.3	4.6
White, Classic Cut, Thick, Hovis*	1 Slice/42g	96	228	7.5	46.3	1.5	2.5
White, Country Maid*	1 Slice/33.2g	76	229	8.5	44.1	2.1	3.0
White, Crusty, Finest, Tesco*	1oz/28g	70	250	8.9	49.0	3.0	2.0
White, Crusty, Gold, Kingsmill*	1 Slice/27g	70	258	9.4	48.5	2.9	2.7
White, Crusty, Hovis*	1 Slice/44g	103	233	8.8	44.3	2.2	2.1
White, Crusty, Sliced Loaf, Tesco*	1 Slice/50g	117	233	7.4	46.0	2.1	2.0
White, Crusty, Sliced, Harvestime*	1 Slice/44g	98	222	6.6	45.6	1.5	1.9
White, Crusty, Sliced, Premium, Budgens*	1 Slice/50g	121	242	8.8	46.9	2.2	2.2
White, Danish, Medium Sliced, Better For You, Morrisons*	1 Slice/17g	42	245	10.2	49.1	1.8	2.2
White, Danish, Soft & Light, Thick Cut, Asda*	1 Slice/26g	60	230	9.0	45.0	1.6	2.1
White, Danish, Tesco*	1 Slice/22g	56	254	9.4	49.7	1.9	2.8
White, Danish, Thick Sliced, Tesco*	2 Slices/47g	105	223	7.4	45.3	1.3	2.6
White, Danish, Warburtons*	1 Slice/25g	61	244	10.8	46.8	1.6	2.8
White, Danish, Weight Watchers*	1 Slice/19g	45	238	10.7	45.6	1.5	2.4
White, Eat Smart, Safeway*	1 Slice/26g	60	230	8.8	45.0	1.8	2.3
White, Extra Thick Sliced, Kingsmill*	1 Slice/58g	135	232	8.8	43.8	2.4	2.8
White, Farmhouse Crusty, Marks & Spencer*	1 Slice/34g	85	250	8.8	48.0	2.6	2.3
White, Farmhouse, Hovis	1 Slice/37g	86	233	8.3	45.9	1.7	2.8
White, Farmhouse, Seeded, Waitrose*	1 Serving/75g	192	256	10.8	40.9	5.5	5.6
White, Farmhouse, Soft, Warburtons*	1 Slice/26g	61	236	9.9	43.4	2.5	2.7
White, Farmhouse, The Best, Safeway*	1 Slice/44.3g	104	237	8.4	47.5	1.5	3.1

BREAD

INFO/WEIGHT	Measure per Measure	KCAL	Nutrition Values per 100g / 100ml KCAL	PROT	CARB	FAT	FIBRE
White, Fibre, Morrisons*	2 Slices/80g	192	240	8.0	48.4	1.7	0.3
White, Floury Batch, Sainsbury's*	1 Serving/62g	166	267	8.0	48.8	4.5	2.3
White, Fried in Blended Oil	1 Slice/28g	141	503	7.9	48.5	32.2	1.6
White, Gluten & Wheat Free, Free From, Sainsbury's*	1 Serving/70g	159	227	1.9	35.5	8.6	1.0
White, Gluten Free, Bakers Delight*	1 Serving/28g	64	227	1.9	35.5	8.6	1.0
White, Gold Seeded, Kingsmill*	1 Slice/44g	108	245	9.7	38.8	5.7	3.5
White, Gold Toastie, Kingsmill*	1 Slice/44g	103	234	9.3	42.3	3.1	0.6
White, Golden, Square Cut, Marks & Spencer*	1 Med Sl/39.5g	86	215	8.9	40.7	2.1	6.1
White, Good Health, Warburtons*	1 Slice/38g	84	220	9.4	41.6	1.8	4.1
White, Great, Hovis*	1 Slice/40g	90	226	8.8	44.4	1.5	2.2
White, Loaf, Crusty, Premium, Warburtons*	1 Slice/28.6g	72	247	10.4	46.1	2.3	2.7
White, Loaf, Danish, Asda*	1 Serving/22.5g	52	236	9.0	45.0	2.2	2.0
White, Loaf, Mini, Medium Sliced, Warburtons*	1 Slice/23.5g	57	239	10.2	44.4	2.5	2.7
White, Low Carb, Sliced, Tesco*	2 Slices/33g	70	211	11.3	36.4	2.2	6.9
White, Medium Sliced	1 Med Slice/39g	93	238	7.5	48.5	1.6	1.8
White, Medium Sliced, Asda*	1 Slice/37g	84	226	7.0	46.0	1.5	2.8
White, Medium Sliced, BGTY, Sainsbury's*	1 Slice/20g	45	225	10.2	43.9	0.9	4.6
White, Medium Sliced, Danish Style, Tesco*	2 Slices/40g	89	223	7.4	45.3	1.3	2.5
White, Medium Sliced, Economy, Sainsbury's*	1 Slice/44g	104	236	7.6	48.6	1.3	1.8
White, Medium Sliced, Hovis*	1 Slice/35g	80	228	7.5	46.3	1.5	2.5
White, Medium Sliced, Keep Fresh, Safeway*	1 Slice/34g	76	224	7.3	44.3	1.9	2.7
White, Medium Sliced, Long Life, Asda*	1 Slice/36g	82	228	8.0	45.0	1.8	2.7
White, Medium Sliced, Longer Life, Co-Op*	1 Slice/44g	99	225	8.0	45.0	2.0	2.0
White, Medium Sliced, Longerlife, Sainsbury's*	1 Slice/36g	87	243	8.3	47.6	2.2	1.7
White, Medium Sliced, Makes Sense, Somerfield*	1 Slice/36.3g	81	226	7.5	46.4	1.2	2.4
White, Medium Sliced, Marks & Spencer*	1 Slice/35g	81	230	7.4	45.9	1.7	2.4
White, Medium Sliced, Mothers Pride*	1 Slice/36g	82	229	8.0	45.6	1.6	3.0
White, Medium Sliced, Nimble*	1 Slice/20g	46	232	9.7	44.3	1.8	2.9
White, Medium Sliced, Sainsbury's*	1 Slice/36g	83	231	8.0	46.4	1.5	2.1
White, Medium Sliced, SmartPrice, Asda*	1 Slice/36g	81	226	7.0	46.0	1.5	2.8
White, Medium Sliced, Soft & Light, Danish, Safeway*	1 Slice/20.2g	47	233	8.7	45.1	2.0	2.2
White, Medium Sliced, Soft, Danish, Somerfield*	1 Slice/21g	48	229	8.6	44.8	1.4	2.4
White, Medium Sliced, Spinaca, Aldi*	1 Slice/25g	59	237	7.2	46.7	1.8	2.3
White, Medium Sliced, Stay Fresh, Tesco*	2 Slices/69g	170	246	8.9	48.1	2.0	0.8
White, Medium Sliced, Superlife, Morrisons*	1 Slice/30g	79	263	9.6	47.4	3.9	2.5
White, Medium Sliced, Tesco*	1 Slice/37g	84	228	8.0	45.5	1.6	3.0
White, Medium Sliced, Value, Tesco*	1 Slice/36g	81	225	7.9	46.1	1.0	2.1
White, Medium Sliced, Weight Watchers*	1 Slice/12g	30	247	12.5	45.2	1.9	3.2
White, Organic, Marks & Spencer*	1 Slice/36g	94	261	7.6	52.5	2.4	2.2
White, Organic, Sainsbury's*	1 Slice/35.9g	84	234	8.9	45.5	1.8	2.3
White, Premium Farmhouse, Lidl*	1 Slice/44g	99	225	7.4	45.4	1.5	2.5
White, Premium Gold, TTD, Sainsbury's*	1 Slice/44g	103	233	8.4	45.6	1.9	2.2
White, Premium, Marks & Spencer*	1 Slice/40.4g	94	235	8.5	45.8	1.9	2.7
White, Sandwich, Bakery, Sainsbury's*	1 Slice/50g	121	242	10.3	49.0	0.6	2.9
White, Sandwich, Kingsmill*	1 Slice/42g	97	232	8.8	43.8	2.4	2.8
White, Scottish, Sunblest*	1 Slice/57g	133	233	10.1	42.3	2.6	2.8
White, Sliced, Brennans*	1 Serving/39g	80	205	8.5	42.0	1.4	2.7
White, Soft Batch, Sliced, Sainsbury's*	1 Slice/44.0g	102	232	8.2	45.4	1.9	2.3
White, Soft Crusty, Marks & Spencer*	1 Slice/25g	64	256	9.3	49.0	2.5	2.4
White, Soft, Batch Loaf, Sliced, Tesco*	1 Slice/50g	117	233	7.5	46.1	2.1	2.1
White, Soft, Farmhouse, Marks & Spencer*	1 Slice/25g	60	239	9.8	42.6	3.3	2.5
White, Soft, Gold, Kingsmill*	1 Slice/47g	111	236	8.9	42.9	3.2	2.8
White, Soft, Medium Slice, Warburtons*	1 Slice/27g	88	326	12.2	61.5	3.3	4.1

B

BREAD

INFO/WEIGHT	Measure	per Measure KCAL	Nutrition Values per 100g / 100ml KCAL	PROT	CARB	FAT	FIBRE
White, Soft, Medium Sliced, Kingsmill*	1 Slice/38g	88	232	8.6	43.8	2.4	2.6
White, Soft, Milk Roll, Warburtons*	1 Slice/18g	46	251	10.8	45.3	3.0	2.8
White, Soft, Organic, Warburtons*	1 Slice/26.7g	62	228	9.7	44.6	3.0	2.6
White, Softgrain, Sliced, Tesco*	1 Med Slice/36g	81	224	7.2	45.5	1.5	3.7
White, Square Cut, Kingsmill*	1 Med Slice/38g	88	232	8.8	43.8	2.4	2.8
White, Square Cut, Medium, Hovis*	1 Med Slice/40g	90	226	8.9	43.7	1.8	2.8
White, Stay Fresh, Tesco*	1 Slice/40g	100	249	8.6	48.3	2.4	1.5
White, Sunblest*	1 Med Slice/33g	77	232	7.4	46.4	1.9	2.1
White, Super Toastie, Warburtons*	1 Serving/57g	134	235	10.1	44.6	1.8	2.7
White, Superior English Quality, Thin Cut, Hovis*	1 Serving/73g	169	232	9.2	42.8	1.5	3.8
White, Thick Sliced, Bakers Gold, Asda*	1 Slice/44g	101	229	8.0	45.0	1.9	2.3
White, Thick Sliced, Budgens*	1 Slice/40g	89	223	7.4	45.3	1.3	2.5
White, Thick Sliced, Co-Op*	1 Slice/43g	99	230	8.0	46.0	2.0	2.0
White, Thick Sliced, Gold, Co-Op*	1 Slice/44g	92	210	10.0	37.0	2.0	7.0
White, Thick Sliced, Golden Sun*	1 Slice/44g	100	228	7.5	46.1	1.5	2.4
White, Thick Sliced, Healthy, Warburtons*	1 Slice/38g	84	222	10.3	41.2	1.8	4.1
White, Thick Sliced, Hovis*	1 Serving/50g	109	218	11.1	38.4	2.0	6.4
White, Thick Sliced, Kingsmill*	1 Slice/42g	98	233	8.8	44.1	2.4	2.5
White, Thick Sliced, Long Life, Somerfield*	1 Slice/44g	100	227	7.5	44.9	1.9	2.4
White, Thick Sliced, Marks & Spencer*	1 Slice/42g	96	228	7.3	46.7	1.3	2.8
White, Thick Sliced, Organic, Tesco*	1 Slice/44g	110	249	7.4	51.3	1.6	2.1
White, Thick Sliced, Premium, Tesco*	1 Slice/44.4g	98	222	8.7	45.2	0.7	1.5
White, Thick Sliced, Sainsbury's*	1 Slice/44g	100	228	7.1	46.4	1.5	2.8
White, Thick Sliced, SmartPrice, Asda*	1 Slice/47g	106	226	7.0	46.0	1.5	2.8
White, Thick Sliced, Square Cut, Asda*	1 Slice/43.9g	101	230	8.0	46.0	1.5	2.1
White, Thick Sliced, Super Toastie, Morrisons*	1 Slice/50g	129	257	8.7	48.9	3.0	2.1
White, Thick Sliced, Tesco*	1 Slice/44g	100	228	7.1	46.4	1.5	2.8
White, Thick Sliced, Value, Tesco*	1 Slice/44g	109	248	8.4	49.3	1.9	1.5
White, Thick Sliced, Warburtons*	1 Slice/28g	65	233	9.8	43.6	2.1	2.7
White, Thin Sliced, Sainsbury's*	1 Slice/29g	66	228	7.1	46.4	1.5	2.8
White, Thin Sliced, Tesco*	2 Slices/59g	135	228	9.5	44.5	1.3	3.4
White, Toast, Gamle Mølle*	1 Slice/32g	83	260	8.0	52.0	2.0	3.0
White, Toasted	1 Med Slice/33g	87	265	9.3	57.1	1.6	1.8
White, Toastie, Kingsmill*	1 Slice/38g	89	234	9.3	42.3	3.1	3.1
White, Toastie, Thick Cut, Hovis*	1 Slice/50g	113	226	8.8	44.4	1.5	2.2
White, Toastie, Thick Sliced, Warburtons*	1 Slice/44.5g	107	238	10.3	44.9	1.9	2.7
White, Weight Watchers*	1 Serving/5g	12	246	12.3	45.1	1.6	3.3
White, Whole, Extra Thick, Kingsmill*	1 Slice/57g	130	228	9.0	42.3	2.5	4.0
White, Whole, Kingsmill*	1 Slice/38g	87	230	9.0	42.9	2.5	3.4
White, Wholesome, Loaf, Sainsbury's*	1 Serving/36g	81	224	9.4	42.5	1.8	4.4
White, Wholesome, Medium Sliced, Premium, Tesco*	1 Slice/36.6g	86	232	8.9	43.9	2.3	4.2
White, Wholesome, Thick Sliced, Tesco*	1 Serving/80g	177	221	10.5	40.5	1.9	4.8
White, With Wheatgerm, Best of Both, Hovis*	1 Slice/40g	89	223	8.8	42.3	2.0	3.8
Whole & White, Kingsmill*	1 Slice/38.2g	87	228	9.0	42.3	2.5	4.0
Whole Grain, Batch, Finest, Tesco*	1 Slice/127g	323	254	9.8	47.7	2.7	4.2
Whole Wheat, Nature's Own*	1 Slice/28g	66	236	14.3	39.3	3.6	10.7
Wholemeal	1 Slice/25g	54	215	9.2	41.6	2.5	5.8
Wholemeal, BGTY, Sainsbury's*	1 Slice/20g	41	207	12.6	36.8	1.0	7.3
Wholemeal, Batch Loaf, Organic, Marks & Spencer*	1 Serving/30g	60	200	10.4	32.1	3.2	7.4
Wholemeal, Batch Loaf, Village Green, Aldi*	1 Slice/30g	67	224	9.8	40.6	2.5	5.8
Wholemeal, Batch, Organic, Waitrose*	1 Slice/40g	88	219	10.0	38.8	2.6	7.2
Wholemeal, Batch, Stoneground, Warburtons*	1 Slice/42g	91	217	9.8	39.3	2.3	7.2
Wholemeal, Bread To Savour, Allinson*	1 Slice/47g	102	216	12.5	34.8	3.0	7.4

B

BREAD

INFO/WEIGHT	Measure	per Measure KCAL	KCAL	PROT	CARB	FAT	FIBRE
Wholemeal, COU, Marks & Spencer*	1 Slice/21g	45	213	13.6	33.7	2.6	7.0
Wholemeal, Country Grain, Hovis*	1 Slice/44.1g	95	216	11.2	36.9	2.5	8.2
Wholemeal, Crusty, Finest, Tesco*	1 Slice/50g	103	206	10.8	37.0	1.7	6.9
Wholemeal, Crusty, Kingsmill*	1 Slice/42g	104	247	11.2	41.1	4.2	7.0
Wholemeal, Danish, Warburtons*	1 Slice/25g	57	229	13.3	38.5	2.4	7.2
Wholemeal, Economy, Sainsbury's*	1 Slice/28g	61	217	10.3	38.4	2.5	6.5
Wholemeal, Family Loaf, Safeway*	1 Slice/45g	96	213	9.5	37.4	2.8	6.0
Wholemeal, Farmhouse Gold, Morrisons*	1 Slice/38g	78	204	9.2	38.3	1.6	6.0
Wholemeal, Farmhouse Soft Golden, Marks & Spencer*	1 Slice/30g	65	215	11.0	35.1	3.1	7.4
Wholemeal, Farmhouse, Hovis*	1 Slice/44g	91	206	10.2	36.6	2.1	5.3
Wholemeal, Farmhouse, Split Top, Hovis*	1 Thick Slice/44g	97	221	11.3	37.1	3.1	6.4
Wholemeal, Fresher For Longer, Sainsbury's*	1 Slice/44.1g	98	222	10.9	36.2	3.7	6.5
Wholemeal, Gold, Kingsmill*	1 Slice/44g	95	217	10.9	36.8	2.9	7.0
Wholemeal, Golden Wheat, Kingsmill*	1 Slice/44g	97	221	10.9	37.8	2.9	6.0
Wholemeal, Good Health, Warburtons*	1 Slice/35.2g	82	233	10.9	41.0	2.7	7.2
Wholemeal, Great Tasting, Warburtons*	1 Serving/42.2g	95	227	10.4	40.0	2.8	6.3
Wholemeal, Hearty, Hovis*	1 Slice/36g	78	217	11.1	38.4	2.1	6.4
Wholemeal, Heavenly, Hovis*	1 Slice/40.1g	87	217	11.4	38.0	2.2	6.5
Wholemeal, Hovis*	1 Med Slice/36g	78	217	11.1	38.4	2.1	6.4
Wholemeal, Keep Fresh, Medium Sliced, Safeway*	1 Slice/37g	75	204	9.1	36.6	2.4	6.2
Wholemeal, Kingsmill*	1 Slice/45g	99	221	10.1	37.6	3.4	6.8
Wholemeal, Loaf, Crusty, Farmhouse, Marks & Spencer*	1 Serving/32.6g	76	230	10.1	40.7	2.7	6.3
Wholemeal, Longer Life, Medium Sliced, Sainsbury's*	1 Slice/36g	73	203	8.6	37.6	2.1	5.1
Wholemeal, Longer Life, Sainsbury's*	1 Med Slice/36g	85	237	10.7	41.0	3.4	6.2
Wholemeal, Longer Life, Thick Slice, Sainsbury's*	1 Slice/45g	101	224	10.6	37.4	3.6	5.9
Wholemeal, Makes Sense, Somerfield*	1 Slice/36g	78	217	10.7	38.6	2.2	6.6
Wholemeal, Marks & Spencer*	1 Med Slice/38g	82	215	11.4	36.0	2.6	7.1
Wholemeal, Medium Cut, Allinson*	1 Slice/36g	78	216	9.5	39.2	2.4	6.5
Wholemeal, Medium Cut, Small Sliced, Allinson*	1 Slice/23g	50	219	10.3	38.3	2.7	6.1
Wholemeal, Medium Sliced, Asda*	1 Slice/36g	80	223	9.0	39.0	3.4	6.0
Wholemeal, Medium Sliced, Fresh For A Week, Asda*	1 Slice/35g	71	202	9.0	36.0	2.4	7.0
Wholemeal, Medium Sliced, Hearty, Hovis*	1 Slice/36g	78	217	11.1	38.4	2.1	6.4
Wholemeal, Medium Sliced, Kingsmill*	1 Slice/38g	87	228	10.1	39.2	3.4	5.2
Wholemeal, Medium Sliced, Longerlife, Sainsbury's*	1 Slice/36g	73	203	8.6	37.6	2.1	5.1
Wholemeal, Medium Sliced, Organic, Asda*	1 Slice/43.3g	93	217	9.0	40.0	2.3	6.0
Wholemeal, Medium Sliced, Organic, Tesco*	2 Slices/53g	111	209	9.2	37.2	2.8	6.0
Wholemeal, Medium Sliced, Premium, Tesco*	2 Slices/72g	141	196	9.8	37.8	0.6	7.2
Wholemeal, Medium Sliced, Safeway*	1 Slice/36g	73	204	9.1	36.6	2.4	6.2
Wholemeal, Medium Sliced, Sainsbury's*	1 Slice/36g	77	214	10.3	37.8	2.4	7.4
Wholemeal, Medium Sliced, Stay Fresh, Somerfield*	1 Slice/36g	72	200	9.2	36.6	1.8	0.5
Wholemeal, Medium Sliced, Stayfresh, Tesco*	1 Slice/36g	84	232	10.5	42.2	2.3	6.3
Wholemeal, Medium Sliced, Tesco*	1 Slice/36g	81	226	9.2	41.6	2.5	5.8
Wholemeal, Medium Sliced, Waitrose*	1 Slice/35.7g	77	213	10.1	37.6	2.4	7.0
Wholemeal, Medium Sliced, Warburtons*	1 Slice/36g	84	234	10.3	40.3	3.5	7.2
Wholemeal, Medium Sliced, Xtra Life, Waitrose*	1 Slice/36g	85	237	10.7	41.0	3.4	6.2
Wholemeal, Medium, Square, Tasty, Kingsmill*	1 Serving/38g	84	221	10.1	37.6	3.4	6.8
Wholemeal, Multigrain, Country, Hovis*	1 Slice/36g	80	222	11.2	37.4	3.1	5.7
Wholemeal, Multigrain, Premium Gold, TTD, Sainsbury's*	1 Slice/44g	106	242	10.2	35.9	6.4	5.3
Wholemeal, Multigrain, Sliced, Finest, Tesco*	1 Serving/50g	123	246	10.1	42.1	4.1	6.5
Wholemeal, Multigrain, Soft Batch, Sainsbury's*	1 Slice/44g	106	242	11.3	34.5	6.5	5.6
Wholemeal, Nimble*	1 Slice/20g	42	209	11.4	37.0	1.7	6.6
Wholemeal, Premium, Marks & Spencer*	1 Med Sl/32.5g	66	200	10.5	32.9	3.1	6.7
Wholemeal, Rathbones*	1 Slice/27g	57	211	9.4	39.2	1.8	7.1

BREAD

INFO/WEIGHT	KCAL	KCAL	PROT	CARB	FAT	FIBRE
Wholemeal, Rustic, Tin, Tesco*	1 Slice/37g	92	249	12.2	44.0	3.5	3.1
Wholemeal, Sandwich, Warburtons*	1 Slice/31g	72	232	10.7	40.2	3.1	7.2
Wholemeal, Savers, Safeway*	1 Slice/36.5g	78	211	8.8	38.2	2.5	1.2
Wholemeal, Sliced, Gluten Free, Glutano*	1 Slice/56g	107	191	7.0	34.0	3.0	0.0
Wholemeal, Sliced, McCambridge*	1 Slice/38g	90	237	7.9	44.7	1.8	0.0
Wholemeal, Sliced, Organic, Warburtons*	1 Slice/27g	65	240	11.5	40.9	3.6	7.2
Wholemeal, Sliced, Premium, Budgens*	1 Slice/45g	101	224	9.3	39.1	3.3	8.2
Wholemeal, Small Sliced, Warburtons*	1 Slice/23.5g	57	239	10.8	41.9	3.1	7.2
Wholemeal, Small, Allinson*	1 Slice/23g	49	213	10.1	37.3	2.6	7.5
Wholemeal, Small, Kingsmill*	1 Slice/25g	56	224	10.7	38.0	3.2	5.8
Wholemeal, Soft Crusty, Marks & Spencer*	1 Slice/25g	58	230	11.4	39.1	3.1	6.5
Wholemeal, Soft, Medium Sliced, Morrisons*	1 Slice/32g	68	214	9.9	38.0	2.5	5.8
Wholemeal, Square, Tasty, Kingsmill*	1 Slice/42g	96	228	10.1	39.2	3.4	5.2
Wholemeal, Stoneground, Organic, Sainsbury's*	1 Slice/29g	61	210	10.2	37.9	1.9	7.8
Wholemeal, Stoneground, Warburtons*	1 Slice/45.8g	100	217	9.9	38.3	2.7	7.1
Wholemeal, Tasty, Kingsmill*	1 Slice/40g	88	221	10.1	37.6	3.4	6.8
Wholemeal, Tesco*	1 Slice/36g	71	198	7.6	37.6	1.9	5.1
Wholemeal, Thick Cut, Allinson*	1 Slice/44g	94	213	10.1	37.3	2.6	7.5
Wholemeal, Thick Sliced Loaf, Tesco*	1 Slice/45g	90	201	8.8	36.4	2.3	5.3
Wholemeal, Thick Sliced, Asda*	1 Slice/45g	97	215	10.0	38.0	2.5	6.0
Wholemeal, Thick Sliced, Bakers Gold, Asda*	1 Slice/44g	99	225	12.0	37.0	3.2	6.0
Wholemeal, Thick Sliced, COU, Marks & Spencer*	1 Slice/26g	56	215	13.6	33.7	2.6	7.0
Wholemeal, Thick Sliced, Hearty, Hovis*	1 Slice/44g	95	217	11.1	38.4	2.1	6.4
Wholemeal, Thick Sliced, Keep Fresh, Safeway*	1 Slice/45g	92	204	9.1	36.6	2.4	6.2
Wholemeal, Thick Sliced, Kingsmill*	1 Slice/42g	96	228	10.1	39.2	3.4	5.2
Wholemeal, Thick Sliced, Organic, Sainsbury's*	1 Slice/44g	92	210	10.0	40.1	1.0	6.7
Wholemeal, Thick Sliced, Organic, Tesco*	1 Slice/44g	98	221	9.3	39.9	2.7	6.1
Wholemeal, Thick Sliced, Organic, Warburtons*	1 Slice/26.5g	57	219	11.0	36.4	3.3	7.2
Wholemeal, Thick Sliced, Premium, Tesco*	1 Serving/44g	95	214	10.0	40.1	1.5	5.7
Wholemeal, Thick Sliced, Sainsbury's*	1 Slice/44g	94	214	10.3	37.8	2.4	7.4
Wholemeal, Thick Sliced, Stay Fresh, Tesco*	1 Slice/44g	96	219	10.3	38.9	2.5	5.3
Wholemeal, Thick Sliced, Waitrose*	1 Slice/44g	111	252	10.9	36.0	7.2	5.8
Wholemeal, Toasted	1 Med Slice/26g	58	224	8.6	42.3	2.2	5.8
Wholemeal, Toastie, Warburtons*	1 Slice/44g	101	230	10.3	40.2	2.9	7.2
Wholemeal, Unsliced, Organic, Doves Farm*	1 Med Slice/35g	73	208	8.5	40.5	2.5	6.4
Wholemeal, Value, Tesco*	1 Slice/36g	78	217	10.3	38.4	2.5	6.5
Wholemeal, Warburtons*	2 Slices/47g	112	239	10.8	41.9	3.1	7.2
Wholemeal, With Kibbled Malted Wheat, Kingsmill*	1 Slice/42g	96	228	10.1	39.2	3.4	5.2
Wholemeal, With Oat Flakes & Seeds, Waitrose*	1 Slice/44.4g	105	238	11.9	33.4	6.3	9.3
Wholemeal, With Pumpkin & Sunflower Seeds, Tesco*	1 Slice/25g	61	243	11.0	33.1	7.4	5.2

BREAD & BUTTER PUDDING

5% Fat, Marks & Spencer*	1 Pudding/237g	367	155	4.4	24.8	4.2	0.4
Asda*	1 Serving/125g	280	224	4.9	24.0	12.0	0.0
Average	1 Portion/190g	304	160	6.2	17.5	7.8	0.3
BGTY, Sainsbury's*	1 Serving/120g	145	121	7.0	19.6	1.6	1.4
COU, Marks & Spencer*	1 Pot/140g	189	135	5.5	24.6	1.7	0.6
Co-Op*	1/2 Pudding/170g	425	250	7.0	28.0	13.0	1.0
Finest, Tesco*	1 Serving/153g	379	248	4.9	24.6	14.4	0.9
GFY, Asda*	1 Serving/125g	153	122	7.0	20.0	1.6	1.3
Good Choice, Iceland*	1 Pudding/129.6g	242	186	6.1	27.7	5.6	2.4
Iceland*	1/2 Pack/160g	413	258	4.7	25.4	16.8	3.4
Individual, Marks & Spencer*	1 Pudding/130.2g	280	215	4.4	21.4	12.6	0.5
Individual, Waitrose*	1 Pudding/116g	247	213	5.4	24.4	10.4	0.3

	Measure INFO/WEIGHT	per Measure KCAL	Nutrition Values per 100g / 100ml				
			KCAL	PROT	CARB	FAT	FIBRE
BREAD & BUTTER PUDDING							
Marks & Spencer*	1 Serving/125g	359	287	5.3	24.1	19.4	0.8
Reduced Fat, Waitrose*	1 Serving/205g	299	146	7.4	23.3	2.6	2.0
Sainsbury's*	1 Pudding/230g	446	194	4.8	21.9	9.7	0.4
BREAD MIX							
Brown, Sunflower, Sainsbury's*	1 Serving/60g	151	251	10.0	38.9	6.1	4.0
Cheese & Onion, Sainsbury's*	1 Serving/100g	311	311	11.9	59.5	2.8	2.6
Ciabatta, Wright's*	1 Serving/45g	154	343	14.2	71.0	3.0	0.0
Crusty White, Made Up, Tesco*	1 Slice/126g	316	251	9.4	49.3	1.8	2.5
Focaccia, Garlic & Herb, Asda*	1 Serving/125g	385	308	11.0	48.0	8.0	3.3
Italian Ciabatta, Sainsbury's*	1 Slice/45g	96	213	8.7	40.0	2.0	2.4
Italian Sun Dried Tomato & Parmesan, Sainsbury's*	1 Serving/100g	247	247	8.1	50.1	1.7	2.5
Mixed Grain, Sainsbury's*	1 Serving/45g	103	228	7.7	46.0	1.5	4.4
White Loaf, Asda*	1 Slice/60g	150	250	10.0	49.0	1.5	3.1
Wholemeal, Crusty, Tesco*	1 Bag/500g	1120	224	9.7	40.7	2.4	7.6
BREADCRUMBS							
Average	1oz/28g	98	350	10.8	74.8	1.9	2.6
BREADFRUIT							
Boiled in Unsalted Water	1oz/28g	33	119	1.6	29.0	0.4	0.0
Canned, Drained	1oz/28g	18	66	0.6	16.4	0.2	1.7
Raw	1oz/28g	27	95	1.3	23.1	0.3	0.0
BREADSTICKS							
Asda*	1 Serving/5g	21	412	12.0	73.0	8.0	2.9
Cheese, Italian, Tesco*	4 Breadsticks/21g	84	399	14.2	67.5	8.0	3.4
Classic, Somerfield*	1 Breadstick/6g	24	396	10.0	82.5	2.9	1.0
Farleys*	1 Serving/12g	50	414	14.0	76.5	5.8	1.1
Grissini, Italian, Sainsbury's*	1 Breadstick/5g	20	408	11.6	72.9	7.8	2.9
Grissini, Thin, With Olive Oil, Forno Bianco*	1 Stick/5g	21	420	11.0	77.0	7.5	0.0
Grissini, Waitrose*	1 Breadstick/6.3g	24	397	12.0	72.5	6.2	3.1
Mini, Wheat & Gluten Free, Free From, Tesco*	1 Stick/2.7g	11	414	4.0	72.1	12.2	2.2
Olive, Italian, Finest, Tesco*	1 Stick/40g	170	424	10.5	65.0	13.6	4.8
Onion, Marks & Spencer*	1 Serving/40g	166	415	12.6	59.6	14.1	4.8
Original, Italian, Tesco*	1 Pack/125g	510	408	11.6	72.9	7.8	2.9
Original, Organic, Kallo*	1 Breadstick/6g	24	393	11.8	69.5	7.6	4.7
Perfectly Balanced, Waitrose*	1 Breadstick/5g	20	378	13.7	77.3	1.6	3.8
Pesto Flavour, Safeway*	1 Stick/6g	24	394	13.4	67.5	7.8	5.2
Plain, Asda*	1 Stick/5g	21	412	12.0	73.0	8.0	2.9
Safeway*	1 Breadstick/6.3g	24	395	12.9	72.7	9.3	4.3
Sesame Seed Grissini, Sainsbury's*	1 Breadstick/5g	21	419	12.7	65.5	11.8	3.2
Sesame Seed, Grissini, Waitrose*	1 Breadstick/5g	21	413	13.7	65.7	10.6	3.0
Tangy Cheese, Tesco*	1oz/28g	121	432	11.9	63.2	14.7	6.2
Thin, Healthy Eating, Primo D'Oro*	1 Breadstick/3g	11	400	10.0	75.0	6.5	1.1
BREAKFAST							
All Day, Kershaws*	1 Pack/280g	392	140	7.3	9.6	8.0	1.6
All Day, With Baked Beans, Heinz*	1 Pack/403g	463	115	5.8	13.3	4.3	2.4
Farmhouse, Ready Meals, Waitrose*	1/2 Pack/250g	385	154	2.9	11.0	10.0	1.2
Pack, Fruit Pudding, Asda*	1 Serving/44g	45	103	1.4	15.0	4.2	0.0
Pack, Lorne, Sausage, Asda*	1 Serving/54g	96	178	6.0	7.0	14.0	0.0
BREAKFAST CEREAL							
Advantage, Weetabix*	1 Serving/30g	105	350	10.2	72.0	2.4	9.0
All Bran Splitz, Kellogg's*	1 Serving/40g	130	325	9.0	69.0	2.0	9.0
All Bran, Apricot Bites, Kellogg's*	1 Serving/45g	129	286	10.0	57.0	2.5	18.0
All Bran, Flakes, Kellogg's*	1 Serving/28g	90	320	10.0	66.0	2.5	15.0
All Bran, Kellogg's	1 Serving/40g	110	275	14.0	48.0	3.0	27.0

BREAKFAST CEREAL

INFO/WEIGHT	Measure per Measure KCAL		KCAL	PROT	CARB	FAT	FIBRE
Almond, Low Carb, Atkins*	1 Serving/30g	100	333	50.0	26.7	5.0	0.0
Alpen*, Blackberry & Apple	1 Serving/40g	140	349	9.2	69.4	3.8	8.3
Alpen*, Caribbean Crunch	1 Serving/40g	155	388	8.8	67.9	9.0	4.6
Alpen*, Crunchy Bran	1 Serving/40g	120	299	11.8	52.3	4.7	24.8
Alpen*, No Added Sugar	1 Serving/40g	142	354	10.5	64.6	6.0	7.7
Alpen*, Nutty Crunch	1 Serving/40g	159	398	10.7	63.6	11.2	6.5
Alpen*, Original	1 Serving/40g	146	365	10.0	66.0	6.8	7.7
Alpen*, Strawberry	1 Serving/40g	144	359	9.4	69.5	4.8	7.9
Alpen*, Wheat Flakes	1 Serving/40g	140	350	10.2	72.0	2.4	9.0
Apple & Cinnamon Flakes, Marks & Spencer*	1 Serving/30g	111	370	6.0	82.7	1.9	3.4
Apple & Cinnamon, Crisp, Sainsbury's*	1 Serving/50g	217	433	6.2	69.1	14.7	3.4
Apple, Balckberry & Raspberry Flakes, GFY, Asda	1 Serving/40g	138	344	9.0	73.0	1.8	11.0
Apricot Bites, Kellogg's*	1 Serving/45g	126	279	11.0	55.0	2.5	19.0
Apricot Wheats, Asda*	1 Serving/50g	165	330	8.0	71.0	1.5	8.0
Apricot Wheats, Whole Grain, Sainsbury's*	1 Serving/50g	165	330	7.8	71.4	1.5	8.0
Apricot Wheats, Whole Grain, Tesco*	1 Serving/40g	130	326	7.6	70.6	1.4	8.0
Balance With Red Fruit, Sainsbury's*	1 Serving/40g	148	369	9.9	78.1	1.9	3.1
Balance, Sainsbury's*	1 Serving/30g	111	370	11.4	77.7	1.5	3.2
Banana & Toffee Crisp, Mornflake*	1 Serving/30g	133	443	5.7	68.8	16.1	5.4
Banana, Papaya & Honey Oat, Crunchy, Waitrose*	1 Serving/40g	170	426	9.6	69.8	12.0	5.5
Barley Crisp, Cocoa, Pertwood Farm*	1 Serving/30g	105	350	8.1	84.0	2.1	9.3
Barley Crisp, Plain, Pertwood Farm*	1 Serving/40g	142	356	9.4	82.7	2.3	8.2
Barley Crisp, With Maple Syrup, Pertwood Farm*	1 Serving/50g	168	335	7.1	86.0	1.7	6.2
Benefit Flakes, Harvest Morn*	1 Serving/40g	148	370	11.4	77.7	1.5	3.2
Berries, Cherries & Flakes, COU, Marks & Spencer*	1 Serving/40g	152	380	8.5	82.2	1.9	3.2
Berry Crunchy, Sainsbury's*	1 Serving/30g	122	408	7.7	67.3	12.0	4.8
Blueberry & Cranberry, Oat Crunchy, Waitrose*	1 Serving/60g	262	437	8.0	67.0	15.2	7.4
Bran Flakes, Asda*	1 Serving/47g	157	333	11.0	65.0	3.2	14.0
Bran Flakes, Co-Op*	1 Serving/30g	99	330	11.0	65.0	3.0	15.0
Bran Flakes, Crunchy Nut, Sainsbury's*	1 Serving/40g	203	508	19.8	85.8	9.5	11.0
Bran Flakes, Harvest Home, Nestle*	1 Serving/30g	99	331	10.2	67.1	2.4	14.1
Bran Flakes, Healthy Living, Tesco*	1 Serving/30g	99	331	10.2	67.1	2.4	14.1
Bran Flakes, Honey & Nut, Safeway*	1 Serving/47g	168	358	9.6	70.0	4.4	11.0
Bran Flakes, Honey Nut, Sainsbury's*	1 Serving/40g	143	358	9.6	70.0	4.4	11.0
Bran Flakes, Honey Nut, Tesco*	1 Serving/40g	143	358	9.6	70.0	4.4	11.0
Bran Flakes, Kellogg's*	1 Serving/30g	97	322	10.0	66.0	2.0	15.0
Bran Flakes, Little Man, Lidl*	1 Serving/30g	99	331	11.0	65.0	3.0	14.5
Bran Flakes, Morrisons*	1 Serving/25g	83	331	11.1	64.6	3.2	14.5
Bran Flakes, Oat With Apple & Raisin, Kellogg's*	1 Serving/40g	140	350	10.0	66.0	5.0	10.0
Bran Flakes, Organic, Sainsbury's*	1 Serving/30g	100	332	10.2	67.4	2.4	14.1
Bran Flakes, Organic, Tesco*	1 Serving/30g	99	330	10.2	67.0	2.4	14.1
Bran Flakes, Somerfield*	1 Serving/50g	166	331	10.2	67.1	2.4	14.1
Bran Flakes, Sultana, Sainsbury's*	1 Serving/30g	157	523	22.0	89.7	8.7	11.7
Bran Flakes, Tesco*	1 Serving/30g	99	331	10.2	67.1	2.4	14.1
Bran Flakes, Value, Tesco*	1 Serving/50g	160	320	11.4	63.2	2.4	17.1
Bran Flakes, Waitrose*	1 Serving/30g	100	333	10.1	67.7	2.4	12.7
Bran Flakes, Whole Grain, Sainsbury's*	1 Serving/30g	99	331	10.2	67.1	2.4	14.1
Bran, Hi Fibre, Tesco*	1 Serving/40g	109	272	14.7	45.5	3.5	27.0
Bran, Natural, Sainsbury's*	1 Serving/30g	64	212	14.7	27.0	5.0	36.0
Cheerios, Honey Nut, Nestle*	1 Serving/40g	150	374	7.0	78.9	3.4	5.2
Cheerios, Nestle*	1 Serving/40g	146	366	8.1	74.6	3.9	6.5
Cheerios, Whole Grain, Nestle*	1 Serving/30g	110	366	8.1	74.6	3.9	6.5
Choc & Nut Crisp, Tesco*	1 Serving/40g	185	462	8.3	62.5	19.9	4.8

B

BREAKFAST CEREAL

	Measure INFO/WEIGHT	per Measure KCAL	Nutrition Values per 100g / 100ml				
			KCAL	PROT	CARB	FAT	FIBRE
Choco Crackles, Morrisons*	1 Serving/30g	115	383	5.5	84.8	2.4	1.9
Choco Crunchies, Tesco*	1 Serving/40g	166	416	7.8	68.4	12.3	4.1
Choco Flakes, Kellogg's*	1 Serving/30g	114	380	5.0	84.0	3.0	2.5
Choco Flakes, Sainsbury's*	1 Serving/30g	111	370	5.5	85.4	0.7	3.0
Choco Flakes, Tesco*	1 Serving/30g	112	374	5.6	86.3	0.7	2.6
Choco Hoops, Asda*	1 Serving/40g	154	385	7.0	79.0	4.5	4.0
Choco Hoops, Kids, Tesco*	1 Serving/30g	116	387	7.6	79.1	4.5	4.5
Choco Snaps, Asda*	1 Serving/30g	115	382	5.0	85.0	2.4	1.9
Choco Snaps, Tesco*	1 Serving/30g	115	383	5.5	84.8	2.4	1.9
Choco Snaps, Value, Tesco*	1 Serving/30g	112	372	7.0	79.7	2.8	3.3
Choco Squares, Asda*	1 Serving/30g	130	434	10.0	67.0	14.0	4.0
Chocolate Cereal, Tesco*	1 Serving/40g	169	423	8.0	66.3	14.0	6.0
Chocolate Crisp, Minis, Weetabix*	1 serving/36g	136	378	9.3	72.3	5.7	7.9
Cinnamon & Apple, Sensations, Asda*	1 Serving/30g	112	373	10.0	72.0	5.0	7.0
Cinnamon Grahams, Nestle*	1 Serving/40g	166	416	4.6	75.1	10.9	4.2
Cinnamon, Puffins, Barbara's Bakery*	1 Serving/30g	100	333	6.7	86.7	3.3	20.0
Clusters, Nestle*	1 Serving/40g	149	372	9.4	70.6	5.8	8.4
Coco Pops Crunchers, Kellogg's*	1 Serving/30g	114	380	7.0	81.0	3.5	3.0
Coco Pops, Kellogg's*	1 Serving/30g	115	383	5.0	84.0	3.0	2.0
Cookie Crunch, Nestle*	1 Serving/40g	154	385	4.6	85.3	2.8	1.8
Corn Flakes, Banana Crunch, Kellogg's*	1 Serving/40g	163	408	6.0	78.0	8.0	3.0
Corn Flakes, Chocolate, Mini Bites, Marks & Spencer*	1 Bite/8g	38	475	6.2	66.5	20.7	1.0
Corn Flakes, Crispy Nut, Asda*	1 Serving/30g	117	390	7.0	81.0	4.2	2.5
Corn Flakes, Crunchy Nut, Kellogg's*	1 Serving/30g	118	392	6.0	83.0	4.0	2.5
Corn Flakes, Harvest Home, Nestle*	1 Serving/25g	92	367	7.3	82.7	0.8	3.6
Corn Flakes, Honey Nut With Cranberries, Tesco*	1 Serving/50g	208	416	7.4	74.4	9.9	3.1
Corn Flakes, Honey Nut, Harvest Home, Nestle*	1 Serving/30g	118	392	7.4	81.1	4.2	2.5
Corn Flakes, Honey Nut, Rumblers*	1 Pack/40g	207	518	17.3	91.3	8.8	3.0
Corn Flakes, Honey Nut, Sainsbury's*	1 Serving/30g	116	387	7.3	80.0	4.2	2.9
Corn Flakes, Honey Nut, Tesco*	1 Serving/30g	118	392	7.4	81.2	4.2	2.5
Corn Flakes, Kellogg's*	1 Serving/30g	112	372	7.0	84.0	0.8	3.0
Corn Flakes, Morrisons*	1 Serving/30g	111	371	7.3	83.8	0.7	3.0
Corn Flakes, Sainsbury's*	1 Serving/25g	92	367	7.3	82.7	0.8	3.6
Corn Flakes, Tesco*	1 Serving/25g	93	371	7.3	83.8	0.7	3.0
Cornflakes, Organic, Lima*	1 Serving/50g	178	355	8.3	77.7	1.0	6.4
Cornflakes, Organic, Whole Earth*	1 Serving/40g	154	386	8.6	84.2	1.0	3.0
Cornflakes, With Semi Skimmed Milk, Bowl, Kellogg's*	1 Serving/30g	170	567	20.0	106.7	8.3	3.0
Counrty Crisp With Whole Raspberries, Jordans*	1 Serving/50g	219	438	7.4	64.6	16.8	6.0
Country Crisp Four Nut Combo, Jordans*	1 Serving/50g	240	480	8.9	54.2	25.3	5.9
Country Crisp Wild About Berries, Jordans*	1 Serving/50g	222	443	7.5	68.0	15.7	5.7
Country Crisp With Strawberries, Jordans*	1 Serving/40g	176	440	7.3	65.3	16.6	6.9
Country Crisp With Whole Raspberries, Jordans*	1 Serving/40g	175	438	7.3	64.6	16.7	6.0
Cranberry Wheats, Tesco*	1 Serving/40g	130	325	7.3	70.9	1.4	7.7
Cranberry Wheats, Whole Grain, Sainsbury's*	1 Serving/50g	163	325	7.3	70.9	1.4	7.7
Cranberry, Cherry & Almond, Dorset Cereals*	1 Serving/25g	89	355	9.2	60.5	8.5	8.4
Crispy Rice & Wheat Flakes, Asda*	1 Serving/50g	185	370	11.0	78.0	1.5	3.2
Crunchy Bran Curls, Weetabix*	1 Serving/40g	120	299	11.8	52.3	4.7	24.8
Crunchy Cereal, Safeway*	1 Serving/45g	207	459	9.2	65.4	17.8	6.3
Crunchy Choco, Crisp & Square, Tesco*	1 Serving/50g	212	423	8.0	66.3	14.0	6.0
Crunchy Chocolate, Carrefour*	1 Serving/40g	176	440	9.0	62.0	17.0	8.0
Crunchy Nut Clusters, Kellogg's*	1 Serving/40g	178	444	7.0	68.0	16.0	4.0
Crunchy Nut Clusters, Milk Chocolate Curls, Kellogg's*	1 Serving/40g	183	458	8.0	66.0	18.0	4.0
Crunchy Nut, Red, Kellogg's*	1 Serving/40g	138	346	10.0	72.0	2.0	9.0

BREAKFAST CEREAL

	Measure INFO/WEIGHT	per Measure KCAL	Nutrition Values per 100g / 100ml				
			KCAL	PROT	CARB	FAT	FIBRE
Crunchy Oat With Raisins, Almonds & Honey, Tesco*	1 Serving/50g	213	425	9.1	62.8	15.3	4.7
Crunchy Oat, Co-Op*	1 Serving/50g	203	405	8.0	64.0	13.0	10.0
Crunchy Oat, Golden Sun, Lidl*	1 Serving/50g	206	411	8.6	65.0	12.9	6.2
Crunchy Rice & Wheat Flakes, Co-Op*	1 Serving/30g	111	370	11.0	78.0	2.0	3.0
Crunchy, Carb Control, Tesco*	1 Serving/35g	174	497	21.5	23.3	35.0	13.4
Eat My Shorts, Kellogg's*	1 Serving/30g	173	577	20.0	103.3	10.0	2.0
Eat Natural*	1 Serving/40g	180	450	12.0	45.0	25.0	6.0
Fibre 1, Nestle*	1 Serving/40g	107	267	10.8	50.2	2.6	30.5
Fibre Bran, Safeway*	1 Serving/48g	124	259	13.3	43.4	3.6	31.0
Fitness & Fruits, Nestle*	1 Serving/40g	147	368	6.6	82.9	1.1	3.9
Fitnesse, Nestle*	1 Serving/30g	111	369	6.3	83.7	1.0	3.7
Flakes & Grains, Exotic Fruit, BGTY, Sainsbury's*	1 Serving/30g	113	377	6.8	76.4	4.9	5.9
Flakes & Orchard Fruits, BGTY, Sainsbury's*	1 Serving/40g	154	385	13.0	80.6	1.2	4.5
Flakes, Multigrain, With Cranberry & Apple, Tesco*	1 Serving/30g	107	357	8.1	75.7	2.4	5.4
Force, Nestle*	1 Serving/40g	138	344	10.6	70.3	2.3	9.2
Four Berry Crisp, Organic, Jordans*	1 Serving/50g	221	442	7.7	67.1	15.8	5.4
Frosted Flakes, Sainsbury's*	1 Serving/30g	112	374	4.9	87.8	0.4	2.4
Frosted Flakes, Tesco*	1 Serving/30g	112	374	4.9	87.8	0.4	2.4
Frosted Wheats, Kellogg's*	1 Serving/30g	105	350	10.0	72.0	2.0	9.0
Frosties, Caramel, Kellogg's*	1 Serving/30g	113	377	5.0	88.0	0.6	2.0
Frosties, Chocolate, Kellogg's*	1 Serving/40g	158	394	5.0	80.0	6.0	3.5
Frosties, Kellogg's*	1 Serving/30g	111	371	4.5	87.0	0.6	2.0
Frosties, Tiger Power, Kellogg's*	1 Serving/40g	147	367	11.0	75.0	2.5	7.0
Fruit & Fibre, Asda*	1 Serving/30g	112	372	9.0	66.0	8.0	8.0
Fruit & Fibre, Flakes, Waitrose*	1 Serving/40g	143	357	8.2	67.2	6.2	9.9
Fruit & Fibre, Kellogg's*	1 Serving/40g	143	358	8.0	68.0	6.0	9.0
Fruit & Fibre, Morrisons*	1 Serving/30g	110	366	8.8	66.5	7.2	8.5
Fruit & Fibre, Organic, Sainsbury's*	1 Serving/40g	147	367	10.0	72.4	4.1	7.8
Fruit & Fibre, Safeway*	1 Serving/40g	143	358	9.0	66.4	6.4	9.0
Fruit & Fibre, Somerfield*	1 Serving/40g	144	361	8.1	68.7	6.0	8.9
Fruit & Fibre, Tesco*	1 Serving/30g	113	375	8.5	66.3	8.4	7.8
Fruit & Fibre, Value, Tesco*	1 Serving/40g	144	359	11.4	65.7	5.6	8.0
Fruit & Fibre, Whole Grain, Sainsbury's*	1 Serving/30g	108	361	8.1	68.7	6.0	8.9
Fruit Nuts & Flakes, Marks & Spencer*	1 Serving/30g	117	391	9.1	69.6	8.5	3.5
Golden Balls, Asda*	1 Serving/30g	112	374	5.0	85.0	1.5	1.5
Golden Grahams, Nestle*	1 Serving/40g	152	381	5.6	81.6	3.6	3.2
Golden Honey Puffs, Tesco*	1 Serving/30g	115	382	6.6	86.3	1.2	3.0
Golden Nuggets, Nestle*	1 Serving/40g	152	381	6.2	87.4	0.7	1.5
Golden Puffs, Sainsbury's*	1 Serving/28g	107	383	6.6	86.3	1.2	3.0
Grape Nuts, Kraft*	1 Serving/30g	104	345	10.5	72.5	1.9	8.6
Harvest Crunch, Nut, Quaker*	1 Serving/40g	184	459	8.0	62.5	19.5	6.0
Harvest Crunch, Real Red Berries, Quaker*	1 Serving/50g	224	447	7.0	66.0	17.0	4.5
Harvest Crunch, Soft Juicy Raisins, Quaker*	1 Serving/50g	221	442	6.0	67.0	16.0	4.0
Hawaiian Crunch, Mornflake*	1 Serving/60g	247	411	8.1	66.8	12.4	6.8
Healthy Flakes, Safeway*	1 Serving/30g	111	371	11.0	78.4	1.5	4.3
High Fibre Bran, Asda*	1 Serving/50g	137	273	13.0	44.0	5.0	29.0
High Fibre Bran, New, Tesco*	1 Serving/30g	73	242	14.0	38.4	3.5	31.0
High Fibre Bran, Sainsbury's*	1 Serving/40g	114	286	13.4	50.7	3.3	23.6
High Fibre Bran, Waitrose*	1 Serving/40g	112	281	14.4	47.2	3.8	26.0
Honey Loops, Kellogg's*	1 Serving/30g	110	367	8.0	77.0	3.0	6.0
Honey Nut & Flakes, Marks & Spencer*	1 Serving/40g	164	411	9.8	73.4	8.7	2.6
Honey Nut Flakes With Red Berries, Somerfield*	1 Serving/30g	126	419	8.6	70.4	11.4	1.9
Honey Nut, Corn Flakes, Somerfield*	1 Serving/30g	118	392	7.4	81.2	4.2	2.5

BREAKFAST CEREAL

	Measure INFO/WEIGHT	per Measure KCAL	KCAL	PROT	CARB	FAT	FIBRE
Honey Raisin & Almond, Crunchy, Waitrose*	1 Serving/40g	170	425	10.5	68.8	12.0	5.7
Hooplas, Sainsbury's*	1 Serving/30g	113	375	6.5	78.6	3.8	4.6
Hoops, Multigrain, Tesco*	1 Serving/30g	113	375	6.5	78.6	3.8	4.6
Hot Cereal, Flax O Meal*	1 Serving/40g	130	325	52.5	2.5	15.0	30.0
Hot Oats, Instant, Tesco*	1 Serving/30g	107	356	11.5	58.8	8.3	8.9
Hunny B's, Kellogg's*	1 Serving/28g	106	379	7.0	78.0	2.5	4.5
Just Right, Kellogg's*	1 Serving/40g	145	362	7.0	77.0	3.0	4.5
Malt Bites, Safeway*	1 Serving/40g	137	343	10.0	69.2	2.9	10.0
Malt Crunchies, Co-Op*	1 Serving/50g	168	335	10.0	69.0	2.0	10.0
Malted Wheaties, Asda*	1 Serving/50g	171	342	10.0	69.0	2.9	10.0
Malted Wheats, Waitrose*	1 Serving/32g	110	343	9.7	71.7	1.9	9.9
Malties, Sainsbury's*	1 Serving/40g	137	343	10.0	69.2	2.9	10.0
Malty Flakes With Peach & Raspberry, BGTY, Sainsbury's*	1 Serving/40g	146	364	10.8	76.4	1.7	3.3
Malty Flakes, Peach Melba, Tesco*	1 Serving/30g	116	385	8.0	79.6	3.8	1.7
Malty Flakes, Tesco*	1 Serving/40g	148	371	11.0	78.4	1.5	4.3
Malty Flakes, With Red Berries, Tesco*	1 Serving/30g	111	369	9.9	78.1	1.9	3.1
Maple & Pecan Crisp, Sainsbury's*	1 Serving/50g	226	452	7.9	61.3	19.5	5.4
Maple & Pecan, Crisp, Tesco*	1 Serving/60g	277	461	8.2	60.6	20.6	6.2
Maple & Pecan, Luxury Crunchy, Jordans*	1 Serving/50g	224	448	9.9	59.9	18.7	6.5
Maple Frosted Flakes, Whole Earth*	1 Serving/30g	113	375	6.2	85.6	1.0	1.6
Mini Crunch, Banana, Weetabix*	1 Serving/36g	134	371	9.0	71.9	5.3	8.3
Mini Crunch, Weetabix*	1 Serving/36g	130	360	9.4	70.4	4.5	7.7
Mini Wheats, Sainsbury's*	1 Serving/45g	157	348	11.8	69.9	2.3	11.8
Minibix, Banana, Weetabix*	1 Serving/40g	148	370	8.8	73.0	5.0	8.1
Minibix, Fruit & Nut, Weetabix*	1 Serving/40g	141	353	8.8	71.2	3.8	8.1
Minibix, Honey, Weetabix*	1 Serving/40g	144	359	8.8	76.1	2.2	0.0
Minibix, Weetabix*	1 Serving/40g	134	335	8.8	71.2	3.8	8.1
Muddles, Kellogg's*	1 Serving/30g	110	368	8.0	76.0	3.5	8.0
Muesli, 12 Fruit & Nut, Sainsbury's*	1 Serving/50g	166	332	8.1	64.2	4.7	7.8
Muesli, Apricot, Traidcraft*	1 Serving/30g	103	344	8.0	68.0	6.0	5.0
Muesli, BGTY, Sainsbury's*	1 Serving/65g	211	324	6.7	70.8	1.6	6.2
Muesli, Base, Nature's Harvest*	1 Serving/50g	179	358	11.0	71.2	5.1	7.4
Muesli, COU, Marks & Spencer*	1 Serving/60g	201	335	7.6	70.2	2.5	8.1
Muesli, Carb Control, Tesco*	1 Serving/35g	154	439	25.0	25.0	26.6	13.8
Muesli, Cranberry & Almond, Dorset*	1 Serving/50g	165	329	10.0	54.8	7.7	7.5
Muesli, Creamy Tropical Fruit, Finest, Tesco*	1 Serving/80g	283	354	7.2	68.8	5.6	6.9
Muesli, Crunchy Bran, Nature's Harvest*	1 Serving/50g	176	352	8.8	62.9	9.9	6.4
Muesli, Crunchy, Organic, Sainsbury's*	1 Serving/40g	168	420	10.6	62.0	14.4	9.2
Muesli, De Luxe, No Added Salt or Sugar, Sainsbury's*	1 Serving/40g	161	403	11.9	57.6	13.9	8.4
Muesli, Dorset Cereals*	1 Serving/70g	256	366	10.8	59.2	9.5	7.4
Muesli, Eat Smart, Safeway*	1 Serving/40g	134	335	8.7	68.6	2.8	7.4
Muesli, Fruit & Bran, Unsweetened, Marks & Spencer*	1 Serving/40g	128	320	8.1	68.0	2.7	9.4
Muesli, Fruit & Nut, 55%, Asda*	1 Serving/40g	151	378	9.0	54.0	14.0	7.0
Muesli, Fruit & Nut, COU, Marks & Spencer*	1 Serving/40g	128	320	7.4	74.5	2.8	7.4
Muesli, Fruit & Nut, Jordans*	1 Serving/50g	189	378	7.3	60.6	11.8	6.7
Muesli, Fruit & Nut, Luxury, Marks & Spencer*	1 Serving/50g	175	349	7.7	62.2	7.7	7.3
Muesli, Fruit & Nut, Marks & Spencer*	1 Serving/40g	128	320	7.4	74.5	2.8	7.4
Muesli, Fruit & Nut, Organic, Marks & Spencer*	1 Serving/50g	167	333	8.2	61.6	6.0	7.6
Muesli, Fruit & Nut, Sainsbury's*	1 Serving/30g	121	402	10.4	51.3	17.2	9.2
Muesli, Fruit & Nut, Tesco*	1 Serving/65g	237	365	7.4	57.9	11.5	8.0
Muesli, Fruit & Nut, Whole Wheat, Organic, Asda*	1 Serving/50g	172	343	10.0	60.0	7.0	7.0
Muesli, Fruit & Spice, Sainsbury's*	1 Serving/50g	184	368	7.4	69.4	6.8	7.7
Muesli, Fruit Sensation, Marks & Spencer*	1 Serving/50g	158	315	6.0	66.0	3.0	7.4

BREAKFAST CEREAL

INFO/WEIGHT	Measure	per Measure KCAL	KCAL	PROT	CARB	FAT	FIBRE
Muesli, Fruit, 55%, Asda*	1 Serving/35g	111	318	6.0	67.0	2.9	7.0
Muesli, Fruit, GFY, Asda*	1 Serving/50g	152	304	8.0	64.0	1.8	10.0
Muesli, Fruit, Luxury, Weight Watchers*	1 Serving/40g	127	318	7.2	67.7	2.0	8.1
Muesli, Fruit, Oat & Wheat Flakes With 45% Fruit, Tesco*	1 Serving/50g	171	342	7.4	67.2	4.8	5.0
Muesli, Fruit, Sainsbury's*	1 Serving/40g	132	330	8.1	64.3	4.5	9.6
Muesli, Fruit, Somerfield*	1 Serving/50g	165	329	6.4	66.5	4.1	6.9
Muesli, Fruit, Tesco*	1 Serving/50g	167	333	7.0	66.0	4.2	6.9
Muesli, Fruit, The Best, Safeway*	1 Serving/40g	138	346	5.3	71.3	4.3	5.0
Muesli, Gluten Free, Nature's Harvest, Holland & Barratt*	1 Serving/60g	234	390	14.1	54.1	13.0	3.3
Muesli, Golden Sun, Lidl*	1 Serving/40g	144	360	8.0	60.0	9.8	7.5
Muesli, Healthy Living, Tesco*	1 Serving/40g	133	333	6.9	71.1	2.3	5.3
Muesli, Less Than 3% Fat, BGTY, Sainsbury's*	1 Serving/40g	128	321	7.3	67.6	2.4	7.5
Muesli, Luxury Fruit, Perfectly Balanced, Waitrose*	1 Serving/50g	162	324	7.1	66.4	3.3	7.0
Muesli, Luxury Fruit, Sainsbury's*	1 Serving/50g	162	324	7.1	66.4	3.3	7.0
Muesli, Luxury Fruit, Waitrose*	1 Serving/30g	101	337	7.7	66.3	4.5	6.9
Muesli, Luxury, Finest, Tesco*	1 Serving/50g	197	394	8.3	60.8	13.1	5.4
Muesli, Luxury, Jordans*	1 Serving/40g	154	384	9.6	58.4	12.5	8.2
Muesli, Luxury, Sainsbury's*	1 Serving/40g	144	359	8.5	57.1	10.7	7.7
Muesli, Mix, The Food Doctor*	1 Serving/50g	196	392	12.1	55.5	14.2	7.1
Muesli, Natural, No Added Sugar Or Salt, Jordans*	1 Serving/40g	138	346	9.6	63.0	6.2	8.6
Muesli, No Added Sugar Or Salt, Organic, Jordans*	1 Serving/30g	106	353	8.9	59.5	8.7	9.0
Muesli, No Added Sugar, Waitrose*	1 Serving/40g	146	364	12.0	64.9	6.3	6.7
Muesli, Orchard Fruit, Luxury, Cape*	1 Serving/30g	98	328	7.6	67.0	2.5	5.7
Muesli, Organic, Waitrose*	1 Serving/50g	179	358	10.8	59.1	8.7	7.8
Muesli, Original, Holland & Barratt*	1 Serving/30g	105	351	11.1	61.2	8.4	7.1
Muesli, Original, Sainsbury's*	1 Serving/60g	226	376	9.3	65.7	8.4	7.1
Muesli, Peach & Vanilla, Sainsbury's*	1 Serving/50g	162	324	7.6	61.4	5.3	7.6
Muesli, Rich, Nature's Harvest*	1 Serving/40g	143	358	10.0	60.5	9.2	7.6
Muesli, Special, Jordans*	1 Serving/40g	144	360	11.6	64.9	6.0	8.2
Muesli, Swiss Style, Co-Op*	1 Serving/40g	148	370	11.0	67.0	6.0	6.0
Muesli, Swiss Style, No Added Salt Or Sugar, Sainsbury's*	1 Serving/40g	143	358	10.7	64.3	6.4	7.0
Muesli, Swiss Style, No Added Salt Or Sugar, Tesco*	1 Serving/30g	106	353	10.9	65.1	5.4	8.2
Muesli, Swiss Style, No Added Sugar or Salt, Asda*	1 Serving/50g	182	363	11.0	64.0	7.0	8.0
Muesli, Swiss Style, No Added Sugar, Somerfield*	1 Serving/50g	180	359	11.0	64.0	6.5	8.0
Muesli, Swiss Style, Sainsbury's*	1 Serving/50g	181	361	9.2	68.1	5.8	7.1
Muesli, Swiss Style, SmartPrice, Asda*	1 Serving/60g	222	370	9.0	70.0	6.0	10.0
Muesli, Swiss Style, Tesco*	1 Serving/40g	147	367	7.3	72.1	5.5	8.7
Muesli, Swiss Style, Waitrose*	1 Serving/40g	146	364	10.2	66.1	6.5	7.6
Muesli, Tropical Fruit, Holland & Barratt*	1 Bowl/60g	197	328	7.5	69.8	3.2	5.1
Muesli, Tropical, Sainsbury's*	1 Serving/50g	183	365	6.5	69.4	6.8	6.4
Muesli, Tropical, Tesco*	1 Serving/50g	173	346	7.8	68.2	4.7	9.1
Muesli, Tropical, Traidcraft*	1 Serving/60g	212	353	7.0	70.0	6.0	4.0
Muesli, Unsweetened Whole Wheat, Safeway*	1 Serving/50g	180	360	7.7	68.0	6.3	7.2
Muesli, Unsweetened, Marks & Spencer*	1 Serving/40g	129	322	8.1	68.0	2.7	9.4
Muesli, Value, Tesco*	1 Serving/50g	171	342	7.5	67.6	4.6	8.6
Muesli, Whole Wheat, Co-Op*	1 Serving/40g	140	350	11.0	61.0	7.0	7.0
Muesli, Whole Wheat, No Added Sugar & Salt, Tesco*	1 Serving/40g	154	386	9.5	59.1	12.4	7.4
Muesli, Whole Wheat, Sainsbury's*	1 Serving/40g	144	359	11.5	60.5	7.9	8.5
Multi Fruit & Flake, COU, Marks & Spencer	1 Serving/39g	142	365	6.5	81.8	1.1	4.0
Multi Fruit & Flake, Perfectly Balanced, Waitrose*	1 Serving/40g	134	335	8.2	68.8	3.0	14.0
Multigrain Flakes With Apple, Eat Smart, Safeway*	1 Serving/45g	160	355	8.0	74.7	2.5	7.0
Multigrain, Balanced Lifestyle, Aldi*	1 Serving/30g	108	360	7.5	77.1	2.4	4.5
Multigrain, Start, Kellogg's*	1 Serving/40g	144	360	8.0	79.0	2.0	6.0

BREAKFAST CEREAL

	Measure INFO/WEIGHT	per Measure KCAL	Nutrition Values per 100g / 100ml KCAL	PROT	CARB	FAT	FIBRE
Natural Wheatgerm, Jordans*	1 Serving/40g	136	340	28.0	36.0	9.3	13.1
Natures Whole Grains, Jordans*	1 Serving/25g	98	390	9.4	61.7	11.7	7.7
Nesquik, Nestle*	1 Serving/30g	118	394	5.0	83.6	4.4	2.4
Nutty Crunch, Deliciously, Marks & Spencer*	1 Serving/50g	238	476	8.8	59.6	22.5	4.4
Oat & Bran Flakes, Sainsbury's*	1 Serving/50g	172	344	12.6	60.0	5.9	15.0
Oat Bran, Crispies, Quaker*	1 Serving/40g	153	383	11.0	69.0	6.5	9.0
Oat Krunchies, Quaker*	1 Serving/30g	118	393	9.5	72.0	7.0	5.5
Oat With Tropical Fruits, Crunchy, Tesco*	1 Serving/35g	157	448	8.7	66.0	16.6	3.2
Oat, Crunchy, Sainsbury's*	1 Serving/50g	227	453	8.2	59.3	20.3	6.6
Oatbran Flakes, Nature's Path*	1 Serving/30g	124	414	8.7	83.0	4.7	6.7
Oatmeal, Instant, Heart To Heart, Kashi*	1 Serving/43g	150	349	7.0	76.7	4.7	9.3
Oatmeal, Quick Oats, Dry, Quaker*	1/3 Cup/30g	114	380	14.0	66.7	6.7	10.0
Oats, Apple Flavour, Instant, Hot, Waitrose*	1 Serving/36g	141	392	8.1	76.4	6.0	6.7
Oats, Apple Flavour, Micro, Tesco*	1 Sachet/36g	128	356	6.8	70.1	5.4	5.4
Oats, Golden Syrup Flavour, Instant, Hot, Waitrose*	1 Serving/39g	153	393	7.8	77.4	5.8	6.0
Oats, Golden Syrup Flavour, Made Up, Micro, Tesco*	1 Serving/199g	226	114	4.0	19.1	2.3	1.2
Oats, Jumbo, Organic, Waitrose*	1 Serving/50g	181	361	11.0	61.1	8.1	7.8
Oats, Orange & Lemon Flavour, Instant, Hot, Waitrose*	1 Sachet/38g	137	361	8.9	68.4	5.8	8.7
Oats, Original, Instant, Hot, Waitrose*	1 Sachet/27g	97	359	11.0	60.4	8.1	8.5
Oats, Ready, Asda*	1 Serving/30g	107	356	12.0	59.0	8.0	9.0
Oats, Tesco*	1 Serving/40g	142	356	11.0	60.0	8.0	8.0
Oatso Easy, Jungle*	1oz/28g	83	296	11.0	45.2	9.0	14.4
Oatso Simple, Apple & Cinnamon, Quaker*	1 Satchet/38g	136	358	8.0	68.0	5.5	2.5
Oatso Simple, Baked Apple Flavour, Quaker*	1 Serving/38g	142	374	8.0	71.0	6.0	5.5
Oatso Simple, Berry Burst, Quaker*	1 Serving/39g	144	370	8.0	70.0	6.0	6.5
Oatso Simple, Country Honey, Quaker*	1 Serving/36g	134	373	8.5	69.0	6.5	6.0
Oatso Simple, Fruit Muesli, Quaker*	1 Sachet/39g	142	364	11.0	60.0	8.5	9.0
Oatso Simple, Golden Syrup Flavour, Quaker*	1 Sacet/39g	145	373	7.5	71.0	6.0	6.0
Oatso Simple, Quaker*	1 Serving/39g	145	372	7.5	71.0	6.0	6.0
Oatso Simple, Toffee Flavour, Quaker*	1 Serving/30g	122	407	6.5	66.0	13.0	5.0
Optimum Power, Nature's Path*	1 Serving/30g	109	363	15.3	60.0	6.7	12.6
Perfect Balance, Weight Watchers*	1 Serving/30g	90	300	7.8	63.3	1.7	15.6
Porridge Flakes, Organic, Barkat*	1 Serving/30g	109	362	8.5	74.1	3.0	0.0
Porridge Oats & Bran, Co-Op*	1 Serving/40g	141	353	12.5	60.0	7.0	12.0
Porridge Oats & Bran, Somerfield*	1 Serving/40g	154	385	12.0	68.0	7.0	0.0
Porridge Oats, Jordans*	1 Serving/40g	145	363	12.5	61.5	7.4	8.0
Porridge Oats, Organic, Evernat*	1 Serving/40g	167	418	13.0	69.0	9.6	7.4
Porridge Oats, Organic, Jordans*	1 Serving/45g	163	363	12.5	61.5	7.4	8.0
Porridge Oats, Organic, Tesco*	1 Serving/28g	100	358	11.0	60.4	8.1	8.5
Porridge Oats, Quaker*	1oz/28g	100	356	11.0	60.0	8.0	4.0
Porridge Oats, Quick & Easy, Morrisons*	1 Serving/28g	103	367	11.8	62.0	8.0	7.0
Porridge Oats, Rolled, Tesco*	1 Serving/50g	180	359	11.0	60.4	8.1	8.5
Porridge Oats, Safeway*	1 Serving/35g	127	364	11.8	62.0	7.6	7.2
Porridge Oats, Scot's, Quaker*	1 Serving/30g	110	368	11.0	62.0	8.0	7.0
Porridge Oats, Scottish, Organic, Sainsbury's*	1 Serving/45g	172	383	10.0	74.4	5.0	7.9
Porridge Oats, Scottish, Tesco*	1 Serving/50g	182	364	11.8	62.0	7.6	7.2
Porridge Oats, SmartPrice, Asda*	1 Serving/50g	178	356	11.0	60.0	8.0	8.0
Porridge Oats, Value, Tesco*	1 Serving/50g	192	384	11.8	68.0	7.2	7.2
Porridge Oats, Whole Rolled, Scottish, TTD, Sainsbury's*	1 Serving/50g	191	381	9.7	74.7	4.8	7.0
Porridge Oats, With Bran, Scottish, Sainsbury's*	1 Serving/50g	190	380	9.6	74.1	5.0	10.3
Porridge Oats, With Wheat Bran, Tesco*	1 Serving/50g	167	334	12.3	55.0	7.2	13.0
Porridge Oats, With Wheatbran, Waitrose*	1 Serving/50g	168	336	11.2	55.8	7.6	13.0
Porridge, Free From, Sainsbury's*	1 Serving/50g	174	348	8.6	72.0	3.0	3.4

	Measure	per Measure	Nutrition Values per 100g / 100ml				
	INFO/WEIGHT	KCAL	KCAL	PROT	CARB	FAT	FIBRE
BREAKFAST CEREAL							
Porridge, Instant, Quaker*	1 Serving/34g	124	364	11.0	60.0	8.5	9.0
Porridge, Multigrain, Jordans*	1 Serving/40g	134	335	10.4	60.9	5.5	10.0
Porridge, Original, Simply Porridge, Asda*	1 Sachet/27g	96	356	11.0	60.0	8.0	8.0
Porridge, Quick, Marks & Spencer*	1 Serving/40g	159	398	15.5	55.1	12.8	5.9
Porridge, Weight Watchers*	1 Pack/220g	114	52	1.1	9.5	1.1	0.9
Precise, Sainsbury's*	1 Serving/40g	148	371	6.4	79.9	2.9	3.5
Puffed Rice, Kallo*	1 Serving/25g	95	380	8.0	80.0	3.0	9.0
Puffed Wheat, Quaker*	1 Serving/15g	49	328	15.3	62.4	1.3	5.6
Puffed Wheat, Tesco*	1 Serving/28g	104	373	13.9	72.2	3.2	5.7
Quaker Oats Crunch, Quaker*	1 Serving/40g	178	445	8.0	66.5	16.0	5.0
Quaker Oats, Quaker*	1 Serving/45g	160	356	11.0	60.0	8.0	9.0
Raisin & Almond, Crunchy, Jordans*	1 Serving/56g	230	411	8.4	66.0	12.5	5.0
Raisin & Coconut, Crunchy, Organic, Jordans*	1 Serving/40g	168	419	8.1	66.3	13.5	6.4
Raisin Wheats, Kellogg's*	1 Serving/30g	96	320	9.0	69.0	2.0	9.0
Raisin Wheats, Sainsbury's*	1 Serving/50g	166	332	8.2	71.5	1.5	8.0
Raisin, Bran Flakes, Asda*	1 Serving/50g	166	331	7.0	69.0	3.0	10.0
Raisin, Honey & Almond Crunch, Asda*	1 Serving/60g	265	442	8.0	62.0	18.0	6.0
Rasberry Crisp, Mornflake*	1 Serving/50g	214	428	6.5	68.2	14.3	6.8
Ready Brek, Banana, Weetabix*	1 Serving/40g	146	365	8.9	68.0	6.4	6.7
Ready Brek, Chocolate, Weetabix*	1 Serving/40g	144	360	9.6	63.7	7.4	8.1
Ready Brek, Oatmeal, Readybrek*	1 Serving/40g	150	375	11.5	58.8	8.3	9.0
Ready Brek, Strawberry, Weetabix*	1 Serving/40g	146	365	8.7	68.6	6.2	6.8
Ready Brek, Weetabix*	1 Serving/40g	142	356	11.6	58.8	8.3	8.9
Red Berries Crisp, Somerfield*	1 serving/30g	134	448	7.3	67.0	16.8	4.3
Red Berry & Almond Luxury Crunch, Jordans*	1 Serving/40g	176	441	8.2	60.5	18.5	6.6
Rice & Wheat Flake, Special Choice, Waitrose*	1 Serving/30g	111	370	11.4	77.7	1.5	3.2
Rice Krispies, Honey, Kellogg's*	1 Serving/30g	114	380	4.0	89.0	0.7	1.0
Rice Krispies, Kellogg's*	1 Serving/30g	114	380	6.0	87.0	1.0	1.0
Rice Pops, Blue Parrot Cafe, Sainsbury's*	1 Serving/30g	111	370	7.2	82.3	1.3	2.2
Rice Pops, Organic, Doves Farm*	1 Serving/30g	107	357	6.8	86.1	0.8	2.0
Rice Pops, Sainsbury's*	1 Serving/30g	113	378	7.4	84.2	1.3	1.5
Rice Snaps, Asda*	1 Serving/28g	105	376	7.0	84.0	1.3	1.5
Rice Snaps, Harvest Home, Nestle*	1 Serving/25g	95	378	7.4	84.2	1.3	1.5
Rice Snaps, Healthy Eating, Tesco*	1 Pack/25g	93	370	7.2	82.3	1.3	2.2
Rice Snaps, Tesco*	1 Serving/30g	113	378	7.3	84.2	1.3	1.5
Ricicles, Kellogg's*	1 Serving/30g	115	384	4.5	90.0	0.7	0.9
Right Balance, Morrisons*	1 Serving/50g	181	362	6.9	78.6	2.2	5.3
Shredded Wheat, Bitesize, Nestle*	1 Serving/45g	158	350	11.8	69.9	2.6	11.9
Shredded Wheat, Fruitful, Nestle*	1 Serving/50g	177	353	8.4	66.9	5.8	10.3
Shredded Wheat, Honey Nut, Nestle*	1 Serving/40g	151	378	10.9	68.8	6.6	10.4
Shredded Wheat, Nestle*	1 Piece/22g	77	350	11.8	69.9	2.6	11.9
Shredded Wheat, Triple Berry, Nestle*	1 Serving/40g	138	344	10.6	70.6	2.1	11.1
Shreddies, Coco, Nestle*	1 Serving/50g	177	353	8.0	76.1	1.9	9.2
Shreddies, Frosted, Kellogg's*	1 Serving/50g	162	323	0.7	78.5	1.8	4.7
Shreddies, Frosted, Nestle*	1 Serving/50g	178	356	7.3	78.5	1.4	8.3
Shreddies, Frosted, Variety Pack, Nestle*	1 Pack/45g	163	363	6.7	81.1	1.3	6.8
Shreddies, Malt Wheats, Tesco*	1 Serving/45g	151	335	8.3	70.7	2.1	9.7
Shreddies, Nestle*	1 Serving/45g	154	343	9.8	71.7	1.9	11.2
Smart Start, Kellogg's*	1 Serving/70g	252	360	6.0	86.0	1.0	4.0
Smoothies, Strawberry, Quaker*	1 Sachet/29g	117	402	6.5	67.0	12.0	5.5
Smoothies, Toffee, Quaker*	1 Serving/30g	122	407	6.5	66.0	13.0	5.0
Special K, Apricot & Peach, Kellogg's*	1 Serving/30g	120	400	8.0	73.0	9.0	2.5
Special K, Choco, Kellogg's*	1 Serving/40g	160	400	14.0	70.0	7.0	3.5

BREAKFAST CEREAL

	Measure INFO/WEIGHT	per Measure KCAL	KCAL	PROT	CARB	FAT	FIBRE
Special K, Kellogg's*	1 Serving/30g	112	373	16.0	75.0	1.0	2.5
Special K, Red Berries, Kellogg's*	1 Serving/30g	111	370	14.0	75.0	1.0	3.0
Start Right, Asda*	1 Serving/40g	150	376	8.0	74.0	6.0	5.0
Strawberry & Almond Crunch, Marks & Spencer*	1 Serving/40g	186	465	8.0	66.0	18.6	4.9
Strawberry & Maltiflakes, COU, Marks & Spencer*	1 Serving/40g	146	365	12.7	73.8	2.3	3.5
Strawberry Crisp, Asda*	1 Serving/30g	134	445	8.0	65.0	17.0	5.0
Strawberry Crisp, Tesco*	1 Serving/50g	200	400	10.2	66.2	10.5	10.2
Sugar Puffs, Quaker*	1 Serving/30g	116	387	6.5	86.5	1.0	3.0
Sultana Bran, Asda*	1 Serving/30g	98	327	9.0	66.0	3.0	11.0
Sultana Bran, Co-Op*	1 Serving/40g	130	325	9.0	66.0	3.0	11.0
Sultana Bran, Healthwise, Kellogg's*	1 Serving/40g	128	320	8.0	68.0	2.0	12.0
Sultana Bran, Healthy Eating, Tesco*	1 Serving/48g	156	326	8.1	69.0	1.9	9.8
Sultana Bran, Healthy Living, Tesco*	1 Serving/30g	87	290	9.8	58.1	2.0	11.7
Sultana Bran, Sainsbury's*	1 Serving/30g	97	324	8.2	68.6	1.9	11.6
Sultana Bran, Waitrose*	1 Serving/30g	97	324	8.2	68.6	1.9	11.6
Superfast Oats, Mornflake*	1 Serving/40g	144	359	11.0	60.4	8.1	8.5
Toasted Multi-Grain Flakes With Apple, Weight Watchers*	1 Serving/30g	97	323	10.4	67.8	1.1	14.4
Triple Chocolate Crisp, Sainsbury's*	1 Serving/40g	180	451	7.7	63.8	18.3	6.0
Tropical Fruit & Bran Multi Flakes, Marks & Spencer*	1 Serving/50g	175	350	7.1	81.2	2.3	7.0
Tropical, Crunchy, Jordans*	1 Serving/40g	169	423	9.0	66.0	13.8	5.0
Tropicana, Weight Watchers*	1 Serving/50g	120	240	5.1	52.0	1.0	7.0
Vanilla, Carb Check, Heinz*	1 Serving/35g	127	362	56.7	27.6	2.7	0.4
Vitality, Asda*	1 Serving/30g	111	370	11.0	78.0	1.5	3.2
Vitality, With Red Fruit, Asda*	1 Serving/30g	110	366	11.0	77.0	1.6	3.8
Vitality, With Tropical Fruit, Asda*	1 Serving/30g	112	373	9.0	73.0	5.0	4.9
Weetabix, Organic, Weetabix*	2 Biscuits/35g	117	335	10.9	66.2	3.0	11.3
Weetos, Weetabix*	1 Serving/30g	115	384	6.2	78.4	5.0	5.6
Wheat Biscuits, Healthy Eating, Tesco*	2 Biscuits/55g	191	348	11.0	70.0	2.7	8.0
Wheat Biscuits, Morrisons*	2 Biscuits/38g	129	340	11.2	67.6	2.7	10.5
Wheat Biscuits, Nature's Own, Organic, Weetabix*	1 Biscuit/17g	58	339	10.3	69.2	2.4	10.4
Wheat Biscuits, Sainsbury's*	1 Biscuit/15g	54	358	13.7	69.5	2.8	7.5
Wheat Biscuits, Value, Tesco*	2 Biscuits/30g	103	342	13.7	69.5	1.0	7.5
Wheat Bisks, Asda*	1 Bisk/19g	64	337	12.0	68.0	1.9	10.0
Whole Wheat Biscuits, Sainsbury's*	2 Biscuits/36g	122	340	11.2	67.6	2.7	10.5
Whole Wheat Biscuits, Waitrose*	2 Biscuits/37g	124	336	11.8	68.0	1.9	10.1
Yoghurt & Raspberry, Crisp, Sainsbury's*	1 Serving/45g	199	442	7.5	66.0	16.4	5.4
Yoghurty, Special K, Kellogg's*	1 Serving/30g	115	383	14.0	75.0	3.0	2.5

BREAKFAST COMPOTE

In Apple Juice, Tesco*	1 Can/300g	219	73	0.4	17.0	0.4	2.1
Sainsbury's*	1 Can/300g	327	109	1.7	24.4	0.5	3.1

BREAKFAST TOPPER

Fruit, Sainsbury's*	1 Dtsp/15g	42	283	2.7	65.6	2.1	4.5
Nut, Sainsbury's*	1 Dtsp/15g	92	615	20.2	19.1	51.0	6.1

BREAM

Sea, Raw	1oz/28g	27	96	17.5	0.0	2.9	0.0

BRESAOLA

Della Valtellina, Sainsbury's*	1 Slice/14g	23	163	34.7	0.1	2.6	0.1
Finest, Tesco*	1 Serving/35g	64	182	36.0	0.5	4.0	0.0
Marks & Spencer*	1oz/28g	56	200	34.6	0.0	6.8	0.0

BROCCOLI

& Cauliflower, Floret Mix, Frozen, Tesco*	1 Serving/150g	50	33	4.0	2.3	0.9	2.2
& Cheese, Morrisons*	1 Pack/350g	406	116	6.2	6.6	7.1	0.8
Baby Courgette & Baby Leeks, Safeway*	1oz/28g	7	24	2.4	2.1	0.8	2.0

INFO/WEIGHT	KCAL	KCAL	PROT	CARB	FAT	FIBRE

BROCCOLI

	Measure / per Measure		Nutrition Values per 100g / 100ml				
	INFO/WEIGHT	KCAL	KCAL	PROT	CARB	FAT	FIBRE
BROCCOLI							
Carrot & Mange Tout, Marks & Spencer*	1oz/28g	10	35	2.9	5.6	0.2	2.1
Cauliflower & Baby Carrots, Safeway*	1 Serving/150g	38	25	2.0	3.0	0.6	2.3
Courgette & Peppers, COU, Marks & Spencer*	1 Pack/283g	156	55	1.7	2.7	4.1	1.7
Green, Boiled, Average	1 Serving/90g	22	24	3.1	1.1	0.8	2.3
Green, Raw, Average	1oz/28g	9	31	3.7	2.1	0.8	2.4
Purple Sprouting, Boiled, Average	1 Serving/90g	17	19	2.1	1.3	0.6	2.3
Purple Sprouting, Raw	1oz/28g	10	35	3.9	2.6	1.1	3.5
BROWNIE							
Cadbury*	1 Serving/36g	145	403	6.1	59.7	15.8	0.0
Chocolate, Chewy, Marks & Spencer*	1 Cake/28.6g	132	455	6.5	59.8	21.1	2.0
Chocolate, Chunky, Marks & Spencer*	1 Serving/30g	126	420	6.3	56.9	18.6	2.5
Chocolate, Fudgy, Marks & Spencer*	1 Brownie/87g	400	460	4.8	56.9	25.2	3.0
Chocolate, Sainsbury's*	1 Brownie/60g	265	442	4.6	55.0	22.6	1.6
Chocolate, Slices, Marks & Spencer*	1 Brownie/36g	158	440	5.3	51.1	24.1	1.3
Chocolate, Tesco*	1oz/28g	123	438	6.6	55.1	21.2	1.5
Chocolate, Topped With M&M's Minis, McVitie's*	1 Cake/92.5g	424	456	4.6	59.4	22.2	0.0
Chocolate, Waitrose*	1 Brownie/45g	192	426	6.3	55.6	19.8	2.7
Pecan & Walnut, Sugar Free, Joseph's*	1 Brownie/26g	150	577	7.7	57.7	26.9	3.9
Praline, Mini, Finest, Tesco*	1 Serving/12g	59	492	4.2	60.0	25.8	0.8
TTD, Sainsbury's*	1 Serving/33g	139	420	4.8	56.5	20.4	1.5
BRUNCHETTA							
Ploughmans, Golden Vale*	1 Serving/90g	267	297	14.4	20.5	17.5	1.4
Red Pepper & Onion, Golden Vale*	1 Pack/90g	266	296	14.6	17.0	19.0	1.3
Soft Cheese & Cranberry, Golden Vale*	1 Serving/95g	200	211	8.2	24.8	9.0	1.3
BRUSCHETTA							
Pane Italia*	1 Serving/75g	367	489	12.4	53.6	25.1	1.4
Safeway*	1/4 Pack/115g	420	365	11.8	65.5	5.8	2.8
Toasted, Olive Oil & Sea Salt, Tesco*	1 Serving/30g	126	420	11.5	58.7	15.5	4.5
BRUSSELS SPROUTS							
& Sweet Chestnuts, Asda*	1 Serving/100g	73	73	3.1	11.0	1.7	4.2
Boiled, Average	1 Med Serving/90g	32	35	3.1	3.2	1.3	3.5
Canned, Drained	1oz/28g	8	28	2.6	2.4	1.0	2.6
Raw, Average	1oz/28g	10	37	3.5	3.3	1.1	3.0
BUBBLE & SQUEAK							
Aunt Bessie's*	1 Serving/100g	145	145	2.7	17.5	7.1	1.3
Fried in Vegetable Oil	1oz/28g	35	124	1.4	9.8	9.1	1.5
Safeway*	1 Serving/200g	160	80	1.8	10.7	3.3	1.4
Tesco*	1/2 Pack/325g	280	86	1.6	11.3	3.9	0.9
Waitrose*	1/2 Pack/225g	216	96	1.6	13.4	4.0	1.8
BUCKWHEAT							
Average	1oz/28g	102	364	8.1	84.9	1.5	2.1
BULGUR WHEAT							
Average	1oz/28g	99	353	9.7	76.3	1.7	0.0
BUNS							
American, Safeway*	1 Bun/60.1g	152	253	8.9	44.5	4.4	3.7
Bath, Marks & Spencer*	1 Bun/71g	217	305	8.3	49.8	8.0	1.9
Bath, Tesco*	1 Bun/80g	262	328	8.0	48.9	11.1	5.8
Belgian, Asda*	1 Bun/133g	464	350	4.8	49.0	15.0	2.2
Belgian, Dairy Cream, Somerfield*	1 Serving/120.8g	401	331	5.2	52.6	11.1	2.0
Belgian, Tesco*	1 Bun/125g	451	361	4.4	56.7	12.9	2.7
Burger, American Style, Sainsbury's*	1 Bun/50g	131	261	10.5	45.6	4.1	3.6
Burger, Cheese & Onion Topped, Finest, Tesco*	1 Serving/105g	309	294	10.2	41.9	9.5	2.8
Burger, Giant, Sainsbury's*	1 Bun/95g	249	262	8.7	45.2	5.2	2.9

B

BUNS

INFO/WEIGHT	Measure per Measure		Nutrition Values per 100g / 100ml				
	Measure	KCAL	KCAL	PROT	CARB	FAT	FIBRE
Burger, Sainsbury's*	1 Bun/56g	162	289	7.8	49.4	6.7	2.4
Burger, Sesame, Sliced, Tesco*	1 Bun/60g	168	280	7.9	47.3	6.6	2.1
Burger, Sliced, Waitrose*	1 Bun/61g	158	264	10.0	47.2	3.9	1.8
Burger, With Sesame Seeds, Co-Op*	1 Bun/55g	143	260	9.0	44.0	5.0	2.0
Caramel Choux, Asda*	1 Serving/100g	421	421	3.6	32.0	31.0	0.3
Chelsea	1 Bun/78g	285	366	7.8	56.1	13.8	1.7
Chelsea, Sainsbury's*	1 Bun/85g	239	281	6.9	51.6	5.2	2.9
Chelsea, Tesco*	1 Bun/85g	269	316	7.9	53.9	7.6	2.3
Currant	1 Bun/60g	178	296	7.6	52.7	7.5	0.0
Currant, Healthy Living, Tesco*	1 Bun/63g	159	252	7.1	50.2	2.5	2.4
Currant, Sainsbury's	1 Bun/72g	197	274	7.0	50.0	5.1	2.8
Currant, Somerfield*	1 Bun/52.7g	150	283	8.0	50.8	5.3	2.4
Custard Choux, Marks & Spencer*	1 Bun/85g	234	275	4.2	15.0	22.0	0.3
Dairy Cream, Somerfield*	1 Bun/98g	304	310	6.0	46.9	10.9	0.0
Fruit, Waitrose*	1 Bun/54g	171	316	7.8	55.7	6.9	1.6
Hevva, Somerfield*	1 Bun/75g	298	397	5.4	57.8	16.0	1.5
Hot Cross	1 Bun/50g	155	310	7.4	58.5	6.8	1.7
Hot Cross, 25% Reduced Fat, Asda*	1 Bun/60.5g	152	253	9.0	49.0	2.3	3.0
Hot Cross, Apple & Cinnamon, Large, Finest, Tesco*	1 Bun/117g	342	292	7.3	49.9	7.0	3.6
Hot Cross, Apple & Cinnamon, Marks & Spencer*	1 Bun/71g	170	240	8.1	46.9	2.1	3.7
Hot Cross, Asda*	1 Bun/60g	190	317	10.0	55.0	6.3	3.3
Hot Cross, BGTY, Sainsbury's*	1 Bun/70g	167	238	7.7	46.6	2.3	4.2
Hot Cross, Chocolate & Raisin, Mini, Tesco*	1 Bun/40g	127	318	8.1	47.0	10.9	2.8
Hot Cross, Chocolate, Mini, Sainsbury's*	1 Bun/39g	127	325	7.7	48.1	11.3	2.5
Hot Cross, Co-Op*	1 Bun/60g	165	275	8.0	47.0	6.0	3.0
Hot Cross, Extra Spicy, Marks & Spencer*	1 Bun/76g	175	230	8.6	44.1	1.9	4.2
Hot Cross, Finest, Tesco*	1 Bun/75g	203	270	6.9	49.0	5.2	2.6
Hot Cross, Fruity, TTD, Sainsbury's*	1 Bun/72g	201	279	6.9	47.9	6.7	3.8
Hot Cross, Golden Wholemeal, 3% Fat, Marks & Spencer*	1 Bun/67g	144	215	8.9	39.6	2.2	6.7
Hot Cross, Golden Wholemeal, Sainsbury's*	1 Bun/65g	180	277	9.9	45.4	6.2	4.3
Hot Cross, Healthy Living, Tesco*	1 Serving/70g	176	251	6.7	50.3	2.7	2.6
Hot Cross, Less Than 3% Fat, Marks & Spencer*	1 Bun/70g	175	250	8.1	49.8	1.8	2.2
Hot Cross, Low Fat, Good Intentions, Somerfield*	1 Bun/50g	135	270	10.0	51.8	2.6	2.8
Hot Cross, Luxury White, Safeway*	1 Bun/75.5g	186	245	8.0	39.4	5.9	3.7
Hot Cross, Luxury, Marks & Spencer*	1 Bun/79g	201	255	8.6	46.2	4.0	2.1
Hot Cross, Mini, Marks & Spencer*	1 Bun/37.3g	91	245	8.5	49.1	1.8	2.2
Hot Cross, Mini, Tesco*	1 Bun/36g	99	274	7.9	48.1	5.5	2.7
Hot Cross, Morrisons*	1 Bun/60g	163	272	8.5	47.4	5.4	3.3
Hot Cross, Perfectly Balanced, Waitrose*	1 Bun/68g	166	244	7.6	48.7	2.1	3.2
Hot Cross, Reduced Fat, GFY, Asda*	1 Bun/67g	149	223	8.0	43.0	2.1	2.4
Hot Cross, Reduced Fat, Waitrose*	1 Bun/67g	171	255	8.1	54.3	2.1	3.3
Hot Cross, Safeway*	1 Bun/65g	174	268	7.9	46.9	5.4	2.2
Hot Cross, Sainsbury's*	1 Bun/70g	180	257	8.5	41.2	6.2	6.8
Hot Cross, Somerfield*	1 Bun/50g	126	252	8.0	43.0	5.3	2.4
Hot Cross, Square, Marks & Spencer*	1 Bun/110.4g	264	240	8.5	49.1	1.8	2.2
Hot Cross, TTD, Sainsbury's*	1 Bun/72g	190	264	7.0	45.7	5.9	4.3
Hot Cross, Tesco*	1 Bun/70g	202	289	6.6	50.0	6.9	2.5
Hot Cross, White, Kingsmill*	1 Bun/24.9g	71	286	7.0	51.1	6.0	3.0
Hot Cross, White, Low Fat, Safeway*	1 Bun/65g	161	248	8.7	47.4	2.6	3.0
Hot Cross, White, Waitrose*	1 Bun/67.5g	175	258	8.1	49.5	3.1	3.9
Hot Cross, Wholemeal, Asda*	1 Bun/69.5g	181	262	9.0	43.0	6.0	6.0
Hot Cross, Wholemeal, Organic, Tesco*	1 Bun/55g	140	254	7.6	44.8	4.9	4.5
Hot Cross, Wholemeal, Tesco*	1 Bun/70g	186	265	9.4	42.6	6.3	5.9

	Measure INFO/WEIGHT	per Measure KCAL	Nutrition Values per 100g / 100ml				
			KCAL	PROT	CARB	FAT	FIBRE
BUNS							
Hot Cross, Wholemeal, Waitrose*	1 Bun/64g	177	276	8.8	45.2	6.7	4.9
Iced & Spiced Soft, Marks & Spencer*	1 Bun/42g	118	280	7.9	55.0	2.9	1.9
Iced Finger, Tesco*	1 Finger/95g	332	349	5.0	55.0	12.1	1.8
Iced Fruit, Marks & Spencer*	1 Bun/95g	285	300	8.5	57.9	4.3	1.3
Iced Lemon, Tesco*	1 Bun/48g	156	325	5.2	56.5	8.7	1.9
Iced, Marks & Spencer*	1 Bun/42g	138	328	8.3	53.7	8.9	2.0
Iced, Tesco*	1 Bun/35g	113	323	7.0	58.9	6.6	2.1
Saffron, Somerfield*	1 Bun/70g	266	380	6.4	50.9	16.7	1.9
Spiced, Carb Control, Tesco*	1 Bun/45g	96	214	17.6	31.4	4.2	9.2
Spiced, Perfectly Balanced, Waitrose*	1 Bun/65g	177	272	8.0	52.3	3.4	2.9
Swiss, Sainsbury's*	1 Bun/90g	314	349	5.1	49.3	14.6	1.3
Swiss, Tesco*	1 Bun/100g	334	334	4.0	52.8	11.9	1.4
Vanilla, Soft Iced, Marks & Spencer*	1 Bun/41g	131	320	8.2	55.5	7.6	1.8
White, Stay Fresh, Tesco*	1 Bun/56g	152	271	7.5	45.5	6.6	0.0
BURGERS							
Aberdeen Angus Beef, Mega, Birds Eye*	1 Burger/101g	279	276	16.3	2.4	22.4	0.1
Aberdeen Angus, Virgin Trains*	1 Serving/240g	695	290	13.5	23.8	15.7	0.0
American Style, Asda*	1 Burger/41.7g	157	374	25.0	10.0	26.0	1.1
American Style, Tesco*	1 Burger/125g	250	200	13.0	20.4	7.3	3.9
BGTY, Sainsbury's*	1 Burger/110g	177	161	20.8	7.1	5.5	1.1
Beef With Onion, Birds Eye*	1 Burger/41g	114	278	15.3	3.5	22.5	0.2
Beef With Onion, Sainsbury's*	1 Burger/42g	102	243	20.7	6.9	14.8	1.0
Beef, & Herb, Finest, Tesco*	1 burger/130g	307	236	15.5	3.1	18.0	2.9
Beef, 100%, Birds Eye*	1 Burger/41g	120	292	17.3	0.0	24.8	0.0
Beef, 100%, Grilled, Tesco*	1 Burger/47g	142	302	31.5	3.8	18.9	4.7
Beef, 100%, Half Pounders, Sainsbury's*	1 Burger/147.6g	463	313	26.0	1.7	22.4	0.2
Beef, 100%, Mega, Birds Eye*	1 Burger/95.6g	281	293	17.3	0.0	24.9	0.0
Beef, 100%, Quarter Pounders, Aldi*	1 Burger/114g	320	282	24.3	0.1	20.5	1.3
Beef, 100%, Quarter Pounders, Birds Eye*	1 Burger/100g	250	250	20.0	0.0	19.0	0.0
Beef, 100%, Quarter Pounders, Prime, Asda*	1 Burger/86g	254	299	26.0	1.6	21.0	0.0
Beef, 100%, Quarter Pounders, Ross*	1 Serving/73.8g	223	301	16.8	1.1	25.5	0.0
Beef, 100%, Sainsbury's*	1 Burger/44g	133	302	21.4	0.9	23.6	0.9
Beef, 100%, Somerfield*	1 Burger/113.5g	329	289	17.0	1.0	24.0	0.0
Beef, 100%, With Seasoning, No Onion, Birds Eye*	1 Burger/41g	134	326	16.1	0.2	29.0	0.0
Beef, 100%, Without Onion, Sainsbury's*	1 Burger/43g	133	308	21.9	0.8	24.1	0.8
Beef, Aberdeen Angus, Asda*	1 Burger/112g	249	222	22.2	6.7	11.9	0.9
Beef, Aberdeen Angus, Marks & Spencer*	1 Burger/142g	298	210	18.3	4.1	13.3	0.1
Beef, Aberdeen Angus, Waitrose*	1 Burger/114g	269	236	18.2	0.3	18.0	0.0
Beef, Asda*	1 Burger/114g	259	227	22.2	5.7	12.8	0.6
Beef, Barbecue, Tesco*	1 Burger/113.5g	259	227	16.4	1.3	17.4	1.2
Beef, Chargrill, Tesco*	1 Burger/113.5g	247	217	17.0	0.8	16.2	2.5
Beef, Farmfoods*	1 Burger/50g	128	255	14.4	5.4	19.6	0.1
Beef, Flame Grilled, Dalepak*	1 Burger/44g	131	304	15.3	2.1	26.0	0.4
Beef, Frozen, Safeway*	1 Burger/44g	123	279	21.3	1.3	20.2	0.0
Beef, Giant Chargrilled, Farmfoods*	1 Burger/170g	352	207	17.3	5.6	12.8	1.2
Beef, Herbs, Finest, Tesco*	1 Burger/170g	284	167	16.9	3.6	9.4	0.3
Beef, In a Bun, Healthy Eating, Tesco*	1 Pack/189g	282	149	13.6	20.7	1.3	2.1
Beef, Mega, Birds Eye*	1 Burger/109g	300	275	14.3	2.7	23.0	0.3
Beef, Morrisons*	1 Burger/56.7g	170	298	12.3	5.5	25.2	0.6
Beef, Organic, Marks & Spencer*	1 Burger/110g	239	217	18.2	0.0	16.0	0.2
Beef, Organic, Tesco*	1 Burger/57g	116	205	16.9	2.1	14.3	1.4
Beef, Quarter Pounder, Asda*	1 Serving/100g	216	216	16.0	4.2	15.0	0.0
Beef, Quarter Pounders, Birds Eye*	1 Burger/139g	386	278	15.3	3.5	22.5	0.2

B

BURGERS

INFO/WEIGHT	Measure	per Measure KCAL	Nutrition Values per 100g / 100ml KCAL	PROT	CARB	FAT	FIBRE
Beef, Quarter Pounders, Farmfoods*	1 Burger/113g	289	256	14.4	5.4	19.6	0.1
Beef, Quarter Pounders, Flame Grilled, Rustlers*	1 Burger/190g	557	293	14.9	24.3	15.1	0.0
Beef, Quarter Pounders, Flame Grilled, Tesco*	1 Burger/88g	246	280	13.1	4.8	23.2	0.8
Beef, Quarter Pounders, Good Intentions, Somerfield*	1 Burger/96.3g	183	191	18.9	1.9	12.0	0.8
Beef, Quarter Pounders, Grilled, Birds Eye*	1 Burger/113.5g	231	203	14.1	2.7	15.0	0.3
Beef, Quarter Pounders, Morrisons*	1 Burger/113.5g	340	298	12.3	5.5	25.2	0.6
Beef, Quarter Pounders, Reduced Fat, Tesco*	1 Burger/95g	171	180	14.0	1.8	13.0	0.8
Beef, Quarter Pounders, Safeway*	1 Burger/100g	227	227	22.2	5.7	12.8	0.6
Beef, Quarter Pounders, Somerfield*	1 Burger/113.9g	319	280	14.7	5.6	22.1	1.2
Beef, Quarter Pounders, Steak Country, Lidl*	1 Burger/68g	188	276	16.3	2.4	22.2	0.1
Beef, Quarter Pounders, Tesco*	1 Burger/113g	292	258	17.8	0.7	20.4	1.3
Beef, Quarter Pounders, With Fresh Onion, Birds Eye*	1 Burger/100g	230	230	16.0	5.9	16.0	0.4
Beef, Quarter Pounders, With Onion, BGTY, Sainsbury's*	1 Burger/83g	171	205	26.6	3.8	9.3	0.9
Beef, Quarter Pounders, With Onion, Sainsbury's*	1 Burger/91.1g	247	271	18.0	5.1	19.8	1.5
Beef, Sainsbury's*	1 Burger/57g	150	267	29.6	1.3	15.9	1.5
Beef, Spicy Jalapeno, Finest, Tesco*	1 Burger/170g	277	163	17.2	2.4	9.4	0.4
Beef, Tesco*	1 Burger/47g	132	281	13.2	4.8	23.2	0.8
Beef, With Onion, Cooked, Ross*	1 Burger/41.2g	116	284	14.7	2.8	23.8	0.4
Beef, With Peppermix, Danish Crown*	1 Burger/100g	250	250	19.0	0.0	19.0	0.0
Beef, With Red Onion & Mustard, Finest, Tesco*	1 Burger/130g	308	237	17.2	0.2	18.6	2.6
Cheeseburger, American, Tesco*	1 Burger/275g	660	240	13.6	24.9	9.6	1.6
Cheeseburger, Bacon, With Bun, Chargrilled, Tesco*	1 Burger/265g	726	274	13.0	19.6	15.9	1.0
Cheeseburger, Micro Snack, Tesco*	1 Serving/115g	309	269	12.6	26.4	12.6	0.0
Cheeseburger, SmartPrice, Asda*	1 Burger/150g	374	249	13.3	28.0	9.3	1.4
Cheeseburger, With Sesame Seed Bun, Tesco*	1 Burger/275g	644	234	12.2	20.1	11.7	2.0
Cheeseburger, Wth Relish, American Style, Tesco*	1 Burger/61.4g	131	215	14.2	17.5	9.8	4.2
Chicken Crunch & Fries, Marks & Spencer*	1 Pack/425g	915	215	8.8	20.8	11.2	2.1
Chicken, Birds Eye*	1 Burger/57g	147	258	13.6	16.8	15.2	0.4
Chicken, Breaded, Asda*	1 Burger/54.8g	145	263	14.0	18.0	15.0	0.0
Chicken, Breaded, Iceland*	1 Burger/57g	173	304	15.8	18.4	18.4	1.2
Chicken, Crispy Crumb, Farmfoods*	1 Burger/242g	707	292	10.5	20.2	18.8	1.1
Chicken, Crunch Crumb, Tesco*	1 Burger/57g	161	282	12.3	15.6	18.9	0.0
Chicken, In Bun, Morrisons*	1 Burger/110g	250	228	12.7	38.1	4.3	3.8
Chicken, Quarter Pounders, Birds Eye*	1 Burger/117g	280	239	13.5	15.2	13.8	0.6
Chicken, Sainsbury's*	1 Serving/46g	115	247	15.6	12.2	15.1	1.3
Chicken, Southern Fried, Sainsbury's*	1 Burger/52g	154	297	12.6	17.2	19.8	1.3
Chicken, Spar*	1 Burger/67g	163	244	16.1	20.8	11.2	1.5
Chicken, With Sesame Seed Bun, Breaded, Tesco*	1 Burger/205g	588	287	10.2	26.2	15.7	2.9
Chilli, Quarter Pounders, Asda*	1 Burger/87.7g	222	252	25.0	2.0	16.0	0.0
Chilli, Quarter Pounders, Farmfoods*	1 Burger/115g	285	248	13.5	2.9	20.3	0.9
Chilli, Quarter Pounders, Iccland*	1 Burger/84g	265	316	18.6	6.5	23.9	0.4
Economy, SmartPrice, Asda*	1 Burger/48.5g	141	293	14.0	12.0	21.0	1.1
Hamburger, Tinned, Westlers*	1 Serving/100g	119	119	5.4	9.7	6.5	0.0
Lamb, Minted, Tesco*	1 Burger/47g	114	240	16.3	0.0	18.4	2.7
Lamb, Quarter Pounders, Birds Eye*	1 Burger/112g	232	207	13.9	3.8	15.1	0.3
Lamb, Quarter Pounders, Farmfoods*	1oz/28g	76	272	12.3	6.6	21.8	1.0
Less Than 7% Fat, Sainsbury's*	1 Burger/102g	164	161	20.8	7.1	5.5	1.1
Low Fat, Iceland*	1 Serving/85g	148	174	27.8	5.0	4.8	1.1
Mushroom & Red Onion, Tesco*	1 Burger/87.1g	135	155	5.4	21.3	5.4	1.6
Nacho, Chicken & Sweetcorn, Asda*	1/2 Pack/143.9g	249	173	14.0	9.0	9.0	2.3
Pork, Quarter Pounders, Birds Eye*	1 Burger/122g	292	239	13.9	3.2	19.0	0.2
Prime Beef, Asda*	1 Burger/45g	123	274	22.0	6.0	18.0	0.6
Quarter Pounder With Cheese & Buns, Sainsbury's*	1 Burger/198g	471	238	15.6	19.1	11.5	1.4

BURGERS

INFO/WEIGHT	Measure	per Measure KCAL	Nutrition Values per 100g / 100ml KCAL	PROT	CARB	FAT	FIBRE
Quarter Pounders, 95% Fat Free, Good Choice, Iceland*	1 Burger/86g	150	174	27.8	5.0	4.8	1.1
Quarter Pounders, Beef, BGTY, Sainsbury's*	1 Serving/97g	161	166	16.9	6.1	8.2	1.0
Quarter Pounders, Big Country*	1 Burger/90g	271	301	22.1	1.8	23.1	0.0
Quarter Pounders, Chargrilled, BGTY, Sainsbury's*	1 Burger/114g	184	161	20.8	7.1	5.5	1.1
Quarter Pounders, Grilled, Healthy Living, Tesco*	1 Burger/88g	135	153	22.3	3.0	5.8	0.6
Quarter Pounders, Healthy Living, Tesco*	1 Burger/114g	188	165	18.7	3.6	8.4	0.6
Quarter Pounders, Highlander*	1 Burger/113.5g	335	295	21.7	4.2	23.2	0.0
Quarter Pounders, Iceland*	1 Burger/83g	253	305	20.4	5.1	22.6	0.6
Quarter Pounders, Marks & Spencer*	1oz/28g	69	247	18.5	3.2	17.9	0.6
Quarter Pounders, Salmon, Tesco*	1 Burger/114g	145	128	15.9	10.6	2.4	1.2
Quarter Pounders, Scotch Beef, Sainsbury's*	1 Burger/113.5g	257	225	22.2	3.5	13.6	0.5
Quarter Pounders, Tuna, Tesco*	1 Burger/114g	132	116	18.8	6.7	1.6	0.9
Salmon, Quarter Pounders, Morrisons*	1 Burger/109.8g	235	214	21.4	5.5	11.8	1.7
Spicy Bean, Dalepak*	1 Burger/118g	243	206	4.6	22.3	10.9	2.6
Spicy Bean, Quarter Pounders, Asda*	1 Serving/108g	257	238	4.5	28.0	12.0	3.0
Spicy Bean, Sainsbury's*	1 Burger/110g	262	240	5.0	27.1	12.4	2.0
Tuna Fish, Quarter Pound, Asda*	1 Burger/113g	212	188	21.0	3.4	10.0	0.0
Tuna, Birds Eye*	1 Burger/50g	125	250	15.0	16.2	14.0	0.8
Tuna, Quarter Pounders, Sainsbury's*	1 Serving/100g	179	179	24.0	10.0	4.8	0.4
Tuna, Sainsbury's*	1 Serving/105g	194	185	20.8	3.4	9.8	1.2
Turkey Cheese, Somerfield*	1oz/28g	79	281	14.0	16.0	18.0	0.0
Turkey Cheeseburgers, Tesco*	1 Burger/105g	252	240	15.4	12.8	14.1	1.3
Turkey, Crispy Crumb, Bernard Matthews*	1 Burger/71g	222	313	11.3	19.3	19.8	0.9
Value, Farmfoods*	1 Burger/49g	138	282	11.4	9.6	22.1	0.9

BURGERS MEAT FREE

INFO/WEIGHT	Measure	per Measure KCAL	KCAL	PROT	CARB	FAT	FIBRE
Asda*	1 Burger/60g	138	230	24.0	11.0	10.0	0.3
Sainsbury's*	1 Burger/57g	92	161	19.6	3.9	7.4	4.8

BURGERS VEGETABLE

INFO/WEIGHT	Measure	per Measure KCAL	KCAL	PROT	CARB	FAT	FIBRE
& Cheese, Tesco*	1 Burger/85g	167	197	7.7	19.5	9.8	1.4
Captains, Birds Eye*	1 Burger/48g	96	200	4.7	25.5	8.8	2.0
Organic, Goodlife*	1 Burger/67.1g	114	170	3.2	26.3	5.8	2.6
Organic, Tesco*	1 Burger/90g	108	120	2.6	17.6	4.3	2.1
Quarter Pounders, Crunchy, Birds Eye*	1 Burger/114g	240	211	4.8	24.9	10.2	1.8
Quarter Pounders, Dalepak*	1 Burger/114g	251	220	4.4	20.8	13.2	2.7
Quarter Pounders, Tesco*	1 Burger/108g	227	211	4.4	20.8	12.2	2.7
Spicy Bean, BGTY, Sainsbury's*	1 Burger/85g	123	145	6.9	23.3	2.7	3.1
Spicy, Asda*	1 Burger/56g	108	193	3.4	20.0	11.0	0.0
With Tofu, Organic, Evernat*	1oz/28g	52	186	7.9	16.9	8.3	0.0

BURGERS VEGETARIAN

INFO/WEIGHT	Measure	per Measure KCAL	KCAL	PROT	CARB	FAT	FIBRE
Bacon, Vegetarian, & Cheese, Tesco*	1 Burger/88g	210	240	6.8	21.4	14.1	1.8
Bean, Mexican Style Quarter Pounders, Tesco*	1 Burger/101g	215	213	4.3	25.0	10.6	2.8
Bean, Quarter Pounders, Mexican Style, Tesco*	1 Burger/101g	215	213	4.3	25.0	10.6	2.8
Chargrilled Style, Safeway*	1 Burger/57g	95	167	18.8	3.7	8.5	4.0
Cheese & Spring Onion, Tesco*	1 Serving/175g	340	194	5.1	18.6	11.0	4.0
Cheese, Tesco*	1 Burger/75g	148	197	7.7	19.5	9.8	1.4
Cheeseburger, Chicken Style, Safeway*	1 Burger/100g	234	234	16.6	11.4	13.5	3.0
Chilli Flavour Brown Rice & Tofu, Cauldron*	1 Burger/75g	185	246	16.2	13.5	14.1	4.3
Flame Grilled, Linda McCartney*	1 Burger/60g	104	174	17.9	13.8	5.2	3.3
Juicy Mushroom & Sweet Onion, Cauldron*	1 Burger/87.5g	99	113	6.4	9.9	5.3	2.7
Mushroom & Red Onion, Tesco*	1 Burger/78g	105	135	4.7	18.6	4.6	1.4
Mushroom, Cauldron*	1 Burger/87.5g	135	153	7.1	15.1	7.1	2.7
Mushroom, Tesco*	1 Burger/87g	145	166	4.0	16.5	9.3	5.0
Quarter Pounders, Beef Style, Sainsbury's*	1 Burger/114g	216	190	20.0	6.0	9.5	2.5

BURGERS VEGETARIAN

	Measure INFO/WEIGHT	per Measure KCAL	Nutrition Values per 100g / 100ml				
			KCAL	PROT	CARB	FAT	FIBRE
Quarter Pounders, Chargrilled, Tesco*	1 Burger/113.5g	187	164	16.0	7.0	8.0	2.5
Quarter Pounders, Healthy Living, Tesco*	1 Burger/102g	117	114	4.0	20.7	1.7	2.0
Spicy Bean, Linda McCartney*	1 Burger/85g	190	223	4.3	26.2	11.2	2.9
Spicy Black Bean, Cauldron*	1 Burger/88g	158	180	10.8	13.4	9.2	5.1
Tesco*	1 Burger/56g	92	164	16.0	7.0	8.0	2.5
Tofu, Savoury, Cauldron*	1 Burger/75g	162	216	14.8	13.2	11.5	3.5
Vegeburger, Linda McCartney*	1 Burger/59g	79	134	22.6	2.9	3.6	1.6
Vegeburger, Retail, Grilled	1oz/28g	55	196	16.6	8.0	11.1	4.2

BUTTER

Brandy, Tesco*	1oz/28g	152	543	0.3	48.3	38.7	0.5
Brandy, With Cognac, Sainsbury's*	1/8 Pot/25g	137	549	0.2	44.1	37.6	0.0
Creamery, Average	1 Serving/10g	74	736	0.5	0.4	81.4	0.0
Fresh, Average	1 Thin Spread/7g	51	735	0.6	0.4	81.3	0.0
Garlic, Somerfield*	1oz/28g	192	686	1.0	2.0	75.0	0.0
Reduced Fat, Fresh, Average	1 Thin Spread/7g	26	368	2.3	1.2	39.4	0.2
Salted, Average	1 Thin Spread/7g	51	729	0.4	0.3	81.1	0.0
Spreadable, Fresh, Average	Thin Spread/7g	51	730	0.4	0.3	80.8	0.0
Spreadable, Reduced Fat, Average	1 Thin Spread/7g	38	540	0.5	0.5	60.0	0.0
With Crushed Garlic, Lurpak*	1 Serving/10g	70	700	1.0	4.0	75.0	0.0

BUTTERMILK

Average	1 Mug/400ml	177	44	4.2	5.9	0.3	0.0

BUTTON SPROUTS

& Chestnuts, Tesco*	1 Serving/100g	80	80	3.1	12.8	1.8	4.1
Raw, Average	1oz/28g	10	37	3.5	2.9	1.3	3.2

BUTTONS

Milk Chocolate, Cadbury*	1 Treat Pack/14g	74	525	7.6	56.2	29.9	0.0
Milk Chocolate, Giant, Cadbury*	1 Button/2.9g	16	525	7.6	56.2	29.9	0.0
Milk Chocolate, Tesco*	1 Bag/70g	359	513	7.1	59.1	27.6	2.1
White Chocolate, Cadbury*	1 Bag/32g	171	535	8.8	56.5	30.3	0.0
White Chocolate, Tesco*	1 Bag/70g	388	554	5.1	58.0	33.5	0.0

	Measure	per Measure	Nutrition Values per 100g / 100ml				
	INFO/WEIGHT	KCAL	KCAL	PROT	CARB	FAT	FIBRE

CABBAGE

& Leek, Crunchy Mix, Ready to Cook, Sainsbury's*	1 Serving/125g	34	27	1.9	3.7	0.5	2.6
Boiled, Average	1 Serving/90g	14	15	1.0	2.2	0.3	1.7
Chinese, Raw	1oz/28g	3	12	1.0	1.4	0.2	1.2
Greens, Trimmed, Average	1oz/28g	8	29	2.9	3.0	0.5	3.4
Mash, Eat Smart, Safeway*	1/2 Pack/225g	146	65	2.0	9.2	1.8	1.7
Medley, Marks & Spencer*	1 Serving/300g	270	90	1.7	2.7	8.2	1.5
Medley, Washed, Ready To Cook, Tesco*	1/2 Pack/75g	23	30	2.3	3.7	0.6	2.8
Raw, Average	1 Serving/100g	21	21	1.3	3.2	0.5	1.9
Red, Average	1 Serving/90g	19	21	1.0	3.7	0.3	2.2
Red, Braised With Red Wine, Marks & Spencer*	1/2 Pack/150g	180	120	1.4	17.1	4.8	1.0
Red, Spiced, Steamer, Sainsbury's*	1/2 Pack/150g	105	70	1.0	10.5	2.2	2.9
Red, With Apple & Cranberry, TTD, Sainsbury's*	1/2 Pack/200g	166	83	1.3	12.8	2.9	1.4
Red, With Apple, Braised, Sainsbury's*	1/2 Pack/117g	91	78	0.8	10.8	3.5	1.7
Red, With Apple, Finest, Tesco*	1/2 Pack/175g	200	114	1.4	14.2	5.7	3.2
Red, With Apple, Frozen, Sainsbury's*	1 Serving/75g	38	50	1.8	10.8	0.0	2.2
Red, With Wine & Cranberies, Waitrose*	1 Serving/200g	210	105	1.2	16.0	4.0	2.3
Savoy, Boiled in Salted Water	1 Serving/90g	15	17	1.1	2.2	0.5	2.0
Savoy, Raw	1 Serving/90g	24	27	2.1	3.9	0.5	3.1
Sweetheart, Tesco*	1 Serving/100g	20	20	1.9	1.6	0.7	2.6
White, Raw, Average	1oz/28g	8	27	1.4	5.0	0.2	2.1

CAKE

Action Man, Birthday, Memory Lane Cakes*	1/12 Portion/83g	322	388	3.0	57.0	16.4	0.8
Alabama Chocolate Fudge, Farmfoods*	1/6 Cake/61g	201	329	4.7	55.7	9.7	2.7
Almond Flavour Slices, GFY, Asda*	1 Slice/25g	67	268	4.0	56.0	3.1	0.7
Almond Flavoured Rounds, Country Garden*	1 Cake/45.4g	181	403	4.3	62.4	14.7	2.3
Almond Slices, Lyons*	1 Slice/26.8g	115	426	7.1	41.3	25.8	1.6
Almond Slices, Mr Kipling*	1 Slice/35g	125	358	3.2	53.1	13.5	1.8
Almond Slices, Sainsbury's*	1 Serving/27g	120	444	5.9	45.9	26.3	1.5
Angel Layer, Tesco*	1 Serving/25g	101	403	4.5	57.4	17.3	0.9
Angel Slices, Mr Kipling*	1 Slice/38g	155	409	2.8	58.9	18.0	0.5
Angel, Asda*	1 Serving/46.1g	184	399	4.5	57.0	17.0	0.9
Angel, Co-Op*	1/8 Cake/35g	131	375	4.0	52.0	17.0	0.7
Angel, Sainsbury's*	1/8 Cake/41g	171	417	4.1	55.7	19.8	0.8
Apple & Cinnamon, Oat Break, Go Ahead, McVitie's*	1 Serving/35g	122	349	5.2	67.2	6.6	2.6
Apple Bakes, Go Ahead, McVitie's*	1 Cake/35g	129	368	2.8	74.7	8.3	1.2
Apple Sponge, Marks & Spencer*	1 Serving/95g	247	260	3.7	30.6	13.9	0.8
Apple, Bramley, & Blackberry Crumble, Marks & Spencer*	1/8 Cake/56g	221	395	4.4	54.1	17.9	1.5
Apple, Home Style, Marks & Spencer*	1 Cake/54g	189	350	5.3	49.4	14.7	1.5
Apricot & Almond, Bakers Delight*	1oz/28g	106	379	5.5	53.2	16.0	1.8
Apricot & Apple, Trimlyne*	1 Cake/50g	134	267	4.3	58.4	2.7	1.9
Assorted Cup, Sainsbury's*	1 Cake/38g	130	341	2.2	69.3	6.1	0.4
Bakewell Slices, Mr Kipling*	1 Slice/36g	150	416	4.2	53.7	20.5	1.0
Bakewell, The Handmade Flapjack Company*	1 Cake/75g	311	415	4.5	47.4	22.8	0.0
Banana & Walnut, Handmade, Boots*	1 Serving/65g	220	338	5.1	48.0	14.0	1.0
Banana Loaf, Organic, Respect*	1 Slice/40g	151	377	3.5	48.7	19.5	0.9
Banana Loaf, Waitrose*	1 Slice/70g	236	337	5.0	55.2	10.7	1.7
Banana, Date & Walnut Slices, BGTY, Sainsbury's*	1 Slice/28g	78	280	5.3	56.1	4.9	2.2
Banana, The Handmade Flapjack Company*	1 Cake/75g	290	387	5.3	59.2	14.4	0.0
Battenberg, Lyons*	1 Serving/26g	112	431	6.9	70.3	13.7	1.3
Battenberg, Mini, Mr Kipling*	1 Serving/35g	138	393	3.7	75.0	8.7	0.9
Best Chocolate Orange Explosion, Safeway*	1 Serving/59g	248	421	4.1	48.8	23.3	0.9
Birthday Present, Tesco*	1 Serving/79g	347	439	3.5	66.6	17.6	0.4
Birthday, Marks & Spencer*	1 Serving/60g	240	400	2.3	70.9	11.9	0.8

CAKE

Measure INFO/WEIGHT	per Measure KCAL	KCAL	PROT	CARB	FAT	FIBRE
		Nutrition Values per 100g / 100ml				

	Measure INFO/WEIGHT	per Measure KCAL	KCAL	PROT	CARB	FAT	FIBRE
Bites, Jaffa Cake Roll, Mini, McVitie's*	1 Cake/15.9g	62	389	3.7	66.7	12.0	1.4
Butterfly, Mr Kipling*	1 Cake/29g	114	392	4.4	43.4	22.2	0.6
Buttons, Cadbury*	1 Cake/25g	110	440	7.2	50.0	22.8	0.0
Cappuccino, Finest, Tesco*	1oz/28g	105	374	2.8	40.4	22.3	0.2
Caramel Shortcake, The Handmade Flapjack Company*	1 Cake/75g	383	511	4.6	54.3	30.6	0.0
Caramel Slice, Marks & Spencer*	1 Slice/64g	304	475	4.9	60.4	25.2	2.6
Caramel, Milk Chocolate, Holly Lane*	1 Cake/25g	110	441	6.9	57.6	20.3	1.1
Carrot & Apple, Safeway*	1 Serving/50g	158	315	3.2	50.4	11.2	0.8
Carrot & Orange Slices, GFY, Asda*	1 Serving/23.1g	77	334	3.4	74.0	2.7	1.0
Carrot & Orange Slices, Good Intentions, Somerfield*	1 Cake/27g	85	315	4.1	68.0	3.0	1.5
Carrot & Orange Slices, Healthy Living, Tesco*	1 Slice/29g	80	276	3.1	56.6	2.8	2.1
Carrot & Orange, Extra Special, Asda*	1/6 Cake/65.0g	240	369	4.7	47.0	18.0	0.9
Carrot & Orange, Finest, Tesco*	1 Serving/50g	171	342	4.1	49.1	14.3	1.0
Carrot & Orange, Safeway*	1 Serving/120g	265	221	4.9	26.8	10.0	0.7
Carrot & Orange, Waitrose*	1/6 Cake/47g	165	350	5.3	46.8	15.7	1.8
Carrot & Pecan, Marks & Spencer*	1 Slice/90.4g	329	365	6.4	48.7	16.2	2.3
Carrot & Walnut, Layered, Asda*	1 Serving/42g	172	409	4.6	55.0	19.0	1.0
Carrot & Walnut, Marks & Spencer*	1/6 Cake/82g	279	340	5.8	34.8	19.5	1.5
Carrot Slices, BGTY, Sainsbury's*	1 Slice/27g	81	313	3.4	68.7	2.7	2.4
Carrot Slices, Weight Watchers*	1 Slice/27g	71	263	3.0	56.7	2.7	1.9
Carrot Wedge, Tesco*	1 Pack/175g	532	304	3.9	36.6	15.8	1.5
Carrot, Entenmann's*	1 Serving/40g	156	391	4.1	47.4	20.5	1.5
Carrot, Marks & Spencer*	1oz/28g	98	350	6.1	34.5	21.0	1.5
Carrot, Organic, Respect*	1 Slice/45g	179	398	3.1	47.4	22.4	1.5
Carrot, The Handmade Flapjack Company*	1 Cake/75g	295	393	6.4	53.0	17.3	0.0
Carrot, Traditional, Farringford Foods*	1oz/28g	115	412	4.4	44.8	25.2	0.0
Carrot, Ultimate, Entenmann's*	1/8 Cake/63.8g	235	367	4.7	51.4	15.8	0.3
Celebration, Sainsbury's*	1/12 Cake/100g	265	265	2.1	43.6	9.2	0.3
Cherry Bakewell Slices, GFY, Asda*	1 Slice/29.1g	96	331	3.3	74.0	2.4	0.7
Cherry Bakewell, Gluten Free, Bakers Delight*	1 Cake/50g	211	422	2.9	66.1	16.3	0.4
Cherry Bakewell, Layer, Asda*	1/8 Cake/50g	210	420	4.4	51.0	22.0	0.6
Cherry Bakewell, Marks & Spencer*	1 Cake/44g	185	420	4.5	61.7	17.7	1.0
Cherry Bakewell, Mini, Sainsbury's*	1 Tart/27.3g	100	370	3.4	62.2	12.0	0.4
Cherry Bakewell, Mr Kipling*	1 Cake/45g	186	414	3.9	59.3	17.9	1.2
Cherry Bakewell, Safeway*	1 Bakewell/47g	203	432	3.5	58.7	20.3	3.9
Cherry Bakewell, Sainsbury's*	1 Cake/46g	200	436	3.1	66.3	17.6	1.4
Cherry Bakewell, Sara Lee*	1/5 Slice/69.9g	228	326	4.1	51.9	11.3	1.4
Cherry Bakewell, Savers, Safeway*	1 Cake/45g	176	391	3.6	60.6	14.9	0.1
Cherry Bakewell, SmartPrice, Asda*	1 Cake/38g	157	413	2.7	60.0	18.0	2.6
Cherry Bakewell, Somerfield*	1 Cake/50g	216	431	3.5	58.7	20.3	3.9
Cherry Bakewell, Tesco*	1 Cake/39g	171	439	3.2	63.3	19.2	1.1
Cherry Bakewell, Waitrose*	1 Tart/43.9g	184	419	3.8	57.4	19.3	2.1
Cherry Bakewell, Weight Watchers*	1 Cake/43g	156	363	3.7	65.1	11.6	3.3
Cherry Genoa, Marks & Spencer*	1oz/28g	99	355	4.5	59.3	10.9	1.6
Cherry, Asda*	1 Slice/37.3g	130	351	4.7	56.0	12.0	0.6
Cherry, Co-Op*	1/8 Cake/47g	190	405	4.0	57.0	18.0	0.8
Cherry, Marks & Spencer*	1 Serving/75g	285	380	5.0	60.6	12.7	0.8
Chewy Fruity Corn Flake, Doves Farm*	1 Bar/40g	155	388	5.8	64.5	14.0	4.5
Chewy Rice Pop & Chocolate, Doves Farm*	1 Bar/35g	156	447	3.9	69.9	20.2	2.3
Chocolate	1oz/28g	128	456	7.4	50.4	26.4	0.0
Chocolate & Brandy Butter, Entenmann's*	1 Portion/38.5g	146	374	3.4	53.5	17.5	2.8
Chocolate & Orange Rolls, Marks & Spencer*	1 Roll/60g	228	380	3.6	27.0	28.4	1.3
Chocolate & Orange Slices, GFY, Asda*	1 Serving/30.2g	95	315	3.2	70.0	2.5	1.3

CAKE

	Measure INFO/WEIGHT	per Measure KCAL	KCAL	PROT	CARB	FAT	FIBRE
			Nutrition Values per 100g / 100ml				
Chocolate Birthday, Asda*	1/10 Cake/61.1g	281	460	6.0	46.0	28.0	0.9
Chocolate Birthday, Marks & Spencer*	1 Serving/68g	279	410	4.5	43.7	24.1	1.3
Chocolate Box, Asda*	1 Serving/60g	263	439	5.0	53.0	23.0	0.7
Chocolate Brownie, Fudge, Entenmann's*	1/8 Cake/55g	168	306	4.0	62.7	4.4	1.5
Chocolate Brownies, Weight Watchers*	1 Serving/47g	143	304	4.8	62.5	3.8	3.2
Chocolate Caramel Mini Bites, Marks & Spencer*	1 Bite/20.7g	97	460	5.6	53.5	24.6	1.6
Chocolate Chip, Co-Op*	1/6 Cake/62.5g	273	440	5.0	44.0	27.0	0.5
Chocolate Chip, The Cake Shop*	1 Cake/35g	178	508	4.7	50.2	31.5	1.1
Chocolate Cup, 5% Fat, Sainsbury's*	1 Cake/38g	133	349	2.5	74.8	4.4	1.7
Chocolate Cup, BGTY, Sainsbury's*	1 Cake/38g	121	318	2.5	66.5	4.6	0.8
Chocolate Cup, Fabulous Bakin' Boys*	1 Cake/40g	182	456	4.0	53.0	26.0	2.0
Chocolate Cup, Lyons*	1 Cake/39g	125	321	2.4	67.5	4.6	0.8
Chocolate Cupcake, COU, Marks & Spencer*	1 Cake/45g	130	290	4.6	62.2	2.8	4.3
Chocolate Egg, Small, Tesco*	1 Cake/31g	132	425	5.4	57.2	20.2	1.7
Chocolate Flavour Slice, Eat Smart, Safeway*	1 Slice/28g	95	340	5.3	73.6	2.4	4.0
Chocolate Flavour Slices, GFY, Asda*	2 Slices/55g	141	257	4.3	54.0	2.6	1.4
Chocolate Flower Pot, Marks & Spencer*	1 Serving/68.6g	297	430	3.8	60.8	19.3	1.5
Chocolate Fudge & Vanilla Cream, Marks & Spencer*	1/6 Cake/69g	306	450	5.2	49.8	26.0	1.3
Chocolate Fudge Slice, Waitrose*	1 Slice/60g	230	383	4.7	54.6	16.2	1.5
Chocolate Fudge, Classic, Marks & Spencer*	1 Serving/70.9g	195	275	2.8	42.8	10.6	1.1
Chocolate Fudge, Entenmann's*	1 Serving/48g	173	361	4.4	51.8	15.1	0.9
Chocolate Fudge, Express, Pizza Express*	1 Serving/300g	395	132	1.3	19.1	5.7	0.0
Chocolate Fudge, Safeway*	1 Serving/93.1g	375	403	4.0	53.2	19.3	1.8
Chocolate Fudge, Sainsbury's*	1/8 Cake/98g	402	410	5.5	47.3	22.3	1.9
Chocolate Fudge, Tea Time Treats, Asda*	1 Cake/37.0g	157	424	3.6	53.0	22.0	1.7
Chocolate Heaven, Extra Special, Asda*	1/6 Cake/65.7g	256	388	4.0	48.0	20.0	1.0
Chocolate Indulgence, Finest, Tesco*	1 Slice/52g	203	390	3.8	47.8	20.4	0.4
Chocolate Loaf, Somerfield*	1oz/28g	111	396	6.0	44.0	22.0	0.0
Chocolate Log, Fresh Cream, Finest, Tesco*	1 Slice/85g	301	354	4.5	43.2	18.1	1.4
Chocolate Orange Slices, BGTY, Sainsbury's*	1 Slice/30g	90	301	3.9	62.8	4.8	1.3
Chocolate Orange Slices, Weight Watchers*	1 Slice/27g	80	297	5.6	63.9	2.1	2.8
Chocolate Orange, Sponge, Asda*	1 Serving/70g	298	425	4.9	42.9	26.0	3.0
Chocolate Party, Marks & Spencer*	1 Serving/60.8g	241	395	4.6	46.9	20.8	1.1
Chocolate Roll, Sainsbury's*	1 Slice/50g	210	420	5.0	54.0	20.4	3.3
Chocolate Sensation, Sainsbury's*	1 Serving/92.0g	320	348	3.7	40.0	19.2	2.3
Chocolate Slice, Go Ahead, McVitie's*	1 Slice/32g	94	293	4.5	49.4	8.2	1.9
Chocolate Slices, Mr Kipling*	1oz/28g	108	386	4.8	50.4	18.3	0.0
Chocolate Sponge Roll, Marks & Spencer*	1/4 Cake/66g	251	380	3.9	50.5	18.4	1.8
Chocolate Sponge, Less Than 5% Fat, Asda*	1 Sponge/110g	198	180	4.4	32.0	3.8	1.1
Chocolate Sponge, Tesco*	1 Serving/35g	129	373	5.3	54.4	14.9	1.5
Chocolate Tiffin, Sainsbury's*	1 Cake/61g	184	301	2.7	29.8	19.0	1.3
Chocolate Truffle, Extra Special, Asda*	1 Serving/103g	402	390	5.0	34.0	26.0	1.8
Chocolate Truffle, Mini, Finest, Tesco*	1 Cake/28g	125	448	5.9	52.9	23.7	0.3
Chocolate Victoria Sponge, Co-Op*	1 Slice/61g	201	330	5.0	42.0	16.0	1.0
Chocolate With Butter Icing	1oz/28g	135	481	5.7	50.9	29.7	0.0
Chocolate, Big, Tesco*	1 Slice/79g	311	396	7.4	54.1	16.7	1.8
Chocolate, Birthday, Tesco*	1 Serving/54g	229	425	5.9	45.5	24.4	2.1
Chocolate, Caterpillar, Tesco*	1 Serving/53g	248	468	5.7	55.3	24.9	1.1
Chocolate, Double Dream, Nestle*	1 Serving/150g	638	425	5.0	44.7	25.1	0.9
Chocolate, Fudge, The Cake Shop*	1 Cake/37.1g	178	480	3.7	50.5	29.2	1.3
Chocolate, Happy Birthday, Tesco*	1 Serving/58g	238	411	6.1	50.8	20.4	2.2
Chocolate, Home Bake, McVitie's*	1oz/28g	99	355	5.7	54.4	14.1	1.4
Chocolate, Iced, Tesco*	1 Serving/40g	158	395	4.7	58.5	15.8	1.8

CAKE

INFO/WEIGHT	Measure per Measure KCAL	KCAL	PROT	CARB	FAT	FIBRE
Chocolate, Large, Happy Birthday, Tesco*	1/18 Cake/63g 249	396	6.2	49.3	19.3	1.8
Chocolate, Low Fat, Safeway*	1 Slice/73.4g 176	241	5.8	45.0	4.8	1.3
Chocolate, Mini Roll, Safeway*	1 Roll/40g 180	450	0.0	53.5	23.9	2.2
Chocolate, Morrisons*	1 Serving/31.5g 157	505	5.3	48.0	32.4	1.2
Chocolate, Part Of Tea Time Selection, Iceland*	1 Cake/31g 144	464	4.5	54.1	25.5	2.0
Chocolate, Party, Tesco*	1 Slice/62g 244	394	4.6	46.3	21.2	0.9
Chocolate, Sainsbury's*	1 Serving/30g 119	395	4.1	52.6	18.5	1.3
Chocolate, Sara Lee*	1/4 Cake/88g 339	385	4.1	54.3	16.8	0.0
Chocolate, Slices, Healthy Eating, Tesco*	1 Slice/25g 79	314	4.7	65.5	2.4	3.7
Chocolate, Smarties*	Per Slice/60g 261	435	5.8	53.8	21.8	0.5
Chocolate, TTD, Sainsbury's*	1 Serving/207g 749	362	4.4	50.9	15.5	1.3
Chocolate, The Handmade Flapjack Company*	1 Cake/75g 303	404	12.5	39.8	21.6	0.0
Chocolate, Thorntons*	1 Serving/87g 408	469	5.2	47.1	28.8	0.6
Chocolate, Triple, Frozen, Majestic*	1/4 Cake/58g 87	150	2.2	14.1	9.4	0.1
Chocolate, Ultimate, TTD, Sainsbury's*	1 Serving/70g 263	375	5.4	51.5	16.4	1.9
Chocolate, Viennese, Marks & Spencer*	1oz/28g 105	375	4.4	54.1	13.6	1.6
Chocolate, White Button, Asda*	1 Cake/30g 117	390	5.0	44.0	21.0	2.0
Chocolate, With White Chocolate, The Cake Shop*	1 Cake/29g 146	503	4.6	49.2	32.0	1.2
Chorley, Asda*	1 Cake/60g 269	449	6.0	59.0	21.0	2.2
Choux Buns, Fresh Cream, Tesco*	1 Bun/95g 340	358	4.9	28.5	24.9	0.9
Choux Buns, Marks & Spencer*	1oz/28g 89	317	5.4	25.6	22.2	0.3
Christmas Slices, Weight Watchers*	1 Slice/40.1g 136	339	4.4	66.0	6.4	3.0
Christmas, Conoisseur, Marks & Spencer*	1 Slice/60g 216	360	4.1	64.7	9.2	3.3
Christmas, Iced, Slices, Tesco*	1 Slice/45g 168	369	2.9	67.6	9.6	1.2
Christmas, Knightsbridge*	1 Slice/50g 189	377	4.3	65.7	10.8	3.2
Christmas, Marks & Spencer*	1 Slice/60g 219	365	3.8	67.3	8.8	2.6
Christmas, Rich Fruit, All Iced, Sainsbury's*	1/16 Cake/85g 307	361	4.0	66.4	8.9	1.5
Christmas, Rich Fruit, Free From, Tesco*	1 Serving/100g 301	301	2.9	56.0	7.3	0.9
Christmas, Rich Fruit, Organic, Tesco*	1 Serving/75.5g 284	374	3.9	67.1	10.0	2.0
Christmas, TTD, Sainsbury's*	1/16 Cake/85g 315	371	3.7	67.1	8.9	1.3
Classic Lemon Drizzle, Marks & Spencer*	1/6 Cake/67.5g 255	375	4.7	55.0	15.3	0.6
Coconut	1 Slice/70g 304	434	6.7	51.2	23.8	2.5
Coconut Delight, Burton's*	1 Cake/25.1g 104	415	4.1	65.0	15.4	1.6
Coconut Macaroons, Sainsbury's*	1 Macaroon/33g 146	441	4.7	63.7	18.6	0.8
Coconut Snowball, Bobby's*	1 Cake/18.3g 78	436	2.2	57.3	22.1	0.0
Coconut Sponge, Mini Classics, Mr Kipling*	1 Cake/38g 155	409	3.7	47.0	22.9	0.9
Coffee & Walnut Slices, Healthy Eating, Tesco*	1 Slice/23g 69	301	4.4	65.7	2.3	2.8
Coffee & Walnut, Classic, Marks & Spencer*	1 Serving/70.8g 309	435	4.3	50.3	24.3	1.6
Coffee & Walnut, Mrs Beeton's*	1 Slice/54g 219	405	3.7	41.4	25.0	0.3
Coffee & Walnut, Somerfield*	1oz/28g 123	440	5.0	46.0	26.0	0.0
Coffee Sponge Roll, Marks & Spencer*	1 Serving/40g 150	375	3.5	51.1	17.3	0.6
Coffee, Entenmann's*	1 Portion/41g 159	388	4.0	54.7	17.3	0.6
Coffee, Iced, Marks & Spencer*	1 Slice/33g 135	410	4.4	54.5	19.6	1.6
Colin The Caterpillar, Marks & Spencer*	1 Slice/60g 234	390	5.3	57.2	21.3	1.3
Country Farmhouse, Waitrose*	1 Serving/80g 308	385	4.7	57.5	15.1	1.4
Country Slices, Good Intentions, Somerfield*	1 Cake/22g 70	318	5.5	70.0	1.8	1.8
Country Slices, Mr Kipling*	1oz/28g 108	385	4.3	56.5	15.7	1.1
Cream Oysters, Marks & Spencer*	1 Oyster/72g 227	315	3.6	27.5	21.2	3.0
Cream Slices, Marks & Spencer*	1 Slice/80g 310	387	2.3	45.7	22.9	0.6
Crispy Fruit Slices, Apple & Sultana, Go Ahead, McVitie's*	1 Slice/14g 54	386	6.0	72.7	7.9	3.3
Crispy Fruit Slices, Forest Fruit, Go Ahead, McVitie's*	1 Biscuit/14g 56	400	5.5	73.0	8.8	3.7
Cup, Marks & Spencer*	1 Cake/55g 195	355	2.8	71.5	6.5	0.5
Custard Slices, Tesco*	1 Slice/108g 320	296	2.4	37.5	15.2	0.5

C

CAKE

	Measure INFO/WEIGHT	per Measure KCAL	Nutrition Values per 100g / 100ml				
			KCAL	PROT	CARB	FAT	FIBRE
D'Oh Nuts, Asda*	1 Cake/50g	186	372	4.0	47.0	19.0	0.0
Date & Walnut Loaf, Sainsbury's*	1/10 Slice/40g	148	371	6.7	40.1	20.4	1.0
Date & Walnut Slices, Healthy Living, Tesco*	1 Slice/24g	74	308	5.4	67.0	2.0	1.4
Date & Walnut, Bakers Delight*	1oz/28g	88	315	5.2	55.5	8.0	1.2
Date & Walnut, Trimlyne*	1 Slice/50g	135	269	5.7	53.8	4.9	1.8
Double Chocolate Ganache, Marks & Spencer*	1/12 Cake/61g	281	460	5.9	46.1	27.6	2.5
Double Chocolate Wedge, Tesco*	1 Piece/100g	416	416	5.0	53.4	20.3	0.9
Dundee, Co-Op*	1/8 Cake/71g	238	335	5.0	53.0	11.0	2.0
Dundee, Somerfield*	1/10 Cake/75g	254	339	5.0	57.0	11.0	0.0
Easter Lemon Bakewells, Morrisons*	1 Cake/45g	186	413	3.1	64.8	15.7	1.8
Eccles	1 Cake/45g	214	475	3.9	59.3	26.4	1.6
Eccles, Weight Watchers*	1 Cake/48g	190	396	4.4	57.5	16.5	2.0
Fairy, Holly Lane*	1 Cake/25.7g	120	460	3.7	52.5	26.1	3.5
Fairy, Iced, Somerfield*	1 Cake/15.1g	59	392	4.9	62.9	13.4	1.4
Fairy, Lemon Iced, Tesco*	1 Cake/24g	94	393	4.4	63.2	13.6	1.1
Fairy, Mini, Kids, Tesco*	1 Cake/12g	54	435	5.3	53.3	22.3	1.1
Fairy, Mini, Tesco*	1 Cake/13g	53	424	6.1	54.6	20.1	1.3
Fairy, Plain, Somerfield*	1 Serving/16g	70	436	6.1	53.7	21.9	1.0
Fairy, Plain, Value, Tesco*	1 Cake/15g	52	348	5.3	62.4	8.6	0.9
Fairy, SmartPrice, Asda*	1 Cake/15g	66	438	6.0	54.0	22.0	1.0
Fairy, Snowman, Christmas, Tesco*	1 Cake/24g	114	471	4.6	49.8	28.1	2.9
Fairy, Strawberry Iced, Tesco*	1 Cake/24g	94	392	4.9	62.9	13.4	1.4
Fairy, Value, Tesco*	1 Cake/16g	70	436	6.1	53.7	21.9	1.0
Fairy, Vanilla Iced, Tesco*	1 Cake/24g	93	388	4.4	65.1	12.2	1.2
Farmhouse Fruit, Bakers Delight*	1oz/28g	107	381	5.2	55.5	15.3	2.1
Farmhouse Loaf, The Handmade Flapjack Company*	1 Cake/75g	274	365	4.5	48.4	17.2	0.0
Farmhouse Slice, Weight Watchers*	1 Slice/23g	73	317	5.5	64.9	4.0	1.3
Figfuls, Go Ahead, McVitie's*	1 Figful/15g	56	365	4.2	76.8	4.6	2.9
Flake, Cadbury*	1 Cake/26g	114	439	6.0	54.1	22.1	0.7
Fondant Fancies, Lemon, Waitrose*	1 Cake/40g	176	441	2.5	67.9	17.7	0.6
Fondant Fancies, Marks & Spencer*	1 Cake/34.5g	148	435	2.4	76.5	13.4	0.5
Fondant Fancies, Sainsbury's*	1 Cake/27g	95	353	2.4	65.7	9.0	0.4
French Fancies, Mr Kipling*	1 Cake/28g	107	381	2.6	70.7	9.7	0.6
Fresh Cream Bramley Apple Sponge, Tesco*	1/6 Slice/43g	130	303	3.6	35.4	16.3	1.0
Fruit & Nut Cluster, Finest, Tesco*	1 Slice/77g	262	338	4.5	50.1	13.3	2.7
Fruit Cake With Marzipan & Icing, Asda*	1/12 Slice/76g	280	369	3.9	68.0	9.0	0.0
Fruit Loaf, Sliced, Sainsbury's*	1 Slice/40g	104	260	8.9	47.9	3.6	2.4
Fruit Loaf, Sultana & Cherry, Sainsbury's*	1 Slice/50g	179	357	2.7	59.0	12.2	1.7
Fruit Slice, Value, Tesco*	1 Slice/22.6g	85	372	4.0	48.7	17.7	1.3
Fruit, Fully Iced, Luxury Rich, Co-Op*	1oz/28g	99	355	3.0	64.0	9.0	4.0
Fruit, Healthy Selection, Somerfield*	1oz/28g	73	260	5.0	55.0	2.0	0.0
Fruit, Parisienne, Rich, Finest, Tesco*	1 Serving/69g	262	380	4.7	55.2	14.1	1.9
Fruit, Plain, Retail	1 Slice/90g	319	354	5.1	57.9	12.9	0.0
Fruit, Rich, Connoisseur, Somerfield*	1oz/28g	91	326	4.0	54.0	10.0	0.0
Fruit, Rich, Iced	1 Slice/70g	249	356	4.1	62.7	11.4	1.7
Fruit, Rich, Retail	1 Slice/70g	225	322	4.9	50.7	12.5	1.7
Fudge Brownie, The Handmade Flapjack Company*	1 Cake/75g	286	381	4.9	62.8	12.3	0.0
Fudgy Chocolate Slices, COU, Marks & Spencer*	1 Slice/36g	95	265	4.6	66.4	2.2	2.1
Genoa, Home Bake, McVitie's*	1oz/28g	107	383	4.7	55.9	15.6	1.4
Genoa, Tesco*	1 Serving/50g	162	324	4.0	58.6	8.2	3.2
Ginger Drizzle, Iced, Co-Op*	1/6 Cake/64.5g	226	350	3.0	58.0	12.0	1.0
Ginger Orange, The Handmade Flapjack Company*	1 Cake/75g	289	385	4.3	46.3	20.3	0.0
Ginger, Marks & Spencer*	1/6 Cake/41g	156	380	6.3	62.3	11.5	1.7

C

CAKE

INFO/WEIGHT	Measure	per Measure KCAL	KCAL	PROT	CARB	FAT	FIBRE
					Nutrition Values per 100g / 100ml		
Glitzy Bag, Birthday, Tesco*	1 Serving/81g	314	388	2.1	75.9	8.5	0.6
Happy Birthday, Sainsbury's*	1 Slice/50g	207	414	2.8	64.5	16.1	0.6
Heavenly Chocolate Brownie, Safeway*	1 Pack/300g	900	300	6.2	38.5	13.4	0.8
Holly Hedgehog, Tesco*	1 Serving/55g	227	413	2.0	69.0	14.3	0.8
Iced Madeira, Sainsbury's*	1/8 Cake/47g	182	388	3.6	61.6	14.1	0.7
Jamaica Ginger With Lemon Filling, McVitie's*	1 Cake/32.9g	143	434	4.0	48.3	25.0	0.8
Jamaica Ginger, McVitie's*	1 Serving/75g	291	388	3.4	61.2	14.4	1.2
Jammy Strawberry Rolls, Mini, Cadbury*	1 Roll/29g	119	411	4.9	59.8	16.5	0.5
Lemon & Orange, Finest, Tesco*	1 Serving/53g	216	410	4.5	52.4	20.3	1.1
Lemon Bakewell, Mr Kipling*	1 Cake/48.0g	195	407	2.6	65.0	15.2	0.7
Lemon Buttercream & Lemon Curd, The Cake Shop*	1 Cake/28g	124	444	3.5	43.4	27.8	0.6
Lemon Cup Cakes, COU, Marks & Spencer*	1 Cake/42.6g	131	305	3.3	68.1	2.1	2.0
Lemon Drizzle Cake, Asda*	1 Serving/50g	150	299	2.8	45.0	12.0	0.4
Lemon Drizzle, Marks & Spencer*	1/6 Cake/63g	230	365	4.2	55.8	13.9	1.4
Lemon Iced Madeira, Co-Op*	1 Cake/290g	1131	390	4.0	53.0	18.0	0.6
Lemon Madeira, Half Moon, Dan Cake*	1 Slice/50g	215	430	3.5	59.0	20.0	0.0
Lemon Slices, BGTY, Sainsbury's*	1 Slice/26.0g	84	323	3.7	74.0	1.4	1.3
Lemon Slices, Eat Smart, Morrisons*	1 Slice/26g	81	312	3.9	68.1	2.7	1.9
Lemon Slices, Mr Kipling*	1oz/28g	117	417	4.1	58.2	16.3	0.0
Lemon Slices, Sponge, Mr Kipling*	1 Slice/30g	119	397	4.1	58.5	16.2	0.0
Lemon Smoothie Bake, Go Ahead, McVitie's*	1 Bar/35g	130	372	3.0	75.1	8.1	1.0
Lemon Tartlette, Go Ahead, McVitie's*	1 Cake/45g	161	357	3.7	67.9	9.5	1.1
Lemon, Entenmann's*	1 Serving/55.6g	214	383	3.7	56.9	15.7	1.1
Lemon, Half Moon, Bobby's*	1/6 Cake/60g	244	406	4.1	55.7	18.4	0.0
Lemon, Home Bake, McVitie's*	1oz/28g	108	384	4.6	53.9	18.2	1.0
Lemon, Low Fat, Weight Watchers*	1 Cake/26g	79	304	3.7	68.8	1.6	3.5
Lemon, Slices, Healthy Eating, Tesco*	1 Slice/26g	86	329	3.4	69.1	2.6	3.0
Lemon, The Handmade Flapjack Company*	1 Cake/75g	312	416	4.5	50.5	21.8	0.0
Leo the Lion, Birthday, Asda*	1 Slice/80.8g	326	402	2.6	62.0	16.0	0.5
Madeira	1 Slice/40g	157	393	5.4	58.4	16.9	0.9
Madeira, All Butter, Sainsbury's*	1 Serving/30g	116	388	5.2	47.4	19.7	0.8
Madeira, Cherry, Tesco*	1/4 Cake/100g	342	342	4.3	55.9	11.2	2.6
Madeira, Iced, Tesco*	1/16 Cake/56g	218	389	2.6	67.2	12.2	0.4
Madeira, Lemon Iced, Tesco*	1 Slice/30g	122	407	4.5	57.8	17.5	0.9
Madeira, Tesco*	1 Serving/50g	197	394	5.5	57.9	15.6	1.2
Magic Roundabout, Dougal, Tesco*	1 Serving/50g	214	428	2.3	68.7	16.0	0.2
Manor House, Mr Kipling*	1 Serving/69.2g	276	400	5.3	49.7	20.0	1.4
Marble, Home Bake, McVitie's*	1oz/28g	115	411	3.7	56.9	18.8	0.9
Marble, Tesco*	1/8 Cake/45g	185	410	4.4	55.9	18.7	1.5
Mini Eggs, Cadbury*	1 Cake/26.2g	109	420	5.3	52.9	21.1	0.0
Mini Rolls, Blackforest, Weight Watchers*	1 Cake/23.8g	90	374	5.3	58.9	14.2	4.4
Mini Rolls, Cadbury*	1 Roll/26g	113	434	5.5	55.6	20.6	0.6
Mini Rolls, Chocolate & Vanilla, Somerfield*	1oz/28g	112	399	5.0	62.0	15.0	0.0
Mini Rolls, Chocolate, Tesco*	1 Roll/31g	135	437	5.2	48.8	24.6	1.3
Mini Rolls, Chocolate, Weight Watchers*	1 Cake/23g	85	371	5.3	61.9	15.0	2.0
Mini Rolls, Easter Selection, Cadbury*	1oz/28g	122	434	5.5	55.6	20.6	0.0
Mini Rolls, Jaffa Cake, McVitie's*	1 Cake/28g	106	379	3.5	67.5	10.5	0.0
Mini Rolls, Juicy Orange, Cadbury*	1 Cake/28g	110	390	5.0	55.0	16.8	0.0
Mini Rolls, Milk Chocolate Orange, Shapers, Boots*	1 Roll/25g	97	386	4.6	64.0	12.0	2.4
Mini Rolls, Milk Chocolate, Cadbury*	1 Roll/27g	120	445	4.4	56.5	22.2	0.0
Mini Rolls, Rolo, Nestle*	1 Cake/29g	111	388	4.8	49.5	19.0	1.0
Orange & Ginger, Oat Break, Go Ahead, McVitie's*	1 Cake/35g	121	347	5.2	67.1	6.4	2.6
Orange Marmalade Loaf, Aldi*	1 Slice/33.0g	88	267	4.5	57.4	2.2	1.8

CAKE

	Measure INFO/WEIGHT	per Measure KCAL	KCAL	PROT	CARB	FAT	FIBRE
Orange Marmalade, Marks & Spencer*	1 Slice/50g	195	390	3.6	53.2	18.3	1.8
Party Bake, Marks & Spencer*	1/15 Cake/59.7g	231	385	4.0	46.6	20.2	0.9
Party, Asda*	1 Serving/56.5g	240	421	2.3	67.0	16.0	0.4
Piece Of Cake, Birthday, Marks & Spencer*	1 Serving/85g	395	465	4.3	39.7	28.7	0.9
Pink Cup Cakes, Marks & Spencer*	1 Cake/39g	160	410	2.5	81.3	8.5	0.6
Raisin, Dernys*	1 Cake/45g	175	388	5.0	54.0	17.0	0.0
Raisin, Tesco*	1 Cake/38g	158	417	5.6	53.8	19.9	1.4
Raspberry Smoothie Bake, Go Ahead, McVitie's*	1 Bar/35g	126	359	3.0	69.8	7.5	2.2
Rich Choc' Roll, Cadbury*	1/6 Portion/39g	149	381	4.8	50.2	15.6	1.0
Rich Chocolate, Christmas, Tesco*	1 Slice/82g	300	367	7.0	47.5	16.5	1.6
Rich Fruit Slices, Free From, Sainsbury's*	1 Slice/40g	144	361	4.5	57.4	12.6	3.7
Rich Fruit, Sainsbury's*	1 Serving/100g	321	321	3.9	57.3	8.5	2.1
Rock	1 Sm Cake/40g	158	396	5.4	60.5	16.4	1.5
Rock, Tesco*	1 Serving/87g	311	357	7.4	60.1	9.7	1.6
Rollers, Culi d'Or*	1 Roll/20.8g	69	330	5.8	50.0	12.0	0.0
Seriously Chocolatey Celebration, Sainsbury's*	1/8 Cake/77g	336	437	6.3	45.0	25.7	0.3
Seriously Chocolatey, Large, Sainsbury's*	1/24 Cake/77g	352	457	5.4	51.0	25.3	3.0
Shrek Birthday, Tesco*	1/16 Cake/72g	248	344	3.3	64.0	12.2	0.5
Snowballs, Chocolate, Tunnock's*	1 Snowball/25g	97	388	3.9	47.0	21.8	0.0
Snowballs, Sainsbury's*	1 Snowball/18g	80	445	2.5	55.6	23.0	3.6
Snowballs, Tesco*	1 Snowball/18g	79	432	2.5	55.8	22.1	5.4
Sponge	1 Slice/53g	243	459	6.4	52.4	26.3	0.9
Sponge With Butter Icing	1 Slice/65g	319	490	4.5	52.4	30.6	0.6
Sponge, Fatless	1 Slice/53g	156	294	10.1	53.0	6.1	0.9
Sponge, Iced, Marks & Spencer*	1 Serving/100g	400	400	3.4	58.4	17.0	1.3
Sponge, Jam Filled	1 Slice/65g	196	302	4.2	64.2	4.9	1.8
Spooky, Birthday, Memory Lane Cakes*	1 Slice/75g	295	393	3.5	50.8	19.5	0.7
St. Clements, Finest, Tesco*	1 Serving/49g	194	395	3.1	47.2	21.5	0.4
Stem Ginger, 96% Fat Free, Trimlyne*	1/4 Cake/62.5g	170	273	4.4	58.1	3.6	1.2
Sticky Toffee Slices, Eat Smart, Safeway*	1 Cake/85g	259	305	3.6	65.8	2.7	1.3
Stollen Slices, Somerfield*	1oz/28g	115	411	7.0	54.0	19.0	0.0
Stollen, Christmas Range, Tesco*	1oz/28g	99	355	5.0	52.9	13.7	1.8
Strawberry Sponge Roll, Marks & Spencer*	1/6 Cake/48.5g	158	330	2.8	58.0	9.5	0.8
Sultana & Cherry Slice, Co-Op*	1oz/28g	87	310	3.0	48.0	12.0	2.0
Sultana & Cherry, Tesco*	1 Cake/37g	124	334	4.7	54.4	10.8	2.5
Sultana, Apple & Cranberry, 99% Fat Free, Trimlyne*,	1/6 Cake/66.6g	130	195	4.6	45.5	0.9	3.3
Sultana, Fair Trade, Co-Op*	1/8 cake/45g	155	345	5.0	60.0	9.0	1.0
Summer Fruit Cream, GFY, Asda*	1 Serving/74.0g	165	223	3.6	41.0	4.9	2.5
Summer Strawberry Bakes, Go Ahead, McVitie's*	1 Bar/35g	128	367	2.7	75.1	8.0	1.0
Swiss Roll	1oz/28g	77	276	7.2	55.5	4.4	0.8
Swiss Roll, Chocolate Flavour, Value, Tesco*	1 Slice/20g	79	394	5.5	49.2	19.5	1.4
Swiss Roll, Chocolate, Individual	1 Roll/26g	88	337	4.3	58.1	11.3	0.0
Swiss Roll, Chocolate, Jumbo, Safeway*	1/12 Roll/35g	129	369	4.1	47.1	18.2	0.9
Swiss Roll, Chocolate, Lyons*	1 Serving/50g	190	379	4.3	47.0	19.3	0.9
Swiss Roll, Chocolate, Mini, Tesco*	1 Roll/22g	87	396	4.6	61.0	14.8	0.0
Swiss Roll, Chocolate, Morrisons*	1/6 Roll/26g	103	401	4.4	56.4	18.9	3.1
Swiss Roll, Chocolate, Somerfield*	1/4 Roll/43.5g	167	384	6.0	55.0	16.0	0.0
Swiss Roll, Chocolate, Value, Tesco*	1 Serving/20g	81	404	5.0	54.1	18.7	2.1
Swiss Roll, Raspberry & Vanilla, Morrisons*	1 Serving/28g	98	350	4.2	61.8	9.5	0.0
Swiss Roll, Raspberry, Lyons*	1 Swiss Roll/175g	485	277	5.2	60.6	1.4	0.0
Swiss Roll, Raspberry, Sainsbury's*	1 Serving/35g	105	301	3.5	67.0	2.1	1.1
Swiss Roll, Raspberry, Somerfield*	1 Swiss Roll/80g	245	306	5.0	66.0	3.0	0.0
Swiss Roll, Raspberry, Tesco*	1 Serving/45g	132	294	3.2	65.4	2.1	1.0

CAKE

INFO/WEIGHT	Measure	per Measure KCAL	KCAL	PROT	CARB	FAT	FIBRE
Swiss Roll, Strawberry, Luxury, Somerfield*	1oz/28g	84	301	4.0	62.0	4.0	0.0
Syrup & Ginger, Tesco*	1 Serving/32g	134	420	4.5	51.4	21.8	0.7
Tangy Lemon Trickle, Marks & Spencer*	1 Slice/75g	281	375	4.7	47.4	18.8	1.1
The Ultimate Carrot Passion, Entenmann's*	1 Slice/52g	206	403	4.6	42.4	24.3	1.0
Toffee & Pecan Loaf, Safeway*	1/6 Cake/62g	225	363	3.6	35.5	22.9	0.5
Toffee & Pecan Slices, Marks & Spencer*	1 Slice/36g	160	445	4.7	54.0	23.7	1.3
Toffee Bakewell, Morrisons*	1 Cake/47g	212	451	3.4	69.5	18.2	1.4
Toffee Bakewell, Tesco*	1 Bakewell/49g	203	414	3.9	63.5	16.1	1.4
Toffee Flavour Slices, Low Fat, Weight Watchers*	1 Slice/27g	80	297	4.2	63.9	2.6	3.2
Toffee Fudge, Entenmann's*	1 Serving/65g	274	421	3.4	53.0	21.7	0.5
Toffee Snap, The Handmade Flapjack Company*	1 Cake/75g	365	487	4.6	62.2	26.1	0.0
Toffee Temptation, Tesco*	1 Slice/67g	228	340	2.9	39.1	19.1	0.3
Toffee, Iced, Tesco*	1 Serving/35g	132	376	3.3	57.2	14.9	1.6
Toffee, Slices, BGTY, Sainsbury's*	1 Slice/27g	88	327	4.3	71.7	2.5	1.8
Toffee, Slices, Healthy Living, Tesco*	1 Cake/24g	76	315	4.5	65.0	2.6	1.6
Toffee, Slices, Value, Tesco*	1 Slice/14g	62	440	4.2	54.9	22.6	0.6
Toffee, The Handmade Flapjack Company*	1 Cake/75g	347	462	5.1	54.0	25.1	0.0
Toffee, Thorntons*	1/6 Cake/70.1g	302	431	4.6	49.2	24.0	0.8
Triple Chocolate, TTD, Sainsbury's*	1/8 Cake/52g	210	412	4.7	42.6	24.7	0.5
Vanilla Sponge, Fresh Cream, Sainsbury's*	1 Slice/50g	152	304	7.5	45.6	10.2	0.4
Victoria Sandwich, Classic, Large, Marks & Spencer*	1/10 Cake/65.8g	261	395	5.1	49.5	19.6	2.3
Victoria Slices, Mr Kipling*	1 Slice/33g	120	366	4.1	53.6	15.0	1.1
Victoria Sponge Sandwich, Somerfield*	1oz/28g	112	400	4.0	53.0	19.0	0.0
Victoria Sponge, Fresh Cream, Tesco*	1 Slice/46.7g	157	334	3.9	40.8	17.3	0.7
Victoria Sponge, Fresh Cream, Value, Tesco*	1 Serving/50g	169	337	4.4	40.7	17.4	0.6
Victoria Sponge, Lemon, Co-Op*	1 Slice/42g	151	360	4.0	44.0	19.0	0.7
Victoria Sponge, Mini, Bobby's*	1 Cake/35g	164	469	4.0	51.3	27.5	0.2
Victoria Sponge, Mini, Mr Kipling*	1 Cake/37g	142	383	3.8	48.7	19.2	0.6
Victoria Sponge, TTD, Sainsbury's*	1 Serving/69g	255	370	4.3	51.4	16.4	1.0
Viennese Whirl, Lemon, Mr Kipling*	1 Cake/28g	115	409	4.2	62.2	15.9	0.7
Viennese Whirl, Mr Kipling*	1 Whirl/28g	139	497	4.1	51.5	30.5	1.2
Viennese Whirl, Tesco*	1 Cake/39g	181	465	4.0	53.2	26.2	1.2
Viennese, Marks & Spencer*	1 Cake/50.5g	252	495	4.1	58.9	28.0	2.8
Walnut & Coffee, Co-Op*	1/4 Cake/65g	254	390	5.0	47.0	20.0	0.7
Walnut Layer, Somerfield*	1/4 Cake/77.5g	295	381	6.0	45.0	20.0	0.0
Walnut, Sandwich, Sainsbury's*	1 Slice/20g	79	393	5.8	53.6	17.3	1.2
Welsh	1oz/28g	121	431	5.6	61.8	19.6	1.5
Wild Blueberry & Apple, Bakers Delight*	1oz/28g	99	354	4.6	48.8	15.6	1.5
Winnie The Pooh Birthday, Disney, Nestle*	1 Serving/100g	361	361	2.4	63.3	10.9	0.5
Xmas Pudding, Tesco*	1 Cake/16.7g	59	349	3.3	60.5	9.3	1.4
Yorkshire Parkin, Bakers Delight*	1oz/28g	111	395	5.1	60.3	14.8	1.5
Yum Yum, Marks & Spencer*	1 Cake/37g	155	420	5.8	42.2	25.6	1.8
Yum Yum, Waitrose*	1 Serving/45g	190	422	5.3	46.9	23.7	1.2
Yum Yums, Tesco*	1 Cake/61g	232	380	6.1	51.6	16.6	1.7

CAKE BAR

INFO/WEIGHT	Measure	per Measure KCAL	KCAL	PROT	CARB	FAT	FIBRE
Blueberry, Trimlyne*	1 Cake/50g	142	283	3.9	64.0	2.2	2.2
Bounty, McVitie's*	1 Cake/36g	166	461	5.1	55.2	24.5	0.0
Caramel, Cadbury*	1 Bar/26g	107	411	6.4	57.0	16.8	0.0
Caramel, Tesco*	1 Cake/26g	103	395	5.1	50.9	12.4	8.2
Choc Chip, Go Ahead, McVitie's*	1 Bar/28g	100	356	6.4	56.9	12.1	1.0
Choc Chip, Mini, Go Ahead, McVitie's	1 Bar/27g	93	343	5.7	55.3	12.1	0.9
Chocolate & Orange, Go Ahead, McVitie's*	1 Cake Bar/33g	109	330	4.3	64.9	6.0	1.0
Chocolate Chip, Healthy Living, Tesco*	1 Serving/37g	109	295	4.8	63.6	2.6	0.6

	Measure	per Measure	Nutrition Values per 100g / 100ml				
	INFO/WEIGHT	KCAL	KCAL	PROT	CARB	FAT	FIBRE
CAKE BAR							
Chocolate Chip, Mr Kipling*	1 Bar/33g	147	444	5.7	45.7	26.5	0.6
Chocolate Chip, Sainsbury's*	1 Cake Bar/25g	108	430	6.1	51.2	22.3	0.6
Chocolate Chip, Tesco*	1 Cake/30g	123	411	7.0	51.4	19.7	2.3
Chocolate Dream, Go Ahead, McVitie's*	1 Bar/36g	141	391	4.6	63.2	13.4	0.9
Chocolate, Asda*	1 Bar/27g	124	461	5.0	63.0	21.0	2.5
Chocolate, Tesco*	1 Serving/26g	113	435	5.2	51.9	23.0	5.4
Crunchie, Cadbury*	1 Cake Bar/32g	147	460	5.9	58.3	22.6	0.0
Double Chocolate, Free From, Sainsbury's*	1 Cake/50.1g	196	391	4.2	58.2	15.7	1.0
Double Chocolate, Free From, Tesco*	1 Serving/45g	179	397	4.6	55.7	17.3	1.1
Dream, Cadbury*	1 Cake bar/37.8g	171	450	4.5	57.2	22.6	0.0
Flake, Cadbury*	1 Cake/22g	97	442	6.5	51.8	23.3	0.5
Fruit & Nut Crisp, Go Ahead, McVitie's*	1 Bar/22g	95	430	5.3	71.3	13.7	1.7
Fudge, Cadbury*	1 Pack/52.4g	218	420	5.7	60.3	17.6	0.0
Galaxy Caramel, McVitie's*	1 Cake/31g	137	441	5.5	57.4	21.1	0.0
Galaxy, McVitie's*	1oz/28g	138	494	5.1	57.5	27.0	0.3
Golden Syrup, McVitie's*	1 Mini Cake/33g	127	385	3.6	60.2	14.4	1.2
Jaffa Cake, McVitie's	1 Bar/31g	116	374	4.8	70.6	8.0	2.1
Jamaica Ginger, McVitie's*	1 Mini Cake/33g	128	388	3.5	60.2	14.7	1.2
Milk Chocolate, Cadbury*	1 Bar/35g	140	401	6.8	48.8	19.8	0.8
Milky Way, McVitie's*	1 Bar/26g	138	530	5.3	53.8	32.6	0.2
Rich Chocolate, Trimlyne*	1 Serving/40g	115	288	5.3	59.3	4.3	2.3
Strawberry & Vanilla, Healthy Eating, Tesco*	1 Serving/42g	124	295	3.7	64.4	2.6	0.8
CAKE MIX							
Cheesecake, Strawberry, Real, Greens*	1 Serving	254	253	3.9	30.6	12.8	0.6
Chocolate, Greens*	1 Cake/1037.6g	3750	361	5.8	54.6	13.3	1.4
Christmas, Mini, Jane Asher*	1oz/28g	104	372	5.2	65.8	12.0	1.3
Dennis, Greens*	1 Cake/17.3g	54	319	4.6	57.8	7.7	0.0
Free From, Sainsbury's*	1 Serving/50g	173	346	1.3	84.4	0.3	2.2
CALAMARI							
Battered With Tartar Sauce Dip, Tesco*	1 Pack/210g	573	273	8.9	15.4	19.5	0.6
Battered, Marks & Spencer*	1 Pack/160g	424	265	14.3	15.8	16.1	0.7
Battered, Young's*	1 Serving/150g	266	177	7.8	13.0	10.4	1.5
Marks & Spencer*	1oz/28g	65	231	13.9	11.5	14.4	0.5
Rings In Batter, Waitrose*	1/2 Pack/85g	227	267	13.9	14.2	17.2	0.6
CALZONE							
Bolognese, Weight Watchers*	1 Calzone/88.1g	178	202	11.7	31.2	3.4	4.3
Cheese & Tomato, Weight Watchers*	1 Calzone/88g	191	217	11.3	33.4	4.3	3.4
Ham & Gruyere, Asda*	1 Serving/280g	661	236	10.0	31.0	8.0	2.7
CAMPINO							
Oranges & Cream, Bendicks*	1oz/28g	116	416	0.1	85.8	8.1	0.0
Strawberries & Cream, Bendicks*	1oz/28g	117	418	0.1	86.2	8.1	0.0
CANAPES							
Caponata, Puff Pastry, Occasions, Sainsbury's*	1 Square/12g	30	249	4.1	22.9	15.7	2.1
CANNELLONI							
Barilla*	1 Pack/250g	875	350	11.5	72.7	1.5	0.0
Beef & Red Wine, Waitrose*	1/2 Pack/170g	355	209	17.5	13.8	9.4	1.0
Beef, BGTY, Sainsbury's*	1 Pack/300g	249	83	5.5	10.1	2.3	1.7
Beef, Finest, Tesco*	1 Serving/300g	480	160	7.3	8.6	10.5	0.7
Beef, Geat Value, Asda*	1 Pack/400g	384	96	6.0	12.0	2.7	1.6
Beef, Healthy Living, Tesco*	1 Pack/340g	323	95	6.4	11.9	2.4	1.5
Beef, Italiano, Tesco*	1 Serving/340g	442	130	5.3	12.4	6.6	0.7
Chicken & Pesto, Italian, Sainsbury's*	1 Pack/450g	675	150	6.1	14.4	7.5	1.1
Findus*	1 Pack/342g	445	130	5.6	11.1	6.7	1.0

C

	Measure INFO/WEIGHT	per Measure KCAL	Nutrition Values per 100g / 100ml				
			KCAL	PROT	CARB	FAT	FIBRE
CANNELLONI							
Five Cheese & Spinach, Finest, Tesco*	1/2 Pack/300g	468	156	7.0	9.6	9.9	1.7
Iceland*	1 Pack/400g	584	146	7.2	13.0	7.2	0.6
Marks & Spencer*	1 Pack/400g	540	135	7.4	7.8	8.1	2.1
Mediterranean Vegetable, Waitrose*	1 Serving/170g	330	194	9.7	18.7	9.0	1.9
Mushroom, Italian, Sainsbury's*	1 Pack/449.6g	599	133	5.2	12.5	6.9	0.5
Parmesan & Basil, Marks & Spencer*	1 Pack/360g	504	140	5.9	11.4	7.9	0.8
Pork, Marks & Spencer*	1 Pack/400g	460	115	6.2	8.7	6.2	1.1
Ricotta & Spinach, Waitrose*	1/2 Pack/225g	288	128	5.9	11.0	6.7	0.8
Ricotta & Spinich, Perfectly Balanced, Waitrose*	1 Pack/350g	312	89	4.1	10.8	3.3	1.1
Roasted Vegetable, Morrisons*	1 Pack/350g	312	89	3.9	12.5	2.5	2.3
Smoked Salmon & Spinach, Sainsbury's*	1 Pack/450g	599	133	5.7	13.5	6.2	0.4
Spinach & Ricotta, BGTY, Sainsbury's*	1 Serving/300g	282	94	4.9	14.7	1.7	1.0
Spinach & Ricotta, COU, Marks & Spencer*	1 Serving/360g	324	90	6.2	10.2	2.7	1.7
Spinach & Ricotta, GFY, Asda*	1 Pack/303g	418	138	6.0	21.0	3.3	0.5
Spinach & Ricotta, Good Intentions, Somerfield*	1 Serving/400g	366	92	5.3	12.2	2.4	2.1
Spinach & Ricotta, Healthy Choice, Asda*	1 Pack/400g	448	112	4.0	15.0	4.0	0.5
Spinach & Ricotta, Healthy Living, Tesco*	1 Pack/340g	316	93	4.3	12.7	2.8	1.6
Spinach & Ricotta, Italian Style, Co-Op*	1 Pack/450g	540	120	5.0	12.0	6.0	2.0
Spinach & Ricotta, Ross*	1 Pack/300g	288	96	3.9	13.2	3.1	1.6
Spinach & Ricotta, Safeway*	1 Pack/401g	565	141	6.5	14.4	6.4	0.4
Spinach & Ricotta, Sainsbury's*	1 Pack/288g	423	147	6.6	12.8	7.7	0.5
Spinach & Ricotta, Somerfield*	1 Pack/300g	393	131	5.0	13.0	7.0	0.0
Spinach & Wild Mushroom, Linda McCartney*	1 Pack/340g	381	112	4.9	14.1	4.0	1.7
Tubes, Dry, Sainsbury's*	2 Tubes/16g	55	357	12.3	73.1	1.7	2.5
Value, Tesco*	1 Serving/250g	320	128	6.6	10.0	6.8	1.4
Vegetarian, Tesco*	1 Pack/400g	552	138	5.3	9.8	8.6	1.5
CAPERS							
Caperberries, Spanish, Waitrose*	1 serving/55g	9	17	1.1	2.1	0.5	2.5
CAPPALLETTI							
Goats Cheese & Red Pesto, Waitrose*	1/2 Pack/125g	374	299	11.6	43.5	8.7	2.2
CAPPELLETTI							
Chicken & Ham, Fresh, Safeway*	1/2 Pack/177g	320	181	9.7	27.7	3.5	1.8
Fresh, Sainsbury's*	1 Serving/125g	294	235	12.9	33.5	5.5	2.7
Meat, Italian, Somerfield*	1/2 Pack/125g	331	265	13.6	38.5	6.3	2.4
Prosciutto, Waitrose*	1/5 Pack/100g	308	308	13.4	51.3	5.5	2.3
With Proscuitto & Grana Padano Cheese, Sainsbury's*	1 Serving/125g	285	228	12.1	29.1	7.0	1.8
CAPRI SUN							
Orange, The Coca Cola Co*	1 Pouch/200ml	90	45	0.0	11.0	0.0	0.0
CARAMAC							
Nestle*	1 Bar/30g	163	563	5.8	54.4	35.8	0.0
CARAMBOLA							
Average	1oz/28g	9	32	0.5	7.3	0.3	1.3
CARAMEL							
Cadbury*	1 Bar/50g	240	480	4.3	61.3	24.3	0.0
Egg, Cadbury*	1 Egg/39g	191	490	4.3	58.9	26.1	0.0
CARIBBEAN TWIST							
Halewood*	500ml	430	86	0.0	13.7	0.0	0.0
CARO							
Instant Beverage, No Caffeine, Nestle*	1 Pot/50g	133	265	5.5	60.0	0.3	0.0
CAROB POWDER							
Average	1 Tsp/2g	3	159	4.9	37.0	0.1	0.0
CARROT & SWEDE							
Diced, For Mashing, Average	1/2 Pack/250g	58	23	0.6	4.7	0.3	1.9

C

	Measure INFO/WEIGHT	per Measure KCAL	Nutrition Values per 100g / 100ml				
			KCAL	PROT	CARB	FAT	FIBRE
CARROT & SWEDE							
Mash, From Supermarket, Average	1 Serving/150g	138	92	1.3	10.4	5.0	1.3
Mash, Healthy Range, Average	1 Serving/150g	98	66	1.3	8.6	2.8	2.1
CARROTS							
& Cauliflower, Marks & Spencer*	1 Serving/335g	74	22	0.6	4.4	0.4	2.3
& Mange Tout, Tendersteam, Marks & Spencer*	1/2 Pack/100g	35	35	2.9	5.6	0.2	2.1
& Peas, Sainsbury's*	1 Serving/200g	100	50	3.3	8.3	0.5	3.8
Baby Corn, & Mange Tout, Safeway*	1 Pack/200g	48	24	2.1	3.2	0.3	0.0
Baby, Canned, Average	1 Can/195g	40	21	0.5	4.2	0.3	2.1
Baby, Fresh, Average	1 Serving/60g	17	29	0.7	5.8	0.3	1.7
Baby, With Fine Beans, Tesco*	1 Pack/200g	58	29	1.3	4.7	0.5	2.3
Batons, & Sliced Runner Beans, Sainsbury's*	1 Serving/200g	40	20	1.0	3.2	0.5	3.2
Batons, Fresh, Average	1/2 Pack/150g	41	28	0.6	5.7	0.3	2.6
Boiled, Average	1oz/28g	6	22	0.6	4.4	0.4	2.3
Canned, Average	1oz/28g	6	22	0.6	4.4	0.3	2.1
Cauliflower & Broccoli, Tesco*	1 Pack/300g	105	35	2.5	4.9	0.6	2.3
Chantenay, Steamer, Sainsbury's*	1/2 Pack/125g	60	48	0.5	7.7	1.7	2.2
Chantenay, Tesco*	1oz/28g	7	24	0.6	4.4	0.4	2.3
Dippers, Marks & Spencer*	1 Serving/130g	195	150	0.9	6.2	13.4	2.1
Dippers, Sainsbury's*	1 Pot/130g	182	140	0.9	5.7	12.5	2.2
Sliced, Canned, Average	1 Serving/180g	36	20	0.7	4.1	0.1	1.5
Sliced, Fresh, Average	1 Serving/60g	17	28	0.7	5.7	0.3	2.0
Whole, Raw, Average	1oz/28g	8	29	0.6	6.3	0.3	2.2
With Parsley & English Butter, Marks & Spencer*	1/2 Pack/100g	65	65	0.6	7.1	3.9	2.4
CASHEW NUTS							
Plain, Average	1/4 Pack/25g	146	585	15.7	18.8	48.9	3.4
Roasted & Salted, Average	1 Serving/50g	306	612	18.8	19.6	51.1	3.1
CASHEWS & PEANUTS							
Honey Roasted, Average	1 Serving/50g	290	579	21.6	26.6	42.9	4.2
CASSAVA							
Baked	1oz/28g	43	155	0.7	40.1	0.2	1.7
Boiled in Unsalted Water	1oz/28g	36	130	0.5	33.5	0.2	1.4
Chips	1oz/28g	99	353	1.8	91.4	0.4	4.0
Gari	1oz/28g	100	358	1.3	92.9	0.5	0.0
Raw	1oz/28g	40	142	0.6	36.8	0.2	1.6
Steamed	1oz/28g	40	142	0.6	36.8	0.2	1.6
CASSEROLE							
Bean, & Lentil, Morrisons*	1 Can/410g	287	70	4.1	12.5	0.4	0.0
Bean, Spicy, BGTY, Sainsbury's*	1 Pack/300g	171	57	3.0	9.1	0.9	4.2
Beef Bourguignon, Finest, Tesco*	1 Serving/300g	258	86	10.8	1.9	3.9	0.8
Beef, & Ale, Finest, Tesco*	1/2 Pack/300g	234	78	11.5	5.0	1.4	1.1
Beef, & Ale, With Dumplings, Sainsbury's*	1 Pack/450g	711	158	7.7	15.4	7.3	0.6
Beef, & Ale, With Mashed Potato, Healthy Living, Tesco*	1 Serving/450g	365	81	5.1	10.9	2.5	0.6
Beef, & Dumplings, Marks & Spencer*	1 Pack/454g	522	115	10.5	7.7	4.7	1.0
Beef, & Dumplings, Safeway*	1 Pack/390g	215	55	1.6	7.5	1.9	1.2
Beef, & Onion, Minced, British Classics, Tesco*	1 Pack/340g	367	108	5.0	9.3	5.6	0.8
Beef, & Red Wine, BGTY, Sainsbury's*	1 Pack/300g	192	64	8.0	6.7	0.6	0.9
Beef, & Vegetable, Ready Meals, Waitrose*	1oz/28g	32	114	4.1	12.8	5.2	0.9
Beef, Diced, Lean, Sainsbury's*	1/2 Pack/250g	340	136	22.5	0.0	5.1	0.0
Beef, Marks & Spencer*	1 Serving/200g	240	120	8.1	9.2	5.7	1.0
Beef, Meal For One, Tesco*	1 Serving/450g	425	94	3.6	10.6	4.2	1.7
Beef, Mini Favourites, Marks & Spencer*	1 Serving/200g	250	125	7.3	9.2	6.7	1.1
Beef, Ready Meals, Marks & Spencer*	1 Meal/454g	622	137	11.1	9.9	6.4	0.7
Beef, Traditional British, TTD, Sainsbury's*	1 Serving/100g	136	136	22.5	0.1	5.1	0.1

CASEROLE

	Measure INFO/WEIGHT	per Measure KCAL	Nutrition Values per 100g / 100ml				
			KCAL	PROT	CARB	FAT	FIBRE
Beef, With Dumplings, Eat Smart, Safeway* ·	1 Pack/390.9g	215	55	1.6	7.3	1.9	1.2
Beef, With Dumplings, GFY, Asda*	1 Pack/400g	416	104	11.0	10.0	2.2	0.9
Beef, With Herb Dumplings, COU, Marks & Spencer*	1/2 Pack/226g	215	95	8.5	9.6	2.3	1.6
Beef, With Herb Potatoes, Tesco*	1 Serving/475g	504	106	6.8	11.5	3.6	1.6
Beef, With Potatoes, Tesco*	1 Pack/475g	470	99	5.0	10.2	4.2	0.7
Chicken, & Asparagus in White Wine, Finest, Tesco*	1 Pack/350.3g	683	195	10.0	11.6	12.1	0.3
Chicken, & Asparagus in White Wine, Tesco*	1/2 Pack/300g	444	148	11.5	7.7	7.9	0.8
Chicken, & Asparagus, Healthy Living, Tesco*	1 Serving/450g	342	76	6.3	8.3	2.3	0.5
Chicken, & Dumplings, Healthy Living, Tesco*	1 Pack/450g	441	98	7.4	11.1	2.7	0.6
Chicken, & Dumplings, Morrisons*	1 Pack/300g	291	97	3.4	11.4	4.2	1.3
Chicken, & Dumplings, Sainsbury's*	1 Serving/450g	612	136	6.8	11.0	7.2	0.6
Chicken, & Herb Dumplings, BGTY, Sainsbury's*	1 Pack/450g	446	99	6.1	9.5	4.1	0.6
Chicken, & Red Wine, Duchy Originals*	1/2 Pack/175g	187	107	14.0	5.1	4.3	1.6
Chicken, & Tomato, Asda*	1/4 Pack/273g	569	208	16.0	2.2	15.0	0.5
Chicken, & Vegetable, Apetito*	1 Pack/330g	286	87	6.3	9.4	3.0	1.6
Chicken, & Vegetable, Long Life, Sainsbury's*	1 Pack/300g	186	62	4.6	7.4	1.5	0.8
Chicken, & White Wine, BGTY, Sainsbury's*	1 Serving/300g	216	72	7.2	5.9	2.2	1.3
Chicken, Catalan, TTD, Sainsbury's*	1/2 Pack/300g	324	108	10.8	4.4	5.2	0.6
Chicken, Fillets, Safeway*	1/2 Pack/172.2g	155	90	15.6	2.9	1.3	0.6
Chicken, GFY, Asda*	1 Pack/400g	316	79	6.0	8.0	2.5	1.4
Chicken, Leek & Mushroom, Tesco*	1 Pack/350g	382	109	4.5	8.6	6.3	1.0
Chicken, Mediterranean, Tesco*	1 Pack/400g	260	65	6.7	4.5	2.3	0.9
Chicken, Mini Favourites, Marks & Spencer*	1 Serving/200g	230	115	7.4	10.9	4.4	0.9
Chicken, Perfectly Balanced, Waitrose*	1 Pack/400g	392	98	6.6	9.8	3.6	1.2
Chicken, With Dumplings, Marks & Spencer*	1/2 Pack/227g	261	115	9.7	9.0	4.4	0.9
Chicken, With Dumplings, Somerfield*	1 Pack/450g	581	129	7.7	9.6	6.6	1.0
Chicken, With Herb Dumplings, COU, Marks & Spencer*	1/2 Pack/227.8g	205	90	10.6	7.2	1.9	0.6
Cowboy, Iceland*	1 Pack/400g	500	125	5.8	10.9	6.5	1.7
Lamb, & Rosemary, BGTY, Sainsbury's*	1 Serving/300g	192	64	7.1	6.8	0.9	0.6
Lamb, & Rosemary, Marks & Spencer*	1 Pack/454g	409	90	9.7	5.5	3.3	1.0
Lamb, BGTY, Sainsbury's*	1 Serving/200g	242	121	20.7	0.1	4.3	0.1
Lamb, Braised, British Classics, Tesco*	1 Pack/350g	333	95	7.5	4.6	5.2	1.2
Lamb, Marks & Spencer*	1 Pack/200g	260	130	6.2	10.6	6.8	1.2
Lamb, With Mint Dumplings, Minced, Sainsbury's*	1 Pack/450g	558	124	5.4	10.4	6.8	1.1
Mushroom, & Onion, Iceland*	1 Pack/400g	272	68	1.3	8.8	3.1	1.9
Pork, Normandy Style, Finest, Tesco*	1 Pack/450g	405	90	7.6	4.1	4.8	2.3
Pork, With Apple & Cider, Safeway*	1 Pack/450g	729	162	8.3	13.4	8.4	1.1
Rabbit	1oz/28g	29	102	11.6	2.6	5.1	0.4
Sausage	1oz/28g	46	165	11.9	5.1	10.9	0.9
Sausage, & Potato, Marks & Spencer*	1 Serving/200g	190	95	3.3	7.5	5.9	0.9
Steak, & Ale, British Classics, Tesco*	1 Serving/100g	93	93	11.2	4.5	3.4	1.1
Steak, & Ale, Sainsbury's*	1 Pack/300g	288	96	10.6	5.6	3.5	0.4
Steak, & Mushroom With Mustard Mash, Finest, Tesco*	1 Pack/550g	523	95	5.9	9.0	3.9	1.1
Steak, & Mushroom, Asda*	1/2 Pack/304.4g	410	135	7.0	4.2	10.0	0.3
Steak, Prime, Sainsbury's*	1oz/28g	34	122	22.6	0.1	3.5	0.1
Vegetable, & Lentil, Granose*	1 Pack/400g	220	55	2.8	7.9	1.4	0.0
Vegetable, Chunky, Marks & Spencer*	1 Bag/450g	90	20	0.7	3.4	0.3	1.4
Vegetable, Country, Sainsbury's*	1 Can/400g	300	75	2.2	11.0	2.5	1.1
Vegetable, Mixed, Safeway*	1 Serving/100g	17	17	0.7	3.0	0.3	2.1
Vegetable, Tesco*	1 Serving/220g	66	30	0.8	6.1	0.3	1.5
Vegetable, With Dumplings, Asda*	1 Pack/350g	343	98	2.7	12.0	4.3	2.1
Vegetable, With Herb Dumplings, COU, Marks & Spencer*	1 Pack/450g	270	60	1.6	10.1	1.2	1.0
Vegetable, With Potato Crush, Safeway*	1 Pack/450g	293	65	1.3	7.7	3.1	2.0

	Measure	per Measure		Nutrition Values per 100g / 100ml			
	INFO/WEIGHT	KCAL	KCAL	PROT	CARB	FAT	FIBRE
CASEROLE							
Venison, Scottish Wild, & Beaujolais, Tesco*	1 Pack/425g	366	86	11.9	4.9	2.1	0.6
CASSEROLE MIX							
Beef Bourguignon, Colman's*	1 Pack/40g	113	283	4.1	65.9	0.4	2.9
Beef, Authentic, Schwartz*	1 Pack/43g	111	257	7.4	54.5	1.0	0.4
Beef, Colman's*	1 Pack/40g	119	297	5.2	67.0	0.6	0.0
Beef, Schwartz*	1/2 Pack/21g	58	276	9.9	53.9	2.3	0.0
Chicken Chasseur, Asda*	1 Pack/80g	273	341	9.0	74.0	1.0	1.4
Chicken, Colman's*	1 Pack/40g	109	272	5.3	60.0	0.7	0.0
Chicken, Schwartz*	1/2 Pack/18g	55	304	10.6	62.8	1.2	0.0
Farmhouse Sausage, Schwartz*	1 Pack/39g	124	317	8.1	64.6	2.9	0.5
Liver & Bacon, Colman's*	1 Pack/40g	116	289	9.3	59.0	1.2	0.0
Peppered Beef, Schwartz*	1 Serving/80g	254	318	8.7	63.1	3.5	0.8
Pork, Colman's*	1 Serving/40g	117	293	5.3	65.5	1.1	3.4
Sausage, Asda*	1/4 Pack/25g	80	321	6.0	65.0	4.1	3.0
Sausage, Colman's*	1 Serving/40g	122	304	8.1	65.7	1.0	5.4
Turkey, Colman's*	1 Pack/50g	148	296	7.2	63.4	1.5	4.9
Vegetable, Co-Op*	1 Serving/100g	30	30	0.8	6.0	0.3	2.0
CATFISH							
Cooked	1 Fillet/87g	199	229	18.0	8.0	13.3	0.7
CAULIFLOWER							
& Broccoli Florets, Tesco*	1oz/28g	9	33	4.0	2.3	0.9	2.2
Boiled, Average	1oz/28g	8	28	2.9	2.1	0.9	1.6
Broccoli & Carrots, Morrisons*	1 Pack/1000g	260	26	2.3	2.1	1.0	0.0
Florets, Peas & Carrots, Frozen, Asda*	1 Serving/100g	37	37	3.0	5.0	0.6	2.8
Peas & Carrots, Birds Eye*	1oz/28g	9	32	2.2	4.8	0.4	2.6
Raw, Average	1oz/28g	9	31	3.3	2.7	0.8	1.6
CAULIFLOWER CHEESE							
& Broccoli, Morrisons*	1 Serving/500g	355	71	3.7	6.6	3.3	0.9
& Broccoli, Sainsbury's*	1 Serving/130g	83	64	4.8	7.6	1.6	2.7
2% Fat, Healthy Eating, Tesco*	1 Pack/400g	164	41	3.8	3.0	1.5	1.9
Asda*	1 Pack/454g	568	125	7.0	4.0	9.0	0.7
BFY, Morrisons*	1 Pack/300g	231	77	4.5	5.4	4.1	1.2
BGTY, Sainsbury's*	1 Pack/403g	238	59	5.4	6.5	1.3	1.0
Birds Eye*	1 Pack/329g	354	108	4.8	7.7	6.4	0.8
COU, Marks & Spencer*	1 Pack/300g	195	65	5.6	3.7	2.6	2.1
Eat Smart, Morrisons*	1 Pack/300g	192	64	4.9	6.7	2.0	1.5
Eat Smart, Safeway*	1 Pack/300g	165	55	4.5	4.0	2.1	1.0
Finest, Tesco*	1 Serving/250g	318	127	6.5	6.1	8.5	0.4
Frozen, Tesco*	1 Pack/400g	224	56	2.9	6.0	2.3	1.3
Great Value, Asda*	1 Pack/396g	352	89	3.9	4.9	6.0	0.8
Healthy Living, Tesco*	1/2 Pack/250g	160	64	6.5	3.8	2.6	1.0
Improved Recipe, Marks & Spencer*	1/2 Pack/225g	214	95	6.4	5.2	5.6	2.4
Made With Semi-Skimmed Milk	1oz/28g	28	100	6.0	5.2	6.4	1.3
Made With Skimmed Milk	1oz/28g	27	97	6.0	5.2	6.0	1.3
Made With Whole Milk	1oz/28g	29	105	6.0	5.2	6.9	1.3
Morrisons*	1 Pack/350g	399	114	5.5	3.8	8.5	1.4
Ross*	1 Pack/300g	300	100	4.9	5.5	6.6	0.1
Sainsbury's*	1 Pack/300g	357	119	6.4	7.8	6.9	0.9
Somerfield*	1 Serving/402.5g	322	80	4.6	3.1	5.5	1.8
TTD, Sainsbury's*	1/2 Pack/150g	252	168	6.9	8.0	12.0	0.9
Vegetarian, Safeway*	1 Serving/150g	138	92	4.7	5.2	5.8	1.4
Waitrose*	1 Pack/450g	419	93	5.0	5.3	5.8	0.9
With Crispy Bacon, Finest, Tesco*	1/3 Pack/166g	211	127	6.5	6.1	8.5	0.4

	Measure INFO/WEIGHT	per Measure KCAL	Nutrition Values per 100g / 100ml				
			KCAL	PROT	CARB	FAT	FIBRE
CAULIFLOWER CHEESE							
With Roasted Potatoes, Marks & Spencer*	1 Pack/200g	290	145	5.4	9.6	9.6	1.2
CAVATELLI							
Egg, Asda*	1 Serving/100g	203	203	9.0	34.0	3.4	3.0
King Prawn & Scallop, Marks & Spencer*	1 Pack/400g	600	150	6.4	18.0	5.6	1.3
CAVIAR							
Average	1oz/28g	26	92	12.0	0.5	4.7	0.0
CELERIAC							
Boiled in Salted Water	1oz/28g	4	15	0.9	1.9	0.5	3.2
CELERY							
Boiled in Salted Water	1 Med Serving/50g	4	8	0.5	0.8	0.3	1.2
Raw, Average	1 Med Stalk/40g	3	8	0.7	1.0	0.2	1.7
CELLANTANI							
Buitoni*	1 Serving/195g	706	362	12.2	74.4	1.7	0.0
CHAMPAGNE							
Average	1 Glass/120ml	89	76	0.3	1.4	0.0	0.0
CHANNA MASALA							
Indian, Sainsbury's*	1 Serving/149g	165	111	4.2	12.4	4.9	3.3
Marks & Spencer*	1 Pack/225g	360	160	5.6	11.2	10.5	8.2
Safeway*	1 Pack/400g	540	135	5.3	16.2	5.4	2.5
CHAPATIS							
Brown Wheat Flour, Waitrose*	1 Chapatis/42g	128	305	8.6	49.4	8.0	4.6
Elephant*	1 Serving/44.9g	129	287	7.5	53.1	6.4	3.2
Gujarati Style, Safeway*	1 Chapatis/40g	111	277	8.1	50.0	4.9	2.8
Indian Style, Asda*	1 Chapatis/43g	95	221	8.0	45.0	1.0	2.9
Made With Fat	1 Chapatis/60g	197	328	8.1	48.3	12.8	0.0
Made Without Fat	1 Chapatis/55g	111	202	7.3	43.7	1.0	0.0
Morrisons*	1 Chapatis/40g	105	269	8.6	49.8	6.9	0.0
Patak's*	1 Chapatis/42g	115	273	9.4	48.8	7.5	0.0
Spicy, Safeway*	1 Chapatis/41g	115	280	8.9	47.6	6.6	4.5
Wholemeal, Patak's*	1 Chapatis/42g	130	310	11.2	44.9	9.5	9.0
CHARD							
Swiss, Boiled in Unsalted Water	1oz/28g	6	20	1.9	3.2	0.1	0.0
Swiss, Raw	1oz/28g	5	19	1.8	2.9	0.2	0.0
CHEDDARS							
Cheese & Ham, Mini, McVitie's*	1 Bag/30g	160	534	11.0	55.5	29.8	2.0
Cheesy Beans, Mini, McVitie's*	1 Serving/30g	155	516	9.3	52.7	29.8	2.5
Peperami, Mini, McVitie's	1 Bag/30g	160	532	9.7	55.2	30.2	2.0
Smokey BBQ, McVitie's*	1 Sm Pack/30g	155	516	9.3	52.8	29.8	2.6
Tangy Salsa, Mini, McVitie's*	1 Bag/50g	266	532	11.0	54.7	29.9	2.1
Totally Cheesy, Crinkly's, Mini, McVitie's*	1 Pack/28g	143	512	9.9	57.0	27.1	1.9
CHEESE							
Ail & Fines Herbes, Boursin*	1oz/28g	116	414	7.0	2.0	42.0	0.0
Alternative To, Vegetarian, Average	1 Serving/30g	110	368	28.2	0.0	28.1	0.0
Appenzellar, Sainsbury's*	1 Serving/25g	97	386	25.4	0.0	31.6	0.0
Applewood, Somerfield*	1oz/28g	119	426	28.0	0.0	35.0	0.0
Asiago, Marks & Spencer*	1oz/28g	105	375	33.0	0.1	27.0	0.0
Babybel, Fromageries Bel*	1 Cheese/20g	62	308	23.0	0.0	24.0	0.0
Babybel, Light, Fromageries Bel*	1 Pack/40g	85	212	26.0	0.0	12.0	0.0
Babybel, Light, Mini, Fromageries Bel*	1 Mini Cheese/20g	43	214	26.5	0.0	12.0	0.0
Babybel, With Cheddar, Mini, Fromageries Bel*	1 Cheese/25g	94	374	25.0	1.0	30.0	0.0
Bavarian Smoked, Processed, Somerfield*	1oz/28g	85	302	29.0	0.0	21.0	0.0
Bavarian, Smoked, With Ham, Sainsbury's*	1 Serving/30g	89	298	19.4	0.8	24.1	0.0
Bleu d' Auvergne, Sainsbury's*	1 Serving/25g	84	335	22.0	2.0	26.5	0.0

C

CHEESE

	Measure INFO/WEIGHT	per Measure KCAL	KCAL	PROT	CARB	FAT	FIBRE
Bresse Bleu, Marks & Spencer*	1oz/28g	99	355	19.0	0.3	31.0	0.0
Brie, Average	1 Serving/25g	74	296	19.7	0.3	24.0	0.0
Brie, Reduced Fat, Average	1 Serving/50g	99	198	23.0	0.8	11.4	0.0
Caerphilly, Average	1 Serving/50g	187	374	23.0	0.1	31.3	0.0
Cambazola, Tesco*	1 Serving/30g	128	425	13.5	0.5	41.0	0.0
Camembert, Average	1 Serving/50g	141	283	20.5	0.1	22.2	0.0
Camembert, Breaded, Average	1 Serving/90g	307	342	16.7	14.3	23.3	0.5
Cantal, French, Sainsbury's*	1 Serving/30g	106	353	23.0	0.1	29.0	0.0
Cantenaar, Marks & Spencer*	1 Serving/28g	84	300	32.2	0.1	19.2	0.0
Chaumes, Marks & Spencer*	1oz/28g	85	305	20.2	1.0	26.0	0.0
Cheddar & Mozzarella, Spicy, Grated, Tesco*	1 Serving/40g	140	350	26.0	2.5	26.2	0.0
Cheddar, Canadian, Average	1 Serving/30g	123	409	25.0	0.1	34.3	0.0
Cheddar, Davidstow, Mature, Average	1 Serving/28g	115	410	25.0	0.1	34.4	0.0
Cheddar, Extra Mature, Average	1 Serving/30g	123	410	25.1	0.1	34.4	0.0
Cheddar, Grated, Average	1 Serving/50g	206	413	24.4	1.5	34.3	0.0
Cheddar, Mature, Average	1 Serving/30g	123	410	25.0	0.1	34.4	0.0
Cheddar, Mature, Grated, Average	1 Serving/28g	113	404	24.7	1.6	33.2	0.0
Cheddar, Mature, Reduced Fat, Average	1 Serving/25g	68	271	30.0	0.1	16.7	0.0
Cheddar, Medium, Average	1 Serving/30g	123	411	24.9	0.2	34.5	0.0
Cheddar, Mild, Average	1 Serving/30g	123	409	25.0	0.1	34.3	0.0
Cheddar, Reduced Fat, Average	1 Serving/30g	76	255	32.2	0.1	14.0	0.0
Cheddar, Smoked, Average	1 Serving/30g	123	411	25.3	0.1	34.4	0.0
Cheddar, West Country Farmhouse, Average	1 Serving/28g	115	410	25.0	0.1	34.4	0.0
Cheddar, Wexford, Average	1 Serving/20g	82	410	25.0	0.1	34.4	0.0
Cheddar, With Caramelised Onion, Sainsbury's*	1 Serving/28g	109	391	22.8	5.1	31.0	0.0
Cheddar, With Caramelised Onion, Tesco*	1 Serving/50g	183	366	21.4	7.1	28.0	0.4
Cheddar, With Onion & Chives, Davidson*	1 Serving/25g	100	400	24.3	0.6	33.3	0.0
Cheddar, With Pickled Onion Relish, Christmas, Tesco*	1/4 Cheese/50g	191	382	23.0	2.7	31.0	0.1
Cheddar, With Winter Berries, Christmas, Tesco*	1oz/28g	106	378	22.9	3.4	30.3	0.2
Cheestrings, Golden Vale*	1 Stick/21g	69	328	28.0	0.0	24.0	0.0
Cheshire	1oz/28g	106	379	24.0	0.1	31.4	0.0
Chevre Pave d'Affinois, Finest, Tesco*	1 Pack/150g	404	269	18.5	0.0	21.7	0.0
Cotswold, Full Fat With Herbs, Somerfield*	1oz/28g	113	405	25.0	0.0	34.0	0.0
Cottage, 1.5% Fat, Perfectly Balanced, Waitrose*	1/2 Pot/125g	108	86	14.3	3.7	1.5	0.3
Cottage, Arla*	1 Serving/25g	23	90	12.0	2.0	4.0	0.0
Cottage, BFY, Morrisons*	1 Pot/125g	110	88	13.0	6.9	0.9	0.0
Cottage, BGTY, Sainsbury's*	1oz/28g	25	91	12.1	8.4	0.9	0.2
Cottage, Crunchy Vegetable, GFY, Asda*	1 Serving/50g	37	74	11.0	4.5	1.3	0.6
Cottage, Danone*	1 Serving/100g	89	89	11.2	2.3	3.9	0.0
Cottage, Garlic & Herb, Diet, Yoplait*	1 Pot/225g	180	80	12.0	3.9	1.9	0.0
Cottage, Healthy Choice, Asda*	1oz/28g	25	88	13.0	4.0	2.0	0.0
Cottage, Less Than 5% Fat, Sainsbury's*	1/2 Pot/125g	131	105	12.3	4.4	4.2	0.0
Cottage, Low Fat, Loseley*	1 Pot/125g	148	118	13.3	2.0	6.0	0.0
Cottage, Low Fat, With Onion & Chive, Safeway*	1 Pot/250g	210	84	12.0	4.2	1.9	0.1
Cottage, Natural	1oz/28g	29	105	12.0	4.0	4.0	0.0
Cottage, Natural, 95% Fat Free, Marks & Spencer*	1oz/28g	28	99	11.6	3.5	4.0	0.0
Cottage, Natural, Asda*	1/4 Pot/113g	118	104	12.0	4.0	4.2	0.0
Cottage, Natural, BGTY, Sainsbury's*	1oz/28g	25	88	13.0	6.9	0.9	0.0
Cottage, Natural, COU, Marks & Spencer*	1/2 Pot/125g	100	80	11.9	3.3	1.8	0.3
Cottage, Natural, Deliciously Creamy, Marks & Spencer	1 Serving/50g	48	95	12.5	4.1	2.9	0.0
Cottage, Natural, Diet Choice, Waitrose*	1oz/28g	27	98	11.4	3.6	4.2	0.0
Cottage, Natural, Eat Smart, Safeway*	1 Pot/115g	93	81	11.8	3.4	1.8	0.3
Cottage, Natural, GFY, Asda*	1 Serving/113g	95	84	13.0	3.9	1.8	0.3

	Measure INFO/WEIGHT	per Measure KCAL	Nutrition Values per 100g / 100ml				
			KCAL	PROT	CARB	FAT	FIBRE
CHEESE							
Cottage, Natural, Healthy Choice, Safeway*	1oz/28g	24	87	12.7	4.0	2.0	0.0
Cottage, Natural, Healthy Living, Tesco*	1 Serving/150g	132	88	14.3	3.4	1.5	0.3
Cottage, Natural, Less Than 5% Fat, Sainsbury's*	1/2 Pot/131g	138	105	12.3	4.4	4.2	0.0
Cottage, Natural, Organic, Loseley*	1 Pot/250g	265	106	13.7	1.5	5.0	0.0
Cottage, Natural, Organic, Sainsbury's*	1 Pot/201g	185	92	12.8	6.3	1.8	0.0
Cottage, Natural, Organic, Tesco*	1/2 Pot/100g	78	78	11.9	3.6	1.8	0.0
Cottage, Natural, Perfectly Balanced, Waitrose*	1/2 Pot/125g	108	86	14.3	3.7	1.5	0.3
Cottage, Natural, SmartPrice, Asda	1/2 Pot/100g	86	86	12.0	4.3	2.0	0.0
Cottage, Natural, Somerfield*	1 Serving/100g	105	105	12.3	4.4	4.2	0.0
Cottage, Natural, Tesco*	1 Serving/50g	49	98	12.4	3.2	3.5	0.4
Cottage, Onion & Chive, Healthy Living, Tesco*	1 Serving/77g	59	77	11.0	4.5	1.7	0.2
Cottage, Onion & Chive, Waitrose*	1 Serving/20g	18	91	10.8	4.9	3.1	0.3
Cottage, Pineapple, Perfectly Balanced, Waitrose*	1 Pot/125g	105	84	10.4	6.7	1.7	0.2
Cottage, Plain	1oz/28g	27	98	13.8	2.1	3.9	0.0
Cottage, Plain, Reduced Fat	1oz/28g	22	78	13.3	3.3	1.4	0.0
Cottage, Red Onion & Garlic, Sainsbury's*	1/2 Tub/125g	91	73	10.4	5.8	0.9	0.6
Cottage, Slimline*	1 Serving/70g	43	62	12.0	3.0	0.2	0.0
Cottage, Stilton & Celery, BGTY, Sainsbury's*	1/2 Pot/125g	99	79	10.8	4.0	2.2	1.5
Cottage, Tropical, Westacre, Aldi*	1 Serving/100g	89	89	13.1	6.4	1.2	1.4
Cottage, Tuna & Sweetcorn, GFY, Asda*	1/2 Pot/113g	104	92	12.4	5.3	2.4	0.3
Cottage, Tuna & Sweetcorn, Morrisons*	1/4 Tub/63g	59	94	12.8	8.2	1.2	0.0
Cottage, Very Low Fat, Nisa Heritage*	1 Tub/227g	193	85	13.8	4.4	1.4	0.0
Cottage, Virtually Fat Free, Longley Farm*	1/2 Pot/125g	84	67	13.4	3.0	0.1	0.0
Cottage, Virtually Fat Free, Sainsbury's*	1oz/28g	22	80	12.9	6.5	0.3	0.0
Cottage, With Black Pepper, Healthy Eating, Tesco*	1 Pot/125g	101	81	12.1	4.0	1.8	0.0
Cottage, With Chargrilled Vegetables, BGTY, Sainsbury's*	1oz/28g	25	88	12.1	7.8	0.9	0.6
Cottage, With Chives, Good Intentions, Somerfield*	1 Pot/125g	101	81	10.8	3.2	2.8	0.0
Cottage, With Chives, Marks & Spencer*	1oz/28g	28	100	11.9	3.5	3.9	0.0
Cottage, With Chives, Somerfield*	1oz/28g	29	105	12.0	5.0	4.0	0.0
Cottage, With Coronation Chicken, BGTY, Sainsbury's*	1oz/28g	25	91	11.3	8.7	1.2	0.1
Cottage, With Cucumber & Mint, BGTY, Sainsbury's*	1/2 Pot/125g	103	82	12.0	6.6	0.9	0.0
Cottage, With Cucumber & Mint, COU, Marks & Spencer*	1 Pot/113g	85	75	11.6	3.1	1.5	0.2
Cottage, With Cucumber & Mint, Healthy Eating, Tesco*	1/2 Pot/125g	91	73	10.7	3.8	1.7	0.1
Cottage, With Lime & Coriander, Low Fat, Safeway*	1/2 Pot/126g	113	90	12.2	5.2	2.0	0.0
Cottage, With Mango & Peach, Healthy Eating, Tesco*	1 Pot/250g	188	75	10.4	4.8	1.6	0.1
Cottage, With Mango & Pineapple, BGTY, Sainsbury's*	1/2 Pot/125g	113	90	10.7	10.4	0.7	0.2
Cottage, With Mango & Pineapple, Morrisons*	1 Pot/125g	113	90	10.7	10.4	0.7	0.0
Cottage, With Mango, COU, Marks & Spencer*	1 Serving/100g	100	100	10.3	11.0	1.1	0.5
Cottage, With Onion & Chive, BGTY, Sainsbury's*	1 Serving/50g	42	83	12.4	6.4	0.9	0.1
Cottage, With Onion & Chive, GFY, Asda*	1 Serving/50g	43	85	12.0	4.4	1.9	0.1
Cottage, With Onion & Chive, Healthy Choice, Safeway*	1 Pot/125g	105	84	12.0	4.2	1.9	0.1
Cottage, With Onion & Chive, Healthy Living, Tesco*	1 Serving/300g	258	86	13.9	3.6	1.5	0.3
Cottage, With Onion & Chive, Tesco*	1 Serving/250g	235	94	10.9	3.7	4.0	0.0
Cottage, With Onion & Chives, Low Fat, Sainsbury's*	1oz/28g	28	99	11.6	4.4	4.0	0.1
Cottage, With Onion & Chives, Marks & Spencer*	1/4 Pot/65g	88	135	10.4	4.0	8.5	0.1
Cottage, With Onions & Chives, BFY, Morrisons*	1oz/28g	23	83	12.4	6.4	0.9	0.0
Cottage, With Peach & Mango, COU, Marks & Spencer*	1 Pot/113g	96	85	9.1	9.7	1.0	0.4
Cottage, With Pineapple, Asda*	1oz/28g	31	109	10.0	8.0	3.9	0.0
Cottage, With Pineapple, BGTY, Sainsbury's*	1oz/28g	24	84	10.5	8.9	0.7	0.1
Cottage, With Pineapple, Balanced Lifestyle, Aldi*	1 Serving/200g	140	70	11.0	4.4	0.9	1.5
Cottage, With Pineapple, GFY, Asda*	1 Pot/227g	193	85	9.0	10.0	1.0	0.5
Cottage, With Pineapple, Good Intentions, Somerfield*	1 Pot/125g	105	84	10.5	8.9	0.7	0.1
Cottage, With Pineapple, Healthy Living, Tesco*	1/2 Pot/125g	116	93	12.3	7.2	1.3	0.4

CHEESE

	Measure INFO/WEIGHT	per Measure KCAL	Nutrition Values per 100g / 100ml KCAL	PROT	CARB	FAT	FIBRE
Cottage, With Pineapple, Less Than 5% Fat, Sainsbury's*	1/2 Pot/125g	121	97	9.9	6.8	3.4	0.1
Cottage, With Pineapple, Low Fat, Waitrose*	1 Serving/40g	34	84	10.4	6.7	1.7	0.2
Cottage, With Pineapple, Tesco*	1 Serving/150g	158	105	9.1	9.8	3.3	0.1
Cottage, With Poached Salmon & Dill, GFY, Asda*	1/3 Pot/75g	65	86	12.0	2.3	2.7	0.6
Cottage, With Prawn & Cucumber, Safeway*	1 Serving/200g	184	92	12.0	4.7	2.5	0.1
Cottage, With Prawn Cocktail, BGTY, Sainsbury's*	1oz/28g	25	91	12.3	8.3	0.9	0.1
Cottage, With Prawn, GFY, Asda*	1oz/28g	22	79	10.0	6.0	1.7	0.3
Cottage, With Prawns, Marks & Spencer*	1 Serving/100g	95	95	13.4	4.3	2.6	0.0
Cottage, With Roasted Vegetables, Low Fat, Safeway*	1 Pot/125g	96	77	10.5	4.3	1.7	1.8
Cottage, With Salmon & Dill, Healthy Eating, Tesco*	1oz/28g	25	89	12.0	4.7	2.5	0.5
Cottage, With Smoked Cheese & Onion, GFY, Asda*	1 Serving/50g	39	78	12.0	3.9	1.6	0.4
Cottage, With Smoked Salmon & Dill, BGTY, Sainsbury's*	1oz/28g	25	89	13.8	6.4	0.9	0.1
Cottage, With Sweet Chilli Chicken, Marks & Spencer*	1 Serving/200g	190	95	13.8	4.7	2.1	0.5
Cottage, With Tomato & Cracked Black Pepper, Asda*	1/2 Pot/113g	86	76	10.0	3.1	2.1	1.3
Cottage, With Tuna & Cucumber, Safeway*	1 Serving/40g	35	87	12.0	3.7	2.5	0.1
Cottage, With Tuna & Pesto, Asda*	1 Serving/170g	184	108	10.0	3.5	6.0	0.7
Cottage, With Tuna & Sweetcorn, Healthy Living, Tesco*	1 Serving/150g	137	91	12.8	4.8	2.1	0.4
Cream	1 Portion/30g	132	439	3.1	0.0	47.4	0.0
Cream, Garlic & Herbs, Light, Boursin*	1 Portion/20g	28	140	12.0	2.5	9.0	0.0
Cream, Reduced Fat, Average	1 Seving/20g	23	117	13.0	4.0	5.3	0.1
Cream, With Onion & Chives, Morrisons*	1 Serving/20g	38	190	11.0	3.0	15.0	0.0
Cream, With Pineapple, Asda*	1 Serving/40g	77	193	8.0	11.0	13.0	0.0
Cream, With Red Peppers & Onion, GFY, Asda*	1 Serving/32.3g	42	130	13.0	6.0	6.0	0.0
Creamy Chaumes, Marks & Spencer*	1oz/28g	80	287	17.6	1.0	23.6	0.0
Creme De Saint Agur, Saint Agur*	1 Serving/75g	214	285	13.5	2.3	24.7	0.0
Danish Blue, Average	1 Serving/30g	106	352	20.8	0.0	29.1	0.0
Demi Pont L'eveque, Finest, Tesco*	1 Serving/46g	138	301	21.1	0.4	23.0	0.0
Dolcelatte, Average	1 Serving/30g	110	366	17.8	0.4	32.3	0.4
Double Gloucester, Average	1 Serving/30g	121	405	24.5	0.1	34.0	0.0
Double Gloucester, With Onion & Chives, Sainsbury's*	1 Serving/30g	110	365	22.2	5.5	28.2	0.0
Doux De Montagne, Average	1 Serving/25g	88	352	22.9	1.5	28.3	0.0
Dubliner, Irish Mature, Kerrygold*	1oz/28g	110	392	26.0	0.2	32.0	0.0
Edam, Average	1 Serving/10g	33	326	25.3	0.0	24.9	0.0
Edam, Dutch, Garlic & Herb Wedge, Asda*	1 Serving/60g	197	329	26.0	0.0	25.0	0.0
Edam, Reduced Fat, Average	1 Serving/30g	69	230	32.4	0.1	11.1	0.0
Edam, Slices, Average	1 Slice/30g	96	320	25.0	0.4	24.1	0.0
Emmental, Average	1 Serving/10g	37	369	28.4	0.0	28.4	0.0
Farmhouse, Healthy Range, Average	1 Serving/30g	78	261	30.4	0.1	15.4	0.0
Feta, Average	1 Serving/30g	79	262	16.3	1.0	21.5	0.0
Feta, With Green Olives, For Salad, Discover*	1oz/28g	75	267	19.0	1.0	21.0	0.0
Feta, With Herbs & Spices, For Salad, Discover*	1oz/28g	75	267	19.0	1.0	21.0	0.0
Feta, With Kalamata Olives, For Salad, Discover*	1oz/28g	75	267	19.0	1.0	21.0	0.0
Feta, With Red Pepper, For Salad, Discover*	1oz/28g	75	267	19.0	1.0	21.0	0.0
For Pizza, Grated, Average	1 Serving/50g	163	326	25.0	1.6	24.4	0.0
Garlic & Parsley Roule, Light, BGTY, Sainsbury's*	1 Pack/100g	176	176	17.6	1.6	11.0	0.0
Garlic Roule With Herbs, Somerfield*	1oz/28g	92	329	10.0	3.0	31.0	0.0
Goats With Roasted Vegetables, Somerfield*	1oz/28g	55	196	8.0	26.0	7.0	0.0
Goats, Average	1 Tsp/10g	26	262	13.8	3.8	21.2	0.0
Goats, Breaded, Bites, Sainsbury's*	1 Bite/24.9g	84	337	13.0	15.1	25.0	0.8
Goats, French, Mild, Average	1 Serving/30g	49	163	11.3	3.0	11.8	0.0
Goats, Premium, Average	1 Serving/30g	98	327	20.5	0.6	26.1	0.0
Goats, Welsh, With Garlic & Chives, Tesco*	1 Serving/32g	93	290	15.1	3.3	24.1	0.1
Goats, Welsh, With Herbs, Sainsbury's*	1 Serving/30g	90	299	15.3	3.6	24.8	0.1

C

CHEESE

INFO/WEIGHT	Measure	per Measure KCAL	KCAL	PROT	CARB	FAT	FIBRE
Gorgonzola, Average	1 Serving/30g	100	334	20.0	0.1	27.0	0.0
Gouda, Average	1 Serving/30g	113	376	24.0	0.0	31.5	0.0
Grana Padano, Italian Cheese, Waitrose*	1 Serving/14g	54	388	33.0	0.0	28.4	0.0
Greek Style, 50% Less Fat, BGTY, Sainsbury's*	1/2 Pack/50g	84	168	24.0	0.1	8.0	0.1
Gruyere	1oz/28g	115	409	27.2	0.0	33.3	0.0
Halloumi, Average	1 Serving/80g	253	316	20.8	1.6	24.7	0.0
Havarti, Danish, Sainsbury's*	1 Serving/100g	426	426	20.0	1.0	38.0	0.0
Italian, Grated, Average	1 Serving/30g	144	481	44.0	1.1	33.4	0.0
Jarlsberg, Tesco*	1 Serving/50g	184	368	28.5	0.0	28.2	0.0
Lancashire	1oz/28g	104	373	23.3	0.1	31.0	0.0
Leerdammer* Wedge	1 Wedge/250g	933	373	28.3	0.0	28.6	0.0
Light Salad, Discover*	1oz/28g	61	216	24.0	1.0	13.0	0.0
Mascarpone, 25% Less Fat, Sainsbury's*	1 Portion/30g	95	316	6.7	4.8	30.0	0.0
Mascarpone, Average	1 Serving/30g	131	437	5.6	4.1	43.6	0.0
Mild, Reduced Fat, Grated, Average	1 Serving/30g	70	235	31.5	2.2	11.1	0.0
Monterey Jack, Shredded, Kraft*	1/4 Cup/28g	101	360	22.0	3.6	28.8	0.0
Morbier, Sainsbury's*	1 Serving/10g	33	330	28.0	0.1	24.2	0.0
Mozzarella & Cheddar, Grated, Tesco*	1 Serving/40g	131	327	25.0	2.5	24.1	0.0
Mozzarella, Average	1 Serving/50g	137	275	21.2	1.2	20.6	0.0
Mozzarella, Reduced Fat, Average	1 Serving/50g	92	184	21.2	1.0	10.3	0.0
Norvegia, Sliced Light, Tine*	1 Slice/10g	27	272	32.0	0.0	16.0	0.0
Parmesan, Average	1 Tbsp/10g	40	401	35.2	0.0	29.4	0.0
Pastrami Flavour, Sandwich, Swiss Processed, Gerber*	2 Slices/25g	87	348	24.0	0.0	28.0	0.0
Pecorino, Italian, Tesco*	1 Serving/30g	119	397	22.0	0.0	33.0	0.0
Poivre, Boursin*	1oz/28g	116	414	7.0	2.0	42.0	0.0
Port Salut, Marks & Spencer*	1oz/28g	90	322	21.0	1.0	26.0	0.0
Provolone Piccante, Sainsbury's*	1 Serving/30g	119	398	25.0	0.2	33.0	0.0
Quark, Average	1 Serving/20g	13	66	11.9	4.0	0.2	0.0
Red Leicester, Average	1 Serving/30g	120	400	23.8	0.1	33.7	0.0
Red Leicester, Reduced Fat, Average	1/4 Pack/75g	196	261	30.2	0.1	15.4	0.0
Ricotta, Average	1 Serving/50g	67	134	9.3	2.9	9.5	0.0
Roquefort	1oz/28g	105	375	19.7	0.0	32.9	0.0
Roule, French, Sainsbury's*	1 Serving/30g	96	321	8.5	3.0	30.5	0.0
Sage Derby	1oz/28g	113	402	24.2	0.1	33.9	0.0
Saint Agur, Marks & Spencer*	1 Serving/25g	91	363	16.0	0.2	33.5	0.0
Selles Sur Cher, TTD, Sainsbury's*	1 Serving/30g	89	296	20.0	0.1	24.0	0.0
Shropshire, Blue, Average	1 Serving/50g	196	391	21.1	0.1	34.3	0.0
Soft, & Creamy With Onions & Garlic, GFY, Asda*	1 Serving/25g	32	126	13.0	5.0	6.0	0.0
Soft, & Creamy With Pineapple, Asda*	1 Serving/32.1g	62	193	8.0	11.0	13.0	0.0
Soft, Creamy, With Onion & Chives, BGTY, Sainsbury's*	1 Serving/20g	23	115	13.5	4.0	5.0	1.0
Soft, Creamy, With Shallots & Chives, BGTY, Sainsbury's*	1 Serving/20g	47	235	5.8	2.2	22.5	0.0
Soft, Double Gloucester, & Chives, Marks & Spencer*	1oz/28g	100	358	20.0	9.2	26.8	0.0
Soft, Extra Light, Average	1 Serving/20g	25	125	14.3	3.6	5.9	0.1
Soft, Fruit & Rum Halo, Discover*	1oz/28g	116	416	8.6	11.7	34.1	0.0
Soft, Full Fat, Average	1 Serving/50g	156	312	8.2	1.7	30.3	0.0
Soft, Garlic & Herb, Extra Light, Healthy Living, Tesco*	1 Serving/50g	63	126	13.5	5.6	5.5	0.0
Soft, Garlic & Herb, Marks & Spencer*	1oz/28g	58	206	8.5	2.7	18.0	0.0
Soft, Garlic & Herb, Medium Fat, Safeway*	1 Serving/10g	20	195	9.3	4.9	15.0	0.0
Soft, Garlic & Herb, Soft & Creamy, Extra Light, Asda*	1/4 Pack/50g	65	130	13.0	6.0	6.0	0.0
Soft, Goats Milk	1oz/28g	55	198	13.1	1.0	15.8	0.0
Soft, Herbs & Garlic, Creamery, Light, Sainsbury's*	1 Serving/30g	54	180	7.2	3.4	15.5	0.3
Soft, Light, Average	1 Serving/30g	54	179	12.1	3.2	13.1	0.0
Soft, Medium Fat, Average	1 Serving/30g	62	207	8.4	3.0	17.9	0.0

C

INFO/WEIGHT	Measure	per Measure KCAL	Nutrition Values per 100g / 100ml				
			KCAL	PROT	CARB	FAT	FIBRE

CHEESE

	Measure	per Measure KCAL	KCAL	PROT	CARB	FAT	FIBRE
Soft, Onion & Chive, Low Fat, BGTY, Sainsbury's*	1 Serving/30g	35	115	13.5	4.0	5.0	1.0
Soft, Orange Halo, Discover*	1oz/28g	110	394	8.1	7.9	35.3	0.0
Soft, Philadelphia, & Breadsticks, Light, Kraft*	1 Portion/50g	119	238	8.5	24.5	12.0	1.1
Soft, Philadelphia, Blue, Kraft*	1 Serving/28g	76	270	6.8	3.4	25.5	0.2
Soft, Philadelphia, Extra Light, Kraft*	1oz/28g	28	101	11.0	3.0	5.0	0.6
Soft, Philadelphia, Garlic & Herb, Light, Kraft*	1oz/28g	50	180	7.2	3.4	15.5	0.2
Soft, Philadelphia, Kraft*	1oz/28g	78	280	6.0	2.5	27.5	0.1
Soft, Philadelphia, Light, Kraft*	1oz/28g	53	190	7.6	3.4	16.0	0.3
Soft, Philadelphia, Light, Snack, Kraft*	1 Pack/50g	123	246	8.4	23.0	13.2	1.6
Soft, Philadelphia, Mini Tubs, Extra Light, Kraft*	1 Mini Tub/35g	39	111	11.0	4.8	5.2	0.0
Soft, Philadelphia, Mini Tubs, Light, Kraft*	1 Tub/35g	57	163	7.1	2.9	14.0	0.0
Soft, Philadelphia, Tomato & Basil, Light, Kraft*	1 Tbsp/20g	38	190	7.6	4.3	16.0	0.5
Soft, Philadelphia, With Chive & Onion, Kraft*	1 Serving/25g	73	290	6.5	6.5	29.0	0.0
Soft, Philadelphia, With Chives, Light, Kraft*	1oz/28g	52	185	7.5	3.4	15.5	0.3
Soft, Philadelphia, With Ham, Light, Kraft*	1oz/28g	52	184	7.9	4.3	15.0	0.2
Soft, Pineapple Halo, Discover*	1oz/28g	107	383	7.0	16.7	30.9	0.0
Soft, Pineapple, Light, Safeway*	1 Serving/25g	48	190	7.6	10.8	12.5	0.0
Soft, With Black Pepper, Light, Sainsbury's*	1/2 Pack/100g	205	205	11.0	3.0	16.5	0.0
Soft, With Cracked Pepper, Marks & Spencer*	1 Serving/40g	44	110	13.0	4.2	4.5	0.3
Soft, With Garlic & Herbs, Full Fat, Deli, Boursin*	1 Serving/28g	84	299	3.5	5.0	29.5	0.0
Soft, With Garlic & Herbs, Sainsbury's*	1 Serving/33g	89	269	6.1	2.7	26.0	0.0
Soft, With Onion & Chives, Extra Light, Tesco*	1 Serving/30g	36	121	12.9	5.0	5.3	0.0
Soft, With Onion & Chives, Marks & Spencer*	1/4 Pack/37.5g	38	100	10.7	4.4	4.7	1.2
Soya	1oz/28g	89	319	18.3	0.0	27.3	0.0
Stilton, Average	1 Serving/30g	123	410	22.4	0.1	35.5	0.0
Stilton, Blue, Average	1 Serving/30g	124	412	22.8	0.1	35.7	0.0
Stilton, White	1oz/28g	101	362	19.9	0.1	31.3	0.0
Stilton, White, & Apricot, Marks & Spencer*	1oz/28g	94	337	13.8	18.5	23.1	0.0
Stilton, White, & Cranberry, Marks & Spencer*	1oz/28g	101	362	18.2	15.5	25.3	0.0
Stilton, White, With Apricot, Somerfield*	1oz/28g	103	369	16.0	8.0	30.0	0.0
Stilton, White, With Cranberries, Tesco*	1 Serving/50g	184	368	15.8	9.5	29.7	0.7
Stilton, White, With Mango & Ginger, Tesco*	1/3 Pack/65g	228	350	13.1	25.8	21.6	0.6
Substitute, Mozzarella Style, Grated, Value, Tesco*	1 Serving/40g	120	300	25.0	2.5	21.1	0.0
Supreme Des Ducs, Ligne Et Plaisir*	1 Serving/50g	100	200	21.0	2.0	12.0	0.0
Taleggio, Tesco*	1 Serving/25g	74	297	18.0	0.0	25.0	0.0
Wensleydale With Cranberries, Sainsbury's*	1 Serving/50g	180	359	20.7	6.4	27.8	0.0
Wensleydale, Average	1 Serving/25g	92	369	22.5	0.1	31.0	0.1

CHEESE ON TOAST

	Measure	per Measure KCAL	KCAL	PROT	CARB	FAT	FIBRE
Average	1oz/28g	106	380	13.8	23.8	26.3	0.7

CHEESE PUFFS

	Measure	per Measure KCAL	KCAL	PROT	CARB	FAT	FIBRE
Cheeky, Tesco*	1 Bag/20g	108	542	6.7	50.2	34.9	0.0
Sainsbury's*	1 Pack/100g	530	530	9.1	51.4	32.0	1.9
Shapers, Boots*	1 Bag/16g	84	523	6.4	59.0	29.0	1.6
SmartPrice, Asda*	1 Bag/18g	92	512	7.0	58.0	28.0	1.3
Value, Tesco*	1 Bag/18g	90	498	7.7	54.1	27.9	1.7

CHEESE SINGLES

	Measure	per Measure KCAL	KCAL	PROT	CARB	FAT	FIBRE
50% Less Fat, BGTY, Sainsbury's*	1 Slice/20g	38	190	18.0	7.0	10.0	0.0
American, 2% Milk, Kraft*	1 Slice/19g	45	237	21.0	5.3	15.8	0.0
Half Fat, Co-Op*	1 Slice/20g	47	235	25.0	7.0	12.0	0.0
Healthy Living, Tesco*	1 Slice/20g	39	195	19.2	7.1	10.0	0.0
Kraft*	1 Single/20g	52	260	13.5	7.6	18.5	0.0
Light, Kraft*	1 Slice/20g	41	205	20.0	6.0	11.0	0.0
Light, Safeway*	1 Slice/20g	38	192	21.2	4.2	10.0	0.0

CHEESE SLICES

INFO/WEIGHT	KCAL	KCAL	PROT	CARB	FAT	FIBRE
40% Less Fat, Iceland*	1 Slice/20.1g	41	204	18.0	6.0	12.0	0.0
97% Fat Free, Kraft*	1 Slice/20g	31	155	23.3	9.9	2.3	0.0
BFY, Morrisons*	1 Slice/20g	39	196	21.0	5.4	10.0	0.0
Bavarian Smoked, Asda*	1 Slice/18g	50	277	17.0	0.4	23.0	0.0
Bettabuy, Morrisons*	1 Slice/17g	47	274	14.0	4.0	22.5	0.0
Cheese Food, Asda*	1 Slice/20g	58	289	18.0	7.0	21.0	0.0
Cheese Food, Sainsbury's*	1 Slice/20g	52	260	14.5	5.4	20.0	0.0
Dairylea*	1 Slice/25g	76	305	13.0	8.0	24.5	0.0
Farmfoods*	1 Slice/17g	49	286	18.0	4.0	22.0	0.0
Half Fat, Asda*	1 Slice/20g	39	194	20.6	5.4	10.0	0.0
Half Fat, Co-Op*	1 Slice/20g	47	235	25.0	7.0	12.0	0.0
Half Fat, Marks & Spencer*	1 Slice/30g	83	277	31.0	0.1	17.0	0.0
Jarlsberg*	1 Slice/15g	54	360	27.0	0.0	27.0	0.0
Kraft*	1 Slice/20g	56	280	13.5	6.6	21.5	0.0
Light & Fine, Milbona*	1 Slice/20g	37	183	19.0	4.3	10.0	0.0
Light, Aldi*	1 Slice/19.9g	41	206	20.1	8.1	10.4	0.9
Light, Dairylea*	1 Slice/22.5g	34	149	15.0	6.3	7.0	0.0
Light, Laughing Cow*	1 Slice/20g	41	203	21.0	6.0	10.5	0.0
Light, Thick, Dairylea*	1 Slice/25g	51	205	17.3	8.6	10.5	0.0
Lightlife, Leerdammer*	1 Slice/20g	55	273	30.6	0.0	16.4	0.0
Low Fat, Healthy Living, Tesco*	1 Slice/27g	52	193	36.1	6.0	2.7	0.0
Mature, Medium Fat, Healthy Eating, Tesco*	1 Slice/30g	78	259	30.9	0.0	15.0	0.0
Reduced Fat, GFY, Asda*	1 Slice/19.9g	38	191	21.0	4.2	10.0	0.0
Safeway*	1 Slice/20.1g	56	279	15.2	7.2	21.0	0.0
SmartPrice, Asda*	1 Slice/16.6g	48	283	14.0	5.0	23.0	0.0
Tesco*	1 Slice/20g	55	275	14.2	7.2	21.0	0.0
Thick, Dairylea*	1 Slice/25g	70	280	13.0	9.5	21.0	0.0
White, 85% Fat Free, Kerry*	1 Slice/20g	54	270	33.0	0.1	15.0	0.0

CHEESE SPREAD

60% Less Fat, Asda*	1 Serving/30g	52	174	16.0	7.3	9.0	0.0
Asda*	1 Serving/33g	92	280	9.0	7.0	24.0	0.0
BFY, Morrisons*	1 Serving/25g	43	172	13.5	6.5	8.5	0.0
BGTY, Sainsbury's*	1 Serving/25g	28	111	11.0	4.3	5.5	0.4
Cheese & Garlic, Primula*	1 Serving/20g	49	247	15.7	4.3	18.6	0.0
Cheese & Salmon With Dill, Primula*	3 Inches/10g	26	261	17.6	3.8	19.5	0.0
Cheez Whiz, Original, Light, 41% Less Fat, Kraft*	2 Tbsp/30g	63	210	15.7	11.7	11.3	0.0
Cream, Light, Sainsbury's*	1 Serving/50g	94	187	7.8	4.1	15.5	0.3
Creamery, Light, Sainsbury's*	1 Serving/25g	46	185	9.0	3.5	15.0	0.0
Dairylea*	1oz/28g	69	245	10.5	6.0	19.5	0.0
Flavoured	1oz/28g	72	258	14.2	4.4	20.5	0.0
Garlic & Herbs, Light, Benecol*	1 Serving/20g	35	174	7.8	4.2	14.0	0.7
Happy Shopper*	1 Serving/30g	64	213	11.0	8.5	15.0	0.0
Healthy Eating, Tesco*	1/4 Pot/25g	47	187	20.0	6.5	9.0	0.0
Kerrygold*	1oz/28g	60	213	11.0	8.5	15.0	0.0
Light, Half Fat, Dairylea*	1 Serving/25g	40	161	12.0	8.2	8.7	0.0
Light, Laughing Cow*	1 Triangle/18g	26	143	13.1	6.3	6.9	0.0
Light, New, Dairylea*	1 Serving/22.5g	34	149	15.0	6.3	7.0	0.0
Light, Primula*	1oz/28g	39	141	18.8	4.1	5.5	0.5
Light, Tub, Dairylea*	1oz/28g	52	186	14.0	7.3	11.0	0.0
Low Fat, Weight Watchers*	1 Serving/50g	56	112	18.1	3.4	2.9	1.2
Mediterranean Soft & Creamy, Extra Light, Asda*	1 Serving/32g	42	130	13.0	6.0	6.0	0.0
Morrisons*	1 Serving/3g	7	225	10.0	7.0	17.5	0.0
Original, Primula*	1oz/28g	72	257	16.0	1.0	21.0	0.0

C

	Measure INFO/WEIGHT	per Measure KCAL	Nutrition Values per 100g / 100ml				
			KCAL	PROT	CARB	FAT	FIBRE
CHEESE SPREAD							
Soft, Low Fat, Marks & Spencer*	1 Pack/100g	111	111	13.0	4.2	4.5	0.3
The Laughing Cow*	1 Portion/17.5g	46	269	10.0	6.5	22.5	0.0
With Chives, Primula*	1oz/28g	71	253	15.0	1.0	21.0	0.0
With Ham, Primula*	1oz/28g	71	253	15.0	1.0	21.0	0.0
With Shrimp, Primula*	1 Tbsp/15g	38	253	15.0	1.0	21.0	0.0
CHEESE STRAWS							
& Bacon, Party, Tesco*	2 Straws/25g	80	321	10.5	23.8	20.4	2.1
Cheddar, Marks & Spencer*	1 Straw/11g	59	535	14.9	40.1	34.9	2.4
Finest, Tesco*	1 Straw/7g	39	558	13.3	41.5	37.6	1.5
Fudges*	1 Serving/10g	53	534	14.9	40.1	34.9	0.0
Homemade Or Bakery, Average	1 Straw/41g	173	422	12.0	24.2	30.7	0.7
Selection, Sainsbury's*	1 Straw/7g	41	558	16.6	34.5	39.3	2.8
Selection, Somerfield*	1 Straw/7g	39	558	13.3	41.5	37.6	1.5
Twists, Tesco*	1 Serving/20g	99	494	14.0	46.4	28.0	4.2
CHEESE STRINGS							
Double Cheese Flavour, The Golden Vale*	1 Stick/21g	69	328	28.0	0.0	24.0	0.0
CHEESE STRIPS							
Dairylea*	1 Pack/21g	72	345	23.5	0.4	27.0	0.0
CHEESE TRIANGLES							
Average	1 Triangle/14g	35	247	10.6	6.6	19.9	0.0
Reduced Fat, Average	1 Triangle/18g	30	170	14.8	7.4	9.0	0.0
CHEESE TWISTS							
All Butter, Marks & Spencer*	1/2 Pack/62.6g	312	495	14.0	46.4	28.0	4.2
Asda*	1 Stick/8g	42	500	14.0	48.0	28.0	5.0
Safeway*	2 Twists/11.8g	60	496	13.6	46.2	28.5	5.6
CHEESECAKE							
American Red White & Blueberry, Sainsbury's*	1/6th/83g	264	318	3.8	35.1	18.5	0.4
Apple & Cinnamon, Baked, Marks & Spencer*	1 Portion/116.4g	389	335	3.7	39.7	18.9	2.1
Apricot, Healthy Living, Tesco*	1 Pot/100g	179	179	4.9	34.7	2.3	1.6
Average	1oz/28g	119	426	3.7	24.6	35.5	0.4
Blackcurrant Swirl, Heinz*	1/5 Portion/87g	241	277	4.1	30.3	15.4	3.6
Blackcurrant, Half Fat, Waitrose*	1 Slice/106g	201	190	3.6	36.0	3.5	4.0
Blackcurrant, Marks & Spencer*	1oz/28g	82	293	3.3	29.4	17.9	0.9
Blackcurrant, Sainsbury's*	1oz/28g	75	267	3.2	29.5	15.1	1.1
Blackcurrant, Value, Tesco*	1 Serving/70g	174	248	2.8	31.4	12.3	1.0
Blueberry & Lemon Flavour Wedges, Sainsbury's*	1 Serving/80g	262	327	5.1	29.2	21.1	1.2
Caramel Swirl, Cadbury*	1 Slice/91g	373	410	6.0	40.1	25.8	0.0
Cherry, BGTY, Sainsbury's*	1 Serving/91g	181	199	4.6	35.5	4.3	0.5
Cherry, Low Fat, Tesco*	1 Serving/91g	185	203	3.4	38.0	4.1	0.9
Chocolate & Hazelnut, Sara Lee*	1 Serving/65g	224	345	6.5	31.2	21.4	1.2
Chocolate & Hazelnut, Gold, Sara Lee*	1 Slice/65g	205	316	5.9	28.7	19.7	1.1
Chocolate & Vanilla, Reduced Fat, Marks & Spencer*	1 Portion/114g	319	280	7.0	37.9	12.0	1.5
Chocolate Brownie, Tesco*	1 Serving/101g	391	387	5.0	36.3	24.6	1.4
Chocolate Chip, Marks & Spencer*	1oz/28g	109	391	5.1	39.7	23.6	0.2
Chocolate Swirl, Deeply Delicious, Heinz*	1/5 Slice/81.5g	221	271	4.6	37.4	11.5	4.7
Chocolate Truffle, Healthy Living, Tesco*	1 Slice/96g	250	260	10.3	23.7	13.8	6.5
Chocolate Truffle, TTD, Sainsbury's*	1 Serving/99g	386	390	4.1	35.2	25.9	4.7
Chocolate, & Irish Cream Liqueur, Tesco*	1 Serving/93g	385	414	5.0	30.7	30.1	0.8
Chocolate, American Style, Asda*	1 Serving/390g	1486	381	5.0	43.0	21.0	6.0
Chocolate, Baked, Ultimate, Entenmann's*	1 Serving/100g	331	331	5.7	34.2	19.0	2.8
Chocolate, Family, Safeway*	1 Serving/100g	385	385	7.2	35.0	23.8	1.6
Chocolate, Marks & Spencer*	1oz/28g	106	380	6.5	40.3	21.5	0.4
Chocolate, Pure Indulgence, Thorntons*	1 Serving/75g	308	410	5.6	44.3	23.4	0.6

CHEESECAKE

INFO/WEIGHT	Measure	per Measure KCAL	Nutrition Values per 100g / 100ml				
			KCAL	PROT	CARB	FAT	FIBRE
Chocolate, Tesco*	1 Serving/91g	317	348	6.2	37.8	19.1	1.5
Chocolate, Weight Watchers*	1 Cheesecake/95g	143	151	7.5	20.7	4.0	0.7
Citrus, Good Choice, Mini, Iceland*	1 Cheesecake/111g	198	178	3.5	31.6	4.2	0.4
Devonshire Strawberry, McVitie's*	1/6 Portion/66g	192	291	4.4	31.8	16.2	3.6
Double Chocolate Wedge, Sainsbury's*	1 Portion/75g	327	436	5.7	29.0	33.0	1.7
Fudge, Tesco*	1 Serving/102g	384	376	4.6	37.5	23.1	0.5
Homestyle Chocolate, Marks & Spencer*	1oz/28g	105	376	6.0	38.0	22.2	0.7
Irish Cream, McVitie's*	1/4 Slice/190g	616	324	4.4	33.0	19.4	0.4
Lemon Creamy & Light, Marks & Spencer*	1/6 Cake/67.5g	238	350	3.5	32.3	20.4	0.4
Lemon Curd, Waitrose*	1/4 Cake/138g	533	386	4.7	28.9	27.9	2.3
Lemon Meringue, Tesco*	1 Wedge/94g	353	375	3.8	30.1	26.6	0.3
Lemon, BGTY, Sainsbury's*	1/6 Cake/71g	142	200	4.4	37.0	3.8	0.5
Lemon, Carb Control, Tesco*	1 Serving/85g	269	316	8.6	9.6	27.1	11.1
Lemon, Marks & Spencer*	1oz/28g	92	330	5.7	38.7	17.1	0.2
Lemon, Sainsbury's*	1 Serving/180g	650	361	4.0	39.9	20.6	1.3
Lemon, Tesco*	1 Slice/93g	315	339	5.2	28.6	22.6	0.3
Lemon, Value, Tesco*	1 Serving/78.6g	222	281	4.3	32.2	15.0	4.2
Mandarin, GFY, Asda*	1 Serving/97g	194	200	4.0	36.0	4.4	0.8
Mandarin, Healthy Choice, Safeway*	1 Serving/92g	189	205	3.8	37.1	4.6	0.4
Mandarin, Low Fat, Tesco*	1 Serving/70g	145	207	3.3	37.0	4.7	1.4
Praline, Asda*	1/8 Cake/62g	226	364	7.0	30.0	24.0	3.2
Raspberry Brulee, Marks & Spencer*	1 Serving/100g	255	255	5.7	29.7	12.9	2.1
Raspberry Rapture, Tesco*	1 Serving/109.5g	332	302	3.8	25.4	20.6	0.6
Raspberry Ripple, Marks & Spencer*	1oz/28g	84	300	5.9	32.8	15.6	0.3
Raspberry Swirl, Heinz*	1 Serving/100g	266	266	3.9	30.1	14.5	2.8
Raspberry, Marks & Spencer*	1 Slice/105g	331	315	5.0	32.2	20.5	1.0
Raspberry, Perfectly Balanced, Waitrose*	1 Serving/106g	212	200	4.0	36.2	3.5	1.7
Rhubarb Crumble, Sainsbury's*	1 Serving/114g	268	235	3.1	34.8	9.3	2.4
Sticky Toffee, Iceland*	1 Pack/116g	331	285	3.8	33.9	14.9	0.1
Sticky Toffee, Tesco*	1 Slice/66g	248	375	4.0	35.3	24.2	0.5
Strawberries & Cream, Finest, Tesco*	1 Serving/104.2g	324	312	4.3	25.3	21.5	0.5
Strawberry Shortcake, Sara Lee*	1/6 Slice/68.2g	229	337	4.9	27.6	23.0	0.5
Strawberry, 95% Fat Free, Marks & Spencer*	1 Slice/98g	187	191	5.1	33.8	4.0	0.3
Strawberry, Finest, Tesco*	1 Slice/113g	383	339	4.8	30.1	22.2	0.9
Strawberry, Fresh, Marks & Spencer*	1/4 Cake/125g	300	240	2.8	23.1	15.4	1.1
Strawberry, Heinz*	1 Pack/245g	588	240	3.4	28.1	12.7	2.4
Strawberry, Sainsbury's*	1 Serving/90g	221	246	3.5	24.4	14.9	4.6
Summerfruit, GFY, Asda*	1/4 Cake/130g	259	199	2.8	36.0	4.7	2.0
The Ultimate New York Baked, Entenmann's*	1 Cake/100g	347	347	4.2	35.7	21.3	0.9
Toffee & Pecan, Wedge, Sainsbury's*	1 Serving/75g	296	395	5.4	28.1	29.0	3.1
Toffee, American Style, Asda*	1 Serving/75g	269	359	4.5	38.0	21.0	3.8
Toffee, Asda*	1 Cake/87g	295	339	4.3	31.0	22.0	3.5
Toffee, Marks & Spencer*	1 Serving/105g	357	340	5.2	37.2	21.5	0.9
Toffee, Tesco*	1 Serving/100g	265	265	4.3	33.1	12.9	0.8
Vanilla Chocolate, Baked, Slice, Sainsbury's*	1 Slice/90g	349	388	5.7	33.8	25.6	2.7
Vanilla, Tesco*	1 Serving/115g	417	363	5.7	29.4	24.7	0.6

CHEETOS

Cheese, Walkers*	1 Bag/24g	120	500	6.5	61.0	26.0	1.3

CHEEZLY

Cheddar Style, Garlic & Herb Flavoured, Redwood Foods*	1 Pack/190g	473	249	3.6	19.4	17.4	0.0
Cream, Garlic & Herb Flavour, Redwood Foods*	1 Pack/113g	360	319	5.8	5.4	30.5	0.0
Cream, Original Flavour, Redwood Foods*	1 Pack/113g	357	316	5.6	4.8	30.5	0.0
Cream, Sour Cream & Chive Flavour, Redwood Foods*	1 Pack/113g	359	318	5.7	5.1	30.5	0.0

	Measure INFO/WEIGHT	per Measure KCAL	Nutrition Values per 100g / 100ml				
			KCAL	PROT	CARB	FAT	FIBRE
CHEEZLY							
Feta Style, In Oil, Redwood Foods*	1 Pack/190g	903	475	2.5	10.6	47.0	0.0
Grated Cheddar Style, Redwood Foods*	1 Pack/150g	242	161	3.1	21.5	7.5	0.0
Mature Cheddar Style, Redwood Foods*	1 Pack/190g	490	258	3.9	19.2	18.4	0.0
Mature Cheddar Style, With Cranberries, Redwood Foods*	1 Pack/190g	454	239	3.2	24.3	14.3	0.0
Nacho Style, Redwood Foods*	1 Pack/190g	321	169	3.3	21.1	7.9	0.0
White Cheddar Style, Redwood Foods*	1 Pack/190g	321	169	3.3	21.1	7.9	0.0
CHERRIES							
Black, In Syrup, Average	1 Serving/242g	160	66	0.6	16.0	0.0	0.7
Dried, Sainsbury's*	2 Tbsp/28g	89	319	3.8	72.4	1.5	6.2
Glace, Average	1oz/28g	79	281	0.4	71.2	0.2	1.1
Raw, Average	1oz/28g	14	49	0.9	11.3	0.1	1.5
Stewed With Sugar	1oz/28g	23	82	0.7	21.0	0.1	0.7
Stewed Without Sugar	1oz/28g	12	42	0.8	10.1	0.1	0.8
CHESTNUTS							
Average	1 Nut/10g	17	170	2.0	36.6	2.7	4.1
CHEWING GUM							
Extra, Peppermint, Sugar Free, Wrigleys*	2 Pieces/4g	6	155	0.0	39.0	0.0	0.0
Spearmint, Wrigleys*	1 Piece/3g	9	295	0.0	73.0	0.0	0.0
CHICK PEAS							
Dried, Average	1oz/28g	89	319	21.7	47.4	5.4	8.0
Dried, Boiled, Average	1 Serving/75g	85	114	7.3	16.4	2.2	2.6
In Salted Water, Canned, Average	1 Can/179g	204	114	7.2	14.9	2.9	4.1
In Water, Canned, Average	1 Can/250g	283	113	7.2	15.3	2.6	4.8
CHICKEN							
Balls, Chinese, Marks & Spencer*	1 Ball/16g	45	280	10.8	29.2	13.6	2.1
Balls, Crispy, Marks & Spencer*	1 Ball/16g	35	220	13.3	23.7	8.1	0.5
Balls, Lemon, Asda*	1 Ball/15g	42	279	14.0	19.0	17.0	1.6
Bites, Battered, Tesco*	1 Pack/200g	440	220	15.2	7.6	14.3	2.0
Bites, Mexican, Somerfield*	1 Pack/227g	508	224	26.0	15.0	7.0	0.0
Bites, Roast, Birds Eye*	5 Bites/80g	160	200	15.0	3.4	13.8	0.1
Bites, Southern Fried, Tesco*	1 Pack/300g	720	240	18.1	16.9	11.1	2.1
Bites, Tikka, Average	1 Serving/50g	96	193	20.7	3.8	10.5	1.9
Breast, Chargrilled, Lemon & Herb, Bernard Matthews*	1 Serving/100g	154	154	23.7	4.7	4.5	0.0
Breast, Chargrilled, Premium, Average	1 Piece/10g	20	197	21.6	1.5	11.2	0.3
Breast, Chargrilled, Sliced, Average	1 Slice/19g	24	124	24.4	0.5	2.7	0.4
Breast, Chunks, Chilli, Safeway*	1 Serving/100g	142	142	22.2	6.3	3.2	0.0
Breast, Diced, Average	1 Serving/188g	215	114	25.0	0.1	2.0	0.1
Breast, Eastern Spices, Birds Eye*	1 Portion/175g	308	176	13.5	3.8	11.9	1.5
Breast, Escalope, Pesto Chargrilled, Marks & Spencer*	1 Serving/100g	135	135	19.6	0.7	6.2	0.6
Breast, Escalope, Plain, Average	1 Serving/100g	110	110	22.3	0.7	2.2	0.5
Breast, Fillets, Breaded, Average	1 Fillet/112g	246	220	17.5	14.0	10.4	1.3
Breast, Fillets, Breaded, Lemon & Pepper, Average	1 Fillet/89g	133	150	22.0	10.1	2.3	1.3
Breast, Fillets, Cajun, Average	1 Fillet/93g	118	127	25.4	3.1	1.5	0.3
Breast, Fillets, Chargrilled, Average	1 Serving/100g	120	120	27.3	0.3	1.1	0.3
Breast, Fillets, Cheesy Salsa, Safeway*	1/2 Pack/163.6g	180	110	17.9	2.2	3.0	1.1
Breast, Fillets, Garlic & Herb Marinated, Mini, Morrisons*	1 Pack/300g	336	112	20.2	4.9	1.0	0.5
Breast, Fillets, Korma Style, Average	1 Serving/100g	132	132	27.4	0.8	2.8	0.6
Breast, Fillets, Lemon Parsley, Marks & Spencer*	1/2 Pack/145g	232	160	14.3	20.7	2.4	4.3
Breast, Fillets, Mini, Raw, Average	1oz/28g	34	121	26.9	0.2	1.5	0.1
Breast, Fillets, Organic, Average	1 Serving/150g	153	102	24.0	0.0	0.8	0.0
Breast, Fillets, Skinless & Boneless, Raw, Average	1 Serving/100g	126	126	25.1	1.2	2.3	0.2
Breast, Fillets, Smokey Maple, Roast, Waitrose*	1 Fillet/96g	140	146	27.9	4.2	2.0	0.1
Breast, Garlic & Herb Flavour, Co-Op*	1 Serving/170g	281	165	19.0	2.0	9.0	0.3

CHICKEN

INFO/WEIGHT	Measure	per Measure KCAL	Nutrition Values per 100g / 100ml				
			KCAL	PROT	CARB	FAT	FIBRE
Breast, Joint, Free Range, Marks & Spencer*	1oz/28g	36	130	22.0	3.9	4.1	0.6
Breast, Joint, Just Cook, Sainsbury's*	1/3 Pack/126g	194	154	22.4	0.1	7.2	0.1
Breast, Joint, Lemon & Tarragon, Finest, Tesco*	1 Serving/175g	247	141	18.8	2.3	6.3	0.2
Breast, Latino Style, Asda*	1 Breast/65g	99	152	27.0	4.1	3.1	0.5
Breast, Lime & Coriander, Summer Eating, Asda*	1/2 Pack/112g	164	146	26.0	1.6	4.0	0.5
Breast, Meat & Skin, Weighed With Bone	1oz/28g	46	165	24.2	0.0	7.6	0.0
Breast, Mediterranean Style Coating, Tesco*	1 Breast/195g	283	145	20.4	0.7	6.7	0.0
Breast, Pieces, Tikka, Average	1 Serving/100g	154	154	28.2	2.8	3.4	0.4
Breast, Roast, Average	1oz/28g	42	149	25.4	1.1	4.7	0.2
Breast, Roast, Sliced, Average	1 Slice/13g	17	139	25.0	1.8	3.5	0.2
Breast, Roast, With Pork Stuffing, Marks & Spencer*	1 Serving/100g	165	165	24.1	3.0	6.5	0.0
Breast, Roll, Average	1 Slice/10g	17	167	16.1	3.2	10.0	0.2
Breast, Sage & Onion, Slices, Sainsbury's*	1 Pack/140g	158	113	23.1	1.0	1.8	0.5
Breast, Sliced, Tex, Mex, Sainsbury's*	1 Serving/140g	185	132	26.7	3.8	1.1	0.0
Breast, Smoked, Sliced, Average	1 Slice/20g	22	110	20.7	0.9	2.6	0.1
Breast, Strips, Raw, Average	1 Serving/280g	358	128	27.1	0.4	2.1	0.3
Breast, Tandoori Style, Average	1 Serving/180g	237	132	22.3	2.3	3.8	1.0
Breast, Tikka, Sliced, Average	1oz/28g	34	120	24.9	2.0	1.7	0.6
Breast, Wafer Thin, Sage & Onion, Bernard Matthews*	1 Serving/25g	30	120	19.8	3.5	3.0	0.0
Breast, With Skin, Raw, Average	1oz/28g	51	181	24.3	4.9	7.2	0.6
Breasts, Honey & Mustard, Birds Eye*	1 Portion/97g	175	180	19.6	4.2	9.4	0.1
Chargrills, Garlic, Birds Eye*	1 Piece/76g	169	222	19.2	1.2	15.6	0.0
Chargrills, Original, Birds Eye*	1 serving/94g	195	208	22.2	2.5	12.1	0.1
Coated, Baked, Tesco*	1 Serving/101g	148	146	13.8	4.6	8.4	0.0
Cooked, Sliced, Average	1 Slice/15g	18	118	22.4	1.6	2.4	0.1
Cracked Pepper, Birds Eye*	1 Portion/94.7g	196	206	21.0	3.9	11.8	0.1
Crispy, Birds Eye*	1 Serving/95g	224	236	15.0	10.2	15.0	0.3
Dippers, Crispy, Average	5 Dippers/93g	231	249	13.2	14.4	15.4	0.6
Dippers, Tikka, Tesco*	1oz/28g	54	193	21.5	5.0	9.7	1.0
Drumsticks, & Thighs, Garlic & Herb, Sainsbury's*	1 Serving/120g	184	153	16.6	1.5	8.9	0.1
Drumsticks, BBQ Flavour, Average	1 Serving/200g	348	174	22.6	3.1	8.0	0.4
Drumsticks, Breaded, Fried, Average	1oz/28g	70	248	19.6	9.9	14.6	0.6
Drumsticks, Chinese Style, Average	1 Drumstick/100g	178	178	22.6	3.6	8.1	0.7
Drumsticks, Roast, Without Skin, Average	1 Serving/100g	163	163	22.6	0.5	7.8	0.2
Drumsticks, Southern Fried, Sainsbury's*	1 Serving/87g	190	218	20.8	11.2	9.9	0.7
Drumsticks, With Skin, Average	1 Drumstick/125g	269	215	22.1	1.8	13.3	0.3
Escalope, Breaded, Average	1 Escalope/128g	361	282	13.4	19.1	16.9	0.7
Escalope, Cheese Topped, Asda*	1 Serving/173.4g	410	237	12.0	18.0	13.0	1.9
Escalope, Lemon & Pepper, Sainsbury's*	1 Serving/143g	428	299	12.8	18.7	19.3	1.9
Escalope, Tomato & Basil, Safeway*	1 Escalope/150g	242	161	21.2	2.2	7.5	1.2
Fillets, Battered, Average	1 Fillet/90g	199	221	16.1	13.3	11.5	0.5
Fillets, Breaded, Average	1 Piece/98g	214	219	14.2	15.9	10.7	1.9
Fillets, Chinese Style, Average	1oz/28g	37	132	24.4	4.6	1.8	0.5
Fillets, Coronation, BGTY, Sainsbury's*	1 Fillet/100g	136	136	27.1	2.4	2.6	1.0
Fillets, Hickory Barbecue & Chilli, BGTY, Sainsbury's*	1 Fillet/100g	133	133	26.9	3.6	1.2	0.9
Fillets, Honey & Maple, Roast, Mini, Waitrose*	1/2 Pack/100g	131	131	23.0	8.6	0.5	1.5
Fillets, Honey & Mustard, Average	1 Serving/100g	138	138	18.4	7.5	3.7	0.8
Fillets, Honey & Mustard, Mini, Marks & Spencer*	1 Serving/105g	142	135	24.9	3.9	2.0	1.3
Fillets, Honey & Mustard, Somerfield*	1 Serving/100g	117	117	22.2	4.9	1.0	1.8
Fillets, Hot & Spicy, Average	1oz/28g	58	206	16.4	10.5	11.0	1.1
Fillets, Lime & Coriander, Mini, Average	1 Fillet/42g	49	118	24.3	2.6	1.3	0.6
Fillets, Mango Salsa, Mini, Sainsbury's*	1/2 Pack/100g	132	132	24.7	5.6	1.2	0.0
Fillets, Mexican Style, Mini, Asda*	1 Serving/100g	127	127	26.0	2.4	1.5	1.0

CHICKEN

INFO/WEIGHT	Measure	per Measure KCAL	KCAL	PROT	CARB	FAT	FIBRE
Fillets, Red Pepper, Mini, BGTY, Sainsbury's*	1 Serving/100g	126	126	26.5	3.7	0.6	0.7
Fillets, Red Thai, Mini, Average	1oz/28g	36	128	21.7	5.5	2.1	0.6
Fillets, Southern Fried, Average	1oz/28g	62	222	16.4	12.2	12.0	1.1
Fillets, Sweet Chilli & Lime, Mini, Marks & Spencer*	1 Serving/210g	284	135	24.5	5.6	1.8	1.1
Fillets, Sweet Chilli, Mini, Sainsbury's*	1/2 Pack/100g	119	119	21.8	5.4	1.1	0.9
Fillets, Tandoori Style, Mini, Average	1 Serving/100g	128	128	24.7	2.6	2.1	0.4
Fillets, Thai, COU, Marks & Spencer*	1 Fillet/120g	160	133	19.5	10.4	1.6	1.3
Fillets, Tikka, Average	1 Serving/100g	141	141	22.4	1.7	5.0	1.1
Fillets, Tikka, Mini, Average	1oz/28g	35	124	25.1	1.3	2.2	1.2
Fillets, Tomato & Basil, Mini, Average	1oz/28g	34	123	23.5	2.5	2.1	0.4
Fingers, Average	1 Serving/75g	188	250	13.7	18.8	13.3	1.2
Garlic Basted, Morrisons*	1 Serving/100g	231	231	23.3	0.7	13.1	0.4
Garlic, Frozen, Tesco*	1 Serving/94.9g	242	255	12.9	14.7	16.1	1.3
Goujons, Breaded, Average	1 Serving/114g	293	258	15.8	15.2	15.0	1.0
Goujons, Breast, Fresh, Average	1oz/28g	36	127	28.0	0.0	1.7	0.0
Goujons, Cracked Black Pepper, American, Asda*	1 Serving/150g	333	222	16.0	8.0	14.0	2.5
Goujons, Garlic & Herb, Breaded, American, Asda*	1/2 Pack/150g	377	251	17.0	12.0	15.0	2.1
Goujons, Hot & Spicy, Sainsbury's*	1/2 Pack/125g	253	202	20.0	13.1	7.7	1.2
Griddlers, BBQ, Mini, Birds Eye*	1/2 Pack/50g	109	217	15.8	6.7	14.1	0.2
Griddles, BBQ, Birds Eye*	1 Serving/48g	105	217	15.8	6.7	14.1	0.2
Honey Roast, Sliced, Average	1 Slice/13g	15	117	21.6	2.2	2.5	0.1
Leg Or Thigh, Hot & Spicy, Average	1oz/28g	50	179	19.4	1.0	10.8	0.4
Leg Portion, Roast, Average	1 Quarter/120g	244	203	21.6	0.3	12.7	0.2
Leg, Meat Only, Stewed, Weighed With Bone & Skin	1oz/28g	52	185	26.3	0.0	8.1	0.0
Leg, With Skin, Raw, Average	1oz/28g	48	172	19.1	0.0	10.4	0.0
Leg, With Skin, Roasted, Average	1oz/28g	66	234	21.5	0.1	16.4	0.0
Light Meat, Raw	1oz/28g	30	106	24.0	0.0	1.1	0.0
Light Meat, Roasted	1oz/28g	43	153	30.2	0.0	3.6	0.0
Meat & Skin Portions, Deep Fried	1oz/28g	73	259	26.9	0.0	16.8	0.0
Meat & Skin, Raw	1oz/28g	64	230	17.6	0.0	17.7	0.0
Meat & Skin, Roasted	1oz/28g	60	216	22.6	0.0	14.0	0.0
Meat, Roasted, Average	1oz/28g	50	177	27.3	0.0	7.5	0.0
Mince, Average	1oz/28g	39	140	20.9	0.1	6.0	0.2
Nuggets, Battered, Average	1 Nugget/20g	50	251	13.5	16.9	14.4	0.9
Nuggets, Breaded, Average	1 Nugget/14g	37	263	14.8	19.8	13.8	1.9
Nuggets, Free From Gluten & Wheat, Sainsbury's*	4 Nuggets/75g	187	251	13.4	19.7	13.2	0.8
O's, Birds Eye*	10 O's/48g	125	260	13.1	14.6	16.6	0.7
Pieces, Garlic, Crunchy, Birds Eye*	1 Piece/99g	259	262	14.4	16.9	15.2	0.9
Pieces, Spicy, Mexican, Birds Eye*	1 Piece/103g	254	247	14.6	16.5	13.6	0.6
Pops, Southern Fried, Tesco*	1 Serving/225g	542	241	13.2	16.7	13.5	1.0
Roast, & Stuffing, Healthy Living, Tesco*	1 Serving/17g	19	111	23.3	1.3	1.4	0.2
Roast, In Sugar Marinade, Marks & Spencer*	1 Portion/200g	370	185	26.4	0.4	8.6	0.1
Seasoned & Basted, Marks & Spencer*	1oz/28g	38	137	17.3	6.7	4.5	0.5
Soy Brasied, Marks & Spencer*	1 Serving/100g	130	130	13.1	3.4	7.0	0.7
Spicy, Fried, Sainsbury's*	1 Serving/150g	414	276	28.8	2.9	16.6	2.1
Steaks, Average	1 Serving/100g	205	205	21.1	9.0	9.4	0.7
Steaks, Garlic & Herb, Tesco*	1 Serving/138g	354	257	14.1	12.2	16.9	1.7
Steaks, Wheat Free & Gluten Free, Sainsbury's*	1 Serving/95g	211	222	11.9	18.6	11.1	0.7
Strips Or Tenders, Chinese Style, Average	1oz/28g	41	145	19.7	8.0	4.1	1.1
Strips, Mexican, Sliced, Marks & Spencer*	1/2 Pack/70g	77	110	24.3	2.3	0.6	0.5
Tenders, Tex Mex, Jumbo, Marks & Spencer*	1 Serving/200g	250	125	22.8	0.7	3.4	0.6
Thigh, Chinese, Forest Farms*	1oz/28g	68	242	20.2	1.4	17.3	9.0
Thigh, Meat & Skin, Average	1 Serving/100g	218	218	21.4	0.0	14.7	0.0

C

	INFO/WEIGHT	KCAL	KCAL	PROT	CARB	FAT	FIBRE
CHICKEN							
Thigh, Meat & Skin, Casseroled	1oz/28g	65	233	21.5	0.0	16.3	0.0
Thigh, Meat Only, Diced, Casseroled	1oz/28g	50	180	25.6	0.0	8.6	0.0
Thigh, Meat Only, Raw, Average	1 Thigh/90g	113	126	19.4	0.0	5.5	0.0
Thigh, Roast, Average	1 Serving/100g	238	238	23.9	0.4	15.7	0.0
Wafer Thin, Average	1 Slice/10g	12	120	19.0	2.8	3.6	0.2
Wafer Thin, Coronation, Sainsbury's*	1/2 Pack/50g	68	135	19.1	4.5	4.5	0.1
Whole, Roast, Average	1oz/28g	59	211	21.2	1.5	13.4	0.2
Whole, Roasted, Sugar & Dextrose Marinade, Tesco*	1 Serving/100g	190	190	22.1	0.1	11.3	0.1
Wing Quarter, Meat Only, Casseroled	1oz/28g	46	164	26.9	0.0	6.3	0.0
Wing, Breaded, Fried, Average	1oz/28g	82	294	18.4	14.0	18.5	0.4
Wing, Meat & Skin, Cooked, Average	1oz/28g	67	241	23.3	1.9	15.6	0.3
Wings, BBQ Flavour, Average	1oz/28g	61	220	20.3	6.6	12.5	0.6
Wings, Chinese Style, Average	1oz/28g	72	256	24.2	5.1	15.5	0.6
Wings, Hickory Smoke Flavour, Nibbles, Sainsbury's*	1 Wing/100g	245	245	23.5	3.5	15.3	0.5
Wings, Hot & Spicy, Average	1oz/28g	65	231	21.9	5.2	13.7	0.9
Wings, Meat & Skin, Raw, Average	1oz/28g	52	184	19.0	0.5	11.8	0.2
CHICKEN &							
Apricot Rice, COU, Marks & Spencer*	1 Pack/400g	360	90	9.4	10.6	0.9	0.7
Asparagus, BGTY, Sainsbury's*	1 Pack/400g	428	107	9.1	14.5	1.4	0.9
Asparagus, In A Champagne Sauce, Finest, Tesco*	1 Pack/500g	615	123	8.8	7.0	6.7	0.9
Asparagus, Long Grain & Wild Rice, BGTY, Sainsbury's*	1 Pack/451g	555	123	9.2	17.1	2.0	0.8
Bacon Parcels, Finest, Tesco*	1 Pack/232.5g	380	163	16.1	3.7	9.3	0.5
Bacon Parcels, Sainsbury's*	1/2 Pack/170g	406	239	21.9	0.1	16.8	0.0
Bacon, Al Forno, Safeway*	1/2 Pack/400g	420	105	6.1	13.3	2.9	1.1
Bacon, Easy Steam, Tesco*	1 Pack/400g	728	182	11.7	13.6	9.1	0.8
Black Bean Noodles, Sainsbury's*	1 Serving/130g	155	119	4.3	23.9	0.7	0.8
Black Bean Sauce, & Egg Fried Rice, BGTY, Sainsbury's*	1 Pack/450g	527	117	7.2	14.7	3.3	0.5
Black Bean, Chinese Takeaway, Tesco*	1 Serving/200g	190	95	8.3	8.0	3.3	0.5
Black Bean, Chinese, Tesco*	1 Pack/350g	382	109	8.9	7.4	4.9	0.7
Black Bean, Tinned, Tesco*	1 Serving/150g	123	82	10.0	7.7	1.3	1.1
Black Bean, With Chinese Rice, COU, Marks & Spencer*	1 Pack/400g	320	80	7.4	7.6	2.4	1.1
Black Bean, With Noodles, Tesco*	1 Pack/475g	470	99	7.6	13.6	1.6	0.2
Black Bean, With Rice, Chinese, Tesco*	1 Serving/450g	459	102	5.3	15.4	2.1	0.5
Black Bean, With Rice, Good Intentions, Somerfield*	1 Pack/400g	352	88	7.0	13.4	0.7	0.6
Black Bean, With Rice, Healthy Living, Tesco*	1 Pack/450g	464	103	6.9	19.6	1.6	0.6
Broccoli, With Rigatoni Pasta, BGTY, Sainsbury's*	1 Pack/450g	590	131	10.5	15.2	3.1	0.7
Cashew Nuts, & Vegetable Rice, COU, Marks & Spencer*	1 Pack/400g	360	90	7.5	9.7	2.6	1.1
Cashew Nuts, Asda*	1 Pack/400g	528	132	8.2	4.2	9.1	0.8
Cashew Nuts, Cantonese, Sainsbury's*	1 Pack/350g	595	170	11.2	9.8	9.6	1.0
Cashew Nuts, Chinese, Sainsbury's*	1 Pack/350g	312	89	7.8	5.7	4.0	1.2
Cashew Nuts, Chinese, Tesco*	1 Pack/350g	378	108	9.5	4.9	5.6	0.6
Cashew Nuts, Easy Steam, Tesco*	1 Serving/400g	460	115	8.7	9.2	4.8	1.0
Cashew Nuts, Marks & Spencer*	1 Pack/300g	300	100	10.3	5.0	4.0	1.2
Cashew Nuts, Oriental, Healthy Living, Tesco*	1 Pack/450g	437	97	7.0	15.1	1.0	0.7
Cashew Nuts, Ready Meals, Waitrose*	1 Pack/400g	416	104	11.3	8.2	2.9	1.0
Cashew Nuts, With Egg Fried Rice, Healthy Living, Tesco*	1 Pack/450g	441	98	8.9	12.7	1.3	1.3
Cashew Nuts, With Egg Fried Rice, Somerfield*	1 Pack/340g	435	128	7.0	13.0	5.0	0.0
Cashew Nuts, With Egg Rice, GFY, Asda*	1 Pack/396g	396	100	7.0	13.0	2.2	1.3
Cashew Nuts, With Rice, Eat Smart, Safeway*	1 Serving/400g	400	100	6.6	12.6	2.3	2.0
Chargrilled Vegetable Roll, Healthy Living, Tesco*	1 Pack/221.1g	336	152	10.1	21.8	2.7	2.3
Chips, BBQ, BGTY, Sainsbury's*	1 Pack/381g	423	111	7.9	15.9	1.8	2.5
Cous Cous, Healthy Eating, Tesco*	1 Pack/351g	263	75	10.3	7.3	0.5	1.4
Cranberry, Perfectly Balanced, Waitrose*	1 Pack/240g	161	67	11.8	4.1	0.4	1.1

	Measure	per Measure		Nutrition Values per 100g / 100ml			
	INFO/WEIGHT	KCAL	KCAL	PROT	CARB	FAT	FIBRE
CHICKEN &							
Fries, Southern Fried Style, Tesco*	1 Pack/500g	930	186	11.5	16.0	8.0	1.4
Fries, Southern Fried, Sainsbury's*	1/2 Pack/250g	563	225	10.5	26.2	8.7	0.8
Gravy, COU, Marks & Spencer*	1 Pack/300g	216	72	7.2	7.8	1.3	1.6
Honey Sauce, For Pancakes, Sainsbury's*	1 Pack/185g	266	144	14.1	15.9	2.7	0.5
King Prawn Special Fried Rice, Finest, Tesco*	1 Pack/450g	734	163	7.7	17.0	7.1	0.7
Mushroom, Chinese, Iceland*	1 Pack/400g	276	69	8.2	3.8	2.3	0.4
Mushroom, Chinese, Sainsbury's*	1/2 Pack/175g	116	66	7.6	4.4	2.0	0.9
Mushroom, Chinese, Tesco*	1 Pack/460g	474	103	5.7	13.8	2.8	1.0
Mushroom, In Oyster Sauce, Tesco*	1 Pack/350g	252	72	8.0	6.3	1.6	0.7
Mushroom, In White Wine Sauce, GFY, Asda*	1 Pack/400g	272	68	6.0	7.0	1.8	1.2
Mushroom, With Egg Fried Rice, Iceland*	1 Pack/500g	410	82	4.9	13.0	1.2	0.7
Mushroom, With Vegetable Rice, BGTY, Sainsbury's*	1 Pack/400g	376	94	6.4	13.0	1.8	0.9
Mushroom, With Vegetable Rice, BGTY, Sainsbury's*	1 Pack/400g	376	94	6.4	13.0	1.8	0.9
Noodles, Chinese Style, Healthy Eating, Tesco*	1 Pack/370g	422	114	8.5	15.9	1.7	1.5
Peppers, In A Black Bean Sauce, Marks & Spencer*	1 Pack/320g	256	80	9.4	7.3	1.5	1.2
Peppers, Marks & Spencer*	1 Serving/240g	264	110	14.7	2.3	4.5	0.6
Pineapple, Chilled, Tesco*	1 Pack/350g	364	104	9.6	11.1	2.4	5.5
Pineapple, With Egg Fried Rice, Healthy Living, Tesco*	1 Pack/450g	414	92	6.0	15.4	0.7	0.6
Pineapple, With Egg Fried Rice, Tesco*	1 Pack/450g	450	100	7.6	12.1	2.4	1.2
Pineapple, With Rice, Healthy Living, Tesco*	1 Pack/450g	401	89	6.6	12.0	1.6	1.0
Pineapple, With Vegetable Rice, Marks & Spencer*	1 Pack/400g	400	100	7.2	13.0	1.9	1.6
Prawn Yaki Udan Noodles, Marks & Spencer*	1 Pack/395g	435	110	8.1	11.9	3.6	0.8
Red Pepper Dressing, Simple Solutions, Tesco*	1 Serving/140g	228	163	19.2	0.1	9.5	0.5
Tomato & Basil, COU, Marks & Spencer*	1/2 Pack/200g	180	90	14.3	3.4	2.3	0.8
Tomato Saag, With Pilau Rice, BGTY, Sainsbury's*	1 Pack/400g	404	101	7.3	15.6	1.0	1.0
Tomato Sauce, With Basil Mash, COU, Marks & Spencer*	1 Pack/400g	360	90	7.9	9.3	2.3	0.9
Vegetable Medley, Chargrilled, Healthy Eating, Tesco*	1 Pack/450g	270	60	6.5	5.8	1.2	0.9
Vegetable Savoury Rice, Safeway*	1/2 Pack/185g	231	125	2.9	25.9	1.1	0.8
White Wine, With Rice, Healthy Eating, Tesco*	1 Pack/450g	450	100	7.1	14.8	1.4	1.0
CHICKEN A L' ORANGE							
Lean Cuisine, Findus*	1 Pack/334g	384	115	5.6	18.0	2.1	0.4
CHICKEN ALFREDO							
BGTY, Sainsbury's*	1 Serving/200g	208	104	18.0	1.9	2.7	0.5
Healthy Living, Tesco*	1 Serving/377g	388	103	9.4	10.6	2.6	0.9
CHICKEN ARRABBIATA							
Al Forno, Sainsbury's*	1 Pack/900g	1026	114	6.5	16.4	2.5	1.4
Bistro, Waitrose*	1/2 Pack/175g	156	89	12.9	2.5	3.0	0.5
Easy Steam, Healthy Living, Tesco*	1 Pack/400g	284	71	8.4	7.6	0.8	1.2
GFY, Asda*	1 Pack/400g	256	64	5.0	9.0	0.9	0.7
Perfectly Balanced, Waitrose*	1 Serving/240g	211	88	12.4	4.0	2.4	0.6
Tesco*	1 Meal/400g	392	98	5.8	12.9	2.5	1.5
CHICKEN BBQ							
& Chips, Sainsbury's*	1 Serving/380g	422	111	7.9	15.9	1.8	2.5
CHICKEN BANG BANG							
Oriental Express*	1/2 Pack/200g	170	85	6.4	11.0	1.7	3.2
Waitrose*	1 Pack/350g	368	105	9.4	5.9	4.9	1.2
CHICKEN BARBECUE							
With Potato Wedges, Eat Smart, Morrisons*	1 Pack/350g	368	105	8.5	14.5	1.4	1.5
CHICKEN BUTTER							
Curry, Fresh, Tesco*	1 Pack/350g	487	139	11.8	7.1	7.0	1.8
Rich & Aromatic, Sainsbury's*	1 Pack/400g	592	148	12.1	4.4	9.1	1.2
Safeway*	1 Pack/350g	473	135	12.0	4.1	7.3	2.5

C

	Measure	per Measure		Nutrition Values per 100g / 100ml			
	INFO/WEIGHT	KCAL	KCAL	PROT	CARB	FAT	FIBRE
CHICKEN CAJUN							
& Pasta, Safeway*	1 Pack/455g	501	110	8.6	10.5	3.4	2.1
& Potato Hash, Healthy Eating, Tesco*	1 Pack/450g	428	95	6.6	11.7	2.4	0.9
& Potato Hash, Healthy Living, Tesco*	1 Pack/450g	414	92	8.0	10.0	2.2	0.9
Fettuccine, Marks & Spencer*	1 Pack/500g	600	120	8.7	11.4	4.4	0.9
Healthy Eating, Tesco*	1 Pack/365g	412	113	7.9	17.3	1.3	0.7
CHICKEN CALIFORNIAN							
Creamy Lime & Wedges, Safeway*	1 Pack/400g	460	115	8.8	9.2	4.5	2.5
CHICKEN CALYPSO							
With Turmeric Rice, BGTY, Sainsbury's*	1 Pack/450g	495	110	6.7	16.3	2.1	1.0
CHICKEN CANTONESE							
& Rice, Sizzler, Tesco*	1 Serving/450g	639	142	7.7	14.9	5.7	0.9
Breast, Fillets, Sainsbury's*	1 Serving/154.1g	168	109	20.3	3.6	1.5	0.6
Chinese, Tesco*	1/2 Pack/175g	196	112	10.3	9.4	3.7	0.4
Honey Pepper, Sainsbury's*	1/2 Pack/175g	124	71	6.6	6.1	2.2	0.9
Honey, Sesame, Sainsbury's*	1/3 Pack/135g	116	86	9.8	5.5	2.7	0.8
CHICKEN CARBONARA							
Steam Cuisine, Marks & Spencer*	1 Pack/400g	560	140	10.4	9.8	6.9	1.2
CHICKEN CARIBBEAN							
Fruity, With Rice & Peas, BGTY, Sainsbury's*	1 Pack/400g	412	103	7.3	14.8	1.6	1.5
Fruity, With Rice & Peas, New, BGTY, Sainsbury's*	1 Pack/400g	352	88	6.9	13.1	0.9	2.2
Somerfield*	1 Pack/400g	554	139	8.7	16.5	4.2	1.7
Style, Breasts, COU, Marks & Spencer*	1 Serving/205g	205	100	14.6	7.3	1.5	1.3
With Potato & Toasted Coconut Rosti, TTD, Sainsbury's*	1/2 Pack/200g	320	160	13.8	9.7	7.3	0.6
CHICKEN CHASSEUR							
& Colcannon, Healthy Eating, Tesco*	1 Serving/450g	329	73	6.4	7.1	2.1	1.0
& Colcannon, Healthy Living, Tesco*	1 Pack/400g	348	87	9.7	6.7	2.4	0.6
BGTY, Sainsbury's*	1 Pack/320g	243	76	6.8	9.5	1.1	1.0
Breast Fillets, Morrisons*	1 Pack/380g	384	101	15.7	2.9	3.0	0.8
Finest, Tesco*	1 Serving/200g	214	107	14.3	2.7	4.3	1.6
With Colcannon, Healthy Living, Tesco*	1 Serving/450g	327	73	6.4	7.1	2.1	1.0
CHICKEN CHILLI							
& Ginger, Breasts, COU, Marks & Spencer*	1 Breast/120g	156	130	19.5	8.6	2.0	1.7
& Lemongrass, With Egg Noodles, BGTY, Sainsbury's*	1 Pack/450g	500	111	10.0	10.2	3.4	1.2
Quick To Cook, BGTY, Sainsbury's*	1 Serving/420g	336	80	7.4	10.2	1.1	1.0
Sweet, & Egg Fried Rice, Healthy Living, Tesco*	1 Serving/450g	446	99	5.7	15.0	1.8	0.4
Sweet, COU, Marks & Spencer*	1 Pack/400g	380	95	9.9	11.0	1.1	1.1
Sweet, Findus*	1 Pack/350g	420	120	6.0	15.0	3.5	1.5
Sweet, Roast, Fillets, Mini, Waitrose*	1 Pack/200g	216	108	23.0	3.8	0.2	0.9
Sweet, With Noodles, Healthy Living, Tesco*	1 Serving/400g	392	98	4.4	17.1	1.3	1.0
With Lime, Breast, Simple Solutions, Tesco*	1 Pack/400g	564	141	22.5	0.8	5.3	1.4
CHICKEN CHINESE							
& Prawns, Sizzler, House Special, Tesco*	1 Serving/450g	684	152	7.5	18.8	5.2	1.2
Battered, With Plum Sauce, Tesco*	1 Pack/350g	648	185	6.7	26.5	5.8	0.8
Crispy Aromatic, Half, Tesco*	1 Serving/233g	524	225	16.3	16.7	10.4	1.2
Oriental Express*	1 Pack/350g	326	93	5.7	15.9	0.7	2.2
Stir Fry, Morrisons*	1 Serving/319g	341	107	5.7	17.0	1.7	1.5
Style Sauce, Breast Fillets, Morrisons*	1/2 pack/200g	162	81	13.5	4.6	1.0	1.2
Style, & Noodles, Healthy Eating, Tesco*	1 Pack/370g	278	75	6.9	9.4	1.1	0.7
Style, GFY, Asda*	1 Serving/200g	220	110	18.0	3.5	2.7	0.5
Sweet Chilli & Garlic, Asda*	1 Serving/400g	436	109	8.0	18.0	0.6	2.1
With Ginger & Spring Onion, Tesco*	1 Serving/350g	299	85	7.6	7.3	2.9	0.6
CHICKEN CIDER							
COU, Marks & Spencer*	1 Pack/400g	300	75	7.2	6.7	2.3	0.8

	Measure	per Measure		Nutrition Values per 100g / 100ml			
	INFO/WEIGHT	KCAL	KCAL	PROT	CARB	FAT	FIBRE
CHICKEN CIDER							
With Colcannon, Perfectly Balanced, Waitrose*	1 Pack/401.1g	353	88	6.2	8.9	3.1	1.1
CHICKEN CORDON BLEU							
Breast, Fillets, Sainsbury's*	1 Serving/150g	304	203	17.5	11.5	9.5	1.6
TTD, Sainsbury's*	1 Fillet/140g	339	242	21.3	14.1	11.2	1.1
Waitrose*	1 Serving/160g	325	203	20.1	9.1	9.6	2.4
CHICKEN CORONATION							
COU, Marks & Spencer*	1oz/28g	34	120	16.3	8.6	2.2	0.7
Marks & Spencer*	1 Serving/200g	420	210	12.6	10.6	13.2	1.3
CHICKEN CURRIED							
With Vegetables, Plumrose*	1 Serving/196g	253	129	5.8	8.0	8.2	0.0
CHICKEN DIJONNAISE							
Steam Cuisine, Marks & Spencer*	1 Pack/400g	320	80	9.6	4.2	2.6	2.0
CHICKEN DINNER							
Breast, With Pork, Sage & Onion Stuffing, Tesco*	1 Serving/180g	277	154	19.4	0.7	8.2	0.5
Kershaws*	1 Pack/350g	210	60	4.3	8.4	1.0	1.2
Tesco*	1 Serving/400g	388	97	9.2	10.9	1.8	1.2
With Gravy, The Crafty Cook*	1 Serving/320g	330	103	5.6	15.3	2.1	1.9
With Stuffing & Roast Potatoes, Tesco*	1 Pack/440g	414	94	7.4	11.6	2.0	1.1
CHICKEN EN CROUTE							
Asda*	1/2 Pack/174g	393	226	14.0	20.0	10.0	1.5
Breast, Tesco*	1 Serving/215g	555	258	9.4	20.4	15.4	0.6
Just Cook, Sainsbury's*	1 Serving/180g	481	267	16.8	15.9	15.1	0.4
CHICKEN ESCALOPE							
Creamy Peppercorn, Sainsbury's*	1 Serving/150g	367	245	13.3	11.2	16.3	1.1
Lemon, & Herb, Waitrose*	1 Serving/200g	202	101	19.2	1.0	2.2	1.4
Sour Cream & Chive, Tesco*	1 Escalope/143g	390	274	13.3	16.1	17.4	2.0
Spinach & Ricotta, Sainsbury's*	1 Escalope/150g	354	236	13.1	11.5	15.3	0.9
Topped With Cheese, Ham & Mushrooms, Asda*	1/2 Pack/149.4g	259	174	25.0	0.6	8.0	0.0
CHICKEN FLORENTINE							
Asda*	1 Serving/200g	322	161	18.0	2.1	9.0	0.9
Finest, Tesco*	1 Serving/225g	297	132	17.6	3.3	5.4	0.7
Healthy Living, Tesco*	1 Pack/400g	340	85	12.1	3.0	2.7	0.9
CHICKEN FORRESTIERE							
Asda*	1 Serving/450g	432	96	8.0	10.0	2.7	2.7
COU, Marks & Spencer*	1 Serving/220g	187	85	14.5	2.2	1.7	0.6
GFY, Asda*	1/2 Pack/225g	205	91	15.0	2.5	2.3	0.3
CHICKEN FU YUNG							
Chinese Takeaway, Tesco*	1 Pack/350g	315	90	5.6	14.5	1.0	0.8
CHICKEN GINGER							
& Lemon, With Apricot Rice, BGTY, Sainsbury's*	1 Pack/401.8g	438	109	9.7	14.5	1.4	0.3
& Lemon, With Basmati Rice, East Smart, Safeway*	1 Pack/395g	395	100	7.3	13.4	1.7	1.4
& Lemon, With Rice, COU, Marks & Spencer*	1 Pack/400g	320	80	7.9	9.7	0.9	2.0
& Plum, With Rice, Perfectly Balanced, Waitrose*	1 Pack/400g	492	123	6.3	23.5	0.5	1.0
& Spring Onion, With Rice, Sharwood's*	1 Pack/375g	347	93	5.1	14.2	1.7	1.7
CHICKEN GLAZED							
Balsamic, Healthy Living, Tesco*	1 Pack/400g	288	72	5.1	10.8	0.9	0.9
CHICKEN HARISSA							
BGTY, Sainsbury's*	1 Serving/250g	211	84	10.4	8.0	1.2	1.5
With Couscous, Perfectly Balanced, Waitrose*	1 Pack/400g	348	87	7.6	9.5	2.0	1.7
CHICKEN HAWAIIAN							
With Rice, Birds Eye*	1 Pack/350g	406	116	5.5	20.2	1.5	0.6
CHICKEN HERB							
Steam Cuisine, Marks & Spencer*	1 Pack/400g	280	70	8.2	6.0	1.6	0.9

C

	Measure INFO/WEIGHT	per Measure KCAL	Nutrition Values per 100g / 100ml KCAL	PROT	CARB	FAT	FIBRE
CHICKEN HONEY & MUSTARD							
Healthy Living, Tesco*	1 Serving/375g	424	113	5.8	17.3	2.3	1.4
Shapers, Boots*	1 Pack/241g	304	126	7.0	19.0	2.4	1.7
With Baby Potatoes, BGTY, Sainsbury's*	1 Pack/450g	392	87	8.5	11.7	0.7	0.8
With Spring Vegetable Rice, SlimFast*	1 Pack/375g	375	100	5.8	15.5	1.4	0.8
With Vegetable Medley, BGTY, Sainsbury's*	1 Pack/400g	288	72	8.4	8.1	0.7	0.8
CHICKEN IN							
A Curry Sauce, Fillets, Safeway*	1 Serving/124g	180	145	17.2	3.9	6.4	0.6
Asparagus Sauce & New Potatoes, Sainsbury's*	1 Pack/495g	545	110	7.4	9.5	4.7	0.9
BBQ Sauce, Breast, Sainsbury's*	1 Serving/170g	199	117	14.5	13.1	0.7	1.3
BBQ Sauce, Breast, Weight Watchers*	1 Pack/339g	336	99	5.8	11.0	3.5	0.9
BBQ Sauce, Chargrilled, Breast, GFY, Asda*	1 Serving/166g	214	129	19.0	5.0	3.7	1.0
BBQ Sauce, GFY, Asda*	1 Pack/380g	414	109	13.0	13.0	0.5	1.3
BBQ Sauce, Weight Watchers*	1 Pack/339g	332	98	5.8	10.8	3.5	0.9
Bacon, Mushroom & Red Wine Sauce, Asda*	1 Serving/151g	145	96	16.0	2.2	2.6	0.5
Barbecue Sauce, COU, Marks & Spencer*	1 Pack/352g	370	105	8.6	13.8	1.6	1.2
Barbeque Sauce, Breasts, COU, Marks & Spencer*	1 Pack/350g	420	120	8.5	20.6	1.9	0.6
Barbeque Sauce, Healthy Eating, Tesco*	1 Breast/170g	177	104	18.3	4.5	1.4	0.9
Black Bean Sauce, & Rice, Morrisons*	1 Pack/400g	408	102	3.9	16.4	2.3	1.2
Black Bean Sauce, Canned, BGTY, Sainsbury's*	1 Can/400g	308	77	9.3	7.9	0.9	0.7
Black Bean Sauce, Chinese Takeaway, Iceland*	1 Pack/400g	348	87	9.3	5.3	3.2	0.7
Black Bean Sauce, Frozen, BGTY, Sainsbury's*	1 Pack/400g	380	95	4.5	16.6	1.1	0.5
Black Bean Sauce, Marks & Spencer*	1 Pack/350g	298	85	8.7	8.0	2.0	1.1
Black Bean Sauce, Sainsbury's*	1 Pack/465g	484	104	5.0	17.3	1.7	0.3
Black Bean Sauce, Somerfield*	1/2 Pack/175g	133	76	10.7	6.1	1.0	1.9
Black Bean Sauce, Tesco*	1 Pack/450g	387	86	7.4	12.4	0.7	1.6
Black Bean Sauce, Tinned, Tesco*	1 Serving/200g	164	82	10.0	7.7	1.3	1.1
Black Bean Sauce, Waitrose*	1 Pack/300g	243	81	10.9	6.6	1.2	0.8
Black Bean Sauce, With Egg Fried Rice, GFY, Asda*	1 Serving/416g	320	77	5.0	12.0	1.0	0.9
Black Bean Sauce, With Egg Fried Rice, Somerfield*	1 Pack/340g	384	113	7.0	13.0	4.0	0.0
Black Bean Sauce, With Noodles, Pro Cuisine*	1 Pack/600g	366	61	5.6	8.5	0.6	0.0
Black Bean Sauce, With Rice, Asda*	1 Pack/400g	500	125	7.0	20.0	1.9	0.6
Black Bean Sauce, With Rice, BGTY, Sainsbury's*	1 Pack/450g	446	99	6.4	16.6	0.8	0.6
Black Bean Sauce, With Rice, Iceland*	1 Pack/400g	388	97	5.1	15.8	1.5	0.8
Black Bean, & Rice, Healthy Eating, Tesco*	1 Pack/450g	387	86	7.4	12.4	0.7	1.6
Black Bean, With Egg Fried Rice, Healthy Living, Tesco*	1 Pack/450g	468	104	6.8	17.1	0.9	0.5
Broccoli & Mushroom, Good Choice, Iceland*	1 Pack/500g	590	118	6.4	18.1	2.2	0.6
Broccoli & Mushroom, With Rice, Healthy Eating, Tesco*	1 Pack/400g	440	110	7.5	17.1	1.2	0.7
Cheese & Bacon, Wrapped, Breast, Tesco*	1 Serving/300g	474	158	20.7	1.2	7.8	0.5
Cheese, Leek & Ham, Breast Fillets, Asda*	1 Serving/190g	291	153	19.0	1.2	8.0	2.0
Cheesy Salsa, Fillets, Safeway*	1/2 Pack/175g	193	110	17.9	2.2	3.0	1.1
Chilli & Lemon Grass With Rice, Sainsbury's*	1 Pack/450g	527	117	6.2	17.4	2.5	0.7
Coriander & Lime Marinade, Chargrilled, Asda*	1/2 Pack/163.4g	285	175	23.0	0.5	9.0	0.0
Coriander, Lime & Chilli Dressing, Fillets, Aldi*	1 Serving/140g	258	184	8.5	11.4	11.6	0.0
Creamy Mushroom Sauce, Healthy Living, Tesco*	1 Pack/400g	296	74	13.2	1.8	1.5	0.5
Creamy Mustard Sauce, GFY, Asda*	1 Pack/400g	468	117	6.0	18.0	2.3	0.4
Creamy Thai Sauce, Somerfield*	1 Pack/440g	748	170	22.0	2.0	8.0	0.0
Creamy Tikka Style Sauce, Tesco*	1 Breast/190g	215	113	15.1	0.7	5.5	0.8
Creamy Tomato & Mascarpone Sauce, Waitrose*	1 Serving/400g	492	123	7.9	9.9	5.8	0.8
Creamy White Wine Sauce, Sainsbury's*	1 Pack/324g	285	88	8.9	4.7	3.7	1.0
Garlic & Cream Sauce, Breast Fillet, Morrisons*	1 Serving/179.5g	261	146	14.9	1.8	8.8	0.6
Garlic & Herbs, Breast, Sainsbury's*	1 Serving/200g	316	158	28.3	5.4	2.6	0.1
Ginger & Chilli With Veg Noodles, COU, Marks & Spencer*	1 Pack/400g	300	75	6.4	10.7	0.6	1.1
Gravy, Breast, Sainsbury's*	1 Box/200g	124	62	11.8	2.9	0.5	0.2

C

CHICKEN IN

INFO/WEIGHT	Measure	per Measure KCAL	Nutrition Values per 100g / 100ml KCAL	PROT	CARB	FAT	FIBRE
Gravy, Chunky, Marks & Spencer*	1 Can/489g	465	95	13.6	1.4	3.9	0.8
Gravy, With Stuffing & Potatoes, British Classics, Tesco*	1 Pack/450.5g	482	107	7.8	12.1	3.0	0.8
Hot Ginger Sauce, With Jasmine Rice, BGTY, Sainsbury's*	1 Pack/400g	400	100	6.6	15.4	1.4	0.5
Hot Ginger Sauce, With Thai Sticky Rice, Sainsbury's*	1 Pack/450g	603	134	6.8	16.3	4.6	0.5
Italian Style Tomato & Herb Sauce, Tesco*	1 Serving/180g	144	80	15.8	1.6	1.2	0.6
Leek & Bacon Sauce, Chilled, Co-Op*	1 Pack/400g	460	115	15.0	2.0	5.0	0.2
Lemon Flavour Sauce, Breast Fillets, Safeway*	1 Fillet/92g	200	217	17.0	16.0	9.4	1.4
Lemon Sauce With Rice, Sainsbury's*	1 Pack/450g	513	114	8.1	17.0	1.5	0.7
Lemon Sauce, Breast, Healthy Eating, Tesco*	1 Pack/385g	385	100	15.9	4.7	1.9	0.5
Mango Ginger Marinade, Breast, Chargrilled, GFY, Asda*	1/2 Pack/190g	234	123	17.0	11.0	1.2	0.5
Mediterranean Sauce, Iceland*	1 Pack/500g	640	128	7.4	21.8	1.2	0.5
Mediterranean Style Sauce, Breasts, BGTY, Sainsbury's*	1/2 Pack/170g	148	87	14.5	2.7	2.0	0.9
Mexican Salsa, Tesco*	1 Pack/320g	368	115	19.5	3.1	2.7	0.6
Mexican Style Sauce, Tesco*	1 Serving/180g	128	71	13.3	2.6	0.8	0.7
Mushroom & Ham Sauce With Rice, BGTY, Sainsbury's*	1 Pack/450g	581	129	9.7	18.9	1.6	0.3
Mushroom & Red Wine Sauce, Breast Fillets, Morrisons*	1 Serving/176.9g	184	104	15.7	4.6	2.5	0.7
Mushroom & White Wine Sauce, Fillets, Morrisons*	1 Serving/190g	243	128	18.8	0.9	5.5	0.5
Mushroom Sauce With Mash, Healthy Living, Tesco*	1 Pack/400g	384	96	9.9	8.0	2.7	0.6
Peppercorn Sauce, GFY, Asda*	1 Serving/399.1g	431	108	6.0	17.0	1.8	0.5
Peppercorn Sauce, Safeway*	1 Pack/395.2g	415	105	8.8	12.2	2.2	1.6
Peppers, Fillets, Sainsbury's*	1 Pack/360g	378	105	13.7	4.2	3.7	1.1
Pesto Style Dressing, Asda*	1 Serving/150g	210	140	18.7	1.3	6.7	0.0
Pesto Style Dressing, Simple Solutions, Tesco*	1 Serving/142g	268	189	20.1	2.5	11.0	1.6
Red Pepper Dressing, Tesco*	1 Serving/140g	228	163	19.2	0.1	9.5	0.5
Red Pepper Sauce, Eat Smart, Safeway*	1 Serving/175g	166	95	18.4	2.3	1.3	1.4
Red Thai Marinade, Breasts, Mini, Healthy Eating, Tesco*	1 Serving/200g	276	138	26.8	2.0	2.5	0.5
Red Thai Sauce, Breasts, Healthy Eating, Tesco*	1 Pack/350g	368	105	17.0	3.1	2.7	0.2
Red Wine & Bacon Sauce, Breast, Somerfield*	1 Breast/150g	131	87	14.0	3.0	2.0	0.0
Red Wine & Mushrooms, Asda*	1/2 Pack/190g	174	92	17.0	1.8	1.9	0.5
Red Wine & Potato Grattin, Healthy Eating, Tesco*	1 Pack/450g	410	91	7.7	8.9	2.7	2.2
Red Wine Sauce, Breast, Tesco*	1 Serving/180g	151	84	15.4	1.6	1.8	0.1
Red Wine Sauce, Fillets, Safeway*	1 Serving/175g	210	120	17.7	2.9	3.9	0.7
Red Wine With Mash, Eat Smart, Safeway*	1 Pack/400g	300	75	9.1	6.1	1.3	1.4
Red Wine, With Mash, Eat Smart, Morrisons*	1 Serving/400g	288	72	9.1	6.1	1.3	1.4
Satay Sauce, Safeway*	1 Serving/250g	363	145	10.5	7.1	8.0	1.4
Shiraz Wine Sauce, Finest, Tesco*	1 Pack/600g	420	70	10.9	2.9	1.6	1.3
Smoky Barbeque Sauce, Tesco*	1 Serving/185g	229	124	16.3	9.9	2.1	1.0
Spicy Chilli Sauce, Topped With Cheese, Breast, Asda*	1/2 Pack/190g	241	127	20.0	3.4	3.7	0.0
Sun Dried Tomato & Basil Sauce, Breast, Iceland*	1 Serving/155.8g	134	86	14.6	3.3	1.6	1.0
Sweet & Sour Sauce, Breasts, Good Choice, Iceland*	1 Pack/340g	350	103	15.3	8.8	0.7	0.8
Sweet & Sour Sauce, GFY, Asda*	1 Pack/400g	548	137	18.0	15.0	0.6	0.2
Sweet & Sour With Noodles, Feeling Great, Findus*	1 Pack/350g	385	110	5.0	17.0	2.5	1.5
Tarragon Sauce, Breast, Glazed, Feeling Great, Findus*	1 Pack/350g	270	77	4.0	10.9	1.9	1.4
Tarragon Sauce, Lean Cuisine*	1 Pack/337.5g	270	80	4.0	11.0	2.0	1.5
Tomato & Basil Sauce, Asda*	1 Breast/189.3g	231	122	22.0	1.2	3.2	2.0
Tomato & Basil Sauce, Breast Fillets, Morrisons*	1/2 Pack/171g	231	135	21.3	2.5	4.4	1.4
Tomato & Basil Sauce, Breast, Fillets, BGTY, Sainsbury's*	1 Fillet/175g	177	101	20.6	1.2	1.5	0.6
Tomato & Basil Sauce, Breast, GFY, Asda*	1 Pack/392g	447	114	12.0	9.0	3.4	1.5
Tomato & Basil Sauce, Chargrilled, Marks & Spencer*	1 Serving/235g	223	95	12.9	2.1	3.8	1.3
Tomato & Basil Sauce, Eat Smart, Safeway*	1 Serving/235.7g	165	70	10.3	2.4	1.6	1.3
Tomato & Basil Sauce, Good Choice, Iceland*	1/2 Pack/170g	153	90	13.3	3.3	2.6	0.6
Tomato & Basil Sauce, Safeway*	1 Serving/175g	201	115	16.7	3.8	3.6	1.1
White Sauce, BGTY, Sainsbury's*	1 Can/200g	250	125	14.5	2.5	6.3	1.0

C

CHICKEN IN

INFO/WEIGHT	Measure	per Measure KCAL	KCAL	PROT	CARB	FAT	FIBRE
White Sauce, Canned, Asda*	1/2 Can/400g	644	161	12.0	3.5	11.0	0.0
White Sauce, Chunky, Marks & Spencer*	1/2 Can/209g	303	145	13.0	3.7	8.6	0.5
White Sauce, Healthy Eating, Tesco*	1 Serving/100g	94	94	12.0	4.8	3.0	0.0
White Sauce, Low Fat, Breast, Safeway*	1 Serving/200g	190	95	11.5	2.1	4.5	0.2
White Wine & Asparagus Panzerotti, Asda*	1/2 Pack/150g	239	159	8.0	28.0	1.7	0.0
White Wine & Mushroom Sauce, Breasts, Asda*	1 Breast/167.9g	217	129	20.0	1.0	5.0	0.4
White Wine & Mushroom Sauce, COU, Marks & Spencer*	1 Serving/400g	400	100	9.6	13.0	1.6	1.3
White Wine & Mushroom Sauce, Marks & Spencer*	1 Serving/200g	260	130	15.6	1.6	6.8	1.0
White Wine & Tarragon Sauce, Breasts, Finest, Tesco*	1/2 Pack/200g	326	163	16.8	1.3	10.1	0.0
White Wine & Tarragon Sauce, Waitrose*	1 Breast/225g	281	125	10.7	3.1	7.7	0.3
White Wine Sauce, Breasts, Tesco*	1 Serving/370g	389	105	16.9	0.8	3.8	0.6
White Wine Sauce, Simple Solutions, Tesco*	1/2 Pack/200g	198	99	19.3	0.9	2.0	0.5
White Wine, With Pasta, Perfectly Balanced, Waitrose*	1 Pack/400g	400	100	8.2	12.1	2.5	2.5
White Wine, With Rice, Eat Smart, Safeway*	1 Serving/400g	400	100	8.9	13.6	1.0	1.1
White Wine, With Rice, Healthy Eating, Tesco*	1 Serving/450g	513	114	7.1	15.3	2.7	0.7
Wild Mushroom Sauce, Breasts, Healthy Living, Tesco*	1 Serving/212g	191	90	15.1	2.1	2.4	1.5
Wild Mushroom Sauce, Extra Special, Asda*	1 Serving/225g	319	142	14.2	2.2	8.4	0.3
Zesty Orange Sauce, Asda*	1 Serving/200g	340	170	16.0	13.0	6.0	0.4
Zesty Orange Sauce, Breast, Asda*	1 Serving/200g	326	163	16.0	9.0	7.0	0.0

CHICKEN INDIAN

INFO/WEIGHT	Measure	per Measure KCAL	KCAL	PROT	CARB	FAT	FIBRE
Style, Fillets, Sainsbury's*	1 Pack/200g	233	112	13.7	4.4	4.4	1.2

CHICKEN ITALIAN

INFO/WEIGHT	Measure	per Measure KCAL	KCAL	PROT	CARB	FAT	FIBRE
Good Choice, Iceland*	1 Pack/400g	388	97	4.7	18.3	0.5	0.6
Iceland*	1 Pack/250g	208	83	13.6	4.8	1.0	0.5
Ready Meal, SlimFast*	1 Pack/375g	390	104	7.1	16.6	1.1	0.4
Style, BGTY, Sainsbury's*	1 Pack/400g	364	91	6.0	14.5	1.1	0.9
Style, Dinner, Asda*	1 Pack/400g	244	61	6.0	7.0	1.0	1.1
Style, Meal, Asda*	1 Pack/408g	241	59	6.0	7.0	0.8	0.8
Style, Sainsbury's*	1/2 Pack/190g	222	117	16.3	3.9	4.0	0.1
With a Spicy Tomato, Chilli & Herb Sauce, SlimFast*	1 Pack/371.4g	390	105	7.1	16.6	1.1	0.4

CHICKEN JEERA

INFO/WEIGHT	Measure	per Measure KCAL	KCAL	PROT	CARB	FAT	FIBRE
Sainsbury's*	1/2 Pack/200.8g	247	123	10.5	4.6	7.0	1.8

CHICKEN KUNG PO

INFO/WEIGHT	Measure	per Measure KCAL	KCAL	PROT	CARB	FAT	FIBRE
Chinese, Tesco*	1 Serving/350g	417	119	8.8	10.2	4.8	0.6
Sainsbury's*	1/2 Pack/175g	131	75	9.2	4.0	2.5	1.0
Waitrose*	1 Pack/350g	319	91	8.2	12.1	1.1	1.2
With Egg Fried Rice, Asda*	1 Pack/450g	689	153	6.0	21.0	5.0	1.0

CHICKEN LAKSA

INFO/WEIGHT	Measure	per Measure KCAL	KCAL	PROT	CARB	FAT	FIBRE
COU, Marks & Spencer*	1 Pack/450g	360	80	7.5	7.0	2.2	1.1

CHICKEN LATTICE

INFO/WEIGHT	Measure	per Measure KCAL	KCAL	PROT	CARB	FAT	FIBRE
With Bacon & Cheese, Birds Eye*	1 Serving/150g	390	260	12.0	18.7	15.3	1.3
With Cheese & Broccoli, Birds Eye*	1 Lattice/134g	385	288	12.6	22.7	16.3	1.1
With Tomato & Basil, Birds Eye*	1 Serving/155g	340	220	10.8	15.7	12.7	1.4

CHICKEN LEMON

INFO/WEIGHT	Measure	per Measure KCAL	KCAL	PROT	CARB	FAT	FIBRE
& Ginger With Apricot Rice, COU, Marks & Spencer*	1 Pack/400g	320	80	7.9	9.7	0.9	2.0
Battered, Cantonese, Sainsbury's*	1 Pack/350g	560	160	10.7	16.6	5.6	0.9
Battered, Chinese Meal For Two, Tesco*	1/2 Portion/175g	294	168	6.6	18.8	7.4	2.0
Battered, Healthy Eating, Tesco*	1 Pack/350g	399	114	8.8	13.9	2.6	0.4
Breast, Fillets, BGTY, Sainsbury's*	1 Fillet/112.5g	195	173	18.4	19.9	2.1	1.9
COU, Marks & Spencer*	1 Pack/150g	150	100	17.9	5.6	0.9	0.8
Cantonese Style, With Egg Fried Rice, Farmfoods*	1 Pack/324g	486	150	4.9	21.8	4.8	0.1
Cantonese, Sainsbury's*	1/2 Pack/140g	217	156	11.0	13.9	6.3	0.6
Chargrilled, COU, Marks & Spencer*	1/2 Pack/175g	158	90	16.1	5.5	0.6	0.9

	Measure INFO/WEIGHT	per Measure KCAL	Nutrition Values per 100g / 100ml				
			KCAL	PROT	CARB	FAT	FIBRE
CHICKEN LEMON							
Chinese, Tesco*	1 Serving/350g	564	161	7.0	26.0	3.2	0.3
Cream, With Rice, Perfectly Balanced, Waitrose*	1 Pack/400g	592	148	7.6	21.7	3.4	0.3
Crispy, Take It Away, Marks & Spencer*	1 Carton/227g	329	145	9.4	19.2	3.4	0.7
Steam Cuisine, COU, Marks & Spencer*	1 Pack/400g	420	105	9.8	11.8	2.2	2.0
Tesco*	1/2 Pack/175g	214	122	11.0	10.1	4.2	0.6
Waitrose*	1 Serving/400g	596	149	12.7	11.7	5.8	0.9
With Rice, Healthy Living, Tesco*	1 Pack/450g	477	106	5.9	14.4	2.7	0.9
With Vegetable Rice, BGTY, Sainsbury's*	1 Pack/400g	428	107	6.5	16.8	1.6	0.8
CHICKEN LUNCH							
Light, French Style, John West*	1 Pack/240.4g	226	94	7.2	6.7	4.3	2.1
Light, Italian Style, John West*	1 Pack/240g	247	103	7.1	9.6	4.1	0.8
CHICKEN MANGO							
Tesco*	1 Pack/455g	687	151	7.3	15.3	6.8	1.2
CHICKEN MEAL							
American, Fillets, Asda*	1 Pack/345g	838	243	9.0	27.0	11.0	2.3
Raost, Marks & Spencer*	1 Pack/250g	375	150	14.6	5.3	7.7	0.1
CHICKEN MEDITERRANEAN							
Style, Somerfield*	1 Pot/215g	455	212	7.4	16.0	13.1	1.0
CHICKEN MEXICAN							
Style, BGTY, Sainsbury's*	1 Serving/260g	255	98	6.9	12.1	2.5	2.2
Style, Combo, Asda*	1 Pack/380g	927	244	19.0	15.0	12.0	0.0
Style, GFY, Asda*	1/2 Pack/200g	256	128	17.0	3.7	5.0	0.3
Style, With Rice, BFY, Morrisons*	1 Pack/400g	360	90	5.1	14.1	1.3	0.8
CHICKEN MOROCCAN							
Style, Sainsbury's*	1/2 Pack/269g	334	124	14.7	10.4	2.6	3.1
Style, With Spicy Cous Cous, BGTY, Sainsbury's*	1 Serving/225g	304	135	9.2	20.6	1.7	0.0
With Apricots & Pine Nuts, TTD, Sainsbury's*	1/2 Pack/200g	210	105	10.6	3.4	5.4	1.3
With Cous Cous & Fruity Sauce, BGTY, Sainsbury's*	1 Pack/400g	440	110	10.0	13.1	2.0	2.6
CHICKEN MUSTARD							
With Creme Fraiche Mash, Perfectly Balanced, Waitrose*	1 Pack/400g	408	102	7.2	9.4	4.0	0.8
With Gratin Potatoes, Healthy Living, Tesco*	1 Pack/450g	464	103	9.0	10.7	2.7	2.5
CHICKEN ORIENTAL							
& Pineapple, Healthy Living, Tesco*	1 Serving/450g	414	92	6.0	15.4	0.7	0.6
SlimFast*	1 Pack/385g	385	100	5.7	18.6	0.6	0.6
With Noodles, Steamfresh, Birds Eye*	1 Meal/399g	335	84	7.1	9.0	2.2	0.3
CHICKEN PAPRIKA							
& Savoury Rice, BGTY, Sainsbury's*	1 Pack/401g	385	96	7.2	15.6	0.5	1.1
COU, Marks & Spencer*	1 Pack/400g	380	95	9.0	11.7	1.6	2.0
With Savoury Vegetables & Rice, BGTY, Sainsbury's*	1 Pack/451g	555	123	7.2	17.8	2.6	0.8
CHICKEN PARMESAN							
& Sun Dried Tomato, Fillets, Mini, Sainsbury's*	1 Pack/200g	278	139	22.1	6.0	2.9	0.5
Sun Dried Tomato, Fillets, BGTY, Sainsbury's*	1/2 Pack/100g	138	138	22.1	6.0	2.9	0.5
With Pasta, Steam Cuisine, Marks & Spencer*	1 Pack/400g	400	100	10.1	8.1	3.0	1.3
CHICKEN PENANG							
Waitrose*	1 Pack/400g	364	91	10.1	6.6	2.7	0.8
CHICKEN PEPPER							
Fry, Sainsbury's*	1 Pack/400g	508	127	15.0	2.9	6.2	1.6
Hot, & Hash, Healthy Living, Tesco*	1 Pack/450g	396	88	7.0	10.7	1.9	1.0
Hot, Tesco*	1 Pack/455g	714	157	7.7	13.4	8.1	1.9
Hot, With Minted Mash, BGTY, Sainsbury's*	1 Serving/450g	333	74	7.3	8.4	1.2	1.3
CHICKEN PEPPERCORN							
BGTY, Sainsbury's*	1 Pack/251.8g	214	85	11.0	4.5	2.6	0.9

C

	Measure INFO/WEIGHT	per Measure KCAL	Nutrition Values per 100g / 100ml				
			KCAL	PROT	CARB	FAT	FIBRE
CHICKEN PICCATA							
Healthy Eating, Tesco*	1 Pack/405g	518	128	15.7	7.7	3.8	0.5
CHICKEN PIRI PIRI							
GFY, Asda*	1 Pack/400g	360	90	4.7	17.0	0.4	0.5
Marks & Spencer*	1 Pack/300g	420	140	10.0	7.3	7.7	1.3
Morrisons*	1 Serving/352g	341	97	11.7	2.3	4.6	2.0
Safeway*	1 Serving/350g	455	130	11.6	4.7	7.0	2.4
Sainsbury's*	1/2 Pack/200g	248	124	14.0	4.8	5.4	0.5
Tesco*	1 Serving/290g	307	106	15.8	1.4	4.1	0.5
With Rice, BGTY, Sainsbury's*	1 Serving/399g	395	99	10.3	11.9	1.1	1.6
CHICKEN PROVENCAL							
Marks & Spencer*	1 Serving/280g	350	125	11.4	4.8	6.8	1.5
CHICKEN RENDANG							
Sainsbury's*	1 Pack/350g	690	197	9.6	5.1	15.3	1.7
CHICKEN ROAST							
In A Pot, Sainsbury's*	1 Pack/450g	477	106	9.6	10.3	2.9	0.7
Meal, Blue Parrot Cafe, Sainsbury's*	1 Pack/285g	259	91	6.9	8.1	3.4	1.5
CHICKEN ROLL							
Broccoli & Mushroom, Sainsbury's*	1/2 Roll/175g	441	252	8.7	24.3	13.3	1.0
Value, Tesco*	1 Slice/13g	30	223	15.4	3.9	16.2	0.1
With Pork, Sage & Onion Stuffing, Value, Tesco*	1 Roll/125g	166	133	9.4	7.8	7.1	0.5
CHICKEN SAFFRON							
& Rice, Marks & Spencer*	1 Pack/400g	360	90	7.6	11.6	1.2	1.1
CHICKEN SALSA							
BGTY, Sainsbury's*	1 Pack/250g	178	71	9.7	4.7	1.5	1.2
Breast, Chunks, Roast, Waitrose*	1oz/28g	36	127	25.9	3.6	1.0	1.1
Mango, Breast, Sainsbury's*	1 Breast/178g	271	152	26.2	6.4	2.4	0.1
CHICKEN SATAY							
Breast, Party Bites, Sainsbury's*	1 Stick/10g	17	168	24.1	6.1	5.2	0.7
Indonesian, Bighams*	1 Serving/240g	314	131	12.2	6.2	6.4	0.6
Oriental, Tesco*	1 Serving/100g	160	160	23.6	5.1	5.0	0.4
Party, Mini, Tesco*	1 Satay/10g	13	133	23.7	3.4	2.8	1.0
Stuffed, Asda*	1/2 Pack/168.1g	242	144	22.0	6.0	3.6	0.8
CHICKEN SICILIAN							
Somerfield*	1 Serving/400g	384	96	7.5	7.8	3.9	1.0
CHICKEN SIZZLER							
Healthy Living, Tesco*	1 Serving/350g	273	78	11.1	3.8	2.0	4.3
CHICKEN SPANISH							
Style, Asda*	1/2 Pack/275.2g	322	117	14.0	4.1	4.9	0.7
CHICKEN SPATCHOCK							
Poussin, Sainsbury's*	1 Serving/122g	168	138	21.1	0.1	5.4	0.2
Salt & Cracked Pepper, Sainsbury's*	1 Serving/122g	168	138	21.1	0.1	5.4	0.2
CHICKEN STUFFED							
Asparagus & Ricotta, With Herb Rice, BGTY, Sainsbury's*	1 Pack/400g	444	111	8.1	13.8	2.6	0.3
Breast, With Mushrooms, Healthy Eating, Tesco*	1 Serving/175g	152	87	16.3	1.5	1.8	0.2
With Moroccan Style Cous Cous, GFY, Asda*	1/2 Pack/180g	259	144	20.0	10.0	2.7	0.0
With Mushrooms, Finest, Tesco*	1 Serving/150g	177	118	15.9	2.0	5.1	0.6
CHICKEN SUPREME							
BGTY, Sainsbury's*	1 Pack/350g	417	119	9.4	17.2	1.4	0.5
Breast, Sainsbury's*	1 Serving/187g	421	225	20.6	0.3	15.8	0.6
With Rice, Asda*	1 Pack/450g	617	137	15.0	3.4	7.0	1.1
With Rice, Birds Eye*	1 Pack/375g	499	133	6.7	19.1	3.3	0.5
With Rice, Healthy Eating, Tesco*	1 Pack/400g	384	96	4.9	15.6	1.6	1.5
With Rice, Weight Watchers*	1 Pack/300g	255	85	5.6	11.9	1.6	0.5

	Measure INFO/WEIGHT	per Measure KCAL	Nutrition Values per 100g / 100ml				
			KCAL	PROT	CARB	FAT	FIBRE
CHICKEN SZECHUAN							
Chilli & Peppercorn, Sainsbury's*	1 Pack/400g	352	88	9.9	3.2	4.0	0.5
Tesco*	1 Pack/350g	385	110	7.2	13.6	3.0	0.3
With Noodles, Sainsbury's*	1 Pack/450g	423	94	6.0	10.4	3.1	0.9
CHICKEN TANDOORI							
GFY, Asda*	1 Pack/420g	420	100	9.0	8.0	3.6	1.4
Healthy Choice, McCain*	1 Pack/270g	297	110	7.5	17.5	1.0	0.0
Masala, & Rice, Healthy Living, Tesco*	1 Serving/450g	410	91	6.6	12.9	1.7	0.6
Masala, Asda*	1 Pack/400g	580	145	7.0	18.0	5.0	1.3
Masala, Indian, Tesco*	1 Serving/350g	431	123	10.2	4.0	7.4	1.8
Masala, Sainsbury's*	1 Pack/400g	536	134	13.2	5.0	6.8	0.5
Safeway*	1 Pack/350g	595	170	13.7	5.7	10.3	1.3
Sizzler, Healthy Eating, Tesco*	1 Serving/350g	273	78	11.1	3.8	2.0	4.3
Sizzler, Morrisons*	1 Pack/350g	434	124	11.0	2.6	7.8	2.2
Sizzler, Sainsbury's*	1 Pack/400g	536	134	12.8	4.3	7.3	1.7
Sizzler, Tesco*	1 Serving/175g	243	139	10.0	10.0	6.6	1.0
Tesco*	1 Serving/175g	198	113	10.6	6.7	4.9	1.0
With Rice, Easy Steam, Tesco*	1 Pack/400g	484	121	8.7	14.7	3.0	0.7
With Spicy Potatoes & Dip, Healthy Eating, Tesco*	1 Pack/370g	322	87	9.7	10.3	0.8	1.3
With Spicy Vegatable Rice, Eat Smart, Safeway*	1 Serving/350g	368	105	9.7	11.1	2.2	7.0
CHICKEN TERIYAKI							
& Noodles, Asda*	1/2 Pack/340g	445	131	9.0	18.0	2.6	0.9
Asda*	1 Pack/360g	299	83	9.1	8.6	1.4	0.8
Japanese, With Ramen Noodles, Sainsbury's*	1 Pack/450g	482	107	6.5	15.5	2.1	0.8
CHICKEN THAI							
Chiang Mai, & Noodles, BGTY, Sainsbury's*	1 Pack/448g	484	108	6.9	11.0	4.0	1.7
Coconut, & Noodles, Marks & Spencer*	1 Pack/400g	320	80	7.2	8.1	1.8	0.7
Green, Fillets, Mini, Sainsbury's*	1/2 Pack/100g	130	130	27.9	0.9	1.6	0.8
Style Marinade, Breast, Chargrilled, GFY, Asda*	1/2 Pack/178g	178	100	17.0	1.3	3.0	0.5
Style, Steam Cuisine, Marks & Spencer*	1 Pack/400g	440	110	8.8	10.4	3.8	1.7
Style, With Noodles, Tesco*	1 Pack/400g	332	83	7.5	9.5	1.7	1.0
With Lemongrass & Rice, SlimFast*	1 Pack/375g	413	110	5.7	18.2	1.3	0.8
With Rice, Steamfresh, Birds Eye*	1 Serving/400g	380	95	6.7	12.7	1.9	0.9
CHICKEN TIKKA							
& Cous Cous, Boots*	1 Pack/160g	307	192	6.2	17.0	11.0	1.3
& Lemon Rice, Deli Meal, Marks & Spencer*	1 Pack/360g	342	95	9.8	10.2	2.0	0.7
& Rice Salad, COU, Marks & Spencer*	1 Pack/390g	351	90	5.9	14.6	0.7	0.6
BGTY, Sainsbury's*	1 Serving/188g	265	141	10.5	21.2	1.6	0.0
Creamy, Breast, Tesco*	1 Breast/190g	215	113	15.1	0.7	5.5	0.8
Pinwheels, BGTY, Sainsbury's*	1 Serving/213.9g	261	122	9.6	16.0	2.2	0.0
With Basmati Rice, GFY, Asda*	1 Pack/400g	592	148	9.0	24.0	1.8	1.6
CHICKEN TOPPED							
With Cheese, Ham & Mushroom, Breast Fillet, Morrisons*	1 Serving/175g	222	127	17.8	0.8	5.8	0.2
With Cheese, Leeks & Ham, Breast, Asda*	1/2 Pack/175g	224	128	20.0	1.7	4.6	0.5
With Ham, Cheese & Mushrooms, Breast, Tesco*	1 serving/350g	445	127	17.8	0.8	5.8	0.2
With Ham, Cheese, & Leek, Tesco*	1 Serving/190g	243	128	17.2	0.8	6.2	0.2
CHICKEN TUSCAN							
Style, Somerfield*	1/2 Pack/175g	222	127	15.7	2.5	5.9	0.2
CHICKEN VEGETARIAN							
Style Pieces, In A White Wine Sauce, Tesco*	1 Serving/430g	542	126	6.2	17.2	3.6	1.2
Style Pieces, Sainsbury's*	1 Pack/375g	754	201	25.5	9.0	7.0	0.6
CHICKEN VINDALOO							
Asda*	1 Pack/411g	649	158	7.0	19.0	6.0	0.0
Indian Takeaway, Tesco*	1 Serving/350g	515	147	7.2	6.3	10.3	1.7

CHICKEN VINDALOO

	Measure INFO/WEIGHT	per Measure KCAL	KCAL	PROT	CARB	FAT	FIBRE
Sainsbury's*	1 Pack/400g	460	115	14.6	4.8	4.2	0.6
Waitrose*	1 Pack/340g	398	117	10.6	6.4	5.4	1.6

CHICKEN WITH

	Measure INFO/WEIGHT	per Measure KCAL	KCAL	PROT	CARB	FAT	FIBRE
A Sea Salt & Black Pepper Crust, Breasts, Asda*	1 Serving/153.7g	186	121	19.0	5.0	2.8	0.0
A Sticky Honey & Chilli Sauce, Breast, Asda*	1 Serving/175g	247	141	20.0	8.0	3.2	0.0
Apricots & Almonds, Healthy Eating, Tesco*	1 Pack/500g	465	93	11.8	7.3	1.9	0.5
Asparagus & Rice, BGTY, Sainsbury's*	1 Pack/400g	428	107	9.1	14.5	1.4	0.9
Bacon & Leeks, GFY, Asda*	1 Pack/400g	328	82	13.0	3.0	2.0	0.6
Bacon & Leeks, With Mashed Potato, BGTY, Sainsbury's*	1 Pack/450g	435	97	8.4	10.1	2.5	0.7
Black Bean Sauce & Noodles, Eat Smart, Safeway*	1 Pack/369g	295	80	7.2	10.5	0.7	1.2
Broccoli & Pesto Pasta, BGTY, Sainsbury's*	1 Pack/300.9g	328	109	10.3	13.2	1.7	2.5
Cheddar & Bacon Filling, Breast, Just Cook, Sainsbury's*	1 Serving/180g	346	192	23.2	6.5	8.1	0.1
Cheese & Bacon, Tesco*	1 Pack/475g	613	129	9.5	9.5	5.9	1.4
Cheese & Chive Sauce, Carb Control, Tesco*	1 Serving/400g	400	100	8.4	2.0	6.4	1.6
Cheese Croutons & Onion, Asda*	1 Serving/200g	200	100	16.0	2.0	3.2	0.9
Cheese, Leek & Bacon, Breasts, Stuffed, Safeway*	1/2 Pack/159.0g	310	195	24.3	1.0	9.9	0.6
Cheesy Salsa, Safeway*	1 Serving/100g	180	180	29.2	3.6	4.9	1.8
Chunky Tomato Sauce, COU, Marks & Spencer*	1 Pack/400g	360	90	7.9	9.3	2.3	0.9
Coriander & Lime, Asda*	1 Serving/105g	122	116	24.0	2.9	0.9	0.2
Cranberry & Orange Stuffing, Sainsbury's*	1 Serving/100g	201	201	23.0	4.1	10.3	0.8
Cranberry Stuffing, Breast, Finest, Tesco*	1/2 Pack/200g	252	126	16.2	9.9	2.4	0.9
Creamy Mushroom Sauce & Mash, Healthy Living, Tesco*	1 Pack/400g	384	96	10.0	8.0	2.7	0.6
Creamy Mushroom Sauce, Eat Smart, Safeway*	1 Serving/250g	213	85	12.8	2.7	2.4	0.9
Garlic & Herbs, Asda*	1 Slice/25g	29	114	23.9	1.1	1.5	0.0
Garlic & Mushrooms, Somerfield*	1/2 Pack/100g	145	145	23.9	0.0	5.5	1.6
Garlic Mushrooms, Asda*	1 Serving/320g	403	126	16.0	2.0	6.0	2.6
Garlic Mushrooms, Breasts, Tesco*	1 Serving/175g	263	150	19.2	0.3	8.0	0.2
Grapes & Asparagus, Sainsbury's*	1/2 Pack/200g	240	120	13.3	1.8	6.6	1.0
Gravy & Stuffing, Breasts, Tesco*	1/2 Pack/173g	257	149	14.4	8.3	6.4	2.2
Gravy & Stuffing, Mini Classics, Tesco*	1 Pack/300g	243	81	5.2	8.1	3.1	1.2
Green Peppers, Black Bean Sauce & Rice, Farmfoods*	1 Meal/324g	408	126	5.5	17.1	3.9	0.4
Gruyere & Smoked Garlic, Breast, TTD, Sainsbury's*	1/2 Pack/200g	444	222	17.3	4.2	15.1	0.1
Ham & Vegetables, Creamy, Eat Smart, Safeway*	1 Pack/370g	241	65	6.5	5.5	1.8	1.4
Ham, Cheese & Mushroom, Breast, Tesco*	1 Serving/175g	222	127	17.8	0.8	5.8	0.2
Hoi Sin Sauce, Ooodles Of Noodles, Oriental Express*	1 Pack/425g	400	94	5.3	13.2	2.2	1.7
Leek & Bacon Sauce, Good Intentions, Somerfield*	1 Pack/400g	284	71	5.4	7.2	2.3	2.9
Leek, Cheese & Bacon, Breasts, Simple Solutions, Tesco*	1 Serving/200g	296	148	17.6	0.5	8.4	0.3
Lemon Grass, Thai Greens & Baby Corn, Sainsbury's*	1 Serving/200g	196	98	10.0	6.9	3.4	1.4
Lime & Coriander Marinade, Chargrilled, Asda*	1 Portion/163.4g	285	175	23.0	0.5	9.0	0.0
Lime & Coriander, Chargrilled, Asda*	1 Serving/190g	352	185	24.0	2.0	9.0	1.1
Lime & Coriander, Easy, Waitrose*	1/2 Pack/168g	203	121	18.9	0.7	4.7	0.5
Lime & Coriander, Marks & Spencer*	1 Pack/140g	168	120	25.8	2.0	1.2	0.3
Lime & Tequila, Asda*	1 Serving/150g	194	129	24.0	4.3	1.8	0.5
Lyonnaise Potatoes, Marks & Spencer*	1/2 Pack/260g	286	110	12.6	8.0	3.1	0.9
Mango Salsa & Potato Wedges, BGTY, Sainsbury's*	1 Pack/400g	336	84	7.0	10.4	1.6	1.5
Mascarpone, Bacon & Roasted Onions, Finest, Tesco*	1 Serving/200g	312	156	14.5	4.7	8.8	0.5
Mushrooauce & Herby Rice, Fillets, Marks & Spencer*	1 Pack/380g	475	125	7.7	12.0	5.1	1.3
Mushroom & Garlic Butter, Breasts, Sainsbury's*	1/2 Pack/180g	388	199	20.0	4.6	10.3	0.1
Mushroom & Garlic, Breast Fillets, Just Cook, Sainsbury's*	1/2 Pack/165.8g	330	199	20.0	4.6	10.3	0.1
Mushroom & Madeira Ragout, TTD, Sainsbury's*	1/2 Pack/225g	218	97	13.6	3.7	3.1	0.1
Mushroom & Tomato Sauce, GFY, Asda*	1 Serving/175g	180	103	19.0	2.0	2.1	2.7
Mushroom Pilaff, BGTY, Sainsbury's*	1 Serving/400g	320	80	8.1	10.5	0.5	1.4
Mushrooms, & Madeira Sauce, Finest, Tesco*	1/2 Pack/200g	318	159	16.5	3.8	8.6	1.1

	Measure INFO/WEIGHT	per Measure KCAL	Nutrition Values per 100g / 100ml				
			KCAL	PROT	CARB	FAT	FIBRE

CHICKEN WITH

	Measure INFO/WEIGHT	per Measure KCAL	KCAL	PROT	CARB	FAT	FIBRE
Mushrooms, In Madeira Sauce, Healthy Eating, Tesco*	1/2 Pack/200g	182	91	15.0	5.4	1.0	0.4
Mushrooms, In Oyster Sauce, Tesco*	1 Pack/350g	189	54	8.0	3.5	0.9	0.8
Olive Oil, Coriander & Lemon, Chargrilled, Sainsbury's*	1 Serving/122g	310	254	22.7	2.2	17.1	0.7
Pancakes & Pluauce, COU, Marks & Spencer*	1 Pack/245g	257	105	7.9	12.7	2.3	0.3
Pancetta & Mozzarella, Finest, Tesco*	1 Serving/150g	297	198	11.6	11.5	11.8	0.9
Pasta & Spicy Arrabbiata Sauce, COU, Marks & Spencer*	1 Pack/360g	252	70	5.2	8.7	1.4	1.3
Penne, Tomato & Basil, Steam Fresh, Birds Eye*	1 Serving/400g	400	100	9.0	12.3	1.6	0.6
Plum Sauce, Battered, Tesco*	1 Serving/175g	324	185	6.7	26.5	5.8	0.8
Plum Tomatoes & Basil, Breasts, Birds Eye*	1 Portion/172.4g	200	116	13.3	5.0	4.7	0.6
Pork, Parsnip Herb Stuffing, Sainsbury's*	1 Serving/100g	181	181	22.9	2.1	9.0	0.7
Pork, Sage & Onion Stuffing, Mini Roasts, Tesco*	1 Serving/240g	353	147	14.7	2.6	8.6	0.2
Pork, Stuffing & Chipolatas, Breast Joint, Tesco*	1/2 Pack/340g	524	154	16.7	3.4	8.2	0.5
Potato & Smoked Bacon Topping, Marks & Spencer*	1 Serving/175g	228	130	17.8	3.2	4.8	1.2
Potato Wedges, BBQ, Eat Smart, Safeway*	1 Pack/350g	368	105	9.6	14.0	0.9	1.8
Prosciutio, Dolcelatte & 3 Cheese Sauce, Asda*	1/2 Pack/195g	355	182	30.0	1.9	6.0	1.2
Rice 'n' Peas, Sainsbury's*	1 Pack/300g	489	163	12.5	14.4	6.1	2.1
Rice, Breast, Chargrilled, Spicy, Asda*	1 Pack/400g	372	93	6.0	16.0	0.6	1.0
Rice, Fiesta, Weight Watchers*	1 Pack/330g	307	93	6.1	12.8	2.0	0.4
Roast Potatoes, & Stuffing, Healthy Living, Tesco*	1 Serving/440g	415	94	7.4	11.6	2.0	1.1
Roast Potatoes, Eat Smart, Morrisons*	1 Serving/380g	346	91	8.5	10.1	1.8	1.5
Roast Potatoes, Eat Smart, Safeway*	1 Serving/363.2g	345	95	8.5	10.1	1.8	1.5
Salsa & Spicy Potato Wedges, GFY, Asda*	1 Pack/400g	332	83	6.0	11.0	1.7	1.8
Spinach & Pasta, Marks & Spencer*	1oz/28g	64	228	9.4	14.0	15.0	1.3
Spinach & Ricotta, Good Food*	1 Serving/300g	281	94	17.3	0.3	2.7	0.3
Spinach, Honey Mustard, American Style, Asda*	1 Serving/240g	394	164	14.0	4.4	10.0	0.3
Stilton & Port Sauce, Breasts, Finest, Tesco*	1 Serving/400g	668	167	18.5	3.9	8.6	0.7
Stuffing & Chipolatas, Joint, Tesco*	1 Serving/187g	338	181	16.2	2.8	11.7	1.9
Stuffing, Breast, TTD, Sainsbury's*	1oz/28g	50	180	21.5	5.2	8.1	0.9
Stuffing, Butter Basted, Co-Op*	1 Slice/23.1g	30	130	21.0	2.0	4.0	1.0
Sun Dried Tomato & Basil Butter, Sainsbury's*	1 Breast/185g	363	196	25.0	2.5	9.5	0.2
Sun Dried Tomato & Basil Sauce, Bistro, Waitrose*	1/2 Pack/175g	254	145	14.2	3.7	8.1	0.3
Sweet Chilli Noodles, Eat Smart, Morrisons*	1 Pack/380g	323	85	6.3	12.7	1.0	1.2
Tagine, Cous Cous, BGTY, Sainsbury's*	1 Pack/450g	626	139	10.1	15.9	3.9	1.5
Tagine, Cous Cous, Perfectly Balanced, Waitrose*	1 Pack/400g	516	129	8.2	16.2	3.5	1.0
Tangy Lemon Sauce, Breasts, Just Cook, Sainsbury's*	1 Serving/164g	244	149	16.2	16.9	1.8	0.1
Tomato & Basil Pasta, Marks & Spencer*	1 Serving/190g	171	90	6.8	10.6	2.1	1.4
Tomato & Basil Sauce, Breasts, Healthy Living, Tesco*	1 Serving/200g	146	73	12.0	3.9	1.1	0.6
Tomato & Basil Sauce, Carb Control, Tesco*	1 Serving/400g	316	79	7.4	1.7	4.7	1.6
Tomato & Basil, GFY, Sainsbury's*	1 Pack/400g	300	75	13.6	3.4	0.8	1.4
Tomato & Basil, Healthy Eating, Tesco*	1 Serving/225g	189	84	11.2	6.1	1.7	1.2
Tomato & Basil, Steam Cuisine, Marks & Spencer*	1 Pack/400g	460	115	9.6	11.6	3.4	2.0
Tomato & Basil, Weight Watchers*	1 Pack/330g	322	98	7.5	14.1	1.2	0.3
Tomato & Herb Sauce, Breasts, Italian Style, Tesco*	1 Breast/180g	144	80	15.8	1.6	1.2	0.6
Tomato & White Wine Sauce, Birds Eye*	1 Pack/382.4g	325	85	9.4	9.7	0.9	0.8
Tomato, Chargrilled, Tesco*	1 Pot/300g	381	127	6.0	14.6	4.9	1.0
Trotolle Pasta, Mediterranean, BGTY, Sainsbury's*	1 Pack/400g	220	55	8.3	3.9	0.7	1.2
White Wine & Tarragon Sauce, Somerfield*	1/2 Pack/136g	163	120	18.1	0.6	5.0	0.6
With Caramelised Peppers, Chargrilled, Marks & Spencer*	1/2 Pack/237g	225	95	12.9	2.1	3.8	1.3
With Cous Cous, Lemon & Herb, Finest, Tesco*	1 Pack/370g	492	133	10.5	11.5	5.0	0.9

CHICORY

	Measure INFO/WEIGHT	per Measure KCAL	KCAL	PROT	CARB	FAT	FIBRE
Average	1 Serving/150g	30	20	0.6	2.8	0.6	0.9

CHILLI

	Measure INFO/WEIGHT	per Measure KCAL	KCAL	PROT	CARB	FAT	FIBRE
& Lemongrass Prawns With Noodles, BGTY, Sainsbury's*	1 Pack/400g	328	82	5.0	13.8	0.7	1.3

CHILLI

	Measure INFO/WEIGHT	per Measure KCAL	KCAL	PROT	CARB	FAT	FIBRE
& Potato Wedges, Good Choice, Iceland*	1 Pack/400g	368	92	5.5	9.8	3.4	1.2
& Potato Wedges, Sainsbury's*	1 Pack/370g	393	106	7.2	10.1	4.1	2.2
& Rice, Birds Eye*	1 Serving/285g	305	107	3.4	17.2	2.7	1.0
& Rice, Frozen, Sainsbury's*	1 Pack/400g	436	109	4.8	18.4	1.9	0.6
& Rice, GFY, Asda*	1 Pack/400g	352	88	5.0	16.0	0.4	1.8
& Rice, Morrisons*	1 Serving/500g	630	126	5.7	18.9	3.1	1.1
& Spicy Wedges, Good Intentions, Somerfield*	1 Serving/400g	340	85	5.6	10.5	2.3	1.1
& Wedges, BBQ, Healthy Living, Tesco*	1 Pack/420g	391	93	5.4	12.2	2.6	1.9
Beef & Chilli Sauce, Chinese Takeaway, Farmfoods*	1oz/28g	66	234	6.7	20.0	13.0	0.3
Beef & Potato Wedges, Superbowl, GFY, Asda*	1 Pack/450g	477	106	6.0	14.0	2.9	1.5
Beef Jacket, Marks & Spencer*	1 Pack/360g	288	80	5.9	9.6	2.0	0.9
Beef, Asda*	1/2 Pack/200g	190	95	7.0	8.0	3.9	1.2
Beef, Crispy, Peking, Sainsbury's*	1 Pack/250g	795	318	11.9	30.7	16.4	0.7
Beef, Crispy, Sainsbury's*	1 Pack/400g	628	157	12.8	4.9	9.6	1.2
Beef, With Rice, GFY, Asda*	1 Serving/402.3g	354	88	4.7	14.0	1.5	0.9
Beef, With Rice, Sainsbury's*	1 Serving/300g	360	120	5.6	20.6	1.7	1.1
Bowl, American Style, Sainsbury's*	1/2 Pack/300g	255	85	8.8	4.6	3.5	2.0
Bowl, Safeway*	1 Pack/300g	327	109	8.8	8.3	4.5	2.7
Chicken Grande, Stagg*	1 Serving/204.9g	168	82	9.7	9.4	0.6	1.6
Chicken With Fettucini, Marks & Spencer*	1 Pack/350g	368	105	7.9	13.9	2.1	1.1
Con Carne & Rice, Co-Op*	1 Pack/300g	195	65	4.0	8.0	2.0	1.0
Con Carne & Rice, Healthy Eating, Tesco*	1 Pack/450g	446	99	9.1	10.9	2.1	1.6
Con Carne & Rice, Healthy Living, Tesco*	1 Pack/450.5g	473	105	5.5	14.8	2.6	1.2
Con Carne & Rice, Somerfield*	1 Pack/500g	490	98	5.0	18.0	1.0	0.0
Con Carne With Potato Wedges, BGTY, Sainsbury's*	1 Serving/400g	336	84	4.6	10.7	2.5	2.4
Con Carne With Rice, BGTY, Sainsbury's*	1 Pack/400g	448	112	6.0	18.8	1.5	1.8
Con Carne With Rice, COU, Marks & Spencer*	1oz/28g	29	105	5.6	15.0	2.3	1.3
Con Carne With Rice, Eat Smart, Safeway*	1 Pack/400g	340	85	5.3	12.2	1.3	1.4
Con Carne With Rice, GFY, Asda*	1 Serving/400g	456	114	6.0	19.0	1.6	0.9
Con Carne With Rice, Healthy Choice, Asda*	1 Pack/400g	412	103	6.0	15.0	2.1	0.9
Con Carne With Rice, Organic, Sainsbury's*	1 Pack/400g	472	118	5.0	18.5	2.7	1.8
Con Carne With Rice, Perfectly Balanced, Waitrose*	1 Pack/400g	508	127	5.6	19.9	2.8	0.9
Con Carne, & Rice, Basics, Sainsbury's*	1 Serving/340g	381	112	4.2	20.3	1.7	0.8
Con Carne, Asda*	1 Can/392g	376	96	7.0	9.0	3.5	0.0
Con Carne, BGTY, Sainsbury's*	1 Serving/377g	430	114	6.9	17.8	1.7	0.8
Con Carne, Baked Bean, Heinz*	1 Can/390g	324	83	7.0	10.3	1.5	2.8
Con Carne, Classic, Stagg*	1 Can/410g	521	127	8.8	8.6	6.4	2.3
Con Carne, Co-Op*	1 Serving/200g	240	120	7.0	15.0	3.3	0.0
Con Carne, Dynamite Hot, Stagg*	1 Serving/250g	310	124	7.6	9.6	6.2	2.5
Con Carne, Frozen, Co-Op*	1 Pack/340g	306	90	6.0	15.0	1.0	1.0
Con Carne, Good Choice, Iceland*	1 Pack/400g	476	119	5.5	21.9	1.0	1.0
Con Carne, Homepride*	1 Can/390g	234	60	2.5	11.2	0.6	0.0
Con Carne, La Caldera, Lidl*	1/4 Can/200g	240	120	6.9	8.6	6.4	0.0
Con Carne, Marks & Spencer*	1 Pack/285g	285	100	8.7	7.4	3.7	2.0
Con Carne, Restaurant, Sainsbury's*	1 Serving/100g	80	80	6.9	7.0	2.7	1.5
Con Carne, Sainsbury's*	1 Pack/376.2g	459	122	7.4	19.6	1.6	1.0
Con Carne, Silverado Beef, Stagg*	1 Can/410g	406	99	7.8	10.9	2.7	1.5
Con Carne, SlimFast*	1 Pack/375g	394	105	5.5	16.2	1.9	1.5
Con Carne, Tesco*	1 Can/392g	463	118	8.0	10.5	4.9	2.4
Con Carne, Tinned, Morrisons*	1 Tin/392g	368	94	8.8	8.0	3.0	2.4
Con Carne, With Rice, Birds Eye*	1 Pack/285g	291	102	3.3	16.6	2.5	0.8
Con Carne, With Rice, Eat Smart, Morrisons*	1 Pack/400g	328	82	5.3	12.2	1.3	1.4
Con Carne, With Rice, Tesco*	1 Serving/480g	600	125	6.8	15.1	4.1	1.7

	Measure	per Measure		Nutrition Values per 100g / 100ml			
	INFO/WEIGHT	KCAL	KCAL	PROT	CARB	FAT	FIBRE

CHILLI

Crispy Beef, Ready Meals, Marks & Spencer*	1oz/28g	74	265	8.9	33.1	10.5	0.7
Extra Hot, Marks & Spencer*	1oz/28g	28	100	8.7	9.1	3.1	1.8
Medium, Uncle Ben's*	1 Jar/500g	305	61	1.8	11.1	0.8	0.0
Mexican Chilli With Potato Wedges, Weight Watchers*	1 Pack/300g	249	83	4.6	9.6	2.9	1.3
Mexican Style, Aldi*	1/2 Can/196g	231	118	8.7	9.2	5.2	2.1
Mixed Vegetable, Tesco*	1 Pack/400g	352	88	3.9	11.0	2.9	3.2
Non Carne, Linda McCartney*	1 Pack/340g	275	81	5.8	9.2	2.3	1.7
Spicy Bean & Vegetable, Safeway*	1 Pack/311g	196	63	3.3	9.6	1.3	2.5
Three Bean & Potato Wedges, Safeway*	1 Pack/415.8g	395	95	3.2	13.1	3.0	3.5
Uncle Ben's*	1oz/28g	17	59	1.8	11.1	0.8	0.0
Vegetable	1oz/28g	16	57	3.0	10.8	0.6	2.6
Vegetable & Rice, BGTY, Sainsbury's*	1 Pack/450g	401	89	3.4	17.8	0.5	2.4
Vegetable & Rice, Good Intentions, Somerfield*	1 Serving/400g	336	84	2.7	15.8	1.1	2.1
Vegetable & Rice, Healthy Eating, Tesco*	1 Pack/450g	392	87	2.8	16.1	1.2	1.5
Vegetable & Rice, Safeway*	1 Pack/500g	530	106	3.4	21.2	0.8	1.7
Vegetable Garden, Stagg*	1 Can/410g	254	62	3.6	10.8	0.5	2.3
Vegetable, Canned, Sainsbury's*	1 Can/400g	368	92	5.1	16.7	0.5	4.9
Vegetable, Chesswood*	1/2 Can/200g	138	69	3.3	13.3	0.3	2.1
Vegetable, Retail	1oz/28g	20	70	4.0	9.4	2.1	0.0
Vegetable, Tinned, GFY, Asda*	1/2 Can/200g	140	70	3.5	12.0	0.9	3.5
Vegetable, Waitrose*	1 Can/392g	227	58	2.9	6.6	2.2	0.0
Wedge Bowl, COU, Marks & Spencer*	1 Pack/400g	380	95	7.2	11.3	2.3	1.8
With Potato Wedges, Healthy Living, Tesco*	1 Pack/400g	304	76	4.1	9.0	2.6	2.7
With Potatoes Wedges, GFY, Asda*	1 Pack/450g	419	93	6.0	12.0	2.3	1.5

CHILLI MEAT FREE

Mexican Style, Asda*	1 Serving/60g	54	90	8.0	12.0	1.1	2.4
Sainsbury's*	1 Pack/400g	308	77	4.0	4.1	5.0	5.2
With Rice, Vegetarian, Tesco*	1 Pack/450g	482	107	4.3	16.1	2.8	2.3

CHINESE LEAVES

Tesco*	1 Serving/100g	18	18	3.5	0.3	0.3	2.6

CHINESE MEAL

For One, GFY, Asda*	1 Pack/570g	946	166	7.0	28.0	2.9	0.0
For One, Safeway*	1 Serving/584g	993	170	5.5	25.8	4.7	1.3
For One, Safeway*	1 Serving/600g	605	101	5.3	17.1	1.2	1.2
For Two, Tesco*	1 Pack/500g	480	96	4.4	16.0	1.6	1.1
House Special, Healthy Living, Tesco*	1 Pack/450g	369	82	6.5	10.5	1.6	1.1
House Special, With Egg Fried Rice, Tesco*	1 Pack/450g	563	125	7.2	19.7	1.9	0.8
My Very Own, Asda*	1 Pack/297g	416	140	7.0	24.0	1.8	0.6

CHINESE TAKEAWAY

Ready Meals, Marks & Spencer*	1oz/28g	38	135	7.5	17.0	4.2	1.1

CHIPLETS

Salt & Vinegar, Marks & Spencer*	1 Bag/35g	170	485	6.4	59.5	25.5	2.4

CHIPS

& Curry Sauce, Tesco*	1 Serving/400g	440	110	2.1	14.1	5.0	1.0
11mm Fresh, Deep Fried, McCain*	1oz/28g	66	235	3.2	31.8	10.6	0.0
14mm Fresh, Deep Fried, McCain*	1oz/28g	59	209	2.7	34.2	6.8	0.0
14mm Friers Choice, Deep Fried, McCain*	1oz/28g	56	199	3.5	29.3	8.0	0.0
3 Way Cook, Somerfield*	1 Serving/96g	145	151	2.5	24.0	5.0	1.6
9/16" Straight Cut Caterpack, Deep Fried, McCain*	1oz/28g	63	225	3.1	32.1	9.4	0.0
Aldi*	1 Serving/50g	65	130	1.9	22.6	3.5	3.3
American Style, Oven, Co-Op*	1 Serving/150g	255	170	2.0	26.0	6.0	3.0
American Style, Oven, Safeway*	1 Serving/125g	288	230	4.1	38.2	6.8	3.0
American Style, Oven, Sainsbury's*	1 Serving/165g	314	190	5.4	23.6	8.3	1.3

CHIPS

INFO/WEIGHT	Measure per Measure KCAL		KCAL	PROT	CARB	FAT	FIBRE
American Style, Southern Fried, Iceland*	1 Serving/100g	251	251	4.0	34.0	11.0	3.0
American Style,Thin, Oven, Tesco*	1 Serving/125g	210	168	2.7	24.6	6.5	2.1
Beefeater, Deep Fried, McCain*	1oz/28g	71	253	3.3	37.7	9.9	0.0
Beefeater, Oven Baked, McCain*	1oz/28g	55	195	4.0	32.2	5.6	0.0
British Classics, Healthy Living, Tesco*	1/2 pack/200g	250	125	2.6	26.9	0.8	1.3
Chip Shop, Average	1 Serving/169g	578	342	4.3	39.8	18.4	3.5
Chippy, Deep Fried, McCain*	1oz/28g	51	182	3.0	27.8	6.5	0.0
Chunky Oven, Harry Ramsden's*	1 Serving/150g	185	123	2.8	19.9	3.6	1.6
Chunky, Baked, Organic, Marks & Spencer*	1 Serving/100g	150	150	1.7	27.1	3.7	2.2
Chunky, COU, Marks & Spencer*	1 Serving/150g	158	105	2.1	20.5	1.6	2.3
Chunky, Eat Smart, Safeway*	1 Serving/158g	150	95	1.6	18.3	1.6	1.4
Chunky, Finest, Tesco*	1 Serving/200g	272	136	2.6	22.4	4.0	1.7
Chunky, Ready To Bake, Marks & Spencer*	1 Serving/200g	310	155	2.2	26.8	4.2	2.0
Crinkle Cut Oven, 5% Fat, McCain*	1 Serving/100g	163	163	2.9	30.2	5.4	2.9
Crinkle Cut, Frozen, Fried in Corn Oil	1oz/28g	81	290	3.6	33.4	16.7	2.2
Crinkle Cut, Marks & Spencer*	1 Serving/150g	270	180	3.3	29.5	5.4	2.4
Crinkle Cut, Oven Baked, McCain*	1oz/28g	51	182	3.3	29.7	5.6	0.0
Crinkle Cut, Oven, Asda*	1 Serving/100g	134	134	2.0	23.0	3.8	8.0
Family Fries Oven, Tesco*	1 Serving/125g	164	131	2.0	22.4	3.7	1.8
Fine Cut, Frozen, Fried in Blended Oil	1oz/28g	102	364	4.5	41.2	21.3	2.4
Fine Cut, Frozen, Fried in Corn Oil	1oz/28g	102	364	4.5	41.2	21.3	2.7
Fried, Average	1 Sm Serving/130g	296	228	4.4	33.3	9.5	1.7
Frying, Crinkle Cut, Tesco*	1 Serving/125g	161	129	2.6	22.2	3.3	1.9
Frying, Value, Tesco*	1 Serving/125g	376	301	4.3	35.4	15.9	2.5
Homefries, Crinkle Cut, Oven Baked, McCain*	1 Serving/225g	448	199	3.2	34.8	6.9	0.0
Homefries, Extra Chunky, McCain*	1 Serving/100g	127	127	2.2	22.5	3.2	0.0
Homefries, Jacket Oven, McCain*	1 Serving/100g	220	220	3.9	37.9	7.4	0.0
Homefries, Straight Cut, Frozen, McCain*	1 Serving/200g	282	141	2.0	26.1	4.4	0.0
Homemade, Fried in Blended Oil	1oz/28g	53	189	3.9	30.1	6.7	2.2
Homemade, Fried in Corn Oil	1oz/28g	53	189	3.9	30.1	6.7	2.2
Homemade, Fried in Dripping	1oz/28g	53	189	3.9	30.1	6.7	2.2
Homestyle Oven, Sainsbury's*	1 Serving/125g	206	165	2.4	29.2	4.3	2.1
Just Bake, Low Fat, Marks & Spencer*	1oz/28g	37	133	2.0	24.7	3.7	1.7
Micro, Asda*	1 Serving/112g	221	197	3.5	30.0	7.0	4.0
Micro, Crinkle Cut, Tesco*	1 Serving/100g	203	203	3.3	29.5	8.0	1.8
Micro, McCain*	1oz/28g	54	194	3.3	27.3	7.9	0.0
Microwave, Cooked	1oz/28g	62	221	3.6	32.1	9.6	2.9
Oven Baked, Crinke Cut, New, McCain*	1oz/28g	55	198	3.5	33.4	5.6	0.0
Oven Baked, McCain*	1oz/28g	48	173	2.8	29.3	4.9	0.0
Oven Baked, Straight Cut, New, McCain*	1oz/28g	51	182	3.6	31.4	4.7	0.0
Oven, 3% Fat, BGTY, Sainsbury's*	1 Serving/165g	185	112	2.4	19.2	2.8	1.9
Oven, 3% Fat, Healthy Living, Tesco*	1 serving/125g	165	132	2.7	23.9	2.8	2.8
Oven, American Style, Champion, Aldi*	1 Serving/200g	372	186	2.2	28.2	7.2	2.0
Oven, BGTY, Sainsbury's*	1oz/28g	42	151	2.7	27.1	3.5	2.1
Oven, Best in the World, Iceland*	1 Serving/175g	333	190	3.4	28.9	6.7	3.5
Oven, Champion, Aldi*	1oz/28g	44	158	2.5	27.0	4.5	0.0
Oven, Chunky, Ross*	1 Serving/100g	177	177	3.1	26.6	6.5	3.9
Oven, Cooked, Value, Tesco*	1 Serving/125g	308	246	4.5	39.5	7.8	2.9
Oven, Crinkle Cut, Oven Baked, Tesco*	1oz/28g	50	180	3.3	29.5	5.4	2.4
Oven, Crinkle Cut, Sainsbury's*	1 Serving/165g	297	180	3.3	29.5	5.5	2.4
Oven, Frozen, Aunt Bessie's*	1 Serving/200g	260	130	2.2	17.6	5.6	2.7
Oven, Frozen, Baked	1oz/28g	45	162	3.2	29.8	4.2	2.0
Oven, Frozen, Healthy Living, Tesco*	1 Serving/125g	133	106	2.1	20.0	1.9	2.3

CHIPS

INFO/WEIGHT		per Measure KCAL	KCAL	PROT	CARB	FAT	FIBRE
Oven, Frozen, McCain*	1oz/28g	39	138	2.5	26.2	4.0	1.9
Oven, Frozen, Value, Tesco*	1 Serving/125g	189	151	2.8	24.7	4.6	1.9
Oven, Good Choice, Iceland*	1 Serving/150g	171	114	2.5	20.3	2.5	1.9
Oven, Healthy Choice, Safeway*	1 Serving/150g	227	151	2.8	27.1	3.5	2.1
Oven, New, BGTY, Sainsbury's*	1 Serving/165g	185	112	2.4	19.2	2.8	1.9
Oven, Organic, Little Big Food Company*	1 Serving/100g	164	164	3.0	28.5	4.2	1.2
Oven, Organic, Waitrose*	1 Serving/165g	233	141	1.5	25.1	3.8	1.6
Oven, Original, McCain*	1 Serving/84g	144	172	3.4	32.4	4.9	2.3
Oven, Steak Cut, Asda*	1 Serving/100g	153	153	2.0	27.0	4.1	2.5
Oven, Steak Cut, Sainsbury's*	1 Serving/165g	266	161	2.6	27.1	4.7	2.8
Oven, Steakhouse, Frozen, Tesco*	1 Serving/125g	165	132	2.7	22.7	3.4	1.7
Oven, Straight Cut, 4% Fat, Healthy Eating, Tesco*,	1oz/28g	35	124	2.3	21.8	3.1	1.9
Oven, Straight Cut, 5% Fat, Sainsbury's*	1 Serving/165g	281	170	3.4	28.0	4.9	2.5
Oven, Straight Cut, BFY, Morrisons*	1 Serving/165g	249	151	2.8	27.1	3.5	2.1
Oven, Straight Cut, Budgens*	1 Portion/180g	205	114	2.3	21.9	1.9	2.7
Oven, Straight Cut, GFY, Asda*	1oz/28g	42	150	2.6	27.0	3.5	2.4
Oven, Straight Cut, Great Value, Asda*	1 Serving/100g	199	199	3.5	35.0	5.0	3.0
Oven, Straight Cut, Healthy Eating, Tesco*	1oz/28g	30	106	2.1	20.0	1.9	2.3
Oven, Straight Cut, Iceland*	1 Serving/100g	197	197	3.6	31.6	6.2	2.3
Oven, Straight Cut, Low Fat, Healthy Living, Tesco*	1 serving/100g	132	132	2.7	23.9	2.8	2.8
Oven, Straight Cut, Nisa Heritage*	1 Av. portion/150g	186	124	1.8	21.3	3.5	0.0
Oven, Straight Cut, Reduced Fat, Tesco*	1 Serving/100g	127	127	2.3	22.7	3.0	2.1
Oven, Straight Cut, Safeway*	1 Serving/125g	226	181	3.6	30.0	5.2	2.5
Oven, Straight Cut, Tesco*	1oz/28g	46	166	2.6	27.8	4.9	1.7
Oven, Straight, Waitrose*	1 Serving/165g	219	133	2.0	23.0	3.7	1.7
Oven, Stringfellows, McCain*	1oz/28g	72	256	4.1	37.0	10.2	0.0
Oven, Thick Cut, Frozen, Baked	1oz/28g	44	157	3.2	27.9	4.4	1.8
Oven, Thin Cut, American Style, Asda*	1 Serving/100g	240	240	3.4	34.0	10.0	3.0
Oven, Weight Watchers*	1 Serving/100g	150	150	2.8	33.7	3.0	5.9
Steak Cut, 3 Way Cook, Somerfield*	1 Serving/200g	294	147	2.4	23.0	5.0	1.5
Steak Cut, Frying, Asda*	1 Serving/96.8g	181	187	2.9	28.0	7.0	2.8
Steak Cut, Oven, Tesco*	1 Serving/165.2g	233	141	2.0	24.4	3.9	2.0
Steak, Cut Frying, Safeway*	1 Serving/125g	289	231	3.3	27.1	12.1	2.2
Steakhouse, Fry, Tesco*	1 Serving/125g	278	222	3.1	25.2	12.1	2.0
Straight Cut, Frozen, Fried in Blended Oil	1oz/28g	76	273	4.1	36.0	13.5	2.4
Straight Cut, Frozen, Fried in Corn Oil	1oz/28g	76	273	4.1	36.0	13.5	2.4
Straight Cut, Low Fat, Tesco*	1 Serving/125g	159	127	2.3	22.7	3.0	2.1
Straight Cut, Microwave Baked, McCain*	1oz/28g	70	251	3.5	35.0	10.7	0.0
Straight Cut, Oven, 5% Less Fat, McCain*	1 serving/100g	172	172	3.4	32.4	4.9	2.3
The Big Chip, Frozen, Tesco*	1 Serving/200g	220	110	1.8	20.3	2.4	2.1
Thick Cut, Caterpack, Deep Fried, McCain*	1oz/28g	60	215	3.1	28.8	9.7	0.0
Thick Cut, Frozen, Fried in Corn Oil	1oz/28g	66	234	3.6	34.0	10.2	2.4
Three Way Cook, Skinny, Co-Op*	1 Serving/100g	175	175	2.0	26.0	7.0	3.0
Vending 3/8" Straight Cut, Deep Fried, McCain*	1oz/28g	62	220	3.3	29.6	9.8	0.0
Waffle, Birds Eye*	1 Serving/75g	156	208	2.5	24.3	11.2	2.6

CHIPSTICKS

Ready Salted, Smiths, Walkers*	1 Bag/22g	105	476	6.8	59.5	23.5	0.0
Salt & Vinegar, Smiths, Walkers*	1 Bag/22g	105	476	6.8	59.5	23.5	0.0

CHIVES

Fresh	1oz/28g	6	23	2.8	1.7	0.6	1.9

CHOC ICES

Average	1 Ice/50g	139	277	3.5	28.1	17.5	0.0
Belgian Milk, Sainsbury's*	1 Serving/80ml	170	212	1.9	21.1	13.4	0.5

C

	Measure INFO/WEIGHT	per Measure KCAL	Nutrition Values per 100g / 100ml				
			KCAL	PROT	CARB	FAT	FIBRE
CHOC ICES							
Chocolate, Real Milk, Sainsbury's*	1 Ice/48.4g	150	312	3.5	30.3	19.7	0.8
Chunky, Wall's*	1 Ice/81g	162	200	2.6	18.9	13.1	0.0
Dark, Sainsbury's*	1 Ice/43.2g	135	315	3.8	25.5	22.0	0.4
Dark, Tesco*	1 Ice/43.4g	136	316	3.0	27.4	21.4	0.7
Light, Safeway*	1 Choc Ice/43.5g	136	310	2.8	25.9	21.6	0.9
Light, Sainsbury's*	1 Ice/43g	135	313	3.2	27.0	21.4	0.3
Light, Tesco*	1 Ice/43g	138	322	3.4	27.1	22.1	0.5
Light, Waitrose*	1 Serving/70ml	141	201	1.7	17.0	14.3	0.3
Mini Mix, Magnum Style, Eis Stern, Lidl*	1 Ice/38.6g	130	334	4.2	29.0	23.0	0.0
Neapolitan Chocolate, Co-Op*	1 Ice/62g	120	194	2.0	16.9	13.2	0.4
Neapolitan, Safeway*	1 Ice/41.4g	119	290	2.6	25.4	19.5	0.3
Real Plain, Sainsbury's*	1 Ice/48.4g	149	310	2.9	29.5	20.0	2.2
Real White, Tesco*	1 Ice/54g	185	343	4.2	27.4	24.1	0.1
Rum & Rasin, Safeway*	1 Ice/45g	136	303	3.3	28.9	19.3	1.1
Safeway*	1 Ice/70g	217	310	2.8	25.9	21.6	0.9
SmartPrice, Asda*	1 Ice/31g	81	262	2.8	20.0	19.0	0.0
Value, Tesco*	1 Ice/31g	87	281	2.6	24.8	19.0	0.6
Vanilla, Co-Op*	1 Ice/70g	130	186	3.6	3.6	17.1	0.0
White Chocolate, Sainsbury's*	1 Choc Ice/48g	140	292	3.8	27.3	18.6	0.1
White, Real, Tesco*	1 Choc Ice/52g	198	381	4.0	26.9	27.6	1.1
CHOCOLATE							
A Darker Shade of Milk, Green & Black's*	1 Serving/20g	108	542	9.5	54.0	32.0	0.0
Animal Bar, Nestle*	1 Bar/19g	97	513	5.8	63.6	26.1	0.0
Assortment, Occasions, Tesco*	1 Serving/150g	705	470	4.6	65.8	20.9	0.5
Bars, Chocolate, Cherry, Lindt*	1 Bar/100g	470	470	4.5	61.7	22.8	0.0
Bars, Chocolate, Pistache, Lindt*	1 Bar/100g	585	585	7.1	48.2	40.6	0.0
Bars, Chocolate, Strawberry, Lindt*	1 Bar/100g	470	470	4.5	61.6	22.8	0.0
Bars, Milk Chocolate, Gold, Lindt*	1 Bar/300g	1605	535	6.6	58.7	31.0	0.0
Bars, Milk Chocolate, Hazelnut, Gold, Lindt*	1 Bar/300g	1665	555	7.9	50.7	36.1	0.0
Bars, Milk Chocolate, Hazelnut, Lindt*	1 Bar/100g	570	570	8.5	47.0	38.8	0.0
Bars, Milk Chocolate, Lindt*	1 Bar/100g	535	535	6.6	57.7	31.0	0.0
Bars, Milk Chocolate, Raisin & Hazelnut, Gold, Lindt*	1 Bar/300g	1590	530	6.8	54.7	31.6	0.0
Bars, Milk Chocolate, Raisin & Hazelnut, Lindt*	1 Bar/ 100g	530	530	3.1	54.7	31.6	0.0
Beans, Coffee, Dark, Solid, Marks & Spencer*	1 Serving/10g	53	532	4.7	42.4	37.6	11.6
Beans, Plain, Carl Brandt, Aldi*	4 Beans/5g	25	501	5.7	54.6	28.9	0.0
Bear, Lindt*	1 Bear/84g	480	572	7.5	57.7	34.6	0.0
Belgian Assortment, Waitrose*	1oz/28g	127	453	6.3	45.5	27.3	3.8
Belgian Dark, Extra Special, Asda*	2 Squares/20g	102	508	11.0	26.0	40.0	16.0
Belgian Milk, TTD, Sainsbury's*	2 Squares/20g	108	540	9.8	50.9	33.0	2.3
Belgian Plain With Ginger, TTD, Sainsbury's*	2 Squares/20g	114	571	7.2	31.2	46.4	10.9
Belgian Plain, Organic, Waitrose*	1 Bar/100g	505	505	9.6	32.0	37.6	5.6
Belgian Seashells, Woolworths*	1 Box/63g	347	550	5.5	52.9	31.1	0.0
Belgian White With Coffee, TTD, Sainsbury's*	2 Squares/20g	110	548	6.5	56.9	32.7	0.0
Belgian White With Lemon, TTD, Sainsbury's*	2 Squares/20g	109	546	5.7	61.2	30.9	0.1
Belgian White, No Added Sugar, Boots*	1 Serving/30g	146	488	6.0	47.8	36.0	7.0
Belgian, Finest, Tesco*	1 Chocolate/12g	62	520	5.9	55.6	28.4	5.2
Belgian, Milk, For Cakes, Luxury, Sainsbury's*	1 Chunk/8g	44	556	7.6	56.5	33.3	1.5
Belgian, Petit Fours, Safeway*	1 Serving/10.5g	53	525	6.2	49.9	33.2	1.8
Belgian, Thins, Extra Special, Asda*	1 Biscuit/8.7g	45	503	7.0	67.0	23.0	0.2
Big Purple One, Nestle*	1 Chocolate/39g	191	489	5.0	60.2	25.4	0.6
Black Magic, Nestle*	1oz/28g	128	456	4.4	62.6	20.8	1.6
Bournville, Cadbury*	1 Bar/50g	250	500	4.0	61.1	26.3	0.0
Bournville, Extra Dark, Cadbury*	1 Square/10g	56	560	8.5	30.8	44.8	0.0

CHOCOLATE

	Measure INFO/WEIGHT	per Measure KCAL	KCAL	PROT	CARB	FAT	FIBRE
Brandy Liqueurs, Asda*	1 Chocolate/8.3g	33	409	4.0	60.0	17.0	0.8
Brazil Nut Assortment, Marks & Spencer*	1oz/28g	163	581	9.6	37.5	45.3	1.5
Bubble Bar, Marks & Spencer*	1 Bar/25g	136	542	9.5	51.8	33.1	2.2
Bunny, Lindt*	1 Bunny/84g	480	572	7.5	57.5	34.6	0.0
Cafe au Lait, Thorntons*	1 Chocolate/16g	77	481	5.3	58.1	25.0	0.6
Cappuccino Bar, Thorntons*	1 Bar/38g	201	529	5.2	49.7	34.7	0.5
Cappuccino Mountain Bar, Marks & Spencer*	1oz/28g	149	533	8.4	52.0	32.5	2.6
Cappuccino, Nestle*	1 Serving/20g	109	545	6.1	56.0	32.9	0.0
Caramels, Milk, Tesco*	1 Sweet/3.3g	15	444	2.7	72.1	16.1	0.1
Chocolat Noir, Lindt*	1/6 Bar/17g	87	510	6.0	50.0	32.0	0.0
Chocolate Favourites, Tesco*	1 Box/454g	2029	447	4.2	64.3	19.2	0.3
Chomp, Cadbury*	1 Treatsize/12g	56	465	3.5	67.9	19.8	0.0
Christmas Tree Decoration, Cadbury*	1 Decoration/12g	60	525	7.6	56.2	29.9	0.0
Chunky Hazelnut Bar, Marks & Spencer*	1 Bar/52g	293	563	8.8	48.1	37.3	1.7
Classic Chocolate Bar, Cadbury*	1 Bar/26g	134	514	6.5	62.3	26.5	0.8
Cocoa, Organic, Green & Black's*	1 Serving/5g	16	321	20.0	13.0	21.0	0.0
Coconut, White, Excellence, Lindt*	1 Square/10g	61	610	6.0	48.0	44.0	0.0
Coins, Milk, Sainsbury's*	1 Coin/5g	26	502	5.5	58.8	27.1	2.5
Continental, Cappuccino, Thorntons*	1 Bar/38.0g	201	529	5.2	49.7	34.7	0.1
Continental, For Home Baking, Luxury, Tesco*	1 Pack/150g	822	548	2.7	27.7	45.1	0.9
Cool & Delicious, Dairy Milk, Cadbury*	1 Bar/21g	110	525	7.6	56.1	30.1	0.0
Cream, Fry's*	1 Serving/50g	215	430	2.6	68.6	15.4	0.0
Creamy Vanilla White, Green & Black's*	1 Serving/20g	115	577	7.5	52.5	37.5	0.0
Credit Card, Solid Milk, Marks & Spencer*	1 Bar/20g	108	540	8.1	54.1	32.4	1.3
Crispy, Sainsbury's*	4 Squares/19g	99	521	9.1	56.9	28.5	2.1
Dairy Milk, Advent Calendar, Cadbury*	1 Piece/4.2g	21	525	7.6	56.1	30.1	0.0
Dairy Milk, Bubbly, Cadbury*	1 Bar/35.2g	184	525	7.6	56.4	29.7	0.0
Dairy Milk, Cadbury*	1 Bar/49g	257	525	7.6	56.1	30.1	0.0
Dairy Milk, Caramel Centre, Cadbury*	1 Square/10g	50	495	5.7	61.1	25.3	0.0
Dairy Milk, Caramel, Cadbury*	1 Bar/50g	240	480	4.9	62.1	23.5	0.0
Dairy Milk, Caramel, Chunk, Cadbury*	1 Chunk/33g	158	480	5.0	63.0	23.0	0.0
Dairy Milk, Crispies, Cadbury*	1 Serving/100g	510	510	7.6	58.6	27.4	0.0
Dairy Milk, Crispies, Chunk, Cadbury*	1 Chunk/31g	158	510	7.6	58.6	27.4	0.0
Dairy Milk, King Size, Cadbury*	1 serving/85g	446	525	7.6	56.4	29.7	0.0
Dairy Milk, Mint Chips, Cadbury*	1 Serving/49g	247	505	6.5	61.2	26.1	0.0
Dairy Milk, Mint Chips, Chunk, Cadbury*	1 Chunk/32g	162	505	6.5	61.2	26.1	0.0
Dairy Milk, Snack Size, Cadbury*	1 Bar/30g	159	530	7.8	57.1	29.9	0.0
Dairy Milk, Turkish Delight, Cadbury*	1 Bar/200g	910	455	5.3	63.0	20.0	0.0
Dairy Milk, Turkish, Cadbury*	1 Serving/100g	455	455	5.3	63.0	20.0	0.0
Dairy Milk, Wafer, Cadbury*	1 Bar/46g	235	510	7.7	57.0	28.0	0.0
Dairy Milk, Whole Nut, Cadbury*	1 Serving/100g	545	545	9.1	48.2	35.2	0.0
Dairy Milk, With Crunchie Bits, Cadbury*	1 bar/200g	1000	500	6.2	63.3	24.4	0.0
Dairy Milk, With Shortcake Biscuit, Cadbury*	1 Square/6g	31	520	7.5	59.0	28.0	0.0
Dark, Bar, Thorntons*	1 Sm Bar/48g	245	511	9.3	31.6	38.8	15.9
Dark, Belgian, Luxury Continental, Sainsbury's*	1 Bar/100g	490	490	11.1	24.2	38.7	7.4
Dark, Co-Op*	1 Bar/50g	253	505	4.0	57.0	29.0	6.0
Dark, Fair Trade, Co-Op*	1 Square/4.7g	25	500	4.0	55.0	29.0	7.0
Dark, Luxury Continental, Sainsbury's*	1/2 Bar/50g	252	504	10.7	25.5	40.0	16.1
Dark, Mint, Thorntons*	1 Box/115g	544	473	4.4	58.8	24.7	5.3
Dark, Orange With Slivered Almonds, Excellence, Lindt*	1 Square/10g	50	500	6.0	46.0	30.0	0.0
Dark, Plain, Tesco*	4 Squares/25g	128	512	4.3	57.2	29.4	6.3
Dark, Raspberry, Ruffles, Jameson's*	1oz/28g	123	441	1.9	65.9	18.9	4.4
Dark, Rich, Tesco*	1 Serving/20g	98	491	5.8	60.0	30.4	0.0

CHOCOLATE

	Measure INFO/WEIGHT	per Measure KCAL	KCAL	PROT	CARB	FAT	FIBRE
Dark, Smooth, Safeway*	4 Squares/25g	128	512	4.3	54.9	29.4	6.3
Dark, TTD, Sainsbury's*	1 Square/10g	57	569	7.2	31.2	46.3	10.9
Dark, Whole Nut, Tesco*	1 Serving/13g	67	539	6.1	48.3	35.7	6.5
Dark, With 70% Cocoa Solids, Organic, Green & Black's*	1 Serving/20g	115	576	7.5	45.5	40.5	0.0
Dark, With Cherries, Green & Black's*	1 Serving/75g	390	520	7.0	57.3	32.8	0.0
Dark, With Hazelnuts & Currants, Green & Black's*	1 Serving/60g	323	539	8.4	51.6	36.4	0.0
Dark, With a Soft Mint Centre, Green & Black's*	4 Squares/30g	136	452	4.8	56.0	23.2	0.0
Darker Shade Of Milk, Organic, Green & Black's*	1 Serving/25g	136	542	9.5	54.0	32.0	0.0
Divine, Milk, Co-Op*	1 Bar/45g	243	540	7.0	57.0	32.0	2.0
Double Blend, Nestle*	1 Rectangle/11g	61	553	7.3	55.9	33.0	0.0
Double Chocolate, Nestle*	1 serving/25g	133	532	9.1	49.4	33.1	0.0
Dream, With Real Strawberries, Cadbury*	1 Bar/45.0g	250	555	4.5	59.6	33.1	0.0
Drops, Plain, Sainsbury's*	1 Serving/125g	638	510	5.3	60.1	27.6	4.0
Egg, Double Cream, Nestle*	1 egg/28.0g	163	582	6.9	49.2	39.7	0.4
Eggs, Party, Mini, Safeway*	1 Egg/20.3g	64	320	11.2	18.4	21.9	0.7
Espresso, Green & Black's*	1 Square/4.4g	22	550	9.7	46.2	41.4	0.0
Excellence, 70%, Lindt*	1 Bar/100g	540	540	8.0	33.0	42.0	0.0
Excellence, 85% Cocoa Solids, Lindt*	1 Square/8.3g	44	530	11.0	32.0	46.0	0.0
Excellence, Extra Creamy, Lindt*	1 Bar/100g	560	560	7.0	51.0	37.0	0.0
Excellence, Macadamia Nut, Lindt*	1 Bar/100g	560	560	7.0	51.0	37.0	0.0
Excellence, Natural Orange, Lindt*	1 Bar/100g	560	560	7.0	50.0	37.0	0.0
Excellence, Natural Vanilla, Lindt*	1 Bar/100g	590	590	6.0	51.0	40.0	0.0
Extremely Chocolatey Mini Bites, Marks & Spencer*	1 Cake/17g	76	445	5.5	51.4	24.6	2.0
Ferrero Rocher, Ferrero*	1 Chocolate/12.5g	74	593	7.0	49.0	41.0	0.0
Florentine, Marks & Spencer*	1 Serving/39g	195	500	7.4	64.5	24.9	1.7
Football, Thorntons*	1 Football/200g	1088	544	7.6	52.9	33.5	1.0
Freddo, Dairy Milk, Cadbury*	1 Frog/20g	105	525	8.0	56.0	30.0	0.0
Fruit & Nut Assortment, Marks & Spencer*	1oz/28g	148	527	7.6	49.8	34.3	1.3
Fruit & Nut, Belgian, Waitrose*	1 Serving/50g	254	508	8.6	54.6	29.2	3.4
Fruit & Nut, Cadbury*	1 Bar/49g	240	490	8.0	55.7	26.3	0.0
Fruit & Nut, Dark, Tesco*	4 Squares/25g	124	494	5.8	54.8	27.9	6.5
Fudge, Keto Bar*	1 Serving/65g	250	385	36.9	36.9	10.8	32.3
Ginger, Dark, Thorntons*	1 Bar/100g	509	509	5.8	44.3	35.1	8.8
Ginger, Traidcraft*	1 Bar/50g	212	424	3.9	68.2	14.8	0.0
Golf Balls, Lindt*	1 Packet/110g	619	563	6.5	53.6	35.9	0.0
Jazz Orange Bar, Thorntons*	1 Bar/56g	304	543	6.8	55.7	32.3	1.2
Kinder Bueno, Ferrero*	1 Twin Bar/43g	245	570	8.5	47.6	38.5	0.0
Kinder Maxi, Ferrero*	1 Bar/21g	116	550	10.0	51.0	34.0	0.0
Kinder Surprise, Ferrero*	1 Egg/20g	110	550	10.0	51.0	34.0	0.4
Kinder, Ferrero*	1 Bar/12.5g	69	550	10.0	51.0	34.0	0.0
Kinder, Riegel, Ferrero*	1 Bar/21g	117	558	10.0	53.0	34.0	0.0
Kitten, Lindt*	1 Kitten/84g	480	572	7.5	57.7	34.6	0.0
Lemon Mousse, Bar, Thorntons*	1oz/28g	141	503	4.1	55.3	29.3	0.0
Light & Whippy, Bite Sized, Sainsbury's*	1 bar/15.0g	66	439	3.3	69.7	16.3	0.1
Limes, Pascall*	1 Sweet/8g	27	333	0.3	77.2	2.5	0.0
Luxury Dark Continental, Tesco*	1 Bar/100g	571	571	11.3	46.5	37.8	0.1
Matchmakers, Mint, Nestle*	1oz/28g	134	477	4.3	69.7	20.1	0.9
Maya Gold, Green & Black's*	1 Bar/20g	110	552	6.0	56.5	33.5	0.0
Milk	1oz/28g	146	520	7.7	56.9	30.7	0.8
Milk & White Belgian, Shells, Waitrose*	1 Serving/15g	77	511	5.0	53.1	31.0	2.8
Milk & White, Winnie The Pooh, Marks & Spencer*	1 Bar/13.9g	76	540	7.9	54.7	32.3	1.0
Milk Caramel, Green & Black's*	1 Serving/20g	92	461	5.9	57.5	22.9	0.0
Milk Chocolate Excellence, Lindt*	1 Bar/100g	570	570	6.6	48.9	39.6	0.0

CHOCOLATE

	Measure INFO/WEIGHT	per Measure KCAL	Nutrition Values per 100g / 100ml				
			KCAL	PROT	CARB	FAT	FIBRE
Milk, Co-Op*	1 Sm Bar/50g	265	530	9.0	55.0	31.0	2.0
Milk, Extra Fine Swiss, Marks & Spencer*	1oz/28g	155	553	8.9	50.4	35.3	2.4
Milk, Extra au Lait, Milch Extra, Lindt*	1/2 Bar/50g	268	535	6.5	57.0	31.0	0.0
Milk, Fair Trade, Co-Op*	4 Squares/19g	106	560	8.0	49.0	37.0	3.0
Milk, Fair Trade, Tesco*	1 Serving/45g	236	524	7.6	56.7	29.6	2.0
Milk, For Home Baking, Luxury, Tesco*	1 Pack/150g	839	559	7.0	51.4	36.2	1.7
Milk, Honey, Traidcraft*	1 Bar/50g	273	545	6.0	54.0	33.0	0.0
Milk, Organic, Green & Black's*	1oz/28g	147	524	9.5	54.0	32.0	0.0
Milk, Organic, Tesco*	1 Serving/25g	140	558	6.3	51.4	36.3	2.3
Milk, Raisins & Hazelnuts, Green & Black's*	1 Serving/20g	109	543	8.5	48.5	35.0	0.0
Milk, Sainsbury's*	4 Squares/25g	133	533	9.2	54.6	30.8	2.2
Milk, Santa, Tesco*	1 Bag/90g	433	481	4.5	61.4	24.2	1.4
Milk, SmartPrice, Asda*	1 Square/6g	32	536	8.0	54.0	32.0	1.8
Milk, Swiss Made, Organic, Traidcraft*	4 Squares/16.6g	94	550	7.0	50.0	34.0	0.0
Milk, Tesco*	1 Serving/25g	133	533	9.5	54.7	30.7	2.2
Milk, Thorntons*	1 Sm Bar/50g	269	538	7.5	54.8	32.0	1.0
Milk, With Biscuit Pieces, Asda*	2 Squares/14g	73	521	8.0	57.0	29.0	1.9
Milk, With Butterscotch, Green & Black's*	1/3 Bar/50g	268	535	8.2	57.5	31.6	0.0
Milk, With Crisped Rice, Dubble*	1 Bar/40g	211	528	6.4	59.6	29.4	0.0
Milk, With Whole Almonds, Green & Black's*	1 Serving/20g	114	572	11.5	41.5	40.0	0.0
Mini Bites, Chunky, Moments, Fox's*	1 Roll/20g	90	450	5.7	52.4	24.6	2.2
Mini Eggs, Milk, Cadbury*	1 Egg/3g	15	485	4.8	67.7	21.8	0.0
Mint Creme, Sainsbury's*	1 Serving/20g	93	467	2.8	62.7	24.5	2.1
Mint Crisp, Cadbury*	1oz/28g	141	505	6.4	70.3	22.2	0.0
Mint Crisp, Sainsbury's*	4 Squares/19g	95	501	5.0	63.7	25.0	3.6
Mint Crisps, Marks & Spencer*	1 Mint/8g	40	494	5.4	54.8	29.6	3.1
Mint Thins, Plain, Safeway*	1 Thin/10g	48	480	2.3	67.5	22.3	0.7
Mint Thins, Waitrose*	1 Thin/5.3g	25	509	4.2	69.6	23.8	0.2
Neapolitans, Terry's*	1oz/28g	146	522	6.0	57.3	29.7	4.1
Nuts About Caramel, Cadbury*	1 Bar/55g	272	495	5.8	56.6	27.4	0.0
Nutty Nougat, Bite Sized, Sainsbury's*	1 bar/23.1g	111	481	7.6	59.0	23.8	0.6
Old Jamaica, Cadbury*	1oz/28g	129	460	5.8	56.9	23.3	0.0
Orange Cream, Cadbury*	1 Bar/51g	217	425	2.6	68.6	15.4	0.0
Orange Cream, Fry's*	1 Bar/50g	210	420	2.8	72.3	13.7	0.0
Orange Mini Bites, Marks & Spencer*	1 Bite/22g	95	430	5.5	54.6	21.6	1.8
Orange Tree, Lidl*	1 Bar/28g	150	537	9.6	53.0	31.8	2.1
Orange, Fair Trade, Divine*	4 Squares/17g	92	541	6.5	57.7	31.5	0.0
Orange, Sainsbury's*	4 Squares/19g	100	531	9.2	54.3	30.7	2.2
Panna Cotta, Raspberry, Marks & Spencer*	1 Bar/36g	190	528	4.7	51.4	33.6	0.3
Peanut Butter Cups, Reese's*	1 Cup/17g	88	518	10.0	55.3	30.6	3.5
Peppermint Cream, Fry's*	1 Bar/51g	217	425	2.6	68.8	15.4	0.0
Peppermint Patty, Hershey*	3 Patties/41g	160	390	2.4	80.5	7.3	0.0
Peppermint, Ritter Sport*	1 Bar/100g	483	483	3.0	60.0	26.0	0.0
Plain	1oz/28g	143	510	5.0	63.5	28.0	2.5
Plain, 72%, Finest, Tesco*	1 Square/10g	60	603	7.7	44.0	44.0	3.7
Plain, Cocoa Solids, Finest, Tesco*	1 Square/10g	58	581	7.7	38.5	44.0	5.8
Plain, Continental, Waitrose*	1 Square/4.1g	22	558	7.7	32.9	44.0	5.9
Plain, Fair Trade, Tesco*	1 Bar/40g	200	501	4.8	53.8	29.6	6.6
Plain, Organic, Tesco*	1 oz/28g	145	519	6.4	44.7	34.9	9.6
Plain, Wholenut, Sainsbury's*	1 Serving/25g	142	567	5.7	54.6	36.2	2.5
Plain, With Hazelnuts, Tesco*	4 Squares/25g	135	539	6.1	48.3	35.7	6.5
Praline, Marks & Spencer*	1 Bar/34g	185	545	7.3	49.6	35.2	3.1
Rafaello, Roche, Ferrero*	1 Sweet/10g	60	600	9.7	35.4	46.6	0.0

CHOCOLATE

INFO/WEIGHT	Measure	per Measure KCAL	KCAL	PROT	CARB	FAT	FIBRE
Rich Dark Fruit & Nut Plain, Sainsbury's*	4 Squares/25g	117	489	5.2	53.9	27.9	5.7
Rich Dark Plain, Co-Op*	1 Bar/200g	1010	505	4.0	57.0	29.0	6.0
Rich Dark Plain, Sainsbury's*	1oz/28g	144	514	3.7	65.0	29.5	0.9
Rico, Organic, Traidcraft*	1 Bar/45g	270	599	7.0	44.1	43.9	0.0
Rocher, Thorntons*	1 Chocolate/15g	76	507	6.8	45.3	33.3	2.0
Roulade, Sainsbury's*	1 Serving/72g	264	367	5.7	36.9	21.8	1.8
Shapes, Easter Friends, Tesco*	1 Chocolate/12.5g	70	540	8.0	52.3	34.2	2.3
Shots, Cadbury*	1 Pack/160g	752	470	5.9	59.7	23.2	0.0
Snaps, Hazelnut, Cadbury*	1 Curl/3.8g	21	520	6.8	57.8	28.8	0.0
Snaps, Milk, Cadbury*	1 Serving/4g	19	510	7.0	58.9	27.5	0.0
Snaps, Orange, Cadbury*	1 Curl/4g	20	510	7.0	58.8	27.4	0.0
Speckled Eggs, Marks & Spencer*	1 Egg/5.7g	26	440	6.6	63.1	18.2	1.5
Swiss Dark Extra Fine, Marks & Spencer*	1 Bar/150g	773	515	6.4	46.7	34.5	9.7
Swiss Milk Chocolate & Hazelnut Bar, Marks & Spencer*	1oz/28g	156	556	6.4	51.9	36.0	3.3
Swiss Milk, Marks & Spencer*	1oz/28g	150	535	5.1	60.9	30.1	1.9
Swiss Mountain Bar, Marks & Spencer*	1 Bar/100g	555	555	6.5	55.2	35.3	0.2
Swiss Mountain Bar, Orange, Marks & Spencer*	1/2 Bar/50g	268	535	8.0	52.2	32.8	3.2
Swiss Plain With Ginger, Waitrose*	4 Squares/17g	88	519	5.3	58.3	29.4	2.0
Swiss White, Bar, Marks & Spencer*	1oz/28g	152	543	8.0	58.3	30.9	0.0
Tasters, Dairy Milk, Cadbury*	1 Bag/45g	239	530	7.6	56.4	30.5	0.0
Taz Chocolate Bar, Cadbury*	1 Bar/25g	121	485	4.8	62.0	24.0	0.0
Teddy, Milk, Thorntons*	1 Teddy/250g	1358	543	7.6	52.6	33.5	1.0
Triple Crunch, Marks & Spencer*	1 Serving/60g	280	467	6.8	66.3	19.4	3.4
Truffle, Belgian, Flaked, Tesco*	1 Truffle/14g	81	575	4.4	52.7	38.5	2.3
Truffle, Dark Chocolate, Balls, Lindor, Lindt*	1 Ball/12g	76	630	3.4	38.5	51.4	0.0
Truffle, French Cocoa Dusted, Sainsbury's*	1 Truffle/10g	57	570	4.0	37.0	45.0	0.0
Turkish Delight, Cadbury*	1 Square/7g	33	477	5.9	61.4	21.8	0.0
Value, Tesco*	4 squares/25.0g	133	531	7.3	55.6	31.0	1.9
White	1oz/28g	148	529	8.0	58.3	30.9	0.0
White, Creamy, Safeway*	4 Squares/21g	113	537	6.9	59.9	29.5	0.0
White, Crispy, Fair Trade, Co-Op*	1/2 Bar/50g	278	555	9.0	51.0	35.0	0.1
White, Double Berry, Nestle*	1/4 Bar/30g	167	556	6.6	54.9	34.5	0.0
White, Nestle*	4 Pieces/40g	220	550	7.5	55.0	32.5	0.0
White, Organic, Green & Black's*	1 Bag/30g	173	577	7.5	52.5	37.5	0.0
White, Organic, Waitrose*	1oz/28g	160	572	6.1	53.9	36.8	0.0
White, SmartPrice, Asda*	1 Serving/25g	137	549	7.0	56.0	33.0	0.0
White, Tesco*	1 serving/25g	134	536	6.8	60.0	30.0	0.0
White, Thorntons*	1 Bar/50g	273	546	6.7	59.4	31.4	0.0
White, Value, Tesco*	1 Serving/10g	55	548	4.7	62.0	31.2	0.0
White, With Honey & Almond Nougat, Toblerone*	1 Serving/25g	133	530	6.2	60.5	29.0	0.2
Whole Nut, Cadbury*	1 Bar/49g	270	550	9.3	48.8	35.2	0.0
Whole Nut, Plain, Belgian, Waitrose*	4 Squares/25g	135	540	6.3	45.4	38.0	7.8
Whole Nut, Sainsbury's*	4 Chunks/25g	142	566	8.5	48.5	37.6	2.6
Wholenut, Milk, Tesco*	1 Serving/25g	129	517	8.7	53.4	33.8	9.0
Wholenut, SmartPrice, Asda*	1/2 Bar/16.4g	90	562	8.0	47.0	38.0	3.3
Wildlife Bar, Cadbury*	1 Bar/21g	109	520	7.8	56.8	29.3	0.0
Winnie The Pooh, Solid Shapes, Marks & Spencer*	1 Chocolate/6g	32	540	8.1	54.1	32.4	1.3
With Almonds, Dark, Organic, Evernat*	1oz/28g	169	604	16.3	37.4	43.2	0.0
With Almonds, Nestle*	1 Square/20g	109	547	9.2	48.7	35.1	0.1
With Ginger, Organic, Green & Black's*	1 Square/10g	52	515	6.6	59.0	31.0	0.0
With Orange & Spices, Green & Black's*	1 Serving/20g	110	552	6.0	56.5	33.5	0.0

CHOCOLATE DRINK

INFO/WEIGHT	Measure	per Measure KCAL	KCAL	PROT	CARB	FAT	FIBRE
Finest, Tesco*	1 Serving/200ml	242	121	4.9	10.7	6.5	0.8

	Measure	per Measure	Nutrition Values per 100g / 100ml				
	INFO/WEIGHT	KCAL	KCAL	PROT	CARB	FAT	FIBRE
CHOCOLATE DRINK							
Flavia*	1 Serving/18g	64	368	15.6	67.2	4.0	0.0
Instant Break, Milk, Cadbury*	4 Tsp/28g	119	425	10.9	64.2	14.0	0.0
Orange, Clipper*	1 Packet/28g	98	350	14.6	69.7	1.5	0.0
Powerup*	1 Serving/325ml	341	105	5.0	14.5	3.0	1.5
CHOCOLATE DROPS							
Plain, Asda*	1 Serving/100g	489	489	7.0	50.0	29.0	10.0
White, For Cooking & Decorating, Sainsbury's*	1oz/28g	152	544	6.5	60.3	30.8	0.0
CHOCOLATE ECLAIRS							
Ashbury, The Sweet Partnership/Childline*	1 Sweet/12g	59	490	4.1	63.1	22.4	0.0
Cadbury*	1 Sweet/8g	36	455	4.5	68.9	17.9	0.0
Co-Op*	1 Sweet/8g	38	480	3.0	71.0	20.0	0.6
Eclair, Marks & Spencer*	1 Sweet/14g	65	465	3.3	69.8	19.3	0.2
Marks & Spencer*	1 Sweet/7g	34	482	1.9	73.9	20.1	0.0
Milk, Sainsbury's*	1 Sweet/8g	33	442	2.1	75.7	14.5	0.5
CHOCOLATE NUTS							
Almonds, Dark Chohcolate Covered, Bolero*	2 Almonds/3g	15	510	2.6	48.8	33.5	0.0
Almonds, In Milk Chocolate, Organic, Green & Black's*	1 Serving/20g	109	547	12.0	46.0	35.0	0.0
Peanuts, Assorted, Thorntons*	1 Bag/140g	785	561	13.8	34.8	40.8	3.6
Peanuts, Belgian Coated, Marks & Spencer*	1 Serving/20g	109	545	14.7	35.6	38.0	5.8
Peanuts, Milk, Tesco*	1 Bag/227g	1221	538	17.5	31.8	37.9	4.4
CHOCOLATE ORANGE							
Bar, Montana*	1 Serving/25g	131	523	7.0	62.2	27.4	0.0
Crunchball, Terry's*	1 Segment/8.7g	47	520	6.9	59.8	28.1	2.0
Dark, Terry's	1 Segment/9g	45	511	4.3	57.0	29.3	6.2
Egg & Spoon, Terry's*	1 Egg/33.9g	196	575	5.5	51.6	38.0	1.7
Milk Bar, Terry's*	1 Bar/40g	212	531	7.2	57.5	30.2	0.4
Milk, Mini Segments, Terry's*	1 Segment/8g	42	527	7.7	57.9	29.4	2.1
Milk, Sandwich Bar, Lyons*	1 Bar/27.5g	144	516	5.0	62.0	29.0	0.0
Milk, Terry's*	1 Orange/175g	915	523	6.5	59.3	28.7	2.2
Oatiz, Sundora*	1 Serving/62.5g	249	396	7.7	61.6	13.3	9.6
Plain, Terry's*	1 Orange/175g	889	508	3.8	56.8	29.4	6.2
Segsations, Terry's*	1 Segsation/8.2g	42	530	5.8	58.5	30.0	2.6
Snowball, Terry's*	1 Segment/8.5g	48	534	6.6	61.3	29.2	0.0
White, Terry's*	1 Segment/11.4g	59	535	6.3	60.9	29.4	0.0
CHOCOLATE RAISINS							
Assorted, Thorntons*	1 Bag/140g	601	429	4.2	58.8	19.7	2.9
Belgian Coated, Marks & Spencer*	1 Bag/100g	450	450	4.3	60.6	20.9	0.8
Californian, Tesco*	1/4 Bag/56.8g	268	472	5.2	66.2	20.7	1.3
Coated, Californian, Marks & Spencer*	1 Bag/130g	520	400	4.3	63.2	14.7	1.9
Marks & Spencer*	1oz/28g	116	414	4.5	66.5	14.6	1.2
Milk, Asda*	1 Serving/28g	127	452	6.0	62.0	20.0	1.2
Milk, Co-Op*	1/2 Bag/100g	420	420	5.0	63.0	17.0	6.0
Milk, Sainsbury's*	1oz/28g	117	418	4.7	62.7	16.5	1.4
Milk, Tesco*	1 Lge Bag/227g	933	411	4.8	63.3	15.4	0.9
CHOCOLATE SPREAD							
Average	1 Tsp/12g	68	569	4.1	57.1	37.6	0.0
Cadbury*	1 Tsp/12g	69	575	4.5	55.0	38.0	0.0
Hazelnut, Asda*	1 Tbsp/15g	86	574	5.0	53.0	38.0	0.0
Hazelnut, Nutella, Ferrero*	1oz/28g	149	533	6.5	57.0	31.0	0.0
Milk, Belgian, Sainsbury's*	1 Serving/10g	56	559	11.9	47.2	35.8	1.4
Milk, SmartPrice, Asda*	1 Tbsp/16g	92	573	4.0	56.0	37.0	2.0
Nutella, Ferrero*	1 Tsp/12g	64	533	6.5	57.0	31.0	0.0
Snickers, Mars*	1 Serving/7g	38	548	8.7	43.3	37.8	0.0

C

	Measure		Nutrition Values per 100g / 100ml				
	INFO/WEIGHT	per Measure KCAL	KCAL	PROT	CARB	FAT	FIBRE
CHOCOLATE SPREAD							
Value, Tesco*	1 Serving/20g	116	581	3.0	54.5	39.0	1.5
With Nuts	1 Tsp/12g	66	549	6.2	60.5	33.0	0.8
CHOCOLATES							
All Gold, Dark, Terry's*	1oz/28g	136	487	3.6	60.9	25.2	4.0
All Gold, Milk, Terry's*	1 Serving/50g	248	496	5.6	61.4	25.2	1.7
Almond Mocca Mousse, Thorntons*	1 Chocolate/14g	76	543	8.5	40.7	37.9	2.9
Alpini, Thorntons*	1 Chocolate/13g	70	538	7.0	54.6	32.3	2.3
Bittermint, Bendicks*	1 Mint/18.2g	74	411	4.4	63.0	17.6	0.0
Cappuccino, Thorntons*	1 Chocolate/13g	70	538	5.9	48.5	36.2	0.8
Caramels, Sainsbury's*	1 Sweet/11.6g	57	490	3.5	69.0	22.2	0.2
Celebrations, Mars*	1 Bounty/8.3g	36	438	0.0	75.0	18.8	0.0
Champagne, Thorntons*	1 Chocolate/16g	76	475	6.9	43.1	29.4	2.5
Chocolate Mousse, Thorntons*	1 Chocolate/13g	67	515	7.5	40.0	36.2	3.1
Coffee Creme, Dark, Thorntons*	1 Chocolate/13g	52	400	3.0	71.5	10.8	0.8
Coffee Creme, Milk, Thorntons*	1 Chocolate/13g	52	400	2.8	74.6	10.0	0.8
Continental, Belgian, Thorntons*	1 Chocolate/13g	67	514	5.8	53.5	30.3	2.9
Continental, Thorntons*	1 Chocolate/15g	76	506	5.6	54.5	29.3	2.7
Country Caramel, Milk, Thorntons*	1 Chocolate/9g	45	500	4.6	62.2	26.7	0.0
Dairy Box, Milk, Nestle*	1 Sm Box/227g	1085	478	5.7	60.8	23.5	0.8
Dark, Elegant, Elizabeth Shaw*	1 Chocolate/8g	38	469	2.9	62.5	23.1	0.0
Dark, Swiss Thins, Lindt*	1 Packet/125g	681	545	4.8	49.2	37.0	0.0
Italian Collection, Amaretto, Marks & Spencer*	1 Chocolate/12.5g	62	480	4.4	59.7	25.1	2.3
Italian Collection, Cappuccino, Marks & Spencer*	1 Bag/100g	545	545	6.3	46.7	37.0	1.8
Italian Collection, Favourites, Marks & Spencer*	1 Chocolate/14g	74	530	5.7	50.4	33.7	1.6
Italian Collection, Panna Cotta, Marks & Spencer*	1 Chocolate/12.8g	71	545	5.3	49.4	36.4	0.1
Liquers, Cognac Truffle, Thorntons*	1 Chocolate/14g	65	464	7.3	40.0	27.1	2.9
Liqueur, Elizabeth Shaw*	1 Chocolate/8g	36	447	2.7	56.5	20.7	0.0
Milk Tray, Cadbury*	1oz/28g	139	495	5.2	60.5	26.0	0.0
Milk, Swiss Thins, Lindt*	1 Packet/125g	688	550	5.8	53.6	34.7	0.0
Mingles, Bendicks*	1 Chocolate/5g	26	528	6.5	55.0	32.9	0.0
Mint Crisp, Bendicks*	1 Mint/7.7g	40	494	5.2	55.0	29.9	0.0
Mint Crisp, Dark, Elizabeth Shaw*	1 Chocolate/6g	27	458	1.9	68.0	20.7	0.0
Mint Crisp, Milk, Elizabeth Shaw*	1 Chocolate/6g	30	493	4.0	70.9	21.4	0.0
Mint Crisp, Thorntons*	1 Chocolate/7g	34	486	7.7	40.0	31.4	4.3
Misshapes, Assorted, Cadbury*	1 Chocolate/8g	41	515	5.2	57.5	29.1	0.0
Orange Crisp, Elizabeth Shaw*	1 Chocolate/6g	29	478	2.9	68.2	21.5	0.0
Praline, Coffee, Thorntons*	1 Chocolate/7g	37	529	7.0	47.1	34.3	2.9
Praline, Hazelnut, Thorntons*	1 Chocolate/5g	27	540	7.0	48.0	36.0	4.0
Praline, Marzipan, Thorntons*	1 Chocolate/14g	63	450	5.9	58.6	21.4	2.1
Praline, Roast Hazelnut, Thorntons*	1 Chocolate/13g	70	538	6.0	51.5	33.8	3.1
Roses, Cadbury*	1oz/28g	136	485	4.8	60.9	24.8	0.0
Strawberrys & Cream, Thorntons*	1 Chocolate/12g	64	533	5.1	54.2	32.5	0.8
Swiss Milk Discs, Marks & Spencer*	1 Disc/5g	28	553	8.9	50.4	35.3	2.4
Swiss Tradition, De Luxe, Lindt*	1 Packet/250g	1388	555	6.3	51.9	36.3	0.0
Swiss Tradition, Mixed, Lindt*	1 Packet/392g	2215	565	6.1	49.8	38.1	0.0
Tartufo, Thorntons*	1 Chocolate/15g	77	513	7.4	40.0	36.0	3.3
Truffle, Amaretto, Thorntons*	1 Chocolate/14g	66	471	5.5	55.0	25.7	2.9
Truffle, Belgian Milk, Waitrose*	1 Serving/14g	72	514	4.3	47.1	34.3	0.0
Truffle, Brandy, Thorntons*	1 Chocolate/14g	68	486	6.1	52.1	27.1	0.7
Truffle, Caramel, Thorntons*	1 Chocolate/14g	67	479	4.2	57.9	25.7	2.1
Truffle, Champagne, Petit, Thorntons*	1 Chocolate/6g	31	517	7.5	48.3	31.7	3.3
Truffle, Champagne, Premier, Thorntons*	1 Chocolate/17g	88	518	6.9	45.3	32.9	2.4
Truffle, Cherry, Thorntons*	1 Chocolate/14g	58	414	4.2	50.7	21.4	1.4

	Measure	per Measure		Nutrition Values per 100g / 100ml				
	INFO/WEIGHT	KCAL		KCAL	PROT	CARB	FAT	FIBRE

CHOCOLATES

	Measure INFO/WEIGHT	per Measure KCAL	KCAL	PROT	CARB	FAT	FIBRE
Truffle, Continental Champagne, Thorntons*	1 Chocolate/16g	78	488	6.1	51.3	28.0	0.6
Truffle, Grand Marnier, Thorntons*	1 Chocolate/15g	77	513	7.2	40.7	34.0	4.0
Truffle, Hazelnut, Balls, Lindor, Lindt*	1 Ball/12g	76	632	5.0	39.1	50.6	0.0
Truffle, Irish Milk Chocolate Cream, Elizabeth Shaw*	1 Chocolate/12g	57	477	3.9	63.4	22.8	0.0
Truffle, Lemon, White, Thorntons*	1 Chocolate/14g	63	450	4.6	64.3	25.0	0.7
Truffle, Milk Chocolate, Balls, Lindor, Lindt*	1 Ball/12g	74	617	4.9	43.1	47.2	0.0
Truffle, Mint, Marks & Spencer*	1 Bar/35g	190	543	6.8	55.9	32.4	1.2
Truffle, Rum	1oz/28g	146	521	6.1	49.7	33.7	1.9
Truffle, Rum, Thorntons*	1 Chocolate/13g	63	485	4.8	58.5	24.6	4.8
Truffle, Selection, Tesco*	1 Chocolate/14g	75	539	5.1	62.0	29.8	0.5
Truffle, Seville, Thorntons*	1 Chocolate/14g	76	543	7.1	53.6	33.6	1.4
Truffle, Swiss, Somerfield*	1 Pack/125g	640	512	4.0	52.0	32.0	0.0
Truffle, Thorntons*	1 Chocolate/7g	33	471	6.0	48.6	27.1	1.4
Truffle, Vanilla, Thorntons*	1 Chocolate/13g	64	492	4.8	57.7	26.9	1.5
Truffle, Viennese, Dark, Thorntons*	1 Chocolate/10g	53	530	5.9	47.0	36.0	3.0
Truffle, Viennese, Milk, Thorntons*	1 Chocolate/10g	56	560	4.9	54.0	36.0	0.0
Truffle, White Chocolate, Balls, Lindor, Lindt*	1 Ball/12g	78	649	5.2	40.2	51.9	0.0
Valentine, Thorntons*	1 Chocolate/11g	60	542	5.7	52.0	34.5	2.1
Winter Selection, Thorntons*	1 Chocolate/10g	51	506	6.2	51.3	30.6	3.8

CHOCOLATINE

	Measure INFO/WEIGHT	per Measure KCAL	KCAL	PROT	CARB	FAT	FIBRE
All Butter, Sainsbury's*	1 Serving/58.1g	241	415	7.9	42.5	23.7	3.3
Mini, Sainsbury's*	1 Serving/30g	120	400	7.7	41.0	23.0	3.3
Sainsbury's*	1 Serving/58g	263	454	8.5	42.3	27.9	2.1

CHOP SUEY

	Measure INFO/WEIGHT	per Measure KCAL	KCAL	PROT	CARB	FAT	FIBRE
Chicken, With Noodles, Sainsbury's*	1 Pack/300g	300	100	5.7	13.6	2.5	1.2

CHOW MEIN

	Measure INFO/WEIGHT	per Measure KCAL	KCAL	PROT	CARB	FAT	FIBRE
Beef, Sainsbury's*	1 Pack/450g	500	111	6.6	15.5	2.5	0.8
Cantonese Chicken, Sainsbury's*	1 Pack/450g	455	101	6.5	11.5	3.2	1.7
Cantonese Vegetable Stir Fry, Sainsbury's*	1/4 Pack/100g	85	85	2.2	10.6	3.8	1.2
Char Sui, Cantonese, Sainsbury's*	1/2 Pack/225g	205	91	5.7	10.0	3.1	1.1
Chicken Stir Fry, Oriental Express*	1 Pack/350g	347	99	5.8	14.9	1.8	2.9
Chicken With Vegetable Spring Roll, Oriental Express*	1 Pack/300g	213	71	5.5	12.4	0.6	1.9
Chicken, Ainsley Harriott*	1 Serving/250g	447	179	14.0	21.2	4.7	2.0
Chicken, Asda*	1 Pack/460g	488	106	5.0	13.0	3.8	2.1
Chicken, BGTY, Sainsbury's*	1 Pack/450g	370	82	6.0	11.4	1.4	1.1
Chicken, COU, Marks & Spencer*	1 Pack/200g	180	90	9.3	8.1	2.3	1.1
Chicken, Cantonese, Sainsbury's*	1/2 Pack/225g	198	88	5.7	11.7	2.0	1.2
Chicken, Chinese Takeaway, Sainsbury's*	1 Pack/316g	338	107	9.1	11.6	2.7	0.7
Chicken, Frozen, Sainsbury's*	1 Pack/403.8g	424	105	6.1	13.4	3.0	0.9
Chicken, Great Value, Asda*	1 Pack/400g	408	102	5.0	14.0	2.9	0.8
Chicken, New Improved Recipe, Sainsbury's*	1 Pack/449g	395	88	5.7	11.7	2.0	1.2
Chicken, New, BGTY, Sainsbury's*	1 Pack/450g	374	83	6.0	11.4	1.4	1.1
Chicken, Oriental Express*	1 Pack/300g	210	70	4.4	13.1	0.6	1.9
Chicken, Oriental, Healthy Living, Tesco*	1 Pack/450g	288	64	7.2	7.6	0.5	3.5
Chicken, Sainsbury's*	1 Serving/400g	364	91	5.2	12.9	2.1	1.0
Chicken, Sizzling Stir Fry, Oriental Express*	1 Pack/375g	360	96	7.3	10.7	2.7	2.2
Chicken, Tesco*	1 Pack/350g	322	92	7.0	10.6	2.4	1.5
Chicken, Waitrose*	1 Serving/400g	384	96	6.0	11.4	2.9	1.3
Chinese Style, Safeway*	1 Serving/150g	167	111	4.0	13.0	4.4	1.1
Noodles, Snack In A Pot, Healthy Living, Tesco*	1 Serving/56g	187	334	7.7	71.1	2.0	3.6
Pork, Perfectly Balanced, Waitrose*	1/2 Pack/310g	332	107	7.6	17.2	0.9	1.6
Special Chinese, Farmfoods*	1 Pack/400g	276	69	4.3	6.7	2.8	0.8
Special, COU, Marks & Spencer*	1 Pack/400g	320	80	7.4	9.9	1.0	1.0

C

	Measure INFO/WEIGHT	per Measure KCAL	Nutrition Values per 100g / 100ml				
			KCAL	PROT	CARB	FAT	FIBRE
CHOW MEIN							
Special, GFY, Asda*	1 Pack/400g	236	59	6.0	8.0	0.3	1.2
Special, Healthy Living, Tesco*	1 Serving/450g	351	78	6.3	10.6	1.2	0.6
Special, Marks & Spencer*	1 Pack/340g	289	85	6.6	8.2	2.7	1.2
Special, Perfectly Balanced, Waitrose*	1 Serving/400g	316	79	7.4	10.0	1.1	0.9
Special, Somerfield*	1 Pot/300g	357	119	6.5	16.2	3.4	0.6
Stir Fry With Veg & Noodles, Somerfield*	1 Serving/200g	234	117	2.8	12.9	6.0	1.3
Stir Fry, Asda*	1 Pack/350g	270	77	2.1	6.0	5.0	0.0
Stir Fry, Somerfield*	1 Pack/300g	474	158	6.0	32.0	1.0	0.0
Stir Fry, Tesco*	1 Pack/500g	335	67	2.5	10.8	1.5	1.0
Vegetable & Cashew Nut, Eat Smart, Safeway*	1 Pack/380g	323	85	7.0	11.4	1.2	1.1
Vegetable, Healthy Eating, Tesco*	1 Pack/350g	221	63	6.8	7.9	0.5	1.3
Vegetable, Take Away, Meal For One, Tesco*	1 Serving/345g	262	76	6.7	7.3	2.2	1.3
Vegetables & Noodles in Sauce, Safeway*	1 Serving/200g	110	55	3.7	9.5	0.2	1.3
CHRISTMAS PUDDING							
Average	1oz/28g	81	291	4.6	49.5	9.7	1.3
BGTY, Sainsbury's*	1 Serving/113g	302	266	2.8	58.2	2.5	4.6
Iceland*	1/4 Pudding/100g	352	352	3.3	63.0	9.6	7.6
Less Than 5% Fat, GFY, Asda*	1/2 Pudding/100g	279	279	2.6	58.0	4.1	1.6
Luxury, Safeway*	1/8 Pudding/114g	316	277	3.1	47.9	8.1	1.3
Luxury, Tesco*	1/4 Pudding/114g	346	305	3.7	50.8	9.7	1.3
Nut Free & Alcohol Free, Healthy Eating, Tesco*	1 Serving/100g	258	258	2.8	55.6	2.7	4.3
Rich Fruit, Laced With Brandy, Tesco*	1 Serving/100g	305	305	3.7	50.8	9.7	1.3
Rich Fruit, Tesco*	1 Serving/114g	331	290	2.4	55.0	5.9	0.0
Sticky Toffee, Tesco*	1/4 Pudding/114g	372	326	2.5	64.5	6.4	0.8
Tesco*	1 Serving/113g	305	270	2.4	55.0	5.9	1.5
Toffee Sauce Coated, Morrisons*	1 Pudding/100g	324	324	2.5	64.5	6.4	0.0
Traditional Style, Asda*	1 Pudding/100g	296	296	2.6	58.0	6.0	1.6
Vintage, Marks & Spencer*	1/8 Pudding/113g	335	295	2.6	59.8	5.6	1.4
With Cider, Value, Tesco*	1 Serving/100g	312	312	2.7	59.6	7.0	3.3
CHUTNEY							
Albert's Victorian, Baxters*	1 Serving/25g	38	150	35.0	6.0	0.1	0.0
Apple, Spiced, TTD, Sainsbury's*	1 Serving/10g	15	153	0.4	36.9	0.4	1.6
Apple, Tomato & Sultana, Tesco*	1 Serving/50g	88	176	1.1	42.4	0.2	1.3
Apricot & Ginger, Safeway*	1 Tsp/15g	24	162	1.4	38.0	0.2	2.0
Apricot, Sharwood's*	1 Tsp/16g	21	131	0.6	32.0	0.1	2.3
Bengal Hot, Sharwood's*	1oz/28g	56	200	0.5	48.7	0.3	1.1
Bengal Spice Mango, Sharwood's*	1 Tsp/5g	12	236	0.5	58.0	0.2	1.2
Caramalised Onion, Sainsbury's*	1 Serving/25g	28	111	1.1	23.5	1.4	1.1
Cranberry & Caramelised Red Onion, Baxters*	1 Serving/20g	31	154	0.3	38.0	0.1	0.3
Flame Roasted Tomato & Pepper, TTD, Sainsbury's*	1 Serving/5g	9	189	1.0	45.3	0.4	1.1
Fruit, Spiced, Baxters*	1 Tsp/16g	23	143	6.0	34.8	0.1	0.0
Fruit, Traditional, Marks & Spencer*	1oz/28g	43	155	0.9	37.2	0.3	1.7
Indian Appetisers, Pot, Waitrose*	1 Pot/158g	330	209	1.8	47.3	1.4	1.8
Lime & Chilli, Geeta's*	1 Serving/25g	69	277	2.0	64.0	1.4	1.9
Major Grey Mango, Patak's*	1oz/28g	71	255	0.4	66.0	0.2	0.7
Mango & Apple, Sharwood's*	1oz/28g	65	233	0.4	57.6	0.1	1.1
Mango & Ginger, Baxters*	1 Jar/320g	598	187	5.0	45.7	0.2	0.9
Mango & Lime, Sharwood's*	1oz/28g	58	206	0.4	50.5	0.3	0.8
Mango, Green Label, Sharwood's*	1 Serving/10g	23	234	0.3	57.8	0.2	0.9
Mango, Hot, Patak's*	1oz/28g	72	258	0.4	67.1	0.2	0.7
Mango, Hot, TTD, Sainsbury's*	1 Tbs/15g	36	240	0.7	54.7	2.0	2.0
Mango, Spicy, Sainsbury's*	1 Tbsp/15g	24	160	0.7	37.0	0.7	1.3
Mango, Sweet	1 Heaped Tsp/16g	30	189	0.7	48.3	0.1	0.0

	Measure	per Measure		Nutrition Values per 100g / 100ml				
	INFO/WEIGHT	KCAL		KCAL	PROT	CARB	FAT	FIBRE
CHUTNEY								
Mango, Tesco*	1 Serving/20g	45		224	0.4	55.5	0.1	1.3
Mixed Fruit	1 Heaped Tsp/16g	25		155	0.6	39.7	0.0	0.0
Onion, TTD, Sainsbury's*	1 Serving/20g	55		277	0.9	67.2	0.5	1.4
Peach Fruit, Sharwood's*	1oz/28g	48		172	0.4	42.3	0.1	0.9
Peach, Spicy, Waitrose*	1 Serving/20g	43		215	1.0	49.0	1.5	1.5
Ploughman's Plum, EPC*	1 Tsp/10g	16		160	1.3	38.1	0.2	1.6
Red Onion & Sherry Vinegar, Sainsbury's*	1 Serving/10g	24		236	0.5	57.1	0.6	1.4
Spicy Fruit, Safeway*	1 Tsp/16g	16		109	0.5	25.5	0.1	0.1
Spicy Mango, Marks & Spencer*	1oz/28g	52		185	0.1	46.1	0.3	1.8
Sweet Mango, Marks & Spencer*	1oz/28g	67		240	0.3	58.8	0.2	1.5
Sweet Mango, Patak's*	1oz/28g	73		259	0.3	67.4	0.1	0.7
Tomato	1 Heaped Tsp/16g	20		128	1.2	31.0	0.2	1.3
Tomato & Red Pepper, Baxters*	1 Jar/312g	512		164	2.0	38.0	0.4	1.5
Tomato, TTD, Sainsbury's*	1 Tbsp/15g	29		193	2.0	44.7	1.3	2.7
Tomato, Waitrose*	1 Pot/100g	195		195	1.3	46.8	0.3	0.0
CIABATTA								
Cheese, & Ham, Asda*	1/4 Bread/74g	231		312	11.6	38.9	12.2	1.2
Chicken Tomato & Basil, Boots*	1 Pack/207g	499		241	11.0	20.0	13.0	3.0
Chicken, & Herb, Shapers, Boots*	1 Pack/168g	290		173	11.9	25.0	2.8	1.7
Tuna, Crunch, Eat Smart, Safeway*	1 Serving/200g	280		140	10.7	21.7	1.1	1.5
CIDER								
Diamond White*	1fl oz/30ml	11		36	0.0	2.6	0.0	0.0
Dry	1 Pint/568ml	205		36	0.0	2.6	0.0	0.0
Dry, French, So Good, Somerfield*	1 Bottle/500ml	150		30	0.0	0.3	0.0	0.0
Dry, Strongbow*	1 Bottle/375ml	161		43	0.0	3.4	0.0	0.0
Low Alcohol	1 Pint/568ml	97		17	0.0	3.6	0.0	0.0
Low Carb, Stowford*	1 Bottle/500ml	140		28	0.0	0.2	0.0	0.0
Magner's*	1/2 Pint/284ml	105		37	0.0	2.0	0.0	0.0
Medium Sweet, Somerfield*	1 Pint/568ml	233		41	0.0	5.0	0.0	0.0
Sweet	1 Pint/568ml	239		42	0.0	4.3	0.0	0.0
Vintage	1 Pint/568ml	574		101	0.0	7.3	0.0	0.0
CINNAMON								
Powder	1 Tsp/3g	8		261	3.9	55.5	3.2	0.0
CLAMS								
In Brine, Average	1oz/28g	22		79	16.0	2.5	0.6	0.0
CLEMENTINES								
Raw, Average	1 Med/60g	23		38	0.9	8.7	0.1	1.2
COCKLES								
Boiled	1 Cockle/4g	2		53	12.0	0.0	0.6	0.0
Bottled in Vinegar, Drained	1oz/28g	17		60	13.3	0.0	0.7	0.0
COCKTAIL								
Bucks Fizz, Premixed, Marks & Spencer*	1 Glass/250ml	152		61	0.0	9.0	0.0	0.0
Grenadine, Oange Juice, Pineapple Juice	1 Serving/200ml	158		79	0.5	19.2	0.1	0.2
Mai Tai, Average	1 Serving/200ml	209		105	0.2	13.9	0.1	0.1
COCOA BUTTER								
Average	1oz/28g	251		896	0.0	0.0	99.5	0.0
COCOA POWDER								
Cadbury*	1 Tbsp/16g	52		322	23.1	10.5	20.8	0.0
Made Up With Semi-Skimmed Milk	1 Mug/227ml	129		57	3.5	7.0	1.9	0.2
Made Up With Skimmed Milk	1 Mug/227ml	100		44	3.5	7.0	0.5	0.0
Made Up With Whole Milk	1 Mug/227ml	173		76	3.4	6.8	4.2	0.2
Valrhona*	1 Tsp/5g	23		450	25.0	45.0	20.0	30.0

C

COCONUT

Item	Measure	per Measure KCAL	KCAL	PROT	CARB	FAT	FIBRE
Creamed, Average	1oz/28g	186	666	6.0	6.7	68.4	7.0
Desiccated	1oz/28g	169	604	5.6	6.4	62.0	13.7
Fresh	1oz/28g	98	351	3.2	3.7	36.0	7.3
Ice	1oz/28g	104	371	1.7	66.7	12.7	2.6
Milk, Amoy*	1oz/28g	39	140	1.9	1.1	17.0	0.0
Milk, BGTY, Sainsbury's*	1/4 Can/100ml	96	96	1.0	3.6	8.6	0.0
Milk, Blue Dragon*	1 Can/400ml	640	160	2.2	2.2	15.7	0.0
Milk, Light, Reduced Fat, Blue Dragon*	1 Can/400ml	408	102	0.9	2.4	9.8	0.0
Milk, Low Fat, Blue Dragon*	1 Can/400ml	272	68	0.7	1.0	6.7	0.0
Milk, Low Fat, Tiger Tiger*	1/2 Tin/200ml	200	100	1.0	0.7	10.0	0.2
Milk, Reduced Fat, Amoy*	1 Serving/100g	115	115	1.2	2.9	11.0	0.0
Milk, Reduced Fat, Bart*	1 Serving/100g	94	94	0.7	3.6	8.6	0.0
Milk, Rich Creamy, Amoy*	1 Can/400ml	684	171	2.0	2.5	17.0	0.0

COD

Item	Measure	per Measure KCAL	KCAL	PROT	CARB	FAT	FIBRE
Baked	1oz/28g	27	96	21.4	0.0	1.2	0.0
Cakes, Big Time, Birds Eye*	1 Cake/114g	223	196	8.3	17.8	10.2	1.0
Captains Coins, Birds Eye*	1 Coin/20g	34	168	10.1	13.3	8.3	0.9
Dried, Salted, Boiled	1oz/28g	39	138	32.5	0.0	0.9	0.0
Fillets, Battered, Average	1 Serving/90g	158	176	12.6	13.0	8.2	1.1
Fillets, Breaded, Average	1 Portion/97g	200	206	13.0	16.7	9.7	1.0
Fillets, Breaded, Chunky, Average	1 Piece/135g	204	151	13.7	10.9	5.9	1.4
Fillets, Breaded, Light, Healthy Range, Average	1 Fillet/135g	209	154	13.6	13.3	5.1	1.2
Fillets, Chunky, Average	1 Fillet/198g	267	135	17.1	8.2	3.7	0.8
Fillets, Skinless & Boneless, Raw, Average	1 Portion/92g	90	98	17.8	2.7	1.7	0.4
Fillets, Smoked, Average	1 Serving/150g	152	101	21.6	0.0	1.6	0.0
In Ovencrisp Crumb, Waitrose*	1 Serving/142g	302	213	11.7	18.3	10.3	0.8
Loins, Average	1 Serving/145g	116	80	17.9	0.1	0.8	0.2
Mediterranean, Perfectly Balanced, Waitrose*	1 Serving/370g	255	69	13.1	1.9	1.0	1.2
Poached	1oz/28g	26	94	20.9	0.0	1.1	0.0
Smoked, Raw	1oz/28g	22	79	18.3	0.0	0.6	0.0
Steaks, Battered, Chip Shop Style, Average	1 Serving/150g	321	214	12.5	14.3	12.0	1.1
Steamed	1oz/28g	23	83	18.6	0.0	0.9	0.0

COD &

Item	Measure	per Measure KCAL	KCAL	PROT	CARB	FAT	FIBRE
Cauliflower Bake, Asda*	1 Pack/400g	492	123	9.5	5.5	7.0	1.0
Cauliflower Cheese, Fillets, Iceland*	1/2 Pack/176g	234	133	12.7	3.3	7.7	1.7
Chips, Oven Baked, Safeway*	1 Pack/250g	523	209	8.4	25.0	8.4	3.5
Parsley Sauce, Frozen, Marks & Spencer*	1 Pack/184g	156	85	11.1	1.9	3.9	1.0
Salmon, Steam Cuisine, COU, Marks & Spencer*	1 Pack/400g	340	85	6.8	8.9	1.8	1.2

COD IN

Item	Measure	per Measure KCAL	KCAL	PROT	CARB	FAT	FIBRE
A Sweet Red Pepper Sauce, Fillets, GFY, Asda*	1/2 Pack/170g	143	84	15.0	2.3	1.6	0.1
Butter Sauce, Portions, Ocean Trader*	1 Pack/150g	137	91	10.3	3.3	4.1	0.1
Butter Sauce, Ross*	1 Serving/150g	126	84	9.1	3.2	3.9	0.1
Butter Sauce, Steaks, Birds Eye*	1 Pack/170g	185	109	9.8	5.0	5.5	0.1
Butter Sauce, Steaks, Frozen, Asda*	1 Pouch/152.3g	163	107	16.0	5.0	2.6	0.8
Butter Sauce, Steaks, Sainsbury's*	1 Serving/170g	184	108	10.5	3.1	5.9	0.3
Butter Sauce, Tesco*	1 Pack/150g	123	82	9.4	2.9	3.6	0.5
Cheese Sauce, BGTY, Sainsbury's*	1 Serving/170g	145	85	12.8	3.1	2.4	0.0
Cheese Sauce, Steaks, Birds Eye*	1 Pack/182g	175	96	10.9	5.2	3.5	0.1
Cheese Sauce, With Vegetables, Healthy Living, Tesco*	1 Pack/450g	276	61	6.5	5.7	1.4	1.6
Mushroom Sauce, BGTY, Sainsbury's*	1 Serving/170g	112	66	9.9	2.8	1.7	0.1
Parsley Sauce, BGTY, Sainsbury's*	1 Pack/170g	143	84	11.4	2.4	3.2	0.3
Parsley Sauce, COU, Marks & Spencer*	1 Pack/185g	130	70	10.6	1.4	2.5	0.6
Parsley Sauce, Fillets, BGTY, Sainsbury's*	1 Pack/351g	316	90	11.6	1.3	4.3	0.7

	Measure	per Measure		Nutrition Values per 100g / 100ml			
	INFO/WEIGHT	KCAL	KCAL	PROT	CARB	FAT	FIBRE

COD IN

	Measure	per Measure KCAL	KCAL	PROT	CARB	FAT	FIBRE
Parsley Sauce, GFY, Asda*	1/2 Pack/149g	124	83	12.0	1.5	3.5	0.6
Parsley Sauce, Portions, Asda*	1 Serving/150g	116	77	11.0	3.8	2.0	0.1
Parsley Sauce, Portions, Ocean Trader*	1 Serving/120g	112	93	9.4	4.0	3.9	0.1
Parsley Sauce, Portions, Sainsbury's*	1 Pack/170g	143	84	11.4	2.4	3.2	0.3
Parsley Sauce, Steaks, Birds Eye*	1 Steak/172g	155	90	10.5	5.6	2.8	0.1
Parsley Sauce, Steaks, Sainsbury's*	1 Serving/150g	126	84	11.4	2.4	3.2	0.3
Parsley Sauce, Tesco*	1 Serving/150g	122	81	10.0	3.3	3.1	0.3

COD MEDITERRANEAN

COU, Marks & Spencer*	1 Pack/400g	320	80	6.5	11.2	0.7	2.3
Style, Fillets, GFY, Asda*	1 Serving/200g	138	69	9.0	2.5	2.5	0.9
Style, Fillets, Herb, Tesco*	1 Serving/115g	163	142	13.8	0.1	9.6	0.1

COD WITH

A Mediterranean Pepper Sauce, Fillets, Waitrose*	1 Pack/370g	241	65	12.2	1.1	1.3	0.9
A Thai Crust, Perfectly Balanced, Waitrose*	1 Pack/280g	249	89	15.1	1.6	2.5	0.6
Mediterranean Butter, Sainsbury's*	1 Pack/170.4g	196	115	17.0	0.1	5.2	0.1
Parma Ham & Sardinian Chick Peas, Marks & Spencer*	1/2 Pack/255g	268	105	9.8	5.3	4.9	0.5
Parsley Sauce, Somerfield*	1 Serving/200g	276	138	13.3	3.3	7.9	0.5
Roasted Vegetables, Marks & Spencer*	1 Serving/280g	238	85	8.0	4.9	3.8	1.7
Salsa & Rosemary Potatoes, BGTY, Sainsbury's*	1 Pack/450g	356	79	4.7	13.1	0.9	1.6
Sunblush Tomato Sauce, GFY, Asda*	1/2 Pack/177.3g	117	66	13.0	0.1	1.5	1.0
Sweet Chilli, COU, Marks & Spencer*	1 Pack/400g	360	90	7.7	13.1	0.5	1.6
Tomato Sauce, Fillets, Asda*	1 Serving/181g	210	116	13.0	2.6	6.0	2.3
Vegetables, Haches, Steaks, Peche Ocean*	1 Serving/200g	184	92	12.0	2.1	3.9	0.0

COD ZESTY

COU, Marks & Spencer*	1 Serving/400g	260	65	7.2	5.2	1.7	1.2

COFFEE

Black	1 Mug/270ml	5	2	0.2	0.3	0.0	0.0
Cafe Latte, Dry, Douwe Egberts*	1 Serving/12g	58	480	10.0	60.0	22.0	0.0
Cafe Vanilla, Nescafe*	1 Sachet/18.5g	82	432	9.7	73.0	11.4	0.0
Cappuccino, Alcafe, Aldi*	1 Sachet/12.5g	49	393	12.5	55.1	13.6	0.0
Cappuccino, Asda*	1 Sachet/15g	60	399	13.0	53.0	15.2	0.9
Cappuccino, Cafe Mocha, Dry, Maxwell House*	1 Serving/23g	100	434	4.3	78.2	10.8	0.0
Cappuccino, Cafe Specials, Dry, Marks & Spencer*	1 Serving/14g	55	395	14.0	59.0	11.5	0.7
Cappuccino, Cappio, Kenco*	1 Sachet/18g	79	439	11.7	73.9	10.6	0.6
Cappuccino, Chocolate, Safeway*	1 Serving/120g	222	185	5.1	32.9	3.7	0.6
Cappuccino, Co-Op*	1 Serving/12.5g	55	440	16.0	64.0	16.0	8.0
Cappuccino, Dry, Maxwell House*	1 Mug/15g	53	350	12.0	64.0	9.6	0.4
Cappuccino, Dry, Waitrose*	1 Sachet/13.2g	57	439	15.1	56.0	17.2	4.4
Cappuccino, For Filter Systems, Kenco*	1 Sachet/6g	23	375	19.0	44.0	13.5	0.0
Cappuccino, Instant, Kenco*	1 Sachet/20g	80	401	13.5	55.7	13.8	0.0
Cappuccino, Instant, Made Up, Maxwell House*	1 Serving/280g	123	44	0.6	5.8	1.9	0.0
Cappuccino, Instant, Unsweetened, Douwe Egberts*	1 Serving/12g	48	400	11.0	53.0	16.0	0.0
Cappuccino, Low Sugar, Tesco*	1 Serving/13g	55	425	18.4	43.3	19.8	0.4
Cappuccino, Marks & Spencer*	1 Serving/164g	66	40	1.5	4.4	1.6	0.1
Cappuccino, Organic Chocolate, Traidcraft*	1 Serving/25g	139	555	7.0	43.0	38.0	0.0
Cappuccino, Original Mugsticks, Maxwell House*	1 Serving/18g	73	406	14.4	52.8	15.6	0.0
Cappuccino, Premium Quality, Ernesto*	1 Sachet/13g	47	372	12.0	71.0	3.0	1.0
Cappuccino, Reduced Sugar, Sainsbury's*	1 Serving/12g	48	418	18.0	41.0	20.0	0.0
Cappuccino, Sachets, Nescafe*	1 Serving/12.5g	52	400	11.2	66.4	9.6	0.0
Cappuccino, Sainsbury's*	1 Serving/12g	49	411	14.9	52.9	15.5	0.4
Cappuccino, Swiss Chocolate, Nescafe*	1 Sachet/20g	81	404	10.5	65.3	11.5	2.9
Cappuccino, Unsweetened Taste, Maxwell House*	1 Serving/15g	65	434	17.4	47.6	19.3	0.3
Cappuccino, Unsweetened, Cappio, Kenco*	1 Serving/18g	73	406	12.2	66.7	10.0	0.6

	Measure INFO/WEIGHT	per Measure KCAL	Nutrition Values per 100g / 100ml				
			KCAL	PROT	CARB	FAT	FIBRE
COFFEE							
Cappuccino, Unsweetened, Dry, Nescafe*	1 Sachet/12g	51	427	14.9	54.7	16.6	0.0
Cappuccino, Whip, Marks & Spencer*	1 Serving/28g	140	500	7.0	57.1	27.0	1.4
Compliment*	1 Serving/14ml	20	143	1.4	6.4	12.9	0.0
Dandelion, Symingtons*	1 Serving/10g	32	320	2.8	79.3	0.0	0.0
Decaffeinated, Gold Blend, Nescafe*	1 Tsp/5g	5	108	14.5	10.0	0.2	11.6
Frappe Iced, Nestle*	1 Serving/25g	96	384	15.0	72.0	4.0	0.5
Ice Mocha Drink, Nescafe, Nestle*	1 Bottle/280ml	160	57	1.1	10.5	1.2	0.0
Infusion, Average With Semi-Skimmed Milk	1 Cup/220ml	14	7	0.6	0.7	0.2	0.0
Infusion, Average With Single Cream	1 Cup/220ml	31	14	0.4	0.3	1.2	0.0
Infusion, Average With Whole Milk	1 Cup/220ml	15	7	0.5	0.5	0.4	0.0
Instant, Decaffeinated, Nescafe*	1 Tsp/5g	5	101	14.9	10.0	0.2	8.4
Instant, Made With Skimmed Milk	1 Serving/270ml	15	6	0.6	0.8	0.0	0.0
Instant, Made With Water & Semi-Skimmed Milk	1 Serving/350ml	25	7	0.4	0.5	0.4	0.0
Latte, 'A' Mocha, Cafe Met*	1 Bottle/290ml	174	60	3.2	9.0	1.4	0.0
Latte, Cafe, Marks & Spencer*	1 Serving/190g	143	75	4.3	8.3	2.8	0.0
Latte, Instant, Skinny, Douwe Egberts*	1 Serving/12g	35	290	11.0	38.0	11.0	29.0
Latte, Nescafe*	1 Sachet/21g	98	469	14.5	52.4	22.5	0.0
Moch'a'Latte, Cafe Met*	1 Bottle/290ml	174	60	3.2	9.0	1.4	0.0
Mocha, Instant, Skinny, Douwe Egberts*	1 Serving/12g	37	308	10.8	40.8	10.8	25.0
Mocha, Sainsbury's*	1 Serving/13g	67	383	14.0	51.0	13.7	1.3
Regular, Ground or Instant	1 Cup (6fl oz)/177g	6	4	0.2	0.7	0.0	0.0
COFFEE MATE							
Lite, Carnation*	1 Serving/5g	20	398	2.5	83.9	6.9	0.0
Lite, Nestle*	2 Tsps/5g	20	398	2.5	83.9	6.9	0.0
Nestle*	2 Tsp/7g	36	520	1.2	60.5	30.3	0.0
COFFEE SUBSTITUTE							
Bambu, A Vogel*	1 Tsp/3g	10	320	3.5	75.3	0.5	0.0
COFFEE WHITENER							
Half Fat, Co-Op*	1 Tsp/5g	22	430	0.9	78.0	13.0	0.0
Light, Asda*	1 Serving/3g	13	433	0.9	78.0	13.0	0.0
Light, Healthy Eating, Tesco*	1 Tsp/6g	27	449	3.5	71.0	16.8	0.0
Light, Tesco*	1 serving/3g	13	429	0.9	77.7	12.7	0.0
Morrisons*	1 Serving/10g	54	535	2.6	57.5	32.8	0.0
Tesco*	1 Tsp/3g	16	533	1.2	61.3	31.4	0.0
COGNAC							
40% Volume	1 Shot/25ml	56	222	0.0	0.0	0.0	0.0
COINTREAU							
Liqueur Specialite De France	1 Serving/37g	80	215	0.0	0.0	0.0	0.0
COLA							
Average	1 Can/330ml	135	41	0.0	10.9	0.0	0.0
Coke, Cherry, The Coca Cola Co*	1fl oz/30ml	13	42	0.0	10.0	0.0	0.0
Coke, Diet, Caffeine Free, The Coca Cola Co*	1 Can/330ml	1	0	0.0	0.1	0.0	0.0
Coke, The Coca Cola Co*	1 Can/330ml	142	43	0.0	10.7	0.0	0.0
Coke, The Coca Cola Co*	1 Can/330ml	142	43	0.0	10.7	0.0	0.0
Coke, Vanilla, The Coca Cola Co*	1 Serving/500ml	215	43	0.0	10.7	0.0	0.0
Coke, With Lemon, Diet, The Coca Cola Co*	1 Can/330ml	5	1	0.0	0.0	0.0	0.0
Coke, With Vanilla, Diet, The Coca Cola Co*	1 Glass/200ml	1	0	0.0	0.1	0.0	0.0
Diet Coke, The Coca Cola Co*	1 Can/330ml	1	0	0.0	0.0	0.0	0.0
Diet, Classic, Sainsbury's*	1 Can/330ml	1	0	0.0	0.0	0.0	0.0
Diet, Just, Asda*	1 Bottle/250ml	1	0	0.0	0.0	0.0	0.0
Diet, Marks & Spencer*	1 Can/330ml	3	1	0.0	0.3	0.0	0.0
Diet, Pepsi*	1 Can/330ml	1	0	0.0	0.0	0.0	0.0
Diet, Tesco*	1 Glass/200ml	2	1	0.1	0.1	0.1	0.0

	Measure	per Measure	Nutrition Values per 100g / 100ml				
	INFO/WEIGHT	KCAL	KCAL	PROT	CARB	FAT	FIBRE
COLA							
Diet, Virgin*	1 Glass/250ml	1	0	0.1	0.1	0.1	0.0
Marks & Spencer*	1 Bottle/500ml	225	45	0.0	11.0	0.0	0.0
Max, Pepsi*	1fl oz/30ml	0	1	0.1	0.1	0.0	0.0
Pepsi*	1 Can/330ml	145	44	0.0	11.1	0.0	0.0
Tesco*	1 Can/330ml	145	44	0.0	10.8	0.0	0.0
Twist, Light, Pepsi*	1 Bottle/500ml	5	1	0.0	0.1	0.0	0.0
Twist, Pepsi*	1 Bottle/500ml	235	47	0.0	11.7	0.0	0.0
COLCANNON							
Co-Op*	1 Pack/500g	325	65	2.0	10.0	2.0	2.0
Healthy Living, Tesco*	1 Serving/250g	188	75	1.7	11.6	2.4	0.9
Potato, Tesco*	1 Serving/250g	223	89	1.6	10.0	4.8	1.4
Sainsbury's*	1 Pack/450g	545	121	2.1	14.1	6.2	1.0
Tesco*	1 Serving/250g	38	15	0.3	2.3	0.5	0.2
Waitrose*	1/2 Pack/150g	138	92	1.7	12.8	3.8	1.4
COLESLAW							
20% Less Fat, Asda*	1 Serving/100g	88	88	1.5	7.0	6.0	1.7
3% Fat, Marks & Spencer*	1oz/28g	47	167	1.3	9.0	14.0	1.4
50% Less Fat, Asda*	1oz/28g	17	61	2.1	6.8	2.8	0.9
99% Fat Free, Kraft*	1 Serving/40ml	50	126	1.0	28.9	1.0	0.0
Apple, Marks & Spencer*	1oz/28g	53	190	1.4	9.2	16.6	1.4
Asda*	1 Serving/100g	190	190	1.0	6.0	18.0	1.4
BFY, Morrisons*	1oz/28g	17	62	1.5	6.7	3.5	0.0
BGTY, Sainsbury's*	1oz/28g	19	69	0.9	6.6	4.3	1.9
Betterbuy, Morrisons*	1 Serving/20g	23	113	0.8	9.2	8.1	0.0
Bryn Wharf Food Co*	1 Serving/90g	109	121	1.4	5.7	10.4	1.8
Budgens*	1 Serving/50g	103	206	1.2	9.5	18.1	2.0
COU, Marks & Spencer*	1/2 Pack/125g	75	60	1.3	7.4	2.7	1.7
Cheese, Co-Op*	1 Serving/125g	344	275	6.0	6.0	25.0	1.0
Cheese, Marks & Spencer*	1 Serving/57g	185	325	4.2	2.0	33.5	1.7
Cheese, Sainsbury's*	1 Pot/125g	230	184	3.7	5.7	16.3	2.6
Chunky, Asda*	1oz/28g	54	194	1.0	7.1	18.0	1.6
Classic, Marks & Spencer*	1 Pot/190g	124	65	1.9	8.8	2.3	1.3
Creamy, 30% Less Fat, Sainsbury's*	1 Serving/30g	38	126	1.0	5.5	11.0	1.4
Creamy, Asda*	1oz/28g	55	195	1.0	7.8	17.7	1.0
Creamy, Healthy Eating, Tesco*	1 Serving/30g	29	95	2.4	6.8	6.4	1.4
Creamy, Sainsbury's*	1oz/28g	69	245	1.3	4.6	24.6	1.6
Creamy, Tesco*	1oz/28g	52	186	1.1	7.6	16.8	1.5
Deli Style, Marks & Spencer*	1/2 Pack/150g	285	190	1.6	3.9	18.5	1.3
Eat Smart, Safeway*	1/4 Pack/50g	30	60	1.8	7.2	2.6	1.9
Finest, Tesco*	1 Serving/50g	107	214	1.2	6.1	20.5	1.6
Fruity, Asda*	1/2 Pot/125g	101	81	1.3	8.0	4.9	1.7
Fruity, Marks & Spencer*	1 Serving/63g	151	240	1.1	8.3	22.7	3.1
GFY, Asda*	1 Serving/50g	28	55	1.3	6.0	2.9	2.3
Garlic & Herb, Asda*	1oz/28g	60	216	1.1	7.2	20.3	1.5
Good Intentions, Somerfield*	1 Serving/50g	36	72	1.6	7.6	3.9	1.5
Half Fat, Safeway*	1 Serving/70g	60	86	1.5	7.4	5.7	1.6
Healthy Choice, Safeway*	1 Pot/250g	215	86	1.5	7.4	5.7	1.6
Healthy Living, Tesco*	1 Serving/60g	51	85	1.3	7.0	5.8	1.6
Heinz*	1oz/28g	38	135	1.6	9.4	10.2	1.2
Less Than 3% Fat, BGTY, Sainsbury's*	1/4 Pot/63.3g	31	49	1.3	6.7	1.9	1.9
Less Than 3% Fat, Marks & Spencer*	1oz/28g	18	65	1.9	8.8	2.3	1.3
Less Than 5% Fat, Marks & Spencer*	1 Serving/225g	169	75	1.8	6.9	4.4	2.8
Light, Morrisons*	1oz/28g	33	118	1.1	8.3	7.8	0.0

	Measure	per Measure	Nutrition Values per 100g / 100ml				
	INFO/WEIGHT	KCAL	KCAL	PROT	CARB	FAT	FIBRE
COLESLAW							
Low Fat Mayonnaise, Tesco*	1oz/28g	18	64	1.4	4.7	4.4	1.4
Luxury, Asda*	1 Serving/50g	109	217	0.9	6.0	21.0	0.0
Luxury, Marks & Spencer*	1oz/28g	43	152	1.0	6.0	13.8	1.0
Organic, Marks & Spencer*	1oz/28g	41	145	1.1	7.3	12.4	1.0
Prawn, Asda*	1oz/28g	54	192	2.4	6.6	17.3	1.4
Premium, Co-Op*	1 Serving/50g	160	320	1.0	3.0	34.0	2.0
Reduced Calorie, Waitrose*	1 Serving/125g	74	59	2.3	5.5	3.1	1.7
Reduced Fat, Asda*	1 Pot/250g	218	87	1.5	6.0	6.3	1.6
Reduced Fat, Healthy Living, Co-Op*	1 Serving/50g	48	95	0.8	8.0	7.0	2.0
Reduced Fat, Sainsbury's*	1/3 Pot/87g	89	102	1.2	7.3	8.0	1.7
Reduced Fat, Traditional, Marks & Spencer*	1oz/28g	57	205	1.1	5.4	20.0	2.8
Sainsbury's*	1/3 Pot/75g	99	132	1.2	6.1	11.4	1.7
Salad, Reduced Fat, 25% Less, Sainsbury's*	1 Serving/250g	333	133	1.1	6.6	11.4	1.6
Savers, Safeway*	1 Serving/114g	122	107	1.1	6.6	8.5	0.0
SmartPrice, Asda*	1oz/28g	30	107	0.8	8.0	8.0	2.0
So Good, Somerfield*	1 Serving/10g	21	210	1.3	6.5	19.9	1.2
Supreme, Waitrose*	1oz/28g	53	190	1.8	4.9	18.1	1.7
TTD, Sainsbury's*	1oz/28g	74	263	1.6	6.1	25.8	1.5
Tesco*	1 Serving/50g	79	158	2.2	5.2	14.3	1.6
The Best, Safeway*	1 Serving/10g	30	296	1.0	7.2	29.2	0.8
Three Cheese, Tesco*	1/2 Pot/125g	230	184	4.0	4.8	16.5	1.2
Traditional, Marks & Spencer*	1 Pack/225g	675	300	1.2	3.9	31.2	1.7
Value, Tesco*	1oz/28g	32	115	1.2	6.8	9.2	1.6
With 60% Less Fat, GFY, Asda*	1 Serving/41g	36	88	1.5	7.0	6.0	1.7
COLESLAW MIX							
Shredded, Waitrose*	1 Serving/100g	29	29	1.1	5.6	0.2	2.2
Tesco*	1 Pack/400g	124	31	1.1	6.2	0.2	2.1
COLEY							
Portions, Raw, Average	1 Portion/92g	75	82	18.4	0.0	0.7	0.0
Steamed	1oz/28g	29	105	23.3	0.0	1.3	0.0
CONCHIGLIE							
Cooked, Average	1 Serving/185g	247	134	4.9	26.7	0.9	0.6
Dry, Average	1 Serving/100g	352	352	12.5	71.6	1.7	2.6
Shells, Dry, Average	1 Serving/100g	346	346	12.3	70.4	1.5	3.0
Whole Wheat, Dry, Average	1 Serving/75g	237	316	12.6	62.0	2.0	10.7
CONCHIGLIONI							
Dry, Waitrose*	1 Serving/75g	256	341	12.5	69.8	1.3	3.7
CONSERVE							
Apricot, Average	1 Tbsp/15g	37	244	0.5	59.3	0.2	1.5
Apricot, Reduced Sugar, Streamline*	1 Tbsp/20g	37	184	0.5	45.0	0.2	0.0
Black Cherry, With Amaretto, Finest, Tesco*	1 Serving/10g	26	261	0.5	64.4	0.1	0.8
Blackcurrant, Average	1 Tbsp/15g	37	245	0.6	60.1	0.1	1.9
Blueberry, Marks & Spencer*	1 Tsp/7.5g	16	206	0.3	51.1	0.1	1.3
Morello Cherry, Waitrose*	1 Tbsp/15g	39	258	0.4	64.2	0.0	1.4
Raspberry, Average	1 Tbsp/15g	37	249	0.6	61.0	0.3	1.3
Red Cherry, Finest, Tesco*	1 Tbsp/15g	42	277	0.6	67.6	0.1	0.8
Rhubarb & Ginger, Marks & Spencer*	1 Tbsp/15g	29	194	0.3	47.9	0.1	1.0
Strawberry, 60% Fruit, Reduced Sugar, Marks & Spencer*	1 Tsp/7g	9	135	0.4	30.1	0.2	1.9
Strawberry, Average	1 Tbsp/15g	37	250	0.4	61.6	0.1	0.5
Yellow Plum & Greengage, TTD, Sainsbury's*	1 Serving/15g	36	243	0.4	60.0	0.1	0.7
CONSOMME							
Average	1oz/28g	3	12	2.9	0.1	0.0	0.0

COOKIES

	Measure INFO/WEIGHT	per Measure KCAL	Nutrition Values per 100g / 100ml KCAL	PROT	CARB	FAT	FIBRE
All Butter Chocolate Chunk, Marks & Spencer*	1 Cookie/26g	130	500	5.2	62.4	25.2	2.6
All Butter Fruity Flapjack, Marks & Spencer*	1 Cookie/24.1g	100	415	4.6	53.4	20.2	4.2
All Butter Melting Moment, Marks & Spencer*	1 Cookie/23.4g	108	470	4.5	51.5	27.5	3.4
All Butter Sultana, Marks & Spencer*	1 Cookie/16g	73	455	5.2	66.0	19.0	2.7
All Butter, Italian Style Sorrento Lemon, Marks & Spencer*	1 Cookie/24g	120	500	4.9	60.4	26.7	2.1
Apple & Raisin, Go Ahead, McVitie's*	1 Cookie/15g	66	443	5.3	76.8	12.7	3.4
Apple Crumble, Marks & Spencer*	1 Cookie/26g	90	345	4.6	76.8	2.0	2.9
Apricot, COU, Marks & Spencer*	1 Cookie/26g	88	340	5.4	75.0	2.4	2.0
Big Milk Chocolate Chunk, Cookie Coach Co*	1 Cookie/35g	174	497	6.2	61.4	25.1	0.0
Bonte Fudge Choc Chip, Patersons*	1 Cookie/5.57g	28	503	6.2	60.1	26.4	2.2
Brazil Nut, Organic, Traidcraft*	1 Cookie/16.6g	93	547	5.8	57.7	32.6	2.1
Butter & Sultana, Sainsbury's*	1 Cookie/13g	61	473	4.5	68.4	20.1	1.6
Cherry Bakewell, COU, Marks & Spencer*	1 Cookie/25.4g	89	355	6.0	77.2	2.5	3.4
Choc Chip & Coconut, Maryland*	1oz/28g	143	512	5.1	62.9	23.7	0.0
Choc Chip & Hazelnut, Maryland*	1oz/28g	140	500	5.4	65.2	24.2	0.0
Choc Chip, Asda*	1 Cookie/11g	56	506	5.0	63.0	26.0	1.8
Choc Chip, Cadbury*	1oz/28g	139	495	6.5	66.1	22.6	0.0
Choc Chip, Giant, Patersons	1 Cookie/60g	296	493	0.1	61.3	25.3	3.2
Choc Chip, Lyons*	1oz/28g	142	506	5.3	68.3	23.5	0.0
Choc Chip, Maryland*	1 Cookie/11g	56	511	6.2	68.0	23.9	0.0
Choc Chunk & Hazelnut, Co-Op*	1 Cookie/17g	89	525	6.0	56.0	31.0	3.0
Choc Chunk & Hazelnut, Luxury, Cadbury*	1oz/28g	146	521	6.3	60.0	28.7	0.0
Choc Chunk, Fabulous Bakin' Boys*	1 Cookie/60g	270	450	5.0	59.0	21.0	3.0
Chocolate & Ginger, The Best, Safeway*	1 Cookie/135g	709	525	5.5	62.0	28.0	2.6
Chocolate & Nut, Organic, Evernat*	1 Cookie/69g	337	489	7.2	64.1	22.6	0.0
Chocolate & Orange, COU, Marks & Spencer*	1 Cookie/25.7g	91	350	5.7	77.2	2.6	3.2
Chocolate & Roasted Hazelnut, TTD, Sainsbury's*	1 Cookie/17g	89	521	6.4	56.3	30.3	2.2
Chocolate Chip & Hazelnut, Asda*	1 Cookie/12g	62	516	6.0	60.0	28.0	0.0
Chocolate Chip & Peanut, Trufree*	1 Cookie/11g	55	496	4.0	66.0	24.0	2.0
Chocolate Chip, BGTY, Sainsbury's*	1 Cookie/16.8g	73	428	4.5	75.6	11.9	2.5
Chocolate Chip, Carb Check, Heinz*	1 Cookie/20g	91	457	7.2	43.1	24.9	7.2
Chocolate Chip, Chips Ahoy*	1 Cookie/11g	55	500	6.0	65.0	25.0	3.0
Chocolate Chip, GFY, Asda*	1 Cookie/10.4g	46	463	5.0	68.0	19.0	3.5
Chocolate Chip, Handbaked, Border*	1 Cookie/15g	72	480	5.9	67.4	22.6	0.0
Chocolate Chip, Low Price, Sainsbury's*	1 Cookie/10.8g	55	500	7.0	70.1	21.3	2.5
Chocolate Chip, Lyons*	1 Cookie/12g	56	483	5.6	66.5	21.6	1.7
Chocolate Chip, Marks & Spencer*	1 Cookie/12g	61	506	6.0	62.1	25.9	1.2
Chocolate Chip, McVitie's*	1 Serving/17g	88	527	5.4	62.4	28.5	2.1
Chocolate Chip, Mini, McVitie's*	1 Pack/50g	260	520	5.7	66.7	25.6	1.9
Chocolate Chip, Mini, Shapers, Boots*	1 Pack/30g	141	471	6.8	70.0	18.0	1.4
Chocolate Chip, Mini, Tesco*	1 Bag/30g	148	493	5.4	64.6	23.7	1.7
Chocolate Chip, Organic, Sainsbury's*	1 Cookie/16.8g	90	530	5.0	61.8	29.2	0.3
Chocolate Chip, Organic, Tesco*	1 Cookie/17g	88	520	0.0	63.3	27.4	2.8
Chocolate Chip, Sainsbury's*	1 Cookie/11g	55	508	6.2	67.0	23.9	1.3
Chocolate Chip, SmartPrice, Asda*	1 Cookie/10g	52	508	5.0	68.0	24.0	0.0
Chocolate Chip, Tesco*	1oz/28g	139	496	5.4	63.6	24.4	2.0
Chocolate Chip, The Decadent, President's Choice*	2 Cookies/31g	159	513	6.1	61.3	26.5	3.5
Chocolate Chip, Value, Tesco*	1 Cookie/11g	56	512	4.8	64.8	26.0	1.6
Chocolate Chunk & Hazelnut, TTD, Sainsbury's*	1 Biscuit/18g	95	529	6.3	53.7	32.2	2.4
Chocolate Chunk & Hazelnut, Tesco*	1 Cookie/22g	118	538	6.2	60.2	30.3	1.9
Chocolate Chunk & Hazelnut, So Good, Somerfield*	1 Cookie/22.3g	117	530	6.3	55.7	31.3	2.4
Chocolate Chunk & Orange, So Good, Somerfield*	1 Cookie/22g	117	525	5.3	60.0	29.3	1.8
Chocolate Chunk, Cadbury*	1 Cookie/22g	119	540	6.5	58.0	31.2	0.0

COOKIES

INFO/WEIGHT	per Measure KCAL	KCAL	PROT	CARB	FAT	FIBRE
Chocolate Chunk, Fresh, Finest, Tesco*	1 Cookie/75g	325	433	5.7	62.4	16.6	2.7
Chocolate Chunk, Quadruple, TTD, Sainsbury's*	1 Cookie/23g	117	509	5.2	57.4	28.7	1.7
Chocolate Coated, Wheatfree, Sunstart*	1 Cookie/20.0g	103	516	5.6	54.4	30.7	4.1
Chocolate Fruit & Nut, Extra Special, Asda*	1 Cookie/24.6g	127	509	6.0	56.0	29.0	2.0
Chocolate Orange, Half Coated, Finest, Tesco*	1 Cookie/22g	107	488	4.9	59.6	25.5	1.2
Chocolate, Belgian, Extra Special, Asda*	1 Cookie/25.8g	139	535	6.0	58.0	31.0	2.0
Chocolate, Half Coated Triple, Finest, Tesco*	1 Cookie/25g	129	517	5.8	58.8	28.7	2.2
Chocolate, Milk, Free From, Tesco*	1 Biscuit/20g	100	500	5.6	50.4	30.7	4.1
Chocolate, Milk, Tesco*	1 Biscuit/20g	100	500	5.6	50.4	30.7	4.1
Chocolate, Quadruple, Sainsbury's*	1 Serving/20g	117	585	6.0	66.5	33.0	1.5
Chocolate, Soft, American Style, Budgens*	1 Cookie/50g	216	431	5.1	60.8	18.6	2.2
Coconut & Raspberry, Gluten Free, Sainsbury's*	1 Cookie/20g	102	511	5.9	56.0	29.3	6.7
Coconut, Gluten-Free, Sainsbury's*	1 Cookie/20g	103	516	5.6	54.4	30.7	4.1
Coconut, TTD, Sainsbury's*	1 Cookie/16.7g	90	527	5.3	60.0	29.5	4.9
Cranberry & Orange, Finest, Tesco*	1 Cookie/25g	108	433	4.2	64.5	17.6	2.9
Cranberry & Orange, Go Ahead, McVitie's*	1 Cookie/17g	77	452	5.3	78.0	13.2	2.4
Cranberry & Orange, Weight Watchers*	2 Cookies/23g	103	448	4.3	72.2	15.7	3.0
Crunchy Muesli, Mini, Shapers, Boots*	1 Pack/30g	134	448	6.7	71.0	15.0	1.8
Dark Treacle, Weight Watchers*	2 Cookies/23g	97	423	5.2	66.7	15.1	1.7
Double Choc Chip, Giant, Patersons*	1 Cookie/60g	293	489	0.3	61.3	25.3	3.7
Double Choc Chip, Mini, Marks & Spencer*	1 Cookie/22g	108	490	5.3	63.6	23.7	1.8
Double Choc Chip, Tesco*	1 Cookie/11g	55	500	4.2	65.3	24.7	3.0
Double Choc Chip, Weight Watchers*	2 Cookies/23g	102	445	4.7	69.7	16.4	5.0
Double Choc, Cadbury*	Per Biscuit/11g	55	485	7.3	64.3	22.2	0.0
Double Choc, Maryland*	1 Cookie/10g	46	510	5.2	64.4	25.7	0.0
Double Chocolate & Walnut, Soft, Tesco*	1 Serving/25g	116	463	5.8	52.1	25.7	4.7
Double Chocolate Chip, Organic, Waitrose*	1 Cookie/18g	96	535	5.1	58.6	31.0	1.9
Double Chocolate Chip, Traidcraft*	1 Cookie/22g	114	520	5.8	64.1	26.7	2.4
Double Chocolate, Premium, Co-Op*	1 Cookie/17g	86	505	5.0	62.0	27.0	2.0
Fruit, Giant, Cookie Coach Co*	1 Cookie/60g	280	466	4.9	62.0	22.0	0.0
Fruity Shewsbury, Giant, Patersons*	1 Cookie/60g	298	496	4.8	62.6	25.4	1.7
Fudge Brownie American Cream, Sainsbury's*	1 Cookie/12g	60	499	4.8	67.9	23.2	2.2
Ginger & Lemon, Weight Watchers*	2 Cookies/23g	104	451	4.2	73.9	15.4	2.2
Ginger Crunch, Hand Baked, Border*	1 Cookie/11.5g	52	470	4.7	71.4	20.4	0.0
Ginger, Free From, Tesco*	1 Serving/20g	97	483	6.5	51.2	28.0	6.8
Ginger, Low Fat, Marks & Spencer*	1 Cookie/23g	82	358	5.1	74.9	4.3	2.4
Ginger, Safeway*	1 Cookie/22g	106	480	4.7	66.5	22.7	2.4
Glace Cherry, Border*	1 Cookie/15.0g	74	493	5.4	64.3	25.6	0.0
Golden Crunch Oatflake Cranberry, TTD, Sainsbury's*	1 Cookie/17g	82	482	5.9	60.0	23.5	3.5
Lemon Meringue, COU, Marks & Spencer*	1 Cookie/25g	89	355	5.6	77.6	2.6	3.0
Lemon Zest, Organic, Doves Farm*	1 Cookie/16.8g	74	435	3.0	57.0	21.5	1.9
Milk Chocolate, Millie's Cookies*	1 Cookie/65g	280	431	4.6	58.5	20.0	1.5
Oat & Cranberry, BGTY, Sainsbury's*	1 Cookie/28g	126	449	6.8	65.0	18.0	5.1
Oat & Raisin, Safeway*	1 Cookie/12g	50	414	7.5	77.5	8.8	0.0
Oat, Giant Jumbo, Patersons*	1 Cookie/60g	299	499	0.4	58.4	27.0	3.2
Oatflake & Honey, Organic, Sainsbury's*	1 Cookie/17g	82	480	6.3	66.0	21.2	2.6
Oatflake & Raisin, Waitrose*	1 Cookie/17g	80	469	5.8	61.7	22.1	4.7
Oatmeal, Chocolate Chip, Chewy, Dad's*	2 Cookies/30g	140	467	6.7	66.7	20.0	3.3
Oreo, Nabisco*	3 Cookies/34g	160	470	6.0	71.0	21.0	3.0
Peanut, Hellema*	1 Cookie/16g	81	509	11.8	47.3	30.3	0.7
Pecan & Maple, Mini, Bronte*	1 Pack/100g	509	509	5.4	60.3	27.3	1.6
Praline Nougatine, Belle France*	1 Cookie/16.6g	86	506	8.0	63.0	25.0	0.0
Raisin & Cinnamon, Low Fat, Marks & Spencer*	1 Cookie/22g	78	355	6.2	73.0	4.1	3.2

	Measure	per Measure	Nutrition Values per 100g / 100ml				

C

	Measure INFO/WEIGHT	per Measure KCAL	Nutrition Values per 100g / 100ml				
			KCAL	PROT	CARB	FAT	FIBRE
COOKIES							
Raspberry Spritz, Heaven Scent*	1 Serving/19g	90	474	5.3	52.6	31.6	0.0
Real Chocolate Chip, Weight Watchers*	2 Cookies/23g	98	427	5.3	66.1	15.7	1.6
Shortbread Rings, Handbaked, Border*	1 Cookie/16.5g	88	520	6.2	61.2	29.5	0.0
Spiced Apple, COU, Marks & Spencer*	1 Cookie/25g	83	330	5.0	72.8	2.5	2.1
Spiced Apple, Marks & Spencer*	1 Cookie/25g	90	360	5.2	75.6	2.8	2.0
Stem Ginger, & Oatflake, TTD, Sainsbury's*	1 Cookie/17g	84	496	4.5	63.4	24.9	1.7
Stem Ginger, BGTY, Sainsbury's*	1 Cookie/17g	73	431	4.5	76.5	11.9	1.7
Stem Ginger, Half Coated, Finest, Tesco*	1 Cookie/25g	127	508	4.4	62.4	26.8	3.6
Stem Ginger, Less Than 5% Fat, Marks & Spencer*	1 Cookie/22g	79	360	6.2	73.9	4.3	3.0
Stem Ginger, Reduced Fat, Waitrose*	1 Cookie/16.7g	76	448	4.5	71.0	16.2	1.6
Stem Ginger, Tesco*	1 Cookie/20g	98	489	4.2	64.0	24.0	2.0
Strawberries & Cream, TTD, Sainsbury's*	1 Cookie/17g	84	504	4.7	62.7	26.0	1.9
Sultana & Cinnamon, Weight Watchers*	2 Cookies/23g	92	398	5.0	67.1	12.1	1.8
Sultana, All Butter, Reduced Fat, Marks & Spencer*	1 Cookie/16.7g	71	420	4.9	68.6	14.2	2.6
Sultana, Soft & Chewy, Sainsbury's*	1 Cookie/25g	104	414	4.4	67.8	13.9	2.5
Tennessee American Style, Stiftung & Co, Lidl*	1 Cookie/19g	96	504	6.0	66.0	24.0	0.0
Toffee, Weight Watchers*	2 Cookies/23g	105	457	4.8	72.2	16.5	2.2
White Chocolate & Raspberry, McVitie's*	1 Cookie/17g	87	512	4.7	64.1	25.9	1.8
White Chocolate & Raspberry, TTD, Sainsbury's*	1 Cookie/77g	372	483	5.9	57.8	25.3	2.6
White Chocolate, Asda*	1 Cookie/54g	256	474	5.0	64.0	22.0	2.1
COQ AU VIN							
Finest, Tesco*	1 Serving/273g	251	92	14.3	0.7	3.6	1.8
Healthy Living, Tesco*	1/2 Pack/200g	172	86	15.2	2.1	1.9	0.4
Marks & Spencer*	1 Serving/295g	398	135	14.2	1.5	7.7	1.0
Perfectly Balanced, Waitrose*	1 Pack/500g	445	89	12.6	2.7	3.1	0.6
Sainsbury's*	1 Pack/400g	484	121	16.8	3.5	4.4	0.2
COQUILLE							
St Jacques, Marks & Spencer*	1 Serving/150g	165	110	5.0	8.8	6.1	1.1
CORDIAL							
Elderflower, Bottle Green*	1 Glass/200ml	46	23	0.0	5.6	0.0	0.0
Elderflower, Undiluted, Waitrose*	1 Cordial/20ml	22	110	0.0	27.5	0.0	0.0
Honey & Lemonbalm, With Chamomile, Bottle Green*	1fl oz/30ml	8	27	0.0	6.8	0.0	0.0
Lime Juice, Concentrated	1floz/30ml	34	112	0.1	29.8	0.0	0.0
Lime Juice, Diluted	1 Glass/250ml	55	22	0.0	6.0	0.0	0.0
Lime, Sainsbury's*	1 serving/50ml	9	18	0.1	4.5	0.1	0.1
Lime, With Aromatic Bitters & Ginger, Sainsbury's*	1 Serving/40ml	12	29	0.0	6.9	0.3	0.3
CORIANDER							
Leaves, Dried	1oz/28g	78	279	21.8	41.7	4.8	0.0
Leaves, Fresh	1oz/28g	6	20	2.4	1.8	0.6	0.0
CORN							
Baby, & Asparagus Tips, Tesco*	1 Pack/150g	38	25	2.6	2.5	0.5	1.9
Baby, & Mange Tout, Tesco*	1 Serving/100g	27	27	2.9	3.3	0.2	2.1
Baby, & Sugar Snap Peas, Safeway*	1/2 Pack/100g	27	27	2.9	3.3	0.2	0.0
Baby, Average	1oz/28g	7	26	2.5	3.1	0.4	1.7
Baby, Fine Beans & Baby Carrots, Tesco*	1 Pack/250g	68	27	1.7	4.0	0.5	2.2
Cobs, Average	1 Serving/75g	44	59	2.1	10.4	1.1	1.0
Cobs, Boiled, Average	1oz/28g	18	66	2.5	11.6	1.4	1.3
Creamed, Green Giant*	1 Can/418g	238	57	1.2	11.9	0.5	3.0
In Brine, For Stir Fry, Braxted Hall*	1 Can/133g	25	19	1.5	3.0	0.0	1.5
CORN CAKES							
Marks & Spencer*	1/2 Pack/85g	238	280	6.4	19.8	20.0	3.4
Organic, Kallo*	1 Cake/5g	16	340	12.7	74.3	4.1	11.2
Thick Slices, Orgran*	1 Cake/11g	42	385	13.2	79.0	3.7	14.2

	Measure INFO/WEIGHT	per Measure KCAL	Nutrition Values per 100g / 100ml				
			KCAL	PROT	CARB	FAT	FIBRE
CORN SNACKS							
American Cheeseburger Flavour, Quarterbacks, Red Mill*	1 Pack/14g	72	512	6.7	54.2	29.8	3.7
Crispy, Bugles*	1 Bag/20g	102	508	4.8	60.7	28.0	1.4
Light Bites, Cheese Flavour, Special K, Kellogg's*	1 Packet/28g	116	416	9.0	77.0	8.0	1.0
Light Bites, Tikka Flavour, Special K, Kellogg's*	1 Packet/28g	116	416	7.0	79.0	8.0	1.5
Light Bites, Tomato & Basil Flavour, Special K, Kellogg's*	1 Packet/28g	116	416	7.0	79.0	8.0	1.5
Paprika Flavour, Shapers, Boots*	1 Pack/13g	64	494	8.7	54.0	27.0	2.2
Rings, Cheese & Onion, Crunchy, Shapers, Boots*	1 Serving/15g	56	374	5.9	81.0	2.9	20.0
Toasted, Holland & Barratt*	1 Serving/100g	412	412	8.1	69.7	12.1	4.0
CORNED BEEF							
Average	1 Slice/35g	75	215	25.9	0.7	12.2	0.0
Lean, Healthy Range, Average	1 Slice/30g	57	191	27.0	1.0	8.7	0.0
Sliced, Premium, Average	1 Slice/31g	69	222	26.6	0.5	12.6	0.0
Slices, Tesco*	1 Slice/35g	69	198	26.4	0.7	10.0	0.0
Spicy, Princes*	1 Serving/100g	195	195	21.0	1.0	12.0	0.0
Waitrose*	1 Slice/35g	72	207	25.3	0.0	12.0	0.0
CORNFLAKE CAKE							
Bobby's*	1/6 Cake/45g	207	461	3.9	65.5	20.4	0.0
CORNFLAKE NEST							
Crunchy Chocolate, Marks & Spencer*	1 Nest/14.7g	71	475	6.3	67.2	20.2	2.2
CORNFLOUR							
Average	1oz/28g	99	355	0.7	86.9	1.2	0.1
COURGETTE							
& Sweetcorn, Fresh 'n' Ready, Sainsbury's*	1oz/28g	12	42	2.3	6.7	0.9	1.3
Boiled In Unsalted Water	1oz/28g	5	19	2.0	2.0	0.4	1.2
Fried, Average	1oz/28g	18	63	2.6	2.6	4.8	1.2
Raw, Average	1oz/28g	5	18	1.8	1.8	0.4	0.9
COUS COUS							
& Chargrilled Vegetables, Marks & Spencer*	1 Serving/200g	200	100	3.9	17.3	1.5	1.6
& Vegetables, Chargrilled, Sainsbury's*	1 Serving/56g	85	152	4.6	25.3	3.6	2.4
& Wok Oriental, Findus*	1/2 Pack/300g	510	170	4.5	19.0	8.5	0.0
Chargrilled Red & Yellow Pepper, Tesco*	1 Pack/200g	212	106	4.6	17.8	1.8	0.5
Chargrilled Vegetable, Morrisons*	1 Serving/225g	227	101	3.3	16.5	2.4	1.3
Chargrilled Vegetables & Olive Oil, Delphi*	1/2 Pot/75g	105	140	3.8	22.5	3.9	1.9
Citrus Kick, Ainsley Harriott*	1/2 Pack/134.3g	184	137	4.3	28.5	0.6	2.4
Cooked, Average	1 Cup/157g	249	159	4.3	31.4	1.9	1.3
Coriander & Lemon, GFY, Asda*	1/2 Pack/145g	189	130	4.2	27.0	0.6	1.8
Coriander & Lemon, Morrisons*	1 Serving/100g	159	159	4.4	27.7	3.4	1.4
Coriander & Lemon, Sainsbury's*	1/2 Pack/165g	200	121	4.8	23.5	0.7	0.8
Dry, Average	1 Serving/50g	178	356	13.7	72.8	1.5	2.6
Garlic & Coriander, Dry, Waitrose*	1 Serving/70g	235	336	11.7	64.2	3.6	6.2
Harissa Style Savoury, Sainsbury's*	1 Serving/260g	434	167	4.7	26.8	4.6	1.3
Hot & Spicy Flavour, Dry, Amazing Grains, Haldane's*	1 Serving/50g	183	365	12.5	67.0	4.2	3.1
Indian Style, Sainsbury's*	1/2 Pack/143g	204	143	4.5	25.1	2.7	1.0
Lemon & Coriander, Cooked, Tesco*	1 Serving/137g	207	151	4.0	28.3	2.4	2.0
Lemon & Coriander, Dry, Tesco*	1 Pack/110g	375	341	11.0	68.2	2.7	6.1
Mediterranean Style, Dry, Tesco*	1 Pack/110g	369	335	11.9	65.1	3.0	5.6
Mediterranean Style, Tesco* Cooked	1 Serving/146g	215	147	4.4	26.5	2.6	1.3
Mediterranean Tomato, GFY, Asda*	1/2 Pack/141g	192	136	5.0	27.0	0.9	1.7
Mediterranean, Safeway*	1/2 Pack/55g	87	158	4.8	25.9	3.9	1.1
Mint & Coriander Flavour, Dry, Amazing Grains, Aldi*	1 Sachet/99g	349	353	12.2	70.0	2.7	3.2
Moroccan Style, Finest, Tesco*	1 Tub/225g	374	166	4.5	26.1	4.9	1.6
Moroccan Style, Sainsbury's*	1/2 Pack/150g	195	130	5.0	21.5	2.7	1.0
Moroccan Sultana & Pine Nuts, Dry, Sammy's*	1 Serving/50g	172	343	12.0	72.0	3.0	6.0

COUS COUS

	Measure INFO/WEIGHT	per Measure KCAL	KCAL	PROT	CARB	FAT	FIBRE
Morroccan Chicken, Shapers, Boots*	1 Serving/218g	311	143	6.9	21.1	3.4	2.4
Mushroom, Morrisons*	1 Serving/100g	164	164	5.7	28.7	3.0	1.7
Mushroom, Safeway*	1 Serving/139g	232	167	4.9	23.9	5.7	1.6
Mushrooms, Onion, Garlic & Herbs, Dry, Tesco*	1/2 Pack/50g	167	333	11.3	66.2	2.6	4.9
Red Pepper & Chilli, Waitrose*	1 Pack/200g	344	172	4.5	23.0	6.9	1.3
Roast Garlic & Olive Oil, Dry, Sammy's*	1 Serving/49.9g	170	339	12.0	71.5	3.0	0.0
Roasted Vegetable, Finest, Tesco*	1 Serving/175g	263	150	4.0	17.4	7.1	1.3
Roasted Vegetables, Waitrose*	1 Serving/200g	328	164	3.9	22.0	6.6	0.9
Salad Bar, BGTY, Sainsbury's*	1 Md Bowl/28g	29	103	3.7	18.5	1.6	0.0
Spice Sensation, Cooked, Ainsley Harriott*	1/2 Pack/100g	123	123	4.3	24.5	0.9	3.4
Spice Sensation, Uncooked, Ainsley Harriott*	1/2 Sachet/50g	166	332	11.6	66.2	2.4	9.2
Spicy Moroccan Chicken & Veg, COU, Marks & Spencer*	1 Pack/400g	380	95	9.1	10.3	1.7	1.9
Spicy Vegetable, GFY, Asda*	1/2 Pack/141g	183	130	5.0	25.0	1.1	2.0
Spicy Vegetable, Morrisons*	1 Serving/50g	85	170	5.1	26.2	5.0	2.9
Spicy, Healthy Living, Tesco*	1 serving/50g	65	130	3.6	25.1	1.7	0.6
Spicy, Safeway*	1 Serving/100g	140	140	3.6	29.8	0.5	1.5
Sun Dried Tomato, & Italian Herbs, Dry, Sammy's*	1 Serving/50g	168	336	12.0	72.0	2.6	6.0
Sun Dried Tomato, Somerfield*	1 Jar/110g	176	160	3.0	25.0	5.0	0.0
Tangy Tomato, Dry, Ainsley Harriott*	1 Serving/50g	166	332	12.2	67.2	1.6	8.8
Tomato & Basil, Made Up, Tesco*	1 Serving/200g	348	174	3.9	21.0	8.3	3.4
Tomato & Onion, Dry, Waitrose*	1/2 Pack/55g	188	342	12.6	64.9	3.6	5.1
Tomato & Vegetable, Snack Pack, Dry, Sammy's*	1 Serving/70g	228	326	12.0	67.9	3.5	6.3
Tomato tango, Ainsley Harriott*	1/2 Pack/132.8g	166	125	4.6	25.3	0.6	3.3
Wild Mushroom & Garlic, Sainsbury's*	1 Serving/166g	239	144	4.2	22.9	4.0	0.6
With Chickpea & Feta, Toasted, TTD, Sainsbury's*	1 Serving/150g	273	182	5.2	12.6	12.3	0.0
With Lemon & Garlic, Dry, Waitrose*	1/2 Pack/55g	188	341	11.8	65.5	3.3	4.5
Zesty Lemon & Coriander, Dry, Sammy's*	1 Serving/50g	171	342	13.0	74.0	2.8	6.0

CRAB

Boiled	1oz/28g	36	128	19.5	0.0	5.5	0.0
Claws, Asda*	1oz/28g	25	89	11.0	9.0	1.0	0.2
Cocktail, Waitrose*	1 Serving/100g	217	217	10.8	3.8	17.6	0.4
Dressed, Average	1 Can/43g	66	154	16.8	4.1	7.9	0.2
Meat, In Brine, Average	1/2 Can/60g	46	76	17.2	0.9	0.4	0.1
Meat, Raw, Average	1oz/28g	28	100	20.8	2.8	0.6	0.0

CRAB CAKES

Goan, Marks & Spencer*	1 Pack/190g	228	120	8.0	12.9	4.0	1.8
Iceland*	1 Serving/18g	52	288	7.2	25.6	18.0	1.3
Marks & Spencer*	1 Pack/170g	340	200	9.5	10.9	12.9	2.2
Tesco*	1 Serving/130g	281	216	11.0	15.4	12.3	1.1

CRAB STICKS

Average	1oz/28g	26	94	9.1	13.9	0.3	0.0

CRACKERBREAD

Golden Wheat, Ryvita*	1 Slice/6g	19	317	8.3	65.0	3.3	3.3
High Fibre, Ryvita*	1oz/28g	90	321	12.6	61.3	2.8	16.8
Multi Grain Rye, Ryvita*	1 Slice/11.1g	37	332	11.0	58.6	6.0	17.3
Original Wheat, Ryvita*	1 Serving/5g	19	380	10.3	76.9	3.5	3.5
Rice, Asda*	1 Serving/5g	19	374	9.1	79.4	2.2	1.9
Sainsbury's*	1 Serving/5g	19	380	10.0	80.0	4.0	2.0
Wholemeal, Ryvita*	1 Slice/5.6g	19	319	10.8	71.5	4.2	6.5

CRACKERS

99% Fat Free, Rakusen's*	1 Cracker/5g	18	366	10.9	83.9	0.9	0.0
Bath Oliver, Jacobs*	1 Cracker/12g	52	432	9.6	67.6	13.7	2.6
Biscuits For Cheese, TTD, Sainsbury's*	1 Cracker/8g	39	493	8.6	61.0	23.8	3.1

CRACKERS

	Measure INFO/WEIGHT	per Measure KCAL	Nutrition Values per 100g / 100ml				
			KCAL	PROT	CARB	FAT	FIBRE
Black Olive, Marks & Spencer*	1 Cracker/4.1g	19	485	8.3	59.4	23.5	4.3
Blazing BBQ, JacoBites, Jacobs*	1 Pack/9g	41	461	5.2	55.8	24.2	1.7
Bombay, Extra Spicy, Pataks, Red Mill*	1 Serving/30g	146	487	1.3	66.0	24.3	0.0
Bran, Jacobs*	1 Cracker/7g	32	454	9.7	62.8	18.2	3.2
Butter Puff, Sainsbury's*	1 Cracker/10g	54	523	10.4	60.7	26.5	2.5
Chapati Chips, Tikka, Medium Spicy, Pataks, Red Mill*	1 Serving/25g	127	508	8.0	56.0	28.0	4.0
Cheddars, Jacobs*	1 Biscuit/4g	19	509	11.6	53.2	27.7	2.7
Cheddars, McVitie's*	1 Cracker/4g	22	543	10.0	55.1	31.3	2.6
Cheese Biscuit Thins, Safeway*	1 Cracker/4g	22	545	11.9	52.6	31.9	2.5
Cheese Melts, Carr's*	1 Cracker/4g	19	468	11.0	58.3	21.2	4.9
Cheese Thins, Asda*	1 Cracker/4g	21	532	12.0	49.0	32.0	0.0
Cheese Thins, Co-Op*	1 Cracker/4g	21	530	12.0	49.0	32.0	3.0
Cheese Thins, Waitrose*	1 Biscuit/4g	21	545	11.9	52.6	31.9	2.5
Cheese, Mini, Shapers, Boots*	1 Serving/23g	97	421	9.4	65.0	14.0	4.6
Cheese, Puff Pastry, Somerfield*	1 Biscuit/4g	21	500	10.6	36.1	34.8	2.1
Chinese, Pop Pan*	2 Crackers/15g	80	533	13.3	53.3	33.3	0.0
Chives, Jacobs*	1 Cracker/6.1g	27	457	9.5	67.5	16.5	2.7
Choice Grain, Jacobs*	1 Cracker/7g	30	435	9.2	65.4	15.2	4.7
Corn Thins, 97% Fat Free, Real Foods*	1 Cracker/6g	19	378	10.2	81.7	3.0	8.6
Corn Thins, Real Foods*	1 Serving/5.8g	25	414	10.3	82.8	3.4	8.6
Cornish Wafer, Jacobs*	1 Cracker/9g	48	528	8.0	54.4	31.2	2.4
Cream	1 Cracker/7g	31	440	9.5	68.3	16.3	2.2
Cream With Flaked Salt, TTD, Sainsbury's*	1 Cracker/7.4g	35	500	8.5	64.8	22.9	2.7
Cream, Asda*	1 Cracker/8g	35	443	10.0	67.0	15.0	0.0
Cream, BFY, Morrisons*	1 Cracker/8g	32	406	10.9	74.4	7.2	2.8
Cream, BGTY, Sainsbury's*	1 Cracker/8g	32	400	10.9	71.7	7.7	3.1
Cream, Choice Grain, Jacobs*	1 Cracker/7g	30	400	9.0	64.5	11.8	7.0
Cream, Half Fat, Safeway*	1 Cracker/8g	32	406	74.4	2.4	7.2	2.9
Cream, Jacobs*	1 Cracker/8g	34	421	9.9	66.8	12.7	4.1
Cream, Lower Fat, Tesco*	1 Cracker/5g	20	393	11.0	72.4	6.6	3.1
Cream, Morrisons*	1 Cracker/8g	36	446	9.6	68.5	14.8	2.7
Cream, Reduced Fat, Tesco*	1 Cracker/8g	31	406	10.9	74.4	7.2	2.8
Cream, Roasted Onion, Jacobs*	1 Cracker/8g	35	441	10.2	66.8	14.8	2.9
Cream, Sainsbury's*	1 Cracker/8.3g	34	422	9.5	66.7	15.2	2.8
Cream, Sun Dried Tomato Flavour, Jacobs*	1 Cracker/8g	35	434	10.2	66.7	14.0	3.0
Cream, Tesco*	1 Cracker/7.7g	34	447	9.0	69.0	15.0	3.0
Crispy Cheese, Marks & Spencer*	1oz/28g	134	478	10.2	57.8	22.6	2.9
Extra Wheatgerm, Hovis*	1 Serving/6g	27	447	10.2	60.0	18.5	4.4
Garden Herbs, Jacobs*	1 Cracker/6g	28	457	9.5	67.5	16.5	2.7
Garlic & Herb, Jacobs*	1 Cracker/100g	450	450	10.0	68.3	16.7	3.3
Glutafin*	1 Serving/11g	52	470	2.4	70.0	20.0	0.7
Harvest Grain, Sainsbury's*	1 Cracker/6g	27	458	8.5	64.5	18.4	4.1
Herb & Onion, 99% Fat Free, Rakusen's*	1 Cracker/4g	14	361	10.0	78.0	1.0	0.0
Herb & Onion, Trufree*	1 Cracker/6g	25	418	2.5	75.0	12.0	10.0
Herb & Spice, Jacobs*	1 Cracker/6g	27	457	9.5	67.5	16.5	2.7
Herbs & Spice Selection, Jacobs*	1 Cracker/6g	27	451	9.5	68.0	15.7	2.7
Italian, Doriano, Doria*	1 Sm Cracker/4g	19	464	9.5	69.8	16.4	0.0
Krackawheat, McVitie's*	1 Cracker/7g	36	515	9.1	62.4	25.4	4.8
Light & Crispy, Sainsbury's*	1 Cracker/11g	42	384	11.3	61.0	10.5	13.0
Lightly Salted, Crispy, Sainsbury's*	1 Cracker/4.7g	27	533	7.8	62.6	27.9	2.1
Lightly Salted, Italian, Jacobs*	1 Cracker/6g	26	429	10.3	67.6	13.0	2.9
Matzo, Rakusen's*	1 Cracker/4g	15	370	8.8	80.2	1.5	4.0
Mediterranean, Jacobs*	1 Cracker/6g	27	450	9.7	66.5	16.1	2.7

CRACKERS	Measure INFO/WEIGHT	per Measure KCAL	Nutrition Values per 100g / 100ml				
			KCAL	PROT	CARB	FAT	FIBRE
Melts, Carr's*	1 Cracker/4g	18	451	10.2	57.0	20.2	5.0
Multigrain, Tesco*	1 Cracker/6g	27	458	8.5	64.5	18.4	4.1
Olive Oil & Oregano, Mediterreaneo, Jacobs*	1 Cracker/6g	25	412	12.4	65.5	11.2	6.0
Oriental Style, Safeway*	1 Serving/25g	88	350	1.5	82.2	1.2	6.2
Oriental, Asda*	1 Serving/30g	115	383	1.7	49.0	20.0	4.3
Passionately Pizza, JacoBites, Jacobs*	1 Pack/150g	708	472	5.7	55.3	25.4	1.7
Peking Spare Rib & Five Spice, Sensations, Walkers*	1 Bag/24g	116	485	1.3	62.0	26.0	3.5
Pesto, Jacobs*	1 Cracker/6g	27	450	9.7	66.5	16.1	2.7
Poppy & Sesame Seed, Sainsbury's*	1 Cracker/4g	21	530	9.6	58.9	28.4	3.4
Poppy & Sesame Thins Savoury, Somerfield*	1oz/28g	147	524	9.0	58.0	28.0	0.0
Poppy & Sesame Thins, Morrisons*	1 Cracker/4g	20	530	9.6	58.9	28.4	0.0
Ritz, Original, Jacobs*	1 Cracker/3g	15	509	6.9	55.8	28.8	2.0
Rye, Organic, Doves Farm*	1 Cracker/7.1g	28	393	7.0	58.4	14.6	8.7
Salt & Black Pepper, Jacobs*	1 Cracker/6g	27	457	9.5	67.5	16.5	2.7
Selection, Finest, Tesco*	1 Serving/30g	136	452	9.6	71.0	14.4	0.0
Sesame & Poppy, Thins, Tesco*	1 Cracker/3.8g	19	507	9.3	54.5	28.0	4.2
Sesame Snaps, Anglo-Dal*	1 Serving/30g	163	542	2.8	61.8	31.5	0.0
Sesame Snaps, In Chocolate, Anglo-Dal*	1 Pack/40g	211	527	9.3	55.6	29.7	0.0
Spicy Indonesian Vegetable, Waitrose*	1 Pack/60g	295	492	1.2	60.6	27.2	2.2
Spicy Vegetable, Tesco*	1 Serving/60g	340	566	2.6	52.4	38.4	1.2
Tangy Malaysian Chutney, Oriental, Sensations, Walkers*	1 Serving/35g	170	485	0.9	62.0	26.0	3.5
Tempting Tandoori, JacoBites, Jacobs*	1 Pack/150g	711	474	5.7	55.5	25.5	1.7
Thai Spicy Vegetable, Sainsbury's*	1 Pack/50g	231	462	7.2	61.5	20.8	2.6
Tuc, Cheese Sandwich, Jacobs*	1 Serving/28g	149	531	8.4	53.8	31.4	0.0
Tuc, Jacobs*	1 Cracker/5g	24	522	7.0	60.5	28.0	2.9
Tuc, McVitie's*	1 Cracker/4g	21	530	7.8	62.2	27.8	2.1
Tuc, Mini, With Sesame Seeds, Jacobs*	5 Biscuits/10g	52	523	9.7	63.1	25.8	3.9
Vegetable, Oriental Snack Selection, Sainsbury's*	1 Cracker/20g	42	209	4.5	26.2	9.6	3.4
Water Biscuit, Carr's*	1 Biscuit/4g	14	350	7.5	62.5	7.5	2.5
Wheaten, Marks & Spencer*	1 Cracker/4.4g	18	450	10.2	57.0	20.2	5.0
Whole Wheat, 100%, Oven Baked, Master, Choices*	7 Crackers/28g	120	429	10.0	75.0	9.6	12.1
Wholemeal, Tesco*	1 Cracker/7g	29	414	9.4	60.6	14.9	10.4
Wholemeal, Organic, Nairn's*	1 Cracker/14g	58	413	9.0	61.4	14.6	8.7
With Onion, Cumin Seed, & Garlic, GFY, Asda*	1 Cracker/6g	22	380	11.0	78.0	2.7	1.7
CRANBERRIES							
& Raisins, Dried, Sweetened, Ocean Spray*	1 Serving/50g	163	326	0.1	80.3	0.5	4.6
Dried, Sweetened, Average	1 Serving/10g	34	335	0.3	81.1	0.8	4.4
Fresh, Raw	1oz/28g	4	15	0.4	3.4	0.1	3.0
CRAYFISH							
Raw	1oz/28g	19	67	14.9	0.0	0.8	0.0
Tails, Chilli & Garlic, Asda*	1 Serving/140g	133	95	16.0	1.1	3.1	0.8
Tails, In Brine, Luxury, The Big Prawn Co*	1/2 Tub/90g	46	51	10.1	1.0	0.7	0.0
CREAM							
Aerosol, Average	1oz/28g	87	309	1.8	6.2	30.9	0.0
Aerosol, Reduced Fat, Average	1 Serving/55ml	33	60	0.6	2.0	5.5	0.0
Brandy, Pourable, With Remy Martin*, Finest, Tesco*	1/2 Pot/125ml	460	368	2.7	19.8	28.4	0.0
Brandy, Really Thick, Finest, Tesco*	1/2 Pot/125ml	579	463	1.3	19.7	39.6	0.0
Brandy, Really Thick, Tesco*	1 Sm Pot/250ml	1163	465	1.4	21.3	39.3	0.0
Clotted, Fresh, Average	1 Serving/28g	162	579	1.6	2.3	62.7	0.0
Double, Average	1 Serving/25ml	110	438	1.8	2.7	46.7	0.0
Double, Reduced Fat, Average	1 Serving/30g	73	243	2.7	5.7	23.3	0.1
Single, Average	1 Serving/50ml	62	123	2.7	4.4	10.5	0.1
Single, Extra Thick, Average	1 Serving/37.5ml	73	192	2.7	4.1	18.4	0.0

	Measure	per Measure	Nutrition Values per 100g / 100ml				
	INFO/WEIGHT	KCAL	KCAL	PROT	CARB	FAT	FIBRE
CREAM							
Soured, Fresh, Average	1 Tbsp/15ml	29	191	2.7	3.9	18.4	0.0
Thick, Sterilised, Average	1 Tbsp/15ml	35	233	2.6	3.6	23.1	0.0
UHT, Double, Average	1 Tbsp/15g	41	275	2.2	7.4	26.3	0.0
UHT, Reduced Fat, Average	1 Serving/25ml	16	62	0.6	2.3	5.7	0.0
UHT, Single, Average	1 Tbsp/15ml	29	194	2.6	4.0	18.8	0.0
Whipping, Average	1 Tbsp/15ml	52	348	2.1	3.2	36.4	0.1
CREAM HORN							
Fresh, Tesco*	1 Horn/57g	244	428	4.1	40.3	27.8	0.3
CREAM SODA							
Traditional Style, Tesco*	1 Can/330ml	139	42	0.0	10.4	0.0	0.0
CREMA CATALANA							
Cafe Culture, Marks & Spencer*	1 Pot/110g	385	350	3.5	12.2	31.7	0.4
CREME BRULEE							
Marks & Spencer*	1 Pot/100g	360	360	3.3	13.0	32.6	0.0
Nestle*	1 Serving/100g	305	305	4.0	14.6	25.6	0.0
Somerfield*	1 Pot/100g	316	316	4.0	15.0	27.0	0.0
CREME CARAMEL							
Asda*	1 Pot/100g	113	113	2.4	20.0	2.6	0.0
Average	1 Carton/128g	140	109	3.0	20.6	2.2	0.0
Carmelle, Greens*	1 Pack/70g	82	117	3.0	17.0	4.0	0.0
La Laitiere*	1 Pot/100g	135	135	5.0	20.0	4.0	0.0
Sainsbury's*	1 Pot/100g	102	102	2.5	21.1	0.9	0.0
SmartPrice, Asda*	1 Pot/100g	87	87	2.5	18.0	0.5	0.0
Tesco*	1 Pot/100g	114	114	2.6	22.4	1.6	0.0
CREME EGG							
Cadbury*	1 Egg/39g	174	445	3.0	71.0	16.0	0.0
CREME FRAICHE							
Average	1 Pot/295g	1067	362	2.2	2.6	38.0	0.0
Cucumber & Mint, Triangles, Sainsbury's*	1 Serving/25g	105	421	11.0	72.3	9.7	2.5
Extra Light, President*	1 Tub/200g	182	91	2.7	8.7	5.0	0.0
Half Fat, Average	1 Dtsp/30g	54	181	3.1	5.5	16.3	0.0
Lemon & Rocket, Sainsbury's*	1 Serving/150g	188	125	2.2	3.0	11.5	0.5
With Courvoisier Cognac, Tesco*	1 tablespoon/15ml	56	372	1.2	16.6	33.4	0.5
CREPES							
Chicken, Asda*	1 Crepe/204.4g	369	181	14.0	11.0	9.0	3.6
Chocolate Filled, Tesco*	1 Crepe/32g	140	438	5.9	62.5	18.1	1.6
Cream Cheese & Onion, Mini, Marks & Spencer*	1 Crepe/2g	10	510	8.3	55.9	28.0	1.0
Lobster, Finest, Tesco*	1 Serving/160g	250	156	10.7	14.0	6.4	1.2
Mushroom, Marks & Spencer*	1 Pack/186g	195	105	5.7	17.1	2.4	2.5
CREVETTES							
Asda*	1oz/28g	11	41	8.6	0.0	0.7	0.0
CRISPBAKES							
Bubble & Squeak, Marks & Spencer*	1 Crispbake/46.5g	78	170	2.7	19.6	8.8	1.5
Cheese & Chive, Sainsbury's*	1 Serving/108g	273	253	7.1	24.5	14.8	1.7
Cheese & Onion, Marks & Spencer*	1 Crispbake/114g	285	250	6.4	19.4	16.2	1.7
Cheese & Onion, Tesco*	1 Crispbake/109g	275	252	7.9	19.6	15.8	2.1
Chicken & Broccoli, Marks & Spencer*	1 Crispbake/114g	225	197	6.1	16.5	11.9	1.9
Dutch, Asda*	1 Toast/10g	39	394	14.0	77.0	3.3	3.9
Dutch, Safeway*	1 Bake/10g	39	394	14.0	77.0	3.3	3.9
Dutch, Tesco*	1 Slice/8g	30	371	17.0	72.0	1.7	4.0
Minced Beef, Marks & Spencer*	1 Crispbake/113g	226	200	10.0	15.6	10.9	1.5
Mushroom & Garlic, Ovenbaked, Iceland*	1 Crispbake/140g	241	172	4.3	23.7	6.7	2.9
Organic, Trimlyne*	1 Bake/10g	38	380	16.0	73.0	2.0	6.0

	Measure INFO/WEIGHT	per Measure KCAL	Nutrition Values per 100g / 100ml				
			KCAL	PROT	CARB	FAT	FIBRE
CRISPBAKES							
Sainsbury's*	1 Serving/9g	35	392	14.5	72.3	5.0	5.8
Spinach, Feta & Soft Cheese, Mini, Safeway*	1 Pack/191.5g	449	235	6.6	20.8	13.4	2.5
Spring Onion & Chive, Sainsbury's*	1 Crispbake/108g	272	253	7.1	24.5	14.8	1.7
Tuna & Sweetcorn, Lakeland*	1 Serving/170g	391	230	11.3	20.1	11.6	0.0
Vegetable, Marks & Spencer*	1 Crispbake/114.3g	160	140	2.8	14.9	7.7	1.8
Vegetable, Sainsbury's*	1 Serving/114g	246	216	2.0	26.2	11.4	2.0
CRISPBREAD							
Bran, Scandinavian, GG*	2 Crispbread/16g	36	223	14.9	29.0	5.3	42.1
Breaks, Ryvita*	1 Crispbread/14.4g	47	333	8.0	69.5	2.5	12.0
Corn, Orgran*	1 Crispbread/5g	18	360	7.5	83.0	1.8	3.0
Crisp N Light, Wasa*	1 Crispbread/7g	24	360	12.0	73.0	2.2	5.3
Currant Crunch, Ryvita*	1oz/28g	94	334	8.7	69.9	2.5	12.8
Dark Rye, Morrisons*	1 Slice/13g	39	300	11.5	61.5	3.1	16.9
Dark Rye, Ryvita*	1 Serving/9g	28	308	8.5	65.0	1.5	18.5
Emmental Cheese & Pumpkin Seed, Dr Kracker*	1 Serving/25g	101	404	20.0	43.2	16.8	15.2
Gluten Free, Dietary Specials*	1 Serving/8g	25	331	6.4	72.9	1.5	0.0
Harvest Wheat, Finn Crisp*	1 Serving/50g	195	390	10.0	72.0	6.7	5.8
Hi-Fibre Rye, Organic, Finn Crisp*	1 Crispbread/12.9g	39	300	10.0	61.0	1.8	18.0
Light, Marks & Spencer*	1 Crispbread/4.2g	14	360	10.7	69.2	4.6	7.6
Light, Ryvita*	1 Slice/5g	19	383	9.8	79.3	3.0	2.6
Milky, Grafschafter*	1 Slice/9g	29	316	11.4	64.0	1.6	15.0
Multigrain, Finn Crisp*	1 Bread/8g	26	320	11.0	58.0	4.7	18.0
Multigrain, Ryvita*	1 Slice/11g	37	332	11.0	58.6	6.0	17.3
Multigrain, Wasa*	1 Crispbread/13g	43	320	12.0	62.0	2.6	14.0
Organic, Trimlyne*	1 Crispbake/10g	38	380	16.0	73.0	2.3	6.0
Original Rye, Wasa*	1 Crispbread/11g	35	315	9.0	67.0	1.4	14.0
Original, Rye, Hi Fibre, Finn Crisp*	1 Serving/14g	43	310	8.7	64.0	2.1	17.0
Original, Rye, Trimlyne*	1 Crispbread/11g	36	325	10.3	65.4	2.5	12.8
Original, Ryvita*	1 Crispbread/9g	34	380	10.3	76.9	3.5	3.5
Pagen*	1 Crispbread/3g	11	370	12.0	65.0	7.0	9.5
Poppyseed, Wasa*	1 Crispbread/13g	46	350	13.0	56.0	8.0	14.0
Provita*	1 Biscuit/6g	26	416	12.5	68.4	9.9	0.0
Rice, & Cracked Pepper, Orgran*	4 Slices/19g	74	388	8.4	81.9	1.8	2.0
Rice, Original, Sakata*	1 Serving/25g	103	410	6.9	88.0	2.6	1.3
Rice, Sakata*	1 Crispbread/25g	26	102	1.7	22.0	0.7	0.3
Rye, Harvest Slims, Finn Crisp*	3 Slices/18g	58	320	11.0	63.0	2.3	16.0
Rye, Original, Ryvita*	1 Crispbread/9g	28	315	8.5	67.2	1.4	16.5
Rye, Somerfield*	1 Crispbread/11g	35	320	9.0	66.0	2.2	13.0
Sesame Rye, Ryvita*	1 Crispbread/9g	30	338	9.5	60.3	6.5	16.5
Sesame, Grafschafter, Lidl*	1 Crispbread/10g	34	337	11.5	58.4	6.4	15.7
Sesame, Ryvita*	1oz/28g	95	339	10.5	58.5	7.0	16.0
Trufree*	1 Crispbread/6g	22	370	6.0	82.0	2.0	1.0
Wheat, Cracottes*	1 Slice/6.9g	26	367	9.8	75.2	3.0	3.2
Whole Grain, Classic, Organic, Dr Karg*	1 Crispbread/25g	89	355	13.4	38.2	16.5	10.2
Wholemeal Rye, Kallo*	1 Crispbread/10g	31	314	9.7	65.0	1.7	15.4
Wholemeal, Light, Allinson*	1 Slice/5g	17	349	11.7	69.7	2.6	11.0
Wholemeal, Organic, Allinson*	1 Crispbread/5g	17	336	14.2	66.0	1.7	12.2
With Currants, Oats & Honey, Ryvita*	1 Crisp/14.8g	50	333	8.0	69.5	2.5	12.0
With Sesame, Spar*	1 Crispbread/15g	62	410	12.0	66.0	11.0	5.0
CRISPS							
Apple, Thyme & Sage, Marks & Spencer*	1 Bag/55g	253	460	5.5	55.3	24.3	6.1
BBQ Chilli & Mesquite, Pan-Fried, TTD, Sainsbury's*	1 Sm Pack/50g	239	478	8.0	51.3	26.7	5.4
Bacon Bites, Eat Smart, Safeway*	1 Bag/12g	41	340	10.8	70.3	1.6	3.5

CRISPS

	Measure INFO/WEIGHT	per Measure KCAL	Nutrition Values per 100g / 100ml				
			KCAL	PROT	CARB	FAT	FIBRE
Bacon Crispies, Sainsbury's*	1 Bag/25g	117	468	19.9	45.8	22.8	4.8
Bacon Flavour Rashers, BGTY, Sainsbury's*	1 Pack/10g	34	340	10.8	70.3	1.6	3.5
Bacon Pillows, Light, Shapers, Boots*	1 Pack/12g	44	367	3.7	83.0	2.3	4.0
Bacon Rashers, Blazin, Tesco*	1 Bag/25g	119	477	15.4	44.7	26.3	4.4
Bacon Rashers, COU, Marks & Spencer*	1 Bag/20g	72	360	9.4	77.5	2.9	3.5
Bacon Rashers, Marks & Spencer*	1 Bag/40g	192	480	8.1	59.9	22.9	2.2
Bacon Rice Bites, Asda*	1 Bag/30g	136	452	7.0	70.0	16.0	0.4
Bacon, Shapers, Boots*	1 Bag/23g	99	431	8.0	66.0	15.0	3.0
Bagels, Sour Cream & Chive, Shapers, Boots*	1 Bag/25g	94	377	9.7	78.0	2.9	1.9
Baked Beans, Walkers*	1 Bag/35g	184	525	6.5	50.0	33.0	4.0
Baked Potato, COU, Marks & Spencer*	1 Bag/25g	88	350	8.5	76.4	2.3	5.7
Banging BBQ, Shots, Walkers*	1 Pack/17.9g	87	485	5.5	60.0	25.0	1.3
Barbecue Beef, Select, Tesco*	1 Pack/25g	134	536	6.4	49.2	34.8	4.4
Barbecue, Handcooked, Tesco*	1 Bag/40g	187	468	6.6	53.8	25.1	5.2
Barbecue, Snack Rite, Aldi*	1 Bag/25g	131	524	5.1	51.3	33.2	0.0
Barbecue, Walkers*	1 Bag/35g	184	525	6.5	50.0	33.0	4.0
Beef & Onion, Asda*	1 Bag/25g	135	539	7.0	49.0	35.0	4.5
Beef & Onion, Morrisons*	1 Pack/25g	131	524	5.9	51.2	32.9	4.2
Beef & Onion, Potato, Marks & Spencer*	1 Bag/24.5g	133	530	6.6	48.2	34.5	5.0
Beef & Onion, Walkers*	1 Bag/35g	184	525	6.5	50.0	33.0	4.0
Beefy, Smiths, Walkers*	1 Bag/25g	133	531	4.3	45.2	37.0	0.0
Beefy, Square, Walkers*	1 Bag/25g	105	420	6.0	59.0	18.0	4.6
Butter & Chive, COU, Marks & Spencer*	1 Bag/26g	95	365	7.7	77.3	1.9	4.6
Chargrilled Chicken Crinkles, Shapers, Boots*	1 Bag/20g	96	482	6.6	60.0	24.0	4.0
Chargrilled Steak, Max, Walkers*	1 Bag/55g	289	525	6.5	50.0	33.0	4.0
Cheddar & Onion, McCoy's*	1 Bag/50g	258	516	7.0	53.2	30.6	3.9
Cheddar & Spring Onion, 35% Less Fat, Sainsbury's*	1 Pack/20g	93	463	6.3	62.4	20.9	0.9
Cheddar, Red Wine & Shallot, TTD, Sainsbury's*	1 Pack/50g	238	476	6.5	55.6	25.2	4.7
Cheese & Branston Pickle Flavour, Walkers*	1 Bag/34.5g	176	510	7.0	49.0	32.0	4.5
Cheese & Chive Flavour, GFY, Asda*	1 Bag/25g	119	476	6.0	59.0	24.0	6.0
Cheese & Chives, Walkers*	1 Bag/35g	186	530	6.5	50.0	33.0	4.1
Cheese & Onion Rings, Shapers, Boots*	1 Pack/15g	56	374	5.9	81.0	2.9	2.0
Cheese & Onion, 30% Less Fat, Sainsbury's*	1 Pack/25g	115	459	7.5	58.1	21.8	5.4
Cheese & Onion, Asda*	1 Bag/25g	133	530	6.0	50.0	34.0	4.5
Cheese & Onion, BGTY, Sainsbury's*	1 Bag/25g	120	479	7.0	57.0	24.8	5.7
Cheese & Onion, Big Eat, Walkers*	1 Bag/55g	289	525	6.5	50.0	33.0	4.0
Cheese & Onion, Crinkle Cut, Low Fat, Waitrose*	1 Bag/25g	123	490	7.7	62.6	23.2	4.7
Cheese & Onion, Flavour Crinkles, Shapers, Boots*	1 Bag/20g	96	482	6.6	60.0	24.0	4.0
Cheese & Onion, GFY, Asda*	1 Pack/26g	122	470	7.0	61.0	22.0	4.2
Cheese & Onion, Golden Wonder*	1 Bag/25g	131	524	6.1	49.2	33.6	2.0
Cheese & Onion, KP*	1 Bag/25g	134	534	6.6	48.7	34.8	4.8
Cheese & Onion, Lites, Walkers*	1 Bag/28g	130	465	7.5	61.0	21.0	5.0
Cheese & Onion, Lower Fat, Asda*	1 Bag/25g	120	481	6.0	58.0	25.0	4.8
Cheese & Onion, Marks & Spencer*	1 Bag/25g	134	535	5.5	48.8	35.5	5.0
Cheese & Onion, Max, Walkers*	1 Bag/55g	289	525	6.5	50.0	33.0	4.0
Cheese & Onion, Morrisons*	1 Bag/30g	152	508	7.1	50.5	30.8	4.6
Cheese & Onion, Organic, Tesco*	1 Bag/25g	129	514	5.2	49.9	32.6	7.0
Cheese & Onion, Potato Heads, Walkers*	1 Pack/23g	105	455	9.0	57.0	21.0	5.0
Cheese & Onion, Sainsbury's*	1 Bag/25g	132	527	4.6	48.8	34.8	3.9
Cheese & Onion, Select, Tesco*	1 Bag/25g	134	535	6.6	48.5	34.9	4.8
Cheese & Onion, Sky Snacks, Safeway*	1 Packet/15g	74	495	4.9	59.8	26.2	3.7
Cheese & Onion, Smiths, Walkers*	1 Bag/25g	133	531	4.3	45.2	37.0	0.0
Cheese & Onion, Snack Rite, Aldi*	1 Bag/25g	132	527	5.3	51.3	33.4	0.0

CRISPS

INFO/WEIGHT	Measure	per Measure KCAL	Nutrition Values per 100g / 100ml KCAL	PROT	CARB	FAT	FIBRE
Cheese & Onion, Square, Smiths, Walkers*	1 Bag/25g	113	452	6.9	62.5	19.4	0.0
Cheese & Onion, Square, Walkers*	1 Bag/25g	106	425	6.5	59.0	18.0	4.4
Cheese & Onion, Tayto*	1 Bag/25g	137	546	4.8	51.9	38.5	0.0
Cheese & Onion, Value, Tesco*	1 Bag/20g	108	541	6.0	48.3	36.0	4.8
Cheese & Onion, Walkers*	1 Bag/35g	184	525	6.5	50.0	33.0	4.0
Cheese Curls, Asda*	1 Bag/14g	74	525	4.2	55.0	32.0	2.2
Cheese Curls, Red Mill*	1/2 Bag/50g	277	553	6.6	50.6	36.0	2.0
Cheese Curls, Shapers, Boots*	1 Pack/13.9g	68	489	4.5	57.0	27.0	2.7
Cheese Flavour Puffs, Morrisons*	1 Bag/25g	136	542	6.7	50.2	34.9	1.1
Cheese Tasters, Marks & Spencer*	1 Sm Bag/30g	156	520	8.6	51.0	31.0	3.2
Cheese XL, Golden Wonder*	1 Bag/30g	155	516	6.2	50.6	32.1	4.2
Cheesy Puffs, Co-Op*	1 Bag/60g	321	535	3.0	54.0	34.0	2.0
Chicken & Thyme, Oven Roasted, Tesco*	1 Pack/150g	728	485	6.5	54.0	27.0	4.5
Chicken & Thyme, Sensations, Oven Roasted, Walkers*	1 Bag/40g	194	485	6.5	54.0	27.0	4.5
Chicken Flavour, Healthy Eating, Tesco*	1 Bag/12g	43	357	5.1	81.0	1.4	3.4
Chicken Tikka Masala, Great British Takeaways, Walkers*	1 Bag/25g	131	525	6.5	50.0	33.0	4.0
Chicken, Firecracker, McCoy's*	1 Bag/35g	177	506	6.2	54.0	29.5	4.0
Chicken, Grilled, Golden Lights, Golden Wonder*	1 Pack/21g	93	443	4.3	66.2	18.1	4.3
Chill, Coriander & Lime, Marks & Spencer*	1 Bag/40g	194	485	6.4	53.6	27.1	5.0
Chinese Sizzling Beef, McCoy's*	1 Bag/35g	178	506	6.9	51.8	30.2	4.0
Chinese Spare Rib, Walkers*	1 Bag/25g	131	525	6.5	50.0	33.0	4.0
Chinese Szechaun Chicken, Hand Cooked, Asda*	1 Serving/50g	254	507	6.0	51.0	31.0	3.4
Cool Cheese Curly, Tesco*	1 Bag/14g	71	510	4.5	51.0	32.0	2.6
Coronation Chicken, Walkers*	1 Bag/25g	131	525	6.5	50.0	33.0	4.0
Cracked Black Pepper Seasoned, TTD, Sainsbury's*	1 Bag/30g	145	484	7.0	54.6	26.4	4.0
Creme Fraiche, Red Onion & Chive, TTD, Sainsbury's*	1 Serving/50g	226	452	7.8	50.8	24.2	6.3
Crinkle Cut, Lower Fat, No Added Salt, Waitrose*	1 Bag/40g	193	483	6.5	58.0	25.0	3.9
Crispy Bacon Bites, Shapers, Boots*	1 Bag/21g	97	464	13.0	58.0	20.0	1.8
Crunchy Claws, Sprinters, Aldi*	1 Serving/30g	152	508	6.0	55.7	29.0	0.0
Double Cheddar & Chives, Deli Style, Brannigans*	1oz/28g	148	529	7.6	49.5	33.4	3.8
Feta Cheese Flavour, Mediterranean, Walkers*	1 Pack/25g	128	510	6.5	49.0	33.0	4.5
Flame Grilled Steak, McCoy's*	1 Bag/50g	252	504	6.4	53.8	29.2	3.9
Four Cheese & Red Onion Sensations, Walkers*	1 Bag/40g	194	485	6.5	54.0	27.0	4.5
Garlic & Herbs Creme Fraiche, Kettle Chips*	1 Bag/50g	249	497	6.0	54.7	28.3	4.2
Greek Kebab, Mediterranean, Walkers*	1 Pack/25g	128	510	6.0	49.0	33.0	4.5
Handcooked, Marks & Spencer*	1 Bag/40g	198	495	5.4	56.9	27.2	4.5
Hint Of Garlic, Doritos*	1 Serving/35g	175	500	7.0	61.0	25.0	3.5
Honey Roast Gammon & English Mustard, Sainsbury's*	1 Serving/50g	236	472	7.2	55.0	-24.8	5.0
Honey Roast Ham, Marks & Spencer*	1 Bag/24.5g	133	530	6.6	49.0	34.1	4.6
Honey Roasted Ham, Sensations, Walkers*	1 Bag/40g	196	490	6.5	55.0	27.0	4.0
Hot & Spicy Salami, Tesco*	1 Bag/50g	216	431	26.2	0.7	35.9	0.0
Lamb & Mint, Sensations, Walkers*	1 Bag/35g	170	485	6.5	54.0	27.0	4.5
Lant Chips, Ikea*	1 Serving/25g	126	505	8.3	55.9	27.6	4.5
Lightly Salted, COU, Marks & Spencer*	1 Bag/26g	91	350	8.5	76.4	2.3	5.7
Lightly Salted, Crinkle Cut, Low Fat, Waitrose*	1 Pack/35g	163	466	5.2	60.1	22.8	5.1
Lightly Salted, Crinkles, Shapers, Boots*	1 Pack/20g	96	482	6.6	60.0	24.0	4.0
Lightly Salted, Golden Lights, Golden Wonder*	1 Bag/21g	92	440	5.1	64.3	18.0	4.3
Lightly Salted, Handcooked, Finest, Tesco*	1/2 Pack/150g	708	472	6.4	52.9	26.1	5.1
Lightly Salted, Kettle Chips*	1 Bag/50g	233	465	6.4	51.5	25.9	6.0
Lightly Salted, Low Fat, Waitrose*	1 Bag/25g	125	500	7.5	61.3	25.0	4.8
Lightly Salted, Traditional Pan Fried, TTD, Sainsbury's*	1 Bag/50g	236	472	6.2	53.6	25.8	5.1
Lightly Sea Salted, Jonathan Crisp*	1 Bag/35g	176	503	6.5	52.0	29.0	5.4
Lightly Sea Salted, Potato Chips, Hand Fried, Burts*	1/4 Bag/50g	252	504	6.4	57.4	27.7	0.0

CRISPS

INFO/WEIGHT	Measure per Measure KCAL	Nutrition Values per 100g / 100ml KCAL	PROT	CARB	FAT	FIBRE
Marmite Flavour, Walkers*	1 Bag/34.5g	176	510	6.5	49.0	32.0	4.0
Mature Cheddar & Chive, Kettle Chips*	1 Serving/50g	239	478	8.1	54.4	25.4	5.0
Mature Cheddar & Shallot, Temptations, Tesco*	1/6 Bag/25g	131	524	6.6	47.4	34.2	4.4
Mediterranean Baked Potato, COU, Marks & Spencer*	1 Pack/25g	90	360	7.6	74.0	2.4	6.8
Mexian Chilli & Chesse, Golden Wonder*	1 Pack/45g	230	511	6.6	50.7	31.3	0.0
Mexican Chilli, McCoy's*	1 Bag/35g	177	511	7.1	52.8	30.2	4.1
Mixed Pepper Flavour Burst, Marks & Spencer*	1 Bag/55g	286	520	6.0	50.1	33.5	4.0
New York Cheddar, Kettle Chips*	1 Bag/50g	242	483	6.7	53.9	26.7	4.5
Nicely Spicy, Shots, Walkers*	1 Bag/18g	87	485	5.5	60.0	25.0	1.5
Paprika, Handcooked, Shapers, Boots*	1 Bag/20g	99	493	7.2	62.0	24.0	5.0
Paprika, Max, Walkers*	1 Bag/29g	152	525	6.5	50.0	33.0	4.0
Paprika, Mini Hoops, Shapers, Boots*	1 Bag/13.0g	64	494	8.7	54.0	27.0	2.2
Parsnip & Black Pepper, Sainsbury's*	1 Serving/35g	166	473	3.2	43.6	31.8	15.2
Pastrami & Cheese, Crinkle, Marks & Spencer*	1 Bag/24.7g	121	485	6.5	61.0	24.0	3.5
Pickled Onion Flavour Rings, BGTY, Sainsbury's*	1 Serving/10g	35	345	5.0	81.7	1.5	3.7
Pickled Onion, Beastie Bites, Asda*	1 Bag/20g	100	498	6.0	60.0	26.0	0.0
Pickled Onion, Golden Wonder*	1 Bag/25g	131	524	5.6	49.0	34.0	2.0
Pickled Onion, Marks & Spencer*	1 Bag/20.3g	69	345	5.0	81.7	1.5	3.7
Pickled Onion, Monster Bites, Sainsbury's*	1 Bag/20g	107	535	5.2	53.5	33.3	1.0
Pickled Onion, Stompers, Morrisons*	1 Pack/25g	129	518	6.1	52.2	31.6	1.3
Pickled Onion, Tesco*	1 Bag/20g	104	520	6.5	50.0	35.0	1.0
Pickled Onion, Walkers*	1 Bag/35g	184	525	6.5	50.0	33.0	4.0
Potato	1oz/28g	148	530	5.7	53.3	34.2	5.3
Potato Sticks, Ready Salted, Marks & Spencer*	1 Packet/40g	210	525	6.5	52.0	33.0	4.0
Potato Triangles, Ready Salted, Sainsbury's*	1/2 Pack/50g	243	486	9.4	59.7	23.4	3.4
Potato, Low Fat	1oz/28g	128	458	6.6	63.5	21.5	5.9
Prawn Cocktail, 30% Less Fat, Sainsbury's*	1 Pack/25g	118	470	6.3	58.9	23.6	5.7
Prawn Cocktail, Asda*	1 Bag/25g	134	535	6.0	49.0	35.0	4.3
Prawn Cocktail, BGTY, Sainsbury's*	1 Bag/25g	118	473	6.3	58.6	23.7	5.7
Prawn Cocktail, Golden Wonder*	1 Bag/25g	130	521	5.8	49.0	33.5	2.0
Prawn Cocktail, KP*	1 Bag/25g	133	531	5.9	48.4	34.9	4.7
Prawn Cocktail, Lites, Shapers, Boots*	1 Bag/21g	92	438	5.1	64.0	18.0	4.1
Prawn Cocktail, Marks & Spencer*	1 Bag/30g	155	515	3.2	60.1	29.3	1.3
Prawn Cocktail, Sainsbury's*	1 Bag/25g	130	521	4.3	47.5	34.9	3.9
Prawn Cocktail, Select, Tesco*	1 Bag/25g	134	535	6.2	49.1	34.9	4.3
Prawn Cocktail, Smiths, Walkers*	1 Bag/25g	133	531	4.3	45.2	37.0	0.0
Prawn Cocktail, Walkers*	1 Bag/35g	184	525	6.5	50.0	33.0	4.0
Prawn Crackers, Tesco*	1 Bag/60g	316	527	3.2	62.8	29.2	0.8
Punchin' Pickled Onion, Beast, Tesco*	1 Bag/20g	104	518	6.1	52.2	31.6	1.3
Punching Paprika, Max, Walkers*	1 Bag/55g	256	465	7.5	61.0	21.0	4.0
Ready Salted Crinkle, Reduced Fat, Marks & Spencer*	1 Bag/40g	190	475	6.5	58.0	24.0	6.5
Ready Salted, 30% Less Fat, Sainsbury's*	1 Serving/25g	122	486	7.3	63.7	22.4	8.2
Ready Salted, BGTY, Sainsbury's*	1 Bag/25g	122	486	6.8	55.7	26.2	6.6
Ready Salted, GFY, Asda*	1 Bag/23g	109	475	7.0	60.0	23.0	4.3
Ready Salted, Golden Wonder*	1 Bag/25g	135	539	5.5	49.9	35.3	2.0
Ready Salted, KP*	1 Bag/24g	131	545	5.6	47.9	36.8	4.9
Ready Salted, Lidl*	1 Bag/25g	139	554	4.9	50.3	37.0	0.0
Ready Salted, Lites, Walkers*	1 Bag/28g	132	470	7.5	60.0	22.0	5.0
Ready Salted, Lower Fat, Asda*	1 Bag/25g	120	481	6.0	58.0	25.0	4.8
Ready Salted, Lower Fat, Sainsbury's*	1 Bag/25g	111	444	7.0	55.0	21.8	5.1
Ready Salted, Marks & Spencer*	1 Bag/25g	136	545	5.6	47.8	36.6	4.9
Ready Salted, McCoy's*	1 Bag/49g	253	517	6.0	52.3	31.5	4.9
Ready Salted, Morrisons*	1 Bag/25g	134	536	4.9	50.9	34.8	4.3

	Measure INFO/WEIGHT	per Measure KCAL	Nutrition Values per 100g / 100ml				
			KCAL	PROT	CARB	FAT	FIBRE
CRISPS							
Ready Salted, Organic, Tesco*	1 Bag/25g	130	520	4.3	49.0	34.1	7.3
Ready Salted, Potato Chips, Tesco*	1 Bag/25g	132	526	5.6	51.7	33.0	3.8
Ready Salted, Potato Squares, Sainsbury's*	1 Bag/50g	192	384	6.5	53.8	15.9	7.8
Ready Salted, Reduced Fat, Tesco*	1 Pack/25g	114	456	6.3	52.0	24.7	5.9
Ready Salted, Sainsbury's*	1 Bag/25g	135	538	4.3	47.4	36.8	4.1
Ready Salted, Savers, Safeway*	1 Packet/20g	110	549	5.6	51.3	35.7	0.0
Ready Salted, Select, Tesco*	1 Bag/25g	136	544	6.2	47.9	36.6	4.5
Ready Salted, SmartPrice, Asda*	1 Bag/20g	111	553	5.0	50.0	37.0	3.0
Ready Salted, Smiths, Walkers*	1 Bag/25g	133	531	4.3	45.2	37.0	0.0
Ready Salted, Snack Rite, Aldi*	1 Bag/25g	136	545	4.9	50.3	36.0	0.0
Ready Salted, Square, Smiths, Walkers*	1 Bag/25g	106	425	6.0	58.0	19.0	4.6
Ready Salted, Squares, Marks & Spencer*	1 Bag/35g	151	430	6.8	63.5	18.1	3.9
Ready Salted, Value, Tesco*	1 Bag/21g	115	548	6.0	50.0	36.0	0.0
Ready Salted, Walkers*	1 Bag/35g	186	530	6.5	49.0	34.0	4.0
Red Leicester & Spring Onion, Marks & Spencer*	1 Bag/40g	194	485	6.2	58.7	27.2	4.9
Roast Beef & Mustard, Thick Cut, Brannigans*	1 Bag/40g	203	507	7.6	51.7	30.0	3.7
Roast Beef, KP*	1 Bag/25g	134	534	6.6	47.5	35.3	4.7
Roast Chicken & Sage Flavour, Marks & Spencer*	1 Bag/25g	135	540	5.9	50.6	34.6	4.6
Roast Chicken Flavour, BGTY, Sainsbury's*	1 Bag/25g	118	473	6.2	58.9	23.6	5.7
Roast Chicken Flavour, Budgens*	1 Bag/25g	129	516	7.3	47.6	33.0	3.6
Roast Chicken, 30% Less Fat, Sainsbury's*	1 Pack/25g	115	460	7.4	58.3	21.9	5.2
Roast Chicken, Golden Wonder*	1 Bag/25g	131	522	6.2	48.6	33.6	2.0
Roast Chicken, Highlander*	1 Bag/25g	139	554	5.3	46.0	38.9	5.1
Roast Chicken, Morrisons*	1 Pack/25g	131	525	5.5	51.7	32.9	4.2
Roast Chicken, Potato Heads, Walkers*	1 Pack/23g	106	460	8.5	58.0	21.0	6.0
Roast Chicken, Select, Tesco*	1 Bag/25g	134	536	6.6	48.6	35.0	4.4
Roast Chicken, Smiths, Walkers*	1 Bag/25g	133	531	4.3	45.2	37.0	0.0
Roast Chicken, Snack Rite, Aldi*	1 Bag/25g	132	526	5.3	51.3	33.3	0.0
Roast Chicken, Walkers*	1 Bag/35g	184	525	6.5	50.0	33.0	4.0
Roast Pork & Apple Sauce, Select, Tesco*	1 Bag/25g	136	544	6.5	50.0	35.3	3.7
Roast Turkey & Paxo, Walkers*	1 Bag/34.5g	184	525	6.4	50.1	33.0	4.1
Salsa With Mesquite, Kettle Chips*	1 Bag/50g	229	458	6.1	54.0	24.3	5.7
Salt & Balsamic Vinegar, Perfectly Balanced, Waitrose*	1 Bag/20g	69	347	4.2	76.4	2.7	5.2
Salt & Black Pepper, Handcooked, Marks & Spencer*	1 Bag/40g	180	450	5.7	55.0	22.9	5.2
Salt & Cracked Black Pepper, Shapers, Boots*	1 Bag/20g	91	453	7.2	57.0	22.0	5.0
Salt & Malt Vinegar Flavour, Sainsbury's*	1 Bag/25g	135	538	4.9	50.3	35.2	2.3
Salt & Malt Vinegar, Hunky Dorys*	1 Serving/30.1g	141	469	6.3	49.3	28.7	0.0
Salt & Malt Vinegar, McCoy's*	1 Bag/50g	256	512	6.8	52.8	30.4	3.9
Salt & Shake, Walkers*	1 Bag/24g	127	530	6.5	49.0	34.0	4.5
Salt & Vinegar Flavour, Asda*	1 Bag/25g	131	522	6.0	48.0	34.0	4.2
Salt & Vinegar Flavour, Half Fat, Marks & Spencer*	1 Bag/40g	168	420	5.8	61.0	17.0	7.7
Salt & Vinegar Fries, COU, Marks & Spencer*	1 Bag/25g	85	340	5.0	80.0	1.6	4.0
Salt & Vinegar, 30% Less Fat, Sainsbury's*	1 Bag/25g	115	458	7.2	58.3	21.8	5.1
Salt & Vinegar, BGTY, Sainsbury's*	1 Bag/25g	121	482	6.5	57.3	25.2	5.2
Salt & Vinegar, Big Eat, Walkers*	1 Bag/55.0g	289	525	6.5	50.0	33.0	4.0
Salt & Vinegar, Crinkle Cut, Low Fat, Waitrose*	1 Bag/25g	121	484	7.1	61.3	23.4	4.5
Salt & Vinegar, Crinkle Cut, Seabrook*	1 Bag/31.8g	182	569	5.4	54.4	36.7	3.9
Salt & Vinegar, Crinkle, Marks & Spencer*	1 Pack/24.7g	121	485	6.5	61.0	24.0	3.5
Salt & Vinegar, Crinkles, Shapers, Boots*	1 Pack/20g	96	482	6.6	60.0	24.0	4.0
Salt & Vinegar, Fish Shapes, Food Explorers, Waitrose*	1 Bag/20g	86	430	2.4	69.1	16.0	1.3
Salt & Vinegar, Fries, Safeway*	1 Bag/20g	75	375	5.1	80.9	1.6	2.3
Salt & Vinegar, GFY, Asda*	1 Bag/26g	120	466	6.0	61.0	22.0	4.1
Salt & Vinegar, Golden Lights, Golden Wonder*	1 Bag/21g	91	435	4.9	64.1	17.8	4.3

CRISPS

Measure INFO/WEIGHT	per Measure KCAL	Nutrition Values per 100g / 100ml				
		KCAL	PROT	CARB	FAT	FIBRE
CRISPS						
Salt & Vinegar, Golden Wonder* — 1 Bag/25g	131	522	5.4	48.5	34.0	2.0
Salt & Vinegar, Healthy Eating, Tesco* — 1 Bag/17g	61	357	3.2	82.4	1.6	3.0
Salt & Vinegar, Hoops, Safeway* — 1 Bag/15g	65	430	4.2	66.3	16.1	5.3
Salt & Vinegar, In Sunflower Oil, Sainsbury's* — 1 Serving/25g	131	524	5.2	49.7	33.8	3.7
Salt & Vinegar, KP* — 1 Bag/25g	133	532	5.5	48.7	35.0	4.7
Salt & Vinegar, Lites, Walkers* — 1 Bag/28g	130	465	7.5	61.0	21.0	4.0
Salt & Vinegar, Lower Fat, Asda* — 1 Bag/25g	120	481	5.0	58.0	25.0	4.8
Salt & Vinegar, Marks & Spencer* — 1 Bag/25g	131	525	5.4	48.8	34.5	4.6
Salt & Vinegar, Max, Walkers* — 1 Bag/55g	289	525	6.5	50.0	33.0	4.0
Salt & Vinegar, Morrisons* — 1 Bag/25g	124	497	7.2	48.7	30.4	4.5
Salt & Vinegar, Reduced Fat, Marks & Spencer* — 1 Bag/40g	190	475	7.0	58.0	24.0	6.5
Salt & Vinegar, Sainsbury's* — 1 Bag/25g	131	522	4.1	46.9	35.3	3.9
Salt & Vinegar, Select, Tesco* — 1 Bag/25g	132	529	5.9	47.8	34.9	4.3
Salt & Vinegar, Smiths, Walkers* — 1 Bag/25g	133	531	4.3	45.2	37.0	0.0
Salt & Vinegar, Square, Smiths, Walkers* — 1 Bag/25g	113	452	6.9	62.5	19.4	0.0
Salt & Vinegar, Square, Walkers* — 1 Bag/25g	105	420	6.0	59.0	18.0	4.5
Salt & Vinegar, Value, Tesco* — 1 Bag/20g	109	547	5.7	47.7	37.0	4.8
Salt & Vinegar, Waitrose* — 1 Bag/25g	134	535	6.2	40.5	34.2	4.3
Salt & Vinegar, Walkers* — 1 Bag/35g	184	525	6.5	50.0	33.0	4.0
Salt Your Own, Jacket, 35% Less Fat, Sainsbury's* — 1 Bag/20g	98	490	7.5	64.5	22.5	9.5
Salt'n'Shake, Smiths, Walkers* — 1 Bag/25g	136	543	4.1	44.2	38.9	0.0
Salted Tubes, Shapers, Boots* — 1 Bag/15g	67	448	5.1	62.0	20.0	3.6
Sausage & Tomato Flavour, Golden Wonder* — 1 Bag/34.5g	177	505	6.1	51.3	30.6	4.5
Sausage & Tomato, Sainsbury's* — 1 Pack/25g	131	525	6.0	49.3	33.8	3.8
Screaming Salt & Vinegar, Max, Walkers* — 1 Bag/55g	256	465	7.5	61.0	21.0	4.0
Sea Salt & Balsamic Vinegar, Kettle Chips* — 1 Bag/50g	234	468	5.6	60.9	24.4	4.4
Sea Salt & Balsamic Vineger, Low Fat, Peak* — 1 Serving/25g	87	348	7.4	76.6	1.4	6.7
Sea Salt & Black Pepper, Highlander* — 1 Serving/25g	141	564	5.6	44.0	38.4	4.8
Sea Salt & Black Pepper, Shapers, Boots* — 1 Bag/19.9g	96	482	6.6	60.0	24.0	4.0
Sea Salt & Cracked Black Pepper, Sensations, Walkers* — 1 Bag/40g	194	485	6.5	54.0	27.0	4.5
Sea Salt & Malt Vinegar, Sensations, Walkers* — 1 Bag/40g	194	485	6.5	54.0	27.0	4.5
Sea Salt & Vinegar, Bagels, Shapers, Boots* — 1 Pack/25g	95	378	11.0	77.0	2.9	3.1
Sea Salt With Crushed Black Peppercorns, Kettle Chips* — 1 Bag/50g	225	449	5.7	55.0	22.9	5.2
Sea Salt, Golden Lights, Golden Wonder* — 1 Serving/21g	94	448	3.9	66.4	18.5	4.4
Sea Salt, Handcooked, Extra Special, Asda* — 1 Pack/31g	149	477	7.0	56.0	25.0	4.1
Sea Salt, Original, Crinkle Cut, Seabrook* — 1 Bag/31.8g	182	569	5.4	54.4	36.7	3.9
Sea Salt, TTD, Sainsbury's* — 1 Serving/50g	236	472	6.2	53.6	25.8	5.2
Sizzling Beef, Spice, McCoy's* — 1 Bag/35g	175	501	6.4	51.7	29.8	4.0
Smoked Ham & Pickle, Thick Cut, Brannigans* — 1 Bag/40g	203	507	7.0	52.8	29.8	3.8
Smokey Bacon, Crinkle, Shapers, Boots* — 1 Pack/20g	96	482	6.6	60.0	24.0	4.0
Smokey Bacon, Seabrook* — 1 Bag/32g	181	569	5.4	54.4	36.7	3.9
Smokey Bacon, Select, Tesco* — 1 Bag/25g	134	536	6.4	49.0	34.9	4.3
Smokey Bacon, Smiths, Walkers* — 1 Bag/25g	133	531	4.3	45.2	37.0	0.0
Smoky Bacon, 30% Lower Fat, Sainsbury's* — 1 Bag/25g	118	471	6.5	58.4	23.6	5.7
Smoky Bacon, Asda* — 1 Bag/25g	133	530	6.0	50.0	34.0	4.5
Smoky Bacon, BGTY, Sainsbury's* — 1 Bag/25g	118	472	6.5	58.5	23.6	5.7
Smoky Bacon, Golden Wonder* — 1 Bag/25g	131	523	5.9	49.1	33.7	2.0
Smoky Bacon, Sainsbury's* — 1 Bag/25g	132	529	5.7	49.5	34.2	4.4
Smoky Bacon, Walkers* — 1 Bag/34g	179	525	6.5	50.0	33.0	4.0
Snax, Tayto* — 1 Pack/17g	82	483	2.4	70.0	21.5	1.6
Sour Cream & Chive Crinkles, Shapers, Boots* — 1 Bag/20g	96	482	6.6	60.0	24.0	4.0
Sour Cream & Chive, Healthy Eating, Tesco* — 1 Bag/19.9g	72	362	6.7	81.1	3.8	3.4
Sour Cream & Chive, Perfectly Balanced, Waitrose* — 1 Pack/20g	69	347	4.4	76.3	2.7	5.2

C

	Measure INFO/WEIGHT	per Measure KCAL	Nutrition Values per 100g / 100ml				
			KCAL	PROT	CARB	FAT	FIBRE
CRISPS							
Sour Cream & Chive, Reduced Fat, Marks & Spencer*	1 Bag/40g	192	480	6.5	60.0	24.0	6.5
Sour Cream & Chives, Jordans*	1 Bag/30g	125	417	7.3	69.9	12.0	2.7
Sour Cream & Onion, Golden Lights, Golden Wonder*	1 Bag/21g	91	435	5.4	64.5	17.2	5.9
Spare Rib Flavour, Chinese, Walkers*	1 Bag/34.5g	184	525	6.5	50.0	33.0	4.0
Spiced Chilli, McCoy's*	1 Bag/35g	175	500	6.1	54.2	28.8	4.2
Spring Onion Flavour, Marks & Spencer*	1 Bag/40g	210	525	5.9	48.7	34.3	5.1
Spring Onion, Seabrook*	1 Bag/32g	182	569	5.4	54.4	36.7	3.9
Stilton & Cranberry, TTD, Sainsbury's*	1 Serving/50g	239	477	6.7	54.6	25.7	4.6
Strawberry Raisin Snack, Fruitwonders, Golden Wonder*	1 Bag/29.5g	115	383	3.8	62.9	12.9	0.0
Sun Dried Tomato & Basil, Jonathan Crisp*	1 Pack/35g	176	503	5.6	52.0	29.0	5.4
Sun Dried Tomato & Chilli, Asda*	1 Pack/150g	701	467	7.0	58.0	23.0	4.1
Sweet & Sour, Great British Takeaways, Walkers*	1 Bag/25g	131	525	6.5	50.0	33.0	4.0
T Bone Steak, Roysters*	1 Bag/31g	160	516	5.7	52.6	31.4	3.6
Tangy Malaysian Chutney, Sensations, Walkers*	1 Bag/24g	116	485	0.9	62.0	26.0	0.0
Tangy Tomato & Red Pepper Salsa, Sensations, Walkers*	1 Bag/35g	168	480	6.5	53.0	27.0	4.5
Tangy Toms, Red Mill*	1 Bag/15g	76	507	6.0	60.0	27.3	0.7
Thai Curry & Coriander, Tyrells*	1 Pack/50g	261	522	6.1	56.5	27.9	5.4
Thai Curry Flavour Curls, Marks & Spencer*	1 Bag/25g	90	360	1.3	82.5	2.5	3.1
Thai Green Curry, TTD, Sainsbury's*	1 Bag/50g	235	470	6.1	55.6	24.8	5.2
Thai Sweet Chicken, McCoy's*	1 Bag/35g	178	509	6.6	53.0	30.1	4.0
Thai Sweet Chilli, Sensations, Walkers*	1 Bag/40g	194	485	6.5	54.0	27.0	4.5
Tomato & Basil, Mediterranean, Walkers*	1 Pack/25g	128	510	6.5	49.0	33.0	4.5
Tomato & Herb, Shapers, Boots*	1 Bag/20g	94	468	3.7	66.0	21.0	3.9
Tomato Ketchup, Walkers*	1 Bag/35g	179	510	6.5	49.0	32.0	4.0
Tomato Sauce, Golden Wonder*	1 Bag/25g	130	521	5.7	49.2	33.5	2.0
Tomato, Olive Oil & Basil, TTD, Sainsbury's*	1 Bag/50g	235	469	7.5	51.4	26.0	5.4
Traditional, Hand Cooked, Finest, Tesco*	1 Bag/150g	708	472	6.4	52.9	26.1	5.1
Tubes, Salt & Vinegar, Healthy Living, Tesco*	1 Bag/17g	61	357	3.2	82.4	1.6	3.0
Vegetable Chips, Mixed Root, Tyrells*	1oz/28g	133	476	5.7	35.4	29.8	12.8
Vegetable, Crunchy, Asda*	1/2 Bag/50g	251	502	1.4	70.0	24.0	6.0
Vegetable, Root, Pan Fried, Sainsbury's*	1/4 Bag/25g	102	407	4.6	36.5	27.0	6.4
Vegetable, Waitrose*	1 Pack/100g	512	512	5.1	35.1	39.0	12.5
Waffles, Bacon Flavour, BGTY, Sainsbury's*	1 Serving/12g	41	345	6.4	79.7	1.4	2.9
Wild Chilli, McCoy's*	1 Bag/50g	255	510	6.0	53.2	30.3	4.8
Wild Paprika Flavour, Croky*	1 Pack/45g	234	521	6.0	58.0	29.0	0.0
Worcester Sauce, Walkers*	1 Bag/25g	131	525	6.4	50.1	33.0	4.1
Worcester Sauce Flavour, Hunky Dorys*	1 Bag/45g	211	469	6.3	49.3	28.7	0.0
Yoghurt & Green Onion, Kettle Chips*	1 Serving/50g	237	473	6.6	54.1	26.1	5.4
CRISPY PANCAKE							
Beef Bolognese, Findus*	1 Pancake/65g	104	160	6.5	25.0	4.0	1.0
Chicken & Bacon, Findus*	1 Pancake/62g	90	145	6.1	23.6	2.8	0.9
Chicken, Bacon & Sweetcorn, Findus*	1 Pancake/63g	101	160	5.8	24.8	4.1	1.1
Minced Beef & Onion, Green Isle*	1 Pancake/60g	140	234	6.0	31.2	9.5	2.7
Minced Beef, Findus*	1 Serving/100g	160	160	6.5	25.0	4.0	1.0
Three Cheeses, Findus*	1 Pancake/62g	118	190	7.0	25.0	6.5	0.9
CROISSANT							
All Butter, BGTY, Sainsbury's*	1 Croissant/44g	176	401	9.8	44.2	20.5	2.2
All Butter, Budgens*	1 Croissant/45g	185	412	7.9	39.7	24.6	3.3
All Butter, Finest, Tesco*	1 Croissant/77g	328	426	8.6	44.9	23.6	1.9
All Butter, Marks & Spencer*	1 Croissant/53.6g	227	420	7.2	44.4	25.0	1.6
All Butter, Mini, Sainsbury's*	1 Croissant/35g	156	446	9.3	38.2	28.4	2.0
All Butter, Mini, Tesco*	1 Croissant/35g	151	430	9.3	45.2	23.5	2.0
All Butter, Reduced Fat, Marks & Spencer*	1 Croissant/54g	181	335	6.8	38.4	16.9	1.5

C

C

CROISSANT

INFO/WEIGHT	Measure	per Measure KCAL	KCAL	PROT	CARB	FAT	FIBRE
All Butter, Reduced Fat, Tesco*	1 Croissant/52g	164	315	7.5	47.4	10.6	1.8
All Butter, Sainsbury's*	1 Croissant/44g	188	428	9.2	42.6	24.5	1.2
All Butter, TTD, Sainsbury's*	1 Croissant/75g	362	483	8.3	40.2	32.1	2.9
All Butter, Tesco*	1 Croissant/77g	297	386	6.5	40.4	22.1	1.9
Average	1 Croissant/50g	180	360	8.3	38.3	20.3	1.6
Butter, Asda*	1 Croissant/46g	191	416	8.0	42.0	24.0	1.9
Butter, GFY, Asda*	1 Croissant/43.5g	151	352	6.0	46.0	16.0	2.0
Butter, Mini, Waitrose*	1 Croissant/35.0g	156	446	9.3	38.2	28.4	2.0
Butter, Part Bake, Morrisons*	1 Croissant/45g	179	397	7.3	49.6	18.8	1.9
Butter, Part Baked, Budgens*	1 Croissant/45g	165	367	7.4	52.7	14.1	2.0
Butter, Part Baked, De Graaf*	1 Croissant/45g	170	378	7.3	45.2	18.7	0.0
Flaky Pastry With A Plain Chocolate Filling, Tesco*	1 Croissant/78g	318	408	6.5	41.0	24.3	2.0
Heart Shaped, Breakfast In Bed, Marks & Spencer*	1 Croissant/53.5g	228	430	8.2	43.7	25.5	1.2
Homebake, Long Life, Stay Fresh Range, Harvestime*	1 Croissant/44g	159	362	7.6	51.9	13.7	1.9
Low Fat, Marks & Spencer*	1 Croissant/45g	180	400	8.2	46.0	20.2	1.8
Mini, Lidl*	1 Croissant/30g	112	373	7.8	48.0	16.6	0.0
Organic, Tesco*	1 Croissant/45g	195	433	8.2	42.0	25.8	2.2
Reduced Fat, Sainsbury's*	1 Croissant/44g	173	393	9.8	49.2	17.5	2.2
Reduced Fat, Waitrose*	1 Croissant/44g	176	401	9.8	44.2	20.5	2.2
Smoked Ham & Cheese, Marks & Spencer*	1 Croissant/105g	341	325	13.4	22.2	21.6	3.9
Wholesome, Sainsbury's*	1 Croissant/44g	192	436	8.8	38.3	27.5	4.0

CROQUETTE

Morrisons*	1 Serving/150g	231	154	3.3	23.1	5.4	1.1
Parsnip, Finest, Tesco*	1 Croquette/37g	77	207	5.9	26.2	8.7	1.3
Potato, Asda*	1 Pack/127g	224	176	2.3	26.0	7.0	1.8
Potato, Bacon & Gruyere, Finest, Tesco*	1 Serving/37g	89	241	8.1	22.3	13.3	1.2
Potato, Birds Eye*	1 Croquette/29g	44	152	2.6	22.6	5.7	1.2
Potato, Crispy, Sainsbury's*	3 Croquettes/125g	245	196	2.5	25.7	9.2	1.9
Potato, Fried in Blended Oil	1oz/28g	60	214	3.7	21.6	13.1	1.3
Potato, Frozen, Tesco*	1 Croquette/30g	58	193	3.7	23.0	9.7	1.0
Potato, Gruyere & Rosemary, TTD, Sainsbury's*	1 Croquette/42g	102	245	5.7	21.8	15.0	1.8
Potato, Marks & Spencer*	1 Serving/125g	206	165	2.4	19.3	8.8	2.2
Potato, Sainsbury's*	1 Croquette/28g	50	180	3.9	23.0	8.0	1.0
Potato, Tesco*	1 Croquette/28g	47	168	1.9	24.5	6.9	1.4
Potato, Waitrose*	1 Croquette/29.9g	47	157	3.0	17.9	8.1	1.5
Vegetable, Sainsbury's*	1 Serving/175g	392	224	5.8	23.3	11.9	2.2

CROUTONS

Cracked Black Pepper & Sea Salt, Safeway*	1 Serving/20g	77	385	11.8	61.6	10.2	4.4
Fresh, Marks & Spencer*	1 Serving/10g	53	530	11.4	50.0	32.8	3.2
Garlic, Waitrose*	1 Serving/40g	209	522	10.8	52.1	30.0	2.7
Herb, Sainsbury's*	1 Serving/15g	64	429	13.4	68.2	11.4	2.8
Italian Salad, Sainsbury's*	1 Pack/40g	204	510	8.5	62.7	25.0	2.5
Migro*	1 Serving/15g	56	375	14.0	72.0	3.0	3.5
Rochelle*	1 Bag/70g	400	572	7.0	49.0	40.0	0.0
Sun Dried Tomato For Salad, Safeway*	1/5 packet/15g	59	395	13.3	59.4	11.5	8.8
Sun Dried Tomato, Sainsbury's*	1/4 Pack/15g	75	497	11.7	55.2	25.5	2.5

CRUDITE

Platter, Sainsbury's*	1 Pack/275g	96	35	1.4	6.6	0.3	1.6

CRUMBLE

Apple & Blackberry, Asda*	1 Serving/175g	427	244	2.7	38.0	9.0	1.2
Apple & Blackberry, Budgens*	1 Serving/240g	821	342	3.7	54.0	13.0	0.6
Apple & Blackberry, Marks & Spencer*	1 Serving/135g	398	295	3.5	44.9	11.2	1.6
Apple & Blackberry, Sainsbury's*	1 Serving/110g	232	211	3.0	37.1	5.6	2.1

CRUMBLE

INFO/WEIGHT	Measure per Measure KCAL	KCAL	PROT	CARB	FAT	FIBRE
Apple & Blackberry, Somerfield*	1 Serving/125g	315	252	3.4	39.4	9.0	2.4
Apple & Blackberry, Tesco*	1 Crumble/335g	667	199	2.6	40.1	3.1	1.9
Apple & Blackberry, With Custard, Somerfield*	1 Serving/120g	324	270	2.3	36.3	12.5	1.1
Apple & Custard, Asda*	1 Serving/125g	250	200	2.3	32.0	7.0	0.0
Apple & Toffee, Weight Watchers*	1 Pot/98g	190	194	1.6	36.6	4.6	0.0
Apple With Custard, Greens*	1 Serving/79g	171	216	1.9	37.0	6.7	1.2
Apple With Custard, Individual, Sainsbury's*	1 Pudding/120g	286	238	2.0	31.4	11.6	2.4
Apple, Co-Op*	1/8 Cake/52g	151	290	4.0	41.0	12.0	2.0
Apple, Dietary Specialists*	1 Pot/240g	497	207	0.9	40.5	5.0	1.1
Apple, Eat Smart, Safeway*	1 Serving/28g	85	305	5.2	64.5	2.4	1.2
Apple, Farmfoods*	1/2 Pack/185g	411	222	2.9	39.3	5.9	2.3
Apple, Frozen, Iceland*	1 Portion/97g	240	247	2.1	36.9	10.1	1.8
Apple, Iceland*	1 Pie/45g	175	389	4.0	58.4	15.6	2.0
Apple, Sara Lee*	1 Serving/200g	606	303	2.3	53.3	9.0	1.2
Apple, Somerfield*	1 Serving/195g	454	233	2.5	36.8	8.4	1.1
Apple, Tesco*	1 Serving/150g	342	228	2.0	33.6	9.5	1.2
Apple, Waitrose*	1 Serving/125g	310	248	2.2	54.5	2.3	1.2
Apple, With Sultanas, Weight Watchers*	1 Dessert/110g	196	178	1.4	34.2	3.9	1.3
Bramley Apple, Favourites, Marks & Spencer*	1 Serving/140g	390	279	4.6	43.2	9.9	1.2
Bramley Apple, Marks & Spencer*	1 Serving/149g	387	260	4.4	40.3	9.2	1.1
Bramley Apple, Sainsbury's*	1 Serving/100g	248	248	2.0	35.4	10.9	2.3
Bramley Apple, Tesco*	1/3 Pack/155g	378	244	2.8	36.7	9.6	1.8
Cauliflower & Camembert, Sainsbury's*	1 Pack/400g	588	147	5.5	6.9	10.8	0.7
Fish & Prawn, Young's*	1 Pie/375g	476	127	5.8	9.7	7.2	1.3
Fruit	1oz/28g	55	198	2.0	34.0	6.9	1.7
Fruit, Wholemeal	1oz/28g	54	193	2.6	31.7	7.1	2.7
Gooseberry, Marks & Spencer*	1 Serving/133g	379	285	3.5	43.3	10.7	1.7
Ocean, Good Choice, Iceland*	1 Pack/340g	377	111	7.2	14.4	2.7	1.1
Ocean, Low Fat, Ross*	1 Crumble/300g	219	73	5.1	11.4	0.8	0.4
Ocean, Young's*	1 Pack/340g	306	90	4.8	11.3	2.8	1.1
Rhubarb, Asda*	1/2 Crumble/200g	460	230	2.4	28.0	12.0	5.0
Rhubarb, Co-Op*	1/4 Crumble/110g	0	245	2.0	42.0	7.0	1.0
Rhubarb, Farmfoods*	1oz/28g	54	192	2.0	35.0	4.9	2.3
Rhubarb, Marks & Spencer*	1 Serving/133g	366	275	3.4	42.6	9.9	1.4
Rhubarb, Sainsbury's*	1 Serving/50g	112	224	3.1	40.4	5.6	1.8
Rhubarb, Somerfield*	1/4 Crumble/130g	281	216	3.0	38.0	6.0	0.0
Rhubarb, Tesco*	1/6 Crumble/117g	228	195	2.8	27.3	8.3	1.7
Rhubarb, With Custard, Sainsbury's*	1 Serving/120g	288	240	2.4	31.4	11.6	2.3
Salmon, Young's*	1 Pie/339g	380	112	4.6	13.0	4.6	0.7
Topping, Sainsbury's*	1 Serving/47g	188	401	5.9	50.3	19.6	5.3

CRUMBLE MIX

INFO/WEIGHT	Measure per Measure KCAL	KCAL	PROT	CARB	FAT	FIBRE
Luxury, Tesco*	1/4 Pack/55g	243	441	5.7	67.9	16.3	3.2

CRUMBLE TOPPING

INFO/WEIGHT	Measure per Measure KCAL	KCAL	PROT	CARB	FAT	FIBRE
Morrisons*	1 Serving/40g	179	448	5.4	69.5	16.5	2.8

CRUMPETS

INFO/WEIGHT	Measure per Measure KCAL	KCAL	PROT	CARB	FAT	FIBRE
Asda*	1 Crumpet/45g	94	208	6.0	44.0	0.9	0.0
Co-Op*	1 Crumpet/55g	102	185	8.0	36.0	1.0	2.0
Finger, Sainsbury's*	1 Crumpet/30g	55	182	7.0	36.6	0.8	1.8
Iceland*	1 Crumpet/46.6g	97	206	6.1	43.8	0.7	1.8
Kwik Save*	1 Crumpet/41.1g	79	192	5.9	39.9	1.0	2.5
Less Than 1% Fat, Warburtons*	1 Crumpet/45.6g	83	181	5.9	31.7	0.7	3.0
Less Than 2% Fat, Marks & Spencer*	1 Crumpet/61g	116	190	8.0	36.9	1.3	2.1
Morning Fresh*	1 Crumpet/20g	36	180	7.3	34.8	1.3	5.2

	Measure INFO/WEIGHT	per Measure KCAL	Nutrition Values per 100g / 100ml				
			KCAL	PROT	CARB	FAT	FIBRE
CRUMPETS							
Morrisons*	1 Crumpet/41g	78	191	6.1	38.6	1.4	0.0
Mothers Pride*	1 Crumpet/48g	90	187	5.6	38.9	1.0	1.7
Perfectly Balanced, Waitrose*	1 Crumpet/55g	94	171	6.1	36.1	0.3	4.4
Premium, Safeway*	1 Crumpet/60g	111	185	7.5	36.3	1.1	2.4
Premium, Sainsbury's*	1 Crumpet/50g	96	191	6.1	38.6	1.4	1.7
Premium, TTD, Sainsbury's*	1 Crumpet/56g	101	180	7.3	34.8	1.3	5.2
Safeway*	1 Crumpet/44g	80	182	7.0	36.6	0.8	1.8
Sainsbury's*	1 Crumpet/46g	93	202	6.4	41.5	1.1	2.8
Scrumptious, Kingsmill*	1 Crumpet/55g	99	180	6.1	37.2	0.8	1.7
SmartPrice, Asda*	1 Crumpet/42g	84	199	6.0	42.0	0.8	1.7
Soldier, Mothers Pride*	1 Crumpet/30g	58	193	7.8	37.1	1.6	1.6
Somerfield*	1 Crumpet/25g	48	192	5.9	39.9	1.0	2.5
Square, Tesco*	1 Crumpet/60g	101	168	6.3	33.8	0.8	2.7
Tesco*	1 Crumpet/46g	92	201	6.0	42.6	0.7	1.8
Toasted	1 Crumpet/40g	80	199	6.7	43.4	1.0	2.0
Toaster, Organic, Waitrose*	1 Crumpet/55g	95	172	7.3	34.4	0.6	4.6
Value, Tesco*	1 Crumpet/35g	59	168	6.4	33.9	0.8	1.8
Waitrose*	1 Crumpet/55g	99	180	7.3	34.8	1.3	5.2
Warburtons*	1 Crumpet/50g	89	178	7.1	35.8	0.7	0.0
CRUNCHERS							
BBQ, Atkins*	1 Bag/28g	100	357	46.4	28.6	10.7	14.3
Nacho Cheese, Atkins*	1 Bag/28g	100	357	46.4	28.6	10.7	10.7
CRUNCHIE							
Cadbury*	1 Std Bar/41g	193	470	4.0	71.5	18.4	0.0
Nuggets, Cadbury*	1 Bag/125g	569	455	3.8	73.1	16.4	0.0
Treat Size, Cadbury*	1 Treat Bar/17g	80	470	4.0	71.5	18.4	0.0
CRUNCHY STICKS							
Ready Salted, Marks & Spencer*	1 Pack/75g	398	530	5.6	52.2	33.0	3.8
Ready Salted, Tesco*	1 Serving/25g	119	475	5.6	60.3	23.5	3.0
Salt & Vinegar, BGTY, Sainsbury's*	1 Bag/15g	51	340	6.0	80.1	1.5	4.1
Salt & Vinegar, Sainsbury's*	1 Bag/25g	119	474	5.9	58.0	24.3	2.4
Salt & Vinegar, Shapers, Boots*	1 Bag/23g	99	430	7.8	66.0	15.0	3.1
Salt & Vinegar, Tesco*	1 Serving/25g	118	470	6.9	55.7	24.4	2.7
CRUSH							
Morello Cherry, Finest, Tesco*	1 Bottle/250ml	115	46	0.0	11.2	0.0	0.0
Orange & Raspberry, Safeway*	1 Serving/100ml	57	57	0.5	13.6	0.1	0.2
Orange & Strawberry, Finest, Tesco*	1 Bottle/250ml	115	46	0.4	10.5	0.1	0.4
Orange, Cool, Diet, Sainsbury's*	1 Can/330ml	10	3	0.1	0.6	0.1	0.1
Pineapple & Grapefruit, No Added Sugar, Morrisons*	1 Glass/250ml	25	10	0.2	1.2	0.0	0.0
CUCUMBER							
Average	1 Serving/14g	1	10	0.7	1.5	0.1	0.6
Crunchies, With A Yoghurt & Mint Dip, Shapers, Boots*	1 Serving/110g	35	32	2.1	3.7	0.9	0.8
CUMIN							
Seeds	1 Tsp/2g	8	375	17.8	33.7	22.7	0.0
CURACAO							
Average	1 Shot/25ml	78	311	0.0	28.3	0.0	0.0
CURLY KALE							
Boiled in Salted Water	1oz/28g	7	24	2.4	1.0	1.1	2.8
Raw	1oz/28g	9	33	3.4	1.4	1.6	3.1
CURLY WURLY							
Cadbury*	1 Bar/28g	126	450	3.5	69.1	17.8	0.0
Squirlies, Cadbury*	1 Squirl/3g	14	450	3.9	69.0	17.8	0.0

	Measure INFO/WEIGHT	per Measure KCAL	Nutrition Values per 100g / 100ml				
			KCAL	PROT	CARB	FAT	FIBRE
CURRANTS							
Average	1oz/28g	75	267	2.3	67.8	0.4	1.9
CURRY							
& Chips, Curry Sauce, Chipped Potatoes, Kershaws*	1 Sering/330g	391	119	10.0	14.0	2.5	2.0
Aubergine	1oz/28g	33	118	1.4	6.2	10.1	1.5
Beef, Hot, Canned, Marks & Spencer*	1 Can/425g	446	105	12.2	2.8	5.1	1.0
Beef, Marks & Spencer*	1oz/28g	34	120	12.2	3.9	6.1	1.0
Beef, Sainsbury's*	1 Serving/400g	552	138	10.7	5.4	8.2	0.9
Beef, SmartPrice, Asda*	1 Serving/392g	223	57	4.0	9.0	0.5	1.0
Beef, Thai, Finest, Tesco*	1 Serving/500g	770	154	9.0	16.5	5.8	1.2
Beef, With Rice, Asda*	1 Pack/406g	547	135	6.0	19.0	3.9	1.2
Beef, With Rice, Birds Eye*	1 Pack/388g	524	135	6.9	20.8	2.8	0.8
Beef, With Rice, Healthy Choice, Asda*	1 Pack/400g	476	119	6.0	18.0	2.6	0.9
Beef, With Rice, Iceland*	1 Pack/400g	404	101	6.7	14.7	1.7	1.0
Beef, With Rice, Morrisons*	1 Serving/400g	480	120	6.0	12.6	5.0	0.6
Beef, With Rice, Tesco*	1 Pack/400g	456	114	4.5	16.7	3.3	0.6
Beef, With Rice, Weight Watchers*	1 Pack/328g	249	76	4.2	12.5	1.0	0.3
Blackeye Bean, Gujerati	1oz/28g	36	127	7.2	16.1	4.4	2.8
Cabbage	1oz/28g	23	82	1.9	8.1	5.0	2.1
Cauliflower & Potato	1oz/28g	17	59	3.4	6.6	2.4	1.8
Chick Pea, Whole	1oz/28g	50	179	9.6	21.3	7.5	4.5
Chick Pea, Whole & Tomato, Punjabi With Vegetable	1oz/28g	31	112	5.6	12.4	4.9	2.9
Chick Pea, Whole, Basic	1oz/28g	30	108	6.0	14.2	3.6	3.3
Chicken, Asda*	1 Can/200g	210	105	10.0	5.0	5.0	0.0
Chicken, COU, Marks & Spencer*	1 Pack/400g	360	90	7.3	13.2	0.9	2.5
Chicken, Canned, Sainsbury's*	1 Serving/100g	136	136	11.1	9.1	6.1	1.0
Chicken, Extra Strong, Marks & Spencer*	1oz/28g	28	100	13.8	2.5	3.9	1.4
Chicken, Frozen, Sainsbury's*	1 Serving/400g	528	132	5.8	18.0	4.1	0.7
Chicken, Green Thai Style, & Sticky Rice, Asda*	1 Pack/450g	585	130	7.0	20.0	2.4	0.1
Chicken, Green Thai, BGTY, Sainsbury's*	1 Pack/400g	316	79	10.6	3.4	2.6	1.9
Chicken, Green Thai, Birds Eye*	1 Pack/450g	536	119	4.7	15.2	4.4	0.3
Chicken, Green Thai, Breasts, Finest, Tesco*	1 Serving/200g	292	146	16.5	2.0	8.0	0.7
Chicken, Green Thai, Marks & Spencer*	1/2 Pack/107g	171	160	12.3	1.8	11.6	0.6
Chicken, Green Thai, Safeway*	1 Pack/350g	490	140	12.5	3.5	8.0	1.4
Chicken, Green Thai, Sainsbury's*	1/2 Pack/200g	264	132	13.0	4.8	6.8	0.9
Chicken, Green Thai, Weight Watchers*	1 Pack/340g	262	77	4.4	10.9	1.7	0.6
Chicken, Hot, Can, Tesco*	1 Can/418g	514	123	9.7	6.9	6.3	0.9
Chicken, Hot, Canned, Asda*	1 Can/398g	501	126	11.0	7.0	6.0	0.5
Chicken, Hot, Tinned, Sainsbury's*	1 Serving/200g	218	109	12.3	6.9	3.6	0.9
Chicken, Kashmiri, Waitrose*	1 Serving/400g	640	160	14.5	5.0	9.1	0.6
Chicken, Medium Hot, Marks & Spencer*	1 Serving/200g	310	155	7.8	14.3	7.1	0.8
Chicken, Mild & Fruity, Breasts, Healthy Eating, Tesco*	2 Breasts/345g	321	93	15.8	4.1	1.5	0.5
Chicken, Mild, Asda*	1/2 Can/189.7g	239	126	11.0	7.0	6.0	0.5
Chicken, Mild, BGTY, Sainsbury's*	1 Serving/200g	184	92	10.0	7.2	2.6	0.5
Chicken, Mild, Marks & Spencer*	1oz/28g	28	100	13.8	2.5	3.9	1.4
Chicken, Mild, Sainsbury's*	1 Can/400g	472	118	10.5	3.5	6.9	1.3
Chicken, Mild, Tinned, Sainsbury's*	1 Serving/200g	214	107	12.7	6.1	3.5	1.1
Chicken, Newgate*	1 Serving/196g	220	112	8.0	6.6	6.0	0.0
Chicken, Red Thai, 97% Fat Free, Birds Eye*	1 Pack/366g	425	116	5.7	19.0	1.9	0.5
Chicken, Red Thai, Asda*	1 Pack/360g	461	128	9.1	5.5	7.7	1.0
Chicken, Red Thai, Healthy Living, Tesco*	1/2 Box/175g	158	90	10.7	5.4	2.8	0.7
Chicken, Red Thai, Sainsbury's*	1 Serving/200g	300	150	14.3	5.5	7.9	1.0
Chicken, Red Thai, Tesco*	1 Serving/175g	215	123	10.5	5.5	6.6	1.4
Chicken, Red Thai, With Fragrant Rice, Somerfield*	1 Pack/340g	503	148	8.0	18.0	5.0	0.0

CURRY

	Measure INFO/WEIGHT	per Measure KCAL	KCAL	PROT	CARB	FAT	FIBRE
Chicken, Red Thai, With Rice, Tesco*	1 Serving/475g	746	157	7.2	16.8	6.8	1.1
Chicken, Reduced Fat, Asda*	1 Pack/400g	476	119	6.0	18.0	2.6	0.9
Chicken, SmartPrice, Asda*	1 Can/392g	282	72	4.0	11.0	1.3	1.0
Chicken, Thai Mango, Sainsbury's*	1/2 Pack/200g	288	144	11.2	4.8	8.9	1.9
Chicken, Thai Peanut, Sainsbury's*	1/2 Pack/200g	314	157	12.8	4.9	9.6	1.2
Chicken, Thai, COU, Marks & Spencer*	1 Pack/400g	320	80	7.2	8.8	1.9	1.0
Chicken, Thai, Tom Yum, Sainsbury's*	1 Pot/400g	416	104	11.1	3.5	5.1	1.9
Chicken, Thai, With Rice, Oriental Express*	1 Pack/340g	303	89	4.1	15.3	1.3	1.2
Chicken, Value, Tesco*	1 Pack/300g	399	133	5.5	15.9	5.2	1.7
Chicken, With Naan Bread, Iceland*	1 Portion/260g	484	186	10.1	22.3	6.3	1.4
Chicken, With Potato Wedges, Healthy Eating, Tesco*	1 Pack/450g	428	95	7.6	10.3	2.7	1.1
Chicken, With Rice, Birds Eye*	1 Pack/380g	494	130	6.4	21.7	2.0	4.0
Chicken, With Rice, Frozen, Tesco*	1 Pack/400g	488	122	4.6	17.2	3.9	0.7
Chicken, With Rice, Fruity, Healthy Living, Tesco*	1 Pack/450g	495	110	6.5	18.2	1.2	1.2
Chicken, With Rice, Hot, Asda*	1 Pack/400g	476	119	5.0	18.0	3.0	1.0
Chicken, With Rice, Malaysian, Bernard Matthews*	1 Pack/400g	512	128	6.1	17.0	3.9	0.0
Chicken, With Rice, Quick Bite, Asda*	1 Serving/300g	294	98	5.0	12.0	3.3	0.5
Chicken, With Rice, Ross*	1 Serving/320g	272	85	3.4	14.7	1.3	0.5
Chicken, With Rice, Sainsbury's*	1 Pack/400g	500	125	5.4	17.5	3.7	0.8
Chicken, With Rice, Tesco*	1 Pack/300g	300	100	5.7	14.4	2.2	0.4
Chicken, With Rice, Weight Watchers*	1 Pack/300g	273	91	4.8	14.3	1.7	0.5
Chicken, With Vegetables, Morrisons*	1 Can/392g	392	100	9.0	7.0	4.0	1.0
Chicken, With Vegetables, Value, Tesco*	1 Serving/196g	123	63	3.1	7.2	2.4	0.7
Chicken, Yellow Thai Style, Healthy Living, Tesco*	1 Pack/450g	504	112	9.3	12.6	2.7	0.5
Chinese Chicken, Oriental Express*	1 Pack/340g	286	84	4.8	16.2	0.6	0.8
Chinese Chicken, With Vegetable Rice, Marks & Spencer*	1 Pack/400g	320	80	7.1	8.4	2.0	1.3
Cod, Red Thai, With Rice, Perfectly Balanced, Waitrose*	1 Pack/400g	360	90	7.5	11.0	1.8	1.0
Courgette & Potato	1oz/28g	24	86	1.9	8.7	5.2	1.2
Dudhi, Kofta	1oz/28g	32	113	2.6	9.4	7.4	2.8
Fish, & Vegetable, Bangladeshi	1oz/28g	33	117	9.1	1.4	8.4	0.5
Fish, Bangladeshi	1oz/28g	35	124	12.2	1.5	7.9	0.3
Fish, Red Thai, Waitrose*	1 Pack/500g	275	55	5.2	3.7	2.2	1.0
Gobi Aloo Sag, Retail	1oz/28g	27	95	2.2	7.1	6.9	1.4
Green Thai, & Rice, GFY, Asda*	1 Pack/400g	356	89	7.0	11.0	1.9	1.6
Green Thai, With Sticky Rice, Healthy Living, Tesco*	1 Pack/450g	518	115	7.7	14.9	2.7	0.6
King Prawn, Coconut & Lime, Sainsbury's*	1/2 Pack/351g	207	59	3.7	5.4	2.5	1.0
King Prawn, Goan, Eat Smart, Safeway*	1 Pack/400g	340	85	3.7	12.7	1.7	2.1
King Prawn, Malay With Rice, Sainsbury's*	1 Pack/400g	608	152	5.0	21.5	5.1	1.4
Lamb, Extra Strong, Marks & Spencer*	1oz/28g	35	125	11.5	4.6	6.9	0.9
Lamb, Kefthedes, Waitrose*	1/2 Pack/200g	294	147	9.0	8.0	8.8	2.1
Lamb, With Rice, Birds Eye*	1 Pack/382g	520	136	5.6	20.8	3.4	0.9
Potato & Pea	1oz/28g	26	92	2.9	13.0	3.8	2.4
Prawn, & Mushroom	1oz/28g	47	168	7.3	2.5	14.4	1.0
Prawn, Frozen, Sainsbury's*	1 Pack/400g	500	125	3.5	19.0	3.9	0.8
Prawn, Malai, Sainsbury's*	1 Serving/171g	299	175	7.7	1.4	15.4	1.1
Prawn, Red Thai Sauce, Young's*	1 Pack/255g	197	77	4.8	6.5	3.4	0.8
Prawn, Red Thai, Sainsbury's*	1 Pack/300g	546	182	6.3	9.4	13.2	1.7
Prawn, Thai, With Jasmine Rice, BGTY, Sainsbury's*	1 Serving/401g	353	88	4.2	14.5	1.5	2.0
Prawn, With Rice, Asda*	1 Pack/400g	420	105	3.5	17.0	2.6	1.1
Prawn, With Rice, Birds Eye*	1 Pack/375g	443	118	3.5	20.6	0.0	0.0
Prawn, With Rice, Iceland*	1 Pack/400g	360	90	3.2	13.8	2.4	0.9
Prawn, With Rice, Morrisons*	1 Serving/400g	484	121	3.2	21.9	2.3	0.9
Red Kidney Bean, Punjabi	1oz/28g	30	106	4.7	10.1	5.6	3.8

	INFO/WEIGHT	KCAL	KCAL	PROT	CARB	FAT	FIBRE
CURRY							
Red Thai, Oriental, Tesco*	1 Pack/350g	508	145	9.8	5.2	9.4	1.1
Red Thai, Safeway*	1 Pack/324g	369	114	10.0	4.8	6.1	1.6
Red Thai, Vegetarian, Tesco*	1 Pack/429ml	588	137	5.4	17.3	5.1	1.6
Red Thai, With Rice, Finest, Tesco*	1 Pack/500g	660	132	8.0	17.8	3.1	0.6
Salmon, Green, Waitrose*	1 Pack/400.7g	581	145	9.1	4.5	10.1	2.7
Vegetable, Asda*	1 Pack/350g	329	94	1.9	8.0	6.0	1.9
Vegetable, Budgens*	1 Pack/350g	249	71	1.8	6.9	4.0	2.2
Vegetable, Canned, Sainsbury's*	1/2 Can/200g	200	100	1.4	9.8	6.1	1.8
Vegetable, Frozen, Mixed Vegetables	1oz/28g	25	88	2.5	6.9	6.1	0.0
Vegetable, Health Eating, Tesco*	1 Pack/350g	280	80	4.5	13.6	0.8	1.3
Vegetable, In Sweet Sauce	1 Serving/330g	162	49	1.4	6.7	2.1	1.3
Vegetable, Indian Meal For One, Tesco*	1 Serving/200g	218	109	2.0	9.0	7.2	1.2
Vegetable, Indian, Tesco*	1 Serving/225g	257	114	2.1	8.6	7.9	1.6
Vegetable, Marks & Spencer*	1 Pack/250g	300	120	2.1	7.1	9.5	2.5
Vegetable, Medium, Tesco*	1 Pack/350g	326	93	2.3	7.1	6.2	1.9
Vegetable, Mild, Tesco*	1 Can/425g	315	74	2.1	10.7	2.5	1.7
Vegetable, Pakistani	1oz/28g	17	60	2.2	8.7	2.6	2.2
Vegetable, Ready Meals, Marks & Spencer*	1 Pack/300g	495	165	2.4	7.2	14.2	2.1
Vegetable, SmartPrice, Asda*	1/2 Can/203g	132	65	2.0	13.0	0.5	1.7
Vegetable, Takeaway	1oz/28g	29	105	2.5	7.6	7.4	0.0
Vegetable, Tesco*	1/2 Can/200g	278	139	3.4	10.5	9.3	3.2
Vegetable, Tinned, Tesco*	1 Can/400g	312	78	2.4	10.5	2.9	1.7
Vegetable, Waitrose*	1 Pack/352g	285	81	3.5	4.9	5.3	2.1
Vegetable, Way to Five, Sainsbury's*	1/2 Pack/344g	227	66	2.5	11.6	1.1	1.4
Vegetable, With Pilau Rice, BGTY, Sainsbury's*	1 Pack/450g	441	98	2.4	16.9	2.3	0.5
Vegetable, With Pilau Rice, Linda McCartney*	1 Pack/339g	224	66	1.6	13.5	0.6	0.5
Vegetable, With Rice, Asda*	1 Pack/392.7g	432	110	2.6	18.0	3.1	1.4
Vegetable, With Rice, Birds Eye*	1 Pack/413.6g	455	110	2.3	19.6	2.3	1.1
Vegetable, With Rice, Healthy Living, Tesco*	1 Pack/450g	486	108	2.7	18.2	2.7	1.1
Vegetable, With Rice, Tesco*	1 Pack/400g	440	110	2.1	18.7	3.0	1.0
Vegetable, With Yoghurt	1oz/28g	17	62	2.6	4.6	4.1	1.4
Vegetable, Yellow Thai, Sainsbury's*	1/2 Pack/200g	256	128	1.7	7.1	10.3	1.5
Vegetable, Yellow, Tesco*	1 Pack/355.6g	324	91	1.9	9.9	4.9	1.4
CURRY LEAVES							
Fresh	1oz/28g	27	97	7.9	13.3	1.3	0.0
CURRY PASTE							
Balti, Patak's*	1 Tbsp/15g	59	393	5.0	20.3	31.8	3.1
Balti, Sharwood's*	1/4 Pack/72.5g	328	453	5.0	19.2	39.6	3.1
Balti, Tomato & Coriander, Patak's*	1 Serving/30g	117	391	4.1	17.2	34.0	2.2
Garam Masala, Cinnamon & Ginger, Hot, Patak's*	1 Tbsp/25g	101	403	3.2	17.9	35.4	0.6
Green Thai, Mild, Sainsbury's*	1 Tbsp/15g	23	156	2.2	14.5	9.9	2.7
Hot, Marks & Spencer*	1oz/28g	69	245	4.2	13.4	19.2	3.3
Hot, Sharwood's*	1oz/28g	123	439	5.1	18.6	38.3	2.6
Korma, Patak's*	1 Tbsp/10g	54	535	4.2	13.0	51.8	2.6
Madras, Patak's*	1/2 Jar/50g	293	586	4.3	21.6	53.6	5.2
Medium, Marks & Spencer*	1oz/28g	64	230	2.5	10.7	19.5	4.9
Medium, Sharwood's*	1oz/28g	122	434	4.5	16.8	38.8	2.7
Mild, Original, Patak's*	1oz/28g	157	559	4.8	16.8	52.5	2.8
Mild, Sharwood's*	1oz/28g	78	279	3.6	17.7	21.5	3.4
Red Thai, Sainsbury's*	1oz/28g	43	154	2.0	8.0	12.0	3.0
Rogan Josh, Patak's*	1 Serving/30g	119	397	4.1	12.7	36.7	5.9
Tandoori, Patak's*	1 Tbsp/25g	28	111	3.1	20.7	1.8	2.6
Tandoori, Sharwood's*	1oz/28g	64	228	5.9	15.5	15.8	1.9

C

	Measure INFO/WEIGHT	per Measure KCAL	Nutrition Values per 100g / 100ml				
			KCAL	PROT	CARB	FAT	FIBRE
CURRY PASTE							
Tikka Masala, Patak's*	1oz/28g	101	361	3.4	16.2	31.4	3.2
Tikka Masala, Sharwood's*	1oz/28g	53	191	3.2	9.9	15.4	2.6
Vindaloo, Patak's*	1 Tbsp/15g	84	557	4.8	16.0	52.6	6.1
CURRY POWDER							
Average	1 Tsp/2g	7	325	12.7	41.8	13.8	0.0
Mixed Flavours	1 Tsp/2g	6	316	13.0	34.7	13.9	0.0
CUSTARD							
Banana, Cow & Gate*	1 Serving/125g	84	67	1.0	13.2	1.2	0.3
Chocolate Flavour, Ambrosia*	1 Pot/150g	177	118	3.0	20.0	2.9	0.7
Chocolate, COU, Marks & Spencer*	1 Pot/140g	147	105	3.1	18.6	2.2	1.0
Dairy Free, Sainsbury's*	1 Serving/250g	210	84	3.0	14.2	1.7	0.2
Instant, Bird's*	1oz/28g	119	425	4.5	76.0	11.5	0.0
Instant, Low Fat, Bird's*	1 Serving/25g	101	405	4.4	78.5	8.3	0.4
Instant, No Added Sugar, Tesco*	1 Serving/Dry/18g	73	406	5.3	77.0	8.5	0.0
Instant, Sainsbury's*	1 Serving/141g	109	77	0.8	14.0	2.0	0.0
Low Fat, Average	1/3 Pot/141g	116	82	2.9	15.0	1.2	0.0
Low Fat, Good Intentions, Somerfield*	1 Serving/106g	82	77	2.3	14.4	1.1	0.2
Mix, Reduced Sugar, Asda*	1 Serving/145ml	103	71	0.7	14.0	1.4	0.1
Pot, Forest Fruits Flavour, Hot 'n' Fruity, Bird's*	1 Pot/174g	171	98	0.9	18.5	2.4	0.1
Pot, Strawberry Flavour, Hot 'n' Fruity, Bird's*	1oz/28g	28	99	1.0	18.5	2.4	0.1
Powder	1oz/28g	99	354	0.6	92.0	0.7	0.1
Powder, Original, Dry, Bird's*	1oz/28g	99	355	0.4	87.0	0.5	0.0
Strawberry Flavoured, Ambrosia*	1 Serving/135g	139	103	2.8	16.7	2.8	0.0
Strawberry Style, Shapers, Boots*	1 Pot/148g	83	56	4.0	8.2	0.8	0.1
Summer, Ambrosia*	1 Pack/500g	490	98	2.7	15.0	3.0	0.0
Toffee Flavour, Ambrosia*	1 Pot/150g	156	104	2.8	17.0	2.8	0.0
Vanilla With Apple Crunch, Ambrosia*	1 Pack/193g	276	143	3.4	22.4	4.5	0.8
Vanilla, COU, Marks & Spencer*	1 Pot/140g	147	105	4.3	16.6	2.5	0.6
Vanilla, Fresh, Waitrose*	1 Serving/100g	214	214	3.2	15.8	15.3	1.1
CUTLETS							
Nut, Goodlife*	1 Serving/88g	248	282	10.2	27.4	14.6	3.0
Nut, Grilled, Cauldron*	1 Cutlet/87g	250	287	10.2	26.8	15.4	4.6
Nut, Retail, Fried in Vegetable Oil	1oz/28g	81	289	4.8	18.7	22.3	1.7
Nut, Retail, Grilled	1oz/28g	59	212	5.1	19.9	13.0	1.8
Vegetable & Nut, Asda*	1 Cutlet/88.4g	295	335	10.0	22.0	23.0	4.6
Vegetable, Nut, Tesco*	1 Serving/88g	271	308	7.7	22.0	21.0	3.5
CUTTLEFISH							
Raw	1oz/28g	20	71	16.1	0.0	0.7	0.0

	Measure INFO/WEIGHT	per Measure KCAL	Nutrition Values per 100g / 100ml				
			KCAL	PROT	CARB	FAT	FIBRE
DAB							
Fillets, Lightly Dusted, Marks & Spencer*	1 Fillet/111.8g	190	170	13.3	8.2	9.1	1.3
Raw	1oz/28g	21	74	15.7	0.0	1.2	0.0
DAIRYLEA DUNKERS							
Jumbo Munch, Dairylea*	1 Serving/50g	150	300	7.2	26.5	18.5	1.2
Salt & Vinegar, Dairylea*	1 Tub/42g	116	275	6.7	17.5	19.5	0.3
Smokey Bacon, Dairylea*	1 Pack/45g	135	300	7.3	24.0	19.5	0.0
DAIRYLEA LUNCHABLES							
Cheese & Pizza Crackers, Dairylea*	1oz/28g	105	375	10.5	24.5	27.0	1.4
Double Cheese, Dairylea*	1 Pack/110g	413	375	18.0	17.0	26.0	0.3
Ham & Cheese Pizza, Dairylea*	1 Pack/97g	247	255	11.5	26.0	11.0	1.6
Harvest Ham, Dairylea*	1 Pack/110g	314	285	16.5	16.5	17.0	0.3
Tasty Chicken, Dairylea*	1 Pack/110g	314	285	17.0	17.5	16.5	0.3
DAMSONS							
Raw, Weighed With Stones	1oz/28g	10	34	0.5	8.6	0.0	1.6
Raw, Weighed Without Stones	1oz/28g	11	38	0.5	9.6	0.0	1.8
DANDELION & BURDOCK							
Original, Ben Shaws*	1 Can/440ml	128	29	0.0	7.0	0.0	0.0
Sparkling, Diet, Morrisons*	1 Glass/200ml	2	1	0.0	0.3	0.0	0.0
DANISH PASTRY							
Apple & Sultana, Tesco*	1 Pastry/72g	293	407	5.4	45.0	22.8	1.4
Apple, Fresh Cream, Sainsbury's*	1 Pastry/67g	248	368	3.1	40.2	21.6	0.4
Cherry, Bar, Sainsbury's*	1/4 Bar/88g	221	252	4.2	33.2	11.4	1.7
Custard Danish Bar, Sara Lee*	1/4 Bar/100g	228	228	6.6	36.1	6.4	0.8
Danish Apple Bar, Sara Lee*	1/6 Bar/70g	160	229	4.3	42.1	5.7	1.7
Danish Twist, Apple & Cinnamon, Entenmann's*	1 Serving/52g	150	288	5.6	62.0	1.9	1.5
Danish Twist, Toasted Pecan, Entenmann's*	1 Slice/48g	171	351	7.0	47.2	15.6	1.4
Pastry	1 Pastry/110g	411	374	5.8	51.3	17.6	1.6
Pecan, Marks & Spencer*	1 Serving/67g	287	428	6.2	45.0	26.0	1.3
DATES							
Dried, Average	1 Date/20g	54	272	2.8	65.4	0.4	4.2
Medjool, Average	1 Date/20g	56	279	2.2	69.3	0.3	4.3
Medjool, Stuffed With Walnuts, Tesco*	2 Dates/40g	98	245	4.4	44.0	5.7	3.4
Raw, Average	1 Date/30g	35	116	1.4	29.1	0.1	1.7
DELI FILLER							
Chinese, Princes*	1 Serving/50g	47	94	3.6	15.6	1.9	0.3
King Prawn & Avocado, Marks & Spencer*	1 Pack/170g	425	250	9.5	1.4	22.8	0.5
Prawn & Mayonnaise, Marks & Spencer*	1 Serving/60g	150	250	11.3	1.0	23.0	0.5
Smoked Salmon & Soft Cheese, Marks & Spencer*	1 Serving/85g	208	245	11.7	3.3	20.4	0.5
DELIGHT							
Blackcurrant, Made Up, Asda*	1 Serving/100g	115	115	3.2	17.0	3.8	0.0
Butterscotch Flavour, No Added Sugar, Tesco*	1/2 Pack/25g	109	434	4.8	66.5	16.5	0.0
Butterscotch, Dessert, Safeway*	1 Pack/69g	302	438	1.8	81.5	11.6	0.3
Chocolate Flavour, Dry, Tesco*	1 Pack/49g	204	417	6.3	63.0	15.5	0.5
Ravishing Raspberry, Made Up, Asda*	1/3 Pack/100g	112	112	3.2	16.0	3.9	0.0
Strawberry Flavour, No Added Sugar, Dry, Tesco*	1/2 Pack/25g	110	440	4.8	67.0	17.0	0.0
Strawberry, Shapers, Boots*	1 Pot/121g	96	79	4.5	13.0	1.0	0.1
DESSERT							
Almond, Naturgreen*	1 Serving/130g	143	110	2.3	14.5	4.8	0.2
Apple Rice, Classic Desserts, Marks & Spencer*	1 Pot/200g	210	105	2.5	20.0	1.7	0.3
Baked Lemon, COU, Marks & Spencer*	1 Serving/100g	140	140	6.8	22.0	2.5	0.8
Baklava	1 Serving/100g	393	393	5.0	46.0	21.0	0.0
Banana Flavour Custard, Ambrosia*	1 Pack/135g	136	101	2.6	16.2	2.9	0.1
Banoffee Layered, Sainsbury's*	1 Pot/115g	270	235	2.2	27.8	12.8	1.0

DESSERT

INFO/WEIGHT	Measure	per Measure KCAL	Nutrition Values per 100g / 100ml KCAL	PROT	CARB	FAT	FIBRE
Banoffee, Frozen, Healthy Living, Tesco*	1 Serving/60g	92	153	2.5	29.9	2.6	0.6
Banoffee, Shape*	1 Pot/120g	175	146	3.3	28.0	2.3	0.5
Banoffee, Weight Watchers*	1 Pot/80g	152	190	4.9	34.3	3.7	1.4
Black Cherry & Chocolate, COU, Marks & Spencer*	1 Pack/115g	132	115	3.6	22.6	1.4	1.2
Black Cherry, Dragana, Waitrose*	1 Pot/125g	236	189	2.1	24.7	9.1	0.5
Black Forest, Tesco*	1 Pot/100g	287	287	3.5	35.8	14.4	2.4
Blackcurrant, Yoghurt & Sorbet, Mini, Eat Smart, Safeway*	1 Pot/75g	90	120	2.2	25.8	0.7	1.8
Blissful Banana, Asda*	1/3 Pack/100g	122	122	3.7	17.0	4.3	0.0
Blueberry Muffin, Tesco*	1 Pot/91g	265	291	2.0	24.5	20.6	3.0
Bounty, Mars*	1 Pot/110g	253	230	5.3	23.2	13.6	0.0
Bread & Butter, Eat Smart, Safeway*	1 Pudding/117g	140	120	5.1	20.4	1.8	0.8
Butterscotch Flavour Whip, Co-Op*	1 Pack/64g	241	377	0.6	93.4	0.1	0.1
Butterscotch, Supreme, Made Up, Sainsbury's*	1/4 Pack/90g	92	102	3.6	13.0	3.9	0.1
Buttons, Cadbury*	1 Pot/100g	295	295	6.4	34.9	14.7	0.0
Cafe Latte, Iced, BGTY, Sainsbury's*	1 Serving/75g	104	139	2.9	23.7	3.6	3.3
Cafe Mocha, COU, Marks & Spencer*	1 Dessert/115g	155	135	5.5	21.8	2.7	1.0
Cappuccino, BGTY, Sainsbury's*	1 Pot/119g	224	188	3.3	25.2	8.1	0.8
Cappuccino, Italian, Co-Op*	1 Pack/90g	257	285	5.0	39.0	12.0	0.1
Caramel, Marks & Spencer*	1oz/28g	41	147	3.9	22.3	4.1	0.0
Catalan Cream, Sainsbury's*	1 Pot/95g	375	395	4.2	11.2	37.0	0.1
Cherry & Chocolate, Eat Smart, Safeway*	1 Serving/100g	150	150	3.2	27.5	2.7	0.1
Cherry & Vanilla, BGTY, Sainsbury's*	1 Pot/115g	225	196	1.6	32.6	6.6	1.0
Chocolait, Luxury, Aldi*	1 Pot/200g	270	135	3.3	18.1	5.5	0.0
Chocolate & Cherry, COU, Marks & Spencer*	1 Pot/130g	156	120	2.6	24.5	1.6	0.9
Chocolate & Coconut, COU, Marks & Spencer*	1 Pot/125g	169	135	3.6	25.6	2.2	0.7
Chocolate & Honeycomb, Weight Watchers*	1 Pot/57.9g	92	159	3.1	26.2	4.3	0.8
Chocolate & Mallow Iced, GFY, Asda*	1 Pot/150ml	143	95	2.0	19.0	1.2	2.3
Chocolate & Mallow, Weight Watchers*	1 Pot/150ml	140	93	2.0	18.7	1.2	2.3
Chocolate & Marshmallow Swirls, Iced, BGTY, Sainsbury's	1/4 Pot/75g	130	173	3.9	33.8	2.5	2.8
Chocolate & Vanilla Caramel, Dairy, Petits Filous, Yoplait*	1 Pot/60g	101	169	4.8	23.6	6.2	0.0
Chocolate Brownie, Marks & Spencer*	1/4 Pack/143.5g	612	425	4.7	39.6	27.5	1.0
Chocolate Creme, Somerfield*	1 Pot/125g	180	144	4.0	22.0	4.0	0.0
Chocolate Dream, Delicious Dessert, Co-Op*	1 Pot/110g	184	167	4.1	22.0	7.0	0.0
Chocolate Fudge Brownie, Tesco*	1 Pot/125g	374	299	4.6	40.2	13.3	1.3
Chocolate Hazelnut, Charolait, Aldi*	1 Serving/200g	270	135	3.3	18.1	5.5	0.0
Chocolate Honeycomb Crisp, COU, Marks & Spencer*	1 Serving/71g	110	155	4.6	27.6	2.9	1.0
Chocolate Mint Crisp, Iced, Marks & Spencer*	1/4 Pot/85.2g	115	135	5.4	21.9	2.9	1.0
Chocolate Mocha, BGTY, Sainsbury's*	1 Pot/100g	115	115	3.8	19.2	2.6	2.8
Chocolate Muffin, COU, Marks & Spencer*	1 Serving/110g	149	135	4.6	26.5	1.9	0.9
Chocolate Muffin, Tesco*	1 Serving/104g	354	340	3.5	35.5	20.4	2.1
Chocolate Orange, Eat Smart, Safeway*	1 Pot/90g	153	170	4.5	32.5	1.9	0.5
Chocolate Profiterole, Sainsbury's*	1/6 Pot/95.0g	192	202	5.4	25.1	8.9	0.8
Chocolate Profiterole, Tesco*	1 Serving/76g	293	386	5.1	26.9	28.7	0.5
Chocolate Toffee, Weight Watchers*	1 Pot/90.1g	164	182	4.9	35.0	3.5	1.8
Chocolate Trifle, Light, Cadbury*	1 Pot/92g	170	185	5.5	23.4	7.5	0.0
Chocolate, BGTY, Sainsbury's*	1 Serving/125g	149	119	3.9	21.4	2.1	1.7
Chocolate, COU, Marks & Spencer*	1 Serving/120g	168	140	5.6	26.4	2.1	1.1
Chocolate, Campina*	1 Pot/125g	186	149	3.2	18.5	6.9	0.0
Chocolate, Frozen, Healthy Eating, Tesco*	1 Serving/52g	68	131	3.5	23.7	2.5	0.9
Chocolate, Healthy Living, Tesco*	1 Pot/95g	87	92	3.7	14.1	2.3	1.1
Chocolate, Supreme, Made Up, Sainsbury's*	1/4 Pack/90g	92	102	3.6	13.0	3.9	0.3
Chocolate, Value, Tesco*	1 Pot/115g	112	97	2.8	15.7	2.6	0.0
Chocolate, Weight Watchers*	1 Serving/82g	145	177	5.2	32.3	3.0	2.9

DESSERT	INFO/WEIGHT	KCAL	KCAL	PROT	CARB	FAT	FIBRE
Creme Caramel, Sainsbury's*	1 Pot/100g	102	102	2.5	21.1	0.9	0.0
Crunchie, Milk Chocolate, Cadbury*	1 Pot/100g	285	285	5.8	37.8	12.5	0.0
Dairy Vanilla Iced, Sainsbury's*	1 Serving/65g	77	119	3.0	19.9	3.0	3.7
Double Chocolate Brownie, Weight Watchers*	1 Serving/82.5g	145	177	5.2	32.3	3.0	2.9
Double Chocolate Fudge, Marks & Spencer*	1 Pot/119g	387	325	3.0	30.6	21.4	1.6
Double Chocolate Heaven, Tesco*	1 pot/140g	249	178	4.5	20.9	8.5	3.4
Double Chocolate, Eat Smart, Safeway*	1 Pot/90g	144	160	3.9	31.0	2.2	2.0
Dreaming of, Cherry Rice, Marks & Spencer*	1 Pot/200g	220	110	2.4	19.7	2.2	0.1
Dreamy Vanilla, BGTY, Sainsbury's*	1 Serving/58g	146	252	3.5	27.6	14.2	5.3
Flake, Milk Chocolate, Cadbury*	1 Pot/100g	290	290	6.3	34.7	14.1	0.0
Fruit & Nut, Cadbury*	1 Pot/100g	285	285	6.4	36.3	12.5	0.0
Galaxy, Mars*	1 Pot/75g	166	221	4.9	22.7	12.3	0.0
Gulabjam Indian, Waitrose*	1 Pot/180g	476	266	4.8	42.9	8.6	0.6
Irish Cream Cafe Latte, COU, Marks & Spencer*	1 Pot/120g	160	133	5.0	24.0	2.2	0.9
Jaffa Cake, COU, Marks & Spencer*	1 Serving/120g	138	115	2.4	20.1	2.6	1.0
Lemon & Sultana Sponge, COU, Marks & Spencer*	1 Pot/130g	169	130	2.8	26.5	1.2	0.5
Lemon Meringue, Weight Watchers*	1 Pot/85g	161	189	2.4	43.1	0.5	0.6
Lemon, Sainsbury's*	1 Pot/115g	136	118	2.8	23.2	1.5	0.9
Lemoncello, Italian, Co-Op*	1 Pot/90g	266	295	3.0	34.0	16.0	0.1
Lemoncillo, Tesco*	1 Pot/100g	273	273	4.2	41.8	9.9	0.8
Luxurious Chocolate Marshmallow, Weight Watchers*	1 Serving/50g	97	194	3.2	34.5	4.7	1.3
Mandarin, COU, Marks & Spencer*	1 Serving/150g	195	130	1.0	22.0	3.8	0.1
Maple & Pecan, American Style, Sainsbury's*	1 Pot/110g	287	261	2.6	30.6	14.2	1.2
Mars, Mars*	1 Pot/110g	215	195	6.0	28.2	6.7	0.7
Natural Rice, Shape*	1 Pot/175g	149	85	3.5	15.4	1.0	0.1
Neapolitan, Frozen, GFY, Asda*	1 Scoop/100g	64	64	1.2	10.0	2.1	0.1
Panna Cotta, BGTY, Sainsbury's*	1 Serving/150g	150	100	2.4	18.2	1.9	1.4
Panna Cotta, Sainsbury's*	1 Pot/100g	304	304	3.0	41.5	15.7	4.0
Passion Fruit & Mango, Weight Watchers*	1/4 Tub/70g	103	147	1.8	29.1	2.6	0.6
Peach & Raspberry, COU, Marks & Spencer*	1 Pot/90g	135	150	2.6	30.5	1.6	1.0
Peach, Iced, So-Lo, Iceland*	1 Lolly/92ml	98	107	2.3	23.5	0.0	2.2
Pineapple & Passionfruit, Marks & Spencer*	1 Pot/100g	130	130	0.8	21.7	3.8	0.3
Profiterole, Marks & Spencer*	1 Pot/61g	209	342	5.5	29.1	22.1	0.5
Pure Bliss, Aldi*	1 Pot/125.4g	158	126	2.5	20.3	3.9	0.2
Raspberry & Chardonnay, COU, Marks & Spencer*	1 Serving/135g	155	115	1.6	25.5	0.5	2.7
Raspberry Flavour Whip, Co-Op*	1 Whip/64g	241	377	1.2	92.5	0.2	0.1
Raspberry Swirl, Iced, Weight Watchers*	1 Scoop/60g	74	124	1.7	23.4	2.5	0.3
Raspberry With Light Lemon Sponge, Weight Watchers*	1 Dessert/85.2g	155	182	3.9	32.0	4.3	1.8
Red Devil, Simpsons, St Ivel*	1oz/28g	38	134	2.8	24.3	2.8	0.4
Rice, Lite, Muller*	1 Pot/150g	116	77	3.5	13.6	0.9	0.0
Rice, Raspberry, Rachel's Organic*	1 Serving/150g	176	117	3.4	20.5	2.4	0.0
Rocky Road, Sainsbury's*	1 Pot/110g	328	298	3.6	26.8	19.6	2.1
Rolo, Nestle*	1 Pot/78g	191	245	3.1	30.3	12.2	0.3
Simply Strawberry, Sainsbury's*	1 Pot/150g	126	84	0.6	19.3	0.1	0.9
Strawberries & Cream, BFY, Morrisons*	1 Serving/200g	244	122	2.2	26.0	1.1	0.1
Strawberry & Rhubarb, COU, Marks & Spencer*	1 Pot/110g	105	95	1.5	20.1	0.7	0.9
Strawberry Flavour, SmartPrice, Asda*	1 Pot/115g	113	98	2.4	17.0	2.3	0.0
Strawberry Flavour, With Cream, Somerfield*	1 Pot/100g	119	119	2.0	16.0	5.0	0.0
Strawberry Panna Cotta, COU, Marks & Spencer*	1 Pot/145g	145	100	2.6	15.7	2.6	0.8
Strawberry, BGTY, Sainsbury's*	1 Pot/115g	133	116	2.7	23.1	1.4	1.3
Strawberry, Healthy Living, Tesco*	1 Pot/122g	94	77	2.7	12.3	1.9	1.1
Strawberry, Supreme, Made Up, Sainsbury's*	1/4 Pack/90g	95	105	3.6	14.0	3.8	0.1
Strawberry, Value, Tesco*	1 Pot/115g	113	98	2.4	16.9	2.3	0.0

D

	Measure INFO/WEIGHT	per Measure KCAL	Nutrition Values per 100g / 100ml				
			KCAL	PROT	CARB	FAT	FIBRE
DESSERT							
Summer Berry, Healthy Living, Tesco*	1 Pot/102g	133	130	2.8	24.5	2.3	1.5
Summer Fruits, COU, Marks & Spencer*	1 Serving/105g	110	105	2.1	21.6	1.1	1.2
Summer Fruits, Marbled Cream, Waitrose*	1 Serving/125g	214	171	2.1	20.2	9.1	1.1
Summer Fruits, Yoghurt, Iced, BGTY, Sainsbury's*	1/4 Pot/85g	105	124	3.3	25.6	0.9	0.5
Supreme, No Added Sugar, Sainsbury's*	1/4 Pack/91g	98	108	3.5	13.6	4.4	0.0
Tantalising Toffee Flavour, Weight Watchers*	1 Serving/57g	93	163	2.7	26.2	4.8	0.2
Tantalising Toffee, COU, Marks & Spencer*	1/4 Pot/85g	145	170	3.1	32.8	2.9	0.5
Toffee & Vanilla, Weight Watchers*	1 Pot/67g	107	159	3.1	34.8	0.8	3.9
Toffee & Walnut, Iced, Free From, Sainsbury's*	1/4 Tub/81g	203	251	3.3	31.6	12.4	0.3
Toffee Apple, Eat Smart, Safeway*	1 Pot/100g	145	145	2.4	29.1	1.7	2.6
Toffee Banana Crunch, Farmfoods*	1/6 Dessert/82g	219	267	2.6	38.5	11.4	0.7
Toffee Chocolate, Weight Watchers*	1 Pot/100g	197	197	4.3	34.9	4.5	2.2
Toffee Flavour & Toffee Sauce, Weight Watchers*	1 Pot/57g	93	163	2.7	26.2	4.8	0.2
Toffee Flavour Custard, Ambrosia*	1 Pack/135g	139	103	2.7	16.4	2.9	0.1
Toffee Flavour Fudge Swirl, Weight Watchers*	1 Pot/57g	82	143	2.5	22.6	4.4	0.4
Toffee Flavoured Dairy, Iced, BGTY, Sainsbury's*	1 Serving/70g	103	147	2.7	24.0	4.5	0.2
Toffee Iced, 3% Fat, Marks & Spencer*	1oz/28g	51	183	3.1	37.2	2.4	0.5
Toffee Muffin, COU, Marks & Spencer*	1 Serving/100g	180	180	3.7	35.8	2.2	0.3
Toffee, BGTY, Sainsbury's*	1 Pot/130g	146	112	3.6	21.4	1.3	0.8
Toffee, Frozen, BGTY, Sainsbury's*	1 Pot/73.8g	96	130	3.3	26.0	1.4	4.2
Toffee, With Biscuit Pieces, Weight Watchers*	1 Pot/57.1g	93	163	2.7	26.2	4.8	0.2
Triple Chocolate Layered, BGTY, Sainsbury's*	1 Pot/105g	147	140	4.2	24.4	2.8	0.5
Triple Chocolate Truffle, Entenmann's*	1 Serving/100g	304	304	4.5	28.4	19.1	2.2
Triple Chocolate, Delice, Sainsbury's*	1 Serving/105g	399	380	3.8	32.4	26.1	0.7
Vanilla & Chocolate Iced, Healthy Living, Tesco*	1 Pot/73g	104	143	3.0	26.9	2.6	0.7
Vanilla & Raspberry Swirl, Weight Watchers*	1 Serving/100ml	81	81	1.5	13.3	2.2	0.2
Vanilla & Strawberry Compote, Weight Watchers*	1 Pot/57g	81	142	2.5	23.4	3.9	0.2
Vanilla & Toffee, Heavenly Swirls, Healthy Living, Tesco*	1 Pot/73g	106	145	2.5	28.1	2.5	0.5
Vanilla Flavour, Iced, Healthy Eating, Tesco*	1 Serving/50g	67	134	3.9	24.1	2.4	4.6
Vanilla Supreme, Sainsbury's*	1 Pot/95g	116	122	3.0	18.0	4.0	0.0
Vanilla With Strawberries Swirl, Weight Watchers*	1 Pot/57g	46	81	1.5	13.3	2.2	0.2
Vanilla, Frozen, BGTY, Sainsbury's*	1 Serving/75g	89	119	3.0	19.9	3.0	3.7
Vanilla, Iced, 3% Fat, Marks & Spencer*	1oz/28g	40	143	3.5	25.9	2.8	0.7
Vanilla, Luxury, Charolait, Aldi*	1 Serving/200g	248	124	3.0	16.6	5.1	0.0
White Chocolate & Raspberry, Tesco*	1 Dessert/88g	180	204	3.4	25.0	10.1	3.1
Wild Blueberry & White Peach, Extra Special, Asda*	1 Pot/120g	180	150	1.8	20.0	7.0	1.0
DESSERT MIX							
Instant Powder, Made Up With Skimmed Milk	1oz/28g	27	97	3.1	14.9	3.2	0.2
Instant Powder, Made Up With Whole Milk	1oz/28g	35	125	3.1	14.8	6.3	0.2
DHAL							
Black Gram	1oz/28g	21	74	4.2	7.0	3.4	1.7
Blackeye Bean, Patak's*	1oz/28g	29	102	3.6	12.4	4.6	1.8
Chick Pea	1oz/28g	42	149	7.4	17.7	6.1	3.8
Chick Pea, Asda*	1 Serving/400g	404	101	4.5	14.0	3.0	3.0
Chick Pea, Sainsbury's*	1/2 Can/200g	432	216	10.8	22.7	9.1	7.1
Lentil, Patak's*	1 Can/283g	156	55	2.8	9.3	1.0	1.0
Lentil, Red Masoor & Tomato With Butter	1oz/28g	26	94	4.0	9.7	4.9	0.9
Lentil, Red Masoor & Vegetable	1oz/28g	31	110	5.8	14.7	3.8	1.8
Lentil, Red Masoor With Vegetable Oil	1oz/28g	48	172	7.6	19.2	7.9	1.8
Lentil, Red Masoor, Punjabi	1oz/28g	39	139	7.2	19.2	4.6	2.0
Lentil, Red Masoorl & Mung Bean	1oz/28g	32	114	4.8	9.9	6.7	1.6
Lentil, Red, Way To Five, Sainsbury's*	1/2 Pack/94g	87	93	5.5	14.4	1.5	1.4
Lentil, Red, Way to Five, Sainsbury's*	1/2 Pack/273.1g	254	93	5.5	14.4	1.5	1.4

D

	Measure INFO/WEIGHT	per Measure KCAL	Nutrition Values per 100g / 100ml				
			KCAL	PROT	CARB	FAT	FIBRE
DHAL							
Lentil, Safeway*	1 Serving/200g	182	91	2.4	10.5	4.4	0.9
Lentil, Tesco*	1 Serving/200g	248	124	5.1	10.6	6.6	2.5
Mung Bean, Bengali	1oz/28g	20	73	4.2	7.4	3.3	1.7
Mung Beans, Dried, Boiled in Unsalted Water	1oz/28g	26	92	7.8	15.3	0.4	0.0
Mung Beans, Dried, Raw	1oz/28g	81	291	26.8	46.3	1.1	0.0
Split Peas, Yellow, Chana, Asda*	1 Serving/275g	300	109	2.6	9.0	7.0	1.8
Tarka, Asda*	1/2 Pack/150g	216	144	6.0	12.0	8.0	6.0
DHANSAK							
Chicken With Bagara Rice, Waitrose*	1 Pack/450g	549	122	8.2	18.2	1.8	1.2
Chicken, Ready Meals, Marks & Spencer*	1oz/28g	50	180	12.4	6.6	11.5	1.6
Vegetable, Sainsbury's*	1 Pack/400g	416	104	2.6	7.2	7.2	1.3
Vegetable, Waitrose*	1 Serving/300g	255	85	3.9	9.8	3.3	2.4
DILL							
Dried	1 Tsp/1g	3	253	19.9	42.2	4.4	13.6
Fresh	1oz/28g	7	25	3.7	0.9	0.8	2.5
DIME							
Terry's*	1oz/28g	154	550	4.6	68.5	33.8	0.6
DIP							
Applewood Cheddar & Onion, Fresh, BGTY, Sainsbury's*	1/2 Pot/85g	85	100	7.3	7.3	4.6	0.5
Aubergine, Fresh, Waitrose*	1 Serving/85g	159	187	2.5	10.5	15.0	1.7
Aubergine, Taverna*	1 Serving/50g	139	277	4.7	11.4	23.6	0.0
Bean & Cheese, Asda*	1 Serving/50g	79	157	7.0	12.0	9.0	1.7
Blue Cheese, Fresh, Sainsbury's*	1/5 Pot/34g	115	337	3.6	3.1	34.5	0.1
Cajun Red Pepper, Sainsbury's*	1 Serving/50g	25	50	1.4	7.0	1.8	1.4
Caramelised Onion & Garlic, Waitrose*	1/2 Pot/85g	389	458	1.7	5.8	47.6	0.5
Celery, Marks & Spencer*	1 Pot/130g	163	125	1.8	4.4	11.0	1.2
Cheddar & Onion, Marks & Spencer*	1oz/28g	88	315	5.1	7.5	29.5	0.5
Cheddar & Spring Onion, Marks & Spencer*	1 Pack/125g	581	465	3.6	4.7	48.3	0.5
Cheese & Bacon With Breadsticks, Weight Watchers*	1 Pack/50g	98	196	16.0	24.0	4.2	1.4
Cheese & Chive, 50% Less Fat, Asda*	1 Pot/125g	261	209	4.5	9.0	17.2	0.0
Cheese & Chive, 50% Less Fat, Morrisons*	1 Serving/50g	86	172	8.8	5.2	12.7	0.2
Cheese & Chive, Asda*	1 Serving/42.5g	192	447	4.9	3.4	46.0	0.0
Cheese & Chive, Classic, Tesco*	1 Serving/32g	164	511	3.3	3.1	54.0	0.1
Cheese & Chive, Fresh, Safeway*	1 Pot/170g	877	516	4.1	3.0	54.2	0.0
Cheese & Chive, Fresh, Sainsbury's*	1oz/28g	109	390	3.9	2.7	40.4	0.0
Cheese & Chive, Healthy Choice, Safeway*	1 Pack/100g	137	137	10.2	6.0	8.0	1.3
Cheese & Chive, Healthy Eating, Tesco*	1 Tsp/10g	23	228	5.7	6.4	19.9	0.0
Cheese & Chive, Healthy Living, Tesco*	1 Serving/43g	93	219	5.4	5.8	19.4	0.1
Cheese & Chive, Healthy Selection, Somerfield*	1oz/28g	67	239	6.0	5.0	22.0	0.0
Cheese & Chive, Marks & Spencer*	1oz/28g	120	430	4.5	3.9	44.1	0.5
Cheese & Chive, Sainsbury's*	1 Pot/300g	1296	432	3.6	4.6	44.5	0.2
Cheese & Chive, Tesco*	1 Pack/170g	811	477	3.3	5.1	49.2	0.1
Cheese & Spring Onion, Weight Watchers*	1 Serving/50g	98	196	16.0	24.0	4.2	1.4
Chilli Cheese, Asda*	1 Serving/50g	131	262	8.0	8.0	22.0	1.1
Chilli Cheese, Max, Walkers*	1 Jar/300g	390	130	3.3	9.4	9.1	0.3
Chilli, Marks & Spencer*	1 Pot/35g	103	295	0.4	73.2	0.2	0.4
Cranberry, Asda*	1/2 Pot/40g	53	132	0.4	29.0	1.6	0.8
Cucumber & Mint, Eat Smart, Safeway*	1/2 Pot/85g	55	65	7.3	4.9	1.3	0.8
Cucumber & Mint, Fresh, Sainsbury's*	1oz/28g	34	123	4.5	3.7	10.0	0.0
Doritos Hot Salsa, Walkers*	1 Jar/326g	130	40	0.9	8.5	0.2	2.2
Doritos Mild Salsa, Walkers*	1oz/28g	11	40	0.9	8.5	0.2	2.2
Feta Cheese, Fresh, Tesco*	1oz/28g	81	288	6.8	7.9	25.5	0.7
Garlic & Herb, Marks & Spencer*	1oz/28g	88	315	2.4	7.1	30.6	0.5

D

DIP

Measure INFO/WEIGHT	per Measure KCAL	Nutrition Values per 100g / 100ml				
		KCAL	PROT	CARB	FAT	FIBRE
Garlic & Herb, Reduced Fat, Marks & Spencer*	1 Serving/10g	10	95	6.0	8.1	4.0	0.5
Garlic & Herb, Tesco*	1/4 Pack/42.5g	260	604	0.9	3.2	65.4	0.3
Garlic Herb & Rocket, Marks & Spencer*	1 Serving/25g	104	415	2.4	4.5	43.0	0.5
Garlic, Olive Oil & Butter, Pizza Express*	1/2 Pot/17g	106	621	1.5	2.8	67.4	0.5
Mature Cheddar Cheese & Chive, Fresh, Waitrose*	1/2 Pot/85g	393	462	5.8	2.4	47.7	1.7
Mexican Bean, Doritos*	1 Tbsp/20g	18	89	2.7	12.1	3.3	2.4
Mustard & Honey, Fresh, Sainsbury's*	1oz/28g	100	356	2.2	5.1	36.3	0.0
Mustard Mash, Marks & Spencer*	1oz/28g	25	90	2.6	12.7	3.1	1.0
Nacho Cheese, Marks & Spencer*	1oz/28g	76	270	9.8	3.8	23.7	0.4
Nacho Cheese, Sainsbury's*	1 Serving/50g	244	487	4.8	3.9	50.2	0.0
Nacho Cheese, Tex Mex, Tesco*	1 Serving/50g	222	444	6.2	3.0	45.3	0.0
Onion & Garlic, 50% Less Fat, Asda*	1oz/28g	59	209	4.5	9.0	17.2	0.0
Onion & Garlic, Classic, Tesco*	1 Serving/30g	133	442	1.7	4.6	46.3	0.2
Onion & Garlic, Fresh, BGTY, Sainsbury's*	1oz/28g	56	201	4.4	4.8	18.2	0.8
Onion & Garlic, GFY, Asda*	1/5 Pot/34g	56	166	2.1	8.0	14.0	0.2
Onion & Garlic, Half Fat, Safeway*	1/2 Pot/85g	170	200	3.2	7.4	17.2	0.1
Onion & Garlic, Healthy Living, Tesco*	1 Serving/42.5g	81	188	2.5	6.3	17.0	0.1
Onion & Garlic, Healthy Selection, Somerfield*	1oz/28g	62	222	3.0	5.0	21.0	0.0
Peanut, Satay Selection, Occasions, Sainsbury's*	1 Serving/2g	4	186	7.1	13.8	11.4	1.1
Pecorino, Basil & Pine Nut, Fresh, Waitrose*	1/2 Pot/85g	338	398	5.1	5.1	39.7	0.0
Red Pepper, Sainsbury's*	1 Pot/100g	103	103	2.3	14.6	4.0	0.0
Roast Onion, Garlic & Rocket, Reduced Fat, Waitrose*	1 Serving/25g	51	202	2.7	5.4	18.8	1.5
Salsa, Chunky Tomato, Tesco*	1 Pot/170g	68	40	1.1	5.9	1.3	1.1
Salsa, Chunky, Fresh, Sainsbury's*	1 Serving/100g	51	51	1.1	7.8	1.7	1.2
Salsa, GFY, Asda*	1 Pot/170g	68	40	1.2	8.0	0.4	1.5
Salsa, Kettle Chips*	1 Serving/25g	10	39	1.7	8.0	0.0	0.0
Salsa, Less Than 5% Fat, Safeway*	1/2 Pot/85g	47	55	1.5	6.1	2.4	0.9
Smoked Salmon & Dill, Fresh, Waitrose*	1/2 Pot/85g	373	439	5.1	4.1	44.7	0.1
Smoked Salmon & Dill, Reduced Fat, Waitrose*	1/2 Pot/85g	184	217	3.9	6.1	19.7	1.1
Sour Cream & Chive, BGTY, Sainsbury's	1oz/28g	46	165	4.9	3.4	14.6	0.7
Sour Cream & Chive, Doritos*	1 Tbsp/20g	64	322	2.5	3.1	33.3	0.1
Sour Cream & Chive, Fresh, Tesco*	1/2 Pot/75g	305	407	2.1	4.1	42.4	0.0
Sour Cream & Chive, Primula*	1oz/28g	97	346	5.0	1.8	35.3	0.0
Sour Cream & Chive, Reduced Fat, Asda*	1oz/28g	55	197	2.3	7.1	17.9	0.1
Sour Cream & Chive, Sainsbury's*	1 Serving/50g	141	282	3.1	5.4	27.5	0.1
Sour Cream, Tesco*	1 Serving/38g	111	297	3.4	3.9	29.8	0.2
Soured Cream & Chive, 95% Fat Free, Marks & Spencer*	1oz/28g	25	90	6.5	9.6	2.8	0.5
Soured Cream & Chive, BGTY, Sainsbury's*	1 Serving/170g	131	77	6.0	6.6	2.9	0.3
Soured Cream & Chive, Classic, Tesco*	1 Serving/25g	81	323	1.7	3.2	33.7	0.2
Soured Cream & Chive, For Skins, Tesco*	1 Serving/12g	36	297	3.4	3.9	29.8	0.2
Soured Cream & Chive, Heathy Living, Tesco*	1 Serving/31g	44	141	3.7	6.0	11.3	0.2
Soured Cream & Chive, Marks & Spencer*	1 Serving/100g	330	330	2.6	5.0	33.5	0.5
Soured Cream & Chive, Morrisons*	1 Serving/100g	317	317	2.6	3.3	32.6	0.0
Soured Cream & Chive, Reduced Fat, Tesco*	1 Serving/85g	159	187	3.6	6.1	16.5	0.4
Spiced Mango, Ginger & Chilli Salsa, Weight Watchers*	1 Serving/56g	48	85	1.0	19.9	0.2	2.6
Spicy Moroccan, BGTY, Sainsbury's*	1/2 Pot/84.8g	56	66	2.1	10.0	2.0	1.7
Sun Dried Tomato, Somerfield*	1oz/28g	155	552	1.0	5.0	59.0	0.0
Sweet & Sour, Marks & Spencer*	1oz/28g	36	130	0.7	31.4	0.1	0.5
Sweet & Zesty, Doritos*	1 Jar/375g	150	40	1.3	8.0	0.5	1.4
Sweet Chilli, Oriental Selection, Waitrose*	1/2 Pot/35.2g	88	250	1.3	59.4	0.8	0.4
Sweet Pepper & Ricotta, Asda*	1 Serving/20g	74	370	1.0	12.0	35.0	0.0
Tangy Barbecue, Marks & Spencer*	1oz/28g	28	100	1.1	22.2	0.6	0.6
Taramasalata, Sainsbury's	1/2 Pot/85g	407	479	4.0	7.5	48.1	0.1

	Measure INFO/WEIGHT	per Measure KCAL	Nutrition Values per 100g / 100ml				
			KCAL	PROT	CARB	FAT	FIBRE
DIP							
Thousand Island, Healthy Living, Tesco*	1 Serving/31g	57	183	2.5	9.6	14.9	0.3
Thousand Island, Marks & Spencer*	1oz/28g	69	245	2.1	9.4	22.2	0.7
Tikka, Classic, Fresh, Healthy Choice, Safeway*	1oz/28g	38	137	10.2	6.0	8.0	1.3
Tomato Ketchip, Asda*	1 Pack/25g	18	71	1.6	16.0	0.1	1.0
Tomato Salsa, Fresh, Waitrose*	1 Serving/50g	24	47	1.5	5.0	2.3	1.7
Tortilla Chips, Cool Flavour, Big, Morrisons*	1/2 Pack/100g	453	453	6.4	57.4	22.0	8.1
Tzatzaki, Somerfield*	1oz/28g	37	131	6.0	3.0	11.0	0.0
Yoghurt & Cucumber Mint, Tesco*	1oz/28g	34	121	7.0	7.2	7.1	0.6
DISCOS							
Cheese & Onion, KP*	1 Pack/28g	144	514	5.4	57.5	29.3	2.9
Pickled Onion, KP*	1 Bag/31g	155	500	3.7	58.6	27.8	2.9
Salt & Vinegar, KP*	1 Bag/31g	158	511	4.8	56.8	29.4	2.6
DOLLY MIXTURES							
Marks & Spencer*	1 Pack/125g	479	383	1.5	90.7	1.5	0.0
Sainsbury's*	1 Serving/10g	40	401	1.4	94.4	1.9	0.1
SmartPrice, Asda*	1 Sweet/2.9g	11	380	0.5	91.0	1.6	0.0
Tesco*	1 Pack/100g	376	376	1.6	88.9	1.5	0.0
DOPIAZA							
Chicken, Safeway*	1 Pack/326g	450	138	10.4	5.3	8.4	1.4
Chicken, Sainsbury's*	1/2 Pack/200g	272	136	13.2	3.1	7.9	0.8
Chicken, Tesco*	1 Pack/350g	448	128	10.8	5.3	7.1	0.6
Chicken, With Pilau Rice, Sharwood's*	1 Pack/375g	473	126	5.3	15.8	4.6	0.8
Chicken, With Pilau Rice, Tesco*	1 Pack/400g	424	106	5.7	12.3	3.8	1.5
Mushroom, Indian, Tesco*	1 Serving/225g	155	69	2.4	5.1	4.4	1.5
Mushroom, Tesco*	1 Pack/350g	291	83	3.0	6.7	4.9	1.3
Mushroom, Waitrose*	1/2 Pack/150g	81	54	2.2	4.3	3.1	2.3
DORITOS							
Chargrilled BBQ, Walkers*	1 Bag/35g	170	485	5.5	59.0	25.0	3.5
Cheesy 3D's, Walkers*	1 Pack/20g	89	445	7.0	68.0	16.0	3.0
Chilli Heatwave, Walkers*	1 Pack/33g	162	490	6.5	58.0	26.0	3.0
Cool Original, Walkers*	1 Bag/40g	202	505	7.5	58.0	27.0	3.0
Cool Spice 3Ds, Walkers*	1 Bag/24g	108	450	8.0	64.0	18.0	4.4
Corn Chips, Cool Original, Doritos*	1 Serving/200g	1010	505	7.5	58.0	27.0	3.0
Dippas, Lightly Salted, Dipping Chips, Doritos*	1 Bag/35g	172	490	7.5	63.0	23.0	3.5
Hint Of Chilli Dippas, Walkers*	1 Bag/35g	173	495	7.0	61.0	25.0	3.5
Hint of Lime, Walkers*	1 Bag/35g	173	495	7.0	60.0	25.0	3.5
Latinos, Mexican Grill, Walkers*	1 Serving/35g	170	485	6.5	59.0	25.0	3.5
Latinos, Sour Cream & Sweet Pepper, Walkers*	1 Pack/40g	194	485	5.5	60.0	25.0	3.5
Lightly Salted Dippas, Walkers*	1 Bag/50g	245	490	7.5	63.0	23.0	3.5
Mexican Hot, Walkers*	1 Bag/40g	202	505	8.0	57.0	27.0	3.5
Tangy Cheese, Walkers*	1 Bag/40g	202	505	8.5	57.0	27.0	3.5
DOUBLE DECKER							
Cadbury*	1 Bar/51g	237	465	5.2	64.9	20.7	0.0
Snack Size, Cadbury*	1 Bar/35.5g	163	465	4.8	64.5	20.9	0.0
With Nuts, Cadbury*	1 Bar/60g	291	485	7.9	58.6	24.5	0.0
DOUGH BALLS							
Cheese & Garlic, Occasions, Sainsbury's*	1 Ball/12g	41	341	10.3	33.4	18.5	2.1
Garlic & Herb, Occasions, Sainsbury's*	1 Ball/12g	41	343	8.4	38.7	17.2	2.2
Garlic, GFY, Asda*	1 Dough Ball/8.4g	20	250	9.0	49.0	2.0	2.0
Garlic, Healthy Living, Tesco*	1 Serving/40g	110	274	8.8	42.0	7.9	2.3
Garlic, Tesco*	1 Serving/10g	40	400	7.0	40.0	23.0	1.0
Garlic, Waitrose*	1 Doughball/11g	38	347	8.5	41.4	16.4	3.3
Pizza Express*	8 Balls/50g	200	400	14.3	85.0	3.2	0.0

D

	Measure INFO/WEIGHT	per Measure KCAL	Nutrition Values per 100g / 100ml				
			KCAL	PROT	CARB	FAT	FIBRE
DOUGH BALLS							
Sainsbury's*	1 Ball/12g	41	343	8.4	38.7	17.2	2.2
With Garlic & Herb Butter, Aldi*	1 Ball/12.3g	44	365	7.7	46.7	18.2	1.8
DOUGHNUTS							
Apple & Custard, Finger, Sainsbury's*	1 Serving/65g	137	210	4.4	27.5	9.2	1.9
Apple & Fresh Cream, Sainsbury's*	1 Doughnut/79g	216	273	5.4	30.5	14.4	1.9
Baked, Healthy Living, Tesco*	1 Doughnut/67g	166	248	6.4	42.2	5.9	1.4
Chocolate, Somerfield*	1 Doughnut/57g	203	356	7.8	43.8	16.6	1.7
Cream & Jam, Assorted Box, Sainsbury's*	1 Finger/71g	229	322	6.2	34.2	17.9	2.2
Cream & Jam, Tesco*	1 Doughnut/90g	288	320	5.4	39.4	15.7	2.0
Custard & Bramley Apple, Sainsbury's*	1 Doughnut/91g	256	282	4.5	34.6	13.9	1.0
Custard, Sainsbury's*	1 Doughnut/70g	172	246	5.1	32.3	10.7	2.3
Custard, Tesco*	1 Doughnut/91g	266	292	4.1	33.4	15.8	1.1
Custard-Filled	1 Doughnut/75g	269	358	6.2	43.3	19.0	0.0
Dairy Cream & Jam, Somerfield*	1 Doughnut/80g	296	370	4.6	35.8	23.1	1.3
Dairy Cream Finger, Safeway*	1 Doughnut/98g	342	349	5.5	36.4	20.1	1.8
Dairy Cream, Marks & Spencer*	1oz/28g	87	310	4.9	40.8	14.1	1.3
Finger, Co-Op*	1 Doughnut/82g	299	365	4.0	45.0	18.0	2.0
Jam	1 Doughnut/75g	252	336	5.7	48.8	14.5	0.0
Jam, American Style, Budgens*	1 Doughnut/46g	127	275	7.1	46.5	6.7	0.0
Jam, Marks & Spencer*	1 Doughnut/49g	141	287	5.0	57.6	4.0	1.3
Jam, Mini, Somerfield*	1 Doughnut/45g	138	307	6.4	50.1	9.0	1.4
Jam, Somerfield*	1 Doughnut/70g	213	304	6.8	47.9	9.5	1.6
Mini Donuts, Crunchie, Cadbury*	1oz/28g	105	375	4.8	49.8	17.0	0.0
Mini, Sainsbury's*	1 Doughnut/14g	53	379	5.2	47.9	18.9	2.1
Ring	1 Doughnut/60g	238	397	6.1	47.2	21.7	0.0
Ring, Iced	1 Doughnut/70g	268	383	4.8	55.1	17.5	0.0
Ring, Waitrose*	1 Doughnut/107g	396	370	4.2	43.5	19.9	0.7
Strawberry Jam & Cream, Sainsbury's	1 Doughnut/80g	299	374	5.3	36.2	23.2	1.3
Toffee, Tesco*	1 Doughnut/75g	235	313	8.0	44.2	11.6	1.6
DOVER SOLE							
Raw	1oz/28g	25	89	18.1	0.0	1.8	0.0
DR PEPPER*							
The Coca Cola Co*	1 Bottle/500ml	210	42	0.0	10.9	0.0	0.0
DRAMBUIE							
39% Volume	1 Shot/25ml	68	272	0.0	0.0	0.0	0.0
DREAM							
Cadbury*	1 Bar/45g	250	555	4.5	59.7	33.3	0.0
Double Fudge, Cadbury*	1oz/28g	139	495	6.3	61.4	25.2	0.0
Snowbites, Cadbury*	1 Serving/31.2g	169	545	3.1	59.7	32.7	0.0
White Chocolate, Cadbury*	1 Piece/8g	44	555	4.5	59.7	33.3	0.0
DREAM TOPPING							
Dry, Bird's*	1oz/28g	193	690	6.7	32.5	58.5	0.5
Made Up, Skimmed Milk, Bird's*	1oz/28g	21	75	2.0	4.8	5.3	0.0
Sugar Free, Dry, Bird's*	1oz/28g	195	695	7.3	30.5	60.5	0.5
DRESSING							
Balsamic Bliss, Ainsley Harriott*	1 Tbsp/15g	41	272	0.8	19.3	21.1	0.0
Balsamic Vinegar & Oregano, Waitrose*	1 Serving/25g	101	404	0.6	8.2	41.0	0.4
Balsamic Vinegar & Smoked Garlic, Safeway*	1 Tbsp/15ml	19	125	0.1	28.3	0.9	0.5
Balsamic Vinegar, Asda*	1 Pack/44ml	121	275	0.9	7.0	27.0	0.0
Balsamic Vinegar, Morrisons*	1 Serving/15ml	17	111	0.1	22.9	1.6	0.1
Balsamic With Garlic & Herbs, Finest, Tesco*	1 Serving/10ml	13	133	0.3	3.4	13.1	0.1
Balsamic With Olive Oil, Pizza Express*	1 Serving/10g	42	421	0.3	10.3	41.2	0.0
Balsamic, Extra Virgin Olive Oil, TTD, Sainsbury's*	1 Tsp/5ml	19	376	0.5	12.8	36.0	0.4

DRESSING

INFO/WEIGHT	Measure per Measure KCAL	KCAL	PROT	CARB	FAT	FIBRE
Balsamic, Marks & Spencer*	1 Tbsp/15g	74	490	0.3	9.7	48.0	0.5
Balsamic, New, Sainsbury's*	1 Tbsp/15g	58	389	0.6	18.3	34.8	0.8
Balsamic, TTD, Sainsbury's*	1 serving/15g	58	389	0.6	18.3	34.8	0.8
Blue Cheese, 60% Less Fat, BGTY, Sainsbury's*	1 Tbsp/15ml	26	172	1.9	7.3	15.1	0.2
Blue Cheese, Fresh, Sainsbury's*	1 Dtsp/10ml	42	423	2.3	0.5	45.7	0.1
Blue Cheese, Healthy Eating, Tesco*	1 Tsp/5g	4	82	4.4	9.0	3.1	0.1
Blue Cheese, Hellmann's*	1 Tbsp/15g	69	459	0.7	6.3	47.2	1.1
Blue Cheese, Low Fat, Weight Watchers*	1oz/28g	17	59	1.5	5.8	3.4	0.0
Blue Cheese, Salad, Waitrose*	1 Serving/50g	265	530	2.1	17.3	50.3	4.1
Blue Cheese, Tesco*	1 Serving/15ml	75	500	2.5	6.9	51.4	0.2
Caesar Salad, Marks & Spencer*	1 Serving/10ml	52	515	1.8	2.2	55.2	0.5
Caesar Salad, Safeway*	1 Serving/25g	122	488	3.7	13.7	48.5	0.1
Caesar Style, GFY, Asda*	1 Sachet/44ml	34	77	5.0	9.0	2.3	0.0
Caesar Style, Kraft*	1 Tbsp/15ml	15	102	2.1	15.0	3.5	0.1
Caesar Style, Low Fat, Weight Watchers*	1 Tsp/6g	4	60	1.6	5.8	3.4	0.0
Caesar, 95% Fat Free, Tesco*	1 Tsp/6g	5	88	4.1	8.9	3.7	0.3
Caesar, Asiago, Briannas	2 Tbsp/30ml	140	467	3.3	3.3	50.0	0.0
Caesar, BGTY, Sainsbury's*	1 Serving/25ml	15	60	3.7	8.5	1.2	1.2
Caesar, Chilled, Reduced Fat, Tesco*	1 Tsp/5ml	13	252	6.5	3.1	23.7	0.1
Caesar, Classic, Sainsbury's*	1 Tsp/5ml	22	442	2.7	4.6	45.9	0.5
Caesar, Finest, Tesco*	1 Tbsp/15ml	72	477	1.9	2.8	50.9	0.2
Caesar, Fresh, Asda*	1 Dtsp/10ml	45	454	2.4	3.2	48.0	0.0
Caesar, Fresh, Marks & Spencer*	1 Tsp/6g	32	525	2.0	1.8	56.4	0.2
Caesar, Fresh, Sainsbury's*	1 Tsp/6g	29	479	3.0	1.1	51.4	0.2
Caesar, Gourmet, Fresh, Waitrose*	1 Tbsp/15ml	72	479	4.5	0.9	50.8	0.5
Caesar, Healthy Living, Tesco*	1 Serving/125ml	93	74	3.0	8.4	2.8	0.2
Caesar, Hellmann's*	1 Tsp/6g	30	499	2.5	4.5	51.7	0.3
Caesar, Light, Kraft*	1 Serving/15ml	15	102	2.1	15.0	3.5	0.1
Caesar, Low Fat, Cardini's*	1 Tsp/6g	7	120	1.0	27.0	1.0	1.0
Caesar, Loyd Grossman*	1 Dtsp/10g	34	342	2.1	7.0	33.9	0.0
Caesar, Luxury, Hellmann's*	1 Teaspoon/4g	20	498	2.5	4.4	51.7	0.3
Caesar, Marks & Spencer*	1 Tsp/6g	31	523	2.0	1.8	56.4	0.2
Caesar, Original, Cardini's*	1 Serving/10g	56	560	2.0	2.0	60.0	0.0
Caesar, Reduced Fat, Marks & Spencer*	1 Tbsp/15ml	30	200	3.5	5.3	18.3	0.5
Caesar, Somerfield*	1 Serving/50ml	274	547	1.3	2.2	59.2	0.0
Caesar, Tesco*	1 Tbsp/15ml	71	475	4.6	2.1	49.8	0.1
Caesar, Weight Watchers*	1 Serving/20g	16	80	3.3	14.7	0.9	0.2
Caesar, With Parmigiano Cheese, Marks & Spencer*	1 Serving/15g	72	480	3.5	3.1	50.4	0.0
Citrus Salad, BGTY, Sainsbury's*	1 Tbsp/15ml	14	90	0.3	14.4	3.1	0.3
Classic French, Fresh, Marks & Spencer*	1 Serving/10ml	52	515	0.6	8.2	53.1	0.2
Classic Italian, Get Dressed, Kraft*	1 Serving/25ml	30	120	0.1	5.6	10.3	0.5
Cream Cheese & Chive, Creamy Ranch, Kraft*	1 Serving/15ml	31	205	1.2	11.0	17.0	0.0
Creamy Caesar, Get Dressed, Kraft*	1 Serving/66.7g	68	102	2.1	15.0	3.5	0.1
Creamy Caesar, Waistline, Crosse & Blackwell*	1 Dtsp/11g	15	135	1.5	11.1	9.2	0.3
Creamy Ranch, 95% Fat Free, Kraft*	1 Tsp/6ml	7	111	1.4	14.5	5.0	0.3
Creamy Roasted Garlic, GFY, Asda*	1 Tbsp/15g	11	70	0.8	8.0	3.9	0.6
Creamy, Waistline, 93% Fat Free, Crosse & Blackwell*	1 Tsp/6g	7	120	1.0	14.4	6.4	0.2
Creme Fraiche, Salad, Kraft*	2 Tbsp/30ml	23	78	0.8	12.5	2.5	0.0
Dijon Honey Mustard, Briannas*	2 Tbsp/30ml	130	433	0.0	20.0	40.0	0.0
Extra Virgin Olive Oil & Balsamic Vinegar, Fresh, Safeway*	1 Serving/20ml	86	432	0.5	6.8	44.7	0.0
Fire Roasted Garlic & Thyme, Tesco*	1 Serving/10ml	45	447	0.9	4.7	47.2	0.0
Fire Roasted Red Pepper, Marks & Spencer*	1 Serving/30g	14	45	0.5	10.7	0.1	0.9
Fire Roasted Tomato Basil, COU, Marks & Spencer*	1 Serving/30g	14	45	0.6	8.1	0.9	1.1

DRESSING

INFO/WEIGHT	Measure	per Measure KCAL	KCAL	PROT	CARB	FAT	FIBRE
For Tuna, Coronation Style, Weight Watchers*	1 Can/80g	122	152	10.2	6.5	9.5	0.6
French Classic, Marks & Spencer*	1 Tbsp/15ml	77	516	0.6	8.2	53.1	0.2
French Salad, Marks & Spencer*	1 Serving/25ml	156	625	0.5	3.8	67.3	0.1
French Style Calorie-Wise Salad, Kraft*	1 Tbsp/15ml	24	160	0.0	18.7	10.7	0.0
French Style, Eat Smart, Safeway*	1 Serving/15ml	22	145	0.7	28.9	2.5	0.7
French Style, Oil Free, Healthy Eating, Tesco*	1 Tbsp/15g	5	30	0.3	6.0	0.2	1.4
French, BGTY, Organic, Sainsbury's*	1 Tbsp/15ml	11	71	0.2	8.3	4.1	0.5
French, BGTY, Sainsbury's*	1 Tbsp/15ml	12	79	1.1	8.8	4.4	0.5
French, COU, Marks & Spencer*	1/3 Bottle/105g	74	70	0.7	11.5	2.6	0.7
French, Chilled, Tesco*	1 Tbsp/15ml	63	421	1.1	15.1	39.6	0.0
French, Classic, Fat Free, Kraft*	1 Tsp/5ml	2	39	0.1	8.7	0.0	0.5
French, Classic, Sainsbury's*	1 Tbsp/15ml	71	473	1.0	5.7	49.6	0.5
French, Fresh, Florette*	1 Bottle/175ml	763	436	0.8	14.1	41.8	0.0
French, Fresh, Healthy Eating, Tesco*	1 Tbsp/15ml	8	56	1.1	6.7	2.8	0.0
French, Fresh, Organic, Sainsbury's*	1 Tbsp/15ml	45	301	0.4	5.5	31.0	0.4
French, Fresh, Safeway*	1 Tbsp/15ml	77	510	1.5	13.8	49.9	0.0
French, Fresh, Sainsbury's*	1 Tbsp/15ml	64	429	0.6	6.6	44.6	0.6
French, GFY, Asda*	1 Tbsp/15g	8	50	0.7	7.0	2.1	0.1
French, Good Intentions, Somerfield*	1 Serving/15ml	12	83	0.7	12.1	3.5	0.3
French, Healthy Living, Tesco*	1 Serving/25ml	14	56	1.1	6.7	2.8	0.0
French, Less Than 3% Fat, Marks & Spencer*	1 Tbsp/15ml	10	68	0.7	11.5	2.6	0.7
French, Luxury, Hellmann's*	1 Tbsp/15g	45	297	0.4	14.9	25.9	0.3
French, Oil Free, Perfectly Balanced, Waitrose*	1 Serving/15ml	11	72	2.2	12.2	1.6	1.1
French, Organic, Marks & Spencer*	1 Tbsp/15g	98	655	0.2	7.5	69.4	0.3
French, Organic, Tesco*	1 Tsp/5ml	23	451	0.6	11.0	44.9	0.2
French, Reduced Fat, Marks & Spencer*	1 Tbsp/15g	11	70	0.7	11.5	2.8	0.7
French, Sainsbury's*	1 Tbsp/15ml	33	219	0.6	9.8	19.1	0.5
French, Tesco*	1 Serving/25ml	110	441	0.7	7.2	44.9	0.2
Garlic & Herb, Perfectly Balanced, Waitrose*	1 Serving/50ml	68	135	0.6	29.9	1.4	0.8
Garlic & Herb, Reduced Calorie, Hellmann's*	1 Tbsp/15ml	35	232	0.6	12.8	19.3	0.4
Green Olive, Marks & Spencer*	1oz/28g	40	144	1.5	2.2	14.4	1.3
Green Thai, Coconut & Lemon Grass, Loyd Grossman*	1oz/28g	49	174	0.2	19.3	10.6	0.5
Green Thai, Finest, Tesco*	1 Bottle/250ml	940	376	0.3	19.1	32.7	0.3
Healthy Choice, Safeway*	1 Tbsp/15ml	4	29	0.2	6.3	0.3	0.0
Herb & Garlic, 5% Fat, Get Dressed, Kraft*	1 Serving/25ml	29	116	1.3	15.5	5.1	0.2
Herb 'n' Garlic, Kraft*	1 Tbsp/15ml	17	116	1.3	15.5	5.1	0.2
Herb, Eat Smart, Safeway*	1 Tbsp/15ml	9	60	0.5	9.5	2.0	0.5
Honey & Mustard, Eat Smart, Safeway*	1 Tbsp/15ml	25	165	0.8	37.5	0.9	0.3
Honey & Mustard, Finest, Tesco*	1 Serving/25ml	72	288	1.7	19.6	22.5	0.7
Honey & Mustard, Fresh, Marks & Spencer*	1 Serving/10ml	43	430	1.7	9.7	42.4	0.5
Honey & Mustard, Fresh, Safeway*	1 Serving/80ml	309	386	1.3	13.4	36.3	0.0
Honey & Mustard, GFY, Asda*	1 Tbsp/15g	13	89	1.5	13.0	3.4	0.8
Honey & Mustard, Healthy Eating, Tesco*	1 Tbsp/15g	12	79	1.5	12.1	2.7	0.9
Honey & Mustard, Healthy Living, Tesco*	1 Serving/15ml	12	82	1.0	13.5	2.7	0.9
Honey & Mustard, Kraft*	1 Serving/30ml	39	131	1.3	19.0	5.0	1.2
Honey & Mustard, Low Fat, Marks & Spencer*	1 Serving/28ml	31	110	1.5	20.0	2.5	0.8
Honey & Mustard, Marks & Spencer*	1 Tbsp/15ml	64	427	1.7	9.7	42.4	0.6
Honey & Mustard, More Than A Dressing, EPC*	1 Tsp/7g	6	91	0.5	21.6	1.0	0.5
Honey & Mustard, Sainsbury's*	1 Serving/10ml	37	366	1.0	15.4	33.0	0.1
Honey & Mustard, Tesco*	1 Serving/10ml	38	378	0.8	13.1	35.8	0.6
Honey, Orange & Mustard, BGTY, Sainsbury's*	1 Tbsp/15ml	16	105	1.8	18.6	2.5	1.8
Hot Lime & Coconut, BGTY, Sainsbury's*	1 Tbsp/15ml	8	51	0.7	5.7	2.9	1.2
Italian Balsamic, Loyd Grossman*	1 Serving/10g	36	357	0.9	13.1	33.5	0.1

DRESSING

	Measure	per Measure		Nutrition Values per 100g / 100ml				
	INFO/WEIGHT	KCAL		KCAL	PROT	CARB	FAT	FIBRE
Italian Salad, Hellmann's*	1 Serving/50g	103		206	0.7	12.8	16.7	0.0
Italian, Marks & Spencer*	1 Tbsp/15ml	62		415	0.9	8.9	41.5	1.0
Italian, Reduced Calorie, Hellmann's*	1 Serving/25ml	65		269	0.5	19.5	20.8	0.3
Italian, Waistline, 99% Fat Free, Crosse & Blackwell*	1 Tsp/6g	2		39	0.7	7.0	0.9	0.3
Lemon & Black Pepper, Good Intentions, Somerfield*	1 Tbsp/15ml	36		241	2.6	10.5	21.0	0.4
Lemon & Cracked Black Pepper, GFY, Asda*	1 Tbsp/15g	9		57	0.2	14.0	0.0	0.3
Lemon & Tarragon, Healthy Eating, Tesco*	1 Serving/10ml	11		113	1.1	21.6	2.4	0.0
Lemon & Watercress, COU, Marks & Spencer*	1 Serving/28g	14		50	0.4	8.5	1.8	0.5
Lemon, Feta & Oregano, Marks & Spencer*	1 Tbsp/15ml	24		160	1.3	8.2	13.4	0.6
Lime & Coriander, EPC*	1 Serving/50g	29		57	0.3	13.3	0.3	0.0
Lime & Coriander, Oil Free, Safeway*	1 Serving/25ml	18		70	1.5	13.2	1.2	0.0
Lime & Coriander, Sainsbury's*	1 Tbsp/15ml	61		409	0.4	10.0	40.8	0.5
Lime Sublime Creamy, Ainsley Harriott*	1 Serving/28g	95		338	0.0	10.0	32.5	0.0
Mayonnaise Style, 90% Fat Free, Weight Watchers*	1 Tsp/11g	14		125	1.7	8.9	9.2	0.0
Mild Mustard, Low Fat, Weight Watchers*	1 Tbsp/10g	6		63	2.0	5.7	3.6	0.0
Miracle Whip, Kraft*	1 Tbsp/15ml	60		400	0.3	11.0	39.0	0.1
Mustard & Dill, Perfectly Balanced, Waitrose*	1 Tbsp/15ml	24		159	1.1	31.5	3.2	1.1
Oil & Lemon	1 Tbsp/15g	97		647	0.3	2.8	70.6	0.0
Olive Oil & Balsamic Vinegar, Sainsbury's*	1 Serving/25ml	104		415	0.9	9.4	41.8	0.2
Olive Oil, Pizza Express*	2 Tsp/5g	29		573	1.4	3.4	63.0	0.0
Orange & Cracked Pepper, Tesco*	1 Tbsp/15ml	17		114	0.5	27.8	0.1	0.3
Orange & Honey, Luxury, Hellmann's*	1 Serving/15ml	17		110	0.8	17.5	3.5	0.8
Parmesan & Peppercorn, Loyd Grossman*	1oz/28g	98		349	2.1	5.9	35.2	0.5
Passion Fruit & Mango, Healthy Eating, Tesco*	1 Tbsp/15ml	25		169	0.6	36.7	2.2	0.4
Pesto, Finest, Tesco*	1 Serving/30ml	108		360	3.5	2.9	37.1	0.9
Porcini Mushroom, TTD, Sainsbury's*	1 Tbsp/15g	46		308	1.3	3.3	32.1	5.4
Provencal Roasted Vegetable, Healthy Eating, Tesco*	1 Serving/10ml	8		75	1.0	12.1	2.5	0.4
Ranch Style, Asda*	1 Serving/44ml	37		85	3.5	9.0	3.9	0.0
Raspberry Balsamic Vinegar, EPC*	1 Serving/50g	34		67	0.4	15.7	0.1	0.6
Red Pepper, Marks & Spencer*	1 Tbsp/15ml	58		385	0.6	7.6	39.2	0.5
Rich Poppy Seed, Briannas*	2 Tbsp/30ml	130		433	0.0	20.0	43.3	0.0
Roasted Red Pepper, TTD, Sainsbury's*	1 Tbsp/15ml	35		235	1.1	14.9	19.0	1.4
Salad Cream Style, Weight Watchers*	1 Tbsp/10g	12		115	1.5	16.2	4.4	0.0
Salad, BGTY, Sainsbury's*	1 Tbsp/15g	21		140	0.8	10.8	9.9	0.3
Salad, Healthy Eating, Tesco*	1 Tbsp/15g	22		144	0.7	14.0	9.5	0.5
Salad, Italian, Light, Calorie-Wise, Kraft*	1 Tbsp/15ml	6		40	0.0	5.3	2.7	0.0
Salad, Italian, Newman's Own*	1 Tbsp/10g	55		545	0.2	1.0	59.8	0.0
Salad, Kickin' Mango, Oil Free, Ainsley Harriott*	1 Tbsp/15ml	14		92	0.1	21.1	0.1	0.0
Salad, Light, Heinz*	1 Serving/9.8g	24		244	1.8	13.5	19.9	0.0
Salad, Low Fat, Weight Watchers*	1 Tbsp/10g	11		106	1.5	15.4	4.3	0.0
Salad, Luxury Caesar, Hellmann's*	1 Serving/10ml	50		498	2.5	4.4	51.7	0.3
Salad, Pizza Express*	1 Serving/5g	29		573	1.4	3.4	63.0	0.0
Salad, Raspberry Balsamic, GFY, Asda*	1 Tbsp/15ml	6		40	0.7	9.3	0.7	1.3
Salad, Sun Dried Tomato & Chilli, Loyd Grossman*	1 Tsp/5g	18		361	0.9	5.3	37.3	0.9
Salad, Thousand Island, Hellmann's*	1oz/28g	97		347	0.9	15.2	31.0	1.0
Salad, Thousand Island, Reduced Calorie, Hellmann's*	1oz/28g	73		259	1.0	19.0	19.4	0.9
Salad, Vinaigrette Style, 95% Fat Free, Asda*	1 Tbsp/15ml	6		42	0.1	10.6	0.0	0.3
Seafood, Marks & Spencer*	1 Tsp/7g	39		555	0.9	4.9	59.3	0.9
Smoked Garlic & Parmesan, Sainsbury's*	1 Serving/20ml	83		415	3.0	4.0	41.1	0.3
Sun Dried Tomato, Safeway*	1 Serving/40ml	126		314	1.1	13.8	28.3	0.0
Sun Dried Tomato, Sainsbury's	1 Serving/15ml	27		179	1.5	10.9	14.4	0.6
Sweet Chilli, COU, Marks & Spencer*	1 Tbsp/15ml	9		60	0.5	14.5	0.5	0.4
Sweetfire Pepper, Healthy Eating, Tesco*	1 Serving/10ml	7		67	0.6	15.7	0.3	0.1

	Measure INFO/WEIGHT	per Measure KCAL	Nutrition Values per 100g / 100ml				
			KCAL	PROT	CARB	FAT	FIBRE
DRESSING							
Texas Ranch, Frank Cooper*	1 Pot/28g	128	457	1.9	9.4	45.8	0.2
Thai Lime & Coriander, EPC*	1 Serving/25g	26	104	1.6	22.3	0.9	1.1
Thousand Island	1 Tsp/6g	19	323	1.1	12.5	30.2	0.4
Thousand Island, BGTY, Sainsbury's*	1 Serving/50g	53	105	1.2	21.6	1.1	2.9
Thousand Island, COU, Marks & Spencer*	1 Serving/30g	26	85	1.4	14.2	2.6	1.1
Thousand Island, Frank Cooper*	1 Pot/28g	122	437	1.2	7.2	44.8	0.3
Thousand Island, Healthy Eating, Tesco*	1 Serving/25ml	47	189	2.9	10.0	15.1	0.0
Thousand Island, Original, Kraft*	1oz/28g	102	365	0.9	19.0	31.5	0.4
Thousand Island, Reduced Calorie	1 Tsp/6g	12	195	0.7	14.7	15.2	0.0
Thousand Island, Tesco*	1 Serving/30ml	130	433	1.0	12.3	42.2	0.0
Tomato & Basil, Fresh, Somerfield*	1 Tbsp/15ml	52	348	2.0	7.0	35.0	0.0
Tomato & Basil, Healthy Living, Tesco*	1/2 Little pot/75ml	41	55	0.8	9.0	1.5	0.5
Tomato & Chipotle, TTD, Sainsbury's*	1 Tbsp/15g	57	381	0.6	6.3	39.3	2.8
Tomato & Herb, Less Than 1% Fat, Asda*	1 Tbsp/15g	6	43	0.7	8.0	0.9	0.4
Tomato & Olive, Eat Smart, Safeway*	1 Tbsp/15ml	15	100	0.7	22.8	0.7	1.8
Tomato & Red Pepper, BGTY, Sainsbury's*	1 Serving/50ml	42	83	1.1	10.0	4.3	0.6
Tomato Basil, Light, Kraft*	1 Serving/15ml	10	68	1.0	14.5	0.4	2.5
True Blue Cheese, Briannas*	2 Tbsp/30ml	120	400	3.3	16.7	36.7	0.0
Tuna Mayonnaise & Sweetcorn Style, Weight Watchers*	1 Can/80g	114	142	11.5	6.2	8.0	0.1
Tuna, Tomato & Herb, Weight Watchers*	1 Can/80g	79	99	11.6	5.1	3.6	0.5
Waistline, Reduced Fat, Crosse & Blackwell*	1oz/28g	29	105	0.8	11.6	6.0	0.3
Whole Grain Dijon Mustard & Honey, Loyd Grossman*	1oz/28g	93	331	1.2	9.9	31.8	1.3
Yoghurt & Mint, GFY, Asda*	1 Tbsp/15ml	9	60	3.9	8.0	1.4	0.0
Yoghurt & Mint, Healthy Living, Tesco*	1 Serving/50g	31	62	4.1	6.9	2.5	0.2
Yoghurt & Mint, Perfectly Balanced, Waitrose*	1 Serving/100ml	130	130	4.6	22.1	2.6	0.7
Yoghurt Mint Cucumber, Marks & Spencer*	1 Tsp/5ml	6	115	1.0	8.7	8.0	0.0
Yogurt & Mint, Safeway*	1 Serving/15ml	54	360	3.3	6.7	35.3	0.0
DRIED FRUIT							
& Nut, The Mix, Whitworths*	1 Pot/90g	341	379	4.1	63.1	14.6	7.3
& Nuts, Marks & Spencer*	1 Serving/28g	126	450	12.4	44.3	25.3	6.0
5 Fruits, Ready To Eat, Sundora*	1/2 Pack/100g	233	233	1.6	58.4	0.4	6.8
Baby Mix, Somerfield*	1 Packet/250g	520	208	3.1	47.2	0.7	5.3
Exotic Mix, Sundora*	1 Sm Pack/50g	138	276	2.3	60.6	2.7	3.8
Exotic, Ready To Eat, Sainsbury's*	1/3 Pack/85g	241	284	0.2	70.6	0.1	2.4
Luxury Mixed, Co-Op*	1 Serving/40g	114	285	2.0	68.0	0.6	4.0
Mix, Taste Of Hawaii, Extra Special, Asda*	1 Serving/100g	314	314	1.7	75.0	0.8	4.4
Mix, Taste Of New England, Asda*	1 Serving/50g	158	316	2.2	74.0	1.2	5.0
Mixed	1 Tbsp/25g	67	268	2.3	68.1	0.4	2.2
Mixed, Albert Heijn*	1 Serving/50g	110	220	2.1	51.0	0.5	0.0
Mixed, Tesco*	1 Tbsp/25g	71	284	2.3	67.9	0.4	2.2
Natural Mix, Positively Healthy, The Food Doctor*	1 Serving/50g	164	328	2.4	77.9	0.7	3.6
Salad, Whitworths*	1 Serving/62g	113	183	2.9	41.8	0.5	6.6
DRIFTER							
Nestle*	1 Finger/31g	143	478	3.7	67.3	21.5	0.8
DRINK MIX							
100% Egg White Powder, Tropicana*	2 Tbsp/20g	66	328	82.0	0.0	0.0	0.0
DRINKING CHOCOLATE							
Cadbury*	3 Heaped Tsp/25g	91	365	6.4	72.4	5.8	0.0
Dry Powder, Cocodirect*	1 Serving/18g	67	372	8.9	65.1	8.4	0.0
Dry, Asda*	1 Serving/30g	111	370	6.0	73.0	6.0	0.0
Dry, Tesco*	3 Tsp/25g	92	368	6.4	72.6	5.8	4.2
Dry, Waitrose*	3 Tsp/12g	48	403	7.2	79.9	6.1	2.9
Granules, Dry, Impress*	1oz/28g	102	365	5.6	77.0	3.7	6.0

	Measure	per Measure		Nutrition Values per 100g / 100ml				
	INFO/WEIGHT	KCAL		KCAL	PROT	CARB	FAT	FIBRE

DRINKING CHOCOLATE
Made Up, BGTY, Sainsbury's*	1 Serving/178.1g	114		64	3.9	11.4	0.2	0.7
Maxpax, Light, Suchard*	1 Cup/10.5g	39		355	20.0	56.0	5.5	9.3
Powder, Made Up With Skimmed Milk	1 Mug/227ml	134		59	3.5	10.8	0.6	0.0
Powder, Made Up With Whole Milk	1 Mug/227ml	204		90	3.4	10.6	4.1	0.0

DRIPPING
Beef	1oz/28g	249		891	0.0	0.0	99.0	0.0

DUCK
Breast, Meat Only, Cooked, Average	1oz/28g	48		173	25.3	1.8	7.1	0.0
Breast, Meat Only, Raw, Average	1 Serving/160g	206		129	22.6	0.1	4.3	0.2
Leg, Meat & Skin, Average	1oz/28g	80		286	17.2	9.5	20.0	0.4
Raw, Meat, Fat & Skin	1oz/28g	109		388	13.1	0.0	37.3	0.0
Roasted, Meat, Fat & Skin	1oz/28g	118		423	20.0	0.0	38.1	0.0
Wings, Chinese Barbecue, Sainsbury's*	1 Serving/175g	430		246	19.4	9.7	14.3	0.0

DUCK &
Orange Sauce, Gressingham Fillets, TTD, Sainsbury's*	1/2 Pack/250g	633		253	24.9	0.1	17.0	1.0
Plum Sauce, Roasted, Sainsbury's*	1/2 Pack/150g	174		116	6.9	16.0	2.5	1.8

DUCK A L' ORANGE
Roast, Marks & Spencer*	1/2 Pack/270g	554		205	12.5	4.1	15.6	0.6

DUCK AROMATIC
Crispy, Asda*	1/3 Pack/165.7g	470		283	19.0	18.0	15.0	0.8
Crispy, Ready Meals, Marks & Spencer*	1 Pack/275g	523		190	13.9	14.0	8.6	2.1
Crispy, Somerfield*	1 Serving/265g	782		295	18.1	14.0	18.5	0.7
Crispy, Tesco*	1 Serving/61g	126		207	14.3	14.3	11.6	0.8
With Plum Sauce, Tesco*	1/2 Pack/250g	350		140	9.3	15.2	4.6	0.3
With a Plum Sauce, Finest, Tesco*	1 Serving/250g	400		160	16.1	11.3	5.6	4.6

DUCK CANTONESE
Style, Roast, Tesco*	1 Pack/300g	375		125	8.2	17.9	2.3	0.5

DUCK IN
A Pluauce, Crispy, Marks & Spencer*	1 Pack/325g	569		175	10.7	11.2	9.6	0.9
Orange Sauce, Iceland*	1 Serving/200g	336		168	11.3	7.4	10.4	1.2
Oriental Sauce, Iceland*	1 Pack/201.1g	352		175	12.0	6.3	11.3	1.5
Red Wine Sauce, Free Range Fillets, Waitrose*	1/2 Pack/250g	378		151	16.4	4.1	7.7	2.2

DUCK PEKING
Crispy, Aromatic, Sainsbury's*	1/2 Pack/300g	1236		412	19.5	0.6	36.9	0.1
Crispy, Cherry Valley*	1 Serving/270g	629		233	14.8	17.5	11.5	0.5

DUCK WITH
Apple & Calvados, Goujons, GFY, Asda*	1 Pack/320g	362		113	16.0	6.0	2.8	0.8
Apple & Calvados Sauce, GFY, Asda*	1 Serving/162g	144		89	13.0	4.2	2.2	1.4
Diuelection, Marks & Spencer*	1 Serving/67g	194		290	7.2	34.8	13.4	2.2
Noodles, Shanghai Roast, Sainsbury's*	1 Pack/450g	581		129	5.6	18.0	3.8	1.2
Orange Sauce, Fillet, Waitrose*	1/2 Pack/250g	418		167	12.0	7.1	9.9	3.9
Pancakes, Shredded, Iceland*	1 Pack/220g	471		214	20.4	27.0	2.7	1.5
Pancakes, With Hoisin Sauce, Marks & Spencer*	1 Pack/80g	136		170	13.0	19.9	4.0	0.9

DUETTO
Pasta, Green & White, Pasta Reale*	1oz/28g	79		281	10.9	49.4	6.0	3.6

DUMPLINGS
Average	1oz/28g	58		208	2.8	24.5	11.7	0.9
Homestyle, Aunt Bessie's*	1 Dumpling/49g	187		382	8.5	39.5	21.1	2.1
Prawn Sui Mai, Marks & Spencer*	1 Serving/25g	29		115	14.6	5.4	3.7	0.6
Prawn, Cantonese, Crispy, Sainsbury's*	1 Dumpling/11g	27		241	9.3	20.9	13.4	1.1

D

EASTER EGG

	Measure INFO/WEIGHT	per Measure KCAL	KCAL	PROT	CARB	FAT	FIBRE
Buttons, Cadbury*	1 Pack/200g	1050	525	7.6	56.1	30.1	0.0
Disney, Nestle*	1 Egg/65g	342	526	6.3	59.7	29.1	0.6
Kit Kat, Chunky, Nestle*	1 Pack/235g	1224	521	5.9	60.3	28.5	0.8
Mars*	1 Serving/62.6g	283	449	4.2	69.0	17.4	0.0
Milk Chocolate, Nestle*	1/2 Egg/42g	205	489	5.0	65.2	23.1	0.5
Milky Bar, Nestle*	1 Egg/40g	182	454	4.2	70.8	17.2	0.0
Smarties, Nestle*	1/2 Egg/37.5g	182	478	4.8	69.6	20.0	0.7

ECLAIR

	Measure INFO/WEIGHT	per Measure KCAL	KCAL	PROT	CARB	FAT	FIBRE
Chocolate, 25% Less Fat, Sainsbury's*	1 Eclair/58g	171	295	6.8	31.1	16.0	1.2
Chocolate, Asda*	1 Eclair/50g	192	383	6.0	20.0	31.0	0.5
Chocolate, Dairy Cream, Co-Op*	1 Eclair/29g	122	420	6.0	23.0	34.0	0.6
Chocolate, Dairy Cream, Safeway*	1 Eclair/27g	101	373	4.1	32.1	26.2	0.4
Chocolate, Fresh Cream, Jumbo, Co-Op*	1 Eclair/94g	357	380	4.0	27.0	28.0	2.0
Chocolate, Fresh Cream, Marks & Spencer*	1 Eclair/62g	242	390	5.2	25.4	29.8	0.6
Chocolate, Fresh Cream, Mini, Tesco*	1 Cake/28g	111	397	4.8	33.6	27.0	0.4
Chocolate, Fresh Cream, Safeway*	1 Eclair/59g	210	356	4.1	24.8	26.7	0.4
Chocolate, Fresh Cream, Sainsbury's*	1 Eclair/59g	218	370	4.4	27.1	27.2	0.5
Chocolate, Fresh, Cream, Tesco*	1 Eclair/66g	281	425	6.3	33.2	29.7	2.1
Chocolate, Healthy Living, Tesco*	1 Serving/77g	192	249	6.8	27.1	12.6	0.9
Chocolate, Mini, Iceland*	1 Eclair/13g	55	426	4.9	21.5	35.6	0.4
Chocolate, Sainsbury's*	1/2 Eclair/30g	104	347	4.0	31.7	22.7	0.3
Chocolate, Tesco*	1 Eclair/66.0g	281	426	6.0	31.1	30.9	1.8
Chocolate, Weight Watchers*	1 Serving/30g	83	278	4.1	36.7	12.7	7.0
Dairy Cream, Safeway*	1 Eclair/59.3g	210	356	4.1	24.9	26.7	0.4

EEL

	Measure INFO/WEIGHT	per Measure KCAL	KCAL	PROT	CARB	FAT	FIBRE
Jellied	1oz/28g	27	98	8.4	0.0	7.1	0.0
Raw	1oz/28g	47	168	16.6	0.0	11.3	0.0

EGGS

	Measure INFO/WEIGHT	per Measure KCAL	KCAL	PROT	CARB	FAT	FIBRE
Dried	1oz/28g	159	568	48.4	0.0	41.6	0.0
Duck, Boiled & Salted	1 Egg/75g	149	198	14.6	0.0	15.5	0.0
Duck, Whole, Raw	1 Egg/75g	122	163	14.3	0.0	11.8	0.0
Free Range, Large, Average	1 Egg/65g	95	147	12.4	0.0	10.8	0.0
Free Range, Medium, Average	1 Serving/56g	82	147	12.3	0.1	10.9	0.0
Fried	1 Med/60g	107	179	13.6	0.0	13.9	0.0
Large, Average	1 Serving/63g	92	147	12.5	0.1	10.8	0.1
Medium, Average	1 Egg/56g	82	148	12.5	0.0	10.8	0.0
Medium, Boiled, Average	1 Size One/67g	98	147	12.5	0.0	10.8	0.0
Poached	1 Med/50g	74	147	12.5	0.0	10.8	0.0
Quail, Whole, Raw	1oz/28g	42	151	12.9	0.0	11.1	0.0
Scrambled	1 Egg/68g	100	147	12.5	0.0	10.8	0.0
Scrambled With Milk	2 Med Egg/120g	296	247	10.7	0.6	22.6	0.0
Turkey, Whole, Raw	1oz/28g	46	165	13.7	0.0	12.2	0.0
White, Dried	1oz/28g	83	295	73.8	0.0	0.0	0.0
Whites, Raw, Average	1oz/28g	12	44	10.0	0.2	0.3	0.0
Whole, Raw	1 Size Three/57g	84	147	12.5	0.0	10.8	0.0
Yolks, Raw	1 Av Yolk/14g	47	339	16.1	0.0	30.5	0.0

ELDERBERRIES

	Measure INFO/WEIGHT	per Measure KCAL	KCAL	PROT	CARB	FAT	FIBRE
Average	1oz/28g	10	35	0.7	7.4	0.5	0.0

ELICHE

	Measure INFO/WEIGHT	per Measure KCAL	KCAL	PROT	CARB	FAT	FIBRE
Pasta, Buitoni*	1 Serving/80g	282	352	11.2	72.6	1.9	0.0

ENCHILADAS

	Measure INFO/WEIGHT	per Measure KCAL	KCAL	PROT	CARB	FAT	FIBRE
Chicken, American, Healthy Living, Tesco*	1 Serving/240g	353	147	10.4	22.5	1.8	1.2
Chicken, Asda*	1 Serving/500g	690	138	10.0	17.0	6.0	1.0

E

	Measure INFO/WEIGHT	per Measure KCAL	Nutrition Values per 100g / 100ml				
			KCAL	PROT	CARB	FAT	FIBRE
ENCHILADAS							
Chicken, In A Spicy Salsa & Bean Sauce, Asda*	1/2 Pack/211.9g	373	176	10.0	16.0	8.0	0.0
Chicken, Marks & Spencer*	1 Serving/225g	405	180	9.2	11.5	10.6	2.2
Chicken, Perfectly Balanced, Waitrose*	1 Pack/450g	482	107	6.9	12.7	3.2	1.1
Chicken, Safeway*	1 Serving/230g	384	167	7.9	22.9	4.9	1.0
Chicken, Value, Tesco*	1 Serving/212g	297	140	7.0	19.3	3.9	1.1
Chilli Beef, Asda*	1 Serving/225g	428	190	12.0	13.0	10.0	1.1
Vegetable, GFY, Asda*	1 Pack/350g	399	114	4.4	14.0	4.5	1.3
ENDIVE							
Raw	1oz/28g	4	13	1.8	1.0	0.2	2.0
ENERGY DRINK							
Burn, The Coca Cola Co*	1fl oz/30ml	13	44	0.0	10.5	0.0	0.0
Lemon, Active Sport, Tesco*	1 Serving/500ml	135	27	0.0	6.5	0.0	0.0
Red Rooster, Hi Energy Mixer, Cott Beverages Ltd*	1 Can/250ml	113	45	0.6	10.3	0.0	0.0
Red Thunder, Aldi*	1 Can/250ml	113	45	0.6	10.3	0.0	0.0
Redcard, Britvic*	1 Can/330ml	96	29	0.1	7.0	0.0	0.0
V, Frucor Beverages*	1 Can/250ml	113	45	0.0	11.2	0.0	0.0
ESCALOPE							
Mushroom, Vegetarian, Creamy, Tesco*	1 Pack/300g	765	255	10.0	20.0	15.0	2.0

E

	Measure INFO/WEIGHT	per Measure KCAL	Nutrition Values per 100g / 100ml				
			KCAL	PROT	CARB	FAT	FIBRE
FAGGOTS							
In Rich Gravy, Iceland*	1 Faggot/81g	116	143	6.5	15.9	6.4	1.1
Mushy Peas & Mash, Sainsbury's*	1 Pack/450g	576	128	6.0	16.3	4.3	1.6
Pork, Mr Brains*	1 Serving/189g	242	128	5.3	11.9	6.6	0.6
FAGOTTINI							
Mushroom, Sainsbury's*	1/2 Pack/155g	339	219	10.2	27.7	7.5	2.7
FAJITA							
Beef, GFY, Asda*	1/2 Pack/208g	354	170	11.0	21.0	4.7	1.6
Chicken With Salsa & Sour Cream Dips, Safeway*	1 Pack/242g	390	161	9.8	16.7	6.1	1.9
Chicken, American Style, Tesco*	1 Pack/275g	388	141	9.5	14.2	5.1	1.0
Chicken, American, Healthy Living, Tesco*	1 Serving/275g	300	109	9.5	12.9	2.2	1.0
Chicken, Asda*	1/2 Pack/225g	371	165	11.0	20.0	4.5	3.5
Chicken, BGTY, Sainsbury's*	1 Pack/299g	446	149	10.1	24.8	2.5	1.7
Chicken, Boots*	1 Pack/223g	448	201	9.1	25.0	7.2	3.9
Chicken, COU, Marks & Spencer*	1 Pack/230g	288	125	10.0	16.5	2.3	1.5
Chicken, Char Grilled Style, Safeway*	1/2 Pack/234.8g	588	250	17.2	40.5	2.3	1.9
Chicken, Eat Smart, Safeway*	1 Serving/248g	290	117	10.6	14.8	1.7	1.6
Chicken, Finest, Tesco*	1 Serving/275g	481	175	12.1	15.9	7.0	0.9
Chicken, GFY, Asda*	1/2 Pack/225g	233	104	9.3	12.9	1.8	2.0
Chicken, Healthy Living, Tesco*	1 Serving/275g	503	183	9.5	31.8	2.0	1.5
Chicken, Just Cook, Sainsbury's*	1/2 Pack/200g	200	100	18.5	3.1	1.5	2.0
Chicken, Marks & Spencer*	1 Pack/230g	345	150	8.6	17.7	5.3	1.0
Chicken, Morrisons*	1 Serving/300g	370	123	7.4	12.2	5.1	1.9
Chicken, Sainsbury's*	1/2 Pack/275g	396	144	9.5	14.5	5.3	1.9
Chicken, Salt Balanced, COU, Marks & Spencer*	1 Pack/230g	253	110	9.5	13.2	2.3	1.7
Chicken, Shapers, Boots*	1 Pack/192g	307	160	9.3	24.0	3.0	1.7
Chicken, Tesco*	1 Serving/275g	349	127	8.6	14.5	3.8	1.0
Chicken, Value, Tesco*	1 Serving/250g	255	102	6.9	13.2	2.4	1.5
Chicken, Weight Watchers*	1 Pack/175g	271	155	8.6	24.1	2.7	1.2
Dinner Kit, With Tortillas, Old El Paso*	1 Serving/163g	559	343	10.0	60.0	7.0	0.0
Gammon Steaks, Tesco*	1 Serving/250g	368	147	17.5	5.3	6.2	0.0
Steak, Marks & Spencer*	1oz/28g	53	190	8.9	17.2	9.1	0.6
Tuna, Eat Smart, Safeway*	1 Pack/263g	302	115	9.7	15.0	1.8	1.4
Tuna, Sainsbury's*	1 Pack/450g	752	167	11.4	18.2	5.4	1.6
Vegetable, Somerfield*	1 Pack/500g	640	128	3.0	17.0	5.0	0.0
Vegetable, Tesco*	1 Wrap/112g	133	119	4.2	14.3	5.0	1.1
FALAFEL							
Cauldron*	1 Falafel/25g	37	149	7.6	15.3	6.4	7.1
Fried in Vegetable Oil	1oz/28g	50	179	6.4	15.6	11.2	3.4
Marks & Spencer*	1 Serving/165g	388	235	8.3	19.2	13.7	8.4
Mini, Marks & Spencer*	1 Falafel/13g	40	310	7.9	28.1	18.4	2.6
Mini, Sainsbury's*	1 Serving/168g	499	297	8.0	26.8	17.6	3.2
Organic, Cauldron*	1 Falafel/25g	55	220	8.0	23.3	10.5	7.6
Vegab Mat AB, Vegab*	1 Falafel/20g	62	309	11.0	28.0	17.0	0.0
Vegetarian, Organic, Waitrose*	1 Felafel/25g	55	220	8.0	23.3	10.5	7.6
FANTA							
Fruit Twist, The Coca Cola Co*	1 Serving/250ml	133	53	0.0	13.0	0.0	0.0
Lemon, The Coca Cola Co*	1 Can/330ml	165	50	0.0	12.0	0.0	0.0
Light, The Coca Cola Co*	1 Glass/250ml	5	2	0.0	0.5	0.0	0.0
Orange, The Coca Cola Co*	1 Can/330ml	142	43	0.0	10.4	0.0	0.0
Orange, Z, The Coca Cola Co*	1 Can/500ml	15	3	0.0	0.5	0.0	0.0
Summer Fruits, Z, The Coca Cola Co*	1fl oz/30ml	1	3	0.0	0.6	0.0	0.0
FARFALLE							
Bows, Dry, Average	1 Serving/75g	265	353	11.4	72.6	1.9	1.9

F

	Measure INFO/WEIGHT	per Measure KCAL	Nutrition Values per 100g / 100ml				
			KCAL	PROT	CARB	FAT	FIBRE
FARFALLE							
Dry, Average	1 Serving/50g	178	357	11.7	73.5	1.8	2.7
Salmon & Broccoli, Eat Smart, Safeway*	1 Pack/380g	361	95	6.4	11.6	2.4	1.1
FARFALLINE							
Bows, Mini, Tesco*	1oz/28g	93	333	13.2	65.6	2.0	2.9
FENNEL							
Florence, Boiled in Salted Water	1oz/28g	3	11	0.9	1.5	0.2	2.3
Florence, Raw	1oz/28g	3	12	0.9	1.8	0.2	2.4
FENUGREEK LEAVES							
Raw	1oz/28g	10	35	4.6	4.8	0.2	0.0
FETTUCINI							
Buitoni*	1oz/28g	101	362	12.2	74.4	1.7	0.0
Cajun Chicken, COU, Marks & Spencer*	1 Pack/350g	370	106	7.9	13.9	2.1	1.1
Chicken Mushroom, GFY, Asda*	1 Pack/400g	359	90	7.3	11.3	1.8	0.7
Garlic Mushroom, GFY, Asda*	1 Pack/450g	347	77	3.3	12.0	1.7	0.9
With Tomato & Mushroom, Easy Cook, Napolina*	1 Pack/120g	461	384	11.8	67.9	7.2	0.0
FIG ROLLS							
Asda*	1 Biscuit/19g	71	372	4.8	68.0	9.0	0.0
Go Ahead, McVitie's*	1 Roll/15g	55	365	4.2	76.8	4.6	2.9
Jacobs*	1 Biscuit/17g	61	357	3.5	67.7	8.0	3.9
Sainsbury's*	1 Biscuit/18g	70	377	4.8	68.3	9.4	2.6
Vitalinea, Jacobs*	1 Biscuit/18g	61	339	3.7	68.2	5.8	3.8
FIGS							
Dried, Average	1 Fruit/14g	32	232	3.6	53.2	1.1	8.7
Raw, Average	1 Fig/35g	16	45	1.3	9.8	0.2	1.5
FIORELLI							
Egg, Marks & Spencer*	1 Serving/100g	355	355	13.9	68.5	2.8	3.0
Mozzarella, Tomato & Basil, Waitrose*	1 Serving/125g	353	282	10.8	38.9	9.3	1.7
FISH							
Balls, Gefilte, Marks & Spencer*	1 Pack/200g	280	140	14.1	11.9	3.9	1.0
Balls, Steamed	1oz/28g	21	74	11.8	5.5	0.5	0.0
Battered, Portion, Ross*	1 Fish/100g	203	203	10.4	16.1	10.8	0.8
Battered, White, Skinless & Boneless, Farmfoods*	1 Serving/122g	238	195	9.3	16.7	10.1	2.3
Breaded, Asda*	1 Serving/150g	351	234	15.0	12.0	14.0	0.5
Breaded, Fishysaurus, Young'uns, Young's*	1 Fishysaurus/70g	143	204	11.4	15.5	10.7	1.5
Breaded, Pollock, Asda*	1 Portion/97g	200	206	12.0	17.0	10.0	1.0
Dried, Small, Ogura*	1 Serving/10g	32	320	69.0	0.3	3.0	0.0
Fillets, Crunch Crumb, Steaks, Birds Eye*	1 Steak/110g	264	240	15.0	18.0	12.0	0.9
Fillets, Garlic & Herb, Young's*	1 Fillet/117.6g	262	222	11.0	16.2	12.6	1.4
Fillets, Lemon & Pepper, Young's*	1 Fillet/130g	283	218	10.3	15.3	12.9	4.3
Fillets, White, Breaded, Tesco*	1 Piece/95g	198	208	10.6	16.9	10.9	1.0
Fillets, White, Breaded, Value, Tesco*	1 serving/100g	192	192	10.6	15.6	9.7	2.2
Fillets, White, Natural, Tesco*	1 Fillet/100g	72	72	16.6	0.0	0.6	0.0
Goujons, Asda*	1 Serving/125g	240	192	12.8	20.8	6.4	0.2
In Batter, Crispy, Birds Eye*	1 Steak/120g	230	192	13.6	11.6	10.1	0.7
In Batter, Light, Iceland*	1 Fillet/120g	230	192	13.6	11.6	10.1	0.7
In Batter, Morrisons*	1 Fish/140g	235	168	14.0	15.0	5.8	0.2
In Batter, Young's*	1 Serving/100g	315	315	14.9	20.4	19.7	0.8
Nuggets, Battered, Farmfoods*	1oz/28g	60	214	10.9	16.0	11.8	0.7
Portion, Chip Shop, Young's*	1 Portion/135g	315	233	11.0	15.1	14.6	0.6
Portions, In Oven Crisp Batter, Value, Tesco*	1 Serving/100g	209	209	11.0	16.4	11.0	2.6
Salted, Chinese, Steamed	1oz/28g	43	155	33.9	0.0	2.2	0.0
Simply, Birds Eye*	1 Serving/123.7g	246	198	12.6	14.2	10.1	0.6
Steaks, Chip Shop, Young's*	1 Portion/100g	198	198	11.0	14.9	10.4	0.9

F

	Measure INFO/WEIGHT	per Measure KCAL	Nutrition Values per 100g / 100ml				
			KCAL	PROT	CARB	FAT	FIBRE
FISH							
Steaks, Skinless & Boneless, Young's*	1 Serving/104.7g	225	214	10.5	16.6	11.8	0.8
Tilapia, Raw, Average	10g	10	95	20.0	0.0	1.0	0.0
White, Tesco*	1 Med Fillet/100g	78	78	16.6	0.0	0.6	0.0
FISH & CHIPS							
Breaded, Budgens*	1 Pack/340g	544	160	8.6	19.3	5.3	1.5
Budgens*	1 Pack/284g	625	220	8.0	24.5	10.0	2.3
Cod, Asda*	1 Serving/279.5g	451	161	8.0	21.0	5.0	1.1
Cod, Healthy Living, Tesco*	1 Pack/400g	492	123	5.3	21.4	1.8	1.7
Cod, Oven Crisp Crumb, Waitrose*	1 Serving/283g	415	147	6.6	17.2	5.7	2.5
Cod, Waitrose*	1 Pack/283g	849	300	14.4	33.7	12.0	4.8
Haddock, Scottish, & Chunky Chips, Marks & Spencer*	1 Pack/343.3g	515	150	7.3	16.0	6.5	2.1
Ross*	1 Serving/250g	415	166	6.2	18.1	7.6	1.6
Tesco*	1 Serving/300g	489	163	5.5	21.2	6.2	1.6
FISH BAKE							
Cheese & Leek, Healthy Living, Tesco*	1 Pack/400g	340	85	11.0	5.8	2.0	0.8
Cheese Pastry, Birds Eye*	1 Piece/171g	390	228	9.3	17.2	13.6	1.9
Haddock & Prawn, COU, Marks & Spencer*	1 Bake/340g	289	85	7.3	7.3	2.8	0.4
Italiano, Birds Eye*	1/2 Pack/205g	180	88	11.5	3.6	3.1	0.3
Mediterranean, Healthy Living, Tesco*	1/2 Pack/200g	158	79	10.3	5.9	1.6	1.4
Vegetable Tuscany, Birds Eye*	1/2 Pack/204.3g	235	115	13.1	4.3	5.0	0.2
FISH CAKES							
Breaded, Sainsbury's*	1 Cake/42g	75	179	10.0	16.2	8.1	0.7
Bubbly Batter, Young's*	1 Fish Cake/44.1g	109	247	7.1	20.5	15.1	1.4
Captain's Coins, Mini, Birds Eye*	1 Fish Cake/20g	34	168	10.1	13.3	8.3	0.9
Cod, & Pancetta, Cafe Culture, Marks & Spencer*	1 Fish Cake/85g	166	195	9.2	7.2	15.5	2.0
Cod, & Parsley, Waitrose*	1 Fish Cake/85g	157	185	10.7	13.1	10.0	2.0
Cod, Asda*	1 Fish Cake/72.2g	163	227	7.0	25.0	11.0	2.3
Cod, Fresh, Asda*	1 Serving/75g	164	219	7.0	23.0	11.0	1.6
Cod, Homemade	1 Fish Cake/50g	121	241	9.3	14.4	16.6	0.7
Cod, In Crunch Crumb, Birds Eye*	1 Fish Cake/52g	85	163	8.8	16.2	7.0	0.7
Cod, Large, Sainsbury's*	1 Fish Cake/90g	176	195	9.5	17.5	9.0	0.8
Cod, Marks & Spencer*	1 Fish Cake/85g	162	190	8.4	15.7	10.1	1.6
Cod, Sainsbury's*	1 Fishcake/39g	75	192	10.8	17.5	8.8	0.8
Cod, Tesco*	1 Fish Cake/49g	110	224	8.9	23.8	10.4	0.2
Cod, Young's*	1 Cake/75g	144	192	7.6	22.1	8.3	1.1
Crab, & Prawn, Thai, Tesco*	1 Fish Cake/115g	269	234	8.8	17.4	14.4	1.2
Crab, Marks & Spencer*	1oz/28g	63	225	8.0	18.0	13.2	1.4
Fried in Blended Oil	1 Fish Cake/50g	109	218	8.6	16.8	13.4	0.0
Frozen	1oz/28g	37	132	8.6	16.7	3.9	0.0
Great Value, Iceland*	1 Fish Cake/42.3g	74	175	9.1	20.3	6.4	1.6
Grilled	1 Fish Cake/50g	77	154	9.9	19.7	4.5	0.0
Haddock, Asda*	1 Fish Cake/88g	181	206	8.0	21.0	10.0	1.5
Haddock, Marks & Spencer*	1 Pack/170g	289	170	8.6	13.7	9.2	1.3
Haddock, Sainsbury's*	1 Fish Cake/90g	173	192	11.7	18.1	8.1	0.7
Haddock, Smoked, Asda*	1 Fish Cake/90g	185	206	10.0	19.0	10.0	1.4
Haddock, Smoked, Frozen, Waitrose*	1 Fish Cake/85g	157	185	11.0	12.4	10.1	2.1
Haddock, Smoked, Marks & Spencer*	1 Cake/85g	153	180	10.6	13.4	9.4	2.6
Haddock, Smoked, Sainsbury's*	1 Fish Cake/63.2g	127	201	11.0	17.8	9.5	2.1
Haddock, Smoked, TTD, Sainsbury's*	1 Cake/115g	232	202	11.6	19.2	8.7	1.0
Haddock, Smoked, Tesco*	1 Fish Cake/90g	197	219	10.3	21.0	10.4	0.2
Haddock, Smoked, Waitrose*	1 Serving/170g	372	219	8.9	19.5	11.7	2.1
Halibut Cod Loin, Finest, Tesco*	1 Serving/115g	213	185	8.8	21.3	7.2	1.4
Halibut, TTD, Sainsbury's*	1 Cake/115g	289	251	10.0	17.6	15.6	1.3

FISH CAKES

	Measure INFO/WEIGHT	per Measure KCAL	KCAL	PROT	CARB	FAT	FIBRE
Makes Sense, Somerfield*	1 Fish Cake/42.2g	70	166	8.2	18.7	6.5	1.5
Marks & Spencer*	1 Fish Cake/80g	180	225	8.0	18.0	13.3	0.0
Prawn, Battered, Asda*	1 Serving/90g	182	202	10.0	15.6	11.1	1.0
Prawn, Chunky, Sainsbury's*	1 Cake/90g	185	205	9.2	20.8	9.4	1.3
Prawn, Sainsbury's*	1 Fish Cake/90g	154	171	10.3	15.6	7.5	0.7
Prawn, Tesco*	1 Fish Cake/90g	209	232	8.2	29.2	9.1	1.8
Ross*	1 Fish Cake/52g	102	196	9.6	18.6	9.2	0.8
Salmon & Haddock, With Lemon & Dill Sauce, Waitrose*	1 Serving/187g	304	163	9.2	9.7	9.7	1.5
Salmon, & Asparagus, Finest, Tesco*	1 Serving/115g	300	261	10.7	19.6	15.5	0.4
Salmon, & Broccoli, Morrisons*	1 Fish Cake/60g	126	210	9.8	17.2	11.9	1.3
Salmon, & Broccoli, With Bubble & Squeak, Safeway*	1 Pack/389g	513	132	3.9	15.0	6.3	1.0
Salmon, & Dill, Waitrose*	1 Fish Cake/85g	179	211	9.1	17.6	11.6	2.2
Salmon, & Tarragon, Waitrose*	1 Fish Cake/85g	179	211	11.9	14.3	11.8	2.2
Salmon, Asda*	1 Fish Cake/86g	215	250	8.0	23.0	14.0	1.4
Salmon, Birds Eye*	1 Fish Cake/50g	84	168	9.5	12.2	9.0	1.4
Salmon, Breaded, Crispy, Frozen, Sainsbury's*	1 Cake/60g	140	234	12.2	13.7	14.5	1.9
Salmon, Chunky, Sainsbury's*	1 Fish Cake/84g	192	228	13.2	15.8	12.5	2.9
Salmon, Homemade	1 Fish Cake/50g	137	273	10.4	14.4	19.7	0.7
Salmon, In Crunch Crumb, Birds Eye*	2 Cakes/99g	214	216	9.7	15.0	13.0	1.4
Salmon, Marks & Spencer*	1 Fish Cake/86g	181	210	9.1	15.1	12.7	1.7
Salmon, Morrisons*	1 Fish Cake/90g	241	268	10.1	27.6	13.1	1.5
Salmon, Sainsbury's*	1 Fish Cake/90g	167	186	13.2	17.4	7.1	1.2
Salmon, Tesco*	1 Fishcake/90g	239	266	11.4	21.3	15.0	0.0
Salmon, With Lemon Butter Sauce, Finest, Tesco*	1 Cake/220g	524	238	7.3	10.9	18.3	1.0
Salmon, With Parsley Sauce, Finest, Tesco*	1/2 Pack/170g	350	206	8.6	11.7	13.9	1.0
SmartPrice, Asda*	1 Fish Cake/41.5g	77	188	7.0	22.0	8.0	0.9
Thai Style, Sainsbury's*	1 Fish Cake/49g	69	141	12.0	13.8	4.2	1.7
Thai, Finest, Tesco*	1 Cake/65g	150	230	7.5	20.3	13.2	1.6
Thai, Frozen, Sainsbury's*	1 Cake/15g	28	187	21.3	9.3	7.3	0.7
Thai, Oriental Selection, Waitrose*	1 Cake/11.2g	18	161	17.8	15.8	3.0	1.5
Thai, Tesco*	4 Cakes/88.9g	148	166	17.4	12.8	5.0	1.1
Tuna, & Red Pepper, Waitrose*	1 Fish Cake/85g	175	206	9.5	15.4	11.8	1.6
Tuna, Asda*	1 Fish Cake/87.2g	171	196	9.0	22.0	8.0	1.3
Tuna, Sainsbury's*	1 Cake/90g	197	219	14.4	26.7	6.1	0.9
Tuna, Tesco*	1 Fishcake/90g	222	247	12.8	25.4	10.5	0.2
Value, Tesco*	1 Fish Cake/40g	74	183	7.1	21.2	7.8	1.2

FISH FINGERS

	Measure INFO/WEIGHT	per Measure KCAL	KCAL	PROT	CARB	FAT	FIBRE
Atlantis*	1 Finger/30g	52	172	12.0	14.0	7.5	0.4
Chip Shop, Young's*	1 Finger/30g	75	251	9.3	16.6	16.4	1.2
Cod, 100% Cod Fillet, Tesco*	1 Finger/30g	53	177	12.4	14.9	7.5	1.4
Cod, Chunky, Tesco*	2 Fingers/80g	140	175	12.3	14.3	7.6	1.6
Cod, Fillet, 100%, Birds Eye*	1 Finger/30g	57	189	13.3	15.5	7.9	0.7
Cod, Fillet, Asda*	1 Finger/31g	66	214	13.0	18.0	10.0	0.0
Cod, Fillet, Waitrose*	1 Finger/30g	55	183	11.9	16.9	7.5	0.7
Cod, Fried in Blended Oil	1 Finger/28g	67	238	13.2	15.5	14.1	0.6
Cod, Frozen	1 Finger/28g	48	170	11.6	14.2	7.8	0.6
Cod, Grilled	1 Finger/28g	56	200	14.3	16.6	8.9	0.7
Economy, Sainsbury's*	1 Finger/26g	51	198	12.6	17.7	8.5	1.3
Farmfoods*	1 Finger/27g	49	183	12.2	15.6	8.0	1.2
Free From, Sainsbury's*	1 Finger/30g	56	188	11.4	18.0	7.8	0.7
Haddock, Fillet, Asda*	1 Finger/30g	62	205	14.0	17.0	9.0	0.0
Haddock, Fillet, Birds Eye*	1 Finger/29g	48	167	12.4	13.2	7.2	0.9
Haddock, In Crunchy Crumb, Morrisons*	1 Finger/30g	57	190	13.1	16.3	8.0	1.1

F

	Measure INFO/WEIGHT	per Measure KCAL	Nutrition Values per 100g / 100ml				
			KCAL	PROT	CARB	FAT	FIBRE
FISH FINGERS							
Hoki, Fillet, Birds Eye*	1 Finger/30g	58	193	12.6	15.6	8.9	0.7
In Batter, Crispy, Birds Eye*	1 Finger/29g	63	218	10.4	15.8	12.6	0.4
Ross*	1 Finger/26g	50	193	10.7	17.7	8.8	0.8
Sainsbury's*	1 Finger/27g	52	194	13.4	16.0	8.5	0.7
SmartPrice, Asda*	1 Finger/25g	46	184	12.0	16.0	8.0	1.1
Value, Tesco*	1 Finger/25g	42	166	11.5	11.9	8.1	1.7
White Fish, Minced, Birds Eye*	1 Finger/25g	47	187	12.7	16.7	7.7	0.7
FISH WITH							
Mushroom, Carrots & Broccoli, Parcel, Birds Eye*	1 Pack/250g	235	94	7.9	3.1	5.6	0.8
FIVE SPICE							
Powder, Sharwood's*	1oz/28g	48	172	12.2	11.6	8.6	23.4
FLAKE							
Cadbury*	1 Std Bar/34g	179	525	7.5	54.7	30.8	0.0
Dipped, Cadbury*	1 Bar/44.3g	233	530	7.0	55.3	31.0	0.0
Luxury, Cadbury*	1 Bar/45g	240	533	7.3	57.8	30.2	0.0
Praline, Cadbury*	1 Bar/38g	201	535	7.7	49.5	34.3	0.0
Snow, Cadbury*	1 Bar/36g	198	550	7.2	60.1	30.9	0.0
FLAN							
Cauliflower Cheese, Safeway*	1 Sm Flan/150g	420	280	7.3	25.0	16.5	2.0
Cauliflower, Cheese & Broccoli, Hot, Sainsbury's*	1/4 Flan/100g	303	303	6.4	24.7	19.8	1.2
Cheese & Onion, Marks & Spencer*	1oz/28g	81	290	6.1	25.1	18.7	1.4
Cheese & Potato, Hot, Tesco*	1/4 Flan/100g	282	282	6.0	20.0	19.7	2.3
Chicken & Smoked Bacon, Hot, Sainsbury's*	1/4 Flan/100g	293	293	10.2	21.5	18.5	1.2
Mediterranean Vegetable, Co-Op*	1/4 Flan/87.5g	189	215	4.0	22.0	12.0	3.0
Mexican Chilli Beef, Safeway*	1 Serving/100g	254	254	6.6	22.5	15.3	2.1
Parsnip, Broccoli & Gruyere, Safeway*	1/2 Flan/200g	534	267	7.0	23.0	16.4	2.8
Pastry, With Fruit	1oz/28g	33	118	1.4	19.3	4.4	0.7
Potato, Cheddar & Onion, Safeway*	1 Serving/150g	420	280	6.4	25.6	16.7	2.7
Smoked Ham Cheese & Leek, Safeway*	1/2 Flan/200g	520	260	8.0	20.0	16.4	2.0
Sponge With Fruit	1oz/28g	31	112	2.8	23.3	1.5	0.6
FLAN CASE							
Sponge, Average	1oz/28g	90	320	7.0	62.5	5.4	0.7
FLAPJACK							
90% Fat Free, Cookie Coach Co*	1 Flapjack/75g	287	383	7.0	66.2	9.9	0.0
All Butter, Blackcurrant Jam, Marks & Spencer*	1 Serving/65g	280	430	4.8	60.5	18.6	2.2
All Butter, Marks & Spencer*	1 Flapjack/31.8g	141	440	6.1	56.1	21.2	4.4
All Butter, Sainsbury's*	1 Flapjack/35g	156	446	5.7	54.5	22.8	2.7
Apple & Raisin, Lite, Crazy Jack*	1 Flapjack70g	227	324	9.8	72.0	2.1	0.0
Apple & Raspberry, Fox's*	1 Flapjack/26g	105	403	4.8	52.5	19.4	3.7
Apple & Sultana, Blackfriars*	1 Flapjack/110g	507	461	5.5	61.0	22.0	0.0
Apple & Sultana, Mr Kipling*	1 Flapjack/27g	123	456	4.6	59.0	22.4	3.6
Apricot & Raisin, Waitrose*	1 Flapjack/38g	143	376	4.7	64.3	11.1	5.8
Apricot, COU, Marks & Spencer*	1oz/28g	96	342	5.4	77.1	2.1	2.0
Apricot, Food To Go, Marks & Spencer*	1 Bar/86g	348	405	4.7	64.4	16.2	4.3
Apricot, Sweet, Shapers, Boots*	1 Flapjack/55g	188	341	5.7	65.0	11.0	4.1
Average	1oz/28g	136	484	4.5	60.4	26.6	2.7
Banana, The Handmade Flapjack Company*	1 Flapjack/90g	379	421	5.3	67.2	14.6	0.0
Belgian Chocolate Dipped, Asda*	1 Serving/67g	321	477	6.0	57.0	25.0	3.2
Black Cherry, Blackfriars*	1 Serving/110g	529	481	5.0	63.0	23.0	0.0
Brazil Nut Cluster, The Handmade Flapjack Company*	1 Flapjack/90g	353	392	6.6	68.7	10.2	0.0
Cappuccino, Blackfriars*	1 Flapjack/110g	481	437	5.0	61.0	25.0	0.0
Caramel Bake, The Handmade Flapjack Company*	1 Flapjack/90g	375	417	6.0	65.6	14.5	0.0
Cherry & Coconut, Blackfriars*	1 Flapjack/110g	490	445	5.0	58.0	21.0	0.0

F

	Measure INFO/WEIGHT	per Measure KCAL	Nutrition Values per 100g / 100ml				
			KCAL	PROT	CARB	FAT	FIBRE
FLAPJACK							
Cherry & Sultana, Cookie Coach Co*	1 Pack/90g	373	414	6.2	58.2	17.3	0.0
Cherry & Sultana, Marks & Spencer*	1oz/28g	111	395	5.4	63.7	13.0	5.1
Chocolate & Hazelnut, Marks & Spencer*	1 Flapjack/71g	330	465	7.3	55.6	25.5	3.8
Chocolate Chip, Boots*	1 Flapjack/75g	313	417	5.6	65.0	15.0	3.5
Chocolate Chunk, Boots*	1 Slice/75g	351	468	5.7	55.0	25.0	3.0
Chocolate Dipped, Marks & Spencer*	1 Flapjack/96g	442	460	6.1	61.3	22.4	3.0
Chocolate Flavour, Blackfriars*	1 Bar/110g	521	474	5.0	61.0	24.0	0.0
Chocolate Special, The Handmade Flapjack Company*	1 Flapjack/90g	392	436	5.7	58.7	19.8	0.0
Chocolate, McVitie's*	1 Flapjack/85g	422	496	6.6	56.6	27.1	3.2
Chocolate, The Handmade Flapjack Company*	1 Flapjack/90g	392	435	6.0	58.6	19.6	0.0
Crazy Raizin, Fabulous Bakin' Boys*	1 Pack/90g	378	420	6.0	60.0	17.0	4.0
Date & Walnut, The Handmade Flapjack Company*	1 Flapjack/90g	360	400	6.1	60.2	15.0	0.0
Fingers, GFY, Asda*	1 Finger/37g	130	350	5.0	60.0	10.0	3.5
Fruit & Nut, Organic, Evernat*	1oz/28g	136	484	4.5	60.4	26.6	0.0
Fruit With Raisins, Boots*	1 Pack/75g	329	439	5.4	57.0	21.0	3.5
Fruit, GFY, Asda*	1 Flapjack/45g	173	384	6.0	72.0	8.0	3.4
Fruit, Mr Kipling*	1 Flapjack/24g	103	430	4.8	51.4	22.9	4.0
Fruit, Tesco*	1 Cake/33g	136	412	5.7	62.0	15.7	4.0
Fruit, Weight Watchers*	1 Slice/30g	106	353	6.0	68.3	6.3	4.7
Fruity, Waitrose*	1 Serving/50g	199	398	6.1	62.9	13.5	3.9
Fudge, Blackfriars*	1 Slice/110g	528	480	5.0	60.0	24.0	0.0
Golden Oaty, Fingers, Fabulous Bakin' Boys*	1 Finger/28g	126	450	5.7	59.6	21.1	3.4
Mini Bites, Marks & Spencer*	1 Bite/14g	70	500	6.4	62.8	25.0	2.6
Mixed Fruit, Fabulous Bakin' Boys*	1 Serving/90g	350	389	5.5	71.0	10.5	4.0
Mixed Fruit, Organic, Evernat*	1oz/28g	136	484	4.5	60.4	26.6	0.0
Organic, Wholebake*	1 Bar/90g	388	431	6.0	59.4	20.8	0.0
Plain, The Handmade Flapjack Company*	1 Flapjack/90g	398	442	5.4	57.1	21.3	0.0
Raspberry Preserve, The Handmade Flapjack Company*	1 Flapjack/90g	311	345	6.4	74.4	2.4	0.0
Raspberry, Fingers, Fabulous Bakin' Boys*	1 Finger/30g	133	443	5.0	61.0	20.0	4.0
Really Raspberry, Fabulous Bakin' Boys*	1 Flapjack/90g	378	420	6.0	60.0	18.0	0.0
Safeway*	1 Flapjack/60g	255	425	5.9	55.1	20.1	2.7
Snickers, McVitie's*	1 Flapjack/65g	320	492	9.5	47.6	29.3	0.0
Sultana, Tesco*	1 Flapjack/50g	173	346	5.0	36.2	20.1	3.7
Syrup, McVitie's*	1 Flapjack/85g	417	490	6.5	56.0	26.7	3.4
Toffee, Finest, Tesco*	1 Piece/35g	156	446	4.9	63.6	19.1	1.3
Toffeemac, The Handmade Flapjack Company*	1 Flapjack/90g	411	457	6.1	59.0	21.9	0.0
Tropical Mix, Reduced Fat, Fabulous Bakin' Boys*	1 Flapjack/90g	347	385	6.0	63.0	12.0	3.0
Weight Watchers*	1 Slice/30g	109	363	6.7	71.0	6.0	4.0
With Sultanas, Tesco*	1 Flapjack/49g	217	442	5.3	57.9	21.0	3.7
Yoghurt Flavour, Blackfriars*	1 Bar/110g	521	474	7.0	58.0	24.0	0.0
FLATBREAD							
BBQ Chicken, Improved, Shapers, Boots*	1 Pack/165.4g	267	162	10.0	25.0	2.3	1.2
BBQ Style Chicken, Shapers, Boots*	1 Serving/108g	187	173	10.0	23.0	4.6	2.8
Cajun Style Chicken, GFY, Asda*	1 Wrap/176.3g	231	131	9.0	21.0	1.2	0.9
Chargrilled Chicken, COU, Marks & Spencer*	1 Pack/163.3g	245	150	10.8	23.0	1.9	5.2
Cheese & Onion Swedish Style, Shapers, Boots*	1 Flatbread/127g	265	209	10.0	24.0	8.1	1.3
Chicken & Black Bean Sauce, Shapers, Boots*	1 Pack/204g	249	122	8.7	20.0	0.8	1.7
Chicken & Mango Salsa, Sainsbury's*	1 Pack/178g	251	141	9.5	22.7	1.4	1.4
Chicken Caesar, Shapers, Boots*	1 Serving/160g	254	159	13.0	22.0	2.1	2.0
Chicken Fajita, Improved, Shapers, Boots*	1 Pack/201.3g	302	150	11.0	21.0	2.6	1.8
Chicken Tikka, BGTY, Sainsbury's*	1 Flatbread/188g	241	128	10.3	18.5	1.4	2.0
Chicken Tikka, Shapers, Boots*	1 Flatbread/164g	269	164	11.0	24.0	2.5	1.5
Chinese Chicken, COU, Marks & Spencer*	1 Flatbread/156g	281	180	13.9	24.3	2.8	2.2

F

	Measure INFO/WEIGHT	per Measure KCAL	Nutrition Values per 100g / 100ml				
			KCAL	PROT	CARB	FAT	FIBRE
FLATBREAD							
Chinese Chicken, Shapers, Boots*	1 Pack/159.3g	273	172	11.0	29.0	1.3	1.8
Feta Cheese, Shapers, Boots*	1 Pack/165.6g	256	154	6.7	23.0	3.9	1.4
Garlic & Herb, Tear & Share, Sainsbury's*	1/4 Flatbread/68g	201	297	10.9	42.5	9.3	3.7
Garlic & Parsley, 50% Less Fat, BGTY, Sainsbury's*	1/4 Bread/62.6g	160	254	9.5	40.3	6.1	3.7
Greek Feta Salad, Boots*	1 Pack/157.5g	242	153	6.4	24.0	3.6	1.2
Greek Style Salad, Waitrose*	1 Pack/171.8g	280	163	7.4	22.3	4.9	3.3
Greek Style, GFY, Asda*	1 Flatbread/165g	256	155	7.0	22.0	4.3	2.1
Houmous Salad, Greek Inspired, Sainsbury's*	1 Pack/177g	313	177	5.5	24.7	6.2	3.3
Italian Chicken, Improved, Shapers, Boots*	1 Pack/151.1g	263	174	11.0	22.0	4.5	1.8
Italian Chicken, Shapers, Boots*	1 Pack/168.4g	265	158	10.0	22.0	3.3	1.3
King Prawn Tikka, Waitrose*	1 Pack/165g	257	156	9.4	25.1	2.0	1.5
Mediterranean Chicken, Ginsters*	1 Pack/167.8g	302	180	10.6	25.5	4.0	0.0
Mediterranean Tuna, Ginsters*	1 Pack/166.9g	297	178	10.3	25.6	3.8	0.0
Mexican Style Chicken, GFY, Asda*	1 Pack/160.7g	242	150	13.0	20.0	2.0	2.5
Peking Duck, Less Than 3% Fat, Shapers, Boots*	1 Pack/155.7g	246	158	7.2	27.0	2.4	1.9
Prawn Korma, Shapers, Boots*	1 Pack/169.0g	267	158	8.8	22.0	3.9	1.3
Rancher's Chicken, COU, Marks & Spencer*	1 Pack/174g	270	155	10.9	23.0	2.0	1.5
Ranchers Chicken, Shapers, Boots*	1 Pack/194.2g	303	156	12.0	22.0	2.2	1.5
Salsa Chicken, Shapers, Boots*	1 Pack/190.7g	329	172	11.0	22.0	4.4	1.6
Spicy Chicken & Salsa, Healthy Living, Tesco	1 Serving/183g	251	137	10.1	21.1	1.4	1.2
Spicy Chicken, Shapers, Boots*	1 Pack/181.4g	291	161	11.0	23.0	2.5	0.0
Spicy Mexican, New, Shapers, Boots*	1 Pack/183.7g	282	153	8.0	24.0	2.7	1.9
Sticky BBQ Style Chicken, Shapers, Boots*	1 Pack/158.4g	273	173	10.0	23.0	4.6	2.8
Tomata & Chilli, Sainsbury's*	1/4 Bread/65g	155	238	11.9	36.9	4.7	2.8
Tomato & Chilli, BGTY, Sainsbury's*	1/4 Bread/100g	155	155	7.7	24.0	3.1	1.8
Tomato & Garlic, Sainsbury's*	1/3 Bread/73g	191	261	8.4	41.7	6.7	3.4
Vegetable & Salsa, Healthy Living, Tesco*	1 Serving/193g	263	136	7.9	22.2	1.8	1.2
FLIPPER DIPPER							
Penguin, McVitie's*	1 Pack/50.1g	267	533	8.2	60.7	28.7	1.5
FLOUR							
Brown, Chapati	1 Tbsp/20g	67	333	11.5	73.7	1.2	0.0
Brown, Wheat	1oz/28g	90	323	12.6	68.5	1.8	6.4
Chick Pea	1oz/28g	88	313	19.7	49.6	5.4	10.7
Corn, Tesco*	1 Serving/90g	316	351	0.4	87.0	0.1	0.1
Millet	1oz/28g	99	354	5.8	75.4	1.7	0.0
Plain, Average	1oz/28g	98	349	10.3	73.8	1.5	2.2
Potato	1oz/28g	92	328	9.1	75.6	0.9	5.7
Rice	1oz/28g	102	366	6.4	80.1	0.8	2.0
Rye, Whole	1oz/28g	94	335	8.2	75.9	2.0	11.7
Soya, Full Fat, Average	1oz/28g	118	422	37.9	19.8	21.8	11.6
Soya, Low Fat	1oz/28g	99	352	45.3	28.2	7.2	13.5
Speciality Gluten Free, Doves Farm*	1 Serving/100g	353	353	4.7	85.2	1.8	2.7
Strong, Brown Bread, Average	1 Serving/100g	311	311	14.0	61.0	1.8	6.4
Strong, Wholemeal, Average	1 Serving/100g	315	315	13.3	60.6	2.2	9.0
Very Strong, White Bread, Allinson*	1 Serving/100g	348	348	13.9	69.0	1.8	3.2
White, Average	1oz/28g	89	319	9.8	66.8	1.0	2.9
White, Chapati,	1 Tbsp/20g	67	335	9.8	77.6	0.5	0.0
White, Self Raising, Average	1oz/28g	94	336	9.9	71.8	1.3	2.9
White, Wheat, Average	1oz/28g	95	341	10.5	76.5	1.4	3.1
Wholemeal, Average	1oz/28g	87	312	12.6	61.9	2.2	9.0
Wholemeal, Self Raising, Tesco*	1oz/28g	89	317	11.5	62.9	2.2	9.0
FLYING SAUCERS							
Asda*	1 Bag/23g	82	355	0.1	83.0	2.5	0.8

F

	Measure INFO/WEIGHT	per Measure KCAL	KCAL	PROT	CARB	FAT	FIBRE
FLYING SAUCERS							
Co-Op*	1 Sweet/1g	4	370	0.5	90.0	1.0	0.6
FLYTE							
Mars*	1 Bar/45g	196	435	3.6	72.3	14.7	0.0
Snacksize, Mars*	1 Bar/22.5g	98	436	3.8	72.5	14.5	0.0
FOOL							
Apricot, BGTY, Sainsbury's*	1 Pot/113g	95	84	3.6	11.4	2.6	0.5
Apricot, Fruit, Tesco*	1 Pot/113g	200	177	2.6	16.4	11.2	0.3
Blackcurrant, Asda*	1 Serving/114g	89	78	3.6	10.0	2.6	0.6
Blackcurrant, BGTY, Sainsbury's*	1 Pot/113g	89	79	3.5	10.4	2.6	0.6
Fruit	1oz/28g	46	163	1.0	20.2	9.3	1.2
Fruit, BFY, Morrisons*	1 Pot/114g	96	84	3.4	10.1	3.4	0.3
Gooseberry, Fruit, BGTY, Sainsbury's*	1 Pot/121g	93	77	2.9	10.0	2.8	0.8
Gooseberry, Fruit, Somerfield*	1 Pot/114g	215	189	3.0	19.0	11.0	0.0
Gooseberry, Perfectly Balanced, Waitrose*	1 Pot/113g	125	111	3.6	18.3	2.6	0.7
Gooseberry, Sainsbury's*	1 Pot/113g	214	189	2.6	19.1	11.4	1.1
Lemon, BFY, Morrisons*	1 Pot/114g	96	84	3.4	10.1	3.4	0.3
Lemon, Fruit, BGTY, Sainsbury's*	1 Pot/113g	94	83	3.4	9.7	3.4	0.3
Lemon, Fruit, Shapers, Boots*	1 Pot/113g	105	93	3.8	11.0	3.8	0.0
Raspberry, Fruit, Tesco*	1 Pot/113g	234	207	2.6	23.6	11.3	0.3
Rhubarb, Fruit, BGTY, Sainsbury's*	1 Pot/120g	91	76	3.5	9.5	2.6	0.3
Rhubarb, Fruit, Somerfield*	1 Pot/114g	201	176	3.0	16.0	11.0	0.0
Rhubarb, Fruit, Waitrose*	1 Pot/114g	182	160	2.7	11.9	11.3	0.3
Rhubarb, Perfectly Balanced, Waitrose*	1 Pot/113g	101	89	3.5	13.0	2.6	0.3
Rhubarb, Sainsbury's*	1 Pot/113g	180	159	2.6	11.5	11.4	0.4
Strawberry, Fruit, BGTY, Sainsbury's*	1 Pot/120g	100	83	3.7	11.1	2.6	0.8
Strawberry, Fruit, Co-Op*	1 Pot/114g	188	165	2.0	18.0	9.0	0.8
Strawberry, Fruit, Shapers, Boots*	1 Pot/112g	90	81	3.5	9.2	3.4	0.3
Strawberry, Fruit, Somerfield*	1 Pot/114g	201	176	3.0	16.0	11.0	0.0
Strawberry, GFY, Asda*	1 Pot/114g	95	83	3.8	11.0	2.6	0.8
Strawberry, Perfectly Balanced, Waitrose*	1 Pot/113g	110	97	3.5	14.9	2.6	0.4
Strawberry, Real Fruit, Safeway*	1 Pot/114g	197	173	2.7	15.4	11.2	0.3
FOR MILK							
Peachy Banana, Robinson's*	1 Serving/50ml	79	158	0.0	39.0	0.0	0.0
Strawberry & Raspberry, Robinson's*	1 Serving/50ml	69	137	0.0	34.0	0.0	0.0
FRANGIPANES							
Tesco*	1 Serving/59g	251	426	4.7	56.6	19.9	0.6
FRANKFURTERS							
Average	1 Frankfurter/42g	123	292	12.0	1.3	26.6	0.0
Meat Free, Asda*	3 Franks/81g	215	266	18.0	3.5	20.0	2.0
Vegetarian, Tivall*	3 Sausages/90g	220	244	18.0	7.0	16.0	3.0
FRAZZLES							
Bacon, Smiths, Walkers*	1 Bag/23g	108	470	8.0	59.0	22.4	0.0
FRENCH FRIES							
Cheese & Onion, Walkers*	1 Bag/22g	95	430	4.8	64.0	17.0	4.2
Fish & Chips, Walkers*	1 Bag/19.0g	79	415	4.2	64.0	16.0	4.3
Ready Salted, Walkers*	1 Bag/22g	97	441	4.5	65.0	18.2	4.1
Salt & Vinegar, BGTY, Sainsbury's*	1 Bag/15g	51	340	6.0	80.1	1.5	4.1
Salt & Vinegar, COU, Marks & Spencer*	1 Bag/25g	88	350	5.1	80.9	1.6	2.3
Salt & Vinegar, Eat Smart, Safeway*	1 Bag/20g	75	375	5.1	80.9	1.6	2.3
Salt & Vinegar, Walkers*	1 Bag/22g	94	425	4.6	64.0	17.0	4.1
Scampi, Smiths, Walkers*	1 Bag/27g	134	496	13.0	52.5	26.0	0.0
Walkers*	1 Pack/22g	94	425	4.5	64.0	17.0	4.1
Worcester Sauce, Walkers*	1 Bag/22g	92	420	5.1	64.0	16.0	4.2

F

	Measure INFO/WEIGHT	per Measure KCAL	Nutrition Values per 100g / 100ml				
			KCAL	PROT	CARB	FAT	FIBRE
FRENCH TOAST							
Asda*	1 Slice/8g	30	381	10.0	74.0	5.0	4.0
Co-Op*	1 Serving/8g	31	385	10.0	72.0	6.0	5.0
Morrisons*	1 Toast/8g	31	393	11.0	72.5	6.6	3.0
Sainsbury's*	1 Serving/8g	31	382	10.0	72.0	6.6	5.0
FRIES							
9/16" Straight Cut Home, Deep Fried, McCain*	1oz/28g	65	233	3.2	32.7	9.9	0.0
9/16" Straight Cut Home, Oven Baked, McCain*	1oz/28g	53	188	3.2	31.5	5.5	0.0
American Style, Frozen, Thin, Tesco*	1 Serving/125g	208	166	2.2	21.1	8.1	1.9
American Style, Slim, Iceland*	1 Serving/100g	187	187	2.4	30.6	6.1	2.4
American, 3 Way Cook, Somerfield*	1oz/28g	43	155	3.0	25.0	5.0	0.0
American, Oven, Asda*	1 Serving/180g	432	240	3.4	34.0	10.0	3.0
Cafe Frites, Marks & Spencer*	1 Pack/200g	440	220	3.0	32.7	8.7	2.4
Crinkle, Home, McCain*	1 Serving/135g	248	184	2.3	25.5	9.0	0.0
Crispy French, McCain*	1 Serving/100g	165	165	2.1	24.3	6.6	0.0
Crispy Savoury Seasoning Southern, McCain*	1 Serving/100g	179	179	2.8	26.4	6.9	0.0
Curly, Southern Style, Tesco*	1 Serving/50g	124	248	3.8	41.7	7.3	3.8
Home Oven Chips, McCain*	1oz/28g	53	188	3.2	31.5	5.5	0.0
Home, Frozen, McCain*	1 Serving/100g	141	141	2.0	26.1	4.4	0.0
Home, Oven Cooked, McCain*	1 Serving/100g	202	202	3.2	37.5	6.1	0.0
Oven, Straight Cut, Morrisons*	1 Serving/100g	149	149	2.8	24.6	4.3	2.6
Seasoned, American Style, Morrisons*	1 Serving/56g	110	197	2.8	26.2	9.0	0.0
Southern Spicy Spiral, Deep Fried, McCain*	1oz/28g	58	208	2.7	26.4	10.2	0.0
Southern Spicy Spiral, Oven Baked, McCain*	1oz/28g	46	165	1.7	24.6	6.6	0.0
Southern, Oven Cook, McCain*	1 Serving/80g	146	182	2.7	26.1	8.4	0.0
Southern, Straight Cut, Oven Baked, McCain*	1oz/28g	74	263	4.1	37.1	10.9	0.0
FRISPS							
Tangy Salt & Vinegar, Frisps*	1 Bag/30g	160	532	5.0	52.6	33.5	2.9
Tasty Cheese & Onion, Frisps*	1 Bag/28g	166	537	5.5	53.2	33.6	3.2
FROMAGE FRAIS							
0% Fat, Vitalinea*	1 Tbsp/28g	14	50	7.4	4.7	0.1	0.0
Apple Pie, Low Fat, Sainsbury's*	1 Pot/90g	108	120	6.7	17.3	2.6	0.3
Apple Strudel, Safeway*	1 Pot/100g	116	116	6.6	14.8	3.4	0.7
Apricot, Makes Sense, Somerfield*	1 Pot/60g	67	112	5.9	13.2	4.0	0.0
Apricot, Tesco*	1 Pot/100g	77	77	6.5	6.0	3.0	1.3
Apricot, Weight Watchers*	1 Pot/100g	47	47	6.2	5.4	0.1	0.2
Bakewell Tart Flavour, BGTY, Sainsbury's*	1 Pot/100g	54	54	7.6	5.5	0.2	1.1
Banana, Organic, Yeo Valley*	1 Pot/90g	118	131	6.6	12.6	6.0	0.2
Banoffee Pie Flavour, Low Fat, Safeway*	1 Pot/100g	135	135	6.8	17.6	4.1	0.2
Banoffee Toffee, Thick & Creamy, Weight Watchers*	1 Pot/100g	59	59	5.2	9.3	0.1	1.0
Banoffee Toffee, Weight Watchers*	1 Pot/100g	64	64	5.7	10.0	0.1	1.1
Black Cherry, Asda*	1 Pot/100g	113	113	4.1	13.0	5.0	0.0
Black Cherry, GFY, Asda*	1 Pot/100g	54	54	6.0	7.0	0.2	0.0
Blackcurrant, GFY, Asda*	1 Pot/100g	43	43	6.0	4.2	0.2	0.0
Blackcurrant, Healthy Living, Tesco*	1 Pot/100g	56	56	6.2	7.4	0.2	0.4
Blue Parrot Cafe, Sainsbury's*	1 Serving/50g	49	98	6.6	11.0	3.1	0.2
Cherries & Chocolate, Finest, Tesco*	1 Serving/165g	299	181	5.4	20.1	8.8	0.7
Cherry Pie Flavour, BGTY, Sainsbury's*	1 Pot/100g	54	54	7.6	5.5	0.2	1.1
Cherry, 0% Fat, Vitalinea, Danone*	1 Serving/150g	89	59	6.1	8.0	0.2	1.6
Chocolate & Orange, Thick & Creamy, Weight Watchers*	1 Pot/100g	59	59	5.2	9.3	0.1	1.0
Chocolate Fudge, Smooth & Creamy, Tesco*	1 Pot/100g	136	136	6.7	13.3	6.2	0.2
Exotic Fruits, Eat Smart, Safeway*	1 Pot/100g	60	60	7.9	6.6	0.2	0.4
Fabby, Loved By Kids, Marks & Spencer*	1 Pot/42.9g	45	105	6.2	12.3	3.7	0.0
Fruit On The Bottom, BFY, Morrisons*	1 Pot/100g	66	66	5.6	10.6	0.2	0.0

F

FROMAGE FRAIS

INFO/WEIGHT		KCAL	KCAL	PROT	CARB	FAT	FIBRE
Fruit, Weight Watchers*	1 Pot/100g	48	48	5.4	6.3	0.1	0.3
Good Intentions, Somerfield*	1 Pot/100g	49	49	7.6	4.5	0.1	0.0
Kids, Yeo Valley*	1 Serving/90g	111	123	6.6	12.6	5.3	0.0
Lemon Pie, Low Fat, Sainsbury's*	1 Pot/90g	108	120	6.7	17.3	2.7	0.2
Lemon Sponge Flavour, BGTY, Sainsbury's*	1 Pot/100g	52	52	7.6	5.0	0.2	1.1
Lemon, Balanced Lifestyle, Aldi*	1 Serving/100g	52	52	5.6	6.6	0.3	0.6
Lemon, COU, Marks & Spencer*	1 Serving/100g	50	50	7.3	5.2	0.1	0.3
Low Fat, Aldi*	1 Pot/100g	52	52	5.4	7.1	0.3	0.7
Mandarin & Orange, Healthy Living, Tesco*	1 Pot/100g	55	55	6.2	7.0	0.2	0.3
Mandarin & Orange, Tesco*	1 Pot/100g	75	75	6.5	5.6	3.0	2.3
Mango & Papaya, Healthy Living, Tesco*	1 Pot/100g	55	55	6.2	7.0	0.2	0.1
Mango, Eat Smart, Safeway*	1 Pot/100g	55	55	7.7	5.1	0.2	1.6
Morello Cherries, Perfectly Balanced, Waitrose*	1/2 Pot/250ml	260	104	2.5	19.1	1.9	1.8
Morrisons*	1 Serving/28g	17	59	9.8	4.8	0.0	0.0
Munch Bunch, Nestle*	1 Pot/42g	50	119	7.6	14.8	2.9	0.0
Natural, Creamy, Co-Op*	1 Pot/200g	204	102	6.1	2.9	7.3	0.0
Natural, Fat Free, Marks & Spencer*	1 Serving/100g	60	60	9.8	4.8	0.1	0.0
Natural, French, Virtually Fat Free, Waitrose*	1 Serving/46g	21	46	7.3	3.7	0.2	0.0
Natural, GFY, Asda*	1oz/28g	13	45	8.0	3.3	0.0	0.0
Natural, Healthy Living, Tesco*	1 Serving/65g	30	46	7.8	3.3	0.2	0.0
Natural, Normandy, BGTY, Sainsbury's*	1 Serving/15g	7	47	7.5	3.9	0.1	0.0
Natural, Virtually Fat Free, Safeway*	1 Serving/50g	23	46	7.3	3.7	0.2	0.0
Normandy, Sainsbury's*	1 Serving/25g	29	116	7.7	3.4	8.1	0.0
Organic, Vrai*	1 Serving/100g	83	83	8.1	4.5	3.6	0.0
Peach & Apricot, Healthy Eating, Tesco*	1 Pot/100g	54	54	6.2	6.8	0.2	0.1
Peach, BGTY, Sainsbury's*	1 Pot/100g	53	53	7.2	5.5	0.2	0.5
Peach, Weight Watchers*	1 Pot/100g	48	48	5.4	6.4	0.1	0.2
Petit Dessert, Co-Op*	1 Pot/60g	74	123	6.3	14.5	4.4	0.0
Petits Filous, Yoplait*	1 Pot/60g	76	127	6.5	14.5	4.7	0.0
Pineapple & Passion Fruit, Healthy Living, Tesco*	1 Pot/100g	55	55	6.2	7.1	0.2	0.1
Pineapple, Eat Smart, Safeway*	1 Pot/100g	60	60	7.9	6.3	0.2	0.3
Plain	1oz/28g	32	113	6.8	5.7	7.1	0.0
Raspberry & Redcurrant, BGTY, Sainsbury's*	1 Pot/100g	51	51	7.4	5.4	0.1	1.6
Raspberry & Strawberry, Weight Watchers*	1 Pot/100g	48	48	5.4	6.2	0.1	0.3
Raspberry, COU, Marks & Spencer*	1 Pot/100g	49	49	7.8	4.9	0.1	0.4
Raspberry, Eat Smart, Safeway*	1 Pot/100g	50	50	7.6	4.5	0.2	1.8
Raspberry, GFY, Asda*	1 Pot/100g	43	43	6.0	4.2	0.2	0.0
Raspberry, Healthy Choice, Asda*	1 Pot/100g	41	41	6.0	3.8	0.2	0.0
Raspberry, Healthy Eating, Tesco*	1 Pot/100g	53	53	6.2	6.6	0.2	0.3
Raspberry, Low Fat, Sainsbury's*	1 Pot/90g	96	107	5.8	15.1	2.6	0.1
Raspberry, Makes Sense, Somerfield*	1 Pot/60g	69	115	5.3	14.8	3.8	0.0
Raspberry, Muller*	1 Pot/50g	68	135	6.1	13.5	6.3	0.0
Raspberry, Organic, Yeo Valley*	1 Pot/100g	127	127	6.1	11.1	6.5	0.4
Raspberry, Value, Tesco*	1 Serving/60g	56	93	7.2	13.5	1.3	0.0
Raspberry, Weight Watchers*	1 Pot/100g	49	49	5.3	6.9	0.1	1.2
Real Fruit, Tesco*	1 Pot/100g	54	54	5.6	7.6	0.1	0.1
Red Cherry, Healthy Eating, Tesco*	1 Pot/100g	55	55	6.2	7.2	0.2	0.1
Red Cherry, Tesco*	1 Pot/100g	75	75	6.5	5.5	3.0	2.3
Rhubarb & Crumble, Low Fat, Sainsbury's*	1 Pot/90g	96	107	6.7	14.1	2.6	0.4
Strawberry & Rasberry, Organic, Yeo Valley*	1 Pot/90g	118	131	6.3	12.9	6.0	0.2
Strawberry Cheesecake, Dessert Selection, Sainsbury's*	1 Pot/90g	95	106	5.8	15.3	2.5	0.1
Strawberry Tart, Sainsbury's*	1 Pot/100g	54	54	7.6	5.5	0.2	1.1
Strawberry, 0% Fat, Vitalinea, Danone*	1 Serving/150g	83	55	6.0	7.4	0.2	1.6

F

F

FROMAGE FRAIS

INFO/WEIGHT	Measure per Measure		Nutrition Values per 100g / 100ml				
		KCAL	KCAL	PROT	CARB	FAT	FIBRE
Strawberry, 99.9% Fat Free, Onken*	1 Serving/50g	46	91	6.9	15.3	0.1	0.0
Strawberry, BGTY, Sainsbury's*	1 Pot/100g	48	48	7.2	4.3	0.2	1.4
Strawberry, BGTY, Sainsbury's*	1 Pot/90g	46	51	7.0	5.8	0.1	1.4
Strawberry, Balanced Lifestyle, Aldi*	1 Serving/100g	52	52	5.4	7.1	0.2	0.7
Strawberry, COU, Marks & Spencer*	1 Pot/100g	50	50	7.7	4.6	0.1	0.5
Strawberry, GFY, Asda*	1 Pot/100g	58	58	6.0	8.0	0.2	0.0
Strawberry, Healthy Eating, Tesco*	1 Pot/100g	54	54	6.2	6.8	0.2	0.1
Strawberry, Low Fat, St Ivel*	1 Pot/100g	69	69	6.9	6.8	1.2	0.0
Strawberry, Organic, Yeo Valley*	1 Pot/90g	116	129	6.3	12.5	6.0	0.2
Strawberry, Puree, Somerfield*	1 Pot/50g	60	120	7.0	14.0	4.0	0.0
Strawberry, Tesco*	1 Pot/100g	75	75	6.5	5.5	3.0	2.5
Strawberry, Thomas The Tank Engine, Yoplait*	1 Pot/50g	51	101	6.8	15.4	1.3	0.0
Strawberry, Value, Tesco*	1 Pot/60g	55	92	7.2	13.0	1.3	0.0
Strawberry, Weight Watchers*	1 Pot/100g	47	47	5.4	6.2	0.1	0.2
Summer Fruits, Weight Watchers*	1 Pot/100g	48	48	5.4	6.3	0.1	0.4
Toffee & Pecan Pie, Smooth & Creamy, Tesco*	1 Pot/100g	148	148	6.9	14.8	6.8	0.2
Toffee, BGTY, Sainsbury's*	1 Pot/100g	60	60	7.2	7.0	0.3	0.2
Toffee, Weight Watchers*	1 Pot/100g	64	64	5.7	10.0	0.1	1.1
Tropical Fruits, BGTY, Sainsbury's*	1 Pot/100g	54	54	7.3	5.8	0.2	0.3
Vanilla Flavour With Fruit, Thick & Fruity, Weight Watchers*	1 Pot/100g	49	49	5.3	6.9	0.0	1.2
Vanilla, Danone*	1 Serving/200g	274	137	5.3	19.6	4.1	0.0
Very Low Fat	1oz/28g	16	58	7.7	6.8	0.2	0.0
Virtually Fat Free, Tesco*	1 Pot/100g	56	56	5.6	8.2	0.1	0.0
Wildlife, Yoplait*	1 Pot/50g	48	96	7.0	14.0	1.3	0.0
With Cereal, Shape Rise, Danone*	1 Serving/165g	205	124	6.5	23.9	1.3	0.5
With Real Fruit Puree, Nestle*	1 Serving/50g	65	130	7.1	18.9	2.7	0.2

FRUIT

INFO/WEIGHT	Measure per Measure		Nutrition Values per 100g / 100ml				
Bites, Apple & Grape, Food Explorers, Waitrose*	1 Pack/80g	44	55	0.4	13.2	0.1	1.4
Black Forest, Shearway*	1oz/28g	12	44	0.7	9.9	0.1	0.0
Citrus Selection, Fresh, Sainsbury's*	1 Pack/240g	79	33	0.9	7.1	0.1	1.6
Collection, Fresh, Marks & Spencer*	1 Pack/240g	108	45	0.6	10.3	0.2	1.3
Deluxe, Fresh, Rindless, Shapers, Boots*	1 Pack/168g	64	38	0.7	8.3	0.2	0.7
Dessert, Sojasun*	1 Pot/135g	105	78	3.5	12.0	1.8	0.0
Exotic, Marks & Spencer*	1 Pack/425g	213	50	0.7	11.8	0.3	0.0
Fantasy, Strawberries & Cranberries, Sundora*	1 Serving/25g	70	280	2.5	67.0	0.6	5.4
Grapefruit & Orange Segments, Breakfast, Del Monte*	1 Can/411g	193	47	1.0	10.2	0.1	1.0
Just Fruit, Shapers, Boots*	1 Pot/140g	60	43	0.6	10.0	0.1	1.5
Melon & Grape Selection, Food To Go, Marks & Spencer*	1oz/28g	10	35	0.5	8.6	0.1	0.7
Melon, Kiwi, & Strawberry, Fully Prepared, Sainsbury's*	1 Pack/245g	74	30	0.8	6.3	0.2	1.3
Mixed, Fresh, Tesco*	1 Pack/200g	70	35	0.8	7.4	0.2	1.4
Mixed, Fruitime, Pieces, Tesco*	1 Can/140g	84	60	0.4	14.0	0.0	1.0
Mixed, Pieces, In Juice, Fruitini*	1 Can/140g	77	55	0.4	13.0	0.1	0.0
Mixed, Pieces, In Orange Jelly, Fruitini*	1 Can/140g	94	67	0.3	15.8	0.1	0.0
Mixed, Tropical, Fruit Express, Del Monte*	1 Pot/185g	89	48	0.2	11.2	0.1	1.2
Mixed, Vine, Crazy Jack*	1 Serving/10g	31	309	2.8	74.0	0.3	4.7
Peaches & Pears, Fruit Express, Del Monte*	1 Serving/185g	87	47	0.4	10.8	0.1	0.9
Pieces, Mixed In Fruit Juice, Fruiyini, Del Monte*	1 Serving/120g	61	51	0.4	12.0	0.1	0.5
Pineapple, Grape & Kiwi, Asda*	1 Serving/200g	98	49	0.6	11.0	0.3	1.7
Pure, Just Apple, Heinz*	1 Jar/128g	60	47	0.4	11.2	0.1	1.8
Seeds & Nuts, Waitrose*	1 Serving/20g	90	452	13.5	36.5	28.0	5.5
Snack Pack, Fresh, Sainsbury's*	1 Serving/120g	54	45	0.1	11.0	0.1	1.3
Snack, Apple & Grape, Blue Parrot Cafe, Sainsbury's*	1 Pack/80g	42	53	0.4	12.5	0.1	2.1
To Go, Del Monte*	1 Can/113g	80	71	0.0	17.7	0.0	0.0

	Measure INFO/WEIGHT	per Measure KCAL	Nutrition Values per 100g / 100ml				
			KCAL	PROT	CARB	FAT	FIBRE
FRUIT							
Tropical Mix, Sainsbury's*	1 Serving/50g	203	406	3.6	54.8	19.2	6.4
Tropical, Fresh, Marks & Spencer*	1 Pack/425g	213	50	0.7	11.8	0.3	2.0
Tropical, In Juice, Dole*	1 Pot/113g	59	52	0.3	14.2	0.0	1.8
Tropical, Tesco*	1 Pack/180g	85	47	0.6	10.8	0.2	1.9
FRUIT & NUT MIX							
Almond, Raisin & berry, Sainsbury's*	1 Bag/50g	189	377	6.1	57.6	14.3	4.2
Cinnamon & Prailine, Christmas, Finest, Tesco*	1/4 Pot/106g	470	442	8.2	45.9	25.1	11.5
Exotic, Waitrose*	1 Serving/50g	207	414	9.0	54.6	17.7	4.6
Luxury, Asda*	1 Serving/50g	226	451	9.0	33.5	30.5	7.4
Organic, Waitrose*	1 Pack/100g	489	489	15.0	33.8	32.6	5.4
Papaya Cranberry, WTF, Sainsbury's*	1 Serving/75g	300	400	4.1	63.1	14.6	7.3
Port & Winter Spice, Perenium, Christmas, Finest, Tesco*	1/4 Pot/90g	379	421	7.8	37.9	26.5	13.9
TTD, Sainsbury's*	1 Bag/250g	900	360	5.1	49.5	15.7	5.9
FRUIT COCKTAIL							
Fresh & Ready, Sainsbury's*	1 Pack/300g	117	39	0.6	9.0	0.1	1.2
In Apple Juice, Asda*	1/3 Can/80g	40	50	0.3	12.0	0.1	1.6
In Fruit Juice, Sainsbury's*	1 Serving/198g	97	49	0.3	11.9	0.1	1.3
In Fruit Juice, Tesco*	1 Serving/255g	148	58	0.5	13.5	0.0	1.4
In Grape Juice, Tesco*	1oz/28g	12	43	0.4	10.0	0.0	1.0
In Juice, Del Monte*	1 Can/415g	203	49	0.4	11.2	0.1	0.0
In Light Syrup, Princes*	1 Serving/206g	64	31	0.4	7.3	0.0	1.0
In Light Syrup, Sainsbury's*	1/2 Can/125g	73	58	0.4	14.0	0.1	1.3
In Pear Juice, Kwik Save*	1 Can/411g	189	46	0.5	11.0	0.0	1.0
In Syrup, Del Monte*	1 Can/420g	315	75	0.4	18.0	0.1	0.0
In Syrup, SmartPrice, Asda*	1 Tin/411g	173	42	0.3	10.0	0.1	1.6
In Syrup, Tesco*	1 Serving/135g	85	63	0.4	15.0	0.0	1.0
In Very Light Syrup, Value, Tesco*	1 Can/410g	123	30	0.4	7.3	0.0	1.0
Light, With Sweeteners, Carrefour*	1 Sm Box/140g	42	30	0.3	7.0	0.1	1.1
No Added Sugar, Asda*	1 Serving/134g	67	50	0.3	12.0	0.1	1.6
Tropical, Asda*	1/2 Can/135g	81	60	0.0	15.0	0.0	1.6
Tropical, In Syrup, Sainsbury's*	1/2 Can/130g	95	73	0.5	17.6	0.1	1.4
Tropical, Morrisons*	1/2 Can/212g	144	68	0.0	17.0	0.0	0.0
Tropical, Safeway*	1/2 Can/214g	154	72	0.5	17.6	0.0	1.4
FRUIT COMPOTE							
& Vanilla Sponge, Weight Watchers*	1 Pack/140.3g	202	144	2.2	29.0	2.1	1.8
Apple, Strawberry & Blackberry, Organic, Yeo Valley*	1/2 Pot/112g	73	65	0.5	15.5	0.1	1.9
Apricot & Prune, Yeo Valley*	1 Pot/225g	207	92	0.6	22.3	0.1	1.6
Black Cherry & Creme Fraiche, Extra Special, Asda*	1 Pot/118g	188	159	1.7	20.0	8.0	0.8
Hartley's*	1 Serving/95g	63	66	0.8	15.5	0.1	2.4
Healthy Eating, Tesco*	1 Pot/140g	113	81	0.9	19.1	0.2	1.6
Orchard Fruits, GFY, Asda*	1 Pot/180g	113	63	0.5	15.0	0.1	0.0
Organic, Yeo Valley*	1oz/28g	13	47	0.5	11.2	0.0	0.0
Spiced, Tesco*	1 Serving/112g	122	109	1.7	24.4	0.5	3.1
Strawberry & Raspberry, Marks & Spencer*	1 Serving/80g	72	90	0.7	23.5	0.1	2.3
Summerfruit, Marks & Spencer*	1/4 Pot/125g	119	95	0.9	22.7	0.6	0.8
FRUIT DRINK							
Alive Tropical Torrent, The Coca Cola Co*	1 Glass/200ml	88	44	0.0	11.0	0.0	0.0
Blackcurrant Bracer, London Fruit & Herb Company*	1 Serving/200ml	4	2	0.0	0.5	0.0	0.0
Infusion, Peach, Lime & Ginger, Marks & Spencer*	1 Serving/250ml	88	35	0.0	8.5	0.0	0.0
FRUIT FILLING							
Apricot, Sainsbury's*	1 Can/400g	316	79	0.5	19.1	0.1	0.9
Black Cherry, Tesco*	1 Serving/100g	110	110	0.4	26.9	0.1	0.4
Bramley Apple, Morton*	1 Serving/197.5g	168	85	0.2	21.1	0.1	0.0

	Measure INFO/WEIGHT	per Measure KCAL	Nutrition Values per 100g / 100ml				
			KCAL	PROT	CARB	FAT	FIBRE
FRUIT FILLING							
Cherry & Amaretto, Asda*	1/4 Pack/100g	105	105	0.9	23.0	0.2	0.0
Red Cherry, Morton*	1 Serving/70g	69	98	0.4	23.9	0.0	0.0
FRUIT FLAKES							
Blackcurrant, Fruit Bowl*	1 Serving/20g	61	307	1.0	79.0	0.3	0.0
Raisins, With A Yogurt Coating, Fruit Bowl*	1 Serving/30g	130	434	2.0	70.5	14.6	0.0
Raspberry, With A Yogurt Coating, Fruit Bowl*	1 Serving/25g	111	443	1.3	72.8	16.5	0.0
Strawberry, Fruit Bowl*	1 Serving/20g	62	310	1.0	79.0	0.3	0.0
Strawberry, With A Yogurt Coating, Fruit Bowl*	1 Serving/25g	111	443	1.3	72.8	16.5	0.0
FRUIT GUMS							
Multi Vitamin, Aldi*	1 Serving/50g	168	336	6.7	76.9	0.2	0.0
No Added Sugar, Boots*	1 Sweet/1.6g	2	88	0.0	22.0	0.0	0.0
Red & Black, Marks & Spencer*	1 Bag/113g	362	320	5.2	75.8	0.1	0.1
Rowntree's*	1 Pack/48g	164	342	4.7	80.8	0.2	0.0
FRUIT LOLLY							
Exotic Fruit, Mini, Healthy Living, Tesco*	1 Lolly/31.3g	41	131	1.0	26.4	2.0	1.0
No Added Sugar, Tesco*	1 Lolly/32.4g	26	80	0.1	20.0	0.0	0.1
FRUIT MEDLEY							
Citrus, Somerfield*	1 Serving/80.6g	25	31	0.6	6.9	0.1	0.4
Dried Fruit Mix, Shapers, Boots*	1 Serving/50g	131	262	3.2	61.0	0.6	5.5
Exotic, Waitrose*	1 Medley/300g	126	42	0.6	9.5	0.2	1.1
Fresh, Marks & Spencer*	1/2 Pack/200g	100	50	0.7	12.3	0.1	1.6
Fresh, Waitrose*	1 Pack/300g	114	38	0.6	8.7	0.1	1.4
Freshly Prepared, Waitrose*	1 Serving/240g	72	30	1.0	6.3	0.1	2.2
In Fresh Orange Juice, Co-Op*	1 Serving/140g	49	35	0.5	9.0	0.0	0.0
Mixed, Fruit Harvest, Whitworths*	1 Pack/50g	166	331	1.8	79.4	0.7	4.8
Raisin, Fruit Harvest, Whitworths*	1 Pack/50g	158	315	1.8	74.4	1.3	4.3
Shapers, Boots*	1 Pack/140g	55	39	0.7	8.6	0.2	1.0
Summer, Waitrose*	1 Bowl/300g	84	28	0.8	5.9	0.1	1.3
Tropical, Soft, Waitrose*	1 Serving/33g	93	283	0.2	70.6	0.0	2.5
FRUIT MIX							
& Seeds, Sainsbury's*	1 Pack/50g	204	408	9.9	51.6	18.9	4.1
Apricot & Passion Fruit, WTF, Sainsbury's*	1/2 Pack/125g	374	299	2.7	70.1	0.2	5.1
Berry, Sainsbury's*	1 Serving/20g	64	319	1.0	78.1	1.9	5.5
Berry, Tesco*	1 Serving/50g	126	252	3.3	60.6	0.7	7.5
Luxury, Sainsbury's*	1 Serving/30g	78	261	1.8	62.3	0.5	2.7
Mango & Cranberry, Way To Five, Sainsbury's*	1 Serving/50g	166	331	1.8	79.4	0.7	4.8
TTD, Sainsbury's*	1 Serving/50g	69	137	0.3	36.4	0.4	1.6
Tropical Dried, & Coconut, Safeway*	1 Pack/50g	185	369	3.0	69.0	9.0	4.3
Tropical, Fresh, Waitrose*	1 Pack/240g	122	51	0.6	11.6	0.2	1.9
FRUIT PUREE							
Apple, & Blueberry, Organix*	1 Pot/100g	54	54	0.4	11.6	0.6	2.5
Apple, & Peach, Organix*	1 Pot/100g	49	49	0.6	11.0	0.3	2.1
Banana, Apple, & Apricot, Organix*	1 Pot/100g	68	68	0.8	15.4	0.4	2.0
FRUIT RUSH							
Rowntree's*	1 Pack/45g	144	319	3.7	75.6	0.2	0.0
FRUIT SALAD							
Autumn, Marks & Spencer*	1 Bowl/400g	220	55	0.4	13.2	0.1	1.8
Chunky, In Grape Juice, Tesco*	1 Serving/135g	63	47	0.4	11.0	0.2	0.8
Citrus, Asda*	1 Serving/265g	88	33	0.9	7.2	0.1	1.5
Classic, Sainsbury's*	1 Serving/600g	228	38	0.0	8.7	0.2	1.8
Dried, Marks & Spencer*	1/2 Pack/125g	269	215	1.8	51.4	0.4	5.9
Dried, Nature's Harvest*	1/2 Pack/125g	231	185	3.1	40.9	1.0	8.0
Exotic, Fully Prepared, Sainsbury's*	1 Serving/200g	74	37	0.6	8.3	0.2	1.3

	Measure	per Measure		Nutrition Values per 100g / 100ml				
	INFO/WEIGHT	KCAL		KCAL	PROT	CARB	FAT	FIBRE
FRUIT SALAD								
Exotic, Safeway*	1/2 Pot/159.6g	75		47	0.6	10.5	0.3	1.1
Exotic, Sainsbury's*	1/2 Tub/200g	80		40	0.6	9.1	0.3	1.0
Exotic, Tesco*	1 Serving/225g	86		38	0.7	8.4	0.2	1.5
Fresh, Asda*	1/2 Pack/200g	86		43	0.7	9.9	0.1	2.1
Fresh, Golden, Asda*	1 Pot/146.8g	69		47	0.6	11.0	0.1	1.6
Fresh, Marks & Spencer*	1oz/28g	13		45	0.6	10.1	0.2	1.3
Fresh, Sainsbury's*	1 Serving/120g	55		46	0.6	10.5	0.2	1.4
Fresh, Seasonal, Asda*	1 Pack/125g	55		44	0.5	10.4	0.1	1.2
Fresh, Sweet, Ripe & Moist, Tesco*	1 Serving/750g	345		46	0.7	10.6	0.1	1.6
Fresh, Tesco*	1oz/28g	13		45	0.6	10.5	0.1	1.4
Fresh, Washed, Ready To Eat, Tesco*	1 Pack/200g	92		46	0.7	10.6	0.1	1.6
Fruit, Mediterranean Style, Shapers, Boots*	1 Pack/141.9g	61		43	0.6	10.0	0.1	1.5
Grapefruit & Orange, Fresh, Marks & Spencer*	1 Serving/250g	88		35	0.9	7.4	0.1	1.6
Grapefruit, Tesco*	1/4 Can/134.5	77		57	0.8	13.5	0.0	0.5
Green, Marks & Spencer*	1 Bowl/400g	200		50	0.6	10.9	0.2	1.2
Homemade	1oz/28g	15		55	0.7	13.8	0.1	1.5
Luxury, Marks & Spencer*	1oz/28g	11		40	0.6	9.2	0.1	1.1
Mediterranean Style, Budgens*	1 Serving/250g	95		38	0.6	8.5	0.2	0.8
Melon, Kiwi, Strawbery, Way to Five, Sainsbury's*	1 Pack/245g	74		30	0.8	6.3	0.2	1.3
Mixed, Food To Go, Marks & Spencer*	1 Pack/400g	400		100	0.9	23.3	0.3	2.8
Mixed, New Improved, Tesco*	1 Pot/225g	79		35	0.8	7.6	0.2	1.2
Mixed, Prepared, Sainsbury's*	1/2 Pack/215g	90		42	0.7	9.4	0.2	1.9
Mixed, Sainsbury's*	1 Pack/400g	176		44	0.7	10.1	0.1	2.1
Mixed, Way To Five, Sainsbury's*	1 Pack/430g	168		39	0.7	8.6	0.2	1.2
Pineapple, Mandarin & Grapefruit, Asda*	1 Serving/200g	86		43	0.6	10.0	0.1	0.0
Sainsbury's*	1 Serving/300g	129		43	0.7	9.9	0.1	2.0
Seasonal, Marks & Spencer*	1 Serving/200g	100		50	0.5	11.8	0.2	2.1
Shapers, Boots*	1 Pack/140g	55		39	0.7	8.6	0.2	1.0
Summer, Sainsbury's*	1 Pack/240g	84		35	0.7	7.8	0.2	1.3
Tropical Fruit, In Light Syrup, Fast Fruit, Safeway*	1 Pot/125g	90		72	0.6	17.2	0.0	1.0
Tropical, Budgens*	1 Pack/250g	128		51	0.6	11.7	0.2	1.8
Tropical, Co-Op*	1 Serving/150g	68		45	0.6	9.0	0.2	1.0
Tropical, Fresh, Asda*	1 Pack/400g	164		41	0.7	9.0	0.2	1.8
Tropical, Fresh, Marks & Spencer*	1 Pack/425g	213		50	0.7	11.8	0.3	2.0
Tropical, Fresh, Sainsbury's*	1 Pack/230g	104		45	0.7	10.2	0.2	2.0
Tropical, Fruit Snacks, Frozen, Sainsbury's*	1 Serving/175g	79		45	0.7	10.4	0.1	1.6
Tropical, In Light Syrup, Passion Fruit Juice, Tesco*	1/2 Can/216g	130		60	0.3	14.1	0.1	1.1
Tropical, Marks & Spencer*	1oz/28g	12		44	0.8	9.6	0.3	1.8
Virgin Trains*	1 Serving/140g	56		40	0.4	10.0	0.1	0.8
Weight Watchers*	1 Serving/135g	50		37	0.2	9.0	0.1	0.7
FRUIT SELECTION								
Fresh, Marks & Spencer*	1 Pack/400g	180		45	0.6	10.1	0.2	1.3
Melon & Grapes, Fresh, Waitrose*	1 Serving/120g	44		37	0.5	8.5	0.1	0.8
New, Shapers, Boots*	1 Pack/160g	72		45	0.6	11.0	0.1	1.8
Shapers, Boots*	1 Pack/235g	96		41	0.5	9.2	0.2	0.8
FRUIT SHOOT								
Apple & Blackcurrant, Robinson's*	1 Bottle/200ml	10		5	0.1	0.8	0.0	0.0
FRUIT SPREAD								
Apricot, Pure, Organic, Whole Earth*	1 Serving/20g	33		167	0.8	40.0	0.4	0.9
Blackcurrant, Carb Check, Heinz*	1 Tbsp/15g	8		54	0.5	12.8	0.1	2.7
High, Blueberry, St Dalfour*	1 Tsp/15g	34		228	0.5	56.0	0.2	2.2
Raspberry, Weight Watchers*	1 Tsp/15g	17		111	0.4	27.1	0.1	0.9
Seville Orange, Weight Watchers*	1 Tsp/15g	17		111	0.2	27.5	0.0	0.3

F

	Measure INFO/WEIGHT	per Measure KCAL	Nutrition Values per 100g / 100ml				
			KCAL	PROT	CARB	FAT	FIBRE
FRUIT SPREAD							
Strawberry, Carb Check, Heinz*	1 Tbsp/15g	8	56	0.3	13.6	0.0	0.5
Strawberry, Weight Watchers*	1 Tsp/15g	17	115	0.2	28.4	0.0	0.4
FU YUNG							
Egg	1oz/28g	67	239	9.9	2.2	20.6	1.3
FUDGE							
All Butter, TTD, Sainsbury's*	1 Pack/125g	536	429	1.3	73.4	14.5	0.0
Average	1oz/28g	123	441	3.3	81.1	13.7	0.0
Butter Tablet, Thorntons*	1oz/28g	116	414	0.9	77.6	11.1	0.0
Butter, Milk, Thorntons*	1 Chocolate/13g	60	462	3.7	68.5	19.2	0.0
Cadbury*	1 Std Bar/25g	110	435	2.5	72.7	14.9	0.0
Cherry & Almond, Thorntons*	1 Bag/100g	464	464	3.2	70.5	19.1	0.4
Chocolate, Thorntons*	1 Bag/100g	459	459	3.1	69.0	19.1	0.6
Clotted Cream, Sainsbury's*	1 Sweet/8g	35	430	1.9	81.5	10.7	0.7
Devon, Somerfield*	1 Pack/250g	1060	424	2.0	78.9	11.1	0.0
Double Chocolate Bar, Marks & Spencer*	1 Bar/43g	202	470	4.2	66.9	21.0	0.7
Maple, TTD, Sainsbury's*	1 Sweet/10g	43	426	1.3	73.0	14.3	0.0
Pure Indulgence, Thorntons*	1 Bar/45g	210	466	1.8	65.9	21.9	0.0
Vanilla, Bar, Marks & Spencer*	1 Bar/43g	205	476	3.7	63.0	23.3	0.4
Vanilla, Tesco*	1 Bag/428g	1832	428	1.8	76.5	12.7	0.0
Vanilla, Thorntons*	1 Bag/100g	465	465	1.8	65.9	21.9	0.0
Vanilla, Whipped, Marks & Spencer*	1 Serving/42.9g	211	490	3.8	65.4	23.9	0.3
FUSE							
Cadbury*	1 Std Bar/49g	238	485	7.6	58.2	24.8	0.0
FUSILLI							
Carb Check, Heinz*	1 Serving/75g	219	292	52.7	15.2	2.3	20.8
Cooked, Average	1 Serving/210g	248	118	4.2	23.8	0.7	1.2
Corn Rice, Free From, Sainsbury's*	1 Serving/75g	262	349	7.6	73.9	2.6	3.6
Dry, Average	1 Serving/90g	316	352	12.3	72.0	1.6	2.2
Fresh, Cooked, Average	1 Serving/200g	329	165	6.4	30.7	1.8	1.8
Fresh, Dry, Average	1 Serving/75g	208	277	10.9	53.4	2.7	2.1
Microwaveable, Express, Dolmio*	1 Serving/220g	299	136	5.3	26.3	1.0	0.0
Tomato, Weight Watchers*	1 Can/388g	198	51	1.9	10.1	0.4	0.8
Tricolore, Dry, Average	1 Serving/75g	264	351	12.2	71.8	1.7	2.7
Tuna, BGTY, Sainsbury's*	1 Pack/400g	304	76	6.0	8.6	2.0	0.5
Whole Wheat, Dry, Average	1 Serving/90g	290	322	13.1	62.3	2.3	9.0
With Chicken & Courgettes, Sainsbury's*	1 Pack/450g	675	150	8.6	14.6	6.4	0.5

	Measure INFO/WEIGHT	per Measure KCAL	Nutrition Values per 100g / 100ml KCAL	PROT	CARB	FAT	FIBRE

GALAXY

	Measure INFO/WEIGHT	per Measure KCAL	KCAL	PROT	CARB	FAT	FIBRE
Amicelli, Mars*	1 Serving/13g	66	507	6.2	59.7	27.1	0.0
Caramel, Mars*	1 Bar/49g	238	485	5.4	60.3	24.7	0.0
Chocolate, Mars*	1 Bar/47g	254	540	6.8	57.0	31.7	0.0
Fruit & Hazelnut, Milk, Mars*	1 Bar/47g	235	501	7.1	55.2	28.0	0.0
Liaison, Mars*	1 Bar/48g	233	485	5.4	60.3	24.7	0.0
Ripple, Mars*	1 Bar/33g	169	528	6.9	59.3	29.3	0.0
Snack Size, Mars*	1 serving/24.5g	135	540	6.8	57.0	31.7	0.0
Swirls, Mars*	1 Bag/150g	747	498	4.9	60.2	26.5	0.0

GAMMON

	Measure INFO/WEIGHT	per Measure KCAL	KCAL	PROT	CARB	FAT	FIBRE
Baked, Hand Carved, Free Range, Waitrose*	1 Slice/37g	50	135	21.5	0.1	5.4	0.0
Breaded, Average	1oz/28g	34	120	22.5	1.0	3.1	0.0
Dry Cured, Ready To Roast, Marks & Spencer*	1/2 Joint/255g	255	100	20.5	0.5	1.5	0.5
Gammon Joint, Raw, Average	1oz/28g	39	138	20.3	0.0	6.3	0.0
Honey & Mustard, Average	1/2 Pack/190g	294	155	19.1	3.6	7.1	0.1
Joint, Applewood Smoked, Tesco*	1 Serving/100g	152	152	17.5	0.2	9.0	0.0
Joint, Boiled, Average	1oz/28g	47	167	25.1	0.4	7.1	0.0
Joint, Raw, Average	1oz/28g	37	138	20.3	0.0	6.3	0.0
Joint, With Honey Glaze, Average	1/4 Joint/113g	165	146	21.4	11.1	1.8	0.0
Joint, With Orange Glaze, Christmas, Finest, Tesco*	1/10 Joint150g	215	143	17.6	2.4	7.0	0.0
Steaks, Average	1 Steak/97.1g	157	161	23.3	0.4	7.4	0.0
Steaks, Healthy Range, Average	1 Serving/110g	107	97	18.0	0.4	3.2	0.2
Steaks, Honey Roast, Average	1 Steak/100g	142	142	21.5	2.3	5.3	0.1
Steaks, Smoked, Average	1 Steak/110g	150	137	22.7	0.1	5.0	0.1
Wiltshire, Traditional British Roast, Marks & Spencer*	1 Serving/70g	133	190	24.7	0.0	9.8	0.0

GAMMON &

	Measure INFO/WEIGHT	per Measure KCAL	KCAL	PROT	CARB	FAT	FIBRE
Pineapple, Roast, Dinner, Iceland*	1 Meal/400g	360	90	6.2	12.7	1.6	1.7

GARAM MASALA

	Measure INFO/WEIGHT	per Measure KCAL	KCAL	PROT	CARB	FAT	FIBRE
Average	1oz/28g	106	379	15.6	45.2	15.1	0.0

GARGANELLI

	Measure INFO/WEIGHT	per Measure KCAL	KCAL	PROT	CARB	FAT	FIBRE
Egg, Dry, Waitrose*	1 Serving/125g	450	360	13.5	66.9	4.2	3.5

GARLIC

	Measure INFO/WEIGHT	per Measure KCAL	KCAL	PROT	CARB	FAT	FIBRE
Minced, Nishaan*	1 Serving/100g	88	88	4.5	10.5	3.1	0.0
Powder	1 Tsp/3g	7	246	18.7	42.7	1.2	9.9
Raw	1 Clove/3g	3	98	7.9	16.3	0.6	4.1
Very Lazy, EPC*	1 Tsp/3g	3	111	6.0	20.9	0.4	3.0

GARLIC PUREE

	Measure INFO/WEIGHT	per Measure KCAL	KCAL	PROT	CARB	FAT	FIBRE
Asda*	1 Tbsp/15g	63	423	2.7	13.0	40.0	6.0
Average	1 Tbsp/18g	61	380	3.5	16.9	33.6	0.0
Co-Op*	1 Teaspoon/5g	18	355	5.0	16.0	30.0	3.0
Sharwood's*	1 Tbsp/18g	9	63	3.4	13.3	0.3	2.4

GATEAU

	Measure INFO/WEIGHT	per Measure KCAL	KCAL	PROT	CARB	FAT	FIBRE
Au Fromage Blanc, Ligne Et Plaisir*	1 Serving/80g	128	160	8.0	26.0	2.6	0.0
Black Forest, Mini, Tesco*	1 Serving/55g	136	247	5.7	35.3	9.2	1.0
Black Forest, Sara Lee*	1 Serving/80g	221	276	3.6	37.9	12.3	1.2
Blackforest, Sainsbury's*	1/8 Gateau/63g	163	259	3.9	27.7	17.1	3.5
Chocolate Layer, Marks & Spencer*	1 Serving/86g	278	323	4.2	35.9	18.3	0.9
Chocolate Orange, Co-Op*	1 Slice/97g	320	330	5.0	37.0	18.0	1.0
Chocolate, Asda*	1 Serving/100g	176	176	2.4	19.0	10.0	0.4
Chocolate, Swirl, Tesco*	1 Serving/83g	230	277	3.8	29.3	16.0	0.2
Coffee, Tesco*	1 Serving/100g	300	300	4.2	32.5	17.0	0.6
Double Chocolate, Light, Sara Lee*	1/5 Gateau/58.6g	140	237	5.7	43.3	4.6	2.0
Double Chocolate, Sara Lee*	1oz/28g	93	331	5.6	41.3	16.5	0.9
Double Chocolate, Tesco*	1 Serving/45g	124	276	4.4	32.1	14.4	2.2

G

	Measure		Nutrition Values per 100g / 100ml				
	INFO/WEIGHT	KCAL	KCAL	PROT	CARB	FAT	FIBRE

GATEAU
Double Strawberry, Sara Lee*	1/8 Slice/199g	533	268	3.2	36.2	12.2	0.6
Ice Cream, Chocolate & Vanilla, Iceland*	1 Serving/130g	252	194	3.3	24.1	9.4	0.6
Lemon & Lime, Marks & Spencer*	1 Serving/100g	295	295	3.2	35.0	15.6	0.3
Orange & Lemon, Iceland*	1 Serving/90g	221	245	2.6	33.8	11.0	0.3
Profiterole, TTD, Sainsbury's*	1/6 Gateau/112g	410	365	3.9	26.2	27.2	1.1
Strawberry, Co-Op*	1 Slice/77g	222	288	5.1	29.2	16.7	1.0
Strawberry, Family Size, Tesco*	1 Serving/84g	197	235	2.9	25.2	13.6	0.6
Swiss, Cadbury*	1/6/60g	228	380	5.2	52.0	16.8	0.9
Toffee Ripple, Sara Lee*	1 Serving/317g	1005	317	4.0	40.2	15.6	0.5
Triple Chocolate, Tesco*	1 Serving/64g	187	292	3.9	31.1	16.9	0.4

GAZPACHO
Average	1oz/28g	13	45	0.8	2.6	3.6	0.6

GELATINE
Average	1oz/28g	95	338	84.4	0.0	0.0	0.0

GEMELLI
Durum Wheat, Tesco*	1 Serving/100g	354	354	13.2	68.5	2.0	2.9

GHEE
Butter	1oz/28g	251	898	0.0	0.0	99.8	0.0
Palm	1oz/28g	251	897	0.0	0.0	99.7	0.0
Vegetable	1oz/28g	251	895	0.0	0.0	99.4	0.0

GHERKINS
Pickled, Average	1 Gherkin/36g	5	14	0.9	2.6	0.1	1.2

GIGLIO
Egg, Tesco*	1 Serving/100g	355	355	14.5	66.4	3.5	2.6

GIN
& Tonic, Premixed, Canned, Gordons*	1 Can/250ml	213	85	0.0	6.7	0.0	0.0
37.5% Volume	1 Shot/25ml	52	207	0.0	0.0	0.0	0.0
40% Volume	1 Shot/25ml	56	222	0.0	0.0	0.0	0.0

GINGER
Crystallised, Nature's Harvest*	1 Tbsp/15g	50	330	0.3	82.0	0.1	16.0
Fresh	1oz/28g	14	49	1.7	9.5	0.7	0.0
Lazy, EPC*	1 Tbsp/10g	2	15	0.2	3.2	0.2	1.5
Root, Raw	1oz/28g	11	38	1.4	7.2	0.6	0.0
Stem, In Sugar Syrup, Sainsbury's*	1oz/28g	76	271	0.2	67.3	0.1	1.4

GINGER ALE
American, Finest, Tesco*	1 Serving/150ml	68	45	0.0	11.0	0.0	0.0
American, Low Calorie, Tesco*	1fl oz/30ml	0	1	0.0	0.0	0.0	0.0
Dry	1 Glass/250ml	38	15	0.0	3.9	0.0	0.0
Dry, Sainsbury's*	1 Glass/250ml	95	38	0.1	9.1	0.1	0.1

GINGER BEER
Tesco*	1 Can/330ml	109	33	0.0	8.2	0.0	0.0

GINGERBREAD
Average	1oz/28g	106	379	5.7	64.7	12.6	1.2
Men, Mini, Marks & Spencer*	1 Biscuit/16.6g	80	470	6.2	63.9	18.6	1.7
Men, Mini, Sainsbury's*	1 Man/12g	56	463	5.7	83.4	11.8	1.5

GLAZE
Balsamic, A Drizzle Of, Waitrose*	1 Serving/15ml	18	122	0.0	26.0	0.0	0.0

GNOCCHI
Aldi*	1 Serving/100g	160	160	3.8	35.6	0.3	0.0
Di Patati, Safeway*	1 Serving/150g	255	170	4.5	37.3	0.3	0.4
Dry, Buitoni*	1 Serving/150g	528	352	11.2	72.6	1.9	0.0
Fresh, Sainsbury's*	1 Serving/100g	152	152	3.8	33.6	0.3	1.4
Plain, Italfresco*	1/2 Pack/200g	296	148	3.3	33.2	0.2	0.1

G

GNOCCHI

Tomato & Mozzarella Filled, Sainsbury's*	1 Serving/125g	205	164	5.7	24.9	4.6	4.6

GOOSE

Meat Only, Roasted	1oz/28g	89	319	29.3	0.0	22.4	0.0
Meat, Fat & Skin, Raw	1oz/28g	101	361	16.5	0.0	32.8	0.0

GOOSEBERRIES

Dessert, Raw	1oz/28g	11	40	0.7	9.2	0.3	2.4

GOULASH

Beef, Bistro Range, Tesco*	1 Pack/450g	545	121	7.9	14.6	3.4	0.6
Beef, Finest, Tesco*	1/2 Pack/300g	297	99	11.6	6.2	3.1	0.6
Beef, With Tagliatelle, COU, Marks & Spencer*	1 Pack/360g	414	115	8.5	14.5	2.3	1.0

GRANOLA

Cranberry & Apple, Good Intentions, Somerfield*	1 Serving/30g	109	363	9.0	71.0	4.8	10.2
Low Fat, Sweet Home Farm*	1 Serving/55g	180	328	7.3	69.0	5.4	9.0

GRAPEFRUIT

In Juice, Average	1oz/28g	13	46	0.5	10.6	0.0	0.4
In Syrup, Average	1oz/28g	19	69	0.5	16.8	0.1	0.5
Raw, Average	1 Med/340g	85	25	0.7	5.7	0.1	1.1
Ruby Red, In Juice, Average	1 Serving/135g	54	40	0.6	9.4	0.1	0.5

GRAPES

Green, Average	1oz/28g	17	62	0.4	15.2	0.1	0.7
Red & Green Selection, Average	1 Bag/80g	50	63	0.4	15.2	0.1	0.9
Red, Average	1 Serving/79g	53	67	0.5	16.5	0.1	0.8

GRATIN

Cauliflower, Findus*	1 Pack/400g	340	85	3.5	7.0	5.0	0.0
Creamy Potato, Marks & Spencer*	1/2 Pack/225g	360	160	2.2	11.9	11.1	0.9
Dauphinoise, Budgens*	1/2 Pack/218g	277	127	3.0	12.5	7.2	2.5
Leek & Carrot, Findus*	1 Pack/400g	440	110	3.5	9.5	6.5	0.0
Potato, Healthy Living, Tesco*	1 Serving/225g	169	75	2.3	11.4	2.2	0.6
Potato, Sainsbury's*	1/2 Pack/450g	896	199	4.4	11.0	15.1	1.0
Spinach & Mushroom, Safeway*	1 Packet/520g	728	140	4.8	10.3	8.4	1.5
Vegetable, Somerfield*	1 Pack/300g	417	139	1.0	5.0	13.0	0.0

GRAVADLAX

Finest, Tesco*	1 Serving/70g	125	178	22.1	0.2	9.9	0.0
Marks & Spencer*	1 Serving/140g	294	210	18.4	5.3	11.4	0.5
Scottish Salmon, Marks & Spencer*	1 Serving/70g	147	210	18.4	5.3	11.4	0.5
TTD, Sainsbury's*	1/4 Pack/35g	64	182	22.9	1.1	9.5	0.6
Waitrose*	1 Serving/65g	124	190	21.8	1.0	11.1	0.4

GRAVY

Beef, Fresh, Sainsbury's*	1 Serving/83ml	47	56	2.4	4.5	3.2	0.6
Beef, Heat Serve, Morrisons*	1 Serving/150g	27	18	0.3	3.9	0.3	0.5
Beef, With Winter Berry Shallot, Made Up, Oxo*	1 Serving/105ml	24	23	0.6	4.3	0.3	0.1
Chips & Onion, Asda*	1 Pack/357.6g	329	92	2.1	15.0	2.6	1.2
For Poultry, Marks & Spencer*	1 Jar/400g	136	34	2.5	5.0	0.4	0.3
Fresh, Somerfield*	1 Pack/300g	69	23	0.0	4.0	1.0	0.0
Granules For Chicken, Dry, Bisto*	1 Serving/4g	12	299	4.4	63.4	3.1	0.5
Granules For Chicken, Made Up, SmartPrice, Asda*	1 Serving/100ml	34	34	0.2	3.0	2.3	0.1
Granules For Meat, Made Up, Asda*	1 Serving/100ml	38	38	0.6	4.0	2.4	0.1
Granules For Meat, Made Up, Sainsbury's*	1 Serving/100ml	37	37	0.4	3.5	2.4	0.1
Granules For Vegetarian Dishes, Dry Weight, Bisto*	1 Serving/50ml	184	367	2.6	59.5	13.2	1.3
Granules With Onion, Dry, Bisto*	1 Serving/4g	15	365	2.9	56.1	14.3	1.8
Granules for Turkey, Dry, Bisto*	1 Serving/4g	15	367	3.3	53.9	15.3	1.2
Granules, Beef, Dry, Tesco*	1 Serving/6g	29	480	5.5	36.4	34.7	1.5
Granules, Beef, Made Up, Tesco*	1 Serving/140ml	49	35	0.3	2.6	2.5	0.1

G

	Measure INFO/WEIGHT	per Measure KCAL	Nutrition Values per 100g / 100ml				
			KCAL	PROT	CARB	FAT	FIBRE
GRAVY							
Granules, Chicken & Hint of Sage & Onion, Oxo*	1 Serving/30g	95	316	11.1	54.2	6.1	0.7
Granules, Chicken, Dry, Oxo*	1oz/28g	83	296	11.1	54.2	4.9	0.7
Granules, Chicken, Made Up, Oxo*	1fl oz/30ml	5	18	0.7	3.3	0.3	0.0
Granules, Chip Shop Curry, Dry Weight, Bisto*	1 Serving/50ml	234	468	4.3	72.6	17.8	2.7
Granules, Dry, Bisto*	1 Serving/10g	38	384	3.1	56.4	16.2	1.5
Granules, Dry, Value, Tesco*	1oz/28g	111	397	3.2	54.4	18.5	1.0
Granules, For Vegetarian Dishes, Made Up, Sainsbury's*	1 Serving/50ml	16	32	0.2	2.8	2.2	0.8
Granules, Instant, Dry	1oz/28g	129	462	4.4	40.6	32.5	0.0
Granules, Instant, Made Up	1oz/28g	10	34	0.3	3.0	2.4	0.0
Granules, Lamb, Made Up, Oxo*	1 Serving/100ml	25	25	0.7	4.3	0.5	0.0
Granules, Made Up, Bisto*	1 Serving/50ml	15	30	0.2	4.2	1.4	0.2
Granules, Made Up, Oxo*	1 Serving/150ml	29	19	0.6	3.4	0.3	0.0
Granules, Onion, Dry, Morrisons*	1 Serving/25g	124	495	3.4	44.0	34.7	0.0
Granules, Onion, Dry, Oxo*	1oz/28g	92	328	8.2	62.3	4.8	0.8
Granules, Onion, Made Up, Bisto*	1 Serving/140ml	39	28	0.2	4.2	1.0	0.2
Granules, Onion, Made Up, Oxo*	1fl oz/30ml	6	20	0.5	3.7	0.3	0.0
Granules, Original, Dry, Oxo*	1oz/28g	88	313	10.2	57.2	4.8	1.0
Granules, Vegetable, Dry, Bisto*	1 Serving/4g	15	367	2.6	59.5	13.2	1.3
Granules, Vegetable, Dry, Oxo*	1oz/28g	88	316	8.4	59.5	4.9	0.9
Granules, Vegetable, Dry, Tesco*	1/2 Pint/20g	94	470	3.8	38.5	33.4	3.7
Granules, Vegetable, Made Up, Bisto*	1 Serving/140ml	39	28	0.2	5.6	0.4	0.2
Granules, Vegetarian, Dry, Bisto*	1 Serving/28g	110	394	2.6	54.9	18.2	1.3
Instant Mix, Dry, BFY, Morrisons*	1 Serving/25g	80	320	3.5	77.0	0.3	1.2
Mix, Instant, Made Up, BGTY, Sainsbury's*	1fl oz/30ml	10	32	0.3	7.4	0.1	0.1
Onion, Fresh, Asda*	1/6 Pot/77g	30	39	1.7	3.3	2.1	0.4
Onion, Fresh, Somerfield*	1 Pack/300g	195	65	1.0	7.0	4.0	0.0
Onion, Rich, Marks & Spencer*	1/2 Pack/150g	60	40	2.0	5.9	1.2	0.3
Onion, TTD, Sainsbury's*	1 serving/100g	78	78	1.3	6.6	5.2	0.8
Powder For Pork, Dry, Best, Bisto*	1 Serving/100g	303	303	5.1	62.3	3.7	0.8
Powder, Dry, Tesco*	1 Serving/20g	57	286	7.2	61.0	1.5	2.0
Powder, Gluten Free, Dry, Allergycare*	1 Tbsp/10g	26	260	0.3	63.8	0.4	0.0
Powder, Made Up, Sainsbury's*	1 Serving/100ml	15	15	0.4	3.2	0.1	0.1
Roast Beef Flavour, Made Up, Best, Bisto*	1 Serving/50ml	13	26	0.4	5.4	0.4	0.2
Roast Beef, Dry, Schwartz*	1 Pack/27g	90	333	12.7	65.2	2.4	0.0
Roast Chicken, Dry, Schwartz*	1 Pack/26g	95	365	10.2	65.7	6.8	0.0
Roast Pork & Sage, Dry, Schwartz	1 Serving/25g	90	359	10.2	65.7	6.2	0.0
Roast Turkey, Dry, Schwartz*	1 Serving/6g	21	355	12.0	60.2	7.4	0.0
GREENGAGES							
Raw, Average	1oz/28g	11	40	0.8	9.5	0.1	2.1
GRILLS							
Bacon & Cheese, Tesco*	1 Grill/78g	222	284	15.0	13.4	18.9	1.2
Cauliflower Cheese, Dalepak*	1 Grill/94g	231	246	4.6	20.0	14.8	2.6
Cheese & Bacon, Danepak*	1 Grill/84.9g	241	284	15.0	13.4	18.9	1.2
Tikka, Organic, Waitrose*	1 Grill/100g	185	185	6.9	18.5	9.3	3.4
Vegetable, Dalepak*	1 Grill/85g	142	167	4.6	22.5	6.5	1.6
Vegetable, Mediterranean, Cauldron*	1 Grill/88g	145	166	5.3	15.8	11.9	6.5
Vegetable, Ross*	1 Grill/114g	252	221	4.3	25.5	11.3	0.9
Vegetable, Tesco*	1 Grill/72.2g	129	179	4.2	18.0	10.0	2.2
Vegetarian, Cauliflower Cheese, Tesco*	1 Serving/92g	232	252	5.0	21.7	16.1	2.8
Vegetarian, Mushroom & Oregano, Organic, Waitrose*	1 Grill/100g	160	160	8.8	12.8	8.2	2.4
GROUSE							
Meat Only, Roasted	1oz/28g	36	128	27.6	0.0	2.0	0.0

	Measure INFO/WEIGHT	per Measure KCAL	Nutrition Values per 100g / 100ml				
			KCAL	PROT	CARB	FAT	FIBRE
GUACAMOLE							
Asda*	1/2 Pot/56.5g	105	184	1.6	4.0	18.0	0.0
Average	1 Tbsp/17g	22	128	1.4	2.2	12.7	2.5
Avocado, Reduced Fat, The Fresh Dip Company*	1 Serving/113g	128	113	2.5	6.1	8.7	2.3
Chunky, Sainsbury's*	1/2 Pot/64.9g	120	185	1.6	3.2	18.4	3.8
Doritos*	1 Tbsp/20g	32	159	1.2	2.6	16.0	0.1
Fresh, Sainsbury's*	1oz/28g	59	210	1.8	5.3	20.2	2.5
GFY, Asda*	1 Pack/113g	144	127	2.8	4.3	11.0	2.2
Reduced Fat, Sainsbury's*	1/2 Pot/65g	87	134	1.5	3.5	12.6	4.0
Reduced Fat, Tesco*	1 Pot/113g	142	126	2.9	5.7	10.2	2.3
Somerfield*	1oz/28g	53	188	2.0	5.0	18.0	0.0
Tesco*	1 Serving/35g	67	190	1.9	4.1	18.4	2.5
GUAVA							
Canned, In Syrup	1oz/28g	17	60	0.4	15.7	0.0	3.0
Raw, Average	1oz/28g	7	25	0.8	4.8	0.5	3.5
GUINEA FOWL							
Boned & Stuffed, Fresh, FayreGame*	1 Serving/325g	650	200	19.1	3.3	12.1	0.5
GUMBO							
Cajun Vegetable, Sainsbury's*	1 Serving/450g	266	59	1.4	7.7	2.5	1.5
Louisiana Chicken, Perfectly Balanced, Waitrose*	1 Serving/235g	207	88	12.2	3.5	2.8	1.3
GUMS							
American Hard, Sainsbury's*	1 Sweet/6g	22	360	0.1	90.0	0.1	0.0
Fruit Salad, Tesco*	6 Sweets/30g	101	335	8.3	73.4	0.5	0.3
Milk Bottles, Bassett's*	1 Pack/25g	88	353	6.2	78.3	1.6	0.0
Milk, Cow, Sainsbury's*	1 Sweet/3g	10	353	6.2	78.3	1.6	0.0
Percy Pig & Pals, Soft, Marks & Spencer*	1 Sweet/7.6g	28	344	5.8	80.0	0.1	0.0

G

	Measure INFO/WEIGHT	per Measure KCAL	Nutrition Values per 100g / 100ml				
			KCAL	PROT	CARB	FAT	FIBRE
HADDOCK							
Fillets, Battered, Average	1oz/28g	64	228	13.4	16.3	12.2	1.1
Fillets, In Breadcrumbs, Average	1oz/28g	57	203	13.5	14.9	9.9	1.2
Fillets, Raw, Average	1oz/28g	22	80	18.0	0.2	0.9	0.0
Fillets, Smoked, Cooked, Average	1 Pack/300g	337	112	21.9	0.4	2.6	0.1
Fillets, Smoked, Raw, Average	1 Pack/227g	194	86	20.3	0.1	0.5	0.2
Flour, Fried in Blended Oil	1oz/28g	39	138	21.1	4.5	4.1	0.2
Goujons, Batter, Crispy, Marks & Spencer*	1 Serving/100g	250	250	11.7	18.5	14.1	0.8
HADDOCK &							
Cauliflower Crunchies, Iceland*	1 Serving/111g	222	200	8.0	15.5	11.8	2.0
Chips, Marks & Spencer*	1oz/28g	52	187	7.0	22.6	7.6	2.1
HADDOCK EN CROUTE							
Young's*	1 Serving/170.1g	432	254	8.0	17.1	16.9	4.3
HADDOCK FLORENTINE							
Eat Smart, Safeway*	1 Serving/250g	200	80	12.0	2.5	1.8	1.3
Healthy Eating, Tesco*	1 Pack/370g	303	82	8.2	10.0	1.0	0.5
HADDOCK IN							
Butter Sauce, Steaks, Young's*	1 Portion/150g	134	89	9.9	4.0	3.7	0.5
Cheese & Chive Sauce, Healthy Eating, Tesco*	1 Pack/360g	284	79	12.7	2.6	2.0	0.1
Cheese & Chive Sauce, Healthy Living, Tesco*	1 Serving/400g	304	76	11.6	2.2	2.3	0.7
Cheese & Chive Sauce, Smoked Fillets, Seafresh*	1 Serving/170g	201	118	14.7	1.2	6.1	0.1
Cheese & Leek Sauce, Fillets, Steamfresh, Birds Eye*	1 Serving/189g	170	90	11.0	2.5	3.9	0.1
Smoked Leek & Cheese Sauce, Asda*	1/2 Pack/200g	232	116	14.0	3.7	5.0	1.5
Tomato Herb Sauce, Fillets, BGTY, Sainsbury's*	1/2 Pack/165g	150	91	12.9	3.6	2.8	0.1
Watercress Sauce, GFY, Asda*	1 Pack/400g	268	67	6.0	7.0	1.7	1.4
HADDOCK RAREBIT							
Smoked, Finest, Tesco*	1 Rarebit/180g	326	181	5.6	19.1	9.2	0.4
HADDOCK TOPPED							
Potato, Cumberland, Marks & Spencer*	1 Pack/300g	390	130	8.2	10.6	6.0	0.4
HADDOCK WITH							
A Rich Cheese Crust, Smoked, Sainsbury's*	1 Serving/199g	295	148	13.0	2.5	9.5	0.9
Broccoli & Cheese, Lakeland*	1 Serving/150g	281	187	10.4	20.6	7.0	0.0
Cheese & Chive, Smoked, GFY, Asda*	1/2 Pack/185.7g	195	105	15.0	3.1	3.6	0.3
Creme Fraiche & Chive Sauce, Smoked, Tesco*	1 Serving/150g	155	103	16.8	2.1	3.1	0.3
HAGGIS							
Neeps & Tatties, Marks & Spencer*	1 Pack/300g	330	110	3.8	12.3	4.8	0.8
Traditional, Average	1 Serving/120g	296	247	12.4	17.2	14.7	1.1
Vegetarian, McSween*	1 serving/100g	216	216	6.6	26.8	10.2	2.4
HAKE							
Fillets, In Breadcrumbs, Average	1oz/28g	66	235	12.9	16.0	13.4	1.0
Goujons, Average	1 Serving/150g	345	230	12.4	18.7	11.9	1.3
Raw, Average	1oz/28g	29	102	20.4	0.0	2.2	0.0
With Tomato & Chilli Salsa, Just Cook, Sainsbury's*	1/2 Pack/180g	112	62	11.4	2.2	0.9	0.0
HALIBUT							
Cooked, Average	1oz/28g	38	135	24.6	0.4	4.0	0.0
Raw	1oz/28g	29	103	21.5	0.0	1.9	0.0
HALIBUT WITH							
Roasted Pepper Sauce, Fillets, Marks & Spencer*	1 Serving/145g	218	150	12.7	2.4	9.9	0.6
HALWA							
Average	1oz/28g	107	381	1.8	68.0	13.2	0.0
HAM							
Applewood Smoked, Average	1 Slice/28g	31	112	21.3	0.6	2.8	0.3
Baked, Average	1 Slice/74g	106	143	21.1	1.8	5.8	0.3
Bavarian, Asda*	1 Slice/15g	18	121	21.4	0.5	3.7	0.0

H

HAM

	Measure INFO/WEIGHT	per Measure KCAL	Nutrition Values per 100g / 100ml				
			KCAL	PROT	CARB	FAT	FIBRE
Beechwood Smoked, Morrisons*	1 Slice/20g	32	160	19.5	0.5	9.0	0.0
Boiled, Average	1 Pack/113g	154	137	20.6	0.6	5.8	0.0
Breaded, Average	1 Slice/37g	57	155	23.1	1.9	6.3	1.6
Breaded, Dry Cured, Average	1 Slice/33g	47	142	22.2	1.4	5.4	0.0
Brunswick, Average	1 Slice/20g	32	160	19.5	0.6	8.8	0.1
Cooked, Sliced, Average	1 Serving/50g	57	115	19.1	0.9	3.9	0.1
Crumbed, Sliced, Average	1 Slice/28g	33	117	21.5	0.9	3.1	0.0
Danish, Average	1 Slice/11g	14	125	18.4	1.1	5.4	0.0
Danish, Lean, Average	1 Slice/15g	14	93	17.9	1.0	1.8	0.0
Dry Cured, Average	1 Slice/18g	26	144	22.4	1.0	5.6	0.2
Dry Cured, Mustard, Slices, TTD, Sainsbury's*	1 Slice/26g	40	153	20.2	1.6	7.3	0.1
Dry Cured, Rosemary &Thyme, Safeway*	1 Slice/28g	37	133	24.8	1.5	3.1	0.0
Extra Lean, Average	1 Slice/11g	10	90	18.0	1.4	1.4	0.0
Gammon, Breaded, Average	1 Serving/25g	31	122	22.0	1.5	3.1	0.0
Gammon, Dry Cured, Average	1 Slice/33g	43	131	22.9	0.4	4.2	0.0
Gammon, Honey Roast, Average	1 Serving/60g	81	135	22.5	0.5	4.8	0.0
Gammon, Mustard, Cured, Waitrose*	1 Slice/45g	54	120	21.4	0.1	4.0	0.0
Gammon, Peppered, Waitrose*	1/3 Pack/36g	51	142	20.7	0.3	6.4	0.0
Gammon, Smoked, Average	1 Slice/43g	59	137	22.3	0.7	4.9	0.2
German Black Forest, Average	1/2 Pack/35g	93	267	27.2	1.3	17.0	0.5
Glazed With Honey & Muscovado Sugar, Waitrose*	1 Slice/21g	25	119	21.3	0.4	3.6	0.0
Honey & Ginger, Roast, Waitrose*	1 Slice/16g	21	134	20.0	0.0	6.0	0.0
Honey & Mustard, Average	1oz/28g	39	140	20.8	4.6	4.3	0.0
Honey Roast, Average	1 Slice/20g	25	123	20.3	1.6	3.8	0.1
Honey Roast, Dry Cured, Average	1 Slice/33g	46	140	22.7	2.3	4.4	0.2
Honey Roast, Lean, Average	1 Serving/25g	28	111	18.2	2.7	3.1	0.0
Honey Roast, Wafer Thin, Average	1 Slice/10g	11	113	17.4	3.7	3.2	0.3
Honey Roast, Wafer Thin, Premium, Average	1 Slice/10g	15	149	22.0	1.6	6.0	0.0
Italian Rostello, Safeway*	1 Serving/60g	78	130	21.0	0.2	5.0	0.0
Joint, Easy Carve, Asda*	1oz/28g	41	146	22.8	1.2	5.9	0.6
Joint, Honey Roast, Asda*	1oz/28g	35	124	23.9	1.7	2.8	0.7
Joint, Roast, Christmas, Tesco*	1/6 Joint/167g	225	135	17.9	1.1	6.5	0.0
Lean, Average	1 Slice/18g	19	104	19.5	1.1	2.4	0.3
Maple Drycure, Asda*	1 Slice/37.1g	53	143	22.0	3.0	4.8	0.0
Oak Smoked, Average	1 Slice/20g	26	130	21.0	1.0	4.7	0.3
On The Bone, Breaded, Somerfield*	1oz/28g	45	161	21.0	0.0	9.0	0.0
Parma, Average	1 Serving/10g	21	213	29.3	0.0	10.6	0.0
Parma, Premium, Average	1 Serving/80g	206	258	27.9	0.3	16.1	0.0
Peppered, Average	1 Slice/12g	13	110	18.5	2.1	2.7	0.0
Peppered, Dry Cured, Average	1 Slice/31g	43	140	23.1	1.3	4.7	0.2
Prosciutto, Average	1 Slice/12g	27	227	28.7	0.1	12.4	0.4
San Daniele, Finest, Tesco*	2 Slices/20g	48	242	30.5	0.5	13.1	0.0
Scrumpy Cured, Tesco*	1 Slice/34g	60	176	27.2	0.9	7.1	0.0
Serrano, Spanish, The Best, Safeway*	1 Packet/70g	153	218	32.0	0.0	10.0	0.0
Smoked, Average	1Slice/18g	21	117	19.7	0.9	3.7	0.0
Smoked, Dry Cured, Average	1 Slice/28g	38	137	23.0	1.5	4.4	0.2
Smoked, Wafer Thin, Average	1 Serving/40g	41	102	17.7	1.2	2.9	0.2
St Clements, Slices, TTD, Sainsbury's*	1 Slice/25g	28	111	21.7	0.6	2.4	0.9
Thick Cut, Average	1 Slice/74g	94	127	22.4	0.6	3.9	0.1
Tinned, Average	1/2 Can/100g	136	136	12.3	2.0	8.8	0.0
Tinned, Lean, Average	1/2 Can/100g	94	94	18.1	0.2	2.3	0.5
Turkey, Average	1 Serving/75g	81	108	15.6	2.8	3.9	0.0
Turkey, Wafer Thin, Average	1 Slice/7g	11	155	17.2	5.9	7.0	0.3

H

	Measure INFO/WEIGHT	per Measure KCAL	Nutrition Values per 100g / 100ml				
			KCAL	PROT	CARB	FAT	FIBRE
HAM							
Wafer Thin, Average	1 Slice/10g	10	101	17.9	1.4	2.6	0.1
Wiltshire, Average	1oz/28g	41	148	23.1	0.0	6.1	0.0
Wiltshire, Orange Marmalade Roasted, Finest, Tesco*	1 Slice/40g	67	167	26.0	2.0	6.1	0.3
HAM VEGETARIAN							
Cheatin', Co, Redwood Foods*	1 Slice/10g	25	247	19.7	8.9	14.7	0.0
HARE							
Raw, Lean Only, Average	1oz/28g	35	125	23.5	0.2	3.5	0.0
Stewed, Lean Only, Average	1oz/28g	48	170	29.5	0.2	5.5	0.0
HARIBO*							
American Hard Gums	1 Pack/175g	630	360	0.3	85.5	1.9	0.2
Build A Burger	1oz/28g	96	344	6.6	79.0	0.2	0.3
Chamallows	1oz/28g	92	330	2.0	80.0	0.0	0.0
Cola Bottles	1 Sm Pack/16g	56	348	7.7	78.9	0.2	0.3
Cola Bottles, Fizzy	1 Med Pack/175g	595	340	6.3	78.3	0.2	0.3
Dinosaurs	1oz/28g	95	340	6.3	78.3	0.2	0.5
Dolly Mixtures	1 Pack/175g	719	411	1.8	90.2	4.8	0.2
Fantasy Mix	1 Sm Pack/100g	344	344	6.6	79.0	0.2	0.3
Fried Eggs/Eggstras	1oz/28g	96	344	6.6	79.0	0.2	0.0
Gold Bears	1 Pack/100g	348	348	7.7	78.9	0.2	0.3
Horror Mix	1 Sm Pack/100g	344	344	6.6	79.0	0.2	0.3
Jelly Babies	1oz/28g	97	348	4.5	82.1	0.2	0.5
Jelly Beans	1 Pack/100g	379	379	0.6	93.8	0.2	0.1
Kiddies Super Mix	1 Pack/100g	344	344	6.6	79.0	0.2	0.3
Liquorice Cream Rock	1oz/28g	107	382	2.3	81.2	5.3	0.3
Liquorice Favourite	1oz/28g	100	357	2.8	78.8	3.0	2.3
Magic Mix	1oz/28g	102	366	5.4	82.0	1.9	0.3
Mao Mix, Stripes	1oz/28g	108	384	1.2	81.7	6.1	0.3
Maoam Stripes	1 Chew/7g	27	384	1.2	81.7	6.1	0.3
Mega Roulette	1oz/28g	97	348	7.7	78.9	0.2	0.3
Mega Roulette Sour	1oz/28g	95	340	6.3	78.3	0.2	0.5
Micro Mix	1oz/28g	106	379	4.7	84.5	2.5	0.4
Milky Mix	1 Pack/175g	607	347	7.1	79.6	0.2	0.4
Mint Imperials	1 Pack/175g	695	397	0.4	98.8	0.5	0.1
Peaches	1oz/28g	98	350	4.3	82.1	0.0	0.0
Pontefract Cakes	1 Pack/200g	612	306	5.3	68.2	1.3	5.6
Shrimps	1oz/28g	99	352	6.1	81.5	0.2	0.1
Snakes	1 snake/8g	28	348	7.7	78.9	0.2	0.3
Starmix	1 Pack/100g	344	344	6.6	79.0	0.2	0.3
Tangfastics	1 Pack/100g	359	359	6.3	78.3	2.3	0.5
Tropifruit	1oz/28g	97	348	4.5	82.1	0.2	0.5
Wine Gums	1 Pack/175g	609	348	0.1	86.4	0.2	0.4
HASH							
Barbecue Beef, COU, Marks & Spencer*	1 Pack/400g	360	90	7.0	14.0	0.4	1.4
Chicken Salsa, Healthy Eating, Tesco*	1 Pack/350g	291	83	4.1	10.6	2.7	1.1
Corned Beef, Apetito*	1 Pack/380g	423	111	3.8	10.3	6.2	1.3
Corned Beef, Asda*	1 Pack/400g	416	104	6.0	12.0	3.6	1.1
Corned Beef, Frozen, Tesco*	1 Serving/400g	348	87	5.7	10.3	2.6	0.7
Corned Beef, Marks & Spencer*	1/2 Pack/320g	368	115	7.6	9.6	5.3	2.8
Corned Beef, Simple, Sainsbury's*	1 Pack/300g	273	91	7.4	8.1	3.2	2.5
Corned Beef, Tesco*	1 Serving/400g	416	104	5.3	14.8	2.6	1.7
Corned Beef, Value, Tesco*	1 Pack/300g	339	113	6.7	12.2	4.2	0.9
Farmhouse, Healthy Living, Tesco*	1 Pack/300g	279	93	3.6	13.6	2.7	1.1
Vegetable & Lentil, Asda*	1 Pack/289g	254	88	3.2	14.0	2.1	0.0

H

INFO/WEIGHT	per Measure KCAL	KCAL	PROT	CARB	FAT	FIBRE

HASH BROWNS

	INFO/WEIGHT	per Measure KCAL	KCAL	PROT	CARB	FAT	FIBRE
Birds Eye*	1 Serving/63g	126	200	2.0	21.9	11.6	1.6
Deep Fried, McCain*	1oz/28g	69	246	2.0	24.3	15.3	0.0
Farmfoods*	1oz/28g	35	124	2.1	18.2	4.7	2.1
Frozen, McCain*	1 Hash Brown/40g	70	174	3.0	24.0	7.3	0.0
Oven Baked, McCain*	1oz/28g	55	196	1.7	25.5	8.6	0.0
Potato, Iceland*	1 Hash Brown/33g	75	227	2.2	27.1	12.2	2.6
Tesco*	1oz/28g	43	154	2.4	20.0	7.2	1.7

HASLET

Somerfield*	1oz/28g	57	205	15.0	10.0	12.0	0.0
Tesco*	1 Slice/15g	36	238	14.4	7.9	16.5	0.3

HAZELNUTS

Average	10 Whole/10g	66	655	15.4	5.8	63.5	6.5
Average	10 Whole/10g	66	655	15.4	5.8	63.5	6.5
Chopped, Average	1 Serving/10g	67	666	16.8	5.7	64.0	6.6

HEART

Ox, Raw	1oz/28g	29	104	18.2	0.0	3.5	0.0
Ox, Stewed	1oz/28g	44	157	27.8	0.0	5.1	0.0
Pig, Raw	1oz/28g	27	97	17.1	0.0	3.2	0.0
Pig, Stewed	1oz/28g	45	162	25.1	0.0	6.8	0.0

HERB CUBES

Basil, Knorr*	1 Cube/10g	47	472	6.1	35.9	33.8	0.6
Parsley & Garlic, Knorr*	1 Cube/10g	42	422	8.6	35.2	27.4	1.8

HERMESETAS

Powdered, Hermes*	1 Tsp/0.78	3	387	1.0	96.8	0.0	0.0
The Classic Sweetener, Hermes*	1 Tablet/0.5g	0	294	14.2	59.3	0.0	0.0

HEROES

Dairy Milk, Whole Nut, Cadbury*	1 Chocolate/11g	60	545	9.1	48.2	35.2	0.0
Fudge, Cadbury*	1 Sweet/10g	44	435	2.5	72.7	14.9	0.0

HERRING

Canned, In Tomato Sauce, Average	1oz/28g	57	204	11.9	4.1	15.5	0.1
Dried, Salted	1oz/28g	47	168	25.3	0.0	7.4	0.0
Fillets, In Mustard & Dill Sauce, John West*	1 Can/190g	426	224	11.7	3.7	18.0	0.1
Fillets, In Olive Oil, Succulent, Princes*	1 Serving/50g	108	215	20.0	0.0	15.0	0.0
Fillets, Raw, Average	1 Herring/100g	185	185	18.4	0.0	12.6	0.0
Grilled	1oz/28g	51	181	20.1	0.0	11.2	0.0
In Horseradish Sauce, John West*	1oz/28g	64	230	13.0	4.0	18.0	0.0
Oatmeal, Fried In Vegetable Oil	1oz/28g	66	234	23.1	1.5	15.1	0.1
Pickled	1oz/28g	59	209	16.7	10.0	11.1	0.0
Rollmop, With Onion, Asda*	1 Rollmop/65g	89	137	13.2	10.3	4.8	0.8
Smoked, Pepper, In Oil, Glyngøre*	1 Can/130g	338	260	21.0	0.0	19.0	0.0

HIGH LIGHTS

Caffe Latte, Made Up, Cadbury*	1 Serving/200g	40	20	1.0	2.5	0.7	0.0
Choc Mint, Made Up, Cadbury*	1 Serving/200ml	40	20	1.0	2.5	0.7	0.3
Chocolate Drink, Dry, Cadbury*	1 Sachet/10g	37	365	17.1	44.7	13.0	0.0
Chocolate Orange, Made Up, Cadbury*	1 Serving/200ml	40	20	1.0	2.3	0.7	0.3
Dairy Fudge, Made Up, Cadbury*	1 Serving/200ml	40	20	1.0	2.8	0.5	0.2
Dark Chocolate, Cadbury*	1 Serving/200ml	35	18	1.3	2.1	0.5	0.0
Espresso, Made Up, Cadbury*	1 Serving/200ml	35	18	1.3	2.0	0.5	0.0
Made Up, Cadbury*	1 Cup/200ml	40	20	1.0	2.5	0.7	0.3
Mint, Cadbury*	1 Serving/200ml	40	20	1.0	2.5	0.7	0.0
Toffee Flavour, Made Up, Cadbury*	1 Serving/200ml	40	20	1.0	2.6	0.7	0.0

HOKI

Grilled	1oz/28g	34	121	24.1	0.0	2.7	0.0

H

	Measure INFO/WEIGHT	per Measure KCAL	Nutrition Values per 100g / 100ml				
			KCAL	PROT	CARB	FAT	FIBRE
HOKI							
In Breadcrumbs, Average	1 Piece/156g	298	191	14.5	13.9	8.9	1.2
Raw	1oz/28g	24	85	16.9	0.0	1.9	0.0
Steaks, In Batter, Crispy, Birds Eye*	1 Steak/123.1g	320	260	12.4	21.3	13.9	0.8
HONEGAR							
Martlet Natural Foods*	1oz/28g	63	225	0.1	60.0	0.0	0.0
HONEY							
Acacia Blossom, Sainsbury's*	1 Serving/24g	81	339	0.1	84.7	0.1	0.3
Acacia, Tesco*	1 Tsp/4g	12	307	0.4	76.4	0.0	0.0
Australian Eucalyptus, Finest, Tesco*	1 Tsp/4g	12	307	0.4	76.4	0.0	0.0
Canadian Clover, TTD, Sainsbury's*	1 Tsp/5g	17	339	0.1	84.7	0.1	0.3
Clear, Runny, Sainsbury's*	1 Serving/15g	51	339	0.1	84.7	0.1	0.3
Florida Orange, Extra Special, Asda*	1 Tbsp/15g	50	334	0.5	83.0	0.0	0.0
Greek, TTD, Sainsbury's*	1 Tbsp/15g	51	339	0.1	84.7	0.0	0.3
Greek, Waitrose*	1 Tsp/6g	18	307	0.4	76.4	0.0	0.0
Manuka Clear, TTD, Sainsbury's*	1 Tsp/5g	17	334	0.3	83.1	0.0	0.0
Mexican, TTD, Sainsbury's*	1 Tbsp/15g	51	339	0.1	84.7	0.1	0.3
Pure, Clear, Average	1 Tbsp/20g	63	314	0.3	79.1	0.0	0.0
Pure, Set, Average	1 Tsp/5g	16	312	0.4	77.6	0.0	0.0
Scottish Heather, Waitrose*	1 Serving/20g	61	307	0.4	76.4	0.0	0.0
Spanish Orange Blossom, Sainsbury's*	1 Tbsp/15g	51	339	0.1	84.7	0.0	0.3
Tasmanian Leatherwood, TTD, Sainsbury's*	1 Serving/6g	20	339	0.1	84.7	0.1	0.3
HOOCH*							
Vodka, (Calculated Estimate)	1 Bottle/330ml	244	74	0.3	5.1	0.0	0.0
HORLICKS							
Low Fat Instant Powder, Made Up With Water	1 Mug/227ml	116	51	2.4	10.1	0.5	0.0
Malted Drink, Light, Horlicks*	1 Sachet/32g	123	384	13.7	73.0	4.1	2.7
Powder, Made Up With Semi-Skimmed Milk	1 Mug/227ml	184	81	4.3	12.9	1.9	0.0
Powder, Made Up With Skimmed Milk	1 Mug/227ml	159	70	4.3	12.9	0.5	0.0
Powder, Made Up With Whole Milk	1 Mug/227ml	225	99	4.2	12.7	3.9	0.0
Snoozoo, Chocolate, Horlicks*	1 Sachet/20g	74	370	8.6	74.2	4.3	4.3
HORSERADISH							
Raw	1 Tsp/5g	3	62	4.5	11.0	0.3	6.2
HOT CHOCOLATE							
Caramel Flavoured, Instant, Dry, Aldi*	1 Serving/11g	40	363	18.5	40.6	14.1	8.5
Chocolate Break, Dry, Tesco*	1 Serving/21g	110	524	7.9	58.9	28.5	1.7
Chocolate Time, Safeway*	1 Serving/30g	123	411	9.4	67.8	11.4	1.8
Drink, Balanced Lifestyle, Camelot, Aldi*	1 Sachet/11g	40	363	18.5	40.6	14.1	0.5
Galaxy, Mars*	1 Mug/28g	115	411	7.0	68.7	12.1	0.0
Horlicks*	1 Serving/32g	128	400	8.8	72.5	8.1	3.8
Impress*	1 Serving/25g	90	360	5.6	76.0	3.6	6.0
Instant Break, Cadbury*	1 Sachet/28g	119	425	10.9	64.2	14.0	0.0
Instant, BGTY, Made Up, Sainsbury's*	1 Sachet/28g	16	56	2.1	10.6	0.6	0.3
Instant, Galaxy*	1 Serving/28g	115	411	7.0	68.7	12.1	0.0
Instant, Tesco*	1 Serving/32g	132	414	8.0	68.3	12.1	0.7
Low Calorie, Somerfield*	1 Sachet/12g	40	330	18.0	48.0	8.0	0.0
Maltesers, Malt Drink, Instant, Made Up, Mars*	1 Serving/220ml	104	47	0.9	7.7	1.4	0.0
Organic, Clipper*	1 Sachet/30g	98	327	13.7	65.0	1.3	0.0
Organic, Green & Black's*	1 Tsp/3g	11	376	7.4	66.8	6.6	0.0
Protein, Easy Body*	1 Serving/20g	74	370	70.7	19.2	1.2	0.0
SlimFast*	1 Serving/59g	203	347	22.2	53.8	4.8	8.4
Toffee Flavour, Good Intentions, Somerfield*	1 Serving/34g	130	381	7.4	77.0	4.8	2.6
Value, Tesco*	1 Serving/32g	132	414	8.0	68.3	12.1	0.7
Velvet, Cadbury*	1 Serving/28g	136	487	8.6	57.8	24.6	2.0

H

	Measure INFO/WEIGHT	per Measure KCAL	Nutrition Values per 100g / 100ml				
			KCAL	PROT	CARB	FAT	FIBRE
HOT DOG							
Sausage, American Style, Average	1 Sausage/75g	180	241	11.6	6.2	19.0	0.0
Sausage, Average	1 Sausage/23g	40	175	10.8	4.3	12.8	0.3
HOT DOG MEAT FREE							
Sainsbury's*	1 Sausage/30g	70	235	17.8	4.2	16.4	1.9
HOT DOG VEGETARIAN							
Tesco*	1 Sausage/30g	81	271	19.0	6.0	19.0	2.0
HOT POT							
Beef, Apetito*	1 Pack/340g	303	89	5.1	10.3	3.1	1.3
Beef, Ross*	1 Pack/322g	254	79	2.5	9.4	3.5	0.4
Beef, Weight Watchers*	1 Pack/320g	270	84	4.7	10.8	2.5	1.1
Chicken & Cider, Ready Meals, Waitrose*	1 Pack/400g	500	125	6.8	12.9	5.1	1.1
Chicken & Mushroom, Healthy Living, Tesco*	1 Serving/450g	369	82	6.3	11.8	1.5	0.5
Chicken, GFY, Asda*	1 Serving/400g	292	73	5.0	10.0	1.4	0.8
Chicken, Healthy Living, Tesco*	1 Pack/400g	348	87	5.0	12.0	2.1	1.8
Chicken, Sainsbury's*	1 Pack/400g	340	85	5.2	9.9	2.8	1.3
Chicken, Weight Watchers*	1 Pack/330g	277	84	5.4	10.1	2.4	0.7
Lamb & Vegetable, Asda*	1 Pot/500g	240	48	4.0	7.0	0.4	0.0
Lamb, Heinz*	1 Pack/340g	337	99	4.9	12.7	3.1	1.7
Lancashire, Asda*	1 Pack/401g	269	67	3.8	10.0	1.3	0.9
Lancashire, Hollands*	1 Serving/250g	340	136	3.6	19.6	4.7	0.0
Lancashire, Sainsbury's*	1/2 Pack/225g	221	98	6.1	9.5	3.9	1.0
Lancashire, Tesco*	1/2 Pack/225g	205	91	6.0	9.7	3.1	0.5
Liver & Bacon, Tesco*	1 Pack/550g	693	126	6.4	12.3	5.7	1.5
Minced Beef & Vegetable, COU, Marks & Spencer*	1 Pack/400g	380	95	10.3	9.0	1.7	2.4
Minced Beef, Asda*	1 Pack/375g	409	109	7.0	10.0	4.6	1.7
Minced Beef, Classic, Sainsbury's*	1 Pack/450g	491	109	6.1	13.4	3.4	1.0
Minced Beef, Long Life, Sainsbury's*	1 Pack/300g	207	69	3.9	10.0	1.5	0.9
Minced Beef, Marks & Spencer*	1/2 Pack/227g	272	120	7.3	11.1	5.0	0.9
Minced Beef, Mini Classic, Tesco*	1 Pack/300g	232	77	3.4	12.6	1.5	1.4
Minced Beef, Mini Favourites, Marks & Spencer*	1 Pack/300g	210	70	5.0	6.4	2.9	2.5
Minced Beef, Sainsbury's*	1 Pack/300g	174	58	3.6	7.0	1.7	2.1
Minced Beef, SmartPrice, Asda*	1 Pack/300g	199	66	3.7	10.0	1.3	0.4
Minced Beef, Tesco*	1 Pack/400g	296	74	4.8	9.7	1.8	1.6
Sausage With Baked Beans, Heinz*	1 Can/340g	354	104	4.6	14.3	3.2	2.4
Sausage, SmartPrice, Asda*	1 Pack/300g	239	80	3.7	11.0	2.3	0.4
Vegetable, Ross*	1 Pack/300g	261	87	2.4	11.7	3.5	2.0
Vegetable, Tesco*	1 Serving/450g	432	96	1.7	11.2	4.9	3.5
Vegetable, Weight Watchers*	1 Pack/335g	228	68	2.6	9.9	1.9	1.5
HOUMOUS							
30% Less Fat, Asda*	1oz/28g	73	259	9.0	13.0	19.0	3.8
BGTY, Sainsbury's*	1 Serving/50g	77	153	6.6	11.7	8.9	6.1
Co-Op*	1 Tbsp/25g	91	365	9.0	14.0	30.0	3.0
Dip, Reduced Fat, Co-Op*	1 Tbsp/25g	63	250	8.0	12.0	19.0	3.0
Extra Virgin Olive Oil, Tesco*	1 Pack/190g	564	297	7.9	11.7	24.3	5.1
Feta, Fresh, Sainsbury's*	1 Serving/100g	292	292	8.0	3.5	27.4	6.7
Fresh, Healthy Choice, Safeway*	1oz/28g	74	264	9.1	13.6	19.2	0.0
Fresh, Reduced Fat, 25% Less Fat, Tesco*	1 Serving/85g	207	244	7.5	12.9	18.1	4.8
Fresh, Tesco*	1oz/28g	87	310	7.4	9.8	26.8	3.4
GFY, Asda*	1/2 Pot/85g	209	246	9.0	12.0	18.0	4.3
Good Intentions, Somerfield*	1/2 Pot/85g	201	236	7.5	12.9	17.2	3.3
Greek, Somerfield*	1 Serving/50g	152	304	7.6	8.2	26.8	5.5
Lemon & Coriander, Sainsbury's*	1/2 Pot/85g	247	291	7.0	9.1	25.1	6.0
Lemon & Coriander, Tesco*	1 Serving/50g	170	340	7.0	12.7	29.0	2.1

H

	Measure INFO/WEIGHT	per Measure KCAL	Nutrition Values per 100g / 100ml				
			KCAL	PROT	CARB	FAT	FIBRE
HOUMOUS							
Light, Morrisons*	1/2 Pack/85g	200	235	7.4	10.9	18.0	0.0
Low Fat, Safeway*	1 Serving/10g	26	258	9.0	12.8	19.0	3.3
Marks & Spencer*	1oz/28g	87	310	7.1	9.5	27.3	3.3
Mixed Olive, Sainsbury's*	1/2 Pot/85g	228	268	6.7	8.4	23.1	7.7
Organic, Marks & Spencer*	1 Serving/42g	139	330	6.9	9.1	29.7	3.3
Organic, Sainsbury's*	1/4 Pot/43g	139	326	6.8	10.7	28.4	3.5
Organic, Tesco*	1 Pot/170g	544	320	6.5	12.3	27.2	2.4
Reduced Fat, Marks & Spencer*	1oz/28g	67	240	7.5	12.9	17.2	3.3
Reduced Fat, Mediterranean Deli, Marks & Spencer*	1 Serving/75g	158	210	7.5	8.3	16.2	9.3
Reduced Fat, Morrisons*	1 Serving/50g	94	188	6.0	14.1	12.6	2.0
Reduced Fat, Safeway*	1 Serving/25g	65	260	9.0	12.5	19.3	3.3
Reduced Fat, Waitrose*	1oz/28g	65	233	7.7	11.1	17.5	4.8
Roasted Red Pepper, 50% Less Fat, Tesco*	1/2 Pot/85g	156	184	7.3	10.9	12.4	9.5
Roasted Red Pepper, BGTY, Sainsbury's*	1 Serving/10g	17	169	6.5	14.4	9.5	6.2
Roasted Red Pepper, Sainsbury's*	1/2 Pot/85.2g	252	297	7.0	7.4	26.6	3.5
Roasted Red Pepper, Tesco*	1 Serving/75g	255	340	7.1	11.1	29.7	2.4
Roasted Vegetable, Sainsbury's*	1 Serving/50g	144	288	6.0	5.0	27.2	7.8
Sainsbury's*	1/2 Pot/85g	244	287	5.9	4.9	27.1	7.8
Spicy Red Pepper, Marks & Spencer*	1/4 Pot/75g	158	210	7.3	14.8	13.7	2.5
Sun Dried Tomato, Chunky, Tesco*	1/2 Pot/95g	322	339	6.7	14.0	28.4	3.3
Waitrose*	1/4 Pot/74.9g	219	292	7.2	6.3	26.4	7.6
HULA HOOPS							
BBQ Beef, KP*	1 Bag/34g	174	513	3.6	60.5	28.5	1.7
Bacon & Ketchup Flavour, KP*	1 Bag/27g	140	517	3.4	56.3	30.9	2.0
Beef & Mustard, KP*	1 Bag/50g	260	519	3.9	55.0	31.5	1.8
Cheese & Onion, KP*	1 Bag/34g	175	514	3.7	60.5	28.6	1.9
Cheese Toastie, KP*	1 Bag/34g	178	523	3.4	56.7	31.4	2.0
Minis, Original, KP*	1 Tub/140g	752	537	3.0	52.9	34.8	1.7
Original, KP*	1 Bag/34g	175	514	3.2	61.5	28.4	1.8
Roast Chicken, KP*	1 Bag/25g	129	514	3.3	61.2	28.5	1.7
Salt & Vinegar, KP*	1 Bag/34g	173	510	3.1	60.4	28.5	1.7
Sizzling Bacon, KP*	1 Bag/34g	175	514	3.2	54.7	31.4	2.1
Totally Cheese Flavour Shoks, KP*	1 Bag/55g	285	519	3.8	54.5	31.8	2.1
HUNGER BREAKS							
The Full Monty, Crosse & Blackwell*	1/2 Can/205g	287	140	8.0	16.3	4.8	4.8

H

ICE CREAM

INFO/WEIGHT	Measure per Measure KCAL	Nutrition Values per 100g / 100ml KCAL	PROT	CARB	FAT	FIBRE
After Dinner, Vanilla, Magnum*	1 Portion/29g	100	344	3.4	31.0	23.0	1.4
After Eight, Nestle*	1 Serving/55.1g	114	207	3.6	27.1	9.4	0.3
Almond Indulgence, Sainsbury's*	1 Serving/120g	286	238	2.8	21.4	15.7	0.6
Baileys, Haagen-Dazs*	1oz/28g	73	260	4.5	22.2	17.1	0.0
Banana, Thorntons*	1oz/28g	63	225	4.0	23.8	12.6	0.0
Bananas Foster, Haagen-Dazs*	1 Serving/125ml	260	208	3.2	22.4	12.0	0.0
Banoffee Fudge, Sainsbury's*	1/8 Pot/67g	119	178	2.8	28.7	5.9	0.2
Banoffee, Criminally Creamy, Co-Op*	1oz/28g	66	235	3.0	26.0	13.0	0.1
Banoffee, Haagen-Dazs*	1 Serving/120ml	274	228	4.0	23.0	13.0	0.0
Belgian Chocolate, Haagen-Dazs*	1oz/28g	89	318	4.6	28.4	20.7	0.0
Berry Nice, Ben & Jerry's*	1 Serving/100g	200	200	0.0	23.0	11.0	0.0
Bounty, Mars*	1oz/28g	77	274	3.3	23.8	18.3	0.0
Bourbon Biscuit, Asda*	1 Dessert/37g	120	324	5.9	48.6	12.2	1.6
Bournville, Cadbury*	1 Bar/120g	258	215	3.5	26.0	11.6	0.0
Brandy, Luxurious, Marks & Spencer*	1 Serving/100g	228	228	3.8	19.1	13.3	0.2
Cappuccino, Thorntons*	1oz/28g	61	218	4.4	20.7	12.9	0.0
Caramel Chew Chew, Ben & Jerry's*	1 Serving/100g	270	270	4.0	28.0	15.0	0.0
Caramel Craze, Organic, Tesco*	1 Serving/100g	253	253	3.3	25.5	15.3	0.0
Caramel, Carte D'or*	2 Boules/50g	106	212	2.6	30.8	8.7	0.0
Cherrylicious, Tesco*	1 Serving/57.7g	122	210	2.8	37.0	5.6	0.2
Chilli Red, Purbeck*	1 Serving/50g	99	198	4.8	18.7	11.5	0.0
Choc Chip Cookie Dough, Ben & Jerry's*	1 Serving/100g	230	230	3.0	23.0	14.0	0.0
Choc Chip, Cookie Dough, Haagen-Dazs*	1oz/28g	74	266	3.8	24.9	16.9	0.0
Choc Chip, Haagen-Dazs*	1oz/28g	80	286	4.7	24.8	18.7	0.0
Chocolate & Caramel, Stick, SlimFast*	1 Ice Cream/55g	87	159	4.1	26.3	4.2	2.2
Chocolate & Marshmallow, Swirl, BGTY, Sainsbury's*	1 Sm Scoop/40g	69	173	3.9	33.8	2.5	2.8
Chocolate & Orange, Organic, Green & Black's*	1 Serving/100g	181	181	3.5	18.3	10.5	1.2
Chocolate Brownie With Walnuts, Haagen-Dazs*	1 Cup/101g	223	221	4.4	21.0	16.2	0.0
Chocolate Chip, Baskin Robbins*	1 Serving/75g	170	227	4.0	24.0	13.3	0.0
Chocolate Flavour, Soft Scoop, Sainsbury's*	1 Serving/70g	122	174	3.1	23.6	7.5	0.3
Chocolate Fudge Swirl, Haagen-Dazs*	1oz/28g	77	276	4.6	25.6	17.2	0.0
Chocolate Honeycomb, COU, Marks & Spencer*	1 Serving/100ml	150	150	3.5	31.5	2.6	0.7
Chocolate Honeycomb, Co-Op*	1/4 Pot/81g	186	230	4.0	26.0	13.0	0.3
Chocolate Midnight Cookies, Haagen-Dazs*	1oz/28g	81	289	4.9	28.7	17.2	0.0
Chocolate Mint Crisp, COU, Marks & Spencer*	1/4 Pot/85.2g	115	135	5.4	21.9	2.9	1.0
Chocolate Orange, Deliciously Dairy, Co-Op*	1oz/28g	55	195	4.0	29.0	7.0	0.8
Chocolate Ripple, Perfectly Balanced, Waitrose*	1 Serving/125ml	205	164	4.8	30.5	2.5	4.1
Chocolate, COU, Marks & Spencer*	1 Serving/140g	231	165	3.9	35.0	2.9	0.8
Chocolate, Dairy, The Best, Safeway*	1 Serving/82.4g	243	296	4.6	28.1	18.3	2.0
Chocolate, Easy Serve, Co-Op*	1oz/28g	46	165	3.0	22.0	7.0	0.3
Chocolate, Haagen-Dazs*	1 Serving/120ml	269	224	4.0	19.0	15.0	0.0
Chocolate, Organic, Green & Black's*	1 Serving/20g	35	176	3.5	18.6	9.8	1.3
Chocolate, Organic, Iceland*	1oz/28g	58	208	4.9	28.6	8.2	0.0
Chocolate, Organic, Marks & Spencer*	1oz/28g	71	255	5.0	24.0	16.0	1.5
Chocolate, Rich, Organic, Sainsbury's*	1 Serving/100g	213	213	4.4	22.6	11.7	1.2
Chocolate, Soft Scoop, Asda*	1 Scoop/47g	84	179	3.7	23.0	8.0	0.0
Chocolate, Soft Scoop, Tesco*	1 Serving/50g	93	186	3.2	25.1	8.1	0.3
Chocolate, Thorntons*	1oz/28g	67	238	4.6	25.1	12.9	0.0
Chocolate, Triple, Sainsbury's*	1 Serving/100g	176	176	3.5	21.7	8.3	0.5
Chocolate, Weight Watchers*	1 Serving/100ml	92	92	1.8	15.2	2.5	0.5
Chocolate, With Chocolate Chips, Milfina, Aldi*	1oz/28g	66	235	3.8	26.7	12.5	0.8
Chocolatino, Tesco*	1 Serving/100g	243	243	4.4	32.2	10.8	0.6
Chunky Chocolate, Giant, Marks & Spencer*	1 Lolly/89.6g	302	335	4.0	28.0	23.0	2.3

ICE CREAM

	Measure INFO/WEIGHT	per Measure KCAL	KCAL	PROT	CARB	FAT	FIBRE
Chunky Monkey, Ben & Jerry's*	1 Serving/100g	280	280	4.0	28.0	17.0	1.0
Coconut, Carte D'or*	1 Serving/100ml	125	125	1.8	14.0	7.1	0.5
Coffee, Finest, Tesco*	1/4 Pot/93g	236	254	4.9	22.5	16.0	0.0
Coffee, Haagen-Dazs*	1 Serving/120ml	271	226	4.1	17.9	15.3	0.0
Coffee, Waitrose*	1 Serving/180ml	256	142	3.2	13.2	8.5	0.0
Cookies & Cream, Haagen-Dazs*	1oz/28g	73	262	4.6	22.6	17.0	0.0
Cornish Clotted, Marks & Spencer*	1 Pot/90g	207	230	2.8	21.8	14.5	0.1
Cornish Dairy, Waitrose*	1 Serving/125ml	161	129	2.3	14.6	6.8	0.0
Cornish Style, Co-Op*	1oz/28g	53	190	4.0	23.0	9.0	0.1
Cornish Vanilla, Organic, Iceland*	1oz/28g	60	214	4.1	21.4	12.4	0.0
Cornish Vanilla, Soft Scoop, Marks & Spencer*	1oz/28g	56	199	3.9	21.8	10.7	0.2
Cornish, Asda*	1 Serving/100ml	100	100	1.8	12.0	5.0	0.0
Cornish, Full Fat, Asda*	1 Serving/100g	204	204	3.5	21.4	11.6	0.1
Creamy Caramella, Tesco*	1 Scoop/60g	134	223	3.8	30.9	9.1	0.6
Creamy Chocolate & Nut, Co-Op*	1oz/28g	66	235	4.0	25.0	13.0	0.5
Crema Di Mascarpone, Carte D'or*	1 Serving/100g	207	207	2.8	29.0	8.9	0.0
Dairy Cornish, Tesco*	1 Serving/49g	112	228	3.2	24.7	12.3	0.1
Dairy Milk, Orange, Cadbury*	1 Serving/120ml	259	216	3.5	26.0	11.6	0.0
Dairy, Flavoured	1oz/28g	50	179	3.5	24.7	8.0	0.0
Dairy, Vanilla	1oz/28g	54	194	3.6	24.4	9.8	0.0
Dark Toffee, Organic, Green & Black's*	1/4 Pot/125ml	193	154	2.8	18.1	7.9	0.1
Date & Almond Cream, Haagen-Dazs*	1 Serving/120ml	254	212	5.0	19.0	13.0	0.0
Demon Chocolate, Marks & Spencer*	1 Serving/79g	208	263	3.7	37.1	11.1	0.6
Double Chocolate, Nestle*	1 Serving/77.5g	250	320	4.8	33.7	18.4	0.0
Dream, Cadbury*	1 Bar/120ml	264	220	3.6	26.0	11.9	0.0
Dulce De Leche, Bar, Haagen-Dazs*	1 Bar/105g	370	352	3.8	32.3	22.9	0.0
Fig & Orange Blossom Honey, Waitrose*	1 Serving/100g	219	219	3.9	24.3	11.8	0.4
Galaxy, Mars*	1 Bar/60ml	203	339	4.7	29.7	22.4	0.0
Get Fruit, Tropical, Solero*	1 Serving/125ml	163	130	1.6	20.6	4.4	0.4
Heavenly Vanilla, Cadbury*	1 Serving/250ml	355	142	2.5	12.8	9.3	0.0
Honey, I'm Home, Ben & Jerry's*	1 Serving/100g	260	260	0.0	28.0	15.0	0.0
Honeycomb Harvest, Mackie's*	1 Serving/100g	209	209	4.0	25.0	10.0	0.0
Knickerbocker Glory	1oz/28g	31	112	1.5	16.4	5.0	0.2
Lemon & White Chocolate, Crackpots, Iceland*	1 Serving/100g	202	202	1.7	29.9	8.4	0.3
Lemon Cream, Dairy, Sainsbury's*	1 Serving/100g	199	199	3.0	25.9	9.3	0.1
Lemon Curd Swirl, Duchy Originals*	1/4 Pot/101g	247	245	3.7	25.8	14.1	0.0
Lemon Curd, Safeway*	1 Serving/100g	185	185	3.0	28.9	8.1	0.2
Lemon Pie, Haagen-Dazs*	1oz/28g	73	262	3.9	24.5	16.3	0.0
Lemon, Haagen-Dazs*	1 Serving/120ml	144	120	0.3	29.3	0.2	0.0
Less Than 5% Fat, Asda*	2 Scoops/80g	111	139	2.7	22.0	4.5	0.0
Light Chocolate Ices, Co-Op*	1 Ice/62g	121	195	2.0	18.0	13.0	0.5
Log, Mint Chocolate, Sainsbury's*	1 Serving/50.75g	100	197	3.0	23.8	10.0	0.2
Luscious Mint Choc Chip, Morrisons*	1 Serving/50g	99	198	2.9	23.1	10.5	0.7
Luxurious Marshallow, Weight Watchers*	1/2 Tub/138g	268	194	3.2	34.5	4.7	1.3
Lychee Cream & Ginger, Haagen-Dazs*	1 Serving/120ml	258	215	3.6	26.1	10.6	0.0
Magic Maple, Marks & Spencer*	1 Ice Cream/93g	259	278	2.9	39.0	12.3	0.6
Magnum Moments, Wall's*	1 Serving/18ml	58	323	4.0	30.0	20.8	0.0
Mango, 98% Fat Free, Bulla*	1 Serving/70g	94	134	4.2	25.4	1.6	0.0
Maple & Walnut, American, Sainsbury's*	1/8 Pot/68g	121	179	3.1	25.6	7.2	0.2
Maple Brazil, Thorntons*	1oz/28g	66	236	4.1	24.4	13.6	0.0
Mars, Mars*	1 Bar/75g	260	346	5.1	37.2	19.7	0.0
Mince Pie, Finest, Tesco*	1/4 Pack/187.5g	478	254	3.9	33.0	11.8	1.1
Mint & Chocolate, Sainsbury's*	1 Serving/80g	154	192	3.4	23.5	9.4	0.4

ICE CREAM

INFO/WEIGHT	Measure per Measure KCAL	KCAL	PROT	CARB	FAT	FIBRE
Mint Choc Chip Soft Scoop, Asda*	1 Serving/46g	86	187	2.9	24.0	9.0	0.3
Mint Crisp, Nestle*	1 Serving/75ml	232	309	2.9	25.5	21.9	0.9
Mint Ripple, Good Choice, Iceland*	1 Scoop/50g	59	117	3.0	21.7	2.1	0.1
Mint, Majestic Luxury, Iceland*	1 Serving/79.8g	270	337	3.8	39.3	18.3	1.3
Mint, Thorntons*	1oz/28g	66	237	4.0	25.0	13.4	0.0
Mocha Coffee Indulgence, Sainsbury's*	1/4 Pot/82g	178	217	3.2	22.1	12.9	0.1
Monster Mint, Sainsbury's*	1/8 Pot/67g	121	180	3.0	26.3	6.9	0.3
Muddy Pigs, Wall's*	1 Serving/150ml	150	100	1.7	12.1	4.9	0.3
Neapolitan, Brick, Tesco*	1 Serving/50g	82	163	3.3	21.9	6.9	0.4
Neapolitan, Organic, Iceland*	1oz/28g	55	196	4.2	26.4	8.2	0.0
Neapolitan, Soft Scoop, Asda*	1 Scoop/47g	82	175	2.8	23.0	8.0	0.2
Neapolitan, Soft Scoop, Marks & Spencer*	1 Scoop/65g	120	185	3.8	23.9	8.2	0.1
Neapolitan, Soft Scoop, Sainsbury's*	1 Serving/75g	124	165	2.8	22.8	6.9	0.2
Neopolitian, Soft Scoop, Tesco*	1 Serving/43g	70	163	3.3	21.9	6.9	0.4
Non-Dairy, Mixes	1oz/28g	51	182	4.1	25.1	7.9	0.0
Non-Dairy, Reduced Calorie	1oz/28g	33	119	3.4	13.7	6.0	0.0
Non-Dairy, Vanilla	1oz/28g	50	178	3.2	23.1	8.7	0.0
One Sweet Whirled, Ben & Jerry's*	1/2 Cup/240ml	280	117	1.7	13.8	6.3	0.0
Panna Cotta, & Raspberry Swirl, Haagen-Dazs*	1 Serving/120ml	250	208	3.2	21.0	12.4	0.0
Panna Cotta, Haagen-Dazs*	1 Serving/120ml	248	207	3.4	18.4	13.3	0.0
Peach Melba, Soft Scoop, Marks & Spencer*	1oz/28g	46	165	2.8	21.4	7.6	0.3
Phish Food, Ben & Jerry's*	1 Serving/100g	280	280	4.0	36.0	13.0	0.0
Picnic, Cadbury*	1 Cone/125ml	258	207	3.4	28.9	9.4	0.3
Pistachio, Haagen-Dazs*	1 Serving/120ml	276	230	4.4	17.7	15.7	0.0
Praline & Chocolate, Thorntons*	1oz/28g	87	309	4.6	21.3	22.9	0.6
Praline, Green & Black's*	1 Sm Pot/100g	191	191	3.5	20.0	10.8	0.9
Pralines & Cream, Haagen-Dazs*	1oz/28g	77	276	4.2	26.2	17.2	0.0
Rage Chocolate With Caramel Sauce, Treats*	1 Ice Cream/60g	177	295	3.3	30.9	17.5	0.0
Raspberries, Clotted Cream, Waitrose*	1 Tub/500ml	790	158	2.9	18.9	7.9	0.1
Raspberry & Shortcake, Co-Op*	1oz/28g	64	230	3.0	23.0	14.0	0.3
Raspberry Ripple Brick, Tesco*	1 Serving/48g	71	148	2.6	20.8	6.0	0.2
Raspberry Ripple, Dairy, Waitrose*	1 Serving/186ml	195	105	1.9	12.3	5.4	0.0
Raspberry Ripple, Soft Scoop, Asda*	1 Scoop/46g	75	164	2.5	25.0	6.0	0.0
Raspberry Ripple, Soft Scoop, Sainsbury's*	1 Serving/75g	128	170	2.6	24.2	7.0	0.3
Raspberry Ripple, Soft Scoop, Tesco*	2 Scoops/50g	79	157	2.5	23.0	6.1	0.2
Raspberry, Easy Serve, Co-Op*	1oz/28g	43	152	2.5	22.3	5.9	0.0
Raspberry, Haagen-Dazs*	1 Serving/120ml	127	106	0.2	25.9	0.2	0.0
Really Creamy After Dinner Mint, Asda*	1 Serving/100g	191	191	3.4	24.0	9.0	0.4
Really Creamy Chocolate, Asda*	1 Serving/100g	227	227	4.1	28.0	11.0	0.4
Really Creamy Lemon Meringue, Asda*	1 Serving/100ml	100	100	1.8	12.0	5.0	0.1
Really Creamy Toffee, Asda*	1 Serving/120ml	146	122	1.8	17.5	5.0	0.1
Rocky Road, Sainsbury's*	1/8 Pot/67g	137	205	3.8	30.9	7.3	1.0
Rolo, Nestle*	1/2 Tub/500ml	1180	236	3.4	31.9	10.5	0.2
Rum & Raisin, Haagen-Dazs*	1 Serving/120ml	264	220	3.4	18.6	14.7	0.0
Rum & Raisin, Organic, Iceland*	1oz/28g	55	195	4.5	28.1	7.2	0.0
Screwball, Asda*	1 Screwball/60.1g	122	203	3.3	25.0	10.0	1.5
Screwball, Co-Op*	1 Lolly/95g	190	200	2.0	31.0	7.0	0.0
Screwball, Morrisons*	1 Screwball/100ml	133	133	2.0	17.0	6.3	0.0
Screwball, Tesco*	1 Screwball/61g	116	190	2.9	25.2	8.6	0.3
Smarties Ice Cream Pot, Nestle	1 Pot	151	218	4.4	33.6	8.2	0.0
Smarties, Nestle*	1 Serving/50g	125	250	3.6	32.3	11.9	0.2
Stem Ginger With Belgian Chocolate, Waitrose*	1 Lolly/109.9g	255	232	2.9	25.5	13.1	1.7
Sticky Toffee, Cream O' Galloway*	1 Serving/30g	80	266	4.7	28.7	14.7	0.0

ICE CREAM

	INFO/WEIGHT	KCAL	KCAL	PROT	CARB	FAT	FIBRE
Strawberries & Cream, Deliciously Dairy, Co-Op*	1oz/28g	46	165	3.0	24.0	6.0	0.3
Strawberry & Cream, Mivvi, Nestle*	1 Serving/60g	118	196	2.6	29.4	7.6	0.2
Strawberry & Cream, Organic, Sainsbury's*	1 Serving/100g	193	193	3.6	22.6	9.8	0.4
Strawberry Cheesecake, Co-Op*	1/6 Pot/86g	163	190	3.0	29.0	7.0	0.2
Strawberry Cheesecake, Haagen-Dazs*	1oz/28g	74	266	3.9	26.5	16.1	0.0
Strawberry, Fromage Frais, Asda*	1 Pot/46g	87	190	3.7	28.0	7.0	0.3
Strawberry, Get Fruit, Solero*	1 Serving/100ml	120	120	1.5	18.8	4.5	1.3
Strawberry, Haagen-Dazs*	1oz/28g	67	241	4.0	21.5	15.5	0.0
Strawberry, Majestic, Luxury, Iceland*	1 Lolly/100g	281	281	2.7	25.8	18.6	0.1
Strawberry, Soft Scoop, Tesco*	1 Serving/45.8g	78	170	2.8	23.1	7.4	0.1
Strawberry, Thorntons*	1oz/28g	52	185	3.2	22.5	9.3	0.1
Strawberry, Weight Watchers*	1 Pot/57g	81	142	2.5	23.4	3.9	0.2
Tantilising Toffee, COU, Marks & Spencer*	1/4 Pot/125ml	125	100	0.6	18.0	2.8	0.0
Terry's Chocolate Orange, Carte D'or*	1 Serving/100g	182	182	2.8	27.0	7.1	0.0
The Full Vermonty, Ben & Jerry's*	1 Serving/100g	280	280	0.0	27.0	18.0	1.0
Tiramisu, Haagen-Dazs*	1 Serving/120ml	303	253	3.8	22.7	16.3	0.0
Toblerone, Carte D'or*	1 Serving/100g	211	211	3.7	29.0	9.1	0.0
Toffee & Biscuit, Weight Watchers*	1 Pot/100ml	93	93	1.5	14.9	2.7	0.1
Toffee & Vanilla, Sainsbury's*	1 Serving/71.2g	146	205	3.1	26.7	9.5	0.1
Toffee Creme, Haagen-Dazs*	1oz/28g	74	265	4.5	26.7	15.6	0.0
Toffee Crunch, Handmade Farmhouse, TTD, Sainsbury's*	1/2 Pot/90g	288	320	2.9	29.7	21.1	0.1
Toffee Fudge, Soft Scoop, Asda*	1 Serving/50g	93	185	2.6	28.0	7.0	0.0
Toffee Ripple, Tesco*	1 Serving/100g	173	173	2.7	24.4	7.2	0.1
Toffee Vanilla, Healthy Eating, Tesco*	1 Serving/73g	106	145	2.5	28.1	2.5	0.5
Toffee, Thorntons*	1oz/28g	61	218	4.1	24.5	11.6	0.0
Totally Toffee, Safeway*	1 Serving/100ml	136	136	1.3	21.1	5.1	0.1
Traditional Cornish Blackberry, Marks & Spencer*	1oz/28g	61	218	2.3	28.0	10.8	0.3
Traditional Cornish Strawberry, Marks & Spencer*	1oz/28g	64	229	2.3	29.7	11.2	0.2
Triple Chocolate, Safeway*	1 Serving/100g	235	235	3.8	30.0	10.8	0.0
Tropical Fruit Sorbet, Waitrose*	1 Lolly/109.8g	90	82	1.5	14.5	2.0	0.2
Tropical, Tesco*	1 Serving/73g	107	148	1.2	26.3	4.3	0.4
Vanilla & Chocolate Swirl, Safeway*	1 Serving/125g	250	200	3.3	26.2	9.1	0.1
Vanilla & Cinnamon, Finest, Tesco*	1 Serving/50g	115	229	3.9	20.2	14.7	0.4
Vanilla & Strawberry, Swirl, Safeway*	1 Serving/100g	190	190	2.9	27.0	7.5	0.2
Vanilla Bean, Purbeck*	1 Serving/100g	198	198	4.8	18.7	11.5	0.0
Vanilla Brick, Co-Op*	1oz/28g	45	160	3.0	21.0	7.0	0.2
Vanilla Caramel Brownie, Haagen-Dazs*	1 Serving/150g	410	273	4.5	26.8	16.5	0.0
Vanilla Caramel Fudge, Ben & Jerry's*	1 Serving/100g	260	260	4.0	28.0	14.0	0.0
Vanilla Choc Fudge, Haagen-Dazs*	1oz/28g	75	267	4.3	23.5	17.2	0.0
Vanilla Flavour, Soft Scoop, Sainsbury's*	1 Serving/70g	111	159	3.0	21.7	6.7	0.1
Vanilla With Strawberry Swirl, Mini Tub, Weight Watchers*	1 Mini Tub/57.0g	81	142	2.5	23.4	3.9	0.2
Vanilla, COU, Marks & Spencer*	1/4 Pot/79g	111	140	1.7	25.9	2.8	0.8
Vanilla, Carte D'or*	1 Serving/100ml	204	204	3.0	28.0	9.0	0.0
Vanilla, Criminally Creamy, Co-Op*	1oz/28g	60	215	3.0	18.0	15.0	0.1
Vanilla, Dairy Milk, Cadbury*	1 Ice Cream/120g	259	216	3.5	26.0	11.6	0.1
Vanilla, Dairy, Finest, Tesco*	1 Serving/92g	227	247	4.5	18.0	17.4	0.3
Vanilla, Dairy, Organic, Yeo Valley*	1 Serving/100g	206	206	4.9	21.3	11.2	0.0
Vanilla, Haagen-Dazs*	1oz/28g	70	250	4.5	19.7	17.1	0.0
Vanilla, Handmade Farmhouse, TTD, Sainsbury's*	1 Serving/100g	252	252	4.2	14.4	19.7	0.0
Vanilla, Light Soft Scoop, 25% Less Fat, Morrisons*	1 Scoop/50g	75	150	2.9	23.2	5.0	0.2
Vanilla, Light, Carte D'or, Wall's*	1 Serving/50g	71	142	2.3	23.0	4.4	0.0
Vanilla, Low Fat, Weight Watchers*	1 Scoop/125ml	75	60	1.1	9.7	1.7	0.1
Vanilla, Organic, Green & Black's*	1 Sm Tub/100ml	164	164	3.5	15.2	9.8	0.1

ICE CREAM

INFO/WEIGHT	per Measure KCAL	KCAL	PROT	CARB	FAT	FIBRE
Vanilla, Organic, Sainsbury's*	1 Serving/85g	176	207	4.3	20.5	12.0	0.1
Vanilla, Organic, Tesco*	1 Serving/100g	237	237	3.7	16.8	17.2	0.0
Vanilla, Pecan, Haagen-Dazs*	1 Serving/120ml	316	263	4.3	17.1	19.6	0.0
Vanilla, Really Creamy, Asda*	1 Serving/50g	98	196	3.5	23.0	10.0	0.1
Vanilla, SmartPrice, Asda*	1 Scoop/40g	55	137	2.8	19.0	6.0	0.2
Vanilla, Soft Scoop, 25% Less Fat, Asda*	1oz/28g	42	149	2.9	23.0	5.0	0.0
Vanilla, Soft Scoop, BGTY, Sainsbury's*	1 Serving/75g	88	117	3.1	22.2	1.7	0.2
Vanilla, Soft Scoop, Light, 94% Fat Free, Wall's*	1 Serving/100ml	80	80	1.4	12.4	2.9	0.1
Vanilla, Soft Scoop, Tesco*	1oz/28g	46	164	3.1	21.8	7.1	0.1
Vanilla, Soft Scoop, Wall's*	2 Scoops/100ml	90	90	1.4	11.2	4.4	0.1
Vanilla, Soft, Non Milk Fat, Waitrose*	1 Serving/125ml	78	62	1.3	8.0	2.7	0.1
Vanilla, Thorntons*	1oz/28g	63	225	4.9	20.5	13.6	0.0
Vanilla, Too Good to be True, Wall's*	1 Serving/50ml	35	70	2.0	14.9	0.4	0.1
Vanilla, Value, Tesco*	1 Serving/56g	77	137	2.8	18.7	5.7	0.2
Vanilla, Waitrose*	1 Serving/100ml	156	156	2.6	12.0	10.8	0.0
Vanilla, Wth Vanilla Pods, Sainsbury's*	1 Serving/100g	195	195	3.5	22.5	10.1	0.1
Vanilletta, Tesco*	1 Serving/46.8g	82	175	4.0	21.6	8.1	0.0
Viennetta, Biscuit Caramel, Wall's*	1/6 Serving/58g	183	315	3.3	27.8	20.9	0.0
Viennetta, Cappuccino, Wall's*	1 Serving/75g	191	255	3.5	22.0	17.0	0.0
Viennetta, Chocolate, Wall's*	1/4 Pot/80g	200	250	4.1	24.0	15.2	0.0
Viennetta, Forest Fruit, Wall's*	1 Serving/98g	265	270	3.4	27.2	16.2	0.0
Viennetta, Mint, Wall's*	1 Serving/80g	204	255	3.4	23.0	16.6	0.0
Viennetta, Selection Brownie, Wall's*	1 Serving/70g	194	277	4.2	28.5	16.2	0.0
Viennetta, Strawberry Cheesecake Biscuit, Wall's*	1 Serving/100g	305	305	3.5	28.1	20.7	0.0
Viennetta, Strawberry, Wall's*	1 Serving/80g	204	255	3.4	22.1	16.8	0.0
Viennetta, Vanilla, Wall's*	1/4 Bar/80gg	204	255	3.3	23.0	16.7	0.0
Virtuous Vanilla & Strawberry, Weight Watchers*	1 Serving/100ml	81	81	1.4	13.3	2.2	0.1
Voluptuous Vanilla, COU, Marks & Spencer*	1 Pot/400g	520	130	4.6	22.0	2.6	0.6
Walnut & Maple, Waitrose*	1 Serving/60g	68	114	1.8	18.2	3.8	0.0
White Vanilla Flavour, Soft Scoop, Sainsbury's*	1oz/28g	38	136	2.9	18.8	5.5	0.2
White Vanilla, Soft Scoop, Tesco*	1oz/28g	46	164	3.1	21.8	7.1	0.1
With Cherry Sauce, Tesco*	1 Serving/57.7g	122	210	2.8	37.0	5.6	0.2
Zesty Lemon Meringue, COU, Marks & Spencer*	1/4 Pot/73g	120	165	2.6	33.0	2.5	0.5

ICE CREAM BAR

Bailey's, Haagen-Dazs*	1oz/28g	86	307	4.1	24.8	21.2	0.0
Choc Chip, Haagen-Dazs*	1oz/28g	90	320	4.3	27.4	21.5	0.0
Chocolate Covered	1oz/28g	90	320	5.0	24.0	23.3	0.0
Chunky Chocolate, Co-Op*	1 Bar/60g	204	340	5.0	35.0	20.0	1.0
Chunky Toffee, Co-Op*	1 Bar/60g	204	340	4.0	34.0	21.0	1.0
Dairy Milk, Fruit & Nut, Cadbury*	1 Bar/74g	178	240	2.2	25.3	14.5	0.0
Dairy Milk, Lolly, Cadbury*	1 Lolly	270	245	2.8	24.2	15.4	0.0
Dream, Cadbury*	1 Serving/118g	260	220	3.6	26.0	11.9	0.0
Feast, Wall's*	1 Bar/60g	190	317	3.3	24.7	22.8	0.0
Maltesers, Mars*	1 Stick/80g	264	330	3.7	33.6	20.2	0.0
Mars, Mars	1 Bar	177	283	3.6	30.1	16.4	0.0
Peanut, Farmfoods*	1 Bar/60ml	187	360	5.3	36.6	21.4	1.2
Racer, Aldi*	1 Bar/59g	194	328	6.0	34.2	18.6	0.0
Snickers, Mars*	1 Bar/67g	250	373	6.0	37.3	22.4	0.0
Toffee Cream, Haagen-Dazs*	1oz/28g	97	345	4.0	31.0	22.0	0.0
Toffee Crisp, Nestle	1 Bar	197	329	3.8	33.4	20.0	0.0
Twix, Mars*	1 Serving/43.5g	231	524	6.9	52.9	32.2	0.0
Yorkie, Nestle	1 Bar	144	359	4.8	36.5	21.6	0.0

	Measure INFO/WEIGHT	per Measure KCAL	Nutrition Values per 100g / 100ml KCAL	PROT	CARB	FAT	FIBRE
ICE CREAM CONE							
Average	1 Cone/75g	140	186	3.5	25.5	8.5	0.0
Blackcurrant, GFY, Asda*	1 Cone/67.2g	161	241	3.0	37.0	9.0	0.1
Carousel Wafer Company*	1 Cone/2g	7	342	12.6	65.0	3.7	0.0
Choc 'n' Nut, Farmfoods*	1 Cone/120ml	183	278	5.0	33.0	14.0	1.0
Chocolate & Nut, Co-Op*	1 Cone/110g	307	279	3.9	31.0	15.5	0.6
Chocolate & Vanilla, Good Choice, Iceland*	1 Cone/110ml	161	146	2.7	22.9	6.5	0.8
Chocolate & Vanilla, Marks & Spencer*	1oz/28g	83	295	4.2	31.8	17.0	0.7
Chocolate Flavour, Somerfield*	1 Cone/110ml	329	299	4.0	38.0	15.0	0.0
Chocolate, Marks & Spencer*	1oz/28g	94	335	4.0	28.0	23.0	2.3
Chocolate, Vanilla & Hazelnut, Sainsbury's*	1 Cone/62g	190	306	4.5	33.9	16.9	0.6
Cone, Haagen-Dazs*	1oz/28g	85	303	4.7	25.5	20.3	0.0
Cornetto, Classico, Wall's	1 Cone	200	205	2.7	19.7	12.9	0.0
Cornetto, Flirt, Choc Chip, With Hazelnut, Wall's*	1 Cone/69.7g	224	320	4.0	40.0	16.0	0.0
Cornetto, GFY, Asda*	1 Cone/67.2g	161	241	3.0	37.0	9.0	0.1
Cornetto, Wall's*	1 Cone/75g	195	260	3.7	34.5	12.9	0.0
Creme Egg, Cadbury*	1 Cone/115ml	270	235	2.9	29.3	11.6	0.0
Dairy Milk, Mint, Cadbury*	1 Cone/115mll	190	165	2.4	21.5	7.7	0.0
Extreme Raspberry, Cornetto, Nestle*	1 Cornetto/88g	220	250	2.5	36.0	10.0	0.2
Flake 99, Cadbury*	1 Cone/125ml	244	195	2.6	23.2	10.0	0.0
Flake 99, Strawberry, Cadbury*	1 Serving/125g	250	200	2.6	27.3	8.7	0.0
Mini, Sainsbury's*	1 Cone/18g	66	366	4.4	39.8	21.0	3.4
Mini, Tesco*	1 Cone/48g	152	316	4.1	31.5	19.3	0.8
Mint Choc Chip, Iceland*	1 Cone/72g	210	292	3.3	40.4	13.0	1.0
Somerfield*	1 Serving/67g	180	268	2.6	38.5	11.5	4.1
Sticky Toffee, Farmfoods*	1 Cone/120ml	177	272	3.2	36.0	12.8	2.0
Strawberry & Vanilla, Asda*	1 Cone/115ml	193	168	1.8	22.6	7.8	0.1
Strawberry & Vanilla, Healthy Living, Tesco*	1 Serving/69g	149	216	3.4	36.4	6.3	1.4
Strawberry & Vanilla, Marks & Spencer*	1oz/28g	81	290	4.2	30.9	16.5	0.7
Strawberry & Vanilla, Sainsbury's*	1 Cone/70g	171	243	3.4	35.6	9.7	1.0
Strawberry & Vanilla, Tesco*	1 Cone/70g	194	277	3.0	35.9	13.5	0.3
Strawberry, BGTY, Sainsbury's*	1 Cone/69g	151	219	2.6	37.5	6.5	1.3
Strawberry, Marks & Spencer*	1oz/28g	74	263	3.5	31.1	14.0	0.4
Toffee Flavoured, Somerfield*	1 Cone/110ml	320	291	4.0	39.0	14.0	0.0
Tropical, GFY, Asda*	1 Cone/100g	135	135	2.6	20.0	5.0	0.3
ICE CREAM ROLL							
Artic	1 Portion/70g	140	200	4.1	33.3	6.6	0.0
Basics, Somerfield*	1/6 Roll/110ml	233	212	4.0	35.0	6.0	0.0
Marks & Spencer*	1oz/28g	60	215	3.6	35.2	6.7	0.0
Mini, Cadbury*	1 Roll/45ml	99	220	3.4	24.3	13.1	0.0
Tesco*	1/4 Roll/57g	131	230	3.7	34.5	8.6	0.4
ICE CREAM SANDWICH							
'Wich, Ben & Jerry's*	1 Serving/117g	350	299	3.4	38.5	15.4	0.9
ICE CREAM STICK							
Chocolate Cookies, Haagen-Dazs*	1 Ice Cream/43g	162	376	4.9	31.8	25.4	0.0
Vanilla Macadamia, Haagen-Dazs*	1 Ice Cream/42g	161	383	4.6	28.7	27.7	0.0
ICE LOLLY							
Assorted, Safeway*	1 Lolly/31ml	26	85	0.0	20.9	0.0	0.1
Baby, Tesco*	1 Lolly/32.4g	26	80	0.1	20.0	0.0	0.1
Berry Burst Sorbet, Sainsbury's*	1 Serving/90ml	93	103	1.1	20.8	1.8	0.7
Blackcurrant Split, Iceland*	1 Lolly/75g	61	81	1.1	12.0	3.2	0.1
Blackcurrant, Dairy Split, Sainsbury's*	1 Lolly/72.7ml	88	121	1.8	20.4	3.6	0.1
Blackcurrant, Real Fruit Juice, Sainsbury's*	1 Lolly/73ml	67	92	0.2	22.8	0.1	0.1
Blackcurrant, Ribena*	1 Lolly/55ml	43	79	0.0	19.2	0.0	0.0

ICE LOLLY

INFO/WEIGHT	Measure	per Measure KCAL	Nutrition Values per 100g / 100ml				
			KCAL	PROT	CARB	FAT	FIBRE
Bournville, Cadbury*	1 Lolly	270	245	2.5	23.2	15.6	0.0
Calippo Shots, Cool Lemon, Wall's*	1oz/28g	8	28	0.1	3.9	1.3	0.0
Calippo Shots, Twisted Berry, Wall's*	1oz/28g	8	28	0.1	4.2	1.2	0.0
Choc & Almond, Mini, Tesco*	1 Lolly/31g	103	331	4.4	24.8	23.8	0.9
Choc Lime Split, Morrisons*	1 Lolly/73ml	120	164	1.6	20.4	8.4	0.1
Chocolate & Vanilla, Sainsbury's*	1 Lolly/40.1g	143	357	3.7	28.7	25.3	2.2
Chocolate, Plain, Mini, Tesco*	1 Lolly/31g	94	304	3.1	24.8	21.4	1.2
Chocolate, Pooh Stick, Nestle*	1 Lolly/40g	36	89	2.1	12.9	3.6	0.0
Cider Refresher, Treats*	1 Lolly/70ml	54	77	0.0	19.2	0.0	0.0
Cola Lickers, Farmfoods*	1 Lolly/56ml	37	68	0.0	17.0	0.0	0.0
Creamy Tropical Sorbet, Sticks, Waitrose*	1 Lolly/85g	100	118	1.9	22.9	2.1	0.8
Elderflower,Tubes, Frozen, Marks & Spencer*	1oz/28g	23	82	0.1	20.5	0.1	0.2
Exotic Fruit, Tesco*	1 Lolly/31.5g	41	131	1.8	26.4	2.0	0.6
Exotic Split, Bars, Marks & Spencer*	1oz/28g	36	127	2.5	25.0	1.9	0.4
Fab, Nestle*	1 Lolly/57g	82	144	0.8	23.7	4.9	0.0
Feast, Chocolate, Mini, Wall's	1 Lolly	185	310	3.2	23.0	22.0	0.0
Feast, Ice Cream, Original, Wall's*	1 Lolly/92ml	296	322	3.5	23.7	23.8	0.0
Feast, Toffee, Mini, Wall's	1 Lolly	180	305	2.9	23.0	22.0	0.0
Fruit Assorted, Basics, Somerfield*	1 Lolly/56ml	32	58	0.0	15.0	0.0	0.0
Fruit Fusion, Mini, Farmfoods*	1 Lolly/45ml	36	79	0.2	19.2	0.1	0.2
Fruit Ices, Made With Orange Juice, Del Monte*	1 Lolly/75ml	79	105	0.5	25.7	0.0	0.0
Fruit Luxury, Mini, Co-Op*	1 Lolly/45g	59	130	2.0	18.0	6.0	0.2
Fruit Split, Asda*	1 Lolly/73.9g	85	115	1.7	19.0	3.6	0.0
Fruit Split, BFY, Morrisons*	1 Lolly/72.5g	50	69	1.6	13.9	0.7	0.1
Fruit Splits, Assorted, Somerfield*	1 Split/73ml	74	102	0.0	18.0	3.0	0.0
Fruit, Assorted, Waitrose*	1 Lolly/73g	59	81	0.0	20.0	0.0	0.1
Fruit, Red, Tesco*	1 Lolly/31.5g	40	128	1.8	25.6	2.0	0.6
Fruity n Freezy, Asda*	1 Lolly/30ml	24	80	0.1	20.0	0.0	0.0
Fruity, Ice Cream, Morrisons*	1 Lolly/73ml	50	69	1.6	13.9	0.7	0.1
Funny Foot, Wall's	1 Lolly	83	102	2.0	12.5	6.0	0.0
Kiwi Burst, Pineapple Sorbet In Kiwi Ice, Sainsbury's*	1 Serving/90ml	76	84	0.1	20.7	0.1	0.4
Lemon & Lime, Mini Bar, Marks & Spencer*	1 Lolly/50g	48	95	0.1	23.6	0.1	0.2
Lemon & Lime, Rocket Split, De Roma*	1 Lolly/60ml	65	108	1.0	16.0	4.3	0.2
Lemon & Lime, Tubes, Frozen, Marks & Spencer*	1oz/28g	27	95	0.1	23.6	0.1	0.2
Lemonade & Cola, Morrisons*	1 Lolly/55ml	36	65	0.0	16.2	0.0	0.0
Mango & Lemon, BGTY, Sainsbury's*	1 Lolly/72g	84	116	0.3	28.1	0.3	0.5
Mango & Passion Fruit, TTD, Sainsbury's*	1 Lolly/73ml	76	104	0.2	25.5	0.1	0.6
Mega Truffle, Nestle*	1 Lolly/71.1g	217	305	3.2	28.0	20.1	0.8
Milk Chocolate & Crisped Wheat, Co-Op*	1 Lolly/110g	259	235	3.0	28.0	12.0	0.7
Milk Flavour, Farmfoods*	1 Lolly/50ml	91	182	2.8	20.1	10.1	0.1
Milky Bar, Nestle*	1 Lolly/45.1g	156	346	4.3	33.2	21.8	0.1
Mini Milk, Chocolate, Wall's*	1 Lolly/24g	29	125	4.1	20.0	3.2	0.0
Mini Milk, Strawberry, Wall's*	1 Lolly/24g	30	130	3.3	19.0	4.1	0.0
Mini Milk, Vanilla, Wall's*	1 Lolly/24g	30	130	3.8	22.0	3.0	0.0
Mint Chocolate, Tesco*	1 Lolly/70g	234	334	3.6	35.4	19.8	1.2
Orange Juice, Asda*	1 Lolly/70g	58	83	0.7	20.0	0.0	0.0
Orange Juice, Bar, Marks & Spencer*	1 Lolly/75g	65	86	0.5	21.0	0.0	0.1
Orange Juice, Freshly Squeezed, Finest, Tesco*	1 Lolly/80ml	89	111	0.7	27.0	0.0	0.0
Orange Juice, Freshly Squeezed, Waitrose*	1 Lolly/73g	88	120	0.6	29.7	0.1	0.0
Orange Juice, Tropicana*	1 Lolly/50g	43	85	0.5	20.7	0.0	0.0
Orange Maid, Nestle*	1 Lolly/73ml	66	91	0.5	21.6	0.0	0.0
Orange, Real Fruit Juice, Sainsbury's*	1 Lolly/73ml	49	67	0.2	16.5	0.1	0.1
Orange, Real Juice, Tesco*	1 Lolly/32g	25	78	0.6	18.7	0.0	0.3

INFO/WEIGHT	Measure per Measure KCAL	Nutrition Values per 100g / 100ml				
		KCAL	PROT	CARB	FAT	FIBRE
ICE LOLLY						
Pineapple, Dairy Split, Sainsbury's*	1 Lolly/72.4ml 84	116	1.8	19.0	3.6	0.1
Pineapple, Real Fruit Juice, Sainsbury's*	1 Lolly/73ml 55	76	0.1	19.0	0.1	0.1
Polar Snappers, Double, Farmfoods*	1 Lolly/60ml 40	66	0.0	16.5	0.0	0.0
Raspberry & Apple, Sainsbury's*	1 Lolly/57ml 39	68	0.1	17.1	0.1	0.1
Raspberry, Real Fruit Juice, Sainsbury's*	1 Lolly/72g 62	86	0.3	21.0	0.1	0.1
Raspberry, Rocket Split, De Roma*	1 Lolly/60ml 65	108	1.0	16.2	4.3	0.2
Real Fruit Juice, Rocket, Blue Parrot Cafe, Sainsbury's*	1 Lolly/58ml 45	77	0.2	19.1	0.0	0.1
Real Fruit, Dairy Split, Sainsbury's*	1 Lolly/73ml 100	137	2.1	22.8	4.2	0.1
Real Orange, Kids, Tesco*	1 Lolly/31.5g 25	78	0.6	18.7	0.0	0.3
Refresher, Bassett's*	1 Lolly/40g 47	117	2.2	22.2	2.2	0.3
Rocket, Co-Op*	1 Lolly/60g 42	70	0.0	17.0	0.0	0.0
Rolo, Nestle*	1 Lolly/75ml 243	324	3.8	36.5	18.8	0.0
Solero, Exotic, Wall's	1 Lolly 104	112	1.5	20.0	3.0	0.0
Solero, Orange Fresh, Wall's	1 Lolly 78	81	0.2	20.0	0.0	0.0
Solero, Red Fruits, Wall's	1 Lollie 99	104	1.3	21.0	2.2	0.0
Strawberries 'n' Cream, Tropicana*	1 Lolly/50g 59	117	1.6	25.0	1.2	0.0
Strawberry & Banana, Smoothies, Sainsbury's*	1 Lolly/60g 100	166	1.5	28.0	5.3	0.2
Strawberry & Vanilla, 99% Fat Free, So-Lo, Iceland*	1 Lolly/92g 98	107	2.3	23.5	0.4	2.2
Strawberry Split, Co-Op*	1 Lolly/71ml 75	105	1.0	17.0	3.0	0.1
Strawberry, Dairy Split, Sainsbury's*	1 Lolly/72.9ml 86	118	1.7	19.8	3.6	0.1
Strawberry, Orange & Pineapple, Rocket, Iceland*	1 Lolly/47g 38	81	0.0	20.2	0.0	0.1
Strawberry, So-Lo, Good Choice, Iceland*	1 Lolly/66.4g 84	128	2.4	25.6	1.8	0.1
Tip Top, Calypso*	1 Lolly/20ml 6	30	0.1	7.1	0.1	0.0
Traffic Light, Co-Op*	1 Lolly/52g 55	105	0.4	25.0	0.8	0.0
Tropical Fruit, Starburst, Mars*	1 Lolly/93ml 94	101	0.3	24.8	0.1	0.0
Tropical, Mmmm, Tesco*	1 Lolly/73g 109	150	1.2	26.6	4.3	0.4
Twister, Wall's*	1 Lolly/80ml 76	95	0.6	18.4	1.9	0.0
Vanilla, Pooh Stick, Nestle*	1 Lolly/40g 34	86	1.9	12.9	3.5	0.0
Vimto*	1 Lolly/73.0ml 84	115	1.3	18.2	4.1	0.1
Wonka Super Sour Tastic, Nestle*	1 Lolly/60ml 84	140	0.0	26.1	3.6	0.0
Zoom, Nestle*	1 Lolly/58.1ml 54	93	0.9	20.6	0.7	0.0
INDIAN MEAL						
Banquet, For One, COU, Marks & Spencer*	1 Pack/500g 400	80	6.7	10.2	1.2	3.1
For One, Asda*	1 Pack/550g 919	167	8.0	18.0	7.0	1.3
For One, Eat Smart, Safeway*	1 Serving/600g 690	115	6.5	16.2	2.6	2.0
For One, GFY, Asda*	1 Serving/495g 644	130	8.0	14.0	4.7	1.0
For One, Healthy Eating, Tesco*	1 Pack/420g 437	104	7.4	14.0	2.1	1.4
For One, Vegetarian, Asda*	1 Pack/500g 789	158	3.2	16.0	9.0	1.4
For Two, Hot, Takeaway, Tesco*	1 Pack/825g 1215	147	6.6	13.6	7.3	1.9
For Two, Menu, Tesco*	1 Serving/537g 811	151	6.3	17.0	6.4	0.8
For Two, Peshwari Naan, Finest, Tesco*	1/2 Pack/200g 612	306	8.3	48.3	8.9	5.2
Takeaway, Ready Meals, Marks & Spencer*	1oz/28g 42	150	6.7	15.3	7.1	1.5
INDIAN MENU						
COU, Marks & Spencer*	1 Pack/550g 413	75	8.4	7.5	1.2	2.1
INDIAN SELECTION						
Snack, Safeway*	1 Serving/170g 347	204	4.0	25.8	9.4	1.9
INSTANT WHIP						
Chocolate Flavour, Dry, Bird's*	1oz/28g 109	390	3.8	80.5	5.9	0.7
Strawberry Flavour, Dry, Bird's*	1oz/28g 112	400	2.5	85.0	5.4	0.4
IRON BRU						
Barrs*	1 Can/330ml 142	43	0.0	10.6	0.0	0.0

I

	Measure	per Measure	Nutrition Values per 100g / 100ml				
	INFO/WEIGHT	KCAL	KCAL	PROT	CARB	FAT	FIBRE
JALFREZI							
Chicken With Basmati Rice, Eat Smart, Safeway*	1 Pack/400g	300	75	6.8	8.5	1.0	1.7
Chicken With Pilau Rice, GFY, Asda*	1 Pack/445.9g	495	111	8.0	14.0	2.5	1.2
Chicken With Pilau Rice, Patak's*	1 Pack/400g	556	139	9.8	14.7	4.6	0.9
Chicken With Pilau Rice, Safeway*	1 Pack/424.2g	700	165	8.1	20.9	5.0	0.8
Chicken With Pilau Rice, Spar*	1 Pack/400g	472	118	6.7	12.0	4.8	1.2
Chicken, & Rice, Healthy Eating, Tesco*	1 Pack/420g	483	115	7.9	17.5	1.6	0.3
Chicken, Asda*	1 Pack/340g	415	122	10.0	7.0	6.0	1.6
Chicken, GFY, Asda*	1 Pack/350g	277	79	11.0	6.0	1.2	0.8
Chicken, Healthy Living, Tesco*	1 Serving/450g	482	107	6.9	18.0	0.8	0.9
Chicken, Hot & Spicy, Sainsbury's*	1/2 Pack/200g	228	114	12.8	2.9	5.7	1.0
Chicken, Indian Takeaway, Tesco*	1 Serving/350g	434	124	7.4	5.7	8.0	1.6
Chicken, Marks & Spencer*	1 Pack/350g	385	110	10.8	4.2	5.7	2.0
Chicken, Medium, GFY, Asda*	1 Pack/644g	972	151	6.0	22.0	4.3	0.9
Chicken, Sainsbury's*	1 Pack/400g	436	109	12.1	3.4	5.2	1.7
Chicken, Tesco*	1 Pack/350g	350	100	9.3	3.5	5.5	1.5
Chicken, With Pilau Rice, BGTY, Sainsbury's*	1 Pack/450g	396	88	6.4	14.3	0.6	2.2
Chicken, With Pilau Rice, Tesco*	1 Pack/460g	506	110	5.3	13.6	3.8	0.9
Chicken, With Rice, Healthy Living, Tesco*	1 Pack/450g	554	123	7.2	21.6	0.9	0.8
Meal For One, Marks & Spencer*	1 Serving/500g	700	140	6.1	13.4	7.0	3.0
Vegetable, Eastern Indian, Sainsbury's*	1 Pack/400g	208	52	3.4	2.0	3.4	1.7
Vegetable, Take Away Menu For 1, BGTY, Sainsbury's*	1 Pack/148g	43	29	1.8	5.4	0.0	2.3
Vegetable, Waitrose*	1 Pack/400g	256	64	2.2	4.7	4.0	3.7
Vegetable, With Rice, Birds Eye*	1 Pack/350g	354	101	2.5	20.2	1.1	1.0
JAM							
Apricot & Peach, 25% Less Sugar, Asda*	1 Tsp/15g	28	184	0.5	45.4	0.1	1.1
Apricot, Average	1 Tbsp/15g	37	248	0.2	61.6	0.0	1.5
Apricot, Reduced Sugar, Average	1 Serving/20g	37	187	0.5	46.0	0.3	0.4
Black Cherry, Average	2 Tbsp/30g	74	247	0.4	61.2	0.3	0.4
Blackberry, Extra Special, Asda*	1 Tbsp/15.3g	29	190	0.9	45.0	0.7	0.0
Blackcurrant, Average	1 Tbsp/15g	38	250	0.2	62.3	0.0	1.0
Blackcurrant, Reduced Sugar, Average	1 Tsp/5.7g	11	178	0.5	44.4	0.2	1.0
Blueberry & Blackberry, Baxters*	1 Tsp/15g	38	252	0.0	63.0	0.0	1.2
Blueberry, St Dalfour*	1 Serving/20g	46	228	0.5	56.0	0.2	2.2
Damson, Extra Fruit, Best, Hartley's*	1 Tsp/5g	12	244	0.2	60.8	0.0	0.0
Golden Peach, Rhapsodie de Fruit, St Dalfour*	2 Tsp/20g	45	227	0.5	56.0	0.1	1.3
Kiwi & Goosberry, 66% Fruit, Asda*	1 Serving/30g	56	187	0.5	45.0	0.5	0.0
Mixed Fruit, Average	1 Tbsp/15g	38	253	0.3	63.5	0.0	0.5
Plum, Tesco*	1 Serving/50g	131	261	0.2	64.4	0.0	0.6
Rasberry, Reduced Sugar, Average	1 Tsp/6.3g	10	160	0.5	39.3	0.2	0.6
Raspberry, Average	1 Tbsp/15.1g	36	239	0.6	58.7	0.1	0.9
Raspberry, Seedless, Average	1 Tsp/10g	26	257	0.5	63.6	0.0	0.3
Rhubarb & Ginger, Baxters*	1 Tsp/15g	32	210	0.0	53.0	0.0	0.6
Strawberry & Redcurrant, Reduced Sugar, Streamline*	1 Tbsp/15g	29	192	0.4	46.8	0.3	0.0
Strawberry, Average	1 Tsp/10g	25	253	0.3	62.8	0.0	0.6
Strawberry, Reduced Sugar, Average	1 Tbsp/15g	28	187	0.4	45.8	0.3	0.2
Wild Blackberry Jelly, Baxters*	1 Tsp/15g	32	210	0.0	53.0	0.0	1.2
JAMBALAYA							
American Style, Tesco*	1 Serving/275g	432	157	7.7	16.0	7.0	0.5
American, Healthy Eating, Tesco*	1 Pack/450g	477	106	6.4	15.5	2.0	0.9
COU, Marks & Spencer*	1 Pack/400g	340	85	6.5	10.8	2.0	0.9
Cajun Chicken, BGTY, Sainsbury's*	1 Pack/400g	364	91	7.7	11.9	1.4	1.1
Chicken, Spicy, Eat Smart, Morrisons*	1 Pack/400g	376	94	6.3	14.0	1.4	1.8
GFY, Asda*	1 Pack/450g	428	95	6.0	12.0	2.5	0.9

J

	Measure INFO/WEIGHT	per Measure KCAL	Nutrition Values per 100g / 100ml				
			KCAL	PROT	CARB	FAT	FIBRE
JAMBALAYA							
Marks & Spencer*	1 Pack/480g	552	115	5.8	14.6	3.5	1.2
Tesco*	1 Pack/550g	765	139	6.9	13.1	6.6	1.1
JELLY							
Blackberry, Unprepared, Morrisons*	1 Serving/20g	52	261	0.3	65.0	0.0	0.0
Blackcurrant, Made Up, Rowntree's*	1/4 Jelly/140ml	100	71	1.4	16.4	0.1	0.0
Blackcurrant, Sugar Free, Unprepared, Rowntree's*	1 Pack/24g	73	305	66.5	0.3	0.0	0.4
Crystals, Orange, Sugar Free, Bird's*	1 Sachet/111/2g	39	335	62.5	6.4	0.9	0.0
Crystals, Strawberry, Tesco*	1 Serving Made/3g	9	303	63.5	12.0	0.1	0.2
Exotic Fruit, Marks & Spencer*	1 Pot/175g	140	80	0.1	18.9	0.2	0.9
Fresh Fruit, Marks & Spencer*	1 Pot/175g	131	75	0.2	18.4	0.1	0.3
Fruit Cocktail, Marks & Spencer*	1oz/28g	31	110	0.4	16.4	4.7	0.3
Fruitini, Del Monte*	1 Serving/120g	78	65	0.3	15.3	0.1	0.5
Lemon & Lime, Sugar Free, Unprepared, Rowntree's*	1oz/28g	85	305	4.5	60.7	0.0	0.0
Lemon, Unprepared, Somerfield*	1 Pack/135g	393	291	6.0	66.0	0.0	0.0
Lime, Made Up, Rowntree's*	1/4 Jelly/140ml	100	71	1.4	16.4	0.1	0.0
Lime, Unprepared, Somerfield*	1 Pack/135g	392	290	6.0	66.0	0.0	0.0
Made With Water	1oz/28g	17	61	1.2	15.1	0.0	0.0
Mandarin & Pineapple, Sainsbury's*	1 Pot/125g	95	76	0.2	18.9	0.1	1.2
Mandarin, Aroma, Marks & Spencer*	1oz/28g	17	60	0.2	14.6	0.0	0.4
Mixed Berry, WTF, Sainsbury's*	1 Serving/160g	112	70	0.7	16.3	0.2	1.5
Orange Flavour, Unprepared, Somerfield*	1 Pack/128g	379	296	5.0	69.0	0.0	0.0
Orange, Quickset, Unprepared, Rowntree's*	1 Serving/1/4 Pint	65	340	0.0	84.0	0.0	3.0
Orange, Sugar Free, Unprepared, Asda*	1 Serving/12g	36	303	63.6	12.0	0.1	0.2
Orange, Unprepared, Rowntree's*	1 Square/11g	33	296	4.4	69.6	0.0	0.0
Pineapple, With Pineapple Pieces, Tesco*	1 Serving/120g	96	80	1.2	18.6	0.1	0.7
Raspberry & Rose, Aroma, Marks & Spencer*	1oz/28g	14	50	0.2	11.9	0.2	0.4
Raspberry Flavour, Sugar Free, Made Up, Rowntree's*	1 Portion/140ml	9	6	1.4	0.1	0.0	0.0
Raspberry Flavour, Tesco*	1 Serving/34g	22	64	1.0	15.0	0.0	0.1
Raspberry, Marks & Spencer*	1 Serving/175g	109	62	0.3	14.6	0.3	0.0
Raspberry, Unprepared, Rowntree's*	1 Serving/135g	405	300	5.6	67.3	0.4	0.0
Strawberry & Raspberry, Sainsbury's*	1/2 Pot/280g	230	82	0.2	20.2	0.0	1.2
Strawberry Flavour, Sugar Free, Made Up, Rowntree's*	1 Serving/140ml	10	7	1.5	0.1	0.0	0.0
Strawberry Flavour, Sugar Free, Unprepared, Rowntree's*	1oz/28g	84	300	64.9	3.0	0.0	0.0
Strawberry, Basics, Unprepared, Somerfield*	1/4 Jelly/32g	95	296	5.0	69.0	0.0	0.0
Strawberry, Unprepared, Somerfield*	1/4 Jelly/33.75g	99	291	6.0	66.0	0.0	0.0
Summer Fruits, Unprepared, Co-Op*	1 Pack/135g	401	297	5.5	68.7	0.1	0.0
Tangerine, Unprepared, Rowntree's*	1 Serving/33g	99	300	5.6	67.3	0.4	0.0
Tropical Fresh Fruit, Eat Smart, Safeway*	1 Serving/185g	120	65	0.6	14.5	0.3	1.1
Tropical Fruit, WTF, Sainsbury's*	1 Serving/160g	144	90	0.3	19.9	1.0	0.9
JELLY BABIES							
Bassett's*	1 Baby/6g	20	335	4.0	79.5	0.0	0.0
Marks & Spencer*	1 Pack/125g	418	334	5.2	78.0	0.0	0.0
Mini, Rowntree's*	1 Small Bag/35g	128	366	4.6	86.9	0.0	0.0
Mini, Waitrose*	1 Bag/125g	370	296	4.3	68.7	0.4	0.0
Sainsbury's*	1 Serving/70g	247	353	4.1	82.5	0.7	0.3
Somerfield*	1 Sweet/6g	21	343	4.7	80.7	0.0	0.0
Tesco*	1 Baby/6g	20	332	5.3	77.4	0.1	0.1
JELLY BEANS							
Asda*	1 Bag/100g	364	364	0.1	90.0	0.4	0.2
Jelly Belly*	35 Beans/40g	140	350	0.0	90.0	0.0	0.0
Marks & Spencer*	1 Bag/113g	407	360	0.1	89.6	0.0	0.0
Rowntree's*	1 Pack/35g	128	367	0.0	91.8	0.0	0.0

J

	Measure INFO/WEIGHT	per Measure KCAL	Nutrition Values per 100g / 100ml KCAL	PROT	CARB	FAT	FIBRE
JELLY BEARS							
Co-Op*	1 Sweet/3g	10	325	6.0	76.0	0.1	0.0
JELLY TOTS							
Rowntree's*	1 Pack/42g	145	346	0.1	86.5	0.0	0.0
JUICE							
Apple & Elderflower, Copella*	1 Glass/250ml	108	43	0.4	10.2	0.1	0.0
Apple & Mango, Average	1 Glass/200ml	108	54	0.3	12.6	0.0	0.1
Apple & Raspberry, Average	1 Serving/200ml	89	45	0.5	10.2	0.1	0.2
Apple, Concentrate, Average	1 Tbsp/15ml	45	302	0.1	73.6	0.2	0.0
Apple, English With Cherry, Cawston Vale*	1 Can/250ml	118	47	0.4	11.6	0.1	0.0
Apple, Pure, Average	1 Glass/100ml	47	47	0.1	11.2	0.0	0.0
Apple, Pure, Organic, Average	1 Serving/200ml	93	46	0.1	11.2	0.1	0.1
Apple, Raspberry, & Grape, Pressed, Sainsbury's*	1 Serving/200ml	92	46	0.3	11.2	0.1	0.5
Apple, Red Grape & Blueberry, Pure, Blends, Del Monte*	1 Serving/250ml	125	50	0.6	11.5	0.0	0.0
Apple, With Calcium, Juice Plus, Tesco*	1 Serving/250ml	118	47	0.1	11.2	0.0	0.0
Apple, With Mango Puree, Safeway*	1 Glass/150ml	80	53	0.3	12.6	0.0	0.0
Breakfast, Sainsbury's*	1 Serving/200ml	94	47	0.7	11.3	0.1	0.3
Carrot, Average	1 Glass/200ml	46	23	0.6	5.2	0.0	0.1
Clementine, Morrisons*	1 Serving/100ml	48	48	0.5	10.9	0.1	0.1
Cranberry & Apple, No Added Sugar, Sainsbury's*	1 Glass/250ml	15	6	0.0	1.5	0.0	0.0
Cranberry & Raspberry, Low Sugar, Sainsbury's*	1 Glass/250ml	10	4	0.1	0.7	0.1	0.1
Cranberry, Average	1 Bottle/250ml	139	56	0.1	13.4	0.1	0.3
Exotic Fruit, Pure, Del Monte*	1 Glass/200ml	96	48	0.3	11.3	0.0	0.0
Exotic Fruit, Waitrose*	1 Glass/175ml	88	50	0.4	11.6	0.0	0.0
Fibre, Tropicana*	1 Serving/200ml	130	65	0.4	15.8	0.0	3.4
Grape & Peach, Don Simon*	1 Serving/200ml	94	47	0.4	11.3	0.0	0.0
Grape & Raspberry, Pressed, Marks & Spencer*	1 Sm Bottle/250ml	138	55	0.4	12.9	0.0	0.1
Grape, Purple, Welch's*	1 Serving/200ml	136	68	0.1	16.5	0.0	0.0
Grape, Red, Average	1 Serving/100ml	62	62	0.2	15.2	0.0	0.0
Grape, White, Average	1 Can/160ml	95	60	0.2	14.3	0.1	0.1
Grapefruit, Low Calorie, Natreen*	1 Sm Glass/100ml	18	18	0.5	3.3	0.5	0.0
Grapefruit, Pink, Average	1 Glass/200ml	81	41	0.6	9.0	0.1	0.2
Lemon, Fresh	1 Tbsp/10ml	1	7	0.3	1.6	0.0	0.1
Lemon, Made With Concentrated Lemon Juice, Tesco*	1 Serving/100ml	10	10	0.4	2.0	0.0	0.0
Lime, Fresh	1 Tsp/5ml	0	9	0.4	1.6	0.1	0.1
Mango & Apple, Copella*	1 Serving/200ml	86	43	0.4	10.1	0.1	0.0
Mango, Canned	1 Glass/200ml	78	39	0.1	9.8	0.2	0.0
Multivitamin, Fruit, Vitafit, Lidl*	1 Glass/200ml	106	53	1.0	12.0	0.0	0.5
Orange & Banana, Sainsbury's*	1 Glass/200ml	108	54	0.7	12.5	0.1	0.3
Orange & Grapefruit, Average	1 Serving/200g	85	42	0.8	9.3	0.1	0.4
Orange & Kiwi Fruit, Tropicana*	1 Serving/175ml	90	51	0.5	12.0	0.0	0.0
Orange & Pineapple, Average	1 Glass/120ml	56	47	0.5	10.5	0.5	0.5
Orange & Raspberry, Average	1fl oz/30ml	15	50	0.6	11.4	0.1	0.2
Orange & Strawberry, Average	1 Serving/125ml	64	51	0.6	10.9	0.4	0.8
Orange Banana & Grapefruit, Marks & Spencer*	1 Serving/250ml	125	50	0.8	11.5	0.2	0.3
Orange With Cranberry Juice, Marks & Spencer*	1 Sm Bottle/250ml	138	55	0.5	14.0	0.5	1.0
Orange, Pure, Smooth, Average	1 Glass/200ml	88	44	0.7	9.8	0.0	0.2
Orange, Pure, With Bits, Average	1 Glass/200ml	90	45	0.6	10.2	0.1	0.1
Orange, Red, Average	1 Glass/250ml	115	46	0.4	10.7	0.0	0.2
Passion Fruit, Average	1 Glass/200ml	94	47	0.8	10.7	0.1	0.0
Pear, Concentrate, Meridian Foods*	1 Serving/45ml	134	298	0.0	74.6	0.0	0.0
Pear, With A Hint Of Ginger, Pressed, Marks & Spencer*	1 Glass/250ml	125	50	0.3	11.7	0.1	0.0
Pineapple & Coconut, Sainsbury's*	1 Glass/250ml	153	61	0.5	11.6	1.4	0.1
Pineapple & Coconut, Tesco*	1 Serving/250ml	123	49	0.2	11.4	0.2	0.0

J

	INFO/WEIGHT	KCAL	KCAL	PROT	CARB	FAT	FIBRE

JUICE

	Measure INFO/WEIGHT	per Measure KCAL	KCAL	PROT	CARB	FAT	FIBRE
Pineapple Mango Crush, Just Juice*	1 Glass/250ml	108	43	0.0	10.6	0.0	0.0
Pineapple, Average	1 Glass/200ml	100	50	0.3	11.7	0.1	0.2
Prune, Average	1 Serving/200ml	123	61	0.6	15.3	0.1	1.8
Raspberry & Black Cherry, Carbonated, Crystal Spring*	1 Glass/200ml	204	102	2.0	7.5	7.1	0.0
Raspberry Cooler, With Mint, Sainsbury's*	1 Serving/250ml	63	25	0.1	6.0	0.1	0.1
Sweet Carrot & Orange, Shapers, Boots*	1 Serving/250ml	100	40	0.9	8.8	0.2	0.4
Tomato, Average	1 Glass/200ml	40	20	0.8	4.0	0.1	0.5
Tropical Fruit, Plenty*	1 Glass/200ml	120	60	0.5	13.7	0.1	0.0
Tropical, Pure, Sainsbury's*	1 Glass/200ml	104	52	0.5	12.0	0.1	0.1
Tropical, Tropics, Tropicana*	1 Serving/250ml	113	45	0.4	11.0	0.0	0.0
Vegetable, Organic, Evernat*	1 Glass/200ml	36	18	0.9	3.5	0.1	0.2
Vegetable, V8*	1/2 Can/165ml	31	19	0.8	3.3	0.5	1.0

JUICE DRINK

	Measure INFO/WEIGHT	per Measure KCAL	KCAL	PROT	CARB	FAT	FIBRE
Apple & Blueberry, The Feel Good Drinks Co*	1 Serving/375ml	163	44	0.1	10.6	0.1	0.0
Apple & Cranberry, Safeway*	1 Serving/250ml	125	50	0.0	12.1	0.0	0.0
Apple & Elderflower, Tesco*	1 Serving/200ml	76	38	0.0	9.4	0.0	0.0
Apple & Raspberry, Tesco*	1 Serving/300ml	138	46	0.0	11.2	0.0	0.0
Apple, Cranberry, & Blueberry, Waitrose*	1 Serving/150ml	75	50	0.1	11.9	0.0	0.1
Berry Blast, 5 Alive*	1 Serving/250ml	133	53	0.0	13.0	0.0	0.0
Blackcurrant, CVit*	1 Glass/200ml	4	2	0.0	0.2	0.0	0.0
Blackcurrant, Kids, Tesco*	1 Serving/250ml	128	51	0.0	12.4	0.0	0.0
Blackcurrant, Purity*	1 Bottle/500ml	265	53	0.0	13.2	0.0	0.0
Cherry, No Added Sugar, Sainsbury's*	1 Carton/250ml	25	10	0.2	1.9	0.0	0.0
Citrus Burst, 5 Alive*	1 Carton/250ml	125	50	0.0	12.8	0.0	0.0
Citrus, Co-Op*	1 Serving/150ml	68	45	0.2	11.0	0.0	0.0
Citrus, Sainsbury's*	1 Serving/200ml	102	51	0.3	12.3	0.1	0.2
Cranberry & Apple, Ocean Spray*	1 Glass/200ml	92	46	0.0	11.1	0.0	0.0
Cranberry & Blackberry, Ocean Spray*	1 Glass/250ml	120	48	0.1	11.3	0.1	0.2
Cranberry & Blackcurrant, Ocean Spray*	1 Bottle/500ml	265	53	0.2	12.7	0.0	0.0
Cranberry & Orange, Healthy Eating, Tesco*	1 Glass/200ml	10	5	0.0	0.8	0.0	0.0
Cranberry & Raspberry, Ocean Spray*	1 Glass/200ml	104	52	0.0	12.7	0.0	0.0
Cranberry & Raspberry, Tesco*	1 Serving/200ml	96	48	0.0	11.6	0.0	0.0
Cranberry, Classic, Ocean Spray*	1 Bottle/500ml	245	49	0.0	11.7	0.0	0.0
Cranberry, Grape & Apple, Ocean Spray*	1 Glass/200ml	108	54	0.1	12.9	0.0	0.0
Cranberry, Juice Burst, Purity*	1 Bottle/500ml	245	49	0.0	12.0	0.0	0.0
Cranberry, Marks & Spencer*	1 Serving/100ml	60	60	0.1	14.3	0.0	0.0
Cranberry, No Added Sugar, Healthy Living, Tesco*	1 Glass/200ml	8	4	0.0	1.1	0.0	0.0
Cranberry, Original, Concentrated, Ocean Spray*	1 Serving/15ml	27	183	0.2	44.1	0.0	0.0
Cranberry, Solevita*	1 Serving/200ml	98	49	0.5	11.7	0.0	0.0
Cranberry, Tesco*	1 Glass/200ml	92	46	0.0	11.1	0.0	0.0
Cranberry, Tropical, Ocean Spray*	1 Glass/200ml	96	48	0.1	11.5	0.0	0.0
Exotic, Tesco*	1 Serving/250ml	128	51	0.1	12.3	0.0	0.0
Forest Fruits, Tesco*	1 Serving/250ml	115	46	0.0	11.1	0.0	0.0
Fruit Cocktail, Sainsbury's*	1 Glass/200ml	94	47	0.2	11.2	0.1	0.1
Grape, Apple & Raspberry, Asda*	1 Glass/200ml	90	45	0.2	11.0	0.0	0.0
Grape, Apple & Raspberry, Co-Op*	1 Serving/150ml	75	50	0.4	12.0	0.0	0.1
Grapefruit & Cranberry, Marks & Spencer*	1 Serving/250ml	125	50	0.2	11.9	0.1	0.0
Grapefruit & Lime, Quest, Marks & Spencer*	1 Bottle/330ml	53	16	0.0	4.0	0.0	0.0
Guava Exotic, Rubicon*	1 Carton/288ml	150	52	0.2	12.8	0.1	0.0
J20, Apple & Mango, Britvic*	1 Bottle/275ml	132	48	0.1	11.3	0.1	0.0
J20, Apple & Raspberry, Britvic*	1 Bottle/275ml	146	53	0.1	13.0	0.1	0.0
J20, Orange & Passion Fruit, Britvic*	1 Bottle/275ml	132	48	0.1	11.3	0.1	0.0
Lemon & Lime, Light, Oasis*	1 Bottle/250ml	7	3	0.0	0.2	0.0	0.0

J

JUICE DRINK

	Measure INFO/WEIGHT	per Measure KCAL	Nutrition Values per 100g / 100ml				
			KCAL	PROT	CARB	FAT	FIBRE
Lemon & Mandarin, Diet, Quest, Marks & Spencer*	1 Bottle/330ml	13	4	0.0	1.0	0.0	0.0
Lemon, The Feel Good Drinks Co*	1 Bottle/171.4ml	78	46	0.1	10.8	0.1	0.0
Lemonade, Asda*	1 Glass/200ml	88	44	0.1	11.0	0.0	0.0
Mango Madness, Snapple*	1 Bottle/227ml	104	46	0.0	12.0	0.0	0.0
Mega Green, Smucker's*	1 Serving/473ml	237	50	0.0	12.5	0.0	0.0
Orange & Banana, Pure, Average	1 Glass/150ml	79	53	0.7	12.1	0.1	0.2
Orange & Mango, Average	1 Bottle/375ml	176	47	0.5	10.7	0.1	0.3
Orange, Caprisun*	1 Pouch/200ml	89	45	0.0	10.8	0.0	0.0
Orange, Carrot & Lemon, Pago*	1 Serving/200g	90	45	0.2	10.5	0.1	0.0
Orange, Fruitish, Spar*	1 Carton/330ml	13	4	0.1	0.8	0.1	0.0
Orange, Healthy Eating, Tesco*	1 Glass/200ml	56	28	0.3	6.1	0.1	0.0
Orange, Juice Burst, Purity*	1 Bottle/500ml	220	44	1.0	10.2	0.0	0.0
Orange, Ribena*	1 Serving/288ml	98	34	0.1	8.1	0.0	0.0
Orange, Sainsbury's*	1 Serving/250ml	18	7	0.1	1.4	0.1	0.1
Orange, Value, Tesco*	1 Glass/250ml	33	13	0.0	3.3	0.0	0.0
Peach & Passionfruit Fruit, Sunmagic*	1 Serving/330ml	172	52	0.3	13.0	0.0	0.1
Pineapple & Coconut, Waitrose*	1 Serving/250ml	125	50	0.2	11.5	0.3	0.2
Pineapple & Grapefruit, Shapers, Boots*	1 Bottle/500ml	10	2	0.1	0.2	0.1	0.0
Pink Grapefruit, Juice Burst, Purity*	1 Bottle/500ml	210	42	0.4	10.0	0.0	0.0
Pomegranate, Pomegreat*	1 Glass/200ml	88	44	0.1	11.1	0.0	0.0
Raspberry & Pear, Tesco*	1 Serving/250ml	118	47	0.0	11.3	0.0	0.0
Summer Fruits, Fresh, Tesco*	1 Glass/250ml	113	45	0.1	10.8	0.1	0.3
Summer Fruits, Oasis*	1 Bottle/500ml	185	37	0.0	9.0	0.0	0.0
Tropical Fruit, Tesco*	1 Glass/250ml	118	47	0.0	11.4	0.0	0.0
Tropical Hit, 5 Alive*	1 Carton/250ml	93	37	0.0	9.3	0.0	0.0
Vimto*	1 Can/330ml	147	45	0.0	11.0	0.0	0.0
White Cranberry & Grape, Oceanspay*	1 Serving/100ml	48	48	0.0	11.6	0.0	0.0
White Cranberry & Lychee, Ocean Spray*	1 Glass/200ml	86	43	0.0	11.5	0.0	0.0
White Grape & Peach, Sainsbury's*	1 Glass/250ml	95	38	0.2	9.0	0.1	0.1

J

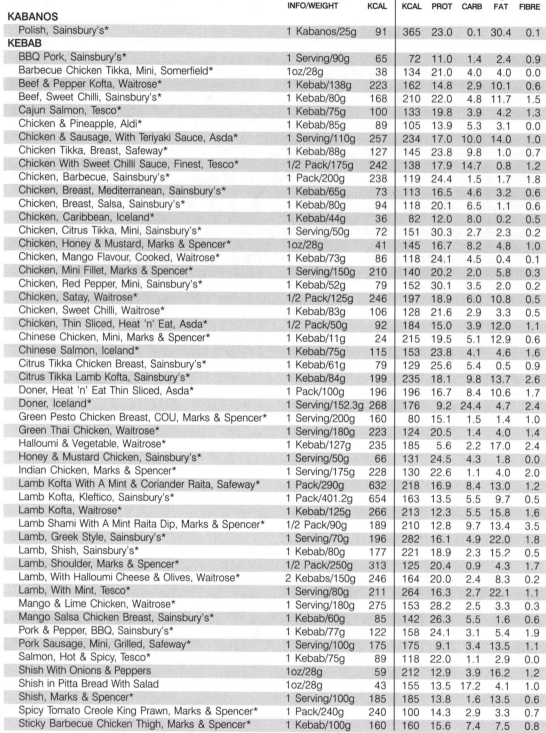

	Measure INFO/WEIGHT	per Measure KCAL	Nutrition Values per 100g / 100ml				
			KCAL	PROT	CARB	FAT	FIBRE
KABANOS							
Polish, Sainsbury's*	1 Kabanos/25g	91	365	23.0	0.1	30.4	0.1
KEBAB							
BBQ Pork, Sainsbury's*	1 Serving/90g	65	72	11.0	1.4	2.4	0.9
Barbecue Chicken Tikka, Mini, Somerfield*	1oz/28g	38	134	21.0	4.0	4.0	0.0
Beef & Pepper Kofta, Waitrose*	1 Kebab/138g	223	162	14.8	2.9	10.1	0.6
Beef, Sweet Chilli, Sainsbury's*	1 Kebab/80g	168	210	22.0	4.8	11.7	1.5
Cajun Salmon, Tesco*	1 Kebab/75g	100	133	19.8	3.9	4.2	1.3
Chicken & Pineapple, Aldi*	1 Kebab/85g	89	105	13.9	5.3	3.1	0.0
Chicken & Sausage, With Teriyaki Sauce, Asda*	1 Serving/110g	257	234	17.0	10.0	14.0	1.0
Chicken Tikka, Breast, Safeway*	1 Kebab/88g	127	145	23.8	9.8	1.0	0.7
Chicken With Sweet Chilli Sauce, Finest, Tesco*	1/2 Pack/175g	242	138	17.9	14.7	0.8	1.2
Chicken, Barbecue, Sainsbury's*	1 Pack/200g	238	119	24.4	1.5	1.7	1.8
Chicken, Breast, Mediterranean, Sainsbury's*	1 Kebab/65g	73	113	16.5	4.6	3.2	0.6
Chicken, Breast, Salsa, Sainsbury's*	1 Kebab/80g	94	118	20.1	6.5	1.1	0.6
Chicken, Caribbean, Iceland*	1 Kebab/44g	36	82	12.0	8.0	0.2	0.5
Chicken, Citrus Tikka, Mini, Sainsbury's*	1 Serving/50g	72	151	30.3	2.7	2.3	0.2
Chicken, Honey & Mustard, Marks & Spencer*	1oz/28g	41	145	16.7	8.2	4.8	0.2
Chicken, Mango Flavour, Cooked, Waitrose*	1 Kebab/73g	86	118	24.1	4.5	0.4	0.1
Chicken, Mini Fillet, Marks & Spencer*	1 Serving/150g	210	140	20.2	2.0	5.8	0.3
Chicken, Red Pepper, Mini, Sainsbury's*	1 Kebab/52g	79	152	30.1	3.5	2.0	0.2
Chicken, Satay, Waitrose*	1/2 Pack/125g	246	197	18.9	6.0	10.8	0.5
Chicken, Sweet Chilli, Waitrose*	1 Kebab/83g	106	128	21.6	2.9	3.3	0.5
Chicken, Thin Sliced, Heat 'n' Eat, Asda*	1/2 Pack/50g	92	184	15.0	3.9	12.0	1.1
Chinese Chicken, Mini, Marks & Spencer*	1 Kebab/11g	24	215	19.5	5.1	12.9	0.6
Chinese Salmon, Iceland*	1 Kebab/75g	115	153	23.8	4.1	4.6	1.6
Citrus Tikka Chicken Breast, Sainsbury's*	1 Kebab/61g	79	129	25.6	5.4	0.5	0.9
Citrus Tikka Lamb Kofta, Sainsbury's*	1 Kebab/84g	199	235	18.1	9.8	13.7	2.6
Doner, Heat 'n' Eat Thin Sliced, Asda*	1 Pack/100g	196	196	16.7	8.4	10.6	1.7
Doner, Iceland*	1 Serving/152.3g	268	176	9.2	24.4	4.7	2.4
Green Pesto Chicken Breast, COU, Marks & Spencer*	1 Serving/200g	160	80	15.1	1.5	1.4	1.0
Green Thai Chicken, Waitrose*	1 Serving/180g	223	124	20.5	1.4	4.0	1.4
Halloumi & Vegetable, Waitrose*	1 Kebab/127g	235	185	5.6	2.2	17.0	2.4
Honey & Mustard Chicken, Sainsbury's*	1 Serving/50g	66	131	24.5	4.3	1.8	0.0
Indian Chicken, Marks & Spencer*	1 Serving/175g	228	130	22.6	1.1	4.0	2.0
Lamb Kofta With A Mint & Coriander Raita, Safeway*	1 Pack/290g	632	218	16.9	8.4	13.0	1.2
Lamb Kofta, Kleftico, Sainsbury's*	1 Pack/401.2g	654	163	13.5	5.5	9.7	0.5
Lamb Kofta, Waitrose*	1 Kebab/125g	266	213	12.3	5.5	15.8	1.6
Lamb Shami With A Mint Raita Dip, Marks & Spencer*	1/2 Pack/90g	189	210	12.8	9.7	13.4	3.5
Lamb, Greek Style, Sainsbury's*	1 Serving/70g	196	282	16.1	4.9	22.0	1.8
Lamb, Shish, Sainsbury's*	1 Kebab/80g	177	221	18.9	2.3	15.2	0.5
Lamb, Shoulder, Marks & Spencer*	1/2 Pack/250g	313	125	20.4	0.9	4.3	1.7
Lamb, With Halloumi Cheese & Olives, Waitrose*	2 Kebabs/150g	246	164	20.0	2.4	8.3	0.2
Lamb, With Mint, Tesco*	1 Serving/80g	211	264	16.3	2.7	22.1	1.1
Mango & Lime Chicken, Waitrose*	1 Serving/180g	275	153	28.2	2.5	3.3	0.3
Mango Salsa Chicken Breast, Sainsbury's*	1 Kebab/60g	85	142	26.3	5.5	1.6	0.6
Pork & Pepper, BBQ, Sainsbury's*	1 Kebab/77g	122	158	24.1	3.1	5.4	1.9
Pork Sausage, Mini, Grilled, Safeway*	1 Serving/100g	175	175	9.1	3.4	13.5	1.1
Salmon, Hot & Spicy, Tesco*	1 Kebab/75g	89	118	22.0	1.1	2.9	0.0
Shish With Onions & Peppers	1oz/28g	59	212	12.9	3.9	16.2	1.2
Shish in Pitta Bread With Salad	1oz/28g	43	155	13.5	17.2	4.1	1.0
Shish, Marks & Spencer*	1 Serving/100g	185	185	13.8	1.6	13.5	0.6
Spicy Tomato Creole King Prawn, Marks & Spencer*	1 Pack/240g	240	100	14.3	2.9	3.3	0.7
Sticky Barbecue Chicken Thigh, Marks & Spencer*	1 Kebab/100g	160	160	15.6	7.4	7.5	0.8

K

INFO/WEIGHT	Measure	per Measure KCAL	Nutrition Values per 100g / 100ml KCAL	PROT	CARB	FAT	FIBRE

KEBAB

	Measure INFO/WEIGHT	per Measure KCAL	KCAL	PROT	CARB	FAT	FIBRE
Sweet Oriental Chicken Breast, COU, Marks & Spencer*	1/2 Pack/200g	220	110	20.8	4.3	1.0	0.1
Sweetcorn, Tesco*	1 Kebab/130g	74	57	2.0	9.9	1.0	0.9
Tandoori, Marks & Spencer*	1oz/28g	34	120	23.3	1.0	2.5	0.0
Thai Style Chicken, Eat Smart, Safeway*	1 Kebab/85g	85	100	15.3	6.4	1.3	1.4
Tiger Prawn, Asda*	1oz/28g	17	59	14.6	0.0	0.1	0.0
Tikka Chicken, Mini, Somerfield*	1oz/28g	38	134	21.0	4.0	4.0	0.0
Tikka, Mini, Marks & Spencer*	1 Kebab/11g	23	205	18.4	4.0	12.7	0.6
Tomato & Basil Chicken, Eat Smart, Safeway*	1 Kebab/71.5g	82	115	18.0	5.0	2.1	1.5
Turkey, Wth Chinese Style Dressing, Sainsbury's*	1 Kebab/5g	84	157	21.4	6.4	5.1	1.7
Vegeatable, Mini, Sainsbury's*	1 Kebab/36g	22	61	2.5	7.4	2.3	2.4
Vegetable, Asda*	1 Kebab/40g	25	63	1.8	4.5	4.3	2.4
Vegetable, Sainsbury's*	1 Kebab/100g	36	36	1.5	6.4	0.5	1.2
Vegetable, Tesco*	1 Kebab/120g	47	39	1.7	6.8	0.6	1.1

KEDGEREE

	Measure INFO/WEIGHT	per Measure KCAL	KCAL	PROT	CARB	FAT	FIBRE
Average	1oz/28g	48	171	15.9	7.8	8.7	0.1
COU, Marks & Spencer*	1 Pack/370g	389	105	7.6	13.7	2.2	2.1
Perfectly Balanced, Waitrose*	1 Pack/400g	368	92	7.0	10.8	2.3	0.6
Seafood Masala, Perfectly Balanced, Waitrose*	1 Pack/400g	380	95	7.5	13.9	1.0	0.6
Smoked Haddock, Big Dish, Marks & Spencer*	1 Pack/450g	585	130	8.5	13.0	5.0	1.9

KETCHUP

	Measure INFO/WEIGHT	per Measure KCAL	KCAL	PROT	CARB	FAT	FIBRE
BBQ, Heinz*	1 Serving/10g	14	137	1.3	31.3	0.3	0.3
Barbeque, Asda*	1 Tbsp/15g	20	136	0.9	33.0	0.0	0.0
Chinese Sweet Chilli, Amoy*	1 Tbsp/15g	33	220	0.4	54.4	0.1	0.0
Tomato, Average	1 Tsp/5g	6	120	1.5	28.1	0.2	0.8
Tomato, Reduced Sugar, Average	1 Tbsp/10g	9	87	2.0	16.9	1.2	0.9
Wicked Orange, Heinz*	1 Serving/11g	12	108	1.0	24.7	0.1	0.6

KIDNEY

	Measure INFO/WEIGHT	per Measure KCAL	KCAL	PROT	CARB	FAT	FIBRE
Lamb, Raw, Average	1oz/28g	44	156	21.5	0.0	7.7	0.0
Ox, Raw	1oz/28g	25	88	17.2	0.0	2.1	0.0
Ox, Stewed	1oz/28g	39	138	24.5	0.0	4.4	0.0
Pig, Fried	1oz/28g	57	202	29.2	0.0	9.5	0.0
Pig, Raw	1oz/28g	24	86	15.5	0.0	2.7	0.0
Pig, Stewed	1oz/28g	43	153	24.4	0.0	6.1	0.0

KIEV

	Measure INFO/WEIGHT	per Measure KCAL	KCAL	PROT	CARB	FAT	FIBRE
Bacon & Cheese, Moy Park*	1 Kiev/142g	342	241	13.4	11.5	15.7	0.8
Cheese & Ham, Tesco*	1 Kiev/142.5g	313	219	13.6	12.4	12.8	1.2
Cheese & Herb, Mini, Bernard Matthews*	1 Kiev/23g	46	199	15.7	12.1	9.8	0.0
Cheese & Mushroom Chicken, Somerfield*	1/2 Pack/142g	294	207	14.0	15.0	11.0	0.0
Cheese, Smoked Ham & Chicken, Sainsbury's*	1 Kiev/136g	299	220	15.9	12.0	12.8	0.3
Chicken & Garlic Butter, Healthy Living, Tesco*	1 Kiev/142.5g	286	200	14.3	9.9	11.5	0.6
Chicken Breast, Garlic Butter, Sun Valley*	1 Kiev/141g	436	309	13.2	11.8	23.2	0.9
Chicken With Garlic Butter, Tesco*	1 Kiev/125g	424	339	8.5	11.0	29.0	1.6
Chicken, BFY, Morrisons*	1 Kiev/134g	304	227	16.1	11.5	13.0	1.0
Chicken, BGTY, Sainsbury's*	1 Kiev/125g	253	202	14.3	11.3	11.1	1.0
Chicken, Bernard Matthews*	1 Kiev/125g	374	299	10.6	13.9	22.3	2.7
Chicken, Breaded, Mini, Family, Bernard Matthews*	1 Kiev/23g	46	199	15.7	12.1	9.8	0.0
Chicken, Breast, Hand Filled, Birds Eye*	1 Kiev/172g	330	192	15.5	9.9	10.0	2.0
Chicken, COU, Marks & Spencer*	1 Kiev/150g	188	125	15.8	10.8	1.8	0.5
Chicken, Cheese & Ham, Tesco*	1 Kiev/142g	338	238	16.3	11.3	14.2	0.6
Chicken, Cheesy Bean, Asda*	1 Kiev/94.0g	202	215	12.0	17.0	11.0	1.9
Chicken, Creamy Garlic, Tesco*	1 Kiev/142g	295	208	12.0	9.3	13.6	1.6
Chicken, Creamy Pepper, Tesco*	1 Kiev/142g	270	190	12.0	10.0	11.0	2.0
Chicken, Creamy Peppercorn, Sun Valley*	1 Kiev/140g	382	273	13.3	13.5	18.5	0.0

K

	Measure INFO/WEIGHT	per Measure KCAL	Nutrition Values per 100g / 100ml				
			KCAL	PROT	CARB	FAT	FIBRE
KIEV							
Chicken, Creamy Peppercorn, Tesco*	1 Kiev/141g	310	220	9.9	11.3	15.0	1.7
Chicken, Finest, Tesco*	1 Kiev/237g	460	194	18.0	9.0	9.5	1.0
Chicken, Garlic & Herb, Reduced Fat, Sainsbury's*	1 Kiev/142g	317	223	15.1	12.1	12.7	0.6
Chicken, Garlic & Herb, Sainsbury's*	1 Kiev/133.5g	318	239	15.0	11.7	14.7	1.3
Chicken, Garlic & Mushroom, Sainsbury's*	1 Kiev/142.4g	345	243	16.2	14.5	13.4	1.4
Chicken, Garlic & Parsley, BGTY, Sainsbury's*	1 Kiev/133g	318	239	15.0	11.7	14.7	1.3
Chicken, Garlic & Parsley, Sainsbury's*	1 Kiev/136.4g	426	313	12.0	9.9	25.4	1.0
Chicken, Garlic Butter, Lower Fat, Asda*	1 Kiev/136g	282	207	13.0	14.0	11.0	0.7
Chicken, Garlic, Asda*	1 Kiev/142.9g	446	312	11.0	13.0	24.0	0.5
Chicken, Garlic, Marks & Spencer*	1 Kiev/150g	375	250	16.5	9.5	16.4	0.5
Chicken, Garlic, Safeway*	1 Kiev/147g	413	281	12.9	11.2	20.5	0.9
Chicken, Ham, & Cheese, Tesco*	1 Serving/143g	325	228	13.5	8.7	15.5	1.9
Chicken, In Crispy Breadcrumbs, Sainsbury's*	1 Kiev/116.5g	311	266	12.8	10.6	19.2	1.1
Chicken, Italian Style, Sainsbury's*	1 Kiev/134.8g	342	253	14.3	12.8	16.1	1.3
Chicken, Tomato & Mozzarella, Tesco*	1 Kiev/143g	339	237	11.4	7.9	17.7	1.4
Chicken, Value, Tesco*	1 Serving/125g	355	284	10.4	11.7	21.7	1.8
Chicken, White Wine & Mushroom, Tesco*	1 Serving/145g	281	194	16.7	10.3	9.5	0.5
Cod & Parsley, Safeway*	1 Kiev/160g	310	194	10.6	17.0	9.2	0.0
Garlic & Parsley, TTD, Sainsbury's*	1 Kiev/150g	371	247	15.7	11.1	15.6	0.8
Garlic Chicken, GFY, Asda*	1 Kiev/138.4g	328	238	14.0	14.0	14.0	0.8
Haddock, & Garlic Butter, Tesco*	1 Kiev/100g	309	309	14.7	17.5	20.0	1.1
Ham & Cheese Chicken, Somerfield*	1/2 Pack/142g	294	207	14.0	14.0	11.0	0.0
Mushroom & Cheese, Oven Baked, Safeway*	1 Kiev/100g	305	305	22.6	14.8	17.3	1.9
Salmon, Fillet, Tesco*	1 Kiev/160g	376	235	13.3	18.0	12.2	2.5
Tikka Chicken, Asda*	1 Kiev/150g	326	217	15.6	15.6	10.2	0.8
KIEV VEGETARIAN							
Cheesy Garlic, Meat Free, Sainsbury's*	1 Kiev/123g	263	214	17.3	10.6	11.4	3.0
Garlic Butter, Tesco*	1 Kiev/142g	462	325	14.4	22.1	19.9	0.8
Garlic Butter, Tivall*	1 Kiev/125g	366	293	15.1	10.8	21.0	2.6
Garlic, Safeway*	1 Kiev/142g	423	298	13.2	20.3	18.2	0.7
Vegetable, Marks & Spencer*	1 Kiev/155g	326	210	4.6	17.8	13.4	2.5
KIPPER							
Baked	1oz/28g	57	205	25.5	0.0	11.4	0.0
Fillets, In Brine, John West*	1 Can/140g	269	192	21.0	0.0	12.0	0.0
Fillets, In Sunflower Oil, John West*	1 Can/140g	321	229	19.0	0.0	17.0	0.0
Fillets, Raw, Average	1 Serving/200g	451	226	17.0	0.0	17.1	0.0
Fillets, With Butter, Farmfoods*	1oz/28g	64	229	17.5	0.0	17.7	0.0
Fillets, With Butter, Scottish, Marks & Spencer*	1 Pack/200g	382	191	16.7	0.0	13.8	0.0
Fillets, With Butter, Scottish, Somerfield*	1 Serving/100g	178	178	16.5	0.0	12.4	0.0
Grilled	1oz/28g	71	255	20.1	0.0	19.4	0.0
Raw	1oz/28g	64	229	17.5	0.0	17.7	0.0
Smoked, Average	1 Serving/150g	322	215	18.9	0.0	15.4	0.0
Smoked, With Butter, Tesco*	1 Serving/200g	446	223	17.0	0.0	17.2	0.0
KIT KAT							
2 Finger, Nestle*	2 Finger Bar/21g	106	507	5.9	62.0	26.1	0.0
4 Fingers, Nestle*	4 Fingers/48g	244	508	6.0	61.5	26.4	1.1
Caramac, 4 Finger, Nestle*	1 serving/48.7g	261	532	5.9	61.9	29.0	0.6
Chunky, Nestle*	1 Bar/55g	283	514	5.6	61.3	27.4	1.0
Chunky, Snack Size, Nestle*	1 Bar/26g	133	513	6.6	60.4	27.2	1.1
Editions, Mango & Passionfruit, Nestle*	1 Serving/45g	225	499	4.7	69.0	23.4	0.0
Editions, Red Berry, Chunky, Nestle*	1 Bar/45g	223	496	4.5	69.5	23.3	0.0
Editions, Seville Orange, Nestle*	1 Bar/45g	223	496	4.6	69.3	23.0	0.8
Kubes, Nestle*	1 Pack/50g	258	515	5.9	60.9	27.5	1.0

	Measure	per Measure	Nutrition Values per 100g / 100ml				
	INFO/WEIGHT	KCAL	KCAL	PROT	CARB	FAT	FIBRE
KIT KAT							
Kubes, Orange, Nestle*	4 Kubes/12.8g	67	514	5.7	61.1	27.4	1.0
Lemon & Yoghurt, Nestle*	1 Pack/45g	240	533	7.3	58.0	29.8	0.4
Low Carb, 2 Finger, Nestle*	1 Pack/21g	92	438	9.2	28.3	31.3	1.3
Low Carb, 4 Finger, Nestle*	1 Finger/11g	46	438	9.2	28.3	31.3	1.3
Mini, Nestle*	1 Bar/15g	75	502	7.5	59.4	26.0	0.0
Mint, Nestle*	4 Finger Bar/48g	244	508	6.0	61.5	26.4	1.1
Orange, 2 Finger, Nestle*	2 Finger Bar/20g	101	507	5.9	62.0	26.1	1.1
White, Nestle*	1 Chunky Bar/53g	276	521	8.3	60.3	27.5	0.7
KIWI FRUIT							
Fresh, Raw	1oz/28g	14	49	1.1	10.6	0.5	1.9
Weighed With Skin	1 Kiwi/60g	25	42	1.0	9.1	0.4	1.6
KOHLRABI							
Boiled in Salted Water	1oz/28g	5	18	1.2	3.1	0.2	1.9
Raw	1oz/28g	6	23	1.6	3.7	0.2	2.2
KORMA							
Chicken & Pilau Rice, BGTY, Sainsbury's*	1 Pack/450g	387	86	8.1	10.8	1.2	1.9
Chicken & Pilau Rice, GFY, Asda*	1 Pack/400g	600	150	8.0	16.0	6.0	1.3
Chicken & Pilau Rice, Good Intentions, Somerfield*	1 Serving/400g	472	118	7.7	15.3	2.9	0.8
Chicken & Pilau Rice, Morrisons*	1 Pack/450g	889	198	9.4	15.9	10.7	1.4
Chicken & Rice, 95% Fat Free, Birds Eye*	1 Pack/370g	444	120	6.2	19.6	1.9	1.1
Chicken & Rice, Easy Steam, BGTY, Sainsbury's*	1 Pack/400g	448	112	7.9	17.1	1.3	0.6
Chicken & Rice, Patak's*	1 Pack/370g	596	161	9.6	13.8	7.4	0.4
Chicken Coconut, Sainsbury's*	1 Pack/400g	664	166	13.0	5.3	10.3	1.6
Chicken Meal, Restaurant, BGTY, Sainsbury's*	1 Serving/201g	223	111	15.0	4.0	4.1	1.2
Chicken With Basmati Rice, Eat Smart, Safeway*	1 Pack/380g	399	105	7.0	13.8	1.9	1.5
Chicken With Pilau Rice, Perfectly Balanced, Waitrose*	1 Pack/400g	528	132	8.9	18.3	2.6	1.1
Chicken With Pilau Rice, Sharwood's*	1 Pack/375g	566	151	6.7	15.4	7.0	0.9
Chicken, & Basmati Rice, Tesco*	1 Pot/350g	588	168	4.3	16.9	9.3	2.3
Chicken, & Pilau Rice, Tesco*	1 Serving/460g	722	157	5.6	11.5	9.8	1.3
Chicken, & Rice, Healthy Eating, Tesco*	1 Pack/420g	487	116	7.2	17.9	1.8	0.3
Chicken, & Rice, Healthy Living, Tesco*	1 Pack/420g	433	103	8.0	14.4	1.5	1.9
Chicken, & Rice, Indian Meal For Two, Sainsbury's*	1 Pack/501g	787	157	6.8	14.3	8.1	3.1
Chicken, & Rice, Indian, Tesco*	1 Serving/550g	996	181	8.9	16.0	9.0	0.6
Chicken, & Rice, Organic, Tesco*	1 Pack/450g	923	205	6.0	21.5	10.6	0.4
Chicken, & Rice, Tesco*	1 Pack/450g	594	132	6.8	13.7	5.5	2.6
Chicken, & White Rice, BGTY, Frozen, Sainsbury's*	1 Pack/375g	341	91	5.6	14.9	1.0	0.5
Chicken, Breast Chunks, Sainsbury's*	1 Serving/227g	354	156	28.0	1.7	4.1	0.8
Chicken, Fresh, Chilled, Tesco*	1 Pack/350g	819	234	13.1	6.3	17.4	2.3
Chicken, Healthy Living, Tesco*	1 Pack/350g	371	106	7.7	15.9	1.2	0.8
Chicken, Indian Meal for 2, Finest, Tesco*	1/2 Pack/200g	348	174	10.3	6.2	12.0	2.5
Chicken, Indian Takeaway For One, Sainsbury's*	1 Serving/300g	498	166	13.0	5.3	10.3	1.6
Chicken, Indian, Take Away, Tesco*	1/2 Pack/175g	299	171	12.2	7.7	10.1	1.7
Chicken, Less Than 3% Fat, Birds Eye*	1 Pack/358g	440	123	6.5	20.4	1.9	0.8
Chicken, Sainsbury's*	1 Pack/400g	580	145	14.1	3.3	8.4	0.7
Chicken, Tesco*	1 Pack/350g	620	177	10.8	6.8	11.8	0.6
Chicken, Vegetable Curry & Rice, Tesco*	1 Pack/450g	495	110	7.1	15.2	2.4	1.4
Chicken, With Coriander & Rice, SlimFast*	1 Pack/375g	394	105	5.7	18.6	0.9	0.7
Chicken, With Peshwari Coriander Rice, Finest, Tesco*	1 Pack/550g	908	165	7.5	13.9	8.8	0.9
Chicken, With Pilau Rice, Asda*	1 Serving/350g	735	210	12.0	9.0	14.0	2.0
Creamy, With Pilau Rice, Safeway*	1 Pack/400g	560	140	5.2	15.8	5.7	2.3
Vegetable & Rice, Tesco*	1 Pack/450g	621	138	2.9	18.3	5.9	1.6
Vegetable, Ready To Cook, Fresh, Sainsbury's*	1/2 Pack/255g	263	103	2.8	7.7	6.8	2.1
Vegetable, Sainsbury's*	1 Serving/200g	302	151	2.7	6.6	12.6	2.2

K

	Measure	per Measure	Nutrition Values per 100g / 100ml				
	INFO/WEIGHT	KCAL	KCAL	PROT	CARB	FAT	FIBRE
KRISPROLLS							
Cracked Wheat, Original, Pagen*	1 Piece/10g	38	380	12.0	67.0	7.0	9.0
Golden Wheat, Pagen*	1 Serving/10g	41	410	11.0	72.0	8.5	4.0
Golden, Pagen*	1 Serving/25g	100	400	11.0	69.0	8.5	5.0
Organic, Bio, Pagen*	1 Serving/12g	46	380	12.0	67.0	7.0	8.0
Whole Grain, Swedish, Pagen*	1 Krisproll/11g	41	370	12.0	65.0	7.0	9.5
KULFI							
Average	1oz/28g	119	424	5.4	11.8	39.9	0.6
KUMQUATS							
Canned, In Syrup	1oz/28g	39	138	0.4	35.4	0.5	1.7
Raw	1oz/28g	12	43	0.9	9.3	0.5	3.8

	Measure INFO/WEIGHT	per Measure KCAL	Nutrition Values per 100g / 100ml				
			KCAL	PROT	CARB	FAT	FIBRE
LACES							
Apple Flavour, Tesco*	5 Laces/15g	52	347	3.6	74.8	3.2	2.1
Strawberry, Fizzy, Somerfield*	1 Pack/100g	380	380	3.0	86.0	2.0	0.0
Strawberry, Tesco*	1 Serving/75g	260	347	3.6	74.8	3.2	2.1
LAGER							
Alcohol Free, Becks*	1 Serving/275ml	55	20	0.7	5.0	0.0	0.0
Amstel, Heineken N V*	1 Pint/568ml	227	40	0.5	3.0	0.0	0.0
Average	1 Pint/568ml	165	29	0.3	0.0	0.0	0.0
Becks*	1 Can/275ml	113	41	0.0	3.0	0.0	0.0
C2, Carling*	1/2 Pint/284ml	80	28	0.0	3.5	0.0	0.0
Export, Carlsberg*	1 Can/440ml	189	43	0.4	4.0	0.0	0.4
Export, Foster's*	1 Pint/568ml	210	37	0.0	2.2	0.0	0.0
Foster's*	1 Pint/568ml	227	40	0.0	3.1	0.0	0.0
German, Low Alcohol, Sainsbury's*	1 Bottle/330ml	92	28	0.4	5.9	0.1	0.1
Grolsch*	1 Sm Can/330ml	145	44	0.0	2.2	0.0	0.0
Heineken*, 5%	1 Bottle/250ml	110	44	0.4	3.4	0.0	0.0
Heineken, Heineken N V*	1 Pint/568ml	256	45	0.5	3.0	0.0	0.0
Kaliber, Guinness*	1 Can/440ml	79	18	0.0	3.8	0.0	0.0
Low Alcohol	1 Can/440ml	44	10	0.2	1.5	0.0	0.0
Organic, Tesco*	1 Bottle/500ml	215	43	0.2	3.5	0.0	0.0
Pills, Holsten*	1 Can/440ml	167	38	0.3	2.4	0.0	0.0
Premium	1 Can/440ml	260	59	0.3	2.4	0.0	0.0
Premium, Co-Op*	1 Can/440ml	132	30	0.4	0.9	0.1	0.0
Premium, French, Biere Speciale, Tesco*	1 Serving/250ml	105	42	0.3	3.3	0.0	0.0
Premium, Tesco*	1 Can/440	229	52	0.4	4.0	0.0	0.0
Shandy, Traditional Style, Asda*	1 Serving/200ml	44	22	0.0	4.6	0.0	0.0
Ultra Low Carb, Michelob*	1 Bottle/275ml	88	32	0.2	0.9	0.0	0.0
Value, Tesco*	1 Can/440ml	75	17	0.2	1.2	0.0	0.0
LAMB							
Chops, Average	1oz/28g	65	231	20.6	0.4	16.4	0.0
Chops, Leg, With Mint Gravy, Tesco*	1 Serving/175g	214	122	15.0	3.2	5.6	1.7
Chops, Leg, With Redcurrant & Rosemary Sauce, Tesco*	1 Pack/325g	605	186	17.6	4.0	11.1	0.5
Chops, Minted, Average	1 Chop/100g	260	260	25.9	5.1	15.1	0.3
Chops, Shoulder, Mango & Mint, Waitrose*	1 Chop/250g	555	222	16.7	2.3	16.2	0.5
Diced, From Supermarket, Healthy Range, Average	1/2 Pack/200g	277	138	24.6	0.1	4.5	0.0
Escalope, Asda*	1 Serving/100g	173	173	32.0	0.0	5.0	0.0
Escalope, British, Healthy Living, Tesco*	1 Piece/95g	105	110	20.1	0.0	3.3	0.0
Fillet, Indian, Somerfield*	1 Pack/300g	570	190	17.0	4.0	12.0	0.0
Grill Steak, Average	1oz/28g	70	251	20.2	4.4	16.9	0.4
Grill Steak, Minted, Sainsbury's*	1 Serving/138g	313	227	24.6	4.0	12.5	1.0
Grill Steak, Prime, Average	1 Steak/63g	197	312	18.5	2.1	25.5	0.1
Grill Steak, Rosemary & Mint, Tesco*	1 Steak/62g	172	277	24.4	5.6	17.6	1.8
Joint, With A Sticky Plum & Orange Glaze, Waitrose*	1 Serving/100g	164	164	13.4	9.8	7.9	3.1
Joint, With Gravy, Tesco*	1 Serving/225g	277	123	14.9	2.8	5.8	0.0
Joint, With Mango & Mint Sauce, Boneless, Asda*	1 Serving/100g	302	302	26.0	0.0	22.0	1.4
Joint, With Mint Gravy, Tesco*	1 Serving/100g	88	88	16.6	1.8	1.7	0.1
Joint, With Rosemary, Tesco*	1 Serving/125g	250	200	17.5	0.8	14.1	0.5
Joint, With Sweet Mint Dressing, Tesco*	1 Serving/50g	97	193	19.9	1.8	11.8	0.6
Leg, Joint, Raw, Average	1 Joint/510g	859	168	20.9	1.4	8.9	0.2
Leg, Roasted, Lean & Fat, Average	1oz/28g	66	237	28.6	0.0	13.6	0.0
Leg, Roasted, Lean, Average	1oz/28g	58	206	29.9	0.0	9.6	0.0
Leg, Steaks, With Mint Glaze & Redcurrant Sauce, Asda*	1/2 Pack/145g	247	170	18.0	11.0	6.0	0.5
Mince, Average	1oz/28g	58	207	17.7	0.5	14.9	0.1
Mince, Extra Lean, Sainsbury's*	1 Serving/225g	324	144	24.1	0.0	5.3	0.1

L

	Measure INFO/WEIGHT	per Measure KCAL	Nutrition Values per 100g / 100ml				
			KCAL	PROT	CARB	FAT	FIBRE
LAMB							
Rack, Raw, Lean & Fat	1oz/28g	79	283	17.3	0.0	23.8	0.0
Rack, Roasted, Lean	1oz/28g	63	225	27.1	0.0	13.0	0.0
Rack, Roasted, Lean & Fat	1oz/28g	102	363	23.0	0.0	30.1	0.0
Rump, With A Mint & Balsamic Vinegar Crust, Waitrose*	1 Serving/151g	236	156	18.1	5.0	7.1	0.0
Shank, Tuscan, Somerfield*	1/2 Shank/200g	350	175	19.0	5.2	8.7	1.5
Shank, With Rosemary Gravy, Sainsbury's*	1 Serving/200g	204	102	13.2	3.1	4.1	0.3
Shoulder, Cooked, Lean & Fat	1oz/28g	84	301	24.4	0.0	22.5	0.0
Shoulder, Raw, Average	1oz/28g	70	249	16.8	0.0	20.2	0.0
Steak, Leg, Raw, Average	1 Steak/150g	169	113	20.1	0.0	3.7	0.0
Steak, Minted, Average	1 Steak/125g	212	170	22.7	3.4	7.2	0.9
Steak, Raw, Average	1 Steak/140g	190	136	21.7	0.2	5.4	0.0
Steaks, With Mint Butter, Leg, Waitrose*	1 Serving/155g	270	174	19.6	0.4	10.5	0.0
Stewing, Raw, Lean & Fat	1oz/28g	57	203	22.5	0.0	12.6	0.0
Stewing, Stewed, Lean	1oz/28g	67	240	26.6	0.0	14.8	0.0
Stewing, Stewed, Lean & Fat	1oz/28g	78	279	24.4	0.0	20.1	0.0
LAMB BRAISED							
& Mash, Tesco*	1 Serving/450g	413	92	6.1	10.7	2.7	0.8
LAMB DINNER							
Roast, Birds Eye*	1 Pack/340g	400	118	7.7	13.2	3.8	1.5
LAMB GREEK							
With Orzo Pasta, Marks & Spencer*	1 Serving/350g	438	125	10.2	9.7	5.0	2.7
LAMB IN							
A Pot, Sainsbury's*	1 Pack/450g	554	123	7.6	14.6	3.8	0.7
A Rich Balsamic Sauce, Shank, Safeway*	1/2 Pack/705g	1304	185	18.0	3.1	11.0	0.9
Gravy, Minted, Roast, Marks & Spencer*	1 Pack/200g	140	70	6.8	6.6	1.5	0.9
Gravy, Roast, Birds Eye*	1 Pack/239g	160	67	8.1	3.8	2.2	0.1
Mint Gravy, Sliced, Sainsbury's*	1 Pack/125g	134	107	15.3	2.9	3.8	0.8
Minted Gravy, Shank, Iceland*	1 Pack/400g	824	206	20.1	1.6	13.2	0.7
LAMB MEAL							
Roast, Ready Meals, Marks & Spencer*	1 Pack/340g	459	135	7.5	14.1	5.7	1.5
LAMB MEDITERRANEAN							
Shanks, Finest, Tesco*	1 Serving/404g	671	166	15.0	6.6	8.8	2.0
LAMB MOROCCAN							
With Cous Cous, Perfectly Balanced, Waitrose*	1 Pack/400g	390	98	7.7	13.6	1.3	2.2
LAMB WITH							
Carrot & Swede Mash, Braised, Eat Smart, Morrisons*	1 Pack/400g	304	76	5.2	8.2	2.3	1.5
Carrot & Swede Mash, Braised, Eat Smart, Safeway*	1 Pack/388g	330	85	7.6	7.4	2.4	1.4
Chunky Vegetables, Braised, Marks & Spencer*	1/2 Pack/425g	808	190	24.7	2.0	9.0	0.7
Cous Cous, Morrocan Style, Tesco*	1 Pack/550g	710	129	6.6	19.6	2.7	1.3
Roasted Vegetables, Shank, Marks & Spencer*	1/2 Pack/420g	660	157	14.9	8.3	7.3	0.7
Rosemary, Ready To Roast, Marks & Spencer*	1 Serving/188g	235	125	17.5	2.0	5.2	0.3
Tagine, Moroccan Style Withss, COU, Marks & Spencer*	1 Pack/400g	380	95	8.2	12.8	1.4	1.7
LARD							
Average	1oz/28g	249	891	0.0	0.0	99.0	0.0
LARDONS							
Smoked, Sainsbury's*	1 Serving/200g	476	238	21.4	0.1	15.4	0.1
LASAGNE							
Al Forno, Marks & Spencer*	1 Pack/330g	528	160	9.6	12.3	8.3	1.4
Asda*	1 Pack/378g	427	113	6.0	11.0	5.0	1.1
Asparagus, Marks & Spencer*	1 Pack/360g	414	115	4.7	12.1	5.2	1.2
BGTY, Sainsbury's*	1 Pack/400g	420	105	5.9	15.5	2.2	0.5
Balsamic Onion & Chicken, Marks & Spencer*	1 Pack/375g	563	150	9.5	12.5	6.7	1.5
Beef & Chunky Vegetable, Healthy Living, Tesco*	1 Pack/340g	354	104	5.9	13.8	2.8	1.2

L

LASAGNE

INFO/WEIGHT	Measure per Measure KCAL	KCAL	PROT	CARB	FAT	FIBRE
Beef, 3% Less Fat, Eat Smart, Safeway*	1 Pack/380g	342	90	5.9	11.1	2.3	1.3
Beef, Asda*	1 Pack/400g	372	93	4.2	11.0	3.6	0.6
Beef, BGTY, Sainsbury's*	1 Pack/400g	352	88	7.8	9.8	2.0	1.4
Beef, Birds Eye*	1 Pack/384g	515	134	7.0	12.5	6.2	0.7
Beef, Chilled, Safeway*	1/2 Pack/325g	452	139	7.5	11.8	5.9	1.2
Beef, Eat Smart, Safeway*	1 Pack/380g	380	100	7.6	10.9	2.7	1.3
Beef, Frozen, Eat Smart, Morrisons*	1 Serving/400g	388	97	7.9	13.6	2.2	0.9
Beef, Frozen, GFY, Asda*	1 Pack/400g	380	95	6.0	12.0	2.6	0.7
Beef, Frozen, Tesco*	1 Pack/400g	492	123	5.7	11.4	6.1	0.7
Beef, GFY, Asda*	1 Pack/350g	385	110	9.0	14.0	2.0	1.0
Beef, Healthy Eating, Tesco*	1 Pack/425g	472	111	5.9	12.4	4.2	1.3
Beef, Less Than 5% Fat, Asda*	1 Pack/400g	460	115	5.0	14.0	4.3	0.6
Beef, Morrisons*	1 Pack/400g	596	149	6.3	11.9	8.4	0.3
Beef, Ready Meals, Waitrose*	1 Pack/325g	471	145	6.7	13.1	7.3	1.4
Beef, Reduced Fat, Waitrose*	1 Pack/325g	345	106	5.5	12.1	4.0	0.8
Beef, TTD, Sainsbury's*	1 Serving/450g	648	144	8.7	10.3	7.5	0.6
Beef, Taste Of Italy, Somerfield*	1/2 Pack/300g	270	90	5.1	11.3	2.7	1.0
Beef, Weight Watchers*	1 Pack/300g	288	96	6.3	9.7	3.4	0.3
Birds Eye*	1 Pack/375g	420	112	6.1	11.6	4.6	0.7
Boiled	1oz/28g	28	100	3.0	22.0	0.6	0.9
Bolognese, Co-Op*	1 Pack/500g	758	152	8.1	13.8	7.1	0.0
COU, Marks & Spencer*	1 Pack/360g	360	100	6.5	11.6	2.7	1.6
Chicken, Italian, Healthy Living, Tesco*	1 Pack/400g	412	103	9.2	13.0	1.6	1.6
Chicken, Italian, Sainsbury's*	1 Pack/450g	549	122	8.4	12.6	4.2	0.5
Chicken, Italiano, Tesco*	1 Serving/450g	491	109	8.6	12.0	3.0	0.6
Chicken, Marks & Spencer*	1 Pack/400g	420	105	7.5	9.7	3.8	1.0
Chicken, Mushroom & Asparagus, Finest, Tesco*	1/2 Pack/300g	396	132	9.2	11.1	5.7	0.6
Chicken, Ready Meals, Waitrose*	1 Pack/300g	411	137	6.3	13.0	6.6	0.9
Chilled, Somerfield*	1 Pack/300g	312	104	6.8	12.2	3.1	1.3
Classic, Deep Filled, Marks & Spencer*	1 Pack/400g	760	190	10.0	11.2	11.9	0.6
Extra Special, Asda*	1/2 Pack/290.9g	416	143	7.0	13.0	7.0	0.3
Family, Marks & Spencer*	1/4 Pack/225g	281	125	10.3	6.9	6.2	1.1
Finest, Tesco*	1/2 Pack/300g	444	148	7.4	11.7	8.0	0.8
Fresh, Findus*	1 Pack/350g	403	115	6.2	11.7	4.5	0.0
Frozen, BGTY, Sainsbury's*	1 Serving/400g	319	80	5.0	10.6	2.0	0.6
Frozen, Safeway*	1 Serving/400g	455	114	6.0	11.8	4.6	0.2
GFY, Asda*	1 Pack/410g	344	84	5.5	11.0	2.0	0.3
Healthy Living, Tesco*	1 Pack/425g	434	102	6.4	13.6	2.5	1.3
Italia, Marks & Spencer*	1 Pack/400g	640	160	8.2	10.7	9.5	0.8
Italian, Healthy Living, Tesco*	1 Serving/430g	409	95	5.0	12.6	2.7	0.5
Italian, Sainsbury's*	1 Pack/450g	639	142	8.7	14.2	5.6	0.6
Italiano, Large, Healthy Living, Tesco*	1/2 Pack/400g	388	97	6.0	12.9	2.4	0.8
Italiano, Tesco*	1 Pack/800g	1144	143	8.4	17.1	4.6	0.5
Layered, Asda*	1 Pack/300g	444	148	5.0	14.0	8.0	0.3
Less Than 3% Fat, Frozen, BGTY, Sainsbury's*	1 Pack/400g	352	88	7.8	9.8	2.0	1.4
Less Than 5% Fat, BFY, Morrisons*	1/2 Pack/350g	227	65	5.9	8.2	2.5	0.7
Marks & Spencer*	1/3 Pack/333g	466	140	8.5	10.4	7.4	0.9
Meat, Somerfield*	1 Pack/600g	768	128	6.0	12.0	6.0	0.0
Mediterranean Vegetable, COU, Marks & Spencer*	1 Pack/360g	306	85	3.4	11.5	2.7	1.4
Mega, Value, Tesco*	1 Pack/600g	726	121	4.7	12.2	5.9	0.5
Pepperoni, Chicago Town*	1 Serving/500g	865	173	4.0	17.4	8.8	0.0
Pizza Express*	1 Serving/350g	514	147	6.2	14.9	6.9	1.4
Ready Meal, Marks & Spencer*	1 Pack/360g	594	165	11.3	11.7	8.2	1.3

L

LASAGNE

	Measure INFO/WEIGHT	per Measure KCAL	Nutrition Values per 100g / 100ml				
			KCAL	PROT	CARB	FAT	FIBRE
Roasted Mushrooms, Safeway*	1 Serving/400g	440	110	3.9	11.2	5.0	1.4
Sainsbury's*	1 Pack/300g	426	142	8.7	14.2	5.6	0.6
Salmon & Spinach, Tesco*	1 Pack/400g	292	73	4.9	10.0	1.5	0.8
Sheets, Dry, Average	1oz/28g	98	349	11.9	72.1	1.5	2.9
Sheets, Fresh, Dry, Average	1 Sheet/21g	56	271	10.9	52.7	2.1	1.9
Sheets, Verdi, Dry, Average	1 Serving/50g	178	356	12.7	71.1	2.3	2.8
Smoked Salmon & Asparagus, Sainsbury's*	1 Pack/350g	665	190	7.9	15.6	10.7	0.7
Spinach & Cheese, Italian, Sainsbury's*	1 Pack/450g	666	148	6.0	15.5	6.8	0.5
Spinach & Ricotta, Asda*	1 Pack/400g	488	122	4.9	12.0	6.0	1.5
Spinach & Ricotta, Finest, Tesco*	1 Pack/350g	585	167	6.1	11.7	10.6	1.2
Triangles With Chicken, COU, Marks & Spencer*	1 Pack/360g	324	90	7.8	11.9	1.8	1.0
Value, Tesco*	1 Pack/500g	680	136	5.3	14.4	6.4	0.5
Vegetable	1oz/28g	29	102	4.1	12.4	4.4	1.0
Vegetable, BGTY, Sainsbury's*	1 Pack/400g	286	72	4.8	9.5	1.6	1.4
Vegetable, Findus*	1 Pack/330g	314	95	4.0	13.0	2.5	0.0
Vegetable, Italian Roasted, Asda*	1 Serving/200g	234	117	2.6	11.0	7.0	0.7
Vegetable, Italian Three Layer, Sainsbury's*	1 Pack/450g	554	123	4.8	14.3	5.2	0.5
Vegetable, Italian, Somerfield*	1 Serving/400g	372	93	3.3	10.0	4.4	1.3
Vegetable, Italiano, Tesco*	1 Pack/410g	328	80	2.9	10.1	3.1	1.0
Vegetable, Luxury Roasted, Safeway*	1 Pack/400g	492	123	3.4	15.8	5.1	1.1
Vegetable, Mediterranean Style, Eat Smart, Safeway*	1 Pack/380g	228	60	3.0	10.1	0.8	1.5
Vegetable, Mediterranean, Linda McCartney*	1 Pack/320g	320	100	5.1	14.6	2.3	2.4
Vegetable, Mediterranean, Waitrose*	1 Pack/351g	397	113	3.7	12.7	5.3	1.0
Vegetable, Two Layered, BGTY, Sainsbury's*	1 Pack/400g	288	72	4.8	9.5	1.6	1.4
Vegetable, Value, Tesco*	1 Pack/500g	410	82	4.1	9.7	3.0	2.3
Vegetable, Weight Watchers*	1 Pack/330g	251	76	3.6	11.8	1.7	0.7

LASAGNE VEGETARIAN

Italiano, Tesco*	1 Serving/410g	385	94	3.1	13.9	2.9	0.8
Linda McCartney*	1 Pack/320g	374	117	7.0	14.2	3.5	1.9
Tesco*	1 Pack/430g	581	135	5.3	13.6	6.6	1.0

LAVERBREAD

Average	1oz/28g	15	52	3.2	1.6	3.7	0.0

LEEKS

Boiled, Average	1oz/28g	6	21	1.2	2.6	0.7	1.7
Creamed, Frozen, Waitrose*	1 Serving/225g	115	51	1.8	5.5	2.4	0.0
Raw, Average	1oz/28g	7	25	1.7	3.7	0.4	2.4
With Sage Butter, Steamer, TTD, Sainsbury's*	1/2 Pack/140g	104	74	1.2	5.9	5.0	2.8

LEMON

Fresh, Raw	1 Slice/5g	0	7	0.3	1.6	0.0	1.7

LEMON CURD

Average	1 Tbsp/15g	44	294	0.7	62.9	4.7	0.1
Luxury, Average	1 Tsp/7g	23	326	2.8	59.7	8.4	0.1

LEMON SOLE

Fillets, Raw, Average	1 Serving/220g	180	82	17.3	0.2	1.3	0.3
Goujons, Average	1 Serving/150g	359	239	13.9	18.5	12.2	1.0
Goujons, With Citrus Mayonnaise, Tesco*	1 Serving/250g	610	244	11.7	19.6	13.2	0.8
In Breadcrumbs, Average	1 Fillet/142g	322	228	13.7	15.7	12.3	1.0
In White Wine, & Herb Butter, Fillets, Marks & Spencer*	1 Pack/220g	385	175	15.1	0.1	12.6	0.0

LEMONADE

7-Up, Light, Britvic*	1 Can/330ml	4	1	0.1	0.2	0.0	0.0
Asda*	1 Glass/250ml	83	33	0.0	8.0	0.0	0.0
Average	1 Glass/250ml	53	21	0.1	5.0	0.1	0.1
Cloudy, Diet, Sainsbury's*	1 Can/330ml	7	2	0.1	0.2	0.1	0.3

L

	Measure INFO/WEIGHT	per Measure KCAL	Nutrition Values per 100g / 100ml				
			KCAL	PROT	CARB	FAT	FIBRE
LEMONADE							
Cloudy, Diet, Tesco*	1 Serving/200ml	6	3	0.0	0.8	0.0	0.0
Cloudy, Sainsbury's*	1 Glass/250ml	118	47	0.1	12.0	0.1	0.1
Cloudy, Waitrose*	1 Glass/250g	125	50	0.0	12.2	0.0	0.0
Diet, Traditional Style, Tesco*	1 Glass/200ml	6	3	0.0	0.8	0.0	0.0
Fresh Squeezed, Marks & Spencer*	1 Bottle/250ml	113	45	0.1	11.8	0.0	0.0
Lime, Safeway*	1 Can/144ml	63	44	0.0	10.6	0.0	0.0
Low Calorie, SmartPrice, Asda*	1 Glass/250ml	1	0	0.0	0.1	0.0	0.0
Organic, Tesco*	1 Can/142ml	61	43	0.0	10.6	0.0	0.0
R White's*	1 Glass/250ml	65	26	0.1	6.2	0.0	0.0
Sainsbury's*	1 Serving/250ml	53	21	0.1	4.9	0.1	0.1
Somerfield*	1/2 Pint/284ml	77	27	0.0	7.0	0.0	0.0
Sparkling, With Spanish Lemon Juice, Waitrose*	1 Serving/250ml	85	34	0.0	8.3	0.0	0.0
Sprite*	1 Bottle/500ml	215	43	0.0	10.5	0.0	0.0
Still, Marks & Spencer*	1 Glass/250ml	5	49	0.1	12.9	0.0	0.0
SunJuice*	1 Serving/250ml	113	45	0.1	12.7	0.0	0.0
Tesco*	1 Glass/200ml	30	15	0.0	3.6	0.0	0.0
Traditional Style, Tesco*	1 Glass/200ml	100	50	0.0	12.3	0.0	0.0
LEMONCELLO							
Asda*	1 Serving/100g	217	217	4.7	27.0	10.0	0.2
LEMONGRASS							
Stalks, Tesco*	1 Stalk/13g	12	99	1.8	25.3	0.5	0.0
LENTILS							
Green & Brown, Whole, Dried, Boiled in Salted Water	1oz/28g	29	105	8.8	16.9	0.7	3.8
Green Or Brown, Dried, Average	1 Serving/50g	151	301	22.8	49.8	1.5	9.6
Green Or Brown, In Water, Tinned, Average	1/2 Can/132g	131	99	8.1	15.4	0.6	3.8
Red, Boiled In Unsalted Water, Average	1oz/28g	28	102	7.6	17.5	0.4	2.6
Red, Dried, Average	1oz/28g	88	315	23.8	53.8	1.3	4.9
LETTUCE							
Chinese Leaf, Tesco*	1 Serving/200g	36	18	3.5	0.3	0.3	2.6
Crest, Sainsbury's*	1/3 Lettuce/33g	5	14	0.8	1.7	0.5	0.0
Curly Leaf, Sainsbury's*	1 Serving/20g	3	14	0.8	1.7	0.5	0.0
Iceberg, Average	1oz/28g	4	13	0.8	1.8	0.3	0.5
Lamb's, Average	1 Serving/25g	4	15	1.4	1.6	0.3	1.0
Leafy, Tesco*	1 Serving/20g	3	14	1.2	1.5	0.4	1.9
Romaine, Average	1 Serving/20g	3	15	0.9	1.7	0.5	0.7
LILT*							
Z	1 Can/330ml	10	3	0.0	0.4	0.0	0.0
LINGUINI							
Asparagas & Ricotta, Sainsbury's*	1 Serving/400g	524	131	3.8	15.8	5.8	2.5
Dry, Average	1 Serving/100g	352	352	13.1	70.0	2.2	2.8
Fresh, Dry, Average	1 Pack/250g	681	273	12.3	51.7	2.6	4.0
King Prawn, Meal for One, Marks & Spencer*	1 Pack/400g	380	95	6.6	13.1	1.7	2.2
Pomodoro, Marks & Spencer*	1 Pack/300g	360	120	4.1	17.6	3.5	1.2
Smoked Salmon, Sainsbury's*	1 Serving/400g	586	147	6.2	14.2	7.2	1.2
Sun Dried Tomato & Chicken, Waitrose*	1 Serving/400g	316	79	7.5	8.0	1.9	3.5
Sun Dried Tomato & Egg, Asda*	1 Serving/200g	324	162	7.0	28.0	2.4	3.9
Tomato & Mushroom, Perfectly Balanced, Waitrose*	1 Pack/350g	294	84	2.2	10.6	3.8	1.0
Vegetable & Ham, BGTY, Sainsbury's*	1 Pack/450g	410	91	4.4	11.7	3.0	0.9
With Prawns & Scallops, BGTY, Sainsbury's*	1 Pack/400g	320	80	6.2	12.7	0.5	0.8
LINSEED							
Seeds, Average	1 Serving/5g	23	464	21.7	18.5	33.5	26.3
LION BAR							
Mini, Nestle*	1 Bar/16g	80	486	4.6	67.7	21.7	0.0

L

	Measure INFO/WEIGHT	per Measure KCAL	Nutrition Values per 100g / 100ml				
			KCAL	PROT	CARB	FAT	FIBRE
LION BAR							
Nestle*	1 Bar/54.9g	279	508	4.9	62.9	26.0	0.0
Peanut, Nestle*	1 Bar/49g	256	522	7.1	56.9	29.6	0.0
LIPOVITAN							
Taisha*	1fl oz/30ml	12	41	0.1	9.6	0.1	0.0
LIQUEURS							
Amaretto, Average	1 Serving/50ml	194	388	0.0	60.0	0.0	0.0
Cream	1 Shot/25ml	81	325	0.0	22.8	16.1	0.0
Grand Marnier*	100ml	268	268	0.0	22.9	0.0	0.0
High Strength	1 Shot/25ml	79	314	0.0	24.4	0.0	0.0
LIQUORICE							
Allsorts, Average	1 Sm Bag/56g	195	349	3.7	76.7	5.2	2.0
Allsorts, Bassett's*	1 Pack/225g	792	352	2.3	75.5	4.5	1.6
Catherine Wheels, Barratt*	1 Serving/19g	54	287	3.8	67.2	0.3	0.0
Comfits, Marks & Spencer*	1oz/28g	100	357	2.4	86.2	0.3	0.7
Organic, Laidback Liquorice*	1 Bar/28g	90	320	4.7	75.0	1.0	3.0
Panda*	1 Bar/32g	109	340	3.8	78.0	0.5	0.0
Red, Fresh, 98% Fat Free, RJ's*	1oz/28g	96	342	3.0	75.0	1.7	0.0
Shapes, Average	1oz/28g	78	278	5.5	65.0	1.4	1.9
Soft Eating, Australia, Darrell Lea*	1 Piece/20g	68	338	2.8	76.1	1.9	0.0
Sweets, Blackcurrant, Tesco*	1 Sweet/8g	32	410	0.0	92.3	3.8	0.0
Twists, Tesco*	1 Serving/63g	186	297	2.7	71.0	0.3	0.7
LIVER							
Calves, Fried	1oz/28g	49	176	22.3	0.0	9.6	0.0
Calves, Raw	1oz/28g	29	104	18.3	0.0	3.4	0.0
Calves, With Fresh Sage Butter, Marks & Spencer*	1 Serving/116.7g	211	180	12.8	10.1	10.7	1.5
Calves, With Garlic Butter, Marks & Spencer*	1oz/28g	56	200	13.3	7.3	13.5	0.4
Chicken, Fried	1oz/28g	47	169	22.1	0.0	8.9	0.0
Chicken, Raw	1oz/28g	26	92	17.7	0.0	2.3	0.0
Lamb's With Onions, Marks & Spencer*	1oz/28g	52	185	14.1	6.8	11.3	0.1
Lamb's, Fried, Average	1oz/28g	66	237	30.1	0.1	12.9	0.1
Lamb's, Raw, Average	1 Serving/125g	171	137	20.3	0.0	6.2	0.0
Ox, Raw	1oz/28g	43	155	21.1	0.0	7.8	0.0
Ox, Stewed	1oz/28g	55	198	24.8	3.6	9.5	0.0
Pig's, Raw	1oz/28g	32	113	21.3	0.0	3.1	0.0
Pig's, Stewed	1 Serving/70g	132	189	25.6	3.6	8.1	0.0
LIVER & BACON							
British Classics, Tesco*	1 Pack/400g	524	131	11.3	5.5	7.1	0.9
Sainsbury's*	1 Serving/250g	303	121	10.9	8.3	4.9	0.4
With Creamy Mash, GFY, Asda*	1 Pack/385.9g	324	84	6.0	10.0	2.2	1.5
With Fresh Mashed Potato, Waitrose*	1 Pack/400g	512	128	6.9	10.2	6.6	0.8
With Mash, Tesco*	1 Serving/450g	432	96	6.9	8.6	3.8	2.8
LIVER & ONIONS							
British Classics, Tesco*	1 Pack/250g	265	106	9.7	5.9	4.8	0.5
Marks & Spencer*	1 Serving/200g	250	125	7.6	10.5	6.0	0.9
LIVER SAUSAGE							
Average	1 Slice/10g	22	216	15.3	4.5	15.2	0.2
LOBSTER							
Boiled	1oz/28g	29	103	22.1	0.0	1.6	0.0
Breaded Squat With Lemon Mayonnaise Dip, Tesco*	1 Pack/210g	506	241	9.0	19.0	14.4	0.5
Breaded, Mini, Sainsbury's*	1 Serving/100g	204	204	8.7	18.8	10.1	1.4
Dressed, John West*	1 Can/43g	45	105	13.0	2.0	5.0	0.0
Dressed, Marks & Spencer*	1oz/28g	76	273	14.3	0.8	23.6	0.1
Half, Marks & Spencer*	1oz/28g	66	235	12.1	2.4	19.6	0.2

L

	Measure INFO/WEIGHT	per Measure KCAL	Nutrition Values per 100g / 100ml				
			KCAL	PROT	CARB	FAT	FIBRE
LOBSTER							
Squat, Young's*	1/2 Pack/125g	246	197	9.8	20.1	8.6	1.1
Tails, Young's*	1 Serving/100g	197	197	9.8	20.1	8.6	1.1
Thermidor, Marks & Spencer*	1 Serving/140g	287	205	10.7	9.7	13.7	0.0
LOGANBERRIES							
Raw	1oz/28g	5	17	1.1	3.4	0.0	2.5
LOLLIPOPS							
Assorted Flavours, Asda*	1 Lolly/7g	27	380	0.0	95.0	0.0	0.0
Chupa Chups*	1 Lolly/18g	44	247	0.0	96.5	1.3	0.0
Cremosa, Sugar Free, Chupa Chups*	1 Lolly/10g	28	275	0.2	92.5	5.4	0.0
Cuore Di Frutta, Chupa Chups*	1 Lolly/10g	25	247	0.0	96.5	1.3	0.0
Marks & Spencer*	1oz/28g	107	383	0.0	95.4	0.0	0.0
LOLLY							
Cookies N Cream, Skinny Cow, Richmond Foods*	1 Lolly/66.9g	89	133	4.7	25.2	1.5	3.6
Fruit, Mini, Tesco*	1 Lolly/31.5g	41	127	1.9	25.7	1.9	0.6
Milk, Blue Parrot Cafe, Sainsbury's*	1 Lolly/30ml	34	113	2.7	18.0	3.3	0.3
Orange N Cream, Tropicana*	1 Lolly/64.5g	84	129	1.4	20.5	4.5	0.3
Sugar Free, Simpkins*	1 Lolly/15g	51	340	0.0	88.0	0.0	0.0
Super Sour, Tesco*	1 Lolly/8.3g	31	385	0.1	95.6	0.2	0.5
LONGANS							
Canned, In Syrup, Drained	1oz/28g	19	67	0.4	17.1	0.3	0.0
LOQUATS							
Raw	1oz/28g	8	28	0.7	6.3	0.2	0.0
LOZENGES							
Original, Victory V*	1 Lozenge/3g	9	350	0.0	91.0	0.0	0.0
LUCOZADE							
Citrus Clear, Energy, SmithKline Beecham*	1 Bottle/380ml	266	70	0.1	17.0	0.0	0.0
Orange Energy Drink, SmithKline Beecham*	1 Bottle/500ml	350	70	0.0	17.2	0.0	0.0
Original, SmithKline Beecham*	1 Bottle/345ml	252	73	0.0	17.9	0.0	0.0
Tropical, SmithKline Beecham*	1 Bottle/380ml	266	70	0.0	17.2	0.0	0.0
LUNCHEON MEAT							
Pork, Average	1oz/28g	81	288	13.3	4.0	24.3	0.0
LYCHEES							
Fresh, Raw	1oz/28g	16	58	0.9	14.3	0.1	0.7
In Juice, Amoy*	1oz/28g	13	46	0.4	10.9	0.0	0.0
In Syrup, Average	1oz/28g	19	69	0.4	17.7	0.0	0.4
Raw, Weighed With Skin & Stone	1oz/28g	10	36	0.5	8.9	0.1	0.4

L

INFO/WEIGHT	Measure per Measure KCAL	Nutrition Values per 100g / 100ml KCAL	PROT	CARB	FAT	FIBRE

M&M'S

	Measure INFO/WEIGHT	per Measure KCAL	KCAL	PROT	CARB	FAT	FIBRE
Mars*	1 Funsize/20g	97	487	4.7	69.6	21.1	0.0
Mini, Mars*	1 Sm Pack/36g	176	489	6.3	63.6	23.2	0.0
Peanut, Mars*	1 Pack/45g	231	514	10.2	57.3	27.1	0.0
Plain, Mars*	1 Pack/48g	240	499	4.1	70.7	20.8	2.1
MACADAMIA NUTS							
Salted	6 Nuts/10g	75	748	7.9	4.8	77.6	5.3
Whole, Unsalted, Sainsbury's*	1 Nut/3g	22	738	9.3	4.7	76.0	5.2
MACARONI							
Dry, Average	1oz/28g	99	354	11.9	73.5	1.7	2.6
MACARONI CHEESE							
Average	1oz/28g	50	178	7.3	13.6	10.8	0.5
BGTY, Sainsbury's*	1 Pack/450g	537	119	5.3	19.4	2.3	1.2
Bettabuy, Morrisons*	1 Serving/205g	229	112	4.3	10.8	5.7	0.4
Birds Eye*	1 Pack/302g	374	124	4.2	15.6	5.0	0.4
Canned	1oz/28g	39	138	4.5	16.4	6.5	0.4
Chilled, GFY, Asda*	1 Pack/442.5g	469	106	6.0	14.0	2.9	1.6
Eat Smart, Safeway*	1 Pack/315g	394	125	6.5	19.2	2.1	0.8
Findus*	1 Pack/360g	576	160	6.3	14.3	8.5	0.0
Finest, Tesco*	1 Serving/500g	1055	211	8.3	20.6	10.6	0.7
Healthy Living, Tesco*	1 Pack/340g	391	115	6.2	18.6	1.8	1.0
Heinz*	1 Can/400g	380	95	3.4	9.8	4.7	0.3
Italian, Tesco*	1 Pack/340g	541	159	6.5	14.2	8.5	2.7
Kraft*	1 Serving/50g	205	410	11.0	47.0	17.5	1.0
Marks & Spencer*	1 Pack/400g	680	170	6.9	12.8	9.9	0.6
New, BGTY, Sainsbury's*	1 Pack/400g	432	108	5.5	17.2	1.9	1.1
Perfectly Balanced, Waitrose*	1 Pack/350g	351	100	6.7	11.4	3.1	0.5
Red Leicester, Heinz*	1 Can/400g	332	83	3.5	11.1	2.7	0.3
Tesco*	1 Can/410g	513	125	4.5	10.1	6.3	0.3
Tinned, Sainsbury's*	1 Can/400g	428	107	5.1	12.2	4.2	0.5
Value, Tesco*	1 Pack/300g	507	169	5.7	18.3	8.1	0.5
Waitrose*	1 Pack/350g	466	133	6.8	5.2	9.4	0.0
MACKEREL							
Fillets, Honey Roast Smoked, Sainsbury's*	1 Serving/100g	349	349	21.5	4.5	27.3	12.4
Fillets, In A Hot Chilli Sauce, Princes*	1 Serving/100g	296	296	13.3	0.0	27.0	0.0
Fillets, In Brine, Average	1 Can/88g	206	234	19.4	0.0	17.4	0.0
Fillets, In Curry Sauce, John West*	1oz/28g	65	233	16.0	4.0	17.0	0.3
Fillets, In Green Peppercorn Sauce, John West*	1 Can/125g	329	263	14.0	4.5	21.0	0.1
Fillets, In Mustard Sauce, Average	1 Can/125g	274	219	14.1	5.4	15.5	0.1
Fillets, In Olive Oil, Average	1 Serving/50g	149	298	18.5	1.0	24.4	0.1
Fillets, In Spicy Tomato Sauce, Average	1oz/28g	56	199	14.3	3.9	14.1	0.0
Fillets, In Sunflower Oil, Average	1 Can/94g	262	279	20.2	0.2	21.9	0.0
Fillets, In Tomato Sauce, Average	1 Can/125g	251	200	14.3	2.7	14.7	0.0
Fillets, In White Wine & Spices, Connetable*	1 Can/120g	169	141	15.5	1.2	8.2	0.0
Fillets, Red Pepper & Onion, Smoked, Asda*	1 Serving/90g	319	354	18.0	0.8	31.0	1.2
Fillets, Smoked, Average	1oz/28g	94	335	19.8	0.5	28.2	0.3
Fried in Blended Oil	1oz/28g	76	272	24.0	0.0	19.5	0.0
Raw, Average	1oz/28g	67	238	19.9	0.0	17.6	0.0
Smoked, Lemon & Parsley, Morrisons*	1/2 Pack/100g	282	282	20.9	4.6	20.0	1.0
Smoked, Peppered, Average	1oz/28g	87	310	20.4	0.3	25.2	0.2
MADRAS							
Beef, Tesco*	1 Pack/460g	616	134	10.6	4.5	8.2	1.2
Chicken & Pilau Rice, Asda*	1 Pack/400g	588	147	8.0	13.0	7.0	1.7
Chicken, & Rice, Indian Meal For Two, Sainsbury's*	1 Pack/501g	702	140	7.4	14.2	6.0	2.7

	Measure INFO/WEIGHT	per Measure KCAL	Nutrition Values per 100g / 100ml				
			KCAL	PROT	CARB	FAT	FIBRE
MADRAS							
Chicken, & Rice, Sainsbury's*	1 Pack/461.3g	572	124	5.9	19.6	2.4	0.7
Chicken, Asda*	1 Serving/350g	431	123	7.0	3.6	9.0	2.3
Chicken, Improved Recipe, Sainsbury's*	1 Pack/400g	468	117	11.7	2.2	6.8	2.8
Chicken, Indian, Sainsbury's*	1 Pack/400g	636	159	13.3	1.8	10.9	2.6
Chicken, Indian, Tesco*	1 Pack/350g	518	148	11.3	5.6	8.9	1.9
Chicken, Tesco*	1 Pack/350g	326	93	10.6	3.6	4.1	0.6
Chicken, Vite Fait*	1 Pack/300g	372	124	14.0	3.5	6.0	0.0
MAGNUM							
Almond, Wall's*	1 Bar/86g	298	346	5.3	28.4	23.2	0.0
Caramel & Nuts Bar, Wall's*	1 Bar/60g	132	220	4.0	19.0	15.0	0.0
Classico, Wall's	1 Lolly	275	250	3.4	25.0	15.0	0.0
Gluttony, Wall's*	1 Lolly/110ml	425	386	4.5	32.7	26.4	0.0
Greed, Wall's*	1 Bar/110ml	307	279	3.6	29.1	16.4	0.0
White, Wall's*	1 Serving/86.5g	255	296	3.8	32.0	17.0	0.0
MAKHANI							
Chicken Tikka & Pilau Rice, BGTY, Sainsbury's*	1 Pack/400g	448	112	8.3	17.5	1.0	1.9
Chicken Tikka, BGTY, Sainsbury's*	1 Pack/251.4g	186	74	11.3	3.0	1.9	1.7
Chicken Tikka, Waitrose*	1 Pack/400g	644	161	13.2	4.2	10.1	1.8
Chicken, Sainsbury's*	1/2 Pack/199.4g	312	157	12.2	2.9	10.7	2.5
King Prawn & Rice, Sainsbury's*	1 Pack/499g	738	148	5.1	15.6	7.2	0.9
Paneer, Ashoka*	1/2 Pouch/150g	283	189	4.7	8.0	15.3	1.0
MALABAR							
Chicken With Pilau Rice, Waitrose*	1 Pack/450g	540	120	7.6	16.1	2.8	1.5
MALTESERS							
Fun Size, Nestle*	1 Serving/20g	97	484	7.8	61.5	22.9	0.0
Mars*	1 Sm Pack/37g	183	494	10.0	61.4	23.1	0.0
White Chocolate, Mars*	1 Pack/37g	186	504	7.9	61.0	25.4	0.0
MANDARIN ORANGES							
Average	1 Sm/50g	18	37	0.9	8.4	0.1	1.3
In Juice, Average	1oz/28g	11	39	0.7	9.0	0.0	0.5
In Light Syrup, Average	1 Can/298g	201	68	0.6	16.0	0.1	0.1
MANGE TOUT							
& Sugar Snap Peas, Tesco*	1 Pack/150g	102	68	7.0	9.2	0.4	3.8
Boiled in Salted Water	1oz/28g	7	26	3.2	3.3	0.1	2.2
Raw, Average	1oz/28g	9	33	3.6	4.2	0.2	1.2
Stir-Fried in Blended Oil	1oz/28g	20	71	3.8	3.5	4.8	2.4
MANGO							
Dried	1 Serving/50g	174	347	1.4	83.1	1.0	4.9
Dried, Unsweetened, Sainsbury's*	1 Bag/75g	246	328	1.9	84.7	1.2	7.2
In Syrup, Average	1oz/28g	22	80	0.3	20.5	0.0	0.9
Pineapple & Passionfruit, Marks & Spencer*	1 Pack/400g	200	50	0.6	10.9	0.2	1.7
Raw, Average	1 Mango/207g	114	55	0.7	13.2	0.2	2.5
MARBLE							
Cadbury*	1 Bar/46g	246	535	8.4	54.8	31.2	0.0
MARGARINE							
Average	1 Thin Spread/7g	51	727	0.1	0.5	81.0	0.0
Butter Style, Average	1 Thin Spread/7g	44	627	0.7	1.1	68.9	0.0
For Baking, Average	1 Thin Spread/7g	42	607	0.2	0.4	67.2	0.0
Olive, Light, GFY, Asda*	1 Thin Spread/4g	14	344	0.1	0.5	38.0	0.0
Olivio*	1 Serving/10g	56	563	0.2	1.0	59.0	0.0
Reduced Fat, Average	1 Thin Spread/7g	25	356	0.6	3.0	38.0	0.0
Soya, Granose*	1oz/28g	209	745	0.1	0.1	82.0	0.0

M

MARINADE

	Measure INFO/WEIGHT	per Measure KCAL	KCAL	PROT	CARB	FAT	FIBRE
Barbecue, COU, Marks & Spencer*	1 Serving/35g	53	150	1.2	35.5	0.2	1.0
Barbecue, In Minutes, Knorr*	1 Pack/110g	337	306	6.2	66.4	1.3	3.4
Cajun Spice, EPC*	1 Serving/50g	94	187	1.3	15.3	13.4	1.6
Chinese, Classic, Sharwood's*	1oz/28g	32	113	1.8	16.1	4.8	1.0
Hickory Dickory Smokey, Ainsley Harriott*	1 Pot/300ml	360	120	0.6	28.1	0.1	0.0
Hot & Spicy Barbecue, Marks & Spencer*	1 Serving/18g	23	130	1.0	31.1	0.3	0.8
Lime & Coriander With Peri Peri, Nando's*	1 Tsp/5g	9	182	0.0	13.1	16.6	0.2
Sticky Barbecue, Tesco*	1/2 Jar/140g	139	99	0.7	23.3	0.3	0.4
Sun Dried Tomato & Basil With Peri-Peri, Nando's*	1 Bottle/270g	319	118	0.1	15.3	9.5	0.8
Sweet Chilli & Garlic, Marks & Spencer*	1 Serving/40g	70	175	0.3	43.2	0.1	0.5
Tequila Chilli Lime, Marks & Spencer*	1 Serving/75ml	116	155	0.6	34.0	1.6	0.5
Thai Coconut, Coriander & Lime, Lea & Perrins*	1oz/28g	45	159	1.3	25.7	6.1	0.0
Tomato & Herb, Lea & Perrins*	1oz/28g	28	100	1.2	24.1	0.5	0.0
Tomato, Basil & Parmesan, Marks & Spencer*	1 Serving/50g	38	75	2.1	10.1	2.5	1.5
White Wine, Garlic & Pepper, Lea & Perrins*	1oz/28g	28	99	0.1	23.7	0.7	0.0

MARJORAM

Dried	1 Tsp/0.6g	3	271	12.7	42.5	7.0	0.0

MARLIN

Smoked, H Forman & Son*	1 Pack/200g	240	120	29.8	0.0	0.1	0.0
Steaks, Chargrilled, Sainsbury's*	1 Serving/240g	367	153	23.6	0.8	6.1	0.6
Steaks, Raw, Sainsbury's*	1 Steak/110g	109	99	24.3	0.0	0.2	0.0

MARMALADE

3 Fruit, Thick Cut, Waitrose*	1 Tspn/15g	39	262	0.4	64.8	0.1	0.7
Christmas Orange & Whisky, Marks & Spencer*	1oz/28g	67	240	0.3	59.5	0.2	1.9
Citrus Shred, Robertson*	1 Tsp/5g	13	253	0.2	63.0	0.0	0.0
Five Fruit, Tesco*	1 Serving/10g	28	278	0.2	68.2	0.1	0.9
Four Citrus Fruits, Thin Cut, TTD, Sainsbury's*	1 Serving/15g	36	242	0.2	60.0	0.1	1.0
Grapefruit & Cranberry, Marks & Spencer*	1 Tsp/15g	36	240	0.3	60.3	0.0	1.5
Grapefruit, Fine Cut, Duerr's	1 Tsp/15g	39	261	0.2	65.0	0.0	0.0
Lemon & Lime, Average	1 Tbsp/20g	53	267	0.2	66.4	0.1	0.4
Lemon Jelly, No Peel, Tesco*	1 Tsp/15g	39	263	0.1	65.0	0.0	0.4
Lemon, With Shred, Average	1 Serving/20g	50	248	0.2	61.6	0.1	0.6
Lime, With Shred, Average	1 Tbsp/15g	39	261	0.2	65.0	0.1	0.4
Orange & Ginger, Average	1 Tbsp/15g	40	264	0.2	65.7	0.1	0.3
Orange & Lemon, Reduced Sugar, Zest*	1 Tsp/6g	12	195	0.3	47.1	0.2	0.0
Orange, Lemon & Grapefruit, Baxters*	1 Tsp/15g	38	252	0.0	63.0	0.0	0.1
Orange, Reduced Sugar, Average	1 Tbsp/15g	26	170	0.4	42.0	0.1	0.6
Orange, Shredless, Average	1 Tsp/10g	26	261	0.2	65.0	0.0	0.1
Orange, Thick Cut, With Drambuie, TTD, Sainsbury's*	1 Serving/15g	36	238	0.3	58.4	0.1	2.7
Orange, With Drambuie, Finest, Tesco*	1 Serving/10g	33	329	0.3	82.0	0.0	0.7
Orange, With Shred, Average	1 Tbsp/15g	39	263	0.2	65.2	0.0	0.3
Pink Grapefruit, Thin Cut, Waitrose*	1 Serving/10g	26	261	0.2	65.0	0.0	0.4
Three Fruit, Diabetic, Thursday Cottage*	1 Serving/5g	8	154	0.4	38.0	0.0	1.0
Three Fruit, Finest, Tesco*	1 Serving/15g	39	262	0.5	63.6	0.2	1.6
Three Fruits, Fresh Fruit, Sainsbury's*	1 Tsp/15g	38	250	0.0	61.3	0.0	0.0

MARMITE

Yeast Extract, Marmite*	1 Tsp/9g	20	219	38.4	19.2	0.1	3.1

MARROW

Boiled, Average	1oz/28g	3	9	0.4	1.6	0.2	0.6
Raw	1oz/28g	3	12	0.5	2.2	0.2	0.5

MARS

Bar, 5 Little Ones, Mars*	1 Piece/8g	38	477	4.5	73.6	18.3	0.0
Bar, Fun Size, Mars*	Fun Size Bar/20g	89	444	3.7	69.7	16.8	1.1

	Measure INFO/WEIGHT	per Measure KCAL	Nutrition Values per 100g / 100ml				
			KCAL	PROT	CARB	FAT	FIBRE
MARS							
Bar, Mars*	1 Std Bar/62.5	281	449	4.2	69.0	17.4	1.2
Delight, Mars*	1 Pack/39.9g	220	551	4.3	54.8	34.9	0.0
MARSHMALLOWS							
Average	1oz/28g	92	327	3.9	83.1	0.0	0.0
Mushy, Mini, Safeway*	1 Serving/30g	98	325	5.5	75.5	0.0	0.0
Pascall*	1 Marshmallow/4.5g	17	335	2.6	80.0	0.0	0.0
Princess*	1oz/28g	88	314	3.4	80.0	0.0	0.0
Sainsbury's*	1 Mallow/7g	23	330	4.1	78.5	0.0	0.5
MARZIPAN							
Bar, Chocolate, Plain, Thorntons*	1 Bar/46g	206	448	5.2	69.1	17.4	2.0
Dark Chocolate, Thorntons*	1 Serving/46g	207	451	5.2	69.4	17.4	2.1
Plain, Average	1oz/28g	115	412	5.9	67.5	14.2	1.7
MASALA							
Prawn, & Rice, Tesco*	1 Pack/475g	656	138	5.2	17.9	5.2	1.2
Prawn, King, Waitrose*	1 Pack/350g	385	110	7.1	3.8	7.4	1.8
Vegetable, Sainsbury's*	1 Pack/400g	388	97	2.1	5.2	7.5	2.5
Vegetable, With Rice, Feeling Great, Findus*	1 Pack/350g	350	100	3.0	18.0	2.0	1.7
MASALA DAL							
Waitrose*	1/2 Pack/150g	164	109	5.9	12.4	4.0	2.8
MASH							
Winter Root, Sainsbury's*	1 Serving/140g	157	112	2.7	22.0	1.5	0.9
MAYONNAISE							
50% Less Fat, GFY, Asda*	1 Tbsp/10g	32	322	0.8	10.0	31.0	0.0
60% Less Fat, BGTY, Sainsbury's*	1 Tbsp/15ml	42	277	0.4	7.3	27.3	0.0
Aioli, Finest, Tesco*	1 Tsp/5g	20	408	0.8	8.5	41.2	0.0
Average	1 Tsp/11g	80	724	1.9	0.2	79.3	0.0
Beolive Roasted Garlic Flavour, Vandemooetele*	1 Serving/15ml	46	305	1.3	11.3	28.2	0.0
Dijonnaise, Hellmann's*	1 Tsp/6g	13	210	2.9	5.1	19.7	0.0
Egg, Reduced Fat, Safeway*	1/2 Pot/85g	136	160	10.2	1.4	12.2	1.6
Egg, Safeway*	1 Serving/50g	121	241	10.4	0.4	22.0	1.0
Extra Light, Hellmann's*	1 Tbsp/15g	16	105	0.5	11.3	6.4	0.2
Finest, Tesco*	1 Dtsp/22g	155	703	1.1	1.5	77.0	0.0
French Style, BGTY, Sainsbury's*	1 Tbsp/15ml	55	366	0.6	7.5	36.9	0.0
French With Course Ground Mustard, Sainsbury's*	1 Serving/15ml	93	618	0.8	1.7	67.3	0.3
French, Sainsbury's*	1 Tsp/6ml	41	678	1.2	2.4	73.6	1.4
Garlic & Herb, Marks & Spencer*	1 Tsp/6g	43	712	3.4	2.4	76.9	0.9
Garlic & Herb, Reduced Calorie, Hellmann's*	1 Serving/25ml	58	233	0.7	13.1	19.3	0.4
Garlic Flavoured, Frank Cooper*	1 Tsp/6g	28	460	2.2	8.8	46.2	0.1
Garlic, Asda*	1 Serving/20g	136	678	1.3	6.0	72.0	0.0
Good Intentions, Somerfield*	1 Serving/30g	93	309	0.5	7.4	30.8	0.0
Half Fat, Healthy Choice, Safeway*	1 Tsp/11g	35	319	0.8	10.8	30.3	0.0
Hellmann's*	1 Tsp/11g	79	722	1.1	1.3	79.1	0.0
Lemon, Waitrose*	1 Tsp/8ml	56	694	1.2	1.3	76.0	5.4
Light Dijon, Benedicta*	1 Tbsp/15g	44	292	0.7	6.7	29.2	0.0
Light, BGTY, Sainsbury's*	1 Tsp/11g	33	296	0.5	7.2	29.3	0.0
Light, Hellmann's*	1 Serving/10g	30	299	0.7	6.7	29.8	0.0
Light, Morrisons*	1 Tsp/11g	32	287	1.4	8.5	27.5	0.0
Light, Organic, Simply Delicious*	1 Tbsp/14g	60	425	1.3	14.5	40.2	0.4
Light, Reduced Calorie, Hellmann's*	1 Serving/15ml	43	285	0.7	6.6	29.4	0.0
Light, Squeezable, Hellmann's*	1 Tbsp/15g	44	295	0.7	6.6	29.4	0.0
Low Fat, Belolive*	1 Serving/15ml	45	298	0.8	11.1	29.0	0.0
Made With Free Range Eggs, Marks & Spencer*	1 Tbsp/15g	108	720	1.1	1.2	78.5	0.0
Mediterranean, Hellmann's*	1 Tsp/11g	79	722	1.1	1.3	79.1	0.0

MAYONNAISE

INFO/WEIGHT	Measure	per Measure KCAL	KCAL	PROT	CARB	FAT	FIBRE
Mild Dijon Mustard, Frank Cooper*	1 Pot/28g	114	406	3.3	9.3	39.5	0.1
Mustard, Safeway*	1 Tbsp/15ml	105	703	1.4	2.1	76.5	0.0
Organic, Evernat*	1 Tsp/11g	83	752	1.3	2.8	81.0	0.0
Organic, Whole Foods*	1 Tbsp/14g	100	714	0.0	7.1	78.6	0.0
Real, Asda*	1 Serving/10g	72	721	1.3	1.2	79.0	0.1
Real, The Big Squeeze, Hellmann's	1 Tbsp/15ml	101	676	1.0	1.2	74.0	0.0
Reduced Calorie	1 Tsp/11g	32	288	1.0	8.2	28.1	0.0
Reduced Calorie, Healthy Selection, Somerfield*	1 Tbsp/15ml	49	326	0.8	9.8	31.5	0.0
Reduced Calorie, Hellmann's*	1 Serving/30g	90	299	0.7	6.7	29.8	0.0
Reduced Calorie, Tesco*	1 Tbsp/15g	49	326	0.8	9.8	31.5	0.0
Reduced Calorie, Waitrose*	1 Tsp/11g	32	287	1.4	8.5	27.5	0.0
Reduced Fat, Safeway*	1 Tbsp/15ml	48	323	0.8	9.7	31.2	0.0
Reduced Fat, Tesco*	1 Tbsp/15ml	44	292	0.8	7.9	28.6	0.0
Sainsbury's*	1 Tsp/11g	75	686	0.4	1.2	75.4	0.0
Tesco*	1 Serving/28g	203	725	1.3	1.2	79.4	0.0
Value, Tesco*	1 Tbsp/15g	73	488	0.8	5.4	51.4	0.0
Vegetarian, Tesco*	1 Tsp/12g	89	738	1.5	0.8	81.0	0.0
Waitrose*	1 Tbsp/15ml	106	709	1.3	0.8	77.8	0.0
Weight Watchers*	1 Tbsp/15g	42	280	1.0	7.3	27.7	0.7
MEAL REPLACEMENT							
Ny-Tro Pro-40, Cool Vanilla, AST Sports Science*	1 Sachet/72g	250	347	55.6	30.6	2.1	2.8
Ny-Tro Pro-40, Creamy Strawberry, AST Sports Science*	1 Sachet/72g	250	347	55.6	30.6	2.1	2.8
MEAT LOAF							
Beef & Pork, Co-Op*	1/4 Loaf/114g	314	275	13.0	7.0	22.0	1.0
Iceland*	1 Serving/150g	332	221	10.8	9.3	15.7	0.9
Somerfield*	1 Pack/454g	867	191	10.0	8.0	13.0	0.0
Turkey & Bacon, Tesco*	1 Serving/225g	401	178	14.7	7.4	9.9	1.1
MEATBALLS							
& Mashed Potato, Tesco*	1 Pack/450g	527	117	4.0	10.4	6.6	1.0
& Pasta, Sainsbury's*	1 Serving/300g	333	111	5.3	15.5	3.1	1.9
Aberdeen Angus In Sauce, Perfectly Balanced, Waitrose*	1/2 Pack/240g	228	95	10.5	6.5	3.0	1.1
Aberdeen Angus, Waitrose*	3 Meatballs/107g	266	249	19.6	2.2	18.0	0.0
Al Forno, Safeway*	1 Pack/450g	684	152	6.0	16.8	6.8	0.4
Beef, Asda*	1 Serving/287g	362	126	11.0	7.0	6.0	0.6
Chicken, In Tomato Sauce, Average	1 Can/392g	580	148	7.7	10.4	8.4	0.0
Galician Style, Cafe Culture, Marks & Spencer*	1/2 Pack/500g	675	135	5.9	13.2	6.7	1.1
Greek, Marks & Spencer*	1 Serving/350g	403	115	7.7	9.1	5.4	1.5
In Bolognese Sauce, Somerfield*	1 Pack/454g	704	155	7.0	7.0	11.0	0.0
In Gravy, Campbell's*	1/2 Can/205g	164	80	5.6	8.6	2.6	0.0
In Sherry Sauce, Tapas, Waitrose*	1 Serving/185g	272	147	18.8	5.9	4.0	1.2
In Tomato Sauce, Canned, Average	1 Can/410g	387	95	5.6	9.9	3.7	0.0
Italian Pork, Al Forno, Sainsbury's*	1 Pack/450g	644	143	6.1	17.6	5.3	1.4
Lemon Chicken With Rice, BGTY, Sainsbury's*	1 Pack/400g	388	97	6.8	12.8	2.1	1.4
Lion's Head, Marks & Spencer*	1 Serving/300g	435	145	10.4	5.1	9.3	1.0
Manhattan Style & Spaghetti, Spicy, Safeway*	1 Pack/450g	540	120	5.7	13.2	4.8	2.0
Marks & Spencer*	1oz/28g	58	208	10.9	10.7	13.5	2.4
Mighty, In Tomato Sauce, Westlers*	1 Tin/400g	424	106	5.8	10.2	4.8	0.0
Roman-Style Sith Basil Mash, COU, Marks & Spencer*	1 Pack/430g	344	80	3.7	10.9	2.2	1.9
Spaghetti, Tesco*	1 Pack/385g	377	98	5.4	9.8	4.2	1.2
Spicy, Marks & Spencer*	1 Pack/400g	540	135	8.8	12.0	6.0	1.4
Swedish, Average	1/4 Pack/88g	198	225	14.0	7.4	15.7	1.3
Turkey, GFY, Asda*	1/2 Pack/330g	333	101	10.0	7.0	3.7	0.0
Vegetarian Style, With Penne, Tesco*	1 Serving/460g	414	90	5.9	11.4	2.3	2.1

	Measure	per Measure	Nutrition Values per 100g / 100ml				
	INFO/WEIGHT	KCAL	KCAL	PROT	CARB	FAT	FIBRE
MEATBALLS VEGETARIAN							
Swedish Style, Sainsbury's*	1 Ball/27g	53	194	21.5	5.5	9.5	4.0
MEDAGLIONI							
Bolognese, Rich Red Wine, Waitrose*	1/2 Pack/125g	266	213	12.5	28.1	5.6	2.6
Cheese & Red Bell Pepper, Eat Smart, Safeway*	1 Serving/125g	175	140	6.3	21.1	2.9	1.0
Roasted Vegetable & Cheese, Safeway*	1/2 Pack/125g	297	238	9.3	34.2	7.0	2.7
MELBA TOAST							
Buitoni*	1 Serving/33g	130	395	12.1	75.5	4.9	4.6
Dutch, Tesco*	1 Serving/20g	75	377	16.0	73.0	2.3	5.0
Dutch, Wheat Bread, Tesco*	1 Pack/20g	80	399	12.8	80.5	2.9	3.9
Organic, Trimlyne*	1 Pack/28g	109	390	13.0	78.0	2.9	5.5
Original, Van Der Meulen*	1 Slice/3g	12	399	12.8	80.5	2.9	3.9
Sainsbury's*	1 Toast/3g	13	399	12.8	80.5	2.9	3.9
With Sesame, Tesco*	1 Slice/3g	11	370	12.8	61.7	8.0	3.8
MELON							
& Grapes, Fresh, Tesco*	1 Pack/400g	132	33	0.5	7.3	0.2	0.6
Canteloupe, Sainsbury's*	1 Serving/100g	19	19	0.6	4.2	0.1	1.0
Galia, Average	1 Serving/240g	60	25	0.8	5.8	0.1	0.2
Honeydew, Raw, Average	1oz/28g	8	30	0.7	6.9	0.1	0.5
MELON MEDLEY							
Average	1 Pack/240g	66	27	0.6	6.0	0.1	0.5
MELT							
Cheese, Chilli, Fresh, Asda*	1 Melt/29g	87	301	6.0	31.0	17.0	0.0
Cheesy Fish, Young's*	1 Pack/340g	418	123	7.6	8.3	6.6	0.9
Chicken, Salsa, Sainsbury's*	1 Pack/400g	516	129	7.2	10.7	6.4	1.6
Chilli With Spicy Potato Wedges, Asda*	1 Pack/450g	540	120	8.0	12.0	4.4	1.2
Mushroom & Broccoli Potato Wedge, Weight Watchers*	1 Pack/310g	285	92	3.1	13.3	3.0	1.0
Salmon & Broccoli Wedge, Weight Watchers*	1 Pack/320g	301	94	5.1	10.2	3.6	0.8
Sausage & Bean, Iceland*	1 Pack/400g	588	147	6.5	17.1	5.8	1.6
Tuna, Go Large, Asda*	1 Roll/175g	509	291	12.0	27.0	15.0	0.0
Tuna, Iceland*	1 Pack/400g	424	106	6.0	11.3	4.2	0.7
Tuna, Marks & Spencer*	1 Pack/218g	621	285	13.0	20.1	17.0	1.0
Vegetable & Potato, Asda*	1 Serving/100g	451	451	17.0	44.0	23.0	6.2
MERINGUE							
Average	1 Portion/8g	30	379	5.3	95.4	0.0	0.0
Bombe, Raspberry & Vanilla, Marks & Spencer*	1 Bombe/100g	155	155	3.4	33.3	1.8	2.6
Chocolate, Waitrose*	1 Meringue/76.8g	342	444	2.6	75.3	14.7	0.5
Coffee Fresh Cream, Asda*	1 Meringue/27.5g	111	396	3.8	57.0	17.0	0.3
Cream, Fresh, Sainsbury's*	1 Meringue/35g	142	407	3.5	65.4	14.6	0.5
Cream, Marks & Spencer*	1 Cake/34.1g	145	425	4.1	52.6	22.2	0.3
Layered, Tesco*	1/5 Meringue/52g	146	280	3.5	63.2	1.5	1.4
Marks & Spencer*	1 Meringue/12g	47	389	5.2	92.0	0.0	0.0
Mini, Marks & Spencer*	1oz/28g	111	395	6.1	91.6	0.0	0.2
Nests, Asda*	1 Nest/15g	57	381	4.9	90.1	0.2	0.1
Nests, Marks & Spencer*	1 Nest/12g	47	395	6.1	91.6	0.0	0.0
Nests, Mini, Tesco*	1 Nest/4g	14	387	3.9	92.8	0.0	0.0
Nests, Safeway*	1 Nest/13.9g	55	395	4.2	93.6	0.1	0.0
Nests, Sainsbury's*	1 Nest/15g	58	387	3.9	92.8	0.0	0.0
Nests, Tesco*	1 Nest/13g	51	387	3.9	92.8	0.1	0.0
Nests, Tropical Fruit, Sainsbury's*	1 Nest/95g	234	246	2.0	42.0	7.8	2.4
Raspberry, Marks & Spencer*	1 Serving/105g	215	205	1.8	20.6	13.1	3.1
Shells, Mini, Asda*	1 Shell/4g	16	388	4.8	92.0	0.1	0.0
Shells, Sainsbury's*	2 Shells/24g	93	387	3.9	92.8	0.0	0.0
Strawberry, COU, Marks & Spencer*	1 Meringue/5.2g	19	385	6.4	90.0	0.1	1.4

	Measure INFO/WEIGHT	per Measure KCAL	Nutrition Values per 100g / 100ml				
			KCAL	PROT	CARB	FAT	FIBRE
MERINGUE							
Summer Fruits, 90% Fat Free, Sara Lee*	1 Meringue/135g	308	228	2.5	35.7	8.5	2.2
Toffee, COU, Marks & Spencer*	1 Mini/5.1g	20	395	5.0	95.3	1.7	0.7
Toffee, Marks & Spencer*	1 Meringue/30g	125	415	4.1	52.2	20.9	0.8
Tropical, Marks & Spencer*	1 Serving/53g	212	400	3.1	37.0	26.9	0.0
MESSICANI							
Egg, Marks & Spencer*	1 Serving/100g	355	355	13.9	68.5	2.8	3.0
MIDGET GEMS							
Marks & Spencer*	1 Bag/113g	367	325	6.3	75.1	0.1	0.0
SmartPrice, Asda*	1 Pack/178g	586	329	6.0	76.0	0.1	0.0
MILK							
Channel Island, Finest, Tesco*	1 Glass/200ml	160	80	3.7	4.7	5.2	0.0
Condensed, Semi Skimmed, Sweetened	1oz/28g	75	267	10.0	60.0	0.2	0.0
Condensed, Skimmed, Unsweetened, Average	1 Sm Can/205g	221	108	7.5	10.5	4.0	0.0
Condensed, Whole, Sweetened	1oz/28g	93	333	8.5	55.5	10.1	0.0
Dried Whole	1oz/28g	137	490	26.3	39.4	26.3	0.0
Dried, Skimmed, Average	1oz/28g	99	355	35.4	52.3	0.9	0.0
Evaporated, Average	1 Serving/85g	136	160	8.2	11.6	9.0	0.0
Evaporated, Reduced Fat, Average	1oz/28g	33	118	7.4	10.5	5.2	0.0
Goats, Pasteurised	1fl oz/30ml	18	60	3.1	4.4	3.5	0.0
Goats, Semi-Skimmed, St Helens Farm*	1 Serving/250ml	109	44	3.0	4.3	1.6	0.0
Low Fat, Calcia Extra Calcium, Unigate*	1fl oz/30ml	14	45	4.3	6.3	0.5	0.0
Rice Dream, Imagine Foods Ltd*	1 Serving/250ml	118	47	0.1	9.4	1.0	0.1
Semi Skimmed, Average	1fl oz/30ml	15	49	3.4	5.0	1.7	0.0
Semi Skimmed, Long Life, Average	1fl oz/30ml	15	49	3.4	5.0	1.7	0.0
Semi Skimmed, Low Lactose, Arla*	1 Glass/125ml	56	45	3.4	5.0	1.5	0.0
Skimmed, Average	1fl oz/28ml	10	34	3.3	5.0	0.1	0.0
Skimmed, UHT, Average	1fl oz/30ml	10	34	3.4	5.0	0.1	0.0
Soya, Flavoured	1floz/30mls	12	40	2.8	3.6	1.7	0.0
Soya, No Added Sugar, Unsweetened, Average	1 Serving/250ml	85	34	3.3	0.9	1.9	0.4
Soya, Sweetened, Average	1 Glass/200ml	94	47	3.4	3.7	2.1	0.4
Soya, Sweetened, Calcium Enriched, Average	1 Glass/200ml	91	46	3.4	3.7	2.0	0.3
Soya, UHT, Non Dairy, Alternative To Milk, Waitrose*	1 Glass/250ml	103	41	3.3	2.7	1.9	0.2
Soya, Vanilla, Organic, Heinz*	1 Serving/200ml	106	53	2.6	6.9	1.6	0.2
Strawberry Flavoured, Tesco*	1 Serving/500ml	370	74	4.4	10.4	1.6	0.3
Whole, Average	1 Serving/200ml	134	67	3.3	4.7	3.9	0.0
MILK DRINK							
Banana Flavour, Sterilised, Low Fat, Gulp*	1 Bottle/500ml	315	63	3.8	9.7	1.0	0.0
Choc O Latte, Cafe Met*	1 Bottle/290ml	203	70	3.5	10.0	1.5	0.0
Chocolate Sterilised Skimmed, Happy Shopper*	1 Bottle/500ml	295	59	3.6	10.4	0.3	0.0
Chocolate, Spar*	1 Serving/500ml	290	58	3.6	10.2	0.3	0.0
Mars Extra Milk Chocolate Caramel, Mars*	1 Bottle/330g	224	68	3.5	12.1	0.3	0.0
Strawberry, Yazoo, Campina*	1 Bottle/500ml	325	65	3.1	10.3	1.3	0.0
MILK SHAKE							
Banana Flavour, Frijj*	1 Bottle/500ml	310	62	3.4	10.1	0.8	0.0
Banana Flavour, Shapers, Boots*	1 Bottle/250ml	201	80	5.6	12.8	0.8	1.9
Banana Flavour, Spar*	1 Bottle/500ml	250	50	3.3	9.1	0.1	0.0
Banana, Yazoo*	1 Bottle/500ml	325	65	3.1	10.3	1.3	0.0
Chocolate Flavour, BGTY, Sainsbury's*	1 Bottle/500ml	290	58	5.3	8.0	0.5	0.9
Chocolate Flavoured, Fresh, Thick, Frijj*	1 Bottle/500ml	350	70	3.5	11.7	1.0	0.0
Chocolate, Asda*	1 Serving/250ml	198	79	4.4	7.0	3.7	0.4
Chocolate, Extreme, Frijj*	1 Bottle/500g	425	85	3.9	12.7	2.1	0.0
Chocolate, Ultra Slim, Tesco*	1 Serving/330ml	223	68	4.2	10.2	1.1	1.4
Measure Up, Asda*	1 Glass/250ml	200	80	6.0	12.0	1.0	2.4

	Measure INFO/WEIGHT	per Measure KCAL	Nutrition Values per 100g / 100ml				
			KCAL	PROT	CARB	FAT	FIBRE
MILK SHAKE							
Mount Caramel, Frijj*	1 Bottle/500ml	360	72	3.4	12.7	0.9	0.0
Powder, Made Up With Semi-Skimmed Milk	1 Serving/250ml	173	69	3.2	11.3	1.6	0.0
Powder, Made Up With Whole Milk	1 Serving/250ml	218	87	3.1	11.1	3.7	0.0
Strawberry Flavour, Thick, Low Fat, Frijj*	1 Bottle/250ml	155	62	3.4	10.1	0.8	0.0
Strawberry, Fresh, Nesquik*	1 Glass/250ml	175	70	3.3	10.4	1.6	0.3
Strawberry, Ultra Slim, Tesco*	1 Serving/330ml	224	68	4.2	10.5	0.9	1.5
Syrup, Crusha*	1 Serving/30ml	37	124	0.0	31.0	0.0	0.0
Syrup, Strawberry, Crusha*	1 Serving/20ml	25	125	0.5	30.0	0.5	0.0
Vanilla Flavour, BGTY, Sainsbury's*	1 Bottle/500ml	230	46	5.3	5.9	0.1	0.4
Vanilla, Frijj*	1 Bottle/500ml	320	64	3.4	10.7	0.8	0.0
Vanilla, Ultra Slim, Tesco*	1 Serving/330ml	224	68	4.2	10.5	0.9	1.5
MILKY BAR							
Buttons, Nestle*	1 Mini Bag/16g	87	542	7.6	57.5	31.3	0.0
Choo, Nestle*	1oz/28g	131	468	4.1	73.2	17.6	0.0
Chunky, Nestle*	1 Bar/40g	217	542	7.6	57.5	31.3	0.0
Crunchies, Nestle*	1 Pack/30g	168	560	7.0	54.9	34.7	0.0
Munchies, Nestle*	1 Serving/70g	392	560	7.0	54.9	34.7	0.1
Nestle*	1 Bar/12g	65	542	7.6	57.5	31.3	0.0
MILKY WAY							
Magic Stars, Mars*	1 Bag/33g	184	557	8.8	51.8	35.0	0.0
Mars*	1 Single Bar/26g	114	440	3.4	74.8	14.1	0.0
MILO							
Nestle*	1 Serving/20g	76	380	8.2	72.9	6.0	4.7
MINCEMEAT							
Average	1oz/28g	77	274	0.6	62.1	4.3	1.3
With Cherries, Almonds & Brandy, Tesco*	1/4 Jar/103g	295	287	1.4	58.8	4.9	1.4
MINSTRELS							
Galaxy, Mars*	1 Pack/42g	209	497	5.3	68.6	22.3	1.1
MINT							
Dried	1oz/28g	78	279	24.8	34.6	4.6	0.0
Fresh	1oz/28g	12	43	3.8	5.3	0.7	0.0
MINTOES							
Morrisons*	1 Sweet/8.1g	33	411	0.1	84.4	8.1	0.0
MINTS							
After Dinner, Dark, Elizabeth Shaw*	1 Chocolate/9g	42	469	2.8	62.5	23.1	0.0
After Dinner, Sainsbury's*	1 Mint/7g	32	456	4.1	62.1	21.2	4.1
After Dinner, Tesco*	1oz/28g	132	471	5.0	70.0	19.0	0.0
After Eight, Nestle*	1 Mint/8g	34	419	2.5	72.9	12.8	1.1
After Eight, Orange, Nestle*	1 Sweet/7g	29	417	2.5	72.6	12.9	1.1
Butter Mintoes, Marks & Spencer*	1 Sweet/9g	35	391	0.0	84.0	6.8	0.0
Butter Mintoes, Tesco*	1 Sweet/7g	24	349	0.0	71.3	7.1	0.0
Clear, Co-Op*	1 Sweet/6g	24	395	0.0	98.0	0.0	0.0
Cream, Luxury, Thorntons*	1 Chocolate/13g	62	477	4.2	62.3	23.8	2.3
Creams, Bassett's*	1 Sweet/11g	40	365	0.0	91.8	0.0	0.0
Curiously Strong, Marks & Spencer*	1 Sweet/1g	4	390	0.4	97.5	0.0	0.0
Everton, Co-Op*	1 Sweet/6g	25	410	0.6	92.0	4.0	0.0
Extra Strong, Trebor*	3 Mints/10g	40	396	0.3	98.8	0.0	0.0
Glacier, Fox's*	1 Mint/5g	19	386	0.0	96.4	0.0	0.0
Humbugs, Asda*	1 Sweet/8g	29	362	0.0	86.0	2.0	0.0
Humbugs, Co-Op*	1 Sweet/8g	34	425	0.6	89.9	7.0	0.0
Humbugs, Marks & Spencer*	1 Sweet/9g	37	407	0.6	91.1	4.4	0.0
Humbugs, Thorntons*	1 Sweet/9g	31	340	1.0	87.8	4.4	0.0
Imperials, Co-Op*	1 Sweet/3g	12	395	0.3	98.0	0.2	0.0

M

	Measure INFO/WEIGHT	per Measure KCAL	Nutrition Values per 100g / 100ml				
			KCAL	PROT	CARB	FAT	FIBRE
MINTS							
Imperials, Marks & Spencer*	1oz/28g	109	391	0.0	97.8	0.0	0.0
Imperials, Sainsbury's*	1 Mint/3g	12	396	0.4	97.9	0.2	0.0
Imperials, Tesco*	1 Mint/3g	12	397	0.6	98.7	0.0	0.0
Mighty, 24-7, Sugar Free, Trebor*	1 Sweet/0.1g	0	277	0.0	94.7	0.0	0.0
Mint Assortment, Marks & Spencer*	1 Sweet/7g	29	414	0.7	85.4	7.7	0.0
Mint Favourites, Bassett's*	1 Sweet/6g	22	367	0.9	77.4	5.9	0.0
Peppermints, Strong, Altoids*	1 Mint/0.8g	4	385	0.5	96.0	0.0	0.0
Soft, Trebor*	1 Pack/48g	182	380	0.0	94.9	0.0	0.0
Softmints, Trebor*	1 Tube/40g	156	391	0.0	93.3	2.0	0.0
MISO							
Average	1oz/28g	57	203	13.3	23.5	6.2	0.0
MIX							
Cheesecake, Original, Made Up, Asda*	1/6 Cake/85g	228	268	4.1	36.0	12.0	1.4
Cheesecake, Tesco*	1 Serving/76g	199	262	4.1	38.0	10.4	1.6
Chinese Curry, Young's*	1 Serving/22g	109	495	8.3	46.4	30.7	0.0
Falafel, Sainsbury's*	1/2 Pack/110g	197	179	7.7	23.5	6.0	5.2
For Fish, Smoked Haddock, Schwartz*	1 Pack/35g	154	440	13.8	46.9	21.9	0.0
For Pork, Somerset, Schwartz*	1 Serving/36g	120	334	8.4	71.6	1.6	0.2
Garlic & Herb, Crust for Cod, Schwartz*	1 Serving/10g	36	359	11.5	72.5	2.6	0.0
MIXED HERBS							
Average	1 Tsp/5g	13	260	13.0	37.5	8.5	6.7
MIXED VEGETABLES							
Bag, Marks & Spencer*	1 Serving/200g	70	35	2.9	5.6	0.2	0.0
Broccoli & Cauliflower Florets, Baby Carrots, Asda*	1 Serving/113g	28	25	2.2	2.6	0.6	2.4
Canned, Drained, Sainsbury's*	1 Can/200g	114	57	3.0	10.6	0.3	2.3
Canned, Re-Heated, Drained	1oz/28g	11	38	1.9	6.1	0.8	1.7
Carrot, Cauliflower, & Broccoli, Tesco*	1/2 Pack/250g	88	35	2.5	4.9	0.6	2.3
Casserole, Frozen, Tesco*	1 Serving/100g	26	26	0.8	4.8	0.4	2.0
Chunky, Frozen, Sainsbury's*	1 Serving/85g	31	37	2.9	4.7	0.7	3.1
Cooked, Tesco*	1 Serving/100g	27	27	2.3	3.2	0.5	2.3
Farmhouse, Four Seasons*	1 Serving/100g	26	26	2.2	2.7	0.7	0.0
Farmhouse, Tesco*	1 Serving/80g	32	40	3.6	4.6	0.8	3.0
Fresh, Asda*	1oz/28g	7	26	1.9	3.0	0.7	1.0
Fresh, Frozen, Tesco*	1 Serving/75g	37	49	2.9	7.9	0.6	3.2
Frozen, Asda*	1 Serving/100g	53	53	3.1	8.0	0.9	4.0
Frozen, Boiled in Salted Water	1oz/28g	12	42	3.3	6.6	0.5	0.0
Frozen, Safeway*	1 Serving/120g	70	58	3.0	9.4	0.9	3.4
Frozen, Sainsbury's*	1 Serving/90g	49	54	2.8	8.4	1.0	3.1
Frozen, Tesco*	1 Serving/100g	49	49	2.9	7.8	0.7	3.2
Frozen, Waitrose*	1 Serving/100g	54	54	3.1	8.7	0.8	3.5
In Salt Water, Tesco*	1/3 Can/65g	34	53	2.6	9.2	0.6	2.7
In Salted Water, Canned, Asda*	1 Serving/65g	31	48	2.6	9.0	0.2	1.7
In Water, Straight to Wok, Amoy*	1/2 Pack/110g	27	25	1.8	3.7	0.3	0.0
Micro, Tesco*	1 Packet/100g	48	48	3.0	7.2	0.8	3.2
Oriental, Marks & Spencer*	1 Serving/250g	50	20	1.6	3.4	0.3	1.6
Peas, Carrots, & Baby Leeks, Prepared, Tesco*	1/2 Pack/130g	57	44	3.1	5.8	0.9	3.5
Ready To Roast, Asda*	1/2 Pack/362g	315	87	1.6	13.0	3.2	2.4
Red Peppers & Courgette, Tesco*	1 Pack/250g	68	27	1.7	3.8	0.5	2.0
Sainsbury's*	1 Serving/230g	55	24	2.1	2.5	0.6	0.0
Seasonal Selection, Tesco*	1 Serving/100g	37	37	1.1	7.2	0.4	2.2
Special, Freshly Frozen, Morrisons*	1 Serving/100g	48	48	3.2	7.2	0.8	0.0
Special, Sainsbury's*	1 Serving/120g	68	57	3.2	8.9	1.0	2.9
Special, Tesco*	1 Serving/125g	62	49	3.3	7.1	0.8	3.5

	Measure INFO/WEIGHT	per Measure KCAL	Nutrition Values per 100g / 100ml				
			KCAL	PROT	CARB	FAT	FIBRE
MIXED VEGETABLES							
Straight to Wok, Water Selection, Amoy*	1/2 Pack/110g	25	23	1.8	3.7	0.3	1.5
Supreme, Frozen, Somerfield*	1 Serving/90g	23	25	1.9	4.3	0.0	3.1
Tesco*	1oz/28g	8	27	1.7	3.8	0.5	2.0
MOLASSES							
Average	1 Tbsp/20g	53	266	0.0	68.8	0.1	0.0
MONKEY NUTS							
Average	1oz/28g	158	565	25.6	8.2	48.0	6.3
MONKFISH							
Grilled	1oz/28g	27	96	22.7	0.0	0.6	0.0
Raw	1oz/28g	18	66	15.7	0.0	0.4	0.0
MONSTER MUNCH							
Baked Bean Flavour, Walkers*	1 Pack/25g	120	480	5.5	58.0	25.0	1.4
Flamin' Hot, Walkers*	1 Bag/25g	123	490	7.0	60.0	25.0	1.5
Pickled Onion, Walkers*	1 Bag/25g	124	495	6.0	62.0	25.0	1.6
Roast Beef, Walkers*	1 Pack/25g	119	475	6.6	58.0	24.0	1.5
Spicy, Walkers*	1 Bag/25g	125	500	5.0	55.0	29.0	1.3
MORNAY							
Broccoli, Somerfield*	1 Meal/400g	372	93	3.5	5.9	6.2	0.5
Cod, Fillets, Sainsbury's*	1 Serving/153g	236	154	15.2	2.2	9.4	0.9
Cod, Sainsbury's*	1 Serving/180g	277	154	15.2	2.2	9.4	0.9
Haddock, COU, Marks & Spencer*	1 Pack/200g	160	80	14.0	0.7	2.5	0.3
Haddock, Iceland*	1/2 Pack/179g	179	100	13.6	4.3	3.2	0.7
Haddock, Meal for One, Marks & Spencer*	1 Pack/400g	340	85	6.6	7.4	3.3	2.3
Haddock, Somerfield*	1 Serving/200g	266	133	13.6	5.1	6.5	0.5
Haddock, Waitrose*	1 Serving/180g	140	78	14.2	1.9	1.6	0.7
Haddock, With Leek Mash, Eat Smart, Safeway*	1 Pack/369.9g	307	83	7.1	7.9	2.5	1.0
Haddock, Young's*	1/2 Pack/190g	236	124	12.1	1.3	7.8	0.6
Salmon, With Broccoli, Weight Watchers*	1 Pack/290g	261	90	9.6	9.0	1.7	0.7
Spinach, Waitrose*	1 Pack/250g	263	105	4.2	4.6	7.7	1.3
MOUSSAKA							
Beef, BGTY, Sainsbury's*	1 Pack/400g	300	75	6.1	6.8	2.6	1.2
Beef, Good Intentions, Somerfield*	1 Pack/400g	364	91	7.1	7.2	3.7	3.3
Beef, Healthy Living, Tesco*	1 Pack/450g	396	88	5.0	10.9	2.7	0.8
COU, Marks & Spencer*	1 Pack/340g	272	80	5.3	8.5	2.9	1.4
Cafe Culture, Marks & Spencer*	1 Serving/375g	619	165	9.2	7.8	10.5	0.8
Eat Smart, Safeway*	1 Pack/400g	380	95	5.2	12.6	2.6	1.2
Lamb, Eat Smart, Safeway*	1 Pack/380g	304	80	6.8	6.4	2.7	1.3
Lamb, Finest, Tesco*	1 Pack/330g	521	158	7.7	9.1	10.1	2.0
Lamb, Sainsbury's*	1 Pack/329.1g	497	151	8.4	7.2	9.8	1.1
Lamb, Tesco*	1 Serving/460g	442	96	3.4	13.2	3.3	0.5
Ready Meals, Waitrose*	1 Pack/300g	492	164	8.2	10.9	9.7	1.7
Vegetable, Marks & Spencer*	1 Pack/300g	345	115	3.3	7.8	7.7	3.1
Vegetable, Ready Meals, Waitrose*	1oz/28g	38	134	3.7	12.3	7.8	2.3
Vegetable, Roasted, Safeway*	1 Pack/365g	365	100	3.7	7.9	5.7	2.9
Vegetarian, Tesco*	1 Pack/300g	489	163	6.4	11.0	10.4	0.9
MOUSSE							
Aero Chocolate, Nestle*	1 Pot/59g	109	185	5.1	21.0	8.9	0.5
Aero Mint, Nestle*	1 Pot/100g	218	218	4.1	23.6	11.9	0.0
Aero Twist Cappuccino & Chocolate, Nestle*	1 Pot/75g	135	180	4.2	16.8	10.8	0.2
Apricot, Lite, Onken*	1 Pot/150g	156	104	4.6	18.0	1.5	0.3
Banoffee, COU, Marks & Spencer*	1 Pot/70g	102	145	2.9	28.8	2.1	1.5
Black Cherry, Lite, Onken*	1 Pot/150g	156	104	4.6	17.9	1.5	0.3
Blackcurrant, Healthy Living, Tesco*	1 Pot/113g	80	71	3.7	8.3	2.6	1.8

MOUSSE

INFO/WEIGHT	Measure per Measure KCAL		Nutrition Values per 100g / 100ml				
			KCAL	PROT	CARB	FAT	FIBRE
Blackcurrant, Onken*	1 Pot/150g	210	140	5.2	14.6	6.8	0.0
Cadbury's Flake, Twinpot, St Ivel*	1 Pot/100g	257	257	5.6	27.4	13.9	0.0
Cadbury's Light Chocolate, St Ivel*	1 Pot/64g	79	123	6.2	17.3	3.2	0.0
Caramel, Meringue, Cadbury*	1 Serving/65g	181	277	4.6	42.4	10.3	1.0
Caramelised Orange, COU, Marks & Spencer*	1 Pot/70g	91	130	2.8	26.3	1.7	3.4
Chocolate	1 Pot/60g	83	139	4.0	19.9	5.4	0.0
Chocolate & Hazelnut Puree, Onken*	1/2 Pot/185g	222	120	3.4	19.5	3.1	0.0
Chocolate & Hazelnut, Onken*	1 Pot/125g	173	138	3.3	17.8	6.0	0.0
Chocolate & Mint, COU, Marks & Spencer*	1 Pot/70g	84	120	6.2	18.7	2.5	1.0
Chocolate & Orange, COU, Marks & Spencer*	1 Pot/70g	77	110	5.9	16.0	2.6	0.9
Chocolate & Vanilla, Weight Watchers*	1 Pot/80g	106	132	4.4	22.2	2.8	0.9
Chocolate Orange, Low Fat, Cadbury*	1 Pot/100g	110	110	5.6	15.1	3.0	0.0
Chocolate With Vanilla Layer, Cadbury*	1 Pot/100g	162	162	4.8	21.9	6.1	0.0
Chocolate, Asda*	1 Pot/61g	134	219	3.7	26.0	10.0	1.0
Chocolate, BGTY, Sainsbury's*	1 Pot/62.5g	82	133	4.9	21.8	2.9	0.5
Chocolate, COU, Marks & Spencer*	1 Pot/70g	81	115	5.8	16.6	2.7	1.0
Chocolate, Finest, Tesco*	1 Pot/82g	321	391	3.7	21.7	32.2	0.0
Chocolate, GFY, Asda*	1 Pot/62.5g	84	134	4.8	23.0	2.5	3.2
Chocolate, Healthy Living, Tesco*	1 Serving/63g	84	135	4.8	23.3	2.5	3.2
Chocolate, Italian Style, Tesco*	1 Pot/90g	243	270	5.0	32.8	13.2	2.4
Chocolate, Less Than 3% Fat, BGTY, Sainsbury's*	1 Pot/63g	85	136	3.8	24.0	2.7	1.1
Chocolate, Light, Cadbury*	1 Pot/55g	69	125	6.2	17.3	3.3	0.0
Chocolate, Organic, Evernat*	1oz/28g	83	296	10.1	21.1	19.1	0.0
Chocolate, Sainsbury's*	1 Pot/62g	122	197	4.0	25.4	8.8	1.1
Chocolate, Shapers, Boots*	1 Pot/70g	97	138	5.3	23.0	2.7	1.7
Chocolate, Somerfield*	1 Pot/60g	115	192	4.3	24.5	8.5	0.0
Chocolate, Tesco*	1 Pot/60g	108	180	3.7	24.0	7.7	1.2
Dream, Cadbury*	1 Pot/53g	100	189	6.0	22.0	8.0	0.0
Fruit Juice, Shape*	1 Pot/100g	115	115	3.5	18.5	2.8	0.0
Layered Lemon, Co-Op*	1 Pot/100g	140	140	3.0	24.0	3.0	0.2
Layered Strawberry, Co-Op*	1 Pot/100g	120	120	3.0	19.0	3.0	0.2
Lemon Fruit Juice, Shape*	1 Pot/100g	116	116	3.5	18.6	2.8	0.0
Lemon, COU, Marks & Spencer*	1 Pot/70g	81	115	2.9	19.4	2.4	3.5
Lemon, Dessert, Sainsbury's*	1 Pot/62.5g	114	182	3.6	20.7	9.4	0.6
Lemon, Eat Smart, Safeway*	1 Pot/70g	95	135	3.4	23.5	2.7	0.4
Lemon, GFY, Asda*	1 Pot/62.5g	58	92	3.6	13.0	2.8	1.7
Lemon, Healthy Living, Tesco*	1 Pot/113g	94	83	3.6	11.3	2.6	0.2
Lemon, Less Than 3% Fat, BGTY, Sainsbury's*	1 Pot/62g	70	113	4.5	17.6	2.8	0.3
Lemon, Less Than 3% Fat, Healthy Eating, Tesco*	1 Pot/60g	57	95	3.4	14.3	2.7	0.7
Lemon, Lite, Onken*	1 Pot/150g	156	104	4.6	18.0	1.6	0.0
Lemon, Onken*	1 Pot/150g	219	146	5.1	15.8	6.9	0.1
Lemon, Tesco*	1 Pot/60g	67	111	3.4	18.2	2.7	0.0
Mars, Eden Vale*	1 Pot/110g	215	195	6.0	28.2	6.7	0.7
Milky Way, Mars*	1 Pot/50g	115	229	4.5	20.0	14.5	0.0
Orange & Lemon, Light, Muller*	1 Pot/150g	147	98	4.3	19.3	0.4	0.0
Orange & Nectarine, Shape*	1 Pot/100g	47	47	3.0	4.9	1.9	0.0
Orange Fruit Juice, Shape*	1 Pot/100g	116	116	3.5	18.5	2.8	0.0
Orange, Mango & Lime, Onken*	1 Pot/150g	207	138	5.1	15.3	6.3	0.1
Peach & Passion Fruit, Perfectly Balanced, Waitrose*	1 Pot/95g	118	124	3.5	21.2	2.8	0.5
Peach, Onken*	1 Pot/150g	200	133	4.8	13.5	6.6	0.0
Peach, Shape*	1 Pot/100g	43	43	3.0	3.9	1.8	0.1
Pineapple, COU, Marks & Spencer*	1 Pot/70g	84	120	3.3	20.7	2.4	3.5
Pineapple, Lite, Onken*	1 Pot/150g	162	108	4.6	19.0	1.5	0.2

	Measure	per Measure	Nutrition Values per 100g / 100ml				
	INFO/WEIGHT	KCAL	KCAL	PROT	CARB	FAT	FIBRE
MOUSSE							
Pineapple, Shape*	1 Pot/100g	43	43	2.9	3.8	1.8	0.1
Plain Chocolate, Low Fat, Nestle*	1 Pot/120g	71	59	2.4	10.4	0.8	0.0
Raspberry Ripple, Value, Tesco*	1 Mousse/47g	70	149	2.1	21.3	6.1	0.1
Raspberry, COU, Marks & Spencer*	1 Pot/70g	81	115	3.0	19.6	2.4	3.9
Raspberry, Lite, Onken*	1 Pot/150g	152	101	4.6	17.3	1.5	1.0
Rhubarb & Vanilla, Onken*	1 Pot/150g	210	140	5.0	15.8	6.3	0.2
Rhubarb, COU, Marks & Spencer*	1 Pot/70g	88	125	2.9	25.7	2.1	4.2
Rhubarb, Lite, Onken*	1 Pot/150g	155	103	4.6	17.8	1.5	0.3
Salmon, Tesco*	1 Mousse/57g	100	177	13.5	2.9	12.4	0.2
Strawberry Fruity, Organic, Sainsbury's*	1 Pot/125g	129	103	6.2	15.7	3.0	3.6
Strawberry, Asda*	1 Pot/64g	107	167	3.5	18.0	9.0	0.2
Strawberry, BGTY, Sainsbury's*	1 Pot/62.5g	64	101	3.4	15.0	2.8	0.2
Strawberry, Eat Smart, Safeway*	1 Pot/70g	95	135	3.2	24.4	2.7	0.5
Strawberry, Healthy Living, Tesco*	1 Pot/114g	90	79	3.8	10.2	2.6	0.8
Strawberry, Light, Muller*	1 Pot/150g	147	98	4.3	19.4	0.4	0.0
Strawberry, Lite, Onken*	1 Pot/150g	153	102	4.6	17.3	1.6	1.1
Strawberry, Low Fat, Waitrose*	1 Pot/95g	112	118	3.2	20.0	2.8	0.6
Strawberry, Morrisons*	1 Pot/62.5g	107	170	3.5	17.6	9.5	0.2
Strawberry, Onken*	1 Pot/150g	204	136	5.1	14.6	6.3	0.1
Strawberry, Safeway*	1 Pot/63g	106	168	3.5	17.3	9.4	0.1
Strawberry, Sainsbury's*	1 Pot/63g	106	168	3.4	17.5	9.4	0.1
Strawberry, Shape*	1 Pot/100g	44	44	3.0	4.0	1.8	0.0
Strawberry, Tesco*	1 Pot/63g	106	169	3.5	17.9	9.3	0.2
Strawberry, Weight Watchers*	1 Pot/90g	124	138	3.0	25.5	2.7	0.5
Summer Fruits, Light, Muller*	1 Pot/149g	143	96	4.3	18.7	0.4	0.0
Tropical Fruits, Light, Muller*	1 Pot/150g	150	101	4.3	20.0	0.4	0.0
Tropical, Eat Smart, Safeway*	1 Pot/90g	122	135	3.3	24.5	2.3	3.2
White Chocolate, Finest, Tesco*	1 Pot/92g	436	474	3.9	30.2	37.5	0.0
MOUSSECAKE							
Lemon, Weight Watchers*	1 Serving/90g	130	144	3.2	26.7	2.7	0.5
Strawberry, Weight Watchers*	1 Serving/90g	124	138	3.0	25.5	2.7	0.5
MOZZARELLA STICKS							
Breaded, With Tomato Dip, D'esir, Aldi*	1 Pack/200g	462	231	12.0	21.0	11.0	0.0
MUFFIN							
All Butter, TTD, Sainsbury's*	1 Muffin/70.1g	183	261	10.7	40.0	6.5	2.7
Apple, Sultana & Cinnamon, GFY, Asda*	1 Muffin/50g	134	268	6.0	53.0	3.5	3.9
Average	1 Muffin/57g	161	283	10.1	49.6	6.3	2.0
Banana & Walnut, The Handmade Flapjack Company*	1 Muffin/135g	520	385	5.3	40.5	22.7	0.0
Berry Burst, Asda*	1 Muffin/60g	139	232	6.2	46.7	2.3	1.7
Blueberry Buster, McVitie's*	1 Muffin/95g	408	429	4.3	49.9	23.6	1.1
Blueberry Mega, The Handmade Flapjack Company*	1 Muffin/135g	562	416	5.1	47.8	22.8	0.0
Blueberry, American Style, Sainsbury's*	1 Muffin/72g	242	336	5.6	40.6	16.8	3.2
Blueberry, Big, Asda*	1 Muffin/105g	342	326	7.5	49.8	10.7	2.3
Blueberry, GFY, Asda*	1 Muffin/58.6g	147	249	6.0	51.0	2.3	3.0
Blueberry, Low Fat, David Powell*	1 Muffin/100g	246	246	6.0	47.9	3.8	0.0
Blueberry, Marks & Spencer*	1 Muffin/75g	282	376	4.8	52.4	16.4	1.2
Blueberry, Martha White*	1 Muffin/38g	170	447	5.3	73.7	11.8	0.0
Blueberry, Mini, Sainsbury's*	1 Serving/28g	82	293	6.3	48.9	8.1	1.9
Blueberry, Mini, Tesco*	1 Muffin/28g	104	370	5.6	43.5	19.3	1.2
Blueberry, Perfectly Balanced, Waitrose*	1 Muffin/100g	225	225	4.6	46.5	2.2	1.8
Blueberry, Sainsbury's*	1 Muffin/75g	242	322	5.4	46.7	12.6	2.2
Blueberry, Tesco*	1 Muffin/70g	259	370	5.6	43.5	19.3	1.2
Blueberry, The Handmade Flapjack Company*	1 Muffin/135g	479	355	4.7	39.9	19.7	0.0

MUFFIN	Measure INFO/WEIGHT	per Measure KCAL	Nutrition Values per 100g / 100ml				
			KCAL	PROT	CARB	FAT	FIBRE
Blueberry, Waitrose*	1 Muffin/65g	239	367	4.7	55.2	14.2	1.7
Blueberry, Weight Watchers*	1 Muffin/65g	172	265	6.4	46.9	5.7	2.6
Blueberry, Wild Canadian, Fabulous Bakin' Boys*	1 Muffin/40g	140	349	4.0	39.0	20.0	1.0
Bran	1 Muffin/57g	155	272	7.8	45.6	7.7	7.7
Bran & Sultana, Weight Watchers*	1 Muffin/60g	144	240	4.5	50.7	2.1	2.3
Cafe Latte, Sainsbury's*	1 Muffin/72g	270	375	5.9	43.6	19.7	2.8
Cappuccino Mega, The Handmade Flapjack Company*	1 Muffin/135g	653	484	14.0	48.4	29.6	0.0
Carrot Cake, Entenmann's*	1 Muffin/105g	344	328	5.1	45.8	15.1	3.0
Carrot Cakelet, The Handmade Flapjack Company*	1 Muffin/135g	479	355	4.0	45.1	17.7	0.0
Carrot, Asda*	1 Muffin/59.2g	137	233	6.0	47.0	2.3	1.6
Cheese & Black Pepper, Sainsbury's*	1 Muffin/65g	142	218	12.9	34.6	2.0	1.2
Cheese, Tesco*	1 Muffin/75g	183	244	12.5	38.1	4.6	2.0
Cherry, The Handmade Flapjack Company*	1 Muffin/135g	500	370	4.6	43.8	19.7	0.0
Cherry Mega, The Handmade Flapjack Company*	1 Muffin/135g	506	375	4.4	44.8	19.8	0.0
Choc Chip, BGTY, Sainsbury's*	1 Muffin/75g	282	376	5.2	51.8	16.4	1.6
Choc Chip, Mini, Weight Watchers*	1 Muffin/15g	47	312	6.6	52.1	8.6	3.1
Chocolate Chip, American Style, Sainsbury's*	1 Muffin/72g	293	407	6.2	49.5	20.5	1.0
Chocolate Chip, Mini, BGTY, Sainsbury's*	1 Muffin/28g	91	324	6.5	55.1	8.7	1.6
Chocolate Chip, Plain, Tesco*	1 Muffin/72g	298	414	5.8	48.8	21.8	1.3
Chocolate Indulgence, McVitie's*	1 Muffin/75g	254	338	5.8	57.9	9.2	1.3
Chocolate, BGTY, Sainsbury's*	1 Muffin/75g	282	376	5.2	51.8	16.4	1.6
Chocolate, Dairy Cream, Safeway*	1 Muffin/109.7g	430	391	7.3	31.9	26.1	3.1
Chocolate, Healthy Living, Tesco*	1 Cake/71g	222	313	6.8	50.4	9.4	1.6
Chocolate, Sainsbury's*	1 Muffin/72.2g	293	407	6.2	49.5	20.5	1.0
Chocolate, The Handmade Flapjack Company*	1 Muffin/135g	527	390	5.3	41.5	22.8	0.0
Christmas, Weight Watchers*	1 Muffin/63g	173	275	6.8	51.1	4.8	3.0
Chunky Choc n Orange, Fabulous Bakin' Boys*	1 Muffin/40g	154	384	5.0	42.0	22.0	1.0
Chunky Chocolate Chip, McVitie's*	1 Muffin/94g	393	418	5.3	50.6	21.6	0.8
Cranberry & White Chocolate, Sainsbury's*	1 Muffin/72g	253	352	5.7	40.7	18.5	1.5
Dairy Cream Lemon, Safeway*	1 Muffin/110g	409	372	4.4	44.5	19.6	0.0
Double Berry Burst, Entenmann's*	1 Muffin/59g	140	238	4.6	50.1	2.1	1.6
Double Choc Chip, Mini, Asda*	1 Muffin/19g	74	390	6.0	51.0	18.0	0.0
Double Choc Chip, Weight Watchers*	1 Muffin/65g	189	291	6.8	47.2	8.3	3.6
Double Chocolate Chip, American Style, Sainsbury's*	1 Muffin/72.0g	290	403	4.8	50.0	20.4	1.9
Double Chocolate Chip, Asda*	1 Serving/105g	420	400	7.4	48.5	19.6	2.7
Double Chocolate Chip, Healthier, Tesco*	1 Muffin/72g	272	378	7.0	51.6	16.0	1.4
Double Chocolate Chip, New, Weight Watchers*	1 Muffin/65g	169	260	3.9	52.2	4.0	1.9
Double Chocolate Chip, Tesco*	1 Muffin/72g	302	419	6.1	48.0	22.5	1.4
Double Chocolate, 95% Fat Free, Entenmann's*	1 Muffin/58g	152	262	2.6	52.3	4.7	1.8
Double Chocolate, Chocolate Chip, Mini, Tesco*	1 Muffin/28g	116	414	6.3	45.7	23.0	1.4
Double Chocolate, Free From, Tesco*	1 Muffin/70g	281	402	4.7	54.8	18.2	1.7
Double Chocolate, Marks & Spencer*	1 Muffin/75g	313	417	5.2	48.7	22.4	1.9
Double Chocolate, Somerfield*	1 Muffin/70g	298	425	6.8	46.5	23.5	0.0
English, Butter, Tesco*	1 Muffin/67.2g	170	253	11.2	39.8	5.4	2.0
English, Marks & Spencer*	1 Muffin/60g	135	225	11.2	43.7	1.9	2.9
Finger, Double Chocolate, Bakers Delight*	1 Muffin/25g	104	416	5.8	56.9	18.4	1.7
Galaxy, McVitie's*	1 Muffin/94.0g	358	381	5.1	45.0	20.1	0.0
Lemon & Blueberry, Tesco*	1 Muffin/110g	411	374	4.0	42.4	20.9	1.1
Lemon & Poppy Seed, Entenmann's*	1 Muffin/105g	417	397	5.6	52.8	19.3	2.5
Lemon & Poppy Seed, Marks & Spencer*	1 Muffin/72g	281	390	6.3	46.1	19.8	1.5
Lemon & Sultana, BGTY, Sainsbury's*	1 Muffin/75g	211	281	4.5	55.6	4.5	1.4
Lemon, Boots*	1 Muffin/110g	424	385	3.6	50.0	19.0	1.3
Magnificent, Kingsmill*	1 Muffin/75g	168	224	9.8	42.3	1.7	2.2

	Measure INFO/WEIGHT	per Measure KCAL	Nutrition Values per 100g / 100ml				
			KCAL	PROT	CARB	FAT	FIBRE
MUFFIN							
Marks & Spencer*	1 Muffin/56g	126	225	11.2	43.7	1.9	2.9
Mini, Tesco*	1 Muffin/28g	120	428	6.4	50.0	22.6	1.2
Mississipi Mud, Sainsbury's*	1 Muffin/72.1g	274	380	5.2	48.6	18.3	4.2
Mixed Fruit, Low Fat, Abbey Bakery*	1 Muffin/35g	93	267	4.5	55.6	4.5	1.4
Oven Bottom, Asda*	1 Muffin/68g	173	255	10.0	50.4	1.5	2.2
Oven Bottom, Tesco*	1 Muffin/68g	173	255	10.0	50.4	1.5	2.2
Oven Bottom, Warburtons*	1 Muffin/69g	175	253	10.9	45.8	2.9	0.0
Plain Choc Chip, Tesco*	1 Muffin/72g	302	419	6.2	48.9	22.1	1.1
Plain Chocolate Chip, Sainsbury's*	1 Muffin/75g	313	423	6.4	51.3	21.4	0.6
Plain, Co-Op*	1 Muffin/60g	150	250	13.3	45.0	1.7	1.7
Plain, Morrisons*	1 Muffin/70g	140	200	8.0	41.4	1.1	0.0
Premium White, Sainsbury's*	1 Muffin/65g	135	208	8.0	41.4	1.1	2.0
Raspberry Cream, Sainsbury's*	1 Muffin/90g	314	349	3.9	33.8	22.0	1.3
Raspberry Injected, The Handmade Flapjack Company*	1 Muffin/135g	564	418	4.5	54.7	20.2	0.0
Raspberry, Perfectly Balanced, Waitrose*	1 Muffin/101g	220	219	4.7	45.4	2.1	3.7
Rolo, Nestle*	1 Muffin/80g	289	361	5.4	44.3	18.0	0.8
Saltana, The Handmade Flapjack Company*	1 Muffin/135g	500	370	4.7	44.8	19.3	0.0
Sausage, Egg & Cheese, American Style, Tesco*	1 Muffin/155g	383	247	12.2	19.9	13.2	1.0
Spiced Fruit, TTD, Sainsbury's*	1 Muffin/70g	181	259	10.1	43.1	5.1	2.3
Spicy Fruit, Sainsbury's*	1 Muffin/63g	140	222	9.6	43.3	1.2	2.7
Strawberry Cakelet, The Handmade Flapjack Company*	1 Muffin/135g	527	390	4.5	43.6	21.9	0.0
Toffee & Pecan, Finest, Tesco*	1 Muffin/127g	551	434	5.4	51.8	22.8	0.9
Toffee Choo Choo, Tesco*	1 Muffin/95g	402	423	6.4	49.1	22.4	1.0
Toffee Mega, The Handmade Flapjack Company*	1 Muffin/135g	567	420	4.5	43.2	25.7	0.0
Toffee Temptation, McVitie's*	1 Muffin/85.5g	295	347	4.7	60.8	9.5	0.8
Toffee, GFY, Asda*	1 Serving/90g	151	168	2.1	34.0	2.6	0.0
Toffee, The Handmade Flapjack Company*	1 Muffin/135g	533	395	4.4	41.2	23.4	0.0
Triple Chocolate, Triumph, Fabulous Bakin' Boys*	1 Muffin/40g	160	400	4.5	42.0	24.0	0.0
Truly Madly Chocolatey, Fabulous Bakin' Boys*	1 Muffin/40g	154	386	5.0	41.0	22.0	2.0
Vanilla & Choc Chip, GFY, Asda*	1 Muffin/58.5g	151	260	7.0	53.0	2.2	1.6
White Chocolate Chunk Lemon, Mini, Marks & Spencer*	1 Muffin/28g	130	464	6.4	55.4	23.9	2.1
White, Finest, Tesco*	1 Muffin/70g	159	227	8.4	45.7	1.2	2.1
White, Marks & Spencer*	1 Muffin/60g	135	225	11.2	43.7	1.9	2.9
White, Sainsbury's*	1 Muffin/72g	164	228	10.0	43.1	1.7	3.0
White, Tesco*	1 Muffin/60g	143	238	10.2	42.0	3.2	2.1
Wholemeal, Organic, Waitrose*	1 Muffin/65g	129	198	12.4	32.9	1.9	7.6
Wholemeal, Tesco*	1 Muffin/65g	137	210	12.9	32.7	3.1	1.9
MUFFIN MIX							
Banana Nut, Betty Crocker*	1 Serving/30g	130	433	6.7	70.0	16.7	0.0
MULBERRIES							
Raw	1oz/28g	10	36	1.3	8.1	0.0	0.0
MULLET							
Grey, Grilled	1oz/28g	42	150	25.7	0.0	5.2	0.0
Grey, Raw	1oz/28g	32	115	19.8	0.0	4.0	0.0
Red, Grilled	1oz/28g	34	121	20.4	0.0	4.4	0.0
Red, Raw	1oz/28g	31	109	18.7	0.0	3.8	0.0
MUNCHIES							
Milky Bar, Nestle*	1 Pack/35g	196	560	7.0	54.9	34.7	0.1
Mint, Nestle*	1 Pack/61g	267	432	3.8	67.5	16.4	0.0
Nestle*	1 Pack/52g	255	490	4.8	63.7	24.0	0.6
MUSHROOMS							
Breaded, Average	1oz/28g	42	152	4.3	20.8	5.7	0.7
Breaded, Garlic, Average	1 Serving/50.3g	91	183	5.2	18.7	9.7	1.7

	Measure INFO/WEIGHT	per Measure KCAL	Nutrition Values per 100g / 100ml				
			KCAL	PROT	CARB	FAT	FIBRE
MUSHROOMS							
Button, Average	1 Serving/50g	7	15	2.3	0.5	0.4	1.2
Chargrilled & Truffle Sauce, The Best, Safeway*	1 Pot/350g	385	110	3.4	5.8	7.6	0.8
Cheesey, Stuffed, Asda*	1 Serving/290g	322	111	4.3	10.0	6.0	0.0
Chestnut, Average	1 Mushroom/63g	8	13	1.8	0.4	0.5	0.6
Chinese, Dried, Raw	1oz/28g	80	284	10.0	59.9	1.8	0.0
Closed Cup, Average	1oz/28g	5	18	2.9	0.5	0.5	0.6
Common, Boiled in Salted Water	1oz/28g	3	11	1.8	0.4	0.3	1.1
Common, Fried, Average	1oz/28g	44	157	2.4	0.3	16.2	1.5
Common, Raw, Average	1oz/28g	4	13	1.9	0.3	0.5	1.1
Creamed, Average	1oz/28g	23	82	1.3	6.8	5.5	0.5
Dried	1oz/28g	45	159	21.8	4.8	6.0	13.3
Flat, Large, Average	1 Mushroom/52g	10	20	3.3	0.5	0.5	0.7
Garlic, Average	1/2 Pack/150g	160	106	2.1	3.7	9.3	1.7
Giant, With Tomatoes & Mozzarella, Marks & Spencer*	1 Serving/145g	218	150	6.3	7.1	10.9	5.5
Hon Shimeji, Sainsbury's*	1oz/28g	6	23	4.0	3.9	0.5	1.1
Oyster, Average	1oz/28g	4	15	1.6	1.7	0.3	1.3
Porcini, Dried, Merchant Gourmet*	1 oz/28g	36	128	12.3	5.0	6.5	0.0
Shiitake, Cooked	1oz/28g	15	55	1.6	12.3	0.2	0.0
Shiitake, Dried, Raw	1oz/28g	83	296	9.6	63.9	1.0	0.0
Sliced, Average	1oz/28g	3	12	1.8	0.4	0.3	1.1
Straw, Canned, Drained	1oz/28g	4	15	2.1	1.2	0.2	0.0
Stuffed, Finest, Tesco*	1 Serving/130g	224	172	4.0	7.4	14.0	1.9
Stuffed, Ready To Roast, Waitrose*	1 Serving/125g	94	75	3.9	6.5	3.7	1.5
Stuffed, With Cheese, Parsley, & Butter, Sainsbury's*	1/2 Pack/110g	246	224	4.1	2.3	22.0	2.6
MUSSELS							
Boiled	1 Mussel/7g	7	104	16.7	3.5	2.7	0.0
Fresh, With Tomato & Garlic, Marks & Spencer*	1 Serving/650g	455	70	7.9	6.5	1.6	0.1
In Garlic Butter Sauce, Average	1/2 Pack/225g	179	80	6.4	2.0	5.1	0.2
In Thai Sauce, Scottish, Waitrose*	1 Serving/250g	135	54	5.4	2.6	2.5	0.6
Pickled, Drained, Average	1oz/28g	32	113	20.0	1.5	2.3	0.0
Raw, Average	1oz/28g	24	87	12.7	3.6	2.5	0.2
Thai Fragrant, Marks & Spencer*	1/2 Pack/325g	358	110	10.6	4.5	5.7	0.1
Vegetable Oil, Smoked, John West*	1oz/28g	58	207	20.0	7.0	11.0	0.0
White Wine Cream Sauce, Cooked, Scottish, Morrisons*	1/2 Pack/250g	263	105	9.0	5.4	5.3	0.5
MUSTARD							
American, French's*	1 Tbsp/15g	27	180	6.0	16.0	12.0	0.0
Cajun, Colman's*	1 Tsp/6g	11	187	7.0	23.0	6.5	2.7
Coarse Grain, Frank Cooper*	1 Tsp/6g	12	206	8.9	17.0	11.4	0.0
Coarse Grain, Organic, Simply Delicious*	1 Tbsp/5g	9	170	8.7	11.5	9.1	2.6
Colman's*	1 Tsp/5ml	9	188	7.0	19.0	9.3	1.6
Dijon, Asda*	1 Tsp/7g	11	163	7.7	6.6	11.1	0.0
Dijon, Frank Cooper*	1 Tsp/6g	11	179	7.2	10.0	12.3	0.0
Dijon, French, Sainsbury's*	1 Tsp/5g	7	139	7.5	3.5	10.5	0.0
Dijon, Marks & Spencer*	1 Tsp/6g	9	153	10.0	7.2	9.5	1.0
Dijon, Organic, Simply Delicious*	1 Serving/10g	17	166	8.2	6.7	10.6	2.6
Dijon, Tesco*	1 Serving/10g	14	141	8.4	6.4	8.2	0.0
English, Colman's*	1 Tsp/10ml	19	188	7.0	19.0	9.3	1.6
English, Marks & Spencer*	1 Tsp/6g	14	226	12.6	8.7	15.9	1.0
English, Powder, Colman's*	1 Tsp/5g	26	518	29.0	24.0	34.0	6.2
English, Tesco*	1 Serving/10g	17	171	7.0	20.2	6.4	0.4
English, With Chillies, Sainsbury's*	1 Tsp/5g	10	204	8.3	18.1	10.9	6.4
French Mild, Colman's*	1 Tsp/6g	6	104	6.3	4.0	7.0	3.8
French, Dark, Sainsbury's*	1 Tsp/5g	4	76	5.1	3.7	4.5	0.0

	Measure INFO/WEIGHT	per Measure KCAL	Nutrition Values per 100g / 100ml				
			KCAL	PROT	CARB	FAT	FIBRE
MUSTARD							
French, Frank Cooper*	1 Tsp/6g	7	113	4.6	7.0	7.4	0.0
German Style, Sainsbury's*	1 Serving/10g	9	92	5.5	2.8	6.5	0.0
Honey, Colman's*	1 Tsp/6g	12	208	7.4	24.0	8.2	0.0
Mayonnaise, BGTY, Sainsbury's*	1 Tsp/6g	9	146	2.9	13.4	8.8	0.5
Peppercorn, Colman's*	1 Tsp/6g	11	182	8.8	12.0	10.0	4.9
Powder	1 Tsp/3.3g	14	452	28.9	20.7	28.7	0.0
Powder, Made Up	1oz/28g	63	226	14.5	10.4	14.4	0.0
Smooth	1 Tsp/8g	11	139	7.1	9.7	8.2	0.0
Sweet Peppers, Colman's*	1 Tsp/6g	13	218	7.9	20.0	11.0	4.9
Tarragon, Tesco*	1 Tbsp/15ml	59	396	0.9	8.6	39.8	0.2
Whole Grain	1 Tsp/8g	11	140	8.2	4.2	10.2	4.9
Whole Grain, Colman's*	1 Tsp/6g	9	157	8.4	12.0	8.4	6.6
MUSTARD							
Whole Grain, Sainsbury's*	1 Tsp/5g	7	137	6.5	4.2	10.5	0.0
MUSTARD							
Whole Grain, Tesco*	1 Tsp/6g	9	153	8.2	8.7	9.5	5.8
Whole Grain, With Green Peppercorns, Finest, Tesco*	1 Serving/20g	41	205	7.9	22.0	9.5	3.3
MUSTARD CRESS							
Raw	1oz/28g	4	13	1.6	0.4	0.6	1.1

	Measure INFO/WEIGHT	per Measure KCAL	Nutrition Values per 100g / 100ml				
			KCAL	PROT	CARB	FAT	FIBRE
NACHOS							
American Chilli Beef, Asda*	1 Serving/200g	208	104	10.0	4.7	5.0	0.8
Cheesy, Morrisons*	1/2 Box/150g	299	199	8.7	20.7	9.0	1.8
Chicken, Safeway*	1/2 Pack/170g	352	207	10.3	15.7	11.4	1.8
Chilli, Sainsbury's*	1/2 Pack/250g	695	278	10.9	29.5	12.9	1.3
Kit, Old El Paso*	1/2 Pack/260g	598	230	4.0	31.0	10.0	0.0
NASI GORENG							
Indonesian, Asda*	1 Pack/360g	778	216	7.4	32.3	6.3	1.3
NECTAR							
Blackcurrant, Vitafit, Lidl*	1fl oz/30ml	17	56	0.3	12.8	0.1	0.0
NECTARINES							
Average	1 Med/140g	53	38	1.3	8.5	0.1	1.2
NESQUIK							
Chocolate Flavour, Dry, Nestle*	3 Tsp/15g	57	377	4.9	82.5	3.0	5.0
Strawberry, Dry, Nestle*	1 Serving/10g	39	390	0.0	96.7	0.5	0.0
NIBBLES							
Cheese & Ham, Sainsbury's*	1/2 Pack/50g	257	514	13.1	54.8	27.1	2.6
NIK NAKS							
Cream 'n' Cheesy, Golden Wonder*	1 Bag/34g	185	545	5.1	56.1	33.4	0.0
Nice 'n' Spicy, Golden Wonder*	1 Bag/34g	184	541	4.7	55.5	33.4	1.0
Rib 'n' Saucy, Golden Wonder*	1 Bag/34g	185	545	5.1	55.7	33.5	1.1
Scampi 'n' Lemon, Golden Wonder*	1 Bag/34g	195	573	5.0	49.6	39.4	1.4
NOODLE BOWL							
Chilli Beef, Healthy Living, Tesco*	1 Bowl/400g	368	92	4.5	15.4	1.4	1.1
Chow Mein, Chicken, Uncle Ben's*	1 Pack/330g	307	93	6.1	13.5	1.4	0.0
Szechuan Style Prawn, Tesco*	1 Bowl/400g	376	94	5.5	17.3	0.3	0.9
NOODLE CUP							
Tom Yum, Hot & Spicy, Tiger Tiger*	1 Pot/90g	407	453	9.5	69.0	15.5	0.2
NOODLES							
& Bean Sprouts, Fresh Ideas, Tesco*	1 Pack/250g	310	124	5.4	19.8	2.6	1.9
Beef Flavour, Instant, Prepared, Heinz*	1 Pack/384g	257	67	2.1	14.4	0.1	0.6
Beef, Shanghai, Chef's Selection, Marks & Spencer*	1 Pack/352g	440	125	6.0	16.2	4.2	1.6
Char Sui, Cantonese, Sainsbury's*	1 Pack/450g	378	84	6.8	10.5	1.6	1.5
Chicken & Red Thai, Easy Steam, Tesco*	1 Serving/400g	556	139	10.3	8.6	7.1	1.1
Chicken Flavour, 3 Minute, Dry, Blue Dragon*	1 Pack/85g	403	475	9.3	61.2	21.4	0.0
Chicken Flavour, Dry, Princes*	1 Pack/85g	395	465	10.0	63.8	18.8	0.0
Chicken Flavour, Instant, Cooked, Sainsbury's*	1 Pack/335g	409	122	2.7	18.0	4.4	0.1
Chicken Flavour, Instant, Value, Tesco*	1 Serving/65g	82	126	3.2	20.7	3.4	0.9
Chicken, Chinese Style, GFY, Asda*	1 Pack/393g	295	75	6.0	9.0	1.7	0.6
Chicken, Chinese, Asda*	1 Pot/302g	305	101	6.0	16.0	1.4	0.8
Chicken, Dry, Heinz*	1 Serving/85g	257	302	9.5	65.3	0.4	2.7
Chicken, Instant, Less Than 1% Fat, Heinz*	1 Pack/385g	258	67	2.1	14.4	0.1	0.6
Chicken, Instant, Prepared, Heinz*	1 Pack/384g	257	67	2.1	14.4	0.1	0.6
Chicken, Snack In A Pot, Dry, Healthy Living, Tesco*	1 Pot/62g	226	363	13.5	73.3	1.8	2.5
Chilli Beef, Finest, Tesco*	1 Pack/450g	486	108	7.7	15.2	1.9	0.9
Chilli Chicken, GFY, Asda*	1 Pack/415g	461	111	6.0	20.0	0.8	1.0
Chilli Chicken, Sweet, Healthy Eating, Tesco*	1 Serving/400g	392	98	4.4	17.1	1.3	1.0
Chilli Chicken, Take Away, Marks & Spencer*	1 Pack/250g	325	130	9.6	15.2	3.1	1.3
Chinese, Egg, Thick, Dry, Sharwood's*	1 Serving/100g	343	343	11.0	70.9	1.8	2.5
Chinese, Stir Fry, Sainsbury's*	1 Serving/100g	185	185	6.0	29.5	4.8	1.5
Chow Mein Flavour, Dry, Princes*	1 Pack/85g	396	466	10.1	64.6	18.6	0.0
Chow Mein, Instant, Made Up, Tesco*	1 Pack/167.5g	255	152	3.8	23.0	5.0	1.2
Chow Mein, Sainsbury's*	1 Pack/125g	136	109	3.9	19.2	1.8	0.8
Chow Mein, Stir Fry, Tesco*	1 Serving/200g	116	58	2.1	9.7	1.2	1.0

NOODLES

INFO/WEIGHT	Measure	per Measure KCAL	Nutrition Values per 100g / 100ml KCAL	PROT	CARB	FAT	FIBRE
Crab Flavour, Dry, 3 Minute, Blue Dragon*	1 Pack/85g	393	463	9.9	62.6	19.2	0.0
Crispy, Dry, Blue Dragon*	1 Box/125g	438	350	2.4	84.0	0.5	0.0
Curry Flavour, Instant, Sainsbury's*	1 Pack/335g	412	123	2.6	17.8	4.6	0.1
Curry Flavour, Instant, Value, Made Up, Tesco*	1 Pack/65g	83	127	3.1	20.3	3.7	0.8
Curry, Instant, Dry, Heinz*	1 Serving/85g	261	307	9.5	66.4	0.4	2.7
Curry, Prepared, Heinz*	1 Pack/85g	58	68	2.1	14.6	0.1	0.6
Dry, Sharwood's*	1 Serving/125g	429	343	11.0	70.9	1.8	2.5
Egg Fried, Cantonese, Safeway*	1oz/28g	29	104	3.4	10.7	5.3	1.1
Egg, & Bean Sprouts, Cooked, Tesco*	1 Pack/250g	238	95	4.4	14.6	2.1	1.5
Egg, Boiled	1oz/28g	17	62	2.2	13.0	0.5	0.6
Egg, Dry	1oz/28g	109	391	12.1	71.7	8.2	2.9
Egg, Ramen, Fresh, The Original Noodle Company*	1 Serving/62.5g	188	298	11.3	57.0	2.7	0.0
Egg, Straight To Wok, Amoy*	1/2 Pack/75g	113	151	4.2	29.0	2.1	1.3
Egg, Tossed In Sesame Oil, Asda*	1/2 Pack/150g	174	116	2.3	11.0	7.0	0.0
Fried	1oz/28g	43	153	1.9	11.3	11.5	0.5
Instant, Express, Dry, Blue Dragon*	1 Serving/75g	338	450	10.0	65.0	17.0	2.0
Instant, Fat Free, Koka*	1 Piece/80g	143	179	6.2	38.5	0.0	1.0
Japanese Udon, Sainsbury's*	1 Serving/150g	210	140	3.9	27.1	1.8	1.2
Medium, Straight To Wok*	1oz/28g	47	169	6.0	24.5	5.2	0.0
Mung Bean, Dry, Amoy*	1oz/28g	95	341	15.9	66.6	1.2	0.0
Oriental Beef & Sweet Red Pepper, Dry, Colman's*	1 Serving/80g	254	317	4.2	73.4	0.7	5.1
Oriental Style, Break, Dry, Asda*	1 Pot/57g	218	382	12.3	80.7	1.2	2.5
Oriental, Chinese, Tesco*	1 Pack/200g	184	92	2.8	14.7	2.5	1.0
Oriental, Snack Pot, Dry, Healthy Living, Tesco*	1 Pot/57g	210	369	14.0	74.4	1.7	2.0
Peking Duck, Shapers, Boots*	1 Pack/280g	395	141	7.2	25.0	1.4	1.8
Plain, Boiled	1oz/28g	17	62	2.4	13.0	0.4	0.7
Plain, Dry	1oz/28g	109	388	11.7	76.1	6.2	2.9
Prawn Satay, Safeway*	1 Serving/400g	460	115	5.3	12.4	4.6	1.8
Prawn, Instant, Made Up, Tesco*	1 Serving/168g	251	150	3.8	21.9	5.2	1.3
Ramen, With Chilli Beef, Marks & Spencer*	1 Pack/484g	532	110	8.1	11.9	3.6	0.8
Rice, Dry, Blue Dragon*	1 Serving/30g	113	376	7.0	84.0	0.0	0.0
Rice, Oriental, Thai, Stir Fry, Dry, Sharwood's*	1 Serving/62.5g	227	361	6.5	86.8	1.0	2.4
Rice, Straight To Wok, Amoy*	1 Serving/75g	87	116	1.6	27.4	0.1	0.0
Rice, Thick, Thai, Dry, Marks & Spencer*	1 Serving/100g	355	355	6.5	80.6	0.7	1.4
Savoury Vegetable, COU, Marks & Spencer*	1 Pack/450g	270	60	2.9	11.5	0.6	1.2
Singapore Spicy, Safeway*	1 Serving/225g	270	120	6.0	14.2	4.3	1.7
Singapore Style, Asda*	1 Pack/400g	688	172	7.0	18.0	8.0	1.0
Singapore, New, Marks & Spencer*	1 Pack/400g	540	135	5.3	14.6	5.9	0.6
Singapore, Sainsbury's*	1 Pack/350g	312	89	6.8	6.1	4.1	2.2
Singapore, Straight To Wok, Amoy*	1 Serving/150g	233	155	4.8	28.4	2.8	0.0
Singapore, Tesco*	1 Pack/350g	389	111	6.3	16.8	2.1	0.7
Special, Chinese Takeaway, Iceland*	1 Pack/340g	422	124	6.5	17.2	3.2	0.6
Spicy Curry Flavour, Dry, Princes*	1 Pack/85g	395	465	9.6	64.1	18.8	0.0
Spicy Thai, Instant, Heinz*	1 Packet/385g	262	68	2.1	14.6	0.1	0.6
Spicy, Sainsbury's*	1 Serving/180g	182	101	10.4	4.5	4.6	0.9
Stir Fry, Tesco*	1 Serving/150g	203	135	5.3	23.0	2.4	1.5
Straight to Wok, Amoy*	1 Pack/180g	272	151	4.2	29.0	2.1	1.3
Straight to Wok, New, Amoy*	1 Serving/150g	240	160	5.8	31.7	1.5	0.0
Super, Bacon, Dry Weight, Batchelors*	1 Pack/100g	457	457	9.8	60.9	19.7	3.2
Super, Barbecue Beef, Made Up, Batchelors*	1 Serving/100g	156	156	3.2	20.9	6.7	1.1
Super, Chicken & Ham, Dry Weight, Batchelors*	1 Pack/100g	472	472	9.4	63.2	20.2	1.5
Super, Chicken & Herb, 98% Fat Free, Batchelors*	1 Serving/85g	291	342	11.0	71.5	1.3	2.6
Super, Chicken Flavour, Dry Weight, Batchelors*	1 Serving/100g	449	449	8.7	60.3	19.2	2.5

N

NOODLES

	INFO/WEIGHT	KCAL	KCAL	PROT	CARB	FAT	FIBRE
Super, Chow Mein Flavour, Made Up, Batchelors*	1 Serving/100g	158	158	3.2	20.9	6.8	1.0
Super, Mild Curry, Dry Weight, Batchelors*	1 Pack/100g	457	457	9.5	60.6	19.7	3.0
Super, Mushroom Flavour, Made Up, Batchelors*	1 Serving/100g	157	157	3.2	20.9	6.8	1.0
Super, Southern Fried Chicken, Made Up, Batchelors*	1 Serving/100g	171	171	3.3	23.2	7.2	0.5
Super, Spiced Beef, 98% Fat Free, Made Up, Batchelors*	1 Pack/271g	235	108	3.3	22.9	0.4	0.9
Super, Spicy Balti, Made Up, Batchelors*	1 Serving/100g	166	166	3.0	21.5	7.5	1.1
Super, Spicy Salsa, Dry Weight, Batchelors*	1 Pack/105g	474	451	7.0	63.8	18.6	1.7
Sweet & Sour, BGTY, Sainsbury's*	1 Serving/100g	112	112	2.3	18.6	3.1	0.0
Sweet Chilli, Wok, Findus*	1 Pack/300g	300	100	3.0	20.0	0.5	0.0
Sweet Thai Chilli Noodles, 98% Fat Free, Batchelors*	1 Serving/270.4g	292	108	3.3	22.8	0.4	0.9
Szechuan Beef Flavour, Dry, Blue Dragon*	1/2 Pack/100g	350	350	10.5	72.3	1.2	0.0
Thai Chicken, Takeaway, Somerfield*	1 Pack/300g	426	142	7.8	16.0	5.6	0.8
Thai Stir Fry Rice, Dry, Sharwood's*	1 Portion/60g	217	361	6.5	86.8	1.0	2.4
Thai Style, GFY, Asda*	1 Pot/237.9g	226	95	3.0	20.0	0.3	0.8
Thai Style, Sainsbury's*	1 Pack/340g	381	112	3.3	19.4	2.3	0.7
Thai, Spicy, Stir Fry, Healthy Living, Tesco*	1/2 Pack/250g	163	65	2.5	8.1	2.5	1.2
Thai, Waitrose*	1 Pack/300g	357	119	6.8	18.4	2.1	1.7
Thread, Fine, Straight To Wok, Amoy*	1 Packet/150g	237	158	5.0	28.7	2.6	0.0
Tiger Prawn, Stir Fry, Tesco*	1 Pack/400g	596	149	6.0	23.0	3.7	2.7
Traditional, Medium, Amoy*	1 Serving/75g	120	160	5.8	31.7	1.5	0.0
Udon Japanese, & Dashi Soup Stock, Yutaka*	1 Pack/230g	290	126	3.0	26.8	0.5	0.0
Udon, New, Amoy*	1 Portion/150g	212	141	4.4	28.8	1.3	0.0
Whole Wheat, Dry, Blue Dragon*	1 Serving/65g	208	320	12.5	63.0	2.0	8.0
Won Ton Flavour, 3 Minute, Dry, Blue Dragon*	1 Serving/80g	370	463	9.1	62.2	19.7	0.0

NOUGAT

Almond & Cherry, Marks & Spencer*	1 Sweet/7g	28	405	4.5	76.0	9.1	1.1
Average	1oz/28g	108	384	4.4	77.3	8.5	0.9
Bassetts & Beyond, Cadbury*	1oz/28g	105	375	4.0	82.0	4.0	0.0
Raspberry & Orange Hazelnut, Thorntons*	1 Chocolate/9g	39	433	4.8	60.0	20.0	2.2
Soft, Bar, Bassett's*	1 Serving/25g	94	375	4.0	82.0	4.0	0.0

NUGGETS

Meat Free, Blue Parrot Cafe, Sainsbury's*	1 Nugget/18g	41	228	17.3	12.5	12.1	3.0
Vegetarian, Safeway*	4 Nuggets/80.1g	161	201	16.3	10.5	10.4	3.6

NURISHMENT

Dunn's River*	1 Serving/420ml	420	100	5.0	14.6	2.6	0.0

NUT ROAST

Average	1oz/28g	99	352	13.3	18.3	25.7	4.2
Courgette & Spiced Tomato, Cauldron*	1 Serving/100g	208	208	11.7	12.5	12.3	4.9
Leek, Cheese & Mushroom, Organic, Cauldron*	1/2 Pack/143g	343	240	13.2	13.2	14.9	4.1
Lentil	1oz/28g	62	222	10.6	18.8	12.1	3.8
Tomato & Courgette, Vegetarian, Organic, Waitrose*	1/2 Pack/142g	295	208	11.7	12.5	12.3	4.9
Vegetarian, Tesco*	1 Serving/160g	218	136	5.4	11.4	7.6	2.0

NUTMEG

Powder	1 Tsp/3g	16	525	5.8	45.3	36.3	0.0

NUTRI-GRAIN

Apple, Kellogg's*	1 Bar/37g	131	353	4.0	66.0	9.0	3.5
Blueberry, Kellogg's*	1 Bar/37g	130	351	4.0	66.0	9.0	4.0
Cappuccino, Kellogg's*	1 Bar/37g	137	370	4.5	66.0	10.0	2.5
Cherry, Kellogg's*	1 Bar/37g	129	348	4.0	67.0	8.0	4.0
Chocolate, Kellogg's*	1 Bar/37g	136	367	4.5	66.0	8.0	4.0
Elevenses, Ginger, Kellogg's*	1 Bar/45g	168	373	5.0	68.0	9.0	3.0
Elevenses, Kellogg's*	1 Bar/45g	162	360	5.0	67.0	8.0	3.5
Minis, Apple, Kellogg's*	1 Pack/45g	158	350	3.5	71.0	7.0	3.5

	Measure INFO/WEIGHT	per Measure KCAL	Nutrition Values per 100g / 100ml				
			KCAL	PROT	CARB	FAT	FIBRE
NUTRI-GRAIN							
Minis, Blueberry, Kellogg's*	1 Bag/45g	163	363	4.0	69.0	9.0	3.5
Minis, Strawberry, Kellogg's*	1 Pack/45g	158	350	4.0	69.0	8.0	3.5
Minis, Strawberry, Yoghurty, Kellogg's*	10g	36	361	4.5	68.0	9.0	3.5
Orange, Kellogg's*	1 Bar/37g	129	349	4.0	65.0	9.0	4.0
Strawberry, Kellogg's*	1 Bar/37g	131	355	4.0	67.0	9.0	3.5
Tangy Orange, Kellogg's*	1 Bar/38g	141	370	5.0	68.0	9.0	4.0
Twists, Forest Fruits & Yoghurt, Kellogg's*	1 Bar/37g	133	360	4.0	69.0	8.0	2.0
Twists, Mixed Fruits, Kellogg's*	1 Bar/37g	133	360	3.5	69.0	8.0	2.0
Twists, Strawberry, Kellogg's*	1 Bar/37g	130	350	4.0	68.0	8.0	3.0
Yoghurty Raspberry, Kellogg's*	1 Bar/37g	134	361	4.5	68.0	9.0	3.5
Yoghurty Strawberry, Kellogg's*	1 Bar/37g	134	361	4.5	68.0	9.0	3.5
NUTS							
Clusters, Sweet Tomato Salsa, Sensations, Walkers*	1 Serving/35g	187	535	14.0	36.0	37.0	5.0
Honey Roasted, Marks & Spencer*	1oz/28g	175	625	18.1	20.5	52.2	5.1
Lemon & Chilli Flavour, Mix, TTD, Sainsbury's*	1 Serving/50g	321	641	20.0	11.2	57.3	5.7
Luxury Assortment, Tesco*	1 Serving/10g	68	676	17.5	6.1	64.6	5.0
Luxury, Organic, Marks & Spencer*	1oz/28g	179	640	21.1	11.6	56.6	6.1
Mixed	1 Pack/40g	243	607	22.9	7.9	54.1	6.0
Mixed, Chopped, Sainsbury's*	1 Serving/100g	605	605	27.1	9.6	50.9	6.0
Mixed, Feast, Eat Natural*	1 Bar/50g	278	556	18.8	28.0	41.0	0.0
Mixed, Honey Roasted, Waitrose*	1 Serving/50g	292	583	17.1	27.5	45.0	5.3
Mixed, Luxury, Unsalted, Somerfield*	1oz/28g	186	663	18.0	10.0	61.0	0.0
Mixed, Marks & Spencer*	1 Serving/25g	166	665	18.2	4.4	63.7	7.4
Mixed, Nature's Harvest*	1 Serving/25g	166	662	16.0	5.6	63.9	5.6
Mixed, Organic, Waitrose*	1oz/28g	179	640	19.3	7.7	59.1	8.4
Mixed, Roasted, Salted, Waitrose*	1 Pack/200g	1252	626	13.7	11.3	58.4	4.4
Mixed, Sainsbury's*	1oz/28g	188	673	18.8	4.6	64.5	5.3
Mixed, Unsalted, Sainsbury's*	1 Serving/50g	311	622	18.5	7.2	57.7	8.7
Natural Assortment, Tesco*	1 Serving/50g	338	676	17.5	6.1	64.6	5.0
Natural, Mixed, Waitrose*	1 Serving/50g	324	648	17.7	6.8	61.1	8.2
Oak Smoke Flavour Selection, Finest, Tesco*	1 Serving/25g	158	633	21.4	11.2	55.8	6.3
Peanuts & Cashews, Honey Roast, Tesco*	1 Serving/25g	145	579	21.6	26.6	42.9	4.2
Roast Salted, Luxury, KP*	1oz/28g	181	646	21.9	10.1	57.6	5.9
Roasted, Salted, Assortment, Luxury, Tesco*	1 Serving/25g	161	643	21.1	9.4	57.9	8.1
Salted, Selection, Sainsbury's*	1 Serving/30g	190	634	20.6	9.7	56.9	8.2
Salted, Selection, TTD, Sainsbury's*	1 Pack/75g	509	678	16.3	8.9	64.2	7.2
Unsalted, Selection, Sainsbury's*	1 Serving/75g	491	655	14.7	5.0	64.0	6.7
NUTS & RAISINS							
Mixed	1 Pack/40g	192	481	14.1	31.5	34.1	4.5
Mixed, KP*	1 Serving/50g	273	546	21.4	24.4	40.3	5.2
Mixed, Natural, Waitrose*	1 Serving/50g	251	501	19.0	26.8	35.3	5.7
Mixed, Nature's Harvest*	1 Serving/50g	232	463	12.4	32.9	33.7	3.4
Mixed, Tesco*	1 Serving/50g	256	512	16.1	31.0	36.0	4.8
Mixed, Unsalted, Sainsbury's*	1oz/28g	143	510	16.2	28.0	37.0	4.8
Peanuts, Average	1 Pack/40g	174	435	15.3	37.5	26.0	4.4
Yoghurt Coated, Waitrose*	1 Serving/50g	264	527	10.9	38.2	36.7	3.0

	Measure INFO/WEIGHT	per Measure KCAL	Nutrition Values per 100g / 100ml				
			KCAL	PROT	CARB	FAT	FIBRE
OATCAKES							
Cheese, Nairn's*	1 Cake/8g	38	471	13.4	54.0	25.1	6.2
Fine, Nairn's*	1 Oatcake/7g	32	455	10.2	62.5	21.9	8.8
Highland, Organic, Sainsbury's*	1 Oatcake/12.5g	59	456	10.2	59.8	19.5	5.5
Nairn's*	1 Oatcake/10g	43	429	11.7	63.5	17.7	7.8
No Wheat, No Sugar, Orgainic, Nairn's*	1 Oatcake/10g	43	423	8.8	70.2	16.0	9.3
Organic, The Village Bakery*	1 Cake/12.5g	59	452	10.9	54.5	21.3	5.6
Retail	1oz/28g	123	441	10.0	63.0	18.3	0.0
Rough Scottish, Sainsbury's*	1 Oatcake/11g	51	462	12.3	59.9	19.3	6.5
Rough With Bran, Walkers*	1 Oatcake/13g	59	454	10.2	53.3	22.2	7.8
Rough, Nairn's*	1 Oatcake/11g	48	436	10.6	64.7	18.2	7.2
Rough, Naturally Nutritious, Nairn's*	1 Cake/11g	46	429	11.7	63.5	17.7	7.8
Rough, Organic, Nairn's*	1 Oatcake/11g	47	428	10.9	57.7	17.0	7.6
Rough, Scottish, Tesco*	1 Oatcake/11g	48	434	12.3	54.8	18.4	6.6
Rough, Traditional, Nairn's*	1 Oatcake/11g	47	429	11.7	63.5	17.7	7.8
Scottish With Cracked Black Pepper, Finest, Tesco*	1 Pack/64g	276	431	11.3	57.6	17.2	9.2
Scottish, Marks & Spencer*	1oz/28g	116	413	9.1	70.0	12.6	8.5
Scottish, Patersons*	1 Cake/12.5g	49	409	11.1	58.6	14.5	8.5
Suncakes*	1 Oatcake/65g	164	252	10.8	44.6	2.9	7.7
Traditional, Marks & Spencer*	1 Cake/11g	49	445	11.0	59.3	18.3	6.6
With Cracked Black Pepper, Walkers*	1 Oatcake/9.5g	39	433	10.4	55.0	19.0	8.5
OATMEAL							
Raw	1oz/28g	112	401	12.4	72.8	8.7	6.8
OATS							
Easy, Original, Sainsbury's*	1 Serving/27g	97	359	11.0	60.4	8.1	8.5
Jumbo, Organic, Evernat*	1oz/28g	117	418	13.0	69.0	9.6	7.4
Porridge, Old Fashioned, Scotts*	1 Serving/45g	160	356	11.0	60.0	8.0	9.0
TTD, Sainsbury's*	1 Serving/40g	152	381	9.7	74.7	4.8	7.0
OCEAN							
Pinks, Asda*	1oz/28g	24	86	10.0	10.0	0.7	0.2
Prawnies, Mini, Asda*	1 Prawnie/11g	9	84	11.0	8.0	0.9	0.5
Snacks, Sainsbury's*	1 Stick/16g	18	113	7.0	21.0	0.1	0.1
Sticks, Average	1 Stick/16g	17	109	7.1	19.9	0.2	0.2
OCTOPUS							
Raw	1oz/28g	23	83	17.9	0.0	1.3	0.0
OIL							
Again & Again, No Cholesterol, Anglia*	1 Tbsp/15ml	124	828	0.0	0.0	92.0	0.0
Avocado, Olivado*	1 Tsp/5ml	40	802	0.0	0.0	88.0	0.0
Black Truffle Grapeseed, Cuisine Perel*	1 Tbsp/15ml	129	857	0.0	7.1	100.0	0.0
Carotino*	1 Tsp/5ml	40	804	0.0	0.0	92.0	0.0
Chilli, Average	1 Tsp/5ml	41	824	0.0	0.0	91.5	0.0
Chinese Stir Fry, Asda*	1 Tbsp/15ml	123	823	0.0	0.0	91.4	0.0
Coconut	1 Tsp/5ml	45	899	0.0	0.0	99.9	0.0
Cod Liver	1 Capsule/1g	9	900	0.0	0.0	100.0	0.0
Corn, Average	1 Tsp/5ml	43	865	0.0	0.0	96.0	0.0
Dipping, Herb, Italian Style, Finest, Tesco*	1 Serving/5g	44	877	0.4	0.9	96.9	0.4
Evening Primrose	1 Serving/1g	9	900	0.0	0.0	100.0	0.0
Fish	1 Serving/1g	9	900	0.0	0.0	100.0	0.0
Flax Seed, Average	1 Tbsp/14ml	116	829	0.0	0.0	92.6	0.0
Fry Light, Bodyline*	4 Sprays/0.8ml	5	522	0.0	0.0	55.2	0.0
Grapeseed, Average	1 Tsp/5ml	43	866	0.1	0.0	96.2	0.0
Groundnut, Average	25ml	206	824	0.0	0.0	91.8	0.0
Hazelnut	1 Tsp/5ml	45	899	0.0	0.0	99.9	0.0
Linseed, Organic, Biona*	1 Serving/10ml	84	837	0.0	0.0	93.0	0.0

	Measure INFO/WEIGHT	per Measure KCAL	Nutrition Values per 100g / 100ml				
			KCAL	PROT	CARB	FAT	FIBRE
OIL							
Olive, Average	1 Serving/5ml	43	855	0.0	0.0	94.9	0.0
Olive, Basil Infused, Tesco*	1 Serving/20ml	180	900	0.0	0.0	100.0	0.0
Olive, Extra Virgin, Average	1 Tbsp/15ml	127	848	0.0	0.0	94.5	0.0
Olive, Extra Virgin, Mist Spray, Belolive*	1fl oz/30ml	150	500	0.0	0.0	55.0	0.0
Olive, Garlic, Average	1 Tbsp/15ml	127	848	0.0	0.0	94.3	0.0
Olive, Lemon Flavoured, Sainsbury's*	1 Tbsp/15ml	123	823	0.1	0.0	91.4	0.1
Olive, Mild, Average	1 Tbsp/15mll	129	862	0.1	0.0	95.7	0.0
Olive, Spray, Fry Light*	5 Sprays/1ml	5	498	0.0	0.0	55.2	0.0
Palm	1 Tsp/5ml	45	899	0.0	0.0	99.9	0.0
Peanut	1 Tsp/5ml	45	899	0.0	0.0	99.9	0.0
Rapeseed, Average	1 Tbsp/15ml	130	864	0.0	0.0	96.0	0.0
Safflower	1 Tsp/5ml	45	899	0.0	0.0	99.9	0.0
Sesame, Average	1 Tsp/5ml	45	892	0.1	0.0	99.9	0.0
Soya	1 Tsp/5ml	45	899	0.0	0.0	99.9	0.0
Stir Fry, Sharwood's*	1fl oz/30ml	269	897	0.0	0.0	99.7	0.0
Sunflower, Average	1 Tbsp/15ml	130	869	0.0	0.0	96.6	0.0
Sunflower, Fry Light Spray	1 Spray/0.2ml	1	522	0.0	0.0	55.2	0.0
Ultimate Blend, Udo's Choice*	1 Capsule/1ml	9	900	1.3	0.0	96.8	0.0
Vegetable, Average	1 Tbsp/15ml	129	858	0.0	0.0	95.3	0.0
Walnut	1 Tsp/5ml	45	899	0.0	0.0	99.9	0.0
Wheatgerm	1 Tsp/5ml	45	899	0.0	0.0	99.9	0.0
OKRA							
Boiled in Unsalted Water	1oz/28g	8	28	2.5	2.7	0.9	3.6
Canned, Drained	1oz/28g	6	21	1.4	2.5	0.7	2.6
Raw	1oz/28g	9	31	2.8	3.0	1.0	4.0
Stir-Fried in Corn Oil	1oz/28g	75	269	4.3	4.4	26.1	6.3
OLIVES							
Black, Pitted, Average	1/2 Jar/82g	135	164	1.0	3.5	16.2	3.1
Green, Garlic Stuffed, Asda*	1 Olive/3.4g	5	174	1.8	3.5	17.0	0.0
Green, Lightly Flavoured With Lemon & Garlic, Attis*	1 Serving/50g	82	164	1.7	2.2	16.5	0.0
Green, Pimiento Stuffed, Somerfield*	1 Olive/3g	4	126	1.0	4.0	12.0	0.0
Green, Pitted, Average	1 Olive/3g	4	130	1.1	0.9	13.3	2.5
Green, Pitted, Stuffed With Anchovies, Sainsbury's*	1 Serving/50g	78	155	1.8	0.6	16.1	3.2
Green, Queen, Sainsbury's*	1 Serving/10g	15	145	1.3	11.0	10.6	2.5
Green, Stuffed With Almonds, Pitted, Waitrose*	1 Serving/50g	90	180	3.8	3.2	16.9	2.5
Kalamata, Greek, Whole, Waitrose*	1 Serving/28g	30	107	1.0	3.8	9.8	3.4
Marinated, Selection, Marks & Spencer*	4 Olives/19.6g	45	225	1.4	3.9	22.6	2.1
Mixed, Marinated, Anti Pasti, Asda*	1 Serving/100g	215	215	1.8	0.7	22.0	3.1
Pimento Stuffed, In Brine, Tesco*	1 Serving/25g	38	153	0.8	0.1	16.4	2.1
Pitted, With Anchovy Paste, Safeway*	1/3 Can/50g	70	139	2.7	0.1	14.2	2.0
OMELETTE							
Cheese & Mushroom, Apetito*	1 Serving/320g	485	152	6.2	14.4	7.8	1.9
Cheese, 2 Egg	1 Omelette/180g	479	266	15.9	0.0	22.6	0.0
Cheese, Findus*	1 Serving/200g	400	200	9.5	14.0	13.0	0.0
Cheese, Tesco*	1 Serving/120g	270	225	11.4	3.7	18.3	0.0
Ham & Mushroom, Farmfoods*	1 Omelette/120g	200	167	8.7	1.8	13.9	0.1
Mushroom & Cheese, Tesco*	1 Omelette/120g	248	207	9.8	1.6	17.9	0.2
Plain, 2 Egg	1 Omelette/120g	229	191	10.9	0.0	16.4	0.0
Spanish	1oz/28g	34	120	5.7	6.2	8.3	1.4
ONION RINGS							
Asda*	1/4 Pack/25g	122	489	6.0	60.0	25.0	2.4
Battered, Asda*	1 Serving/100g	343	343	3.8	31.0	22.7	1.7
Battered, Oven Baked, Tesco*	1 Serving/50g	110	219	3.9	28.4	10.0	3.5

ONION RINGS

INFO/WEIGHT	KCAL	KCAL	PROT	CARB	FAT	FIBRE
Breadcrumbs, Tesco*	1 Serving/100g	294	294	4.3	34.1	15.6	2.3
Breaded, Asda*	1 Serving/10g	29	289	4.4	34.0	15.0	2.7
Breaded, Safeway*	1 Serving/44.7g	132	293	4.4	34.2	15.4	2.7
COU, Marks & Spencer*	1oz/28g	95	340	4.7	80.7	1.5	3.7
Hot & Spicy, Sainsbury's*	1 Serving/50g	159	318	4.9	36.2	17.1	4.8
Maize Snacks, Sainsbury's*	1/2 Pack/50g	240	479	8.5	57.8	23.8	3.9
Marks & Spencer*	1 Pack/40g	186	465	5.2	62.1	21.5	4.3
Oven Crisp Batter, Tesco*	1 Onion Ring/17g	40	236	4.2	24.8	13.3	2.5
Pickled, BGTY, Sainsbury's*	1 Bag/10g	35	345	5.0	81.7	1.5	3.7
Pickled, COU, Marks & Spencer*	1 Bag/20g	69	345	5.0	81.7	1.5	3.7
Pickled, Healthy Eating, Tesco*	1 Pack/15g	51	340	6.2	74.7	1.8	6.5
Red Mill*	1 Bag/50g	243	486	8.3	58.5	24.3	2.2
Tesco*	1 Serving/16g	77	481	7.5	58.1	24.4	11.9
Value, Tesco*	1 Bag/16g	77	482	7.6	58.3	24.3	2.5

ONIONS

Baked	1oz/28g	29	103	3.5	22.3	0.6	3.9
Boiled in Unsalted Water	1oz/28g	5	17	0.6	3.7	0.1	0.7
Dried, Raw	1oz/28g	88	313	10.2	68.6	1.7	12.1
Fried, Average	1oz/28g	46	164	2.3	14.1	11.2	3.1
Pickled, Average	1oz/28g	6	23	0.8	4.9	0.1	0.7
Raw, Average	1 Med Onion/90g	28	31	1.3	6.0	0.2	1.4
Red, Raw, Average	1 Onion/50g	18	37	1.2	7.9	0.2	1.5

OPTIONS*

Belgian Chocolate, Instant	1 Serving/11g	40	363	12.4	54.9	10.4	7.5
Belgian, Ovaltine	3 Tsp/11g	40	363	12.4	54.9	10.4	7.5
Caribbean Coconut	1 Serving/40g	146	364	15.1	50.7	11.2	0.0
Choca Mocha Drink	1 Sachet/11g	39	359	14.1	50.1	11.4	7.0
Chocolate Au Lait Drink	1 Sachet/10g	36	355	11.8	54.5	10.0	7.3
Diet Friendly	1 Sachet/11ml	40	364	14.3	50.6	11.6	7.1
Irish Cream	1 Sachet/10.9g	39	357	13.9	50.0	11.3	8.1
Irish Cream Drink	1 Sachet/10g	36	357	13.9	50.0	11.3	8.1
Mint Drink	1 Sachet/10g	37	365	15.0	50.6	11.4	7.1
Mint, Made Up	1 Serving/200ml	40	20	0.8	2.8	0.7	0.4
Orange Flavour	1 Serving/11ml	40	364	14.2	50.8	11.6	7.1
Outrageous Orange Drink	1 Sachet/10g	36	364	14.2	50.8	11.6	7.1
Outrageous Orange Flavour	1 Serving/11g	40	367	15.3	50.8	11.4	0.0
Pleasure	1 Sachet/18g	68	377	16.7	48.4	13.0	7.8
Toffee Drink	1 Sachet/13g	52	400	10.5	68.9	9.2	0.0
Turkish Delight Drink	1 Sachet/11g	40	364	15.1	50.4	11.3	7.2
Wicked White Chocolate	1 Sachet/11g	45	412	10.9	63.9	12.5	16.3

ORANGE DRINK

Active Sport, Tesco*	1 Bottle/500ml	135	27	0.0	6.5	0.0	0.0
Sparkling, Diet, Tesco*	1 Glass/250ml	8	3	0.1	0.5	0.1	0.0
Sparkling, Florida, Marks & Spencer*	1 Serving/500ml	250	50	0.0	12.5	0.0	0.0
Sparkling, Shapers, Boots*	1 Bottle/500ml	15	3	0.1	0.4	0.1	0.0

ORANGES

Fresh, Raw	1 Med/160g	59	37	1.1	8.5	0.1	1.7
Ruby Red, Tesco*	1 Orange/130g	51	39	1.1	8.5	0.1	1.7
Weighed With Peel & Pips	1oz/28g	7	26	0.8	5.9	0.1	1.2

OREGANO

Dried, Ground	1 Tsp/1g	3	306	11.0	49.5	10.3	0.0
Fresh	1oz/28g	18	66	2.2	9.7	2.0	0.0

INFO/WEIGHT	Measure	per Measure KCAL	Nutrition Values per 100g / 100ml				
			KCAL	PROT	CARB	FAT	FIBRE
OVALTINE*							
Hi Malt, Light, Instant Drink	1 Sachet/20g	72	358	9.1	67.1	5.9	2.8
Powder, Made Up With Semi-Skimmed Milk	1 Mug/227ml	179	79	3.9	13.0	1.7	0.0
Powder, Made Up With Whole Milk	1 Mug/227ml	220	97	3.8	12.9	3.8	0.0
OXTAIL							
Raw	1oz/28g	48	171	20.0	0.0	10.1	0.0
Stewed	1oz/28g	68	243	30.5	0.0	13.4	0.0
OYSTERS							
Raw	1oz/28g	18	65	10.8	2.7	1.3	0.0
in Vegetable Oil, Smoked, John West*	1oz/28g	64	230	16.0	10.0	14.0	0.0

	Measure INFO/WEIGHT	per Measure KCAL	Nutrition Values per 100g / 100ml				
			KCAL	PROT	CARB	FAT	FIBRE
PAELLA							
Big Dish Chicken & Chorizo, Marks & Spencer*	1 Pack/450g	630	140	7.9	18.4	3.9	1.6
Bistro, Waitrose*	1 Serving/300g	534	178	7.4	22.2	6.6	0.7
Chicken & Chorizo, Asda*	1 Pack/390g	484	124	10.0	16.0	2.2	2.6
Chicken & Vegetable, Healthy Living, Tesco*	1 Pack/450g	441	98	9.7	11.8	1.3	1.1
Chicken, Healthy Living, Tesco*	1 Pack/400g	432	108	6.7	19.2	0.5	1.7
Chicken, Steam Pack, Healthy Eating, Tesco*	1 Pack/350g	291	83	8.1	11.8	0.4	7.0
Chicken, Tesco*	1 Serving/475g	575	121	7.9	15.7	3.0	1.6
Enjoy, Birds Eye*	1 Pack/500g	620	124	7.7	16.2	3.2	0.6
Seafood, Finest, Tesco*	1 Pack/400g	756	189	6.8	27.2	5.9	1.0
Seafood, Sainsbury's*	1 Pack/400g	504	126	8.3	20.3	1.3	0.6
Spanish, TTD, Sainsbury's*	1/2 Dish/350g	448	128	7.9	15.9	3.6	0.2
TTD, Sainsbury's*	1 Pack/375g	386	103	8.3	16.9	0.2	3.1
Tesco*	1 Serving/460g	584	127	4.6	18.9	3.7	1.0
Vegetable, Waitrose*	1 Serving/174g	202	116	2.2	22.7	1.8	1.5
With Prawns, Chicken, Cod & Salmon, Sainsbury's*	1 Pack/750g	773	103	8.3	16.9	0.2	3.1
PAIN AU CHOCOLAT							
All Butter, Finest, Tesco*	1 Pain/78g	310	398	7.6	45.3	20.7	2.9
Extra Special, Asda*	1oz/28g	113	405	8.0	46.0	21.0	3.3
Marks & Spencer*	1 Pain/60g	210	350	5.9	38.0	19.2	1.6
Mini, Asda*	1 Chocolat/22.8g	97	421	9.0	49.0	21.0	2.2
Mini, Waitrose*	1 Serving/35g	159	454	8.5	42.3	27.9	2.1
Sainsbury's*	1 Serving/58g	241	415	7.9	42.5	23.7	3.3
Tesco*	1 Pain/56g	235	420	7.0	46.5	22.9	1.4
PAIN AU RAISIN							
Asda*	1 Pain/110g	421	383	7.0	46.0	19.0	2.5
Marks & Spencer*	1 Pain/74.1g	215	290	5.3	38.7	12.8	1.2
PAK CHOI							
Tesco*	1 Serving/100g	11	11	1.0	1.4	0.2	1.2
PAKORA							
Bhajia, Onion, Fried in Vegetable Oil	1oz/28g	76	271	9.8	26.2	14.7	5.5
Bhajia, Potato Carrot & Pea, Fried in Vegetable Oil	1oz/28g	100	357	10.9	28.8	22.6	6.1
Bhajia, Vegetable, Retail	1oz/28g	66	235	6.4	21.4	14.7	3.6
Potato & Spinach, Mini, Indian Snack Selection, Waitrose*	1 Pakora/21g	56	266	5.4	17.0	19.6	4.5
Prawn, Indian Appetisers, Waitrose*	1 Pakora/21g	35	165	16.8	5.9	8.2	1.5
Sainsbury's*	1 Pakora/55g	166	302	7.3	26.8	18.3	1.1
Spinach, Mini, Indian Selection, Somerfield*	1 Serving/22g	61	277	6.2	26.9	16.1	4.9
Vegetable, Indian Selection, Party, Co-Op*	1 Pakora/23g	47	205	6.0	28.0	7.0	4.0
Vegetable, Indian Starter Selection, Marks & Spencer*	1 Pakora/23g	61	265	6.3	19.6	18.1	2.9
Vegetable, Mini, Tesco*	1 Pakora/21g	36	173	6.0	16.8	9.1	4.9
Vegetable, Somerfield*	1 Pakora/15g	46	305	7.0	19.0	23.0	0.0
PANCAKE							
Apple & Sultana, Marks & Spencer*	1 Serving/80g	160	200	2.2	30.2	7.9	1.2
Apple, GFY, Asda*	1 Pancake/85g	114	134	4.2	24.0	2.5	1.0
Aunt Bessie's*	1 Pancake/60g	90	150	6.1	24.6	3.1	1.1
Bramley Apple, Sainsbury's*	1 Pancake/85g	114	134	4.2	23.6	2.5	1.0
Cherry, GFY, Asda*	1 Serving/206g	206	100	1.9	18.9	1.8	1.8
Chinatown, Asda*	1 Pancake/10g	34	335	10.9	51.7	9.2	2.4
Chinese Roll, Farmfoods*	1 Roll/88g	125	142	4.3	21.6	4.3	1.0
Chinese Style, Cherry Valley*	1 Pancake/8g	25	310	9.2	54.7	6.0	0.0
Chocolate, Marks & Spencer*	1 Pancake/80g	125	156	3.1	22.1	6.1	0.3
For Duck, Sainsbury's*	1 Pancake/50g	141	281	8.7	47.3	6.4	2.1
For Honey Chicken, Sainsbury's*	1 Pack/50g	146	293	8.0	51.6	6.1	5.3
Healthy Living, Tesco*	1 Panceake/30g	74	246	7.3	49.9	1.9	1.5

P

	Measure INFO/WEIGHT	per Measure KCAL	Nutrition Values per 100g / 100ml KCAL	PROT	CARB	FAT	FIBRE
PANCAKE							
Irish, Marks & Spencer*	1 Pancake/35g	85	243	7.1	53.8	1.4	1.3
Lemon, Marks & Spencer*	1 Pancake/38.3g	89	235	4.5	38.5	7.2	2.8
Maple & Raisin, Marks & Spencer*	1 Pancake/32.7g	89	269	6.5	49.7	5.4	2.2
Mini, For Kids, Tesco*	1 Pancake/16g	45	283	6.6	51.7	5.5	1.3
Morello Cherry, Iceland*	1 Pancake/129g	204	158	3.1	29.8	2.9	2.9
Morrisons*	1 Pancake/60g	133	221	8.4	37.3	5.0	1.5
North Staffordshire Oatcakes Ltd*	1 Pancake/71g	166	234	5.0	40.9	6.1	1.0
Perfect, Kingmill	1 Pancake/26.9g	71	264	6.2	49.7	4.5	1.2
Plain, Sainsbury's*	1 Pancake/63g	144	228	8.4	37.3	5.0	1.5
Raisin & Lemon, Tesco*	1 Pancake/36g	99	275	5.8	49.3	6.1	2.7
Sainsbury's*	2 Pancakes/92g	256	278	6.1	46.8	7.4	1.8
Savoury, Made With Skimmed Milk	1oz/28g	70	249	6.4	24.1	14.7	0.8
Savoury, Made With Whole Milk	1oz/28g	76	273	6.3	24.0	17.5	0.8
Scotch	1 Pancake/50g	146	292	5.8	43.6	11.7	1.4
Scotch, BGTY, Sainsbury's*	1 Pancake/30g	76	252	5.3	48.5	4.1	1.3
Scotch, Healthy Living, Tesco*	1 Pancake/30g	74	246	7.3	49.9	1.9	1.5
Scotch, Sainsbury's	1 Pancake/30g	98	337	7.5	54.4	9.9	1.6
Scotch, SmartPrice, Asda*	1 Pancake/35g	107	305	7.0	49.0	9.0	1.4
Sultana & Syrup Scotch, Sainsbury's*	1 Pancake/35g	113	322	6.7	55.2	8.3	1.7
Sweet, Made With Skimmed Milk	1oz/28g	78	280	6.0	35.1	13.8	0.8
Sweet, Made With Whole Milk	1oz/28g	84	301	5.9	35.0	16.2	0.8
Sweet, Raspberry Ripple Sauce, Findus*	1 Pancake/38.1g	80	210	3.9	37.1	4.7	0.9
Syrup, Tesco*	2 Pancakes/60g	175	291	7.0	48.4	7.7	1.9
Toffee Apple, Marks & Spencer*	1 Pancake/88.9g	160	180	2.2	32.6	4.7	1.5
Traditional, Tesco*	1 Pancake/62g	137	221	8.4	35.6	5.0	1.5
Vegetable Roll	1 Roll/85g	185	218	6.6	21.0	12.5	0.0
Warburtons*	1 Serving/28g	64	230	6.3	37.7	6.0	0.0
With Golden Syrup, Value, Tesco*	1 Pancake/27g	72	265	4.7	47.4	6.3	1.5
With Maple Sauce & Fromage Frais, BGTY, Sainsbury's*	1 Serving/100g	163	163	5.0	30.0	2.5	0.8
With Syrup, American Style, Large, Tesco*	2 Pancakes/76g	204	268	5.1	54.2	3.4	0.9
PANCAKE MIX							
Buttermilk, Krusteaz*	3 Pancakes/16.2g	56	352	11.3	66.0	4.7	3.4
Fresh, Marks & Spencer*	1 Pancake/38.3g	89	235	7.5	22.4	13.1	0.5
Traditional, Asda*	1 Pack/256g	545	213	6.0	27.0	9.0	1.8
PANCETTA							
Average	1/2 Pack/65g	212	327	17.0	0.1	28.7	0.1
Italian, Tesco*	1/2 Pack/60g	191	318	20.5	0.5	26.0	0.0
Smoked, Sainsbury's*	1 Slice/7g	23	345	18.8	0.1	30.0	0.1
PANEER							
Matar, Ashoka*	1/2 Pack/150g	183	122	5.3	10.0	6.7	2.0
PANINI							
Bacon, British Midland*	1 Serving/150g	273	182	9.1	21.6	6.6	0.0
Mozzarella & Tomato, Marks & Spencer*	1 Serving/176g	484	275	11.3	21.3	16.2	2.1
Tuna & Sweetcorn, Tesco*	1 Serving/250g	559	224	12.0	29.3	6.6	1.4
PAPAYA							
Dried, Strips, Tropical Wholefoods*	1 Strip/10g	310	310	3.9	71.4	0.9	1.5
Dried, Sweetened, Tesco*	4 Pieces/25g	59	235	0.4	56.3	0.9	2.9
Pieces, Nature's Harvest*	1 Serving/50g	178	355	0.2	85.4	0.0	2.6
Unripe, Raw, Weighed With Seeds & Skin	1oz/28g	8	27	0.9	5.5	0.1	1.5
PAPPADS							
Green Chilli & Garlic, Sharwood's*	1oz/28g	75	267	19.9	43.3	1.6	9.7
PAPPARDELLE							
Basil, Fresh, Sainsbury's*	1 Serving/240g	281	117	5.0	21.2	1.4	2.0

P

	Measure INFO/WEIGHT	per Measure KCAL	KCAL	PROT	CARB	FAT	FIBRE
PAPPARDELLE							
Buitoni*	1 Serving/65g	242	373	15.0	67.5	4.8	0.0
Chilli, Fresh, Sainsbury's*	1 Serving/250g	303	121	5.7	20.7	1.7	2.0
Cracked Black Pepper, Safeway*	1 Bowl/120g	173	144	5.7	26.5	1.8	1.9
Egg, Dry, Average	1 Serving/100g	364	364	14.1	68.5	3.7	2.1
Egg, Fresh, Waitrose*	1/4 Pack/125g	350	280	12.9	51.0	2.7	1.9
Salmon, COU, Marks & Spencer*	1 Pack/358g	340	95	6.3	13.0	1.9	0.8
PAPRIKA							
Average	1 Tsp/2g	6	289	14.8	34.9	13.0	0.0
PARATHA							
Average	1oz/28g	90	322	8.0	43.2	14.3	4.0
PARCELS							
Basil & Parmesan, Fresh, Sainsbury's*	1 Pack/250g	550	220	10.0	26.4	8.3	3.3
Beef Steak, Sainsbury's*	1/2 Pack/226g	488	216	12.2	6.6	15.6	1.0
Cheese & Ham, Sainsbury's*	1 Pack/250g	445	178	7.4	19.9	7.6	1.5
Chilli Beef, Tex Mex Feast, Asda*	1 Parcel/25g	68	270	9.0	27.0	14.0	2.1
Filo, Brie & Cranberry, Tesco*	1 Parcel/22g	82	373	9.5	29.3	24.2	1.5
Filo, Mushroom Leek & Gruyere, Finest, Tesco*	1 Serving/160g	490	306	6.8	20.4	22.0	0.9
Filo, Mushroom, Savoury, Creamy, Somerfield*	1oz/28g	86	308	5.0	24.0	21.0	0.0
Smoked Salmon, Sainsbury's*	1 Pack/115g	269	234	15.8	3.5	17.6	0.2
Sun Dried Tomato & Wild Mushrooml, The Best, Safeway*	1 Parcel/181g	483	267	8.8	41.8	7.2	4.2
Tomato & Mozarella, Fresh, Sainsbury's*	1 Serving/175g	340	194	7.5	23.0	8.0	3.4
Turkey Breast, With Cheddar Cheese & Chive, Asda*	1 Parcel/140g	242	173	23.0	4.6	7.0	0.9
With Cheese & Sweet Pepper Sauce, Egg, Somerfield*	1/2 Pack/125g	349	279	12.4	30.7	11.8	2.2
PARSLEY							
Dried	1 Tsp/1.3g	2	181	15.8	14.5	7.0	26.9
Fresh	1oz/28g	10	34	3.0	2.7	1.3	5.0
PARSNIP							
Boiled, Average	1oz/28g	18	66	1.6	12.9	1.2	4.7
Fragrant, Tesco*	1 Serving/50g	34	67	1.8	12.5	1.1	4.6
Honey Roasted, Tesco*	1 Serving/125g	203	162	1.9	20.0	8.2	2.2
Raw, Average	1oz/28g	19	66	1.8	12.5	1.1	4.6
PARTRIDGE							
Meat Only, Roasted	1oz/28g	59	212	36.7	0.0	7.2	0.0
PASANDA							
Chicken, Marks & Spencer*	1/2 Pack/150g	240	160	11.3	3.8	10.9	1.3
Chicken, Sainsbury's*	1 Serving/200g	368	184	14.7	3.4	12.4	2.3
Chicken, Waitrose*	1oz/28g	52	185	14.8	3.8	12.3	1.1
Chicken, With Pilau Rice, Healthy Living, Tesco*	1 Pack/440g	466	106	5.7	15.2	2.5	0.9
PASSION FRUIT							
Raw, Fresh	1 Fruit/15g	5	36	2.6	5.8	0.4	3.3
Weighed With Skin	1oz/28g	6	22	1.7	3.5	0.2	2.0
PASTA							
& Chargrilled Mushrooms, Finest, Tesco*	1 Pot/200g	404	202	5.4	16.7	12.5	1.3
& Flame Grilled Chicken, Marks & Spencer*	1 Pack/180g	414	230	8.2	17.5	14.0	0.8
& Roasted Vegetables, Waitrose*	1oz/28g	43	154	2.4	14.2	9.7	1.0
Amori, Waitrose*	1 Serving/200g	754	377	10.8	82.8	0.3	0.0
Bean & Tuna, BGTY, Sainsbury's*	1 Serving/200g	176	88	7.3	12.6	0.9	2.8
Blue Cheese, Bacon & Spinach, Marks & Spencer*	1 Pack/400g	640	160	6.5	13.8	8.5	0.7
Boccoletti, Dried, Sainsbury's*	1 Serving/125g	446	357	12.3	73.1	1.7	2.5
Carbonara, With Cheese & Bacon, SlimFast*	1 Serving/70g	240	343	22.7	48.9	6.3	5.7
Chargrilled Chicken Salsa, Healthy Eating, Tesco*	1 Pack/450g	396	88	7.3	11.7	1.3	1.0
Chargrilled Chicken, Asda*	1 Serving/250g	538	215	7.0	22.0	11.0	1.7
Cheese & Broccoli, Tubes, Tesco*	1 Serving/202g	319	158	5.0	19.1	6.9	2.3

PASTA

	Measure INFO/WEIGHT	per Measure KCAL	Nutrition Values per 100g / 100ml KCAL	PROT	CARB	FAT	FIBRE
Cheese & Ham, Shapers, Boots*	1 Pack/76g	220	289	23.7	34.2	6.5	6.5
Cheesy Spirals, Curly Whirly, Asda*	1/3 Pack/200g	214	107	6.0	15.0	2.6	0.5
Chicken & Green Pesto, Healthy Living, Tesco*	1 Serving/376g	440	117	8.3	18.5	1.2	1.4
Chicken & Ham, Easy Steam, Tesco*	1 Pack/400g	572	143	9.8	11.2	6.6	0.6
Chicken & Mushroom, Pasta & Sauce, Dry, Tesco*	1 Pack/120g	427	356	16.0	65.0	3.6	3.9
Chicken & Pineapple, Shapers, Boots*	1 Pack/221g	210	95	5.4	15.0	1.5	0.9
Chicken & Roasted Tomato, Healthy Living, Tesco*	1 Serving/374g	426	114	7.4	16.7	1.9	1.3
Chicken & Spinach, Waitrose*	1 Pack/350g	483	138	7.0	14.0	6.0	0.8
Chicken & Tomato, Classic, Mini, Tesco*	1 Pack/300g	165	55	6.6	1.7	2.4	1.7
Chicken & Vegetable, Mediterranean, Waitrose*	1 Serving/400g	375	94	7.5	10.5	2.3	2.2
Chicken, Cheese, & Bacon, Italiano, Tesco*	1 Pack/400g	680	170	10.9	13.7	8.0	1.2
Chicken, Tomato & Basil, Healthy Living, Tesco*	1 Pack/400g	264	66	7.9	7.5	0.5	1.1
Chicken, Tomato & Herb, Easy Steam, Tesco*	1 Serving/400g	528	132	8.9	10.2	6.2	1.3
Chicken, Tomato & Mascarpone, Heathly Living, Tesco*	1 Pack/450g	504	112	7.5	14.8	2.5	1.1
Chicken, Tomato, & Basil, Asda*	1 Pack/400g	474	119	6.5	17.5	2.5	1.2
Chicken, Tomato, & Mascarpone, Italiano, Tesco*	1 Pack/400g	572	143	7.4	14.3	6.2	1.3
Creamy Garlic Mushroom, Healthy Living, Tesco*	1 Serving/100g	106	106	3.6	14.6	3.7	1.1
Creamy Mushroom, Sainsbury's*	1 Serving/63g	148	237	4.5	21.7	14.6	1.2
Elicoidali, Waitrose*	1 Serving/200g	682	341	11.5	70.7	1.3	3.7
Fagottini, Wild Mushroom, Sainsbury's*	1/2 Pack/125g	274	219	10.2	27.7	7.5	2.7
Florentina, With Broccoli & Spinach, SlimFast*	1 Serving/71g	239	336	23.0	50.5	4.6	5.8
Garlic Mushroom Filled, Extra Special, Asda*	1 Serving/125g	224	179	8.0	21.0	7.0	2.5
Honey & Mustard Chicken, Somerfield*	1 Serving/200g	280	140	8.5	18.0	3.7	1.0
Lumache, Tesco*	1 Serving/100g	345	345	13.2	68.5	2.0	2.9
Meat Feast, Italian, Sainsbury's*	1 Pack/450g	509	113	7.4	11.8	4.0	0.6
Parcels, Basil & Parmesan, Fresh, Sainsbury's*	1 Serving/162g	357	220	10.0	26.4	8.3	3.3
Parcels, Tomato & Mozarella, Sainsbury's*	1 Serving/175g	340	194	7.5	23.0	8.0	3.4
Pepper & Tomato, Asda*	1 Serving/250g	340	136	3.2	15.0	7.0	2.4
Pomodoro, With Tomato & Herbs, SlimFast*	1 Serving/71g	235	331	21.5	51.5	4.3	6.0
Riccioli, Buitoni*	1 Serving/75g	264	352	11.2	72.6	1.9	0.0
Sausage & Tomato, Italiano, Tesco*	1 Serving/450g	680	151	5.7	18.8	5.9	1.6
Seafood, Retail	1oz/28g	31	110	8.9	7.6	4.8	0.4
Stuffed Mushroom & Emmental, Sainsbury's*	1 Pack/250g	650	260	11.3	33.5	9.2	3.7
Sundried Tomato, Sainsbury's*	1 Serving/50g	197	393	4.5	13.4	35.7	6.2
Tomato & Bacon, Value, Tesco*	1 Pack/300g	300	100	4.0	17.8	1.4	1.1
Tomato & Basil Chicken, Boots*	1 Serving/320g	621	194	9.0	19.0	9.0	1.4
Tomato & Mascapone, Tesco*	1 Pack/400g	468	117	9.7	10.3	4.1	0.9
Tomato & Mascarpone, GFY, Asda*	1/2 Can/200g	128	64	2.1	9.0	2.2	0.0
Tomato & Onion, Shells, Tesco*	1 Serving/193g	643	333	12.5	67.1	1.6	6.3
Tomato & Pepper, Fireroast, Finest, Tesco*	1 Serving/200g	384	192	3.9	19.4	11.0	1.4
Tomato & Pepper, GFY, Asda*	1 Pack/400g	344	86	3.1	14.0	1.9	1.1
Tuna & Sweetcorn, Sainsbury's*	1 Pasta/300g	327	109	6.7	14.7	2.6	1.4
Twists, With Tuna, Balanced Lifestyle, Aldi*	1 Can/400g	264	66	4.8	7.8	1.7	1.7
Twists, With Tuna, Italian, Weight Watchers*	1 Can/385g	239	62	4.3	8.2	1.4	0.6
Vegetable, Creamy, BGTY, Sainsbury's*	1 Pack/400g	348	87	4.0	14.3	1.5	1.9
Wheat Free, Delverde*	1 Serving/63g	229	366	0.5	86.9	1.9	1.2
PASTA 'N' SAUCE							
Bolognese Flavour, Dry, Batchelors*	1 Pack/126g	459	364	14.0	71.9	2.3	5.2
Carbonara Flavour, Dry, Batchelors*	1 Pack/120g	463	386	14.3	71.0	5.0	3.1
Cheese & Broccoli Sauce Mix, Made Up, Sainsbury's*	1 Pack/120g	164	137	4.2	17.2	5.7	1.1
Cheese & Broccoli, Made Up, SmartPrice, Asda*	1 Serving/120g	198	165	4.6	21.0	7.0	2.1
Cheese, Leek & Ham, Dry, Batchelors*	1 Pack/126g	478	379	14.1	68.3	5.5	2.3
Chicken & Mushroom, Dry, Batchelors*	1 Pack/126g	455	361	12.4	73.5	2.0	2.7

	Measure INFO/WEIGHT	per Measure KCAL	Nutrition Values per 100g / 100ml				
			KCAL	PROT	CARB	FAT	FIBRE
PASTA 'N' SAUCE							
Chicken & Mushroom, Made Up, Morrisons*	1 Pack/110g	166	151	5.0	20.3	5.6	2.1
Chicken & Mushroom, Made Up, SmartPrice, Asda*	1 Pack/110g	183	166	5.0	23.0	6.0	2.2
Chicken & Roasted Garlic Flavour, Dry, Batchelors*	1/2 Pack/60g	223	372	12.6	73.8	2.9	3.4
Creamy Tikka Masala, Dry, Batchelors*	1 Pack/122.1g	426	349	12.7	69.5	2.2	4.4
Creamy Tomato & Mushroom, Dry, Batchelors*	1 Pack/125g	458	366	13.0	71.0	3.3	3.2
Macaroni Cheese, Dry, Batchelors*	1 Pack/108g	408	378	17.2	63.6	6.1	2.8
Mild Cheese & Brocolli, Dry, Batchelors*	1 Pack/123g	456	371	13.5	69.0	4.5	2.8
Mushroom & Wine, Dry, Batchelors*	1 Pack/132g	498	377	12.0	71.3	4.9	2.5
Tomato & Bacon Flavour, Dry, Batchelors*	1 Pack/134g	476	355	13.0	70.0	2.6	3.0
Tomato & Mascarpone, BGTY, Sainsbury's*	1 Pack/380g	555	146	6.6	25.6	1.9	1.3
Tomato Onion & Herb Flavour, Dry, Batchelors*	1 Pack/135g	470	348	13.2	64.5	4.1	5.8
Tomato, Onion & Herb, Made Up, Morrisons*	1 Serving/110g	141	128	3.2	18.7	4.5	2.3
PASTA ALFREDO							
Tesco*	1 Pack/450g	621	138	10.5	14.9	4.0	0.6
PASTA BAKE							
Aberdeen Angus Meatball, Waitrose*	1/2 Pack/350.3g	501	143	5.2	12.5	8.0	0.9
Bacon & Leek, Tesco*	1 Pack/450g	774	172	8.1	16.1	8.3	2.0
Bolognese, Asda*	1 Serving/375g	799	213	10.0	14.0	13.0	0.5
Bolognese, Finest, Tesco*	1 Serving/250g	375	150	7.3	16.1	6.3	1.1
Bolognese, Italian, Healthy Living, Tesco*	1 Serving/450g	482	107	7.0	15.1	2.1	1.0
Bolognese, Italiano, Tesco*	1/3 Pack/284g	409	144	8.7	15.7	5.1	2.3
Cheese & Bacon, Fresh Italian, Asda*	1 Serving/250g	265	106	0.0	2.6	8.0	0.5
Cheese & Broccoli, Fish Bakes, Birds Eye*	1/2 Pack/200g	264	132	12.5	6.1	6.4	0.3
Cheese & Tomato, Italiano, Tesco*	1 Bake/300g	354	118	3.9	16.1	4.2	1.0
Cheese & Tomato, Tesco*	1 Pack/400g	388	97	3.4	17.8	1.4	1.2
Chicken & Bacon, Italiano, Tesco*	1 Pack/800g	1288	161	7.7	16.9	7.0	0.5
Chicken & Bacon, Tesco*	1oz/28g	46	166	6.9	19.3	6.8	0.5
Chicken & Broccoli, Pasta Presto, Findus*	1 Pack/321g	449	140	7.5	12.0	7.0	0.0
Chicken & Broccoli, Weight Watchers*	1 Bake/305g	290	95	6.0	14.2	1.5	0.9
Chicken & Courgette, Asda*	1/2 Pack/387.3g	519	134	6.0	14.0	6.0	0.6
Chicken & Mushroom, Waitrose*	1 Pack/400g	532	133	6.7	9.1	7.7	0.8
Chicken & Roast Mushroom, Healthy Living, Tesco*	1 Pack/390g	413	106	8.6	17.6	0.1	1.3
Chicken & Spinach, GFY, Asda*	1 Pack/400g	380	95	5.0	13.0	2.6	0.7
Chicken & Spinach, Safeway*	1 Serving/383g	440	115	6.9	12.0	4.0	1.2
Chicken & Spinach, Sainsbury's*	1 Pack/340g	286	84	4.9	10.0	2.7	0.6
Chicken & Sweetcorn, Eat Smart, Safeway*	1 Pack/400g	380	95	6.5	13.0	1.8	1.8
Chicken & Vegetable, Healthy Living, Tesco*	1 Serving/400g	336	84	6.1	13.1	0.8	1.4
Chicken, BGTY, Sainsbury's*	1 Pack/400g	376	94	8.2	12.4	1.3	0.9
Chicken, GFY, Asda*	1 Pack/400g	356	89	5.0	13.0	1.9	0.6
Chicken, Healthy Living, Tesco*	1 Pack/400g	336	84	6.1	13.1	0.8	1.4
Chicken, Italiano, Tesco*	1 Serving/190g	219	115	8.4	11.2	4.1	3.1
Chicken, Mushroom & Leek, Healthy Eating, Tesco*	1 Pack/450g	468	104	8.6	11.9	2.5	1.4
Chicken, Somerfield*	1 Pack/300g	351	117	8.0	8.0	6.0	0.0
Chicken, Tesco*	1 Serving/400g	376	94	8.2	12.4	1.3	0.9
Chicken, Tomato, & Mascarpone, Tesco*	1 Serving/400g	448	112	8.0	15.2	2.1	1.7
Chilli & Cheese, American Style, Tesco*	1 Pack/425g	638	150	6.8	21.8	3.9	1.5
Creamy Ham & Mushroom, Homepride*	1 Pack/425g	489	115	1.8	2.8	10.7	0.0
Creamy Mushroom, Dolmio*	1/2 Jar/245g	267	109	1.1	5.5	9.2	0.0
Creamy Tomato, Dolmio*	1 Serving/125g	141	113	2.3	8.4	7.2	0.0
Findus*	1 Pack/320g	448	140	7.5	12.0	7.0	0.0
Ham & Broccoli, Asda*	1 Pack/340g	309	91	3.4	10.0	4.1	0.5
Ham & Mushroom, Italiano, Tesco*	1 Pack/425g	646	152	5.8	21.3	4.8	1.7
Italian Bolognese, Asda*	1 Serving/300g	429	143	8.0	12.0	7.0	2.0

P

	Measure INFO/WEIGHT	per Measure KCAL	Nutrition Values per 100g / 100ml				
			KCAL	PROT	CARB	FAT	FIBRE
PASTA BAKE							
Italian Creamy Tomato & Bacon, Asda*	1 Serving/125g	131	105	2.0	3.9	9.0	0.6
Leek & Bacon, Morrisons*	1 Pack/400.7g	553	138	4.8	9.9	9.0	0.2
Meatball, Tesco*	1 Pack/400g	576	144	5.9	19.3	4.8	0.5
Mediterranean Style, Tesco*	1 Pack/450g	423	94	2.9	19.6	0.4	2.0
Mushroom, Creamy, Asda*	1/4 Jar/118g	204	173	1.8	3.3	17.0	0.5
Penne Mozzarella, Tesco*	1 Pack/340g	408	120	4.7	19.7	2.5	0.6
Pepperoni & Ham, Tesco*	1/2 Pack/425g	502	118	8.9	19.3	0.6	2.5
Roast Vegetable, Eat Smart, Safeway*	1 Pack/330g	380	115	3.8	19.6	1.9	1.3
Spicy Tomato & Pepperoni, Asda*	1 Pack/440g	431	98	1.1	10.0	6.0	1.2
Three Bean, Asda*	1/4 Jar/124.7g	188	150	2.4	8.0	12.0	1.3
Tomato & Cheese, Dolmio*	1 Serving/125g	69	55	2.2	8.8	1.2	0.0
Tomato & Herb, Asda*	1 Jar/436g	715	164	1.8	10.0	13.0	1.2
Tomato & Mozzarella, Healthy Living, Tesco*	1 Serving/385g	358	93	3.8	14.6	2.2	0.7
Tomato & Mozzarella, Italiano, Tesco*	1 Pack/340g	398	117	4.8	18.9	2.5	1.7
Tuna & Sweetcorn, Asda*	1 Serving/250g	333	133	5.0	8.0	9.0	0.9
Tuna & Tomat & Fish Sauce, Schwartz*	1 Jar/315g	246	78	2.6	12.1	2.2	0.0
Tuna & Tomato, BGTY, Sainsbury's*	1 Pack/450g	554	123	8.7	12.6	4.2	0.4
Tuna, BGTY, Sainsbury's*	1 Serving/400g	368	92	7.6	11.9	1.5	1.8
Tuna, COU, Marks & Spencer*	1 Pack/360g	378	105	8.0	13.4	2.0	1.1
Tuna, Good Intentions, Somerfield*	1 Serving/400g	400	100	5.9	14.5	2.1	1.2
Tuna, Healthy Living, Tesco*	1 Serving/400g	360	90	8.3	10.7	1.5	0.9
Tuna, Italian, Healthy Living, Tesco*	1 Pack/500g	475	95	7.1	13.5	1.4	1.5
Tuna, Lean Cuisine*	1 Pack/345.5g	380	110	5.0	16.0	2.5	1.5
Tuna, Somerfield*	1 Bake/300g	411	137	9.0	10.0	7.0	0.0
Tuna, Tesco*	1oz/28g	36	129	6.9	11.7	6.1	0.9
Vegetable, Asda*	1 Serving/300g	231	77	2.4	9.0	3.5	0.8
Vegetable, Findus*	1 Pack/330.8g	430	130	6.0	13.0	6.5	0.0
Vegetable, Marks & Spencer*	1 Pack/350g	455	130	4.8	14.6	5.7	1.6
Vegetable, Mediterranean, Healthy Living, Tesco*	1 Serving/450g	374	83	2.9	16.0	0.8	1.5
Vegetable, Mediterranean, Tesco*	1 Serving/450g	495	110	4.3	12.9	4.6	1.3
Vegetable, Tesco*	1 Pack/380g	467	123	5.6	12.6	5.6	1.6
PASTA BREAK							
Cheese & Ham, Unprepared, Asda*	1 Pot/63g	257	408	11.1	58.7	14.3	0.0
Chicken & Herb, Prepared, Knorr*	1 Pot/347g	382	110	3.7	16.5	3.3	0.9
Chicken & Mushroom Flavour, Prepared, Asda*	1 Pot/231g	254	110	2.7	19.0	2.6	0.0
Tomato & Herb, Unprepared, Asda*	1 Pot/66g	180	273	7.1	57.6	1.5	0.0
PASTA IN							
A Rich Tomato & Mushroom Sauce, Spirals, Tesco*	1 Serving/217g	326	150	4.6	18.8	6.3	2.5
Herb Sauce, Sainsbury's*	1 Pack/420g	441	105	3.5	22.4	0.2	0.8
PASTA MEAL							
Tomato & Basil, Shapers, Boots*	1 Serving/76g	214	282	22.4	38.2	4.3	6.8
PASTA QUILLS							
Dry, Average	1 Serving/75g	257	342	12.0	72.3	1.2	2.0
Gluten Free, Salute*	1 Serving/75g	269	359	7.5	78.1	1.9	0.0
Whole Wheat, Morrisons*	1 Serving/100g	362	362	12.5	71.2	2.5	0.0
PASTA SALAD							
& Mixed Leaf, With Basil Pesto Dressing, Tesco*	1 Pack/220g	528	240	4.7	16.9	17.1	0.7
BBQ Bean, Tesco*	1 Pack/850g	1139	134	3.6	18.5	5.1	1.8
BBQ Chicken, Positive Eating, Scottish Slimmers*	1 Serving/239.8g	223	93	6.4	14.0	1.8	1.3
Basil & Parmesan, Tesco*	1 Serving/50g	65	130	4.3	20.2	3.6	0.6
Big Penne, Honey & Mustard Chicken, Marks & Spencer*	1 Pack/380g	646	170	8.1	17.7	7.2	2.6
Caesar & Santa Tomatoes, Marks & Spencer*	1 Serving/220g	495	225	5.2	15.9	15.3	0.8
Carbonara, Waitrose*	1oz/28g	72	257	5.4	8.1	22.6	0.5

PASTA SALAD

	Measure INFO/WEIGHT	per Measure KCAL	KCAL	PROT	CARB	FAT	FIBRE
Chargrilled Chicken, Marks & Spencer*	1 Serving/190g	285	150	9.6	23.6	2.9	1.6
Chargrilled Vegetables & Tomato, Shapers, Boots*	1 Pack/175g	187	107	2.8	17.0	3.1	1.5
Cheese, With Mayonnaise & Vinaigrette, Sainsbury's*	1/4 Pot/50g	125	249	6.1	17.0	17.3	1.7
Cherry Tomato & Rocket, Healthy Eating, Tesco*	1 Salad/225g	223	99	3.2	15.8	2.5	1.0
Chicken & Smoked Bacon, Marks & Spencer*	1 Salad/380g	817	215	7.5	19.0	12.3	1.9
Chicken & Sweetcorn, Eat Smart, Safeway*	1 Serving/200g	230	115	7.5	16.3	1.8	1.0
Chicken Caesar, Asda*	1 Pack/300g	537	179	8.0	21.0	7.0	1.5
Chicken Caesar, Ginsters*	1 Pack/220g	504	229	7.5	13.6	16.1	0.0
Chilli & Cheese, Sainsbury's*	1 Serving/300g	384	128	4.3	15.5	5.6	0.3
Crayfish, Rocket & Lemon, Finest, Tesco*	1 Serving/250g	728	291	8.9	28.0	15.9	4.2
Crayfish, Shapers, Boots*	1 Pack/280.2g	269	96	6.0	13.0	2.3	0.7
Farfalle, Prawns Tomatoes & Cucumber, Sainsbury's*	1 Serving/260g	270	104	4.5	10.9	4.7	0.7
Feta Cheese, Sun Blush Tomatoes, Marks & Spencer*	1 Serving/190g	361	190	5.5	17.2	11.1	2.1
Fire Roast Tomato & Red Pepper, Finest, Tesco*	1 Pack/200g	328	164	4.1	15.5	9.5	2.1
Fire Roasted Tomato, So Good, Somerfield*	1/2 Pack/100g	199	199	4.4	21.6	10.6	1.5
Garlic Mushroom, Salad Bar, Asda*	1oz/28g	59	212	2.5	12.5	16.9	0.8
Goats Cheese, & Mixed Pepper, Sainsbury's*	1 Pack/200g	366	183	6.4	18.2	9.4	1.5
Ham & Pineapple, Salad Bar, Asda*	1oz/28g	62	221	3.3	15.6	16.2	1.4
Ham, Sainsbury's*	1 Pot/250g	610	244	4.1	13.4	19.3	0.8
Honey & Mustard Chicken, Marks & Spencer*	1 Serving/190g	304	160	8.7	26.7	2.5	1.5
Honey & Mustard Chicken, Sainsbury's*	1 Pack/260g	447	172	7.3	16.9	8.3	1.4
Italian Style, Sainsbury's*	1/3 Pot/84g	129	153	3.5	20.5	6.3	1.4
Italian, Bowl, Sainsbury's*	1 Serving/210g	309	147	3.1	16.9	7.4	1.9
Lime & Coriander Chicken, Marks & Spencer*	1 Serving/190g	371	195	7.6	14.4	12.2	0.6
Mediterranean Chicken, Waitrose*	1 Serving/200g	314	157	7.0	16.9	6.8	2.1
Mediterranean Style, Layered, Waitrose*	1 Pot/275g	190	69	2.6	11.8	1.3	1.0
Mediterranean Tuna, Shapers, Boots*	1 Serving/239g	232	97	6.2	15.0	1.3	0.9
Mediterranean Vegetable & Bean, BGTY, Sainsbury's*	1 Serving/66g	53	80	3.2	12.5	1.9	2.8
Mediterranean, Good Intentions, Somerfield*	1 Pack/250g	290	116	2.8	19.8	2.8	1.1
Mozzarella & Plum Tomatoes, COU, Marks & Spencer*	1 Bowl/255g	204	80	4.6	11.5	1.6	1.7
Mozzarella & Roasted Tomato, TTD, Sainsbury's*	1 Serving/50g	78	156	5.7	16.3	7.6	0.0
Mozzarella & Sun Dried Tomato, Waitrose*	1 Serving/150g	312	208	5.8	18.8	12.2	1.3
Oven Roasted Tomato and Olive, TTD, Sainsbury's*	1 Serving/50g	88	176	5.2	22.1	7.4	0.0
Pepper, Healthy Eating, Tesco*	1 Salad/210g	139	66	2.4	13.3	0.4	1.0
Pepper, Side, Tesco*	1 Serving/46g	56	122	2.4	13.0	6.5	1.3
Pesto, Spinach, & Pine Nut, Sainsbury's*	1 Box/200g	496	248	5.7	18.2	16.8	0.0
Poached Salmon, Marks & Spencer*	1 Serving/200g	340	170	7.8	16.2	8.4	1.4
Poached Salmon, Sainsbury's*	1 Serving/200g	472	236	6.7	17.9	15.3	12.0
Prawn Cocktail, Improved, Shapers, Boots*	1 Pack/248.5g	256	103	5.0	15.0	2.7	1.6
Prawn, COU, Marks & Spencer*	1 Pack/274g	260	95	5.1	16.4	1.5	0.9
Prawn, Shapers, Boots*	1 Pot/250g	250	100	4.1	14.0	3.1	0.4
Ready To Eat, Somerfield*	1/2 Pack/123g	175	142	2.8	17.1	6.9	1.6
Roast Chicken & Pesto, Shaker, Sainsbury's*	1 Box/224g	253	113	8.2	12.3	3.4	0.0
Roast Garlic Mushroom, TTD, Sainsbury's*	1 Pot/200g	358	179	5.1	19.8	8.8	0.0
Roasted Mushroom, Spinach & Tarragon, Tesco*	1 Pot/200g	216	108	4.3	17.2	2.4	0.8
Roasted Vegetable, Waitrose*	1 Pack/190g	270	142	6.8	18.2	4.6	1.1
Sainsbury's*	1/2 Pack/160g	235	147	3.2	20.0	6.0	1.5
Salmon, Marks & Spencer*	1 Serving/380g	817	215	6.8	12.7	15.2	0.7
Spicy Chicken, Geo Adams*	1 Pack/230g	580	252	5.1	14.9	19.1	2.9
Spicy Chilli Pesto, Sainsbury's*	1/4 Pot/62.5g	171	272	3.8	20.1	19.6	1.6
Spinach & Nuts, Marks & Spencer*	1oz/28g	64	229	6.9	18.2	15.0	1.6
Sun Dried Tomato Dressing, Sainsbury's*	1 Pack/320g	442	138	3.7	20.8	4.4	3.6
Sweetcorn & Pepper, GFY, Asda*	1 Serving/175g	68	39	1.9	7.0	0.4	0.0

	Measure INFO/WEIGHT	per Measure KCAL	Nutrition Values per 100g / 100ml				
			KCAL	PROT	CARB	FAT	FIBRE
PASTA SALAD							
Three Cheese, Tesco*	1 Serving/300g	633	211	7.5	14.4	13.7	2.8
Tiger Prawn & Tomato, GFY, Asda*	1 Serving/200g	250	125	4.6	20.0	2.9	2.0
Tiger Prawn, Waitrose*	1 Serving/225g	545	242	5.4	16.7	17.1	0.4
Tomato & Basil Chicken, Marks & Spencer*	1 Serving/279g	446	160	7.0	14.8	7.9	1.8
Tomato & Basil With Red & Green Pepper, Sainsbury's*	1/4 Pot/63g	89	141	3.2	16.4	6.9	3.8
Tomato & Basil, Marks & Spencer*	1 Pot/225g	484	215	2.9	15.0	15.9	1.2
Tomato & Basil, Perfectly Balanced, Waitrose*	1 Serving/100g	97	97	3.7	16.8	1.7	0.0
Tomato & Basil, Pot, Healthy Living, Tesco*	1 Pot/200g	242	121	2.0	22.1	2.7	2.2
Tomato & Basil, Sainsbury's*	1 Serving/250g	383	153	3.5	20.5	6.3	1.4
Tomato & Chargrilled Vegetable, Tesco*	1 Serving/200g	248	124	3.7	18.6	3.9	1.4
Tomato & Mozzarella, Leaf, Shapers, Boots*	1 Pack/185g	356	192	5.1	16.0	12.0	2.5
Tomato & Mozzarella, Sainsbury's*	1 Pack/200g	440	220	7.5	22.2	11.3	1.3
Tomato & Pepper, Healthy Living, Tesco*	1 Serving/100g	81	81	2.6	13.9	1.6	1.4
Tomato & Tuna, Snack, Sainsbury's*	1 Serving/200g	238	119	5.3	21.7	1.2	0.0
Tomato, Bacon & Cheese, Ginsters*	1 Pack/220g	381	173	7.4	15.6	9.0	0.0
Tuna & Spinach, COU, Marks & Spencer*	1 Pack/270g	257	95	6.8	14.3	1.8	3.8
Tuna & Sweetcorn, COU, Marks & Spencer*	1 Pack/200g	210	105	7.1	18.3	0.9	1.2
Tuna & Sweetcorn, Healthy Eating, Tesco*	1 Pot/200g	230	115	5.7	17.0	2.7	1.3
Tuna & Sweetcorn, Sainsbury's*	1 Serving/100g	111	111	7.1	18.3	1.2	1.2
Tuna Nicoise, Waitrose*	1 Pot/190g	306	161	5.1	14.9	9.0	1.1
Tuna, Arrabiatta, BGTY, Sainsbury's*	1 Serving/200g	196	98	6.8	14.7	1.3	0.0
Tuna, Mediterranean, Johnsons*	1 Serving/225g	148	66	2.8	7.5	2.8	0.9
Tuna, Perfectly Balanced, Waitrose*	1 Tub/190g	181	95	7.0	11.5	2.3	1.1
Tuna, Tesco*	1 Pot/300g	399	133	6.2	10.5	7.3	0.0
Vegetable, Healthy Selection, Somerfield*	1 Pot/200g	180	90	2.8	19.6	0.0	0.7
Vegetable, Somerfield*	1 Salad/200g	288	144	3.0	20.0	6.0	0.0
Wild Mushroom, TTD, Sainsbury's*	1 Serving/259g	464	179	4.6	16.6	10.5	1.5
With Avocado & Cherry Tomatoes, Marks & Spencer*	1 Pack/185g	259	140	2.9	13.9	8.0	1.2
With Italian Style Chicken, Weight Watchers*	1 Pack/185g	237	128	6.7	22.9	1.1	0.7
With Spinach & Pine Nuts, Marks & Spencer*	1 Pack/205g	440	215	7.9	26.6	8.4	2.2
PASTA SAUCE							
Amatriciana, Asda*	1 Jar/320g	496	155	4.4	5.0	13.0	1.0
Amatriciana, Fresh, Safeway*	1/2 Pot/175g	89	51	2.5	5.6	2.1	1.2
Amatriciana, Fresh, Sainsbury's*	1/2 Pot/150g	69	46	3.5	3.6	1.9	1.3
Amatriciana, Italiano, Tesco*	1/2 Pot/175g	124	71	4.1	5.3	3.8	0.9
Amatriciana, Tesco*	1 Serving/175g	109	62	2.3	4.0	4.1	0.7
Arrabbiata, BGTY, Sainsbury's*	1 Jar/150g	107	71	1.3	7.6	3.9	0.7
Arrabbiata, Barilla*	1 Serving/100g	47	47	1.5	3.5	3.0	0.0
Arrabbiata, Fresh, Tesco*	1 Serving/110ml	29	26	0.7	3.7	0.9	0.9
Arrabbiata, GFY, Asda*	1 Serving/350g	133	38	1.1	6.0	1.1	0.0
Arrabbiata, Italian, Waitrose*	1 Jar/320g	102	32	1.6	5.6	0.3	0.0
Arrabbiata, Italiano, Tesco*	1/2 Pot/175g	65	37	1.7	6.1	0.6	1.0
Arrabbiata, Marks & Spencer*	1 Jar/320g	240	75	1.2	6.2	5.3	0.8
Arrabbiata, Sainsbury's*	1oz/28g	13	45	1.4	3.3	2.9	1.6
Aubergine & Pepper, Sacla*	1/2 Pot/95g	238	250	1.8	5.6	24.5	0.0
Basil & Oregano For Bolognese, Ragu*	1 Serving/200g	76	38	2.0	7.6	0.0	0.8
Beef Bolognese, Fresh, Asda*	1/4 Pot/82g	78	95	4.3	3.4	7.3	0.4
Bolognese With Beef, Tesco*	1/2 Can/213g	179	84	4.9	5.5	4.7	0.0
Bolognese, Carb Check, Heinz*	1 Serving/150g	80	53	3.8	3.6	2.6	0.4
Bolognese, Dolmio*	1/4 Jar/175g	91	52	1.8	10.3	0.0	0.0
Bolognese, Finest, Tesco*	1 Serving/175g	170	97	7.0	3.8	6.1	0.5
Bolognese, Fresh, Sainsbury's*	1/2 Pot/150g	120	80	6.0	4.7	4.1	1.2
Bolognese, Fresh, Waitrose*	1 Pot/350g	277	79	5.1	5.3	4.2	0.7

PASTA SAUCE

INFO/WEIGHT	Measure per Measure KCAL	KCAL	PROT	CARB	FAT	FIBRE
Bolognese, Italiano, Tesco*	1 Serving/175g	194	111	5.9	4.8	7.5	0.8
Bolognese, Marks & Spencer*	1 Jar/100g	115	115	7.0	10.8	4.9	1.2
Bolognese, Mediterranean Vegetable, Chunky, Dolmio*	1/2 Jar/250g	138	55	1.3	8.8	1.6	0.0
Bolognese, Organic, Seeds Of Change*	1 Jar/530g	313	59	1.5	10.5	1.2	1.2
Bolognese, Original, Asda*	1 Serving/157.5g	73	46	1.4	7.0	1.4	0.8
Bolognese, Original, Light, Dolmio*	1 Serving/125g	48	38	1.6	7.8	0.1	0.0
Bolognese, Original, Sainsbury's*	1/4 Jar/136g	90	66	1.9	9.9	2.1	1.3
Bolognese, SmartPrice, Asda*	1/2 Jar/226g	88	39	0.9	7.0	0.8	0.6
Bolognese, Tesco*	1 Serving/175g	100	57	4.2	4.0	2.6	0.8
Bolognese, Traditional, Ragu	1 Jar/515g	345	67	2.0	9.9	2.1	1.2
Cacciatore, Fresh, Sainsbury's*	1/2 Pot/150g	152	101	5.4	8.1	5.9	1.5
Carbonara, 50% Less Fat, Asda*	1/2 Pot/175g	170	97	4.8	6.0	6.0	0.6
Carbonara, Asda*	1/2 Pot/175g	359	205	7.0	6.0	17.0	0.1
Carbonara, BGTY, Sainsbury's*	1/2 Pack/165g	225	136	6.3	23.4	1.9	1.0
Carbonara, Dolmio*	1 Serving/150g	224	149	3.4	4.2	13.2	0.0
Carbonara, Italiano, Tesco*	1 Pot/350g	613	175	5.8	6.1	14.1	0.0
Carbonara, Tesco*	1 Jar/315g	501	159	3.2	6.8	13.2	0.1
Carbonara, With Cheese & Bacon, BGTY, Sainsbury's*	1 Serving/150g	138	92	5.5	10.1	3.3	1.5
Chargrilled Vegetable With Extra Virgin Olive Oil, Bertolli*	1/2 Jar/250g	150	60	2.1	8.7	1.9	2.4
Cheery Tomato & Roasted Pepper, Asda*	1 Jar/171.7g	91	53	1.5	5.0	3.0	2.4
Cheese & Bacon Bake, Homepride*	1oz/28g	27	95	2.0	2.5	8.6	0.0
Cheese & Tuna, Safeway*	1 Serving/175g	175	100	6.9	4.8	5.7	0.6
Cheese, Fresh, Perfectly Balanced, Waitrose*	1/2 Pot/175g	144	82	6.1	7.9	2.9	0.5
Cherry Tomato & Basil, Sacla*	1 Serving/96g	90	94	1.2	5.3	7.4	0.0
Chilli With Jalapeno Peppers, Seeds Of Change*	1 Jar/350g	322	92	3.6	16.0	1.5	2.2
Chunky Vegetable, Asda*	1 Serving/250g	123	49	1.4	7.0	1.7	1.2
Cirio Pomodoro*	1 Serving/200g	116	58	1.4	8.4	2.3	0.0
Cream & Mushroom, Marks & Spencer*	1oz/28g	45	160	1.5	6.6	14.3	0.6
Creamy Mushroom, Chicken Tonight*	1/4 Jar/125g	110	88	0.7	2.8	8.2	0.4
Creamy Mushroom, Dolmio*	1 Pack/150g	167	111	1.3	3.7	10.0	0.0
Creamy Mushroom, Express, Dolmio*	1 Serving/150g	161	107	1.4	3.8	9.6	0.0
Creamy Mustard, Dry, Colman's*	1 Pack/29g	108	374	11.0	46.0	16.0	0.0
Creamy Pepper & Mushroom, Dry, Colman's*	1 Pack/25g	82	327	8.1	56.0	9.1	0.0
Creamy Tomato & Bacon Bake, Homepride*	1 Serving/110g	99	90	1.9	6.5	6.3	0.0
Creamy Tomato & Basil, BGTY, Sainsbury's*	1/2 Jar/250g	173	69	1.7	7.6	3.6	1.0
Creamy Tomato & Herb Bake, Homepride*	1 Jar/455g	464	102	2.0	7.5	7.1	0.0
Creamy Tomato, Carb Check, Heinz*	1 Serving/150g	92	61	2.0	4.2	4.0	0.5
Extra Mushrooms Bolognese, Dolmio*	1 Jar/500g	235	47	1.6	9.3	0.1	0.0
Extra Spicy Bolognese, Dolmio*	1 Serving/250g	133	53	1.7	9.2	1.1	0.0
Fiorentina, Fresh, Sainsbury's*	1/2 Pot/157g	165	105	3.2	4.3	8.4	0.9
Five Cheese, Italiano, Tesco*	1/2 Tub/175g	271	155	6.8	6.0	11.5	0.0
Four Cheese, Asda*	1/2 Jar/155g	242	156	3.5	3.9	14.0	0.1
Four Cheese, BGTY, Sainsbury's*	1 Serving/150g	104	69	2.9	5.5	4.0	0.1
Four Cheese, Fresh, Asda*	1/2 Pot/162g	309	191	5.4	2.2	17.8	0.5
Four Cheese, GFY, Asda*	1/2 Pot/175g	144	82	4.0	6.3	4.6	0.5
Four Cheese, Loyd Grossman*	1 Jar/350g	476	136	2.6	4.6	11.9	0.0
Four Cheese, Sainsbury's*	1 Serving/150g	296	197	6.6	4.5	17.0	0.8
Garlic & Chilli, Slow Roasted, Seeds Of Change*	1/2 Jar/175g	158	90	1.7	8.7	5.3	2.0
Garlic, Perfectly Balanced, Waitrose*	1 Jar/440g	330	75	2.3	12.7	1.7	2.3
Grilled Vegetable With Extra Virgin Olive Oil, Bertolli*	1/2 Jar/250g	150	60	2.1	8.7	1.9	2.4
Ham & Mushroom, Creamy, Stir & Serve, Homepride*	1 Serving/92g	124	135	1.8	5.5	11.7	0.0
Hot & Spicy, Morrisons*	1 Serving/130g	82	63	1.3	9.3	2.4	1.0
Hot Pepper & Mozzarella, Stir Through, Sacla*	1/2 Jar/95g	229	241	4.7	7.2	21.5	0.0

PASTA SAUCE

INFO/WEIGHT	Measure per Measure KCAL	KCAL	PROT	CARB	FAT	FIBRE
Hot, Heinz*	1 Serving/200g	120	60	1.2	5.7	3.6	0.9
Italian Cheese, Finest, Tesco*	1/2 Pot/175g	172	98	4.8	8.4	5.1	0.0
Italian Mushroom, Sainsbury's*	1 Serving/85g	56	66	2.0	9.8	2.1	1.7
Italian Style, Princes*	1 Jar/475g	404	85	1.7	16.0	1.6	1.2
Italian Tomato & Herb, For Pasta, Sainsbury's*	1/2 Jar/146g	102	70	2.0	11.1	2.0	1.4
Italian Tomato & Smoked Bacon, Stir-In, Safeway*	1/2 Jar/75g	152	203	2.9	7.3	18.0	1.2
Italian, Tomato, Mushroom & Pancetta, Sainsbury's*	1/2 Jar/75g	125	167	2.2	6.1	14.9	1.3
Italian, Vongole, Waitrose*	1 Serving/175g	116	66	4.2	5.2	3.2	0.7
Layered Tomato & Mozarella, Finest, Tesco*	1 Jar/160g	232	145	6.6	6.9	10.1	0.7
Leek & Bacon, Safeway*	1/2 Pot/170.6g	145	85	4.0	5.7	4.9	0.5
Mediterrainean Vegetable Pasta, Tesco*	1 Serving/166g	95	57	1.4	9.0	1.7	1.2
Mediterranean Sizzling, Homepride*	1 Serving/96g	83	86	0.9	6.3	6.4	0.0
Mediterranean Tomato, Asda*	1 Jar/500g	285	57	1.5	10.0	1.2	0.0
Mediterranean Vegetable, Rustico, Bertolli*	1/2 Jar/160g	141	88	1.7	4.1	7.2	0.7
Mediterranean Vegetable, Seeds Of Change*	1 Serving/100g	89	89	1.7	7.8	5.6	2.1
Mediterranean, BGTY, Sainsbury's*	1oz/28g	23	82	1.9	9.0	4.3	1.4
Mediterranean, Fresh, Waitrose*	1 Pot/350g	214	61	1.4	5.0	3.9	2.4
Mushroom & Garlic, 98% Fat Free, Homepride*	1 Jar/450g	230	51	1.1	8.9	1.4	0.5
Mushroom & Garlic, Deliciously Good, Homepride*	1/3 Jar/147g	109	74	0.9	6.9	4.8	0.3
Mushroom & Marsala Wine, Sacla*	1/2 Pot/85g	165	194	2.2	3.9	18.8	0.0
Mushroom & Mascarpone, Healthy Eating, Tesco*	1/2 Jar/175g	86	49	2.1	5.3	2.2	0.3
Mushroom & White Wine, Knorr*	1oz/28g	27	98	1.0	4.0	8.0	0.0
Mushroom, Dry, Colman's*	1 Pack/27g	97	358	14.0	53.0	9.7	0.0
Mushroom, Fresh, Waitrose*	1 Serving/175g	142	81	1.6	5.7	5.7	0.5
Mushroom, GFY, Asda*	1 Serving/175g	112	64	2.7	7.0	2.8	0.0
Mushroom, Microwaveable, Dolmio*	1 Serving/150g	161	107	1.4	3.8	9.6	0.0
Mushroom, Perfectly Balanced, Waitrose*	1 Jar/440g	330	75	2.6	11.8	1.9	2.2
Mushroom, Sainsbury's*	1 Serving/100g	66	66	2.0	9.8	2.1	1.7
Mushroom, Tesco*	1/4 Jar/188g	90	48	1.4	6.8	1.7	1.0
Napoletana, BGTY, Sainsbury's*	1/2 Pot/151g	71	47	1.2	5.0	2.5	1.3
Napoletana, Fresh, Asda*	1 Pot/330g	149	45	1.4	5.0	2.2	2.8
Napoletana, Fresh, Sainsbury's*	1oz/28g	25	91	1.9	7.9	5.8	1.1
Napoletana, GFY, Asda*	1 Serving/175g	58	33	1.0	5.0	1.0	0.0
Napoletana, Sainsbury's*	1/2 Pot/150g	126	84	1.9	6.6	5.6	0.9
Napoletana, Tesco*	1 serving/175g	110	63	1.5	7.2	3.1	1.1
Olive & Tomato, Sacla*	1 Serving/95g	87	92	1.3	3.6	8.0	0.0
Olive, Barilla*	1 Serving/100g	92	92	1.5	10.3	5.0	0.0
Onion & Garlic Bolognese, Extra, Dolmio*	1 Serving/125g	66	53	1.7	9.0	1.0	0.0
Onion & Garlic For Bolognese, Ragu*	1 Serving/125g	80	64	2.2	11.4	1.1	1.2
Onion & Garlic, Tesco*	1 Serving/225g	83	37	1.2	7.6	0.3	0.8
Original, BFY, Morrisons*	1/3 Jar/200g	100	50	1.6	10.6	0.1	1.2
Original, For Bolognese, Ragu*	1 Jar/525g	268	51	1.7	10.7	0.1	1.0
Original, Healthy Eating, Tesco*	1 Jar/455g	155	34	1.2	6.5	0.1	0.8
Original, Tesco*	1 Jar/300g	111	37	1.1	6.8	0.6	0.9
Original, With Tomato & Onions, BFY, Morrisons*	1 Serving/125g	51	41	1.4	6.3	1.1	1.2
Original, With Tomatoes & Onions, Morrisons*	1 Serving/100g	64	64	1.2	9.3	2.5	1.0
Oven Roasted Vegetables, Stir In, Dolmio*	packet/150g	201	134	1.5	8.7	10.3	0.0
Pepper & Tomato, Marks & Spencer*	1 Jar/320g	224	70	1.6	6.1	4.2	0.9
Porcini Mushroom & Pepperoni, Asda*	1/2 Jar/140g	158	113	3.8	11.0	6.0	0.0
Porcini Mushroom Stir In, BGTY, Sainsbury's*	1/2 Jar/75g	57	76	3.8	5.7	4.2	1.9
Primavera, Fresh, Morrisons*	1/2 Pot/175g	152	87	2.4	6.1	5.9	0.0
Puttanesca, Italian, Waitrose*	1 Jar/350g	195	56	1.5	6.1	2.8	1.3
Puttanesca, Loyd Grossman*	1oz/28g	25	90	1.7	6.8	6.2	0.9

PASTA SAUCE

	Measure INFO/WEIGHT	per Measure KCAL	Nutrition Values per 100g / 100ml KCAL	PROT	CARB	FAT	FIBRE
Puttanesca, Sainsbury's*	1 Serving/110g	132	120	2.0	8.1	8.8	0.0
Puttanesca, The Best, Safeway*	1 Serving/170g	139	82	1.0	5.6	6.2	0.0
Red Pepper & Plum, Finest, Tesco*	1 Serving/63g	109	173	3.7	14.0	11.4	5.4
Red Pepper Tomato, Finest, Tesco*	1 serving/145g	117	81	1.2	6.8	5.4	2.2
Roasted Red Pepper & Tomato, Finest, Tesco*	1 Serving/145g	117	81	1.2	6.8	5.4	2.2
Roasted Vegetable, & Olive, TTD, Sainsbury's*	1/2 Pot/150g	84	56	1.7	6.9	2.4	2.0
Roasted Vegetable, GFY, Asda*	1/2 a pot/175g	84	48	1.3	7.0	1.6	0.5
Roasted Vegetable, Microwaveable, Dolmio*	1/2 Pack/190g	103	54	1.4	7.6	2.0	0.0
Roasted Vegetable, Sainsbury's*	1/2 Pot/151g	103	68	1.6	6.7	3.9	0.4
Roasted Vegetable, Tesco*	1 Pack/175g	114	65	1.5	8.0	3.0	0.8
Roasted Vegetables & Tuna, BGTY, Sainsbury's*	1/2 Pot/150g	74	49	3.5	4.5	1.9	3.1
Romano, Aldi*	1 Serving/235g	141	60	1.7	8.8	2.0	1.1
Salsina With Onions & Garlic, Valfrutta*	1 Serving/150g	36	24	1.6	4.5	0.0	1.4
Scotch Salmon & Lemon, The Best, Safeway*	1 serving/175g	271	155	7.6	4.6	11.6	0.9
Siciliana, Sainsbury's*	1/3 Jar/113g	168	149	1.8	6.2	13.0	0.0
Sliced Mushroom, Tesco*	1 Jar/460g	161	35	1.3	7.0	0.2	0.8
Smoky Bacon, Loyd Grossman*	1oz/28g	27	98	3.1	5.4	7.2	0.7
Spicy Italian Chilli, Express, Dolmio*	1 serving/170g	87	51	1.5	7.5	1.6	0.0
Spicy Italian Chilli, Microwaveable, Dolmio*	1 Sachet/170g	92	54	1.4	7.6	2.0	0.0
Spicy Pepper & Tomato, Sacla*	1/2 Jar/95g	132	139	1.4	6.8	11.8	0.0
Spicy Pepper, Tesco*	1 Jar/500g	245	49	1.7	8.4	1.0	1.0
Spicy Red Pepper & Vegetable, Asda*	1 Pot/350g	182	52	1.2	5.0	3.0	1.1
Spicy Roasted Garlic, Seeds Of Change*	1 Serving/195g	123	63	1.5	9.7	2.0	1.2
Spicy Tomato, Asda*	1 serving/155g	76	49	1.5	8.0	1.2	1.0
Spicy With Peppers, Tesco*	1 Jar/455g	177	39	1.2	7.9	0.3	1.1
Spinach & Ricotta, Asda*	half a pot/175g	175	100	3.2	6.0	7.0	0.5
Spinach & Ricotta, BGTY, Sainsbury's*	1 Serving/150g	74	49	2.7	3.4	2.7	2.2
Spinach & Ricotta, Stir Through, Sacla*	1/2 Jar/95g	196	206	3.7	3.7	19.6	0.0
Stir & Serve, Homepride*	1 Bottle/480g	187	39	1.2	6.0	1.2	0.0
Sun Dried Tomato & Basil, Free From, Sainsbury's*	1/2 Jar/172.2g	124	72	2.9	8.7	2.8	1.5
Sun Dried Tomato & Garlic, Sacla*	1 Serving/95g	177	186	3.0	10.3	14.7	0.0
Sun Dried Tomato & Olive Oil, Loyd Grossman*	1oz/28g	52	187	0.8	10.3	15.8	0.3
Sun Dried Tomato & Roasted Garlic, Discovery*	1 Serving/100g	102	102	1.8	19.2	2.0	0.0
Sun Dried Tomato, Asda*	1/2 Jar/158.7g	165	104	1.9	6.0	8.0	1.5
Sun Dried Tomato, Garlic & Basil, Finest, Tesco*	1 Serving/72.5g	123	168	2.0	6.8	14.8	2.9
Sun Dried Tomato, Stir In, Light, Dolmio*	1 Serving/75g	62	83	1.7	9.8	4.7	0.0
Sun Ripened Tomato & Basil, Dolmio*	1 Serving/150g	117	78	1.3	7.9	4.6	0.0
Sun Ripened Tomato & Basil, Microwaveable, Dolmio*	1/2 Pack/190g	106	56	1.4	7.9	2.1	0.0
Sundried Tomato & Basil, Organic, Seeds Of Change*	1/2 Jar/100g	155	155	1.6	7.7	13.1	0.0
Sundried Tomato & Garlic, Marks & Spencer*	1/2 Jar/95g	147	155	2.9	4.4	13.7	0.8
Sweet Pepper, Dolmio*	1 Serving/150g	239	159	1.6	8.8	13.4	0.0
Sweet Red Pepper, Loyd Grossman*	1oz/28g	24	87	1.7	7.3	5.6	1.2
Three Cheeses, Co-Op*	1 Pack/300g	405	135	6.0	6.0	9.0	0.1
Tomato & Aubergine, TTD, Sainsbury's*	1 Serving/150g	107	71	2.1	7.7	3.5	2.0
Tomato & Basil, Bertolli*	1 Serving/250g	118	47	1.5	7.9	1.1	1.6
Tomato & Basil, Carb Check, Heinz*	1 Serving/150g	84	56	1.5	4.4	3.6	0.6
Tomato & Basil, Dolmio*	1 Serving/170g	95	56	1.4	7.9	2.1	0.0
Tomato & Basil, Loyd Grossman*	1/2 Jar/175g	152	87	1.7	7.3	5.6	1.2
Tomato & Basil, Organic, Pasta Reale*	1 Pack/300g	216	72	1.0	5.1	5.3	0.4
Tomato & Basil, Organic, Seeds Of Change*	1 Jar/390g	234	60	1.4	8.5	2.2	1.1
Tomato & Black Olive, Carb Control, Tesco*	1 Serving/110g	74	67	1.3	6.0	4.3	2.3
Tomato & Chargrilled Vegetable, Loyd Grossman*	1 Serving/150g	134	89	1.8	7.9	5.6	0.9
Tomato & Chilli, Loyd Grossman*	1/2 Jar/175g	154	88	1.7	7.3	5.7	0.9

PASTA SAUCE

	Measure INFO/WEIGHT	per Measure KCAL	Nutrition Values per 100g / 100ml KCAL	PROT	CARB	FAT	FIBRE
Tomato & Chilli, Pour Over, Marks & Spencer*	1/2 Jar/165g	124	75	1.2	6.2	5.3	0.8
Tomato & Chunky Mushroom, Dolmio*	1 Pack/475g	323	68	1.2	7.6	3.7	0.0
Tomato & Chunky Vegetable, Asda*	1/2 Jar/280g	143	51	1.4	8.0	1.5	0.5
Tomato & Creme Fraiche, Perfectly Balanced, Waitrose*	1/2 Pot/177g	85	48	1.8	7.1	1.3	2.0
Tomato & Herb, Co-Op*	1 Serving/125g	75	60	1.0	9.0	2.0	1.0
Tomato & Herb, Organic, Marks & Spencer*	1 Jar/320g	176	55	1.1	6.8	2.6	1.8
Tomato & Herb, Organic, Meridian Foods*	1/2 Jar/220g	141	64	1.6	8.1	2.8	1.1
Tomato & Herb, Organic, Sainsbury's*	1 Serving/75g	38	51	1.2	6.6	2.0	0.5
Tomato & Herb, Perfectly Balanced, Waitrose*	1/2 Pot/175g	86	49	1.2	5.3	2.6	0.9
Tomato & Herb, With Extra Garlic, Sainsbury's*	1/2 Pot/150g	62	41	1.4	6.3	1.1	1.6
Tomato & Marscapone, Fresh, Waitrose*	1 Serving/175ml	184	105	1.9	5.5	8.4	1.1
Tomato & Mascapone, Italiano, Tesco*	1/2 Pot/175g	168	96	2.8	5.5	7.0	0.7
Tomato & Mascapone, Sainsbury's*	1/2 Pot/150g	137	91	2.1	5.9	6.6	1.2
Tomato & Mascarpone, BGTY, Sainsbury's*	1/2 Pot/150g	75	50	2.0	3.6	3.0	3.6
Tomato & Mascarpone, Finest, Tesco*	1 Serving/175g	135	77	2.7	5.4	5.0	0.8
Tomato & Mascarpone, Fresh, Sainsbury's*	1 Serving/150g	177	118	2.2	4.2	10.3	1.1
Tomato & Mascarpone, Pasta Reale*	1 Pack/300g	318	106	2.9	5.9	7.9	0.5
Tomato & Mascarpone, Sacla*	1/2 Jar/95g	161	169	2.2	6.2	15.0	0.0
Tomato & Mascarpone, Tesco*	1 Serving/175g	194	111	2.8	5.4	8.7	0.6
Tomato & Mushroom, Asda*	1 Serving/127g	71	56	1.8	8.0	1.9	1.2
Tomato & Mushroom, Organic, Sainsbury's*	1 Serving/150g	87	58	1.6	7.1	2.6	1.5
Tomato & Olives, La Doria*	1 Jar/90g	76	84	1.2	5.0	6.6	0.0
Tomato & Parmesan, Seeds Of Change*	1 Serving/150g	101	67	2.5	7.8	2.9	1.1
Tomato & Roasted Garlic, Loyd Grossman*	1/2 Jar/175g	161	92	2.0	8.8	5.5	0.8
Tomato & Smokey Bacon, Dolmio*	1 Pot/150g	240	160	5.5	5.8	13.1	0.0
Tomato & Spicy Sausages, Marks & Spencer*	1 Jar/330g	215	65	4.0	5.5	3.0	0.8
Tomato & Tuna, Loyd Grossman*	1/2 Jar/175g	154	88	4.4	7.5	4.4	0.8
Tomato & Wild Mushroom, Waitrose*	1 Serving/175g	65	37	1.7	6.0	0.7	0.9
Tomato And Chilli, Pour Over, Marks & Spencer*	1 Serving/110g	77	70	1.3	7.6	3.8	1.8
Tomato Bacon, Stir & Serve, Homepride*	1 Serving/96g	81	84	2.7	8.1	4.5	0.0
Tomato Red Wine Shallots, Bertolli*	1/2 Jar/250g	113	45	1.7	7.2	1.7	1.5
Tomato With Herbs & Garlic, Italian, Safeway*	1 Serving/120g	73	61	1.9	8.7	2.1	1.3
Tomato With Herbs Buon Appetito, Princes*	1 Jar/475g	214	45	0.7	9.6	0.4	0.0
Tomato With Mushrooms, Italian, Safeway*	1/2 Jar/235g	146	62	2.0	8.8	2.1	1.9
Tomato With Onions & Garlic, Italian, Safeway*	1 Serving/50g	35	69	2.3	10.2	2.1	1.8
Tomato, Bacon & Mushroom, Asda*	1/2 Pot/50g	33	66	2.5	6.0	3.6	0.0
Tomato, Basil & Parmesan Stir In, BGTY, Sainsbury's*	1 Serving/75g	69	92	2.9	7.8	5.5	1.0
Tomato, Black Olive, Caper, Finest, Tesco*	1 serving/145g	146	101	1.5	6.4	7.7	3.3
Tomato, Blue Parrot Cafe, Sainsbury's*	1/3 Jar/63g	91	144	3.6	11.5	9.3	1.9
Tomato, Chilli & Onion, Bertolli*	1 Serving/100g	49	49	1.8	6.7	1.7	1.8
Tomato, Garlic & Chilli, Finest, Tesco*	1 serving/145g	199	137	2.0	7.1	11.2	3.4
Tomato, Kalamata Olive & Pine Nut, The Best, Safeway*	1/2 Pot/175g	158	90	1.7	5.0	6.7	1.9
Tomato, Low Price, Sainsbury's*	1 Jar/440g	220	50	0.6	10.1	0.7	0.4
Tomato, Organic, Evernat*	1oz/28g	18	64	2.8	10.2	1.3	0.0
Tomato, Pepper & Herb, Somerfield*	1 Serving/186g	233	125	3.0	17.4	4.8	0.8
Tomato, Roasted Garlic & Mushroom, Bertolli*	1 Jar/500g	255	51	1.9	6.4	2.0	1.5
Tomato, Romano & Garlic, Bertolli*	1/4 Jar/181g	127	70	2.9	7.6	3.0	1.7
Vegetable, Chunky, Tesco*	1 Jar/455g	155	34	1.2	7.0	0.2	1.0
Veneziana, Marks & Spencer*	1/2 Jar/140g	196	140	5.7	5.5	10.7	1.6
Vine Ripened Tomato & Aromatic Basil, Discovery*	1 Serving/125g	161	129	1.8	14.3	7.2	0.0
Vine Ripened Tomato & Black Olive, Bertolli*	1/2 Jar/92.5g	146	157	2.3	7.3	13.3	0.0
Whole Cherry Tomato & Red Chilli, Sacla*	1 Serving/96g	85	89	1.5	6.2	6.5	0.1
Whole Cherry Tomato & Roasted Pepper, Sacla*	1/2 Jar/145g	93	64	1.5	5.2	4.1	0.0

P

	Measure INFO/WEIGHT	per Measure KCAL	Nutrition Values per 100g / 100ml				
			KCAL	PROT	CARB	FAT	FIBRE
PASTA SAUCE							
Wild Mushroom & Herb, Seeds Of Change*	1 Serving/190g	103	54	1.6	8.8	1.4	1.2
PASTA SHAPES							
Dried, Tesco*	1 Serving/100g	345	345	13.2	68.5	2.0	2.9
Economy, Sainsbury's*	1oz/28g	97	346	12.0	72.2	1.0	2.3
In A Cheese & Broccoli Sauce, Tesco*	1 Serving/84g	317	377	13.1	66.2	6.6	4.1
In Rich Chicken, Garilc & Wine Sauce, Tesco*	1 Pack/110g	393	357	14.0	66.1	4.1	4.2
Postman Pat, HP*	1 Can/410g	279	68	1.8	14.3	0.4	0.7
Sabrina, In Tomato Sauce, Heinz*	1 Serving/200g	104	52	1.7	10.9	0.2	0.5
Scooby Doo, HP*	1 Can/410g	279	68	1.8	14.3	0.4	0.7
Teletubbies, Heinz*	1 Can/400g	244	61	2.0	12.3	0.4	0.6
Tesco*, Cooked	1 Serving/260g	356	137	5.1	26.3	0.8	1.1
PASTA SHELLS							
Dry, Average	1 Serving/75g	265	353	11.1	71.8	2.0	2.0
Egg, Fresh, Average	1 Serving/125g	344	275	11.5	49.8	2.9	3.5
In Bolognese Sauce, Weight Watchers*	1 Pack/395g	280	71	5.2	9.6	1.3	0.7
PASTA SNACK							
Cheese & Ham, Pot, Tesco*	1 Serving/208g	254	122	3.4	17.9	4.1	1.5
Cheese & Ham, Tubes, Made Up To Instructions, Tesco*	1 Serving/214g	312	146	4.9	19.5	5.4	2.6
Chicken & Smoked Bacon, Sainsbury's*	1 Pack/190g	490	258	7.2	14.1	19.2	0.0
Chicken, Morrisons*	1 Pack/250g	285	114	3.3	19.3	2.7	0.0
Chicken, With Sweetcorn & Mushroom, Pot, Tesco*	1 Pot/216g	238	110	3.0	18.5	2.7	0.7
Creamy Cheese, Mug Shot, Asda*	1 Serving/250g	273	109	2.5	19.0	2.5	1.8
Ham & Mushroom, Tesco*	1 Pack/300g	618	206	4.2	15.0	14.3	1.1
Tomato & Herb, In A Pot, Dry, Tesco*	1 Pot/59g	207	352	11.8	70.7	2.4	2.6
Tomato & Herb, Morrisons*	1 Pot/247g	247	100	3.1	19.5	1.1	0.0
PASTA SPIRALS							
Co-Op*	1 Serving/100g	350	350	12.0	73.0	1.0	3.0
Glutenfree, Glutano*	1oz/28g	100	357	4.0	83.0	1.0	0.0
PASTA TWIRLS							
Asda*	1 Serving/50g	173	346	12.0	71.0	1.5	3.0
Tri-Colour, Sainsbury's*	1 Serving/75g	268	357	12.3	73.1	1.7	2.5
PASTA TWISTS							
Dry, Average	1oz/28g	99	354	12.3	71.8	1.5	2.2
Wheat & Gluten Free, Glutafin*	1 Serving/75g	263	350	8.0	75.0	2.0	0.1
Whole Wheat, Dry, Tesco*	1 Serving/75g	242	322	12.5	62.5	2.5	10.0
PASTA WITH							
Chargrilled Vegetables & Tomatoes, BGTY, Sainsbury's*	1 Serving/100g	96	96	2.9	17.4	1.6	0.0
Cheese & Tomato, Al Forno, Sainsbury's*	1/2 Pack/499g	749	150	5.5	18.9	5.8	1.8
Chicken, Spicy BBQ, Healthy Living, Tesco*	1 Serving/440g	471	107	5.7	17.2	1.7	0.7
Meatballs, Puglian Style, Marks & Spencer*	1/2 Pack/500g	600	120	5.5	12.5	5.3	1.2
Meatballs, Sainsbury's*	1 Can/300g	339	113	6.6	10.6	4.9	1.6
Prawns & Tomatoes, COU, Marks & Spencer*	1 Serving/270g	243	90	5.4	13.9	1.3	1.3
Rcasted Vegetables & Goats Cheese, Marks & Spencer*	1 Pack/360g	576	160	5.3	19.0	6.8	1.2
Salmon & Broccoli, Lemon Dressed, Sainsbury's*	1 Serving/300g	486	162	6.9	20.4	5.9	2.1
Spicy Chicken, Sainsbury's*	1 Pot/300g	489	163	7.1	20.1	6.1	2.3
Tuna & Roasted Peppers, Marks & Spencer*	1 Serving/220g	308	140	9.1	17.7	3.9	0.9
PASTE							
BBQ Bean, Princes*	1 Serving/33g	35	106	5.7	19.8	0.4	0.0
BBQ Chicken, Princes*	1oz/28g	69	246	14.3	9.5	16.8	0.0
Bacon & Tomato, Tesco*	1 Serving/20g	46	232	14.0	3.4	18.0	0.1
Beef, Princes*	1 Serving/18g	40	220	14.4	5.2	15.8	0.0
Beef, Sainsbury's*	1 Jar/75g	142	189	16.0	1.5	13.2	1.4
Chicken & Ham, Princes*	1 Jar/100g	233	233	13.6	2.8	18.6	0.0

	Measure INFO/WEIGHT	per Measure KCAL	Nutrition Values per 100g / 100ml				
			KCAL	PROT	CARB	FAT	FIBRE
PASTE							
Chicken & Ham, Tesco*	1 Serving/19g	44	231	12.5	1.4	19.5	0.0
Chicken & Mushroom, Princes*	1 Serving/50g	94	187	17.1	5.0	11.0	0.0
Chicken & Stuffing, Asda*	1/2 Jar/35g	71	203	16.0	3.3	14.0	0.0
Chicken & Stuffing, Princes*	1 Jar/100g	229	229	15.7	3.3	17.0	0.0
Chicken, Asda*	Thin Spread/7g	13	184	16.0	0.8	13.0	0.0
Chicken, Princes*	Thin Spread/9g	22	240	12.6	5.6	18.5	0.0
Chicken, Tesco*	1 Serving/12g	30	248	14.8	2.3	20.0	0.1
Chicken, Value, Tesco*	Thin Spread/9g	18	196	15.1	1.8	14.3	0.1
Crab, Princes*	1 Pot/35g	36	104	13.4	4.8	3.5	0.0
Crab, Sainsbury's*	1 Thick Spread/5g	6	115	16.5	1.7	4.7	0.5
Crab, Tesco*	1 Jar/75g	89	119	14.0	4.6	5.0	0.1
Salmon & Shrimp, Tesco*	1 Jar/75g	83	111	15.1	5.0	3.4	0.1
Salmon, Princes*	1 Serving/30g	59	195	13.5	6.5	12.8	0.0
Salmon, Value, Tesco*	1 Serving/10g	17	165	14.0	4.6	10.1	0.8
Sardine & Tomato, Princes*	1 Jar/75g	110	146	15.4	5.0	7.2	0.0
Sardine & Tomato, Sainsbury's*	1 Mini Pot/35g	60	170	16.9	1.2	10.8	1.3
Sardine & Tomato, Tesco*	1 Jar/75g	98	130	14.6	4.8	5.8	0.1
Smokey Bacon, Princes*	1 Serving/30g	60	199	17.3	5.4	12.0	0.0
Sun Dried Tomato, Average	1 Heaped Tsp/10g	39	385	3.2	13.9	35.2	0.0
Tomato, Average	1 Tbsp/20g	19	96	5.0	19.2	0.2	1.5
Tuna & Mayonnaise, Princes*	1 Pot/75g	158	210	16.6	1.3	15.4	0.0
Tuna & Mayonnaise, Sainsbury's*	1 Tbsp/17g	41	242	19.2	0.6	18.1	1.6
Tuna & Mayonnaise, Tesco*	1 Serving/15g	31	209	14.9	2.1	15.7	0.1
Vegetable, Sainsbury's*	1 Serving/17g	26	154	7.4	5.9	11.2	3.4
PASTILLES							
Fruit, Average	1 Tube/33g	108	327	2.8	84.2	0.0	0.0
Fruit, Rowntree's*	1 Tube/53g	186	351	4.4	83.7	0.0	0.0
Wine, Maynards*	1 Pack/52g	161	310	3.9	72.1	0.0	0.0
PASTRAMI							
American Style, Morrisons*	1 Slice/10g	11	114	22.2	2.5	1.7	0.8
Asda*	1 Serving/10g	10	105	24.0	0.3	0.9	0.0
Beef, Average	1 Serving/40g	51	128	23.1	1.1	3.6	0.2
British, Waitrose*	1 Pack/80g	92	115	21.8	0.9	2.7	0.0
Turkey, Average	1/2 Packet/35g	38	107	21.8	1.7	1.5	0.5
PASTRY							
Case, From Supermarket, Average	1 Case/230g	1081	470	5.8	55.9	25.6	1.2
Cherry & Custard, Danish Bar, Tesco*	1 Bar/350g	910	260	3.5	29.9	14.0	7.7
Choux, Cooked	1oz/28g	91	325	8.5	29.8	19.8	1.2
Choux, Raw	1oz/28g	59	211	5.5	19.4	12.9	0.8
Filo, Average	1 Sheet/45g	137	304	9.0	61.4	2.7	0.9
Flaky, Chinese	1oz/28g	110	392	5.4	59.3	16.4	0.0
Flaky, Cooked	1oz/28g	157	560	5.6	45.9	40.6	1.8
Flaky, Raw	1oz/28g	119	424	4.2	34.8	30.7	1.4
Flan Case	1oz/28g	152	544	7.1	56.7	33.6	1.8
Greek	1oz/28g	90	322	4.7	40.0	17.0	0.0
Puff, Fresh, Sainsbury's*	1/2 Pack/250g	1113	445	5.4	28.8	34.3	1.3
Rice, Spring Roll, TY Foods*	1oz/28g	53	190	5.0	36.0	4.0	0.0
Shortcrust, Cooked	1oz/28g	146	521	6.6	54.2	32.3	2.2
Shortcrust, Raw, Average	1oz/28g	127	453	5.6	44.0	29.1	1.3
Wholemeal, Cooked	1oz/28g	140	499	8.9	44.6	32.9	6.3
Wholemeal, Raw	1oz/28g	121	431	7.7	38.5	28.4	5.4
PASTRY MIX							
Short Crust, Somerfield*	1oz/28g	134	479	7.0	49.0	28.0	0.0

	Measure INFO/WEIGHT	per Measure KCAL	Nutrition Values per 100g / 100ml				
			KCAL	PROT	CARB	FAT	FIBRE

PASTY

	Measure INFO/WEIGHT	per Measure KCAL	KCAL	PROT	CARB	FAT	FIBRE
Bite Size Pasties, Food To Go, Sainsbury's*	1 Serving/60g	226	377	8.2	31.2	24.4	1.5
Cheese & Onion, Freshbake*	1 Pastry/135g	368	272	5.6	25.5	16.6	1.1
Cheese & Onion, Geo Adams*	1 Pasty/150g	420	280	6.9	27.9	15.6	1.1
Cheese & Onion, Sainsbury's*	1 Serving/150g	486	324	7.4	24.5	21.8	1.3
Cheese & Onion, Somerfield*	1 Pasty/145g	419	289	7.0	24.0	18.0	0.0
Cheese & Onion, Tesco*	1 Pasty/150g	416	277	5.9	23.7	17.6	2.2
Cheese & Onion, Waitrose*	1 Pasty/70g	233	333	8.0	24.7	20.9	1.7
Chicken & Vegetable, Proper Cornish Ltd	1 Pasty/255g	671	263	7.4	30.2	13.6	2.4
Corned Beef, Mega, Marks & Spencer*	1oz/28g	87	310	9.5	22.3	20.2	0.9
Cornish Roaster, Ginsters*	1 Pasty/130g	417	321	8.5	29.9	18.6	1.3
Cornish, Asda*	1 Pasty/100g	287	287	7.0	22.0	19.0	1.2
Cornish, BGTY, Sainsbury's*	1 Pasty/135g	308	228	7.7	28.2	9.4	1.6
Cornish, Cheese & Onion, Ginsters*	1 Pasty/130g	511	393	10.4	30.7	25.4	2.3
Cornish, Chicken & Bacon, Ginsters*	1 Pasty/227g	574	253	6.9	22.2	15.2	0.8
Cornish, Marks & Spencer*	1 Pasty/150g	480	320	6.5	27.3	20.3	1.5
Cornish, Mega, Marks & Spencer*	1oz/28g	84	300	6.0	18.7	22.1	1.2
Cornish, Mini, Marks & Spencer*	1 Pastie/72g	227	315	6.7	21.0	22.6	1.0
Cornish, Mini, Sainsbury's*	1 Pasty/70g	280	400	7.3	28.1	28.7	1.5
Cornish, Mini, Tesco*	1 Pasty/24g	66	274	5.6	23.2	17.7	0.5
Cornish, Original, Ginsters*	1 Pasty/227g	568	250	6.0	19.0	15.8	1.1
Cornish, Pork Farms*	1 Pasty/250g	673	269	7.7	22.8	16.3	0.0
Cornish, Sainsbury's*	1 Pasty/150g	489	326	6.7	26.6	21.4	2.0
Cornish, SmartPrice, Asda*	1 Pasty/94g	286	304	8.0	32.0	16.0	1.7
Cornish, Tesco*	1 Pasty/150g	467	311	6.8	21.9	21.8	1.6
Cornish, Traditional Style, Geo Adams*	1 Pasty/165g	488	296	7.1	25.4	18.4	1.3
Cornish, Value, Tesco*	1 Pasty/150g	425	283	6.7	24.2	17.7	2.2
Steak & Onion, Marks & Spencer*	1 Pasty/164g	459	280	8.7	19.2	18.8	1.4
Tandoori & Vegetable, Holland & Barratt*	1 Pack/110g	232	211	4.3	29.4	8.5	1.8
Vegetable	1oz/28g	77	274	4.1	33.3	14.9	1.9
Vegetable, Hand Crimped, Waitrose*	1 Pasty/200g	454	227	4.5	26.8	11.3	2.2
Vegetarian, Cornish, Linda McCartney*	1 Pasty/170g	420	247	5.2	25.5	13.8	1.5

PATE

	Measure INFO/WEIGHT	per Measure KCAL	KCAL	PROT	CARB	FAT	FIBRE
Apricot, Asda*	1 Serving/50g	156	312	12.0	3.0	28.0	0.0
Ardennes, 50% Less Fat, BGTY, Sainsbury's*	1 Serving/28g	48	171	18.0	2.2	10.0	0.0
Ardennes, Asda*	1 Serving/50g	143	286	13.9	3.6	24.0	1.3
Ardennes, BGTY, Sainsbury's*	1 Serving/50g	85	169	16.7	2.4	10.3	0.1
Ardennes, Healthy Living, Tesco*	1 Serving/50g	116	231	14.6	7.7	15.8	1.5
Ardennes, Reduced Fat, Good Intentions, Somerfield*	1 Serving/50g	98	195	16.4	2.6	13.2	1.6
Ardennes, Reduced Fat, Safeway*	1 Serving/50g	97	194	18.5	3.1	11.9	0.1
Ardennes, Reduced Fat, Waitrose*	1/4 Pack/42g	94	224	15.4	2.6	16.9	0.5
Ardennes, Sainsbury's*	1 Serving/20g	60	299	16.5	2.1	24.9	0.1
Ardennes, Tesco*	1 Tbsp/15g	53	354	13.3	0.5	33.2	1.2
Ardennes, With Bacon, Tesco*	1/2 Pack/85g	232	273	11.5	3.8	24.1	1.3
Asparagus, Sainsbury's*	1/2 Pot/57g	88	153	3.4	5.4	13.1	1.0
Breton Course Country With Apricots, Sainsbury's*	1 Serving/21g	60	285	13.5	7.0	22.5	0.5
Brie & Cranberry, Marks & Spencer*	1 Serving/55g	193	350	6.0	7.3	33.3	1.5
Brussels & Garlic, Reduced Fat, Tesco*	1 Serving/65g	135	208	16.2	8.1	12.3	0.6
Brussels & Mushroom, 25% Less Fat, Asda*	1 Serving/40g	88	220	14.0	2.7	17.0	0.0
Brussels With Garlic, Asda*	1 Serving/50g	170	340	10.7	4.0	31.3	2.5
Brussels With Wild Mushrooms, The Best, Safeway*	1 oz/28g	89	319	11.6	2.9	29.0	1.0
Brussels, 25% Less Fat, Morrisons*	1/4 Pack/42.5g	107	249	14.2	0.7	20.6	0.0
Brussels, Asda*	1 Serving/50g	175	350	10.7	4.4	32.2	1.7
Brussels, BGTY, 50% Less Fat, Sainsbury's*	1 Serving/100g	223	223	14.6	5.1	16.0	0.1

PATE

INFO/WEIGHT	Measure	per Measure KCAL	KCAL	PROT	CARB	FAT	FIBRE
			Nutrition Values per 100g / 100ml				
Brussels, Fat Reduced, Somerfield*	1 Serving/50g	96	192	14.0	2.0	14.0	0.0
Brussels, Healthy Living, Tesco*	1 Serving/29g	66	229	14.4	8.4	15.3	1.3
Brussels, Marks & Spencer*	1 Pot/170g	519	305	13.3	2.8	26.6	1.0
Brussels, Reduced Fat, Asda*	1 Serving/44g	88	199	15.0	2.1	15.0	1.9
Brussels, Reduced Fat, Waitrose*	1 Serving/40g	92	229	13.2	2.4	18.5	0.5
Brussels, Sainsbury's*	1 Pack/170g	663	390	10.6	1.1	38.2	0.1
Brussels, Sanpareil*	1/4 Pack/37g	121	326	13.0	1.0	30.0	0.0
Brussels, Smooth, Safeway*	1 Pack/170g	553	325	11.5	3.9	29.3	1.6
Brussels, Tesco*	1 Serving/28g	92	330	11.0	3.0	30.5	1.1
Brussels, With Forest Mushroom, Co-Op*	1 Serving/57g	180	315	12.0	2.0	29.0	1.0
Brussels, With Herbs, Tesco*	1 Serving/25g	87	347	8.4	6.4	32.6	1.5
Carrot, Ginger & Spring Onion, Marks & Spencer*	1 Serving/50g	73	145	1.5	9.6	11.0	0.9
Celery, Stilton & Walnut, Waitrose*	1 Pot/115g	294	256	9.0	3.2	23.0	2.2
Chargrilled Vegetable, BGTY, Sainsbury's*	1/2 Pot/57.3g	43	75	4.9	10.8	1.3	2.7
Chick Pea & Black Olive, Cauldron*	1 Pot/113g	203	180	6.2	15.6	10.3	4.5
Chicken & Brandy, Morrisons*	1 Serving/44g	133	303	10.8	4.3	26.9	0.8
Chicken Liver & Brandy, Asda*	1 Serving/50g	177	353	9.0	5.5	32.8	3.2
Chicken Liver Parfait, TTD, Sainsbury's*	1 Serving/20g	72	359	8.0	2.0	35.0	0.5
Chicken Liver With Brandy, Tesco*	1oz/28g	82	293	11.8	3.5	25.8	1.4
Chicken Liver, BGTY, Sainsbury's*	1 Serving/30g	64	214	11.5	6.0	16.0	0.5
Chicken Liver, Marks & Spencer*	1oz/28g	79	281	14.0	1.9	24.1	0.1
Chicken Liver, Organic, Waitrose*	1/2 Tub/87.5g	205	233	12.6	1.8	18.4	1.4
Chicken Liver, With Madeira, Sainsbury's*	1 Serving/30g	84	279	13.1	1.9	24.3	0.0
Chickpea, Fragrant Moroccan, Organic, Cauldron*	1 Tsp/15g	27	177	4.9	9.4	13.3	11.8
Coarse Farmhouse, Organic, Sainsbury's*	1 Serving/56g	138	246	13.3	3.7	19.7	0.8
Coarse Pork Liver With Garlic, Asda*	1 Pack/40g	130	326	13.0	1.0	30.0	0.0
Crab, Waitrose*	1oz/28g	59	209	14.5	0.5	16.6	0.0
De Campagne, Sainsbury's*	1 Serving/55g	129	235	16.3	1.4	18.2	0.0
Duck & Champagne, Luxury, Marks & Spencer*	1oz/28g	106	380	8.3	8.3	35.2	7.8
Duck & Orange, Marks & Spencer*	1oz/28g	88	315	10.6	2.8	29.0	0.5
Duck & Orange, Tesco*	1 Serving/20g	71	357	8.4	3.5	34.4	0.5
Duck & Truffle Medallions, Marks & Spencer*	1 Slice/25g	91	365	9.0	4.8	35.0	1.4
Duck Liver With Champagne & Truffles, TTD, Sainsbury's*	1 Serving/50g	212	423	8.2	2.5	42.2	0.0
Farmhouse Mushroom, Asda*	1 Serving/50g	126	252	13.0	5.0	20.0	0.7
Farmhouse Style, Finest, Tesco*	1 Serving/28g	83	295	11.9	3.6	25.9	1.0
Farmhouse Style, Marks & Spencer*	1/4 Pack/42g	90	215	14.4	1.9	16.9	1.2
Farmhouse Style, Weight Watchers*	1 Serving/36.8g	49	133	14.8	5.5	5.7	0.5
Farmhouse With Christmas Ale, Sainsbury's*	1oz/28g	67	239	15.4	1.6	19.1	0.0
Farmhouse With Herbes de Provence, Tesco*	1 Serving/50g	137	273	13.9	5.4	21.6	1.0
Farmhouse With Mushrooms & Garlic, Tesco*	1 Serving/90g	257	285	13.8	0.6	25.3	1.3
Forestiere, Marks & Spencer*	1 Serving/20g	61	305	11.5	4.2	26.6	1.4
Garlic & Herb Yeast, Tartex*	1 Serving/10g	23	230	7.0	10.0	18.0	0.0
Herb, Organic, Suma*	1 Serving/25g	59	234	12.0	6.0	18.0	0.0
Isle of Skye Smoked Salmon, TTD, Sainsbury's*	1/2 Pot/58g	161	277	16.5	0.8	23.1	0.1
Kipper, Waitrose*	1/4 Tub/28g	105	370	16.8	2.0	32.7	0.6
Liver & Bacon, Tesco*	1 Serving/10g	28	276	12.9	4.3	23.0	0.4
Liver & Pork, Healthy Eating, Tesco*	1 Serving/28g	64	229	14.4	8.4	15.3	1.3
Liver Spreading, Somerfield*	1oz/28g	77	275	14.0	3.0	23.0	0.0
Liver, Value, Tesco*	1 Serving/50g	151	302	13.0	4.1	26.0	0.5
Luxury Orkney Crab, Castle MacLellan*	1 Serving/15g	27	178	11.1	9.2	10.7	0.8
Mackerel, Smoked	1oz/28g	103	368	13.4	1.3	34.4	0.0
Mackerel, Tesco*	1 Serving/29g	102	353	14.3	0.5	32.6	0.0
Mediterranean Roast Vegetable, Tesco*	1 Serving/28g	31	112	2.4	4.3	9.4	1.2

PATE

INFO/WEIGHT	Measure per Measure KCAL	Nutrition Values per 100g / 100ml				
		KCAL	PROT	CARB	FAT	FIBRE
Mexican Red Pepper & Wild Chilli Organic Yeast, Tartex*	1 Pot/50g	99	198	6.4	7.0	16.0	0.0
Mushroom & Herb, Somerfield*	1oz/28g	81	289	4.0	8.0	27.0	0.0
Mushroom & Tarragon, Cauldron*	1oz/28g	43	155	2.8	5.5	13.5	1.4
Mushroom, BGTY, Sainsbury's*	1/2 Pot/58g	29	50	4.6	6.7	0.5	3.0
Mushroom, Marks & Spencer*	1 Pot/115g	224	195	4.2	4.8	17.5	1.3
Mushroom, Organic, Cauldron*	1oz/28g	33	119	2.8	4.3	10.1	1.0
Mushroom, Roast, Tesco*	1/2 Pack/58g	91	159	3.2	7.8	12.8	0.5
Mushroom, Sainsbury's*	1oz/28g	47	168	3.1	5.9	15.2	1.3
Mushroom, Tesco*	1oz/28g	39	138	3.3	9.8	9.5	1.0
Pheasant, TTD, Sainsbury's*	1/6 Pack/28g	59	212	15.4	3.9	15.0	0.8
Poached Salmon & Watercress, Tesco*	1 Serving/25g	60	238	19.2	0.4	17.7	0.2
Pork & Garlic, Somerfield*	1oz/28g	83	295	14.0	3.0	25.0	0.0
Pork & Mushroom, Somerfield*	1oz/28g	95	339	11.0	3.0	31.0	0.0
Pork With Port & Cranberry, Tesco*	1 Serving/28g	83	296	12.1	4.3	25.6	0.6
Pork, With Apple & Cider, Sainsbury's*	1 Serving/50g	152	303	12.5	6.3	25.3	1.1
Pork, With Peppercorns, Tesco*	1 Serving/28g	84	300	12.9	1.4	26.8	0.7
Red Pepper, Marks & Spencer*	1oz/28g	52	185	3.0	6.6	16.2	0.9
Rich Roasted Vegetable & Feta, Cauldron*	1 Pack/115g	147	128	5.3	13.0	7.5	3.3
Ricotta, Subdried Tomato & Basil, Princes*	1 Jar/110g	343	312	5.2	8.3	28.7	0.0
Roasted Carrot, Ginger & Spring Onion, Marks & Spencer*	1 Serving/50g	73	145	1.5	9.6	11.0	0.9
Roasted Red Pepper & Houmous, Princes*	1/4 Jar/27g	32	120	4.6	12.4	5.8	0.0
Roasted Red Pepper, Oven Roasted, Castle MacLellan*	1oz/28g	46	163	3.3	8.2	13.5	0.8
Roasted Red Pepper, Princes*	1 Serving/35g	47	135	4.8	17.6	5.0	0.0
Roasted Vegetable, COU, Marks & Spencer*	1 Pot/115g	86	75	6.2	9.1	1.5	1.4
Salmon Dill, Princes*	1 Serving/70g	124	177	15.4	4.0	11.1	0.5
Salmon, Organic, Marks & Spencer*	1oz/28g	76	270	16.9	0.0	22.5	0.0
Salmon, Smoked, Marks & Spencer*	1oz/28g	74	265	16.9	0.0	22.0	0.0
Salsa, Princes*	1 Serving/25g	21	84	3.6	16.7	0.3	0.0
Scottish Smoked Salmon, Castle MacLellan*	1/4 Tub/28g	62	220	13.5	5.6	16.0	0.0
Scottish Smoked Salmon, Marks & Spencer*	1 Serving/30g	81	270	17.0	0.2	22.3	0.0
Smoked Duck, With Cranberry Coulis, TTD, Sainsbury's*	1 Serving/62g	174	280	10.7	9.3	22.2	1.0
Smoked Mackerel, Sainsbury's*	1/2 Pot/57g	215	378	14.2	0.8	35.3	0.0
Smoked Mackerel, Scottish, Marks & Spencer*	1/2 Pot/57.5g	160	275	15.9	0.6	23.2	0.1
Smoked Salmon, Healthy Living, Tesco*	1 Serving/28g	43	154	16.6	3.4	8.2	0.0
Smoked Salmon, Scottish, Healthy Living, Tesco*	1 Serving/68g	80	118	15.3	1.1	5.8	0.5
Smoked Salmon, Waitrose*	1/2 Pot/56g	122	217	17.7	1.5	15.6	0.6
Smoked Trout, Waitrose*	1/2 Pot/56g	130	232	15.8	0.9	18.4	0.6
Spiced Parsnip & Carrot, Organic, Asda*	1/2 Pot/58g	63	109	3.7	10.0	6.0	2.6
Spicy Bean, BGTY, Sainsbury's*	1/2 Pot/58g	56	97	5.0	15.1	1.9	5.4
Spicy Bean, Princes*	1/2 Pot/55g	46	84	3.6	16.7	0.3	0.0
Spicy Bean, Weight Watchers*	1 Serving/37g	33	89	5.7	12.9	1.6	4.2
Spicy Mexican, Organic, Waitrose*	1 Serving/50g	58	115	6.2	8.6	6.2	3.5
Spinach & Soft Cheese, Cauldron*	1 Pack/113g	209	185	5.1	6.8	15.4	2.3
Spinach, Parmesan & Almond, Cauldron*	1/3 Pack/38g	66	173	7.2	6.3	13.2	2.3
Spinach, Soft Cheese & Onion, Co-Op*	1oz/28g	48	170	5.0	3.0	15.0	4.0
Sweet Roasted Parsnip & Carrot, Cauldron*	1 Serving/60g	64	107	3.7	9.8	5.9	2.6
Tofu, Spicy Mexican, Organic, GranoVita*	1 Serving/50g	112	224	4.0	7.0	20.0	0.0
Tomato, Lentil & Basil, Cauldron*	1oz/28g	43	154	7.5	15.6	6.8	1.5
Tomato, Organic, GranoVita*	1 Tsp/5g	11	215	5.0	6.0	19.0	0.0
Tuna With Butter & Lemon Juice, Sainsbury's*	1/2 Pot/58g	209	360	19.0	0.1	31.6	0.3
Tuna, Marks & Spencer*	1oz/28g	99	355	18.0	0.0	31.3	0.0
Tuna, Tesco*	1 Pack/115g	332	289	19.8	0.3	23.2	0.2
Vegetable	1oz/28g	48	173	7.5	5.9	13.4	0.0

P

	Measure INFO/WEIGHT	per Measure KCAL	Nutrition Values per 100g / 100ml				
			KCAL	PROT	CARB	FAT	FIBRE
PATE							
Vegetable, Cauldron*	1 Pack/112.8g	220	195	9.2	14.1	11.3	4.4
Yeast With Mushrooms, Organic, Tartex*	1oz/28g	56	200	7.0	7.0	16.0	0.0
Yeast With Red & Green Peppers, Vessen*	1 Pot/50g	111	222	6.0	9.0	18.0	0.0
Yeast, Wild Mushroom, GranoVita*	1oz/28g	60	213	10.0	5.0	17.0	0.0
PAVLOVA							
Bucks Fizz Mini Champagne, Co-Op*	1 Pavlova/19g	62	325	3.0	38.0	18.0	0.5
Mandarin, Mini, Iceland*	1 Pavlova/22.0g	59	268	2.1	37.9	12.0	1.7
Raspberry & Lemon, Asda*	1 Serving/43.4g	101	235	2.8	46.0	4.4	0.5
Raspberry, Individual, Marks & Spencer*	1 Pavlova/65g	133	205	4.0	41.8	2.4	0.2
Raspberry, Marks & Spencer*	1 Serving/84g	193	230	2.3	33.3	9.6	0.3
Raspberry, Sara Lee*	1/6 Slice/55.4g	167	303	2.7	38.5	15.3	1.1
Raspberry, Tesco*	1 Serving/65g	191	294	2.7	41.8	12.9	1.1
Sticky Toffee, Sainsbury's*	1/6 Pack/61g	249	415	3.7	63.1	16.4	0.9
Strawberry & Champagne, Mini, Co-Op*	1 Pavlova/19g	65	340	3.0	40.0	19.0	0.8
Strawberry, COU, Marks & Spencer*	1 Pot/95g	147	155	2.4	30.5	2.4	0.8
Toffee Pecan, Marks & Spencer*	1oz/28g	118	420	3.9	41.5	26.6	0.4
Toffee, Mini, Iceland*	1 Pavlova/19.3g	67	353	3.0	51.5	15.0	1.9
PAW-PAW							
Raw, Fresh	1oz/28g	10	36	0.5	8.8	0.1	2.2
Raw, Weighed With Skin & Pips	1oz/28g	8	27	0.4	6.6	0.1	1.7
PEACHES							
Dried, Average	1 Pack/250g	473	189	2.6	45.0	0.7	6.9
In Fruit Juice, Average	1oz/28g	13	47	0.5	11.2	0.0	0.7
In Syrup, Average	1oz/28g	19	67	0.4	16.3	0.1	0.4
Pieces In Strawberry Jelly, Fruitini*	1 Can/140g	91	65	0.3	15.3	0.1	0.0
Raw, Average	1oz/28g	9	32	1.0	7.2	0.1	1.4
PEANUT BUTTER							
Creamy, Smooth, Sun Pat*	1 Tsp/15g	93	620	24.0	17.5	50.2	6.1
Crunchy, Harvest Spread*	1 Tbsp/25g	148	592	23.6	12.5	49.7	6.9
Crunchy, No Added Sugar, Whole Earth*	1 Tsp/10g	59	592	24.9	10.1	50.2	7.3
Crunchy, Organic, Evernat*	1 Tsp/10g	64	641	29.0	13.0	53.0	7.0
Crunchy, Organic, No Added Sugar, Waitrose*	1 Tbsp/12g	71	592	24.9	10.1	50.2	7.3
Crunchy, Original Style, Whole Earth*	1 Serving/20g	118	592	24.9	10.1	50.2	7.3
Crunchy, Original, Sun Pat*	1 Tsp/10g	60	600	27.0	14.5	48.2	6.8
Crunchy, Sainsbury's*	1 Tsp/10g	59	594	23.2	12.0	50.2	6.7
Crunchy, Tesco*	1 Tsp/10g	61	614	27.8	12.0	50.5	6.5
Crunchy, Value, Tesco*	1 Serving/20g	121	606	22.5	11.6	52.2	5.7
Extra Crunchy, Sun Pat*	1 Serving/10g	62	615	25.1	16.3	50.2	6.3
GFY, Asda*	1 Tsp/15g	80	531	28.0	31.0	35.0	0.0
Kraft*	1 Serving/10g	56	557	17.0	37.8	38.0	0.0
Organic, Rapunzel*	1 Tsp/5g	31	613	29.0	4.5	53.0	0.0
Organic, Whole Earth*	1 Serving/5g	30	595	24.6	9.9	50.8	7.1
SmartPrice, Asda*	1 Tbsp/15g	87	582	23.0	10.0	50.0	6.0
Smooth	1 Tsp/10g	62	623	22.6	13.1	53.7	5.4
Smooth, 25% Less Fat, Tesco*	1 Serving/30g	159	529	22.6	30.7	35.1	6.7
Smooth, BGTY, Sainsbury's*	1 Tsp/10g	53	533	22.6	31.7	35.1	6.7
Smooth, Light, Kraft*	1 Tsp/20g	114	571	16.3	40.1	38.6	0.0
Smooth, Organic, Meridian Foods*	1 Serving/10g	61	612	31.2	12.2	48.7	6.5
Smooth, Organic, Tesco*	1 Tbsp/15g	89	596	23.3	12.4	50.3	6.8
Smooth, Organic, Waitrose*	1 Serving/12g	71	595	24.6	9.9	50.8	7.1
Smooth, Sun Pat*	1 Serving/20g	117	585	27.9	14.4	46.3	7.1
Smooth, Tesco*	1 Tsp/10g	61	614	27.8	12.0	50.5	6.5
Stripy, Sun Pat*	1 Tsp/10g	62	617	13.0	35.0	47.0	3.0

P

	Measure INFO/WEIGHT	per Measure KCAL	Nutrition Values per 100g / 100ml				
			KCAL	PROT	CARB	FAT	FIBRE
PEANUT BUTTER							
Whole Grain	1 Tsp/10g	61	606	24.9	7.7	53.1	6.0
Wholenut, Sainsbury's*	1 Tbsp/15g	90	598	24.2	9.8	51.3	7.0
Wholenut, Tesco*	1 Tsp/5g	30	590	24.9	10.1	50.0	6.3
PEANUT SHOOTS							
Sainsbury's*	1 Pack/80g	177	221	10.6	4.1	16.9	2.5
Without Oil, Sainsbury's*	1 Serving/80g	48	60	10.6	4.1	0.0	2.5
PEANUTS							
Chilli, Average	1/2 Pack/50g	303	605	28.2	9.3	50.6	6.8
Dry Roasted, Average	1 Serving/20g	117	587	25.7	11.5	48.8	6.5
Honey Roasted, Average	1oz/28g	169	605	26.9	23.6	47.1	5.5
Plain, Average	10 Whole/10g	59	592	24.7	11.0	50.0	6.3
Roast, Salted, Average	10 Nuts/12g	74	614	27.8	7.9	52.4	4.9
Salted, Average	10 Peanuts/6g	37	609	27.0	8.3	52.1	5.4
PEARL BARLEY							
Boiled	1oz/28g	34	120	2.7	27.6	0.6	0.0
Raw	1oz/28g	101	360	7.9	83.6	1.7	0.0
PEARS							
Comice, Raw, Weighed With Core	1 Med/170g	56	33	0.3	8.5	0.0	2.0
Conference, Average	1oz/28g	14	49	0.3	11.6	0.2	2.3
Dessert, Green, Sainsbury's*	1 Pear/135g	53	39	0.3	9.2	0.1	2.0
Dried, Average	1oz/28g	57	204	1.9	48.4	0.5	9.7
In Fruit Juice, Average	1 Serving/225g	102	45	0.3	10.9	0.0	1.2
In Syrup, Average	1oz/28g	16	58	0.2	14.4	0.1	1.4
Prickly, Raw, Fresh	1oz/28g	14	49	0.7	11.5	0.3	0.0
Raw, Average	1oz/28g	11	38	0.3	9.1	0.1	1.4
Red, Tesco*	1 Pear/180g	65	36	0.4	8.3	0.1	2.2
William, Raw	1 Med/170g	58	34	0.4	8.3	0.1	2.2
PEAS							
& Sweetcorn, Fresh, Marks & Spencer*	1oz/28g	21	75	4.8	11.4	1.5	3.0
Dried, Raw	1oz/28g	85	303	21.6	52.0	2.4	13.0
Frozen, Average	1 Serving/85g	55	64	5.4	9.0	0.8	4.9
Frozen, Boiled, Average	1 Serving/75g	51	68	6.0	9.4	0.9	5.1
Garden, Canned, No Sugar Or Salt, Average	1 Can/80g	36	45	4.4	6.0	0.4	2.8
Garden, Canned, With Sugar & Salt, Average	1 Serving/90g	59	66	5.3	9.3	0.7	5.1
Garden, Frozen, Average	1 Serving/90g	66	74	6.3	9.8	1.1	3.3
Garden, Minted, Average	1 Serving/113g	84	74	6.3	9.7	1.1	5.9
Hand Shelled, & Baby Leeks, Sainsbury's*	1 Serving/120g	59	49	4.0	5.8	1.2	3.3
Marrowfat, Average	1 Sm Can/160g	140	88	6.4	14.3	0.6	3.9
Mushy, Average	1 Can/200g	173	86	6.2	14.3	0.5	2.2
Processed, Canned, Average	1 Sm Can/220g	176	80	6.1	12.3	0.8	3.7
Sugar Snap, Average	1oz/28g	10	34	3.3	4.9	0.2	1.4
Summer Sweet, Green Giant*	3/4 Cup/175ml	107	61	3.4	11.0	0.4	0.0
PEASE PUDDING							
Canned, Re-Heated, Drained	1oz/28g	26	93	6.8	16.1	0.6	1.8
PECAN NUTS							
Average	3 Nuts/18g	125	693	10.1	5.7	70.1	4.7
PECORINO ROMANO							
Tesco*	1 Serving/100g	366	366	28.5	0.0	28.0	0.0
PENNE							
Arrabbiata, BGTY, Sainsbury's*	1 Pack/450g	414	92	2.9	16.5	1.6	1.9
Chicken & Red Wine, Italiana, Weight Watchers*	1 Pack/395g	249	63	3.7	10.1	0.7	0.6
Chicken & Tomato, Italian, Sainsbury's*	1/2 Pack/350g	473	135	7.6	19.0	3.2	1.6
Chilli & Garlic, Asda*	1 Serving/75g	260	346	12.0	71.0	1.5	3.0

	Measure INFO/WEIGHT	per Measure KCAL	Nutrition Values per 100g / 100ml				
			KCAL	PROT	CARB	FAT	FIBRE
PENNE							
Cooked, Average	1 Serving/185g	244	132	4.7	26.7	0.7	1.1
Corn, Free From, Dry, Sainsbury's*	1 Serving/100g	348	348	7.6	74.2	2.3	5.2
Creamy Mushroom, Tesco*	1/2 Pack/200g	288	144	4.5	17.4	6.4	3.3
Creamy Sun Dried Tomato & Mascarpone, Somerfield*	1 Pack/500g	775	155	5.0	21.0	6.0	0.0
Dry, Average	1 Serving/100g	352	352	12.4	71.3	1.9	2.7
Egg, Fresh, Average	1 Serving/125g	353	282	11.1	52.2	3.2	2.0
Free From, Tesco*	1 Serving/100g	340	340	8.0	72.5	2.0	2.5
Fresh, Dry, Average	1 Serving/125g	223	178	7.3	32.2	1.9	1.6
Hickory Steak, American, Sainsbury's*	1 Pack/450g	545	121	6.5	19.8	1.8	1.5
Hickory Steak, Marks & Spencer*	1 Pack/400g	540	135	6.9	19.3	3.1	1.3
In Tomato & Basil Sauce, Sainsbury's*	1/2 Pack/110g	118	107	3.6	21.8	0.6	1.1
Leek & Bacon, Al Forno, Asda*	1/2 Pack/300g	531	177	5.0	10.0	13.0	0.5
Mediterranean, Healthy Living, Tesco*	1 Pack/400g	296	74	2.9	9.6	2.7	1.5
Mozzarella, Safeway*	1 Serving/400g	480	120	5.2	16.3	3.8	1.5
Napoletana Chicken, BFY, Morrisons*	1 Pack/350g	252	72	6.4	7.2	1.6	0.2
Organic, Dry, Average	1 Serving/100g	352	352	12.4	71.6	1.8	1.9
Rigate, Dry, Average	1 Serving/50g	177	353	12.3	72.1	1.8	1.8
Roasted Red Pepper, GFY, Asda*	1 Pack/400g	212	53	1.9	10.0	0.6	0.8
Tomato & Basil Sauce, Asda*	1/2 Pack/314g	185	59	0.8	6.0	3.5	2.0
Tomato & Vegtable, Heinz*	1 Serving/300g	135	45	1.7	8.3	0.6	0.7
Tuna, Tomato & Olive, Asda*	1 Pack/340g	173	51	4.2	4.2	1.9	0.6
Wheat, Gluten, Milk & Egg Free, Dry, Trufree*	1 Serving/75g	263	350	8.0	75.0	2.0	0.0
With Chilli & Red Peppers, Asda*	1 Can/400g	224	56	1.3	10.0	1.2	0.6
With Roasted Vegetables, Waitrose*	1 Pack/400g	424	106	2.8	15.0	3.9	0.8
PENNETTE							
Tricolore, Sainsbury's*	1 Serving/100g	357	357	12.3	73.1	1.7	2.5
PEPERAMI*							
Hot	1oz/28g	155	554	19.0	2.5	52.0	1.2
Mini	1 stick/10.1g	54	536	22.0	1.7	49.0	0.1
Original	1oz/28g	150	536	22.0	1.7	49.0	0.1
PEPPER							
Cayenne, Ground	1 Tsp/1.8g	6	318	12.0	31.7	17.3	0.0
Frank Cooper*	1 Serving/1g	1	68	12.2	0.0	2.1	0.0
PEPPERONI							
Ready To Eat, Average	1 Pack/50g	204	407	21.2	2.7	34.6	0.2
PEPPERS							
Capsicum, Green, Boiled in Salted Water	1oz/28g	5	18	1.0	2.6	0.5	1.8
Capsicum, Green, Raw	1oz/28g	4	15	0.8	2.6	0.3	1.6
Capsicum, Red, Boiled in Salted Water	1oz/28g	10	34	1.1	7.0	0.4	1.7
Capsicum, Red, Raw	1oz/28g	9	32	1.0	6.4	0.4	1.6
Capsicum, Yellow, Raw	1oz/28g	7	26	1.2	5.3	0.2	1.7
Chilli, Green, Raw	1 Med Pepper/13g	4	40	2.0	9.5	0.2	1.5
Chilli, Green, Very Lazy, EPC*	1 Serving/10g	11	114	4.2	15.3	4.0	0.5
Chilli, Mixed, Raw, Tesco*	1 Chili/13g	3	27	1.8	4.2	0.3	1.6
Green, Filled, Tesco*	1 Pepper/150g	117	78	2.6	9.0	3.5	0.7
Italian Style, Sainsbury's*	1 serving/150g	161	107	3.5	14.1	5.0	2.1
Jalapeno, Co-Op*	1oz/28g	74	265	5.0	31.0	13.0	0.9
Mixed Bag, From Supermarket, Average	1oz/28g	7	25	1.0	4.5	0.4	1.7
Red, Filled With Feta, COU, Marks & Spencer*	1 Pepper/153.8g	200	130	4.1	12.4	7.2	0.6
Roasted Red & Yellow, in Oil, Marks & Spencer*	1 Serving/40g	34	85	1.1	4.4	6.9	3.5
Stuffed With Rice	1oz/28g	24	85	1.5	15.4	2.4	1.3
Stuffed With Vegetables, Cheese Topping	1oz/28g	31	111	3.4	9.8	6.7	1.5
Stuffed, Fresh, Asda*	1 Pepper/150g	144	96	3.8	9.0	5.0	1.2

P

	Measure	per Measure	Nutrition Values per 100g / 100ml				
	INFO/WEIGHT	KCAL	KCAL	PROT	CARB	FAT	FIBRE
PEPPERS							
Stuffed, Perfectly Balanced, Waitrose*	1 Pack/300g	243	81	3.0	11.8	2.4	1.3
Stuffed, Ready To Roast, Waitrose*	1 Serving/150g	129	86	3.6	10.5	3.3	2.3
Stuffed, Sainsbury's*	1 Serving/137g	169	123	3.3	11.8	6.9	1.0
Stuffed, Yellow, Italian, Ready to Roast, Sainsbury's*	1 Pack/136g	144	106	5.3	9.9	5.0	1.3
Sweet, Raw	1 Serving/100g	16	16	0.8	2.6	0.3	1.6
Sweet, Tinned, Sainsbury's*	1/2 Can/125g	45	36	1.1	7.0	0.4	1.7
PERNOD*							
19% Volume	1 Shot/50	65	130	0.0	0.0	0.0	0.0
PETIT POIS							
& Baby Carrots, Tesco*	1 Serving/110g	63	57	3.0	11.2	0.0	3.0
& Sugarsnap Peas, & Baby Corn, Asda*	1 Serving/120g	50	42	3.2	7.0	0.0	2.9
Average	1 Serving/65g	34	53	5.0	6.8	0.7	3.5
In Water, Sugar & Salt Added, Sainsbury's*	1/2 Tin/140g	81	58	4.0	9.4	0.5	2.0
PHEASANT							
Meat Only, Roasted	1oz/28g	62	220	27.9	0.0	12.0	0.0
Meat Only, Roasted, Weighed With Bone	1oz/28g	32	114	14.5	0.0	6.2	0.0
Stuffed, Easy Carve, Finest, Tesco*	1 Serving/200g	540	270	23.2	2.2	18.7	0.9
PICCALILLI							
Dijon, Sainsbury's*	1 Dtsp/15.4g	14	91	1.8	19.0	0.9	0.7
Haywards*	1 Serving/28g	18	66	1.4	13.9	0.5	0.0
Sainsbury's*	1 Dtsp/15g	9	60	1.8	11.9	0.6	0.7
Sandwich, Tesco*	1 Serving/20g	19	93	0.6	21.5	0.5	0.7
Sweet, Asda*	1 Tbsp/15g	17	112	0.5	27.0	0.2	0.6
Tesco*	1 Serving/50g	51	102	0.5	17.8	3.6	2.0
Three Mustard, Finest, Tesco*	1 Serving/30g	40	134	1.3	30.7	0.7	1.0
PICKLE							
Branston, Crosse & Blackwell*	1 Tsp/10g	11	109	0.8	26.1	0.2	1.1
Brinjal, Patak's*	1 Tsp/16g	59	367	2.2	34.6	24.4	0.9
Chilli Tomato, Patak's*	1oz/28g	27	95	2.5	16.0	3.2	1.5
Chilli, Branston*	1 Tsp/16g	21	130	0.7	30.0	0.7	1.5
Chilli, Patak's*	1 Tsp/16g	52	325	4.3	1.3	33.7	0.0
Dill, Cucumbers, Safeway*	1oz/28g	5	19	0.9	3.5	0.2	0.0
Garlic, Patak's*	1 Tsp/16g	42	261	3.6	20.0	18.5	1.6
Lime, Hot, Patak's*	1 Tsp/16g	31	194	2.2	4.0	18.7	0.4
Lime, Marks & Spencer*	1 Tsp/16g	34	215	0.8	42.5	4.8	2.4
Lime, Oily	1oz/28g	50	178	1.9	8.3	15.5	0.0
Lime, Sharwood's*	1 Tsp/16g	24	152	2.2	15.0	9.3	2.9
Mango, Hot, Patak's*	1 Tsp/16g	43	270	2.3	7.4	25.7	1.9
Mild Mustard, Heinz*	1 Tbsp/10g	13	129	2.2	25.7	1.3	0.9
Mixed, Drained, Haywards*	1/2 Jar/120g	22	18	1.4	2.4	0.3	0.0
Mixed, Patak's*	1 Serving/30g	78	259	2.3	4.7	25.7	0.8
Original, Tesco*	1 Tsp/25g	33	132	0.8	30.4	0.2	1.1
Sandwich, Branston*	1 Tsp/10g	14	140	0.7	34.2	0.3	1.3
Sandwich, Tesco*	1 Serving/5g	7	138	1.0	33.1	0.2	1.0
Smooth, Branston*	1 Serving/13g	18	139	0.6	34.0	0.1	1.4
Spicy, Branston*	1 Heaped Tsp/15g	21	140	0.7	34.7	0.3	1.3
Sweet	1 Tsp/10g	14	141	0.6	36.0	0.1	1.2
Sweet Harvest, Asda*	1 Serving/25g	39	154	0.8	37.0	0.3	0.8
Sweet, Frank Cooper*	1 Pot/20g	21	104	0.5	25.3	0.1	0.8
Sweet, Hartley's*	1 Tsp/16g	7	140	0.5	36.2	0.0	0.0
Sweet, Low Price, Sainsbury's*	1 serving/23g	23	98	0.7	23.2	0.3	0.7
Sweet, Value, Tesco*	1 Serving/10g	10	96	0.6	23.0	0.2	0.7
Tangy, Sandwich, Heinz*	1 Tsp/10g	13	134	0.7	31.4	0.2	0.9

	Measure INFO/WEIGHT	per Measure KCAL	Nutrition Values per 100g / 100ml				
			KCAL	PROT	CARB	FAT	FIBRE
PICKLE							
Tomato, Tangy, Heinz*	1 Tsp/10g	10	102	2.0	22.0	0.3	1.5
PICKLES							
Mixed, Salad Bar, Asda*	1oz/28g	11	40	0.5	9.2	0.1	0.0
Red Cabbage, Asda*	1 Serving/50g	16	32	1.6	6.0	0.1	0.0
PICNIC							
Cadbury*	1 Bar/48g	228	475	7.5	58.3	23.6	0.0
PIE							
Admiral's, Ross*	1 Pie/340g	357	105	4.8	10.9	4.6	0.7
Admiral, Young's*	1 Pie/340g	357	105	4.6	10.7	4.9	0.7
Apple & Blackberry, Lattice Topped, BGTY, Sainsbury's*	1/4 Serving/100g	256	256	2.8	44.4	7.5	3.1
Apple & Blackberry, Shortcrust, Marks & Spencer*	1 Serving/142g	469	330	4.3	50.2	12.5	1.1
Apple & Blackberry, Tesco*	1 Serving/106g	287	271	4.2	38.4	11.2	1.7
Apple & Blackcurrant, Mr Kipling*	1 Pie/66g	228	346	3.4	53.9	13.0	1.6
Apple Meringue, Frozen, Sara Lee*	1/6 Slice/74g	179	242	2.7	37.9	8.8	1.5
Apple, & Blackberry, Fruit, Finest, Tesco*	1 Pie/95g	265	279	13.7	29.3	11.9	2.8
Apple, American, Iceland*	1 Portion/92g	258	280	4.8	39.2	11.6	2.2
Apple, Asda*	1/4 Pack/106.7g	288	269	3.6	39.0	11.0	1.7
Apple, Bramley, Free From, Tesco*	1 Pie/60g	185	309	2.5	55.4	8.6	1.4
Apple, Bramley, Individual, Sainsbury's*	1 Pie/53.7g	166	307	3.6	52.2	9.3	1.3
Apple, Bramley, Individual, Tesco*	1 Pie/61g	210	344	3.4	53.1	13.0	1.5
Apple, Bramley, Large, Tesco*	1/8 Slice/87g	224	257	3.8	37.4	10.2	1.7
Apple, Cooked, Speedibake*	1 Serving/120g	340	283	3.4	38.5	12.8	1.5
Apple, Deep Filled, Sainsbury's*	1/4 Pie/137g	374	273	3.8	35.6	12.8	1.6
Apple, Individual, Somerfield*	1 Pie/47.2g	178	379	3.5	53.2	16.9	1.3
Apple, Low Price, Sainsbury's*	1/4 Pie/103g	291	283	4.4	33.5	14.6	1.3
Apple, McVitie's*	1 Slice/117g	316	270	3.0	39.0	11.0	2.0
Apple, Pastry Top & Bottom	1oz/28g	74	266	2.9	35.8	13.3	1.7
Apple, Puff Pastry, Marks & Spencer*	1 Pie/135g	338	250	2.4	31.3	12.7	1.0
Apple, Ready Baked, Sara Lee*	1/6 Pie/89.9g	249	277	2.8	35.4	13.8	1.2
Apple, Ready to Bake, TTD, Sainsbury's*	1/6 Pie/125g	353	282	3.2	38.2	12.9	0.7
Apple, Sainsbury's*	1/6/118g	314	266	3.4	37.1	11.5	0.6
Apple, SmartPrice, Asda*	1 Serving/47g	178	379	3.5	53.0	17.0	1.3
Apple, Tesco*	1 Pie/47g	191	406	3.3	59.4	17.2	1.5
Apple, Value, Tesco*	1 Pie/47g	179	381	3.4	53.2	17.0	1.3
Apricot Fruit, GFY, Asda*	1 Serving/52g	162	311	3.3	52.0	10.0	0.0
Banoffee Cream, American Dream, Heinz*	1/6 Pie/70g	239	342	3.7	33.7	21.4	3.9
Banoffee Cream, American Dream, McVitie's*	1 Portion/70g	277	396	4.3	36.7	25.5	0.8
Banoffee, Sainsbury's*	1 Pie/104g	383	368	3.7	37.1	22.8	0.7
Banoffee, Tesco*	1 Pie/112g	381	340	3.7	45.4	15.9	1.2
Beef & Kidney, Farmfoods*	1oz/28g	68	242	5.6	23.9	13.8	1.1
Beef & Vegetable, MacDougalls, McDougalls*	1/4 Pie/114g	292	256	5.3	20.6	16.9	0.3
Beef Steak, Aberdeen Angus, Top Crust, Waitrose*	1/2 Pie/280g	476	170	10.0	13.4	8.6	4.1
Beef, Lean, BGTY, Sainsbury's*	1 Serving/212g	280	132	7.3	12.2	6.0	1.5
Beef, Sainsbury's*	1 Pie/209.8g	536	255	10.3	21.2	14.3	2.0
Blackberry & Apple, Sara Lee*	1 Serving/100g	272	272	2.9	34.0	13.9	0.0
Blackcurrant, Deep Filled, Sainsbury's*	1 Slice/137g	440	321	5.8	42.6	14.1	2.2
Blackcurrant, Shortcrust, Marks & Spencer*	1 Pie/142g	412	290	3.9	45.6	10.1	1.3
Bramley Apple & Blackberry, Marks & Spencer*	1/4 Pie/146g	380	260	3.4	39.8	9.9	1.3
Bramley Apple & Custard, Lattice Topped, Mr Kipling*	1 Pie/64g	236	369	3.8	53.7	15.4	1.1
Bramley Apple & Damson, Marks & Spencer*	1/4 Pie/142.3g	369	260	3.3	39.7	9.8	2.1
Bramley Apple, Deep Filled, Mr Kipling*	1 Pie/66g	220	333	3.4	50.7	13.0	1.3
Bramley Apple, Deep Filled, Sainsbury's*	1/6 Pie/120g	329	274	3.7	38.0	11.9	1.9
Bramley Apple, Individual, Mr Kipling*	1 Pie/66g	228	346	3.3	53.9	13.0	1.3

P

PIE

INFO/WEIGHT	Measure	per Measure KCAL	KCAL	PROT	CARB	FAT	FIBRE
Bramley Apple, Less Than 10% fat, Sainsbury's*	1 Pie/53.7g	166	307	3.6	52.2	9.3	1.3
Bramley Apple, Marks & Spencer*	1 Pie/55g	184	335	2.9	57.6	11.7	1.6
Bramley Apple, Reduced Fat, Asda*	1 Pie/56g	176	314	3.3	55.1	9.4	1.3
Bramley Apple, Somerfield*	1/6 Pie/70.2g	193	275	3.5	34.0	12.8	2.4
Cheese & Onion, Hollands*	1 Pie/200g	516	258	6.3	30.9	12.2	0.0
Cheese & Potato	1oz/28g	39	139	4.8	12.6	8.1	0.7
Cherry Bakewell Meringue, Sara Lee*	1 Slice/69.9g	228	326	4.1	51.9	11.3	1.4
Cherry, Deep Filled, Somerfield*	1/6 Pie/90g	259	288	3.0	41.0	12.0	0.0
Cherry, Sainsbury's*	1 Serving/117g	325	278	3.9	39.6	11.6	1.7
Cherry, Shortcrust, Marks & Spencer*	1 Pie/142g	412	290	3.6	43.4	10.9	0.8
Cherry, Tesco*	1 Serving/106g	294	277	4.0	38.3	12.0	1.8
Chicken & Asparagus, Lattice, Waitrose*	1 Serving/100g	295	295	7.4	22.3	19.6	1.8
Chicken & Asparagus, McDougalls*	1 Serving/170g	394	232	7.4	21.6	12.9	1.5
Chicken & Asparagus, Tesco*	1 Serving/170g	468	275	8.3	22.4	16.9	0.8
Chicken & Bacon, Filo Pastry, Finest, Tesco*	1 Serving/160g	362	226	11.3	18.9	11.7	1.7
Chicken & Bacon, Puff Pastry, Deep Fill, Sainsbury's*	1/3 Pie/200g	532	266	9.1	19.1	17.0	1.3
Chicken & Bacon, Shortcrust Pastry, Tesco*	1 Pie/600g	1632	272	7.6	22.2	17.0	0.2
Chicken & Bacon, With Cheese Sauce, Tesco*	1 Serving/200g	540	270	12.0	17.6	16.8	0.8
Chicken & Basil, Marks & Spencer*	1oz/28g	59	210	8.9	17.0	11.9	1.1
Chicken & Broccoli Lattice, Sainsbury's*	1/2 Pie/192g	520	271	9.3	22.4	16.0	0.9
Chicken & Broccoli Potato, Top, Asda*	1 Pack/400g	319	80	5.3	10.8	1.8	0.7
Chicken & Broccoli, BGTY, Sainsbury's*	1 Pack/490g	377	77	6.9	7.7	2.1	1.9
Chicken & Broccoli, COU, Marks & Spencer*	1 Serving/320g	272	85	8.1	8.8	1.9	1.3
Chicken & Broccoli, Cumberland, Tesco*	1 Pie/450g	482	107	7.0	8.8	4.9	1.0
Chicken & Broccoli, Eat Smart, Safeway*	1 Pack/400g	320	80	6.9	8.5	2.0	1.2
Chicken & Broccoli, GFY, Asda*	1 Pack/400g	340	85	7.0	9.0	2.3	0.5
Chicken & Broccoli, Good Intentions, Somerfield*	1 Pack/450g	383	85	6.8	10.5	1.8	0.5
Chicken & Broccoli, Healthy Living, Tesco*	1 Pie/400g	387	86	5.4	9.9	2.7	0.7
Chicken & Broccoli, Lattice, Tesco*	1/2 Pie/200g	496	248	8.5	18.9	15.4	2.1
Chicken & Gravy, Deep Fill, Asda*	1 Serving/130g	371	285	10.0	23.0	17.0	0.8
Chicken & Gravy, Healthy Living, Tesco*	1 Serving/450g	284	63	5.0	8.3	1.5	1.5
Chicken & Gravy, Puff Pastry, Deep Fill, Sainsbury's*	1 Pie/250g	575	230	9.1	20.9	12.3	1.9
Chicken & Gravy, Shortcrust Pastry, Sainsbury's*	1 Serving/250g	638	255	8.0	24.1	14.1	1.0
Chicken & Gravy, Shortcrust Pastry, Tesco*	1 Pie/250g	618	247	6.8	23.9	13.8	1.0
Chicken & Ham, Deep Filled, Sainsbury's*	1 Pie/210g	594	283	8.0	23.0	17.7	1.0
Chicken & Ham, Safeway*	1 Pie/134.7g	385	285	9.2	23.0	17.4	1.3
Chicken & Ham, Sainsbury's*	1 Pie/128g	461	360	11.0	28.5	22.4	2.0
Chicken & Ham, Tesco*	1 Serving/113g	293	259	9.4	20.2	15.6	1.2
Chicken & Leek, Deep Filled, Puff Pastry, Sainsbury's*	1/3 Pie/451g	1109	246	10.1	18.7	14.5	1.5
Chicken & Mushroom, Asda*	1 Pie/ 150g	444	296	7.7	25.4	18.2	1.0
Chicken & Mushroom, British Classics, Tesco*	1 Serving/150g	398	265	6.5	25.2	15.4	2.5
Chicken & Mushroom, Favourites, Morrisons*	1/4 Pie/352g	989	281	7.2	23.8	17.4	0.9
Chicken & Mushroom, Fray Bentos*	1 Pie/425g	684	161	6.7	11.5	9.5	0.0
Chicken & Mushroom, Luxury, Marks & Spencer*	1/2 Pie/275g	880	320	9.9	20.0	22.5	1.0
Chicken & Mushroom, Premium, Tesco*	1/4 Pie/170g	406	239	8.5	20.2	13.8	0.9
Chicken & Mushroom, Puff Pastry, Birds Eye*	1 Pie/152.0g	415	273	11.9	24.9	14.0	1.6
Chicken & Mushroom, Puff Pastry, Sainsbury's*	1 Pie/150g	450	300	7.8	29.6	16.7	0.9
Chicken & Mushroom, Tesco*	1 Pie/150g	375	250	8.5	22.4	14.1	1.5
Chicken & Vegetable, Individual, Somerfield*	1 Pie/142g	382	269	7.6	24.8	15.5	1.3
Chicken & Vegetable, Kids, Tesco*	1 Serving/235g	235	100	5.9	9.1	4.5	0.7
Chicken & Vegetable, Perfectly Balanced, Waitrose*	1 Serving/375g	285	76	5.1	10.8	1.4	1.3
Chicken & Vegetable, Potato Topped, Somerfield*	1 Pack/350g	270	77	3.7	8.8	3.0	2.0
Chicken & Vegetable, Value, Tesco*	1 Pie/150g	378	252	8.0	21.9	14.7	1.3

	Measure INFO/WEIGHT	per Measure KCAL	Nutrition Values per 100g / 100ml KCAL	PROT	CARB	FAT	FIBRE
PIE							
Chicken & Wiltshire Ham, Finest, Tesco*	1 Pie/250g	660	264	11.5	18.7	15.5	0.8
Chicken Cottage, Tesco*	1 Pack/400g	344	86	3.1	11.7	3.0	1.2
Chicken, Aunt Bessie's*	1/4 Pie/200g	452	226	9.5	22.3	11.0	1.3
Chicken, Bacon & Cheddar Cheese, Lattice, Birds Eye*	1 Lattice/157g	460	293	13.4	21.0	17.3	1.5
Chicken, Birds Eye*	1 Pie/158g	493	312	8.3	26.1	19.4	2.5
Chicken, Broccoli & White Wine, Waitrose*	1 Serving/200g	605	303	12.6	17.7	20.3	2.3
Chicken, Cheese & Bacon, Healthy Living, Tesco*	1 Pack/450g	401	89	6.2	10.0	2.7	0.1
Chicken, Cheese & Brocolli Lattice, Birds Eye*	1 Lattice/150g	380	253	10.3	18.4	14.8	1.0
Chicken, Cheese & Leek Lattice, Sun Valley*	1 Lattice/125g	315	252	15.2	8.6	17.5	1.0
Chicken, Deep Filled, Puff Pastry, Sainsbury's*	1 Pie/210g	538	256	10.0	19.9	15.2	3.1
Chicken, Eat Smart, Safeway*	1 Pack/400g	340	85	8.2	9.0	1.7	1.2
Chicken, Finest, Tesco*	1 Pie/250g	615	246	10.7	21.9	12.9	1.2
Chicken, Individual Shortcrust, Asda*	1 Pie/175g	534	305	10.0	28.0	17.0	1.0
Chicken, Individual, Birds Eye*	1 Pie/155g	473	305	8.7	25.6	18.6	1.9
Chicken, Leek & Ham, Morrisons*	1 Serving/113g	305	270	8.8	25.7	14.7	1.1
Chicken, Puff Pastry, Tesco*	1/4 Pie/114g	250	220	8.6	21.3	11.2	1.4
Chicken, Roast, Puff Pastry, Deep Fill, Asda*	1/2 Pie/259g	739	285	10.0	23.0	17.0	0.8
Chicken, Short Crust, Marks & Spencer*	1 Pie/170g	510	300	9.7	26.2	17.4	1.7
Chocolate, Mini, Waitrose*	1 Pie/24.0g	109	455	5.3	51.4	25.3	1.7
Cod & Prawn, Marks & Spencer*	1oz/28g	43	155	10.6	8.7	8.9	0.7
Cod & Smoked Haddock, COU, Marks & Spencer*	1 Serving/300g	240	80	6.1	9.0	2.4	1.2
Cottage, Aberdeen Angus, Finest, Tesco*	1/2 Pie/360g	403	112	8.2	8.4	5.1	0.7
Cottage, Asda*	1 Pie/300g	324	108	7.0	9.0	4.2	0.7
Cottage, British Classics, Tesco*	1/2 Pie/475g	480	101	4.7	11.6	4.0	0.6
Cottage, British, Tesco*	1 Serving/500g	515	103	5.2	11.2	4.2	0.6
Cottage, Classic British, Sainsbury's*	1 Pack/450g	500	111	6.3	11.1	4.6	0.6
Cottage, Fresh, Marks & Spencer*	1 Pie/400g	460	115	6.8	9.9	5.6	0.6
Cottage, Frozen, Asda*	1 Serving/121g	146	121	4.8	12.0	6.0	0.6
Cottage, GFY, Asda*	1 Pack/414g	323	78	6.0	10.0	1.5	0.5
Cottage, Good Intentions, Somerfield*	1 Serving/300g	261	87	6.2	11.0	2.0	1.2
Cottage, Healthy Living, Tesco*	1 Pack/400g	300	75	2.6	11.2	2.2	0.7
Cottage, Large, Tesco*	1 Pack/475g	575	121	5.5	10.8	6.2	0.5
Cottage, Luxury, Marks & Spencer*	1/2 Pack/310g	403	130	7.7	9.5	6.9	1.6
Cottage, Meal for One, Marks & Spencer*	1 Pack/445g	356	80	4.7	7.1	3.7	1.2
Cottage, Meatfree, Sainsbury's*	1 Pack/400g	364	91	4.4	11.7	3.0	0.7
Cottage, Ross*	1 Pack/320g	240	75	3.0	10.9	2.2	0.3
Cottage, Safeway*	1 Serving/400g	1000	250	13.6	38.8	4.3	7.8
Cottage, Sainsbury's*	1 Pack/300g	297	99	6.4	10.7	3.4	1.1
Cottage, SmartPrice, Asda*	1 Pie/159g	149	94	3.1	12.0	3.7	0.7
Cottage, Tesco*	1 Pie/300g	300	100	3.3	12.5	4.1	0.5
Cottage, Vegetarian, Tesco*	1 Pack/450g	446	99	4.9	8.0	5.2	1.8
Cottage, Weight Watchers*	1 Pack/320g	230	72	3.8	11.3	1.2	0.5
Country, Vegetarian, Tesco*	1 Pie/142g	381	268	5.6	27.3	15.2	1.2
Cumberland Fish, Healthy Living, Tesco*	1 Serving/450g	396	88	6.0	10.0	2.7	0.8
Cumberland, Asda*	1 Serving/300g	402	134	10.0	10.0	6.0	0.9
Cumberland, BGTY, Sainsbury's*	1 Pack/450g	360	80	5.3	10.1	2.0	1.6
Cumberland, Beef, Healthy Living, Tesco*	1 Pack/500g	460	92	5.0	11.8	2.7	0.9
Cumberland, British Classics, Tesco*	1 Pack/500g	545	109	5.0	12.4	4.3	0.6
Cumberland, GFY, Asda*	1 Pack/400g	384	96	7.0	12.0	2.2	0.1
Cumberland, Healthy Living, Tesco*	1 Pie/500g	430	86	4.5	10.8	2.7	1.2
Cumberland, Marks & Spencer*	1 Pie/195g	312	160	6.9	10.1	10.4	1.1
Cumberland, Tesco*	1 Pie/500g	575	115	6.3	10.9	5.1	1.3
Festive, BGTY, Sainsbury's*	1 Pie/58g	222	383	6.2	69.9	8.7	2.6

PIE

INFO/WEIGHT	Measure	per Measure KCAL	Nutrition Values per 100g / 100ml KCAL	PROT	CARB	FAT	FIBRE
Fish	1 Serving/250g	263	105	8.0	12.3	3.0	0.7
Fish & Prawn, Perfectly Balanced, Waitrose*	1 Serving/375g	379	101	6.8	10.4	3.6	0.7
Fish With Cheese, Ross*	1 Pack/300g	321	107	4.7	12.0	4.5	0.8
Fish With Vegetables, Ross*	1 Pack/300g	255	85	4.4	10.2	2.9	1.3
Fish, Asda*	1 Pack/338g	426	126	5.0	13.0	6.0	1.1
Fish, BFY, Morrisons*	1 Pack/350g	301	86	5.0	10.0	2.9	0.9
Fish, Creamy, Finest, Tesco*	1 Serving/300g	438	146	10.3	5.7	9.1	0.8
Fish, Cumberland, BGTY, Sainsbury's*	1/2 Pack/245g	186	76	6.0	9.5	1.6	1.7
Fish, Frozen, Asda*	1 Pie/400g	504	126	5.0	13.0	6.0	1.1
Fish, GFY, Asda*	1 Pack/356.4g	360	101	6.0	14.0	2.3	0.9
Fish, Healthy Living, Tesco*	1 Pack/400g	316	79	4.0	10.8	2.2	1.7
Fish, Luxury, Cafe Culture, Marks & Spencer*	1 Pack/660g	627	95	7.1	7.8	4.0	1.1
Fish, Luxury, Marks & Spencer*	1 Pack/300g	330	110	7.3	7.6	5.6	1.5
Fish, Mashed Potato Topped, Asda*	1/4 Pie/257g	306	119	6.0	8.0	7.0	0.5
Fish, Topped With Potato, GFY, Asda*	1 Pack/450g	414	92	6.0	9.0	3.6	1.1
Fish, With Grated Cheddar, Asda*	1/4 Pie/250g	263	105	7.0	8.0	5.0	1.0
Fisherman's, Asda*	1 Serving/300g	429	143	7.0	13.0	7.0	0.0
Fisherman's, Healthy Options, Asda*	1 Pie/406g	337	83	5.0	10.0	2.5	0.9
Fisherman's, Marks & Spencer*	1 Pie/248g	335	135	9.3	9.8	6.4	0.3
Fisherman's, Perfectly Balanced, Waitrose*	1 Pack/376g	380	101	6.8	10.4	3.6	0.7
Fisherman's, Sainsbury's*	1 Pack/300g	195	65	3.9	9.7	1.2	1.2
Fisherman's, Tesco*	1 Pie/400g	400	100	4.2	9.8	4.9	1.1
Fisherman's, Young's*	1 Pack/375g	499	133	6.2	11.2	7.0	0.8
Fishermans, Perfectly Balanced, Waitrose*	1 Serving/400g	436	109	8.1	12.8	2.8	0.9
Fruit, Pastry Top & Bottom	1oz/28g	73	260	3.0	34.0	13.3	1.8
Gala, Tesco*	1 Serving/70g	241	344	10.6	24.5	25.2	0.0
Haddock & Broccoli, Marks & Spencer*	1 Serving/250g	263	105	8.1	9.3	4.0	0.5
Haddock Cumberland, Marks & Spencer*	1 Pie/300g	345	115	7.8	10.1	4.7	0.7
Haddock, Eat Smart, Safeway*	1 Pack/400g	300	75	5.2	10.0	1.4	1.0
Key Lime, Sainsbury's*	1/4 Pie/80g	280	350	4.2	51.8	14.0	0.7
Lamb & Mint, Tesco*	1/4 Pack/150g	413	275	5.9	23.6	17.4	1.6
Lamb Shepherd's, Waitrose*	1 Pie/350g	448	128	7.1	10.5	6.4	1.0
Lemon Meringue	1oz/28g	89	319	4.5	45.9	14.4	0.7
Lemon Meringue, 90% Fat Free, Sara Lee*	1/6 Slice/75g	204	273	2.4	46.1	8.9	0.9
Lemon Meringue, Lyons*	1 Serving/100g	310	310	0.0	45.9	14.4	0.0
Lemon Meringue, Mr Kipling*	1 Cake/51g	184	360	2.9	59.9	12.1	3.0
Lemon Meringue, Sainsbury's*	1/4 Pie/110g	351	319	2.3	57.3	9.0	0.5
Lemon Meringue, Sara Lee*	1oz/28g	77	276	2.6	46.6	9.2	0.9
Lemon Meringue, Tesco*	1 Pie/385g	989	257	4.0	43.7	7.3	0.5
Lemon Meringue, Weight Watchers*	1 Serving/85g	161	189	2.4	43.1	0.5	0.6
Mariner's, Ross*	1 Pie/340g	435	128	5.0	13.9	5.9	1.0
Mashed Potato Topped Cumberland, Marks & Spencer*	1/3 Pack/300g	360	120	5.8	9.6	5.9	1.0
Meat & Potato, Shortcrust, Co-Op*	1/4 Pie/137g	403	294	7.3	23.3	19.1	1.4
Meat & Potato, Tesco*	1 Serving/150g	414	276	5.1	23.6	17.9	1.6
Meat & Potato, Value, Tesco*	1 Pie/95g	274	288	6.9	23.8	18.4	3.5
Meat, Freshbake*	1 Pie/48.6g	153	313	6.6	23.2	21.6	1.0
Mince Puff, Tesco*	1 Cake/25g	105	420	3.3	62.0	17.6	2.0
Mince, Asda*	1 Pie/53.4g	202	382	3.8	58.0	15.0	1.5
Mince, Brandy Rich, Mini, TTD, Sainsbury's*	1 pie/24.9g	98	390	3.1	60.4	14.6	2.0
Mince, Christmas, Sainsbury's*	1 Pie/37g	147	397	4.5	58.0	16.3	2.6
Mince, Deep Filled, Tesco*	1 Pie/57g	212	370	3.8	57.5	13.9	1.5
Mince, Dusted, Mini, Finest, Tesco*	1 Pie/20g	76	379	7.3	62.9	12.2	5.0
Mince, Extra Special, Asda*	1 Pie/59.5g	243	405	3.4	64.0	15.0	2.5

PIE

INFO/WEIGHT	Measure	per Measure KCAL	Nutrition Values per 100g / 100ml KCAL	PROT	CARB	FAT	FIBRE
Mince, Finest, Tesco*	1 Pie/61g	234	384	4.3	59.9	14.1	2.7
Mince, Free From, Tesco*	1 Pie/60g	188	314	2.0	58.4	8.0	4.8
Mince, Iced Top, Asda*	1 Pie/57g	214	375	2.8	61.0	12.0	1.1
Mince, Iced top, Tesco*	1 Serving/52g	202	387	2.8	65.7	12.5	1.1
Mince, Individual	1 Pie/48g	203	423	4.3	59.0	20.4	2.1
Mince, Lattice, Marks & Spencer*	1 Pie/51g	204	400	4.4	58.0	16.8	4.1
Mince, Luxury, Deep Filled, Marks & Spencer*	1 Pie/65g	234	360	4.3	55.0	13.8	3.8
Mince, Merry, Mr Kipling*	1 Pie/62g	233	374	3.7	58.6	13.9	1.5
Mince, Mini, Marks & Spencer*	1 Pie/27.6g	106	380	4.3	57.8	14.6	4.0
Mince, Mini, Waitrose*	1 Pie/30g	150	501	5.7	51.3	30.3	1.7
Mince, Mr Kipling*	1 Pie/62g	231	372	3.8	56.8	14.4	1.5
Mince, Organic, Sainsbury's*	1 Pie/46.1g	177	384	5.0	54.5	16.2	5.6
Mince, Shortcrust, Waitrose*	1 Pie/54.5g	212	385	3.6	60.0	14.6	20.9
Mince, Somerfield*	1oz/28g	111	398	4.0	56.0	17.0	0.0
Mince, Star Motif, Mini, Finest, Tesco*	1 Pie/20g	75	377	4.2	62.8	12.1	3.6
Mince, Tesco*	1 Pie/47g	180	383	3.9	54.7	16.5	1.5
Mince, Topped With Nibbed Almonds, Mini, Finest, Tesco*	1 Pie/20g	77	383	4.9	59.0	14.1	3.4
Mince, Value, Tesco*	1 Pie/45g	185	410	4.3	58.4	17.7	1.6
Minced Beef & Onion, Aberdeen Angus, Somerfield*	1 Serving/240g	732	305	8.6	25.8	18.6	1.0
Minced Beef & Onion, Birds Eye*	1 Pie/145g	419	289	7.1	26.3	17.3	0.7
Minced Beef & Onion, Denny's*	1 Sm Pie/140g	288	206	6.1	17.3	14.1	0.0
Minced Beef & Onion, Sainsbury's*	1 Pie/150g	410	273	6.8	27.8	15.0	0.9
Minced Beef & Onion, Tesco*	1 Pie/150g	455	303	5.7	27.4	19.0	1.7
Minced Beef & Vegetable, Pot, Marks & Spencer*	1/3 Pie/183g	366	200	7.8	9.1	14.5	7.1
Minced Beef, Aberdeen Angus, Marks & Spencer*	1/4 Pie/137g	349	255	9.3	19.3	15.6	3.0
Minced Beef, Plate, Marks & Spencer*	1oz/28g	71	253	7.6	20.7	16.0	2.0
Minced Steak & Onion, Sainsbury's*	1/3 Pie/172.9g	524	303	11.7	24.8	17.4	2.0
Mississippi Mud, Tesco*	1 Serving/104g	399	384	5.3	33.1	25.6	1.8
Moroccan, Filo, Marks & Spencer*	1 Serving/125g	181	145	4.9	16.4	6.5	2.6
Mushroom & Parsley Potato, Waitrose*	1 Pack/350g	347	99	2.5	10.9	5.0	1.2
Ocean, BGTY, Sainsbury's*	1 Pack/350g	285	81	6.3	11.1	1.3	0.8
Ocean, Basics, Sainsbury's*	1 Serving/302g	196	65	3.9	9.7	1.2	1.2
Ocean, Frozen, BGTY, Sainsbury's*	1 Pack/350g	319	91	7.0	12.4	1.5	0.9
Ocean, Marks & Spencer*	1 Pie/650g	532	95	8.2	7.6	3.5	0.9
Ocean, Weight Watchers*	1 Pack/295g	221	75	4.7	10.4	1.6	0.5
Ocean, With Cod, Weight Watchers*	1 Pack/295g	251	85	5.4	10.0	2.6	0.8
Ocean, With White Fish, Weight Watchers*	1 Pack/295g	221	75	4.7	10.4	1.6	0.5
Ocean, Young's*	1 Serving/187.5g	250	133	6.2	11.2	7.0	0.8
Pork, & Egg, Marks & Spencer*	1/4 Pie/108g	379	351	9.7	19.8	25.9	0.8
Pork, & Pickle, Pork Farms*	1 Pie/50g	185	370	8.5	30.1	24.0	0.0
Pork, Buffet, Bowyers*	1 Pie/60g	217	362	10.4	24.9	24.5	0.0
Pork, Buffet, Mini, Somerfield*	1 Pie/70g	292	418	10.8	29.5	28.5	0.2
Pork, Cheese & Pickle, Mini, Tesco*	1 Pie/49g	191	389	9.2	29.3	26.1	1.2
Pork, Crusty Bake, Mini, Sainsbury's*	1 Pie/43g	165	384	11.5	26.0	26.0	1.5
Pork, Crusty Bake, Sainsbury's*	1 Pie/75g	293	390	10.5	27.0	26.7	1.0
Pork, Geo Adams*	1 Pie/125g	488	390	11.8	23.1	27.8	0.9
Pork, Medium, Pork Farms*	1/6 Pie/51g	188	369	10.2	20.8	27.2	0.0
Pork, Melton Mowbray, Cured, Mini, Marks & Spencer*	1 Pie/50g	193	385	9.8	32.6	24.4	1.0
Pork, Melton Mowbray, Ginsters*	1 Pie/75g	317	423	12.3	25.2	30.3	0.9
Pork, Melton Mowbray, Individual, Sainsbury's*	1 Pie/75g	296	395	10.2	26.1	27.7	2.4
Pork, Melton Mowbray, Lattice, Sainsbury's*	1 Serving/100g	342	342	10.8	21.7	23.6	1.2
Pork, Melton Mowbray, Medium, Somerfield*	1/4 Pie/70g	275	393	11.0	27.0	27.0	0.0
Pork, Melton Mowbray, Mini, Finest, Tesco*	1 Pie/50g	180	359	12.1	26.6	22.7	0.9

P

PIE

INFO/WEIGHT	per Measure KCAL	KCAL	PROT	CARB	FAT	FIBRE
Pork, Melton Mowbray, Mini, Tesco*	1 Pie/50g	196	392	12.6	20.8	28.7	2.9
Pork, Melton Mowbray, Tesco*	1 Sm Pie/148g	679	459	10.0	29.0	33.7	1.3
Pork, Melton Mowbray, Uncured, Small, Tesco*	1 Pie/140g	465	332	11.2	24.4	21.1	2.4
Pork, Melton, Mini, Pork Farms*	1 Pie/50g	200	399	8.9	26.2	29.2	0.0
Pork, Mini, Christmas, Tesco*	1 Pie/50g	195	389	10.7	26.3	26.8	2.3
Pork, Mini, Tesco*	1 Pie/45g	162	359	10.2	25.9	23.8	1.0
Rhubarb, Sara Lee*	1 Serving/89.6g	225	250	2.9	28.7	13.8	1.3
Roast Chicken & Vegetable, Pot, Marks & Spencer*	1/3 Pie/183g	366	200	7.7	13.5	12.5	4.5
Roast Chicken, COU, Marks & Spencer*	1 Pack/320g	272	85	9.4	9.7	1.0	0.8
Roast Chicken, Marks & Spencer*	1 Serving/170g	451	265	9.9	23.4	14.4	1.0
Roast Chicken, Sainsbury's*	1/3 Pie/173g	535	311	10.5	27.2	17.8	0.9
Roast Chicken, Shortcrust, Sainsbury's*	1 Pie/200g	1012	506	19.2	44.4	28.0	2.4
Salmon & Broccoli Lattice, Marks & Spencer*	1/3 Lattice/120g	300	250	8.7	14.9	17.4	4.4
Salmon & Broccoli, Birds Eye*	1 Pie/351g	449	128	6.6	11.4	6.2	0.7
Salmon & Broccoli, Filo Pastry, Finest, Tesco*	1 Pie/170g	386	227	7.9	18.9	13.3	2.1
Salmon & Broccoli, Healthy Living, Tesco*	1 Serving/450g	306	68	6.7	8.6	0.7	1.1
Salmon & Broccoli, Premium, Tesco*	1 Serving/170g	425	250	6.1	17.7	17.2	0.7
Salmon Cottage, Sainsbury's*	1 Pack/218g	159	73	4.6	10.4	1.4	1.3
Salmon, Value, Tesco*	1 Pack/300g	312	104	4.5	11.3	4.5	1.0
Sausage & Onion, Lattice, Puff Pastry, Tesco*	1 Serving/133g	408	307	9.4	21.7	20.3	4.0
Sausage & Onion, Tesco*	1 Pack/300g	333	111	2.3	11.7	6.1	0.5
Scotch, Co-Op*	1 Pie/132g	408	309	7.3	27.3	18.9	1.5
Scottish Steak, Topcrust Puff Pastry, Marks & Spencer*	1 Portion/240g	432	180	13.1	12.1	8.5	0.7
Shepherd's	1oz/28g	31	112	6.0	9.3	5.9	0.7
Shepherd's, Asda*	1 Pie/153g	193	126	5.0	13.0	6.0	0.8
Shepherd's, BGTY, Sainsbury's*	1 Pack/300g	225	75	3.6	10.2	2.2	1.7
Shepherd's, Baked Bean Cuisine, Heinz*	1 Pie/340g	299	88	4.1	11.6	2.8	1.5
Shepherd's, British Classics, Tesco*	1 Pack/500g	715	143	4.8	10.5	9.1	1.4
Shepherd's, COU, Marks & Spencer*	1 Pack/300g	210	70	5.2	8.6	1.3	1.6
Shepherd's, Classic British, Sainsbury's*	1 Pack/450g	500	111	6.6	10.8	4.6	0.7
Shepherd's, Finest, Tesco*	1 Pack/350g	364	104	7.2	9.5	4.1	0.6
Shepherd's, Frozen, Tesco*	1 Pack/400g	508	127	4.2	11.7	7.1	1.0
Shepherd's, Great Value, Asda*	1 Pack/400g	376	94	4.7	12.0	3.0	0.6
Shepherd's, Mashed Potato Topped, Marks & Spencer*	1/2 Pack/200g	200	100	5.4	9.6	4.5	1.2
Shepherd's, Sainsbury's*	1 Pie/300g	225	75	3.6	10.2	2.2	1.7
Shepherd's, Tesco*	1 Pie/400g	380	95	6.0	10.5	3.2	0.7
Shepherd's, Weight Watchers*	1 Pack/326g	290	89	5.8	12.7	1.5	0.8
Shepherd's, Welsh Hill Lamb, Marks & Spencer*	1/2 Pack/310g	295	95	5.4	10.2	3.5	1.5
Shepherd's, With Lamb, Weight Watchers*	1 Pack/320g	234	73	3.8	11.6	1.2	0.5
Smoked Haddock, Eat Smart, Safeway*	1 Pack/400g	376	94	8.1	10.1	2.4	1.2
Steak & Ale, British Classics, Tesco*	1 Serving/150g	380	253	7.8	22.8	14.5	3.3
Steak & Ale, Deep Filled, Somerfield*	1 Pie/200g	550	275	12.0	22.0	16.0	0.0
Steak & Ale, Fray Bentos*	1 Pie/425g	697	164	7.6	13.0	9.1	0.0
Steak & Ale, Sainsbury's*	1 Serving/190g	445	234	8.3	22.6	12.3	0.9
Steak & Guinness, Sainsbury's*	1/4 Pie/137g	399	291	8.7	22.2	18.6	1.0
Steak & Kidney, Birds Eye*	1 Pie/146g	447	306	9.0	23.7	19.5	2.3
Steak & Kidney, Deep Fill, Sainsbury's*	1/2 Pie/125g	314	251	8.4	21.0	14.9	2.0
Steak & Kidney, Individual	1 Pie/200g	646	323	9.1	25.6	21.2	0.9
Steak & Kidney, Marks & Spencer*	1 Serving/170g	459	270	8.8	24.7	15.1	1.3
Steak & Kidney, Premium, Tesco*	1 Serving/170g	428	252	9.9	18.3	15.5	1.2
Steak & Kidney, Princes*	1/2 Pack/212g	379	179	8.8	14.8	9.4	0.0
Steak & Kidney, Puff Pastry, Sainsbury's*	1 Pie/150g	423	282	8.2	26.9	15.7	0.9
Steak & Kidney, Tesco*	1 Pie/250g	638	255	8.7	21.5	14.9	1.0

P

	Measure INFO/WEIGHT	per Measure KCAL	Nutrition Values per 100g / 100ml				
			KCAL	PROT	CARB	FAT	FIBRE
PIE							
Steak & Kidney, Tinned, Fray Bentos*	1/2 Pie/212g	346	163	8.2	12.9	8.8	0.0
Steak & Mushroom, Birds Eye*	1 Pie/142g	389	274	7.5	22.7	17.0	2.0
Steak & Mushroom, Deep Fill, Asda*	1/3 Pie/175g	476	272	11.0	21.0	16.0	1.1
Steak & Mushroom, Finest, Tesco*	1 Pie/250g	640	256	9.2	21.9	14.6	1.1
Steak & Mushroom, Healthy Eating, Tesco*	1 Serving/200g	380	190	10.5	24.2	5.7	1.9
Steak & Mushroom, McDougalls*	1 Pack/340g	779	229	9.0	10.0	17.0	1.0
Steak & Mushroom, Sainsbury's*	1/4 Pie/130g	372	286	8.6	26.0	16.4	1.0
Steak & Mushroom, Tesco*	1 Pie/142g	410	289	7.1	22.5	18.9	1.2
Steak & Onion, Minced, Aberdeen Angus, Tesco*	1/2 Pie/300g	897	299	9.4	22.1	19.2	0.7
Steak & Potato, Asda*	1/3 Pie/173g	442	255	6.9	23.1	15.0	0.9
Steak & Red Wine, Puff Pastry, Pub, Sainsbury's*	1 Pie/240g	497	207	7.2	16.8	12.3	2.1
Steak, Au Gratin, Tesco*	1 Pack/450g	594	132	8.7	10.7	6.0	1.1
Steak, British Classics, Tesco*	1 Pie/150g	429	286	8.3	21.0	18.8	4.0
Steak, Classic British, Shortcrust Pastry, Sainsbury's*	1/4 Pie/130g	519	299	9.9	27.1	16.8	0.9
Steak, Individual, Tesco*	1 Pie/150g	492	328	8.1	25.4	21.6	1.2
Steak, Large, Glenfell*	1/4 Pie/170g	445	262	6.8	21.8	16.4	1.0
Steak, Marks & Spencer*	1oz/28g	64	230	10.0	19.0	12.7	1.2
Steak, Mini, Asda*	1 Serving/67g	117	176	9.0	17.0	8.0	0.9
Steak, Mushroom & Ale, Topcrust, Waitrose*	1 Pie/250g	500	200	11.1	12.2	11.8	1.1
Steak, Puff Pastry, Deep Filled, Sainsbury's*	1 Pie/210g	536	255	10.3	21.2	14.3	2.0
Steak, Safeway*	1/4 Pie/130g	381	293	9.4	27.4	16.2	1.1
Steak, Scotch, Bells*	1 Serving/150g	378	252	13.6	18.6	13.5	0.7
Steak, Short Crust, Sainsbury's*	1/4 Pie/131g	392	299	9.9	27.1	16.8	0.9
Steak, Shortcrust Pastry, Finest, Tesco*	1 Pie/250g	660	264	10.9	21.2	15.1	0.8
Steak, Shortcrust Pastry, Tesco*	1/3 Pie/300g	693	231	10.7	21.9	11.2	1.0
Steak, Tesco*	1 Serving/205g	556	271	7.2	23.3	16.5	1.4
Summer Fruits, Orchard Tree, Aldi*	1/8 Pie/75g	242	323	3.0	46.6	13.8	1.2
Teviot, Minced Beef, Morrisons*	1/2 Pie/250g	383	153	8.0	14.5	6.9	1.6
Tuna & Sweetcorn, Healthy Living, Tesco*	1 Pack/450g	392	87	7.1	8.6	2.7	2.0
Turkey & Ham, Farmfoods*	1 Pie/147g	404	275	8.6	26.5	14.9	1.4
Turkey & Ham, Shortcrust, Marks & Spencer*	1/3 Pie/183g	494	270	11.9	19.5	15.9	1.0
Vegetable	1oz/28g	42	151	3.0	18.9	7.6	1.5
Vegetable & Cheese, Asda*	1 Pie/131g	346	264	6.0	24.0	16.0	1.8
Vegetable, Healthy Eating, Tesco*	1 Pack/450g	360	80	2.7	11.1	2.7	0.8
Vegetarian, Deep Country, Linda McCartney*	1 Pie/176g	375	213	5.5	25.1	10.0	3.4
Vegetarian, Shepherd's, Linda McCartney*	1 Pack/340g	284	84	3.7	12.3	2.2	2.3
Vegetarian, Vegetable Cumberland, Marks & Spencer*	1/2 Pack/211.1g	190	90	2.8	13.4	2.6	1.6
Welsh Lamb, Sainsbury's*	1/4 Pie/120g	290	242	9.1	19.2	14.3	0.8
West Country Chicken, Sainsbury's*	1 Serving/240g	614	256	11.9	17.1	15.6	2.1
PIE FILLING							
Apple, Sainsbury's*	1 Serving/75g	67	89	0.1	22.1	0.1	1.0
Black Cherry, Fruit, Sainsbury's*	1 Serving/100g	73	73	0.3	17.7	0.1	0.3
Blackcurrant, Fruit, Sainsbury's*	1 Serving/100g	82	82	0.4	20.0	0.1	1.6
Cherry	1oz/28g	23	82	0.4	21.5	0.0	0.4
Fruit	1oz/28g	22	77	0.4	20.1	0.0	1.0
Lemon, Sainsbury's*	1 Sachet/280g	218	78	0.1	18.6	0.4	0.0
Summer Fruits, Fruit, Tesco*	1 Can/385g	377	98	0.4	24.1	0.0	0.9
PIGEON							
Meat Only, Roasted	1oz/28g	52	187	29.0	0.0	7.9	0.0
Meat Only, Roasted, Weighed With Bone	1oz/28g	25	88	13.6	0.0	3.7	0.0
PIKELETS							
Free from, Tesco*	1 Serving/30g	58	194	2.8	36.2	4.3	1.4
Less Than 2% Fat, Marks & Spencer*	1 Pikelet/35g	70	200	7.3	39.1	1.3	1.6

	Measure INFO/WEIGHT	per Measure KCAL	Nutrition Values per 100g / 100ml				
			KCAL	PROT	CARB	FAT	FIBRE
PIKELETS							
Tesco*	1 Pikelet/35g	68	193	5.8	40.9	0.7	1.7
PILAF							
Forest Mushroom & Pine Nut, Bistro, Waitrose*	1 Serving/225g	338	150	7.0	15.8	6.5	1.5
With Tomato	1oz/28g	40	144	2.5	28.0	3.3	0.4
PILCHARDS							
Fillets, In Tomato Sauce, Average	1 Can/120g	158	132	16.2	2.2	6.5	0.1
Fillets, In Virgin Olive OIl, Glenryck*	1 Serving/92g	223	242	23.3	2.0	15.7	0.0
In Brine, Average	1/2 Can/77g	114	148	20.8	0.0	7.3	0.0
PIMMS*							
& Lemonade, Premixed, Canned	1 Can/250ml	167	67	0.0	9.4	0.0	0.0
19% Volume	1fl oz/30ml	44	146	0.0	0.0	0.0	0.0
PINE NUTS							
Average	1oz/28g	195	695	15.7	3.9	68.6	1.9
PINEAPPLE							
& Papaya, Dried, Garden Gang, Asda*	1 Pack/50g	142	283	2.8	64.0	1.7	8.0
Dried, Tropical Wholefoods*	1 Slice/10g	355	355	1.8	84.2	1.2	8.6
Dried, Unsweetened, Sainsbury's*	1 Bag/75g	255	340	1.7	84.7	2.0	6.0
In Juice, Average	1 Can/106g	57	53	0.3	12.9	0.0	0.6
In Syrup, Average	1 Can/240g	158	66	0.3	16.1	0.0	0.8
Mango & Passion Fruit, Fresh, Marks & Spencer*	1 Serving/134g	67	50	0.7	10.8	0.2	1.8
Pieces, Yoghurt Coated, Holland & Barratt*	1 Pack/100g	344	344	2.1	46.8	19.3	0.6
Raw, Average	1 Serving/200g	99	49	0.4	11.6	0.2	0.9
PINK GRAPEFRUIT							
In Natural Juice, Waitrose*	1 Serving/100g	32	32	0.6	7.3	0.0	0.4
Segments, Waitrose*	1/4 Can/134ml	43	32	0.6	7.3	0.0	0.4
PINK GRAPEFRUIT JUICE							
100% Pure Squeezed, Sainsbury's*	1 Serving/150ml	59	39	0.5	9.2	0.1	0.3
PISTACHIO NUTS							
Plain, Average	1 Serving/15g	91	607	20.6	8.4	54.5	7.1
Roasted & Salted, Average	1 Serving/25g	152	608	19.6	9.9	54.5	6.1
PITTA BREAD							
Coronation Chicken, COU, Marks & Spencer*	1 Serving/207g	269	130	9.2	20.4	1.2	2.0
Sweet Chilli Chicken, Shapers, Boots*	1 Pack/177.5g	246	138	9.2	19.0	2.8	2.2
PIZZA							
American Hot, Chicargo Town, Chicago Town*	1 Pizza/170g	445	262	8.2	30.8	11.8	0.9
American Hot, Pizza Express, Sainsbury's*	1/2 Pizza/147g	281	191	9.9	28.2	4.4	1.4
BBQ Chicken Stuffed Crust, Asda*	1/2 Pizza/245g	613	250	13.0	27.0	10.0	2.7
BBQ Chicken, Chicago Town*	1 Pizza/172.4g	373	217	7.0	30.9	7.3	1.0
BBQ Chicken, Stonebaked, Tesco*	1/2 Pizza/158g	285	180	10.5	20.9	6.0	3.9
BBQ Chicken, Thin & Crispy, Sainsbury's*	1/2 Pizza/147g	384	261	13.8	33.1	8.2	1.6
BBQ Chicken, Thin & Crispy, Tesco*	1 Serving/165g	355	215	11.9	31.6	4.5	1.2
BBQ Chicken, Weight Watchers*	1 Pizza/224g	412	184	11.5	26.5	3.5	2.7
Bacon & Mushroom Pizzeria, Sainsbury's*	1 Pizza/355g	880	248	11.7	34.5	7.0	3.7
Bacon & Mushroom, Deep Pan, Big Bite, Goodfella's*	1/4 Pizza/104g	241	232	11.3	27.3	8.6	3.6
Bacon & Mushroom, Stone Bake, Marks & Spencer*	1 Pizza/375g	750	200	9.9	27.2	6.4	1.6
Bacon & Mushroom, Stonebaked, Tesco*	1 Serving/157g	352	224	10.5	24.3	9.4	3.3
Bacon & Mushroom, Thin & Crispy, Sainsbury's*	1/2 Pizza/150g	396	264	12.9	29.2	10.6	1.7
Bacon & Mushroom, Thin Crust, Tesco*	1 Serving/163g	395	243	13.1	23.6	10.7	2.0
Bacon, Mushroom & Tomato, Deep Pan, Loaded, Tesco*	1/2 Pizza/219g	464	212	9.3	30.6	5.8	1.5
Bacon, Mushroom & Tomato, Healthy Living, Tesco*	1 Pizza/231g	395	171	10.6	25.9	2.7	1.5
Bacon, Mushroom & Tomato, Stonebaked, Tesco*	1 Serving/173g	351	203	9.9	24.1	7.4	2.0
Balsamic Roast Vegetable & Mozzarella, Sainsbury's*	1/2 Pizza/200g	444	222	8.5	29.4	7.8	2.4
Bianca, Bistro, Waitrose*	1/2 Pizza/207g	618	298	12.9	26.2	15.7	2.3

PIZZA

	Measure INFO/WEIGHT	per Measure KCAL	Nutrition Values per 100g / 100ml KCAL	PROT	CARB	FAT	FIBRE
Big American, Dr Oetker*	1 Serving/225g	572	254	9.7	28.9	11.0	0.0
Bistro Caramelised Onion, Feta & Rosemary, Waitrose*	1/2 Pizza/229.9g	607	264	8.6	26.1	13.9	2.4
Bistro Cheese & Tomato, Waitrose*	1/2 Pizza/205g	488	238	10.0	27.6	9.7	1.2
Bistro Salami & Pepperoni, Waitrose*	1/2 Pizza/190g	492	259	12.9	28.8	10.2	1.5
Cajun Chicken, BGTY, Sainsbury's*	1/2 Pizza/165g	363	220	11.0	36.0	3.6	1.7
Cajun Chicken, Pizzatilla, Marks & Spencer*	1/2 Pizza/240g	636	265	10.5	21.8	15.1	1.3
Cajun Chicken, Sainsbury's*	1/2 Pizza/146g	285	195	12.9	31.8	1.8	2.6
Cajun Style Chicken, Stonebaked, Tesco*	1 Pizza/561g	1318	235	11.9	24.8	9.8	1.4
Calzone Speciale, Ristorante, Dr Oetker*	1/2 Pizza/145g	378	261	11.5	22.1	16.0	0.0
Capricciosa, Pizza Express*	1 Serving/300g	753	251	13.6	29.1	9.8	0.0
Caprina, Pizza Express*	1 Pizza/300g	635	212	8.0	31.0	7.3	0.0
Charged Up Chilli Beef, Goodfella's*	1/2 Pizza/357g	857	240	12.8	26.4	9.2	1.6
Chargrilled Chicken & Bacon, Pizzeria, Sainsbury's*	1/2 Pizza/181g	554	306	12.8	35.4	12.6	1.2
Chargrilled Chicken & Vegetable, GFY, Asda*	1/2 Pizza/166g	355	214	13.0	36.0	2.0	2.0
Chargrilled Chicken & Vegetable, Low Fat, Bertorelli*	1 Pizza/180g	439	244	14.2	39.3	4.4	2.3
Chargrilled Chicken, Thin & Crispy, Asda*	1 Pizza/373g	780	209	9.0	32.0	5.0	1.6
Chargrilled Vegetable, COU, Marks & Spencer*	1 Pizza/294g	397	135	6.0	23.4	2.4	1.9
Chargrilled Vegetable, Eat Smart, Safeway*	1 Pizza/206g	361	175	10.2	27.6	2.1	2.6
Chargrilled Vegetable, Frozen, BGTY, Sainsbury's*	1 Pizza/290g	548	189	10.2	26.7	4.6	3.0
Chargrilled Vegetable, Healthy Eating, Tesco*	1/2 Pizza/143g	320	224	10.4	39.6	2.7	1.1
Chargrilled Vegetable, Thin & Crispy, GFY, Asda*	1 Serving/188.3g	290	154	6.0	28.0	2.0	3.1
Cheese & Onion, Tesco*	1 Serving/22g	56	255	10.5	32.7	9.1	2.7
Cheese & Tomato	1oz/28g	66	237	9.1	25.2	11.8	1.4
Cheese & Tomato French Bread, Findus*	1 Piece/143g	322	225	9.4	29.0	8.1	0.0
Cheese & Tomato Range, Italiano, Tesco*	1 Pizza/380g	969	255	11.4	31.7	9.2	3.3
Cheese & Tomato Slice, Ross*	1 Slice/77g	148	192	6.5	22.2	8.6	2.0
Cheese & Tomato Thin & Crispy, Stonebaked, Tesco*	1 Pizza/155g	355	229	11.6	28.1	7.8	1.3
Cheese & Tomato, Basics, Somerfield*	1 Serving/80g	194	242	9.7	35.1	7.0	1.9
Cheese & Tomato, Blue Parrot Cafe, Sainsbury's*	1/4 Pizza/87.5g	218	248	12.7	29.5	8.8	1.2
Cheese & Tomato, Deep & Crispy, Tesco*	1oz/28g	65	231	10.8	31.7	6.8	1.2
Cheese & Tomato, Deep Pan, Goodfella's*	1/4 Pizza/102.4g	258	253	11.5	29.6	10.5	3.7
Cheese & Tomato, Deep Pan, Sainsbury's*	1 Pizza/182g	470	258	11.7	33.1	8.7	1.9
Cheese & Tomato, Eat Smart, Safeway*	1 Pizza/165g	355	215	11.5	40.1	0.7	1.9
Cheese & Tomato, Economy, Sainsbury's*	1 Pizza/60g	142	237	11.2	34.1	6.2	1.8
Cheese & Tomato, French Bread, Co-Op*	1 Pizza/135g	270	200	9.0	27.0	6.0	2.0
Cheese & Tomato, Frozen, Sainsbury's*	1 Serving/122g	300	246	13.7	28.0	8.8	3.0
Cheese & Tomato, Healthy Eating, Tesco*	1 Serving/100g	211	211	11.9	35.5	2.4	1.6
Cheese & Tomato, Kids, Tesco*	1 Pizza/95g	219	231	11.5	33.9	5.5	1.9
Cheese & Tomato, Micro, McCain*	1 Slice/135g	420	311	11.7	29.5	16.2	0.0
Cheese & Tomato, Mini, Bruschetta, Iceland*	1 Pizza/33.5g	64	188	8.0	23.0	7.0	2.1
Cheese & Tomato, Mini, Marks & Spencer*	1 Pizza/95g	233	245	10.0	38.7	5.8	1.6
Cheese & Tomato, Piccadella, Tesco*	1 Pizza/295g	684	232	9.1	24.8	10.6	1.5
Cheese & Tomato, Retail, Frozen	1oz/28g	70	250	7.5	32.9	10.7	1.4
Cheese & Tomato, Sainsbury's*	1 Pizza/247g	706	286	13.7	35.4	9.9	2.4
Cheese & Tomato, Small, Tesco*	1 Pizza/102g	226	222	9.5	31.9	6.3	1.2
Cheese & Tomato, SmartPrice, Asda*	1 Pizza/125g	336	269	8.0	39.0	9.0	2.1
Cheese & Tomato, Square, Sainsbury's*	1 Square/160g	435	272	14.0	37.6	7.3	2.1
Cheese & Tomato, Stonebaked, Co-Op*	1 Pizza/325g	699	215	10.0	26.0	8.0	3.0
Cheese & Tomato, Stonebaked, Thin & Crispy, Tesco*	1/2 Pizza/161g	388	241	11.6	29.4	8.6	2.1
Cheese & Tomato, Thin & Crispy, Asda*	1 Pizza/366g	827	226	11.0	23.0	10.0	2.0
Cheese & Tomato, Thin & Crispy, Organic, Tesco*	1/2 Pizza/147g	369	251	10.6	30.1	9.8	1.3
Cheese & Tomato, Thin & Crispy, Sainsbury's*	1 Serving/135g	344	255	14.9	32.2	7.4	5.0
Cheese & Tomato, Thin & Crispy, Stonebaked, Tesco*	1/3 Pizza/212g	509	240	10.1	29.2	9.2	1.4

PIZZA

INFO/WEIGHT	Measure	per Measure KCAL	KCAL	PROT	CARB	FAT	FIBRE
Cheese & Tomato, Thin & Crispy, Waitrose*	1/2 Pizza/140g	350	250	11.2	24.6	11.4	2.2
Cheese & Tomato, Value, Tesco*	1 Serving/140g	319	228	10.0	28.7	8.1	2.4
Cheese Feast, Big Fill, Somerfield*	1 Pizza/430g	1135	264	13.0	28.0	11.0	0.0
Cheese Feast, Deep Pan, Asda*	1/2 Pizza/210g	422	201	13.0	17.0	9.0	2.3
Cheese Suprema, Freschetta, Schwan's*	1/2 Pizza/150g	392	261	12.4	32.4	9.3	1.8
Cheese Supreme, New Recipe, Goodfella's*	1/4 Pizza/102g	269	264	12.3	31.2	10.0	2.2
Cheese Triple, Chicago Town*	1 Serving/170g	418	246	9.9	27.6	10.7	0.0
Cheese, Onion & Garlic, Pizzeria, Waitrose*	1/2 Pizza/245.2g	684	279	10.8	29.8	11.8	2.5
Cheese, Stuffed, Crust, Sainsbury's*	1 Pizza/525g	1428	272	14.0	31.5	10.0	2.0
Cheese, Thin & Crispy, Goodfella's*	1 Serving/275g	729	265	15.7	27.6	10.1	1.8
Cheese, Three, Slice, Microwaveable, Tesco*	1 Slice/160g	486	304	13.3	36.7	11.7	1.6
Cheesefeast, Deep & Crispy 12", Takeaway, Iceland*	1 Slice/132g	342	259	13.1	32.8	8.4	1.5
Chesse & Tomato, Kids Crew, Iceland*	1 Pizza/89.9g	204	227	9.6	32.4	6.5	1.2
Chicken & Bacon Carbonara, Thin Crust, Italian, Asda*	1 Pizza/492g	1156	235	12.0	31.0	7.0	3.4
Chicken & Bacon, Loaded, Tesco*	1 Serving/258g	622	241	12.8	25.4	9.8	1.9
Chicken & Bacon, Sainsbury's*	1 Serving/125g	358	286	14.5	27.9	12.9	2.3
Chicken & Maple Bacon Carbonara, Asda*	1/2 Pizza/195g	484	248	11.0	33.0	8.0	2.2
Chicken & Pesto, Californian Style, Asda*	1/2 Pizza/234.8g	533	227	10.0	31.0	7.0	2.0
Chicken & Red Pepper Tapenade, TTD, Sainsbury's*	1/4 Pizza/39.0g	103	264	12.3	25.5	12.5	2.1
Chicken & Red Pepper, Healthy Eating, Tesco*	1 Pizza/260g	608	234	12.7	40.1	2.5	0.7
Chicken & Spinach, Eat Smart, Safeway*	1 Pizza/165g	322	195	19.0	24.0	2.1	2.5
Chicken & Sweetcorn, Stonebaked, Tesco*	1 Serving/177g	354	200	11.9	26.0	5.4	2.0
Chicken & Vegetable, Chargrill, Italiano, Tesco*	1/2 Pizza/184g	383	208	10.6	23.3	8.0	2.4
Chicken & Vegetable, Stone Baked, GFY, Asda*	1/2 Pizza/160.8g	349	217	13.0	36.0	2.3	1.7
Chicken Arrabbiata, Marks & Spencer*	1 Pizza/325g	618	190	11.6	26.5	4.2	1.1
Chicken Arrabiata, Sainsbury's*	1/2 Pizza/191.4g	443	232	12.1	31.4	6.4	1.7
Chicken Provencal, Goodfella's*	1/2 Pizza/142.5g	389	272	13.7	25.9	12.6	2.1
Chicken Salsa, Healthy Living, Tesco*	1/2 Pizza/169g	269	159	11.1	24.0	2.1	2.2
Chicken Tikka, Stonebaked, Tesco*	1 Serving/153g	326	213	10.7	27.3	6.8	1.3
Chicken, Thin & Crispy, Somerfield*	1/2 Pizza/159g	356	224	11.1	29.0	7.1	2.9
Chilli Beef, Stone Bake, Marks & Spencer*	1 Pizza/395g	790	200	9.6	26.7	5.8	1.9
Chorizo & CherryBell Peppers, TTD, Sainsbury's*	1/2 Pizza/194.7g	589	302	13.8	33.0	12.8	2.2
Chorizo & Sweet Pepper, Stonebaked, Safeway*	1 Serving/190g	466	245	9.9	35.5	6.8	3.8
Cream Cheese & Pepperonata, Calzone, Waitrose*	1/2 Pizza/165g	383	232	7.0	29.4	9.6	1.5
Deep South, Chicago Town*	1 Pizza/171g	363	212	6.9	30.0	7.1	0.0
Delicata Four Season Ultra Thin, TTD, Sainsbury's*	1/2 Pizza/168g	445	265	13.3	24.3	12.9	2.3
Delicia, Mediterranean, Goodfella's*	1/2 Pizza/150.2g	371	247	9.1	25.3	12.2	2.1
Double Cheese, Chicago Town*	1 Pizza/405g	932	230	11.7	30.6	6.7	0.0
Double Cheese, Square Snacks, Food Explorer, Waitrose*	1 Pizza/145.5g	415	286	12.4	40.2	7.5	1.9
Easy Cheesy, Deep Pan, Chicago Town*	1/2 Pizza/547g	1455	266	11.4	30.9	10.8	1.7
Fajita Chicken, COU, Marks & Spencer*	1 Pizza/255g	434	170	9.9	25.5	2.4	1.2
Fajita Vegetable, BGTY, Sainsbury's*	1 Pizza/214g	366	171	8.9	30.8	1.4	2.9
Farmhouse, Tesco*	1/2 Pizza/190g	353	186	9.7	20.3	7.4	2.7
Fingers & Curly Fries, Marks & Spencer*	1 Pack/211.8g	360	170	7.9	22.9	4.9	1.6
Fingers, McCain*	1 Finger/33g	76	230	11.8	28.9	7.5	0.0
Fire Roasted Pepper, Sainsbury's*	1 Pizza/344g	605	176	5.3	35.3	1.5	1.6
Fire Roasted Peppers & Vegetables, Waitrose*	1/2 Pizza/235g	442	188	9.8	21.3	7.1	2.7
Five Cheese & Pepperoni, Deep & Crispy, Waitrose*	1/3 Pizza/200g	560	280	11.7	32.3	11.6	1.3
Flamed Chicken & Vegetables, BGTY, Sainsbury's*	1 Pizza/260g	660	254	14.2	39.3	4.4	2.3
Flamin' Hot, Deep Dish, Chicago Town*	1 Pizza/170g	454	267	8.6	31.1	12.0	0.0
Focaccia Tomato & Black Olive, TTD, Sainsbury's*	1/2 Pizza/222g	515	232	9.3	28.7	8.9	2.9
Four Cheese & Tomato, Pizzatilla, Marks & Spencer*	1 Serving/69.3g	224	324	10.5	26.0	19.9	1.5
Four Cheese, Deep Pan, Tesco*	1/2 Pizza/253g	638	252	15.7	27.0	9.0	2.6

PIZZA

	Measure INFO/WEIGHT	per Measure KCAL	Nutrition Values per 100g / 100ml KCAL	PROT	CARB	FAT	FIBRE
Four Cheese, Finest, Tesco*	1/2 Pizza/230g	575	250	12.1	29.8	9.2	1.3
Four Cheese, Freschetta, Schwan's*	1/4 Slice/75g	205	273	11.3	34.8	9.8	1.4
Four Cheese, Italian, Somerfield*	1/2 Pizza/175g	488	279	13.5	39.1	7.6	2.2
Four Cheese, Thin & Crispy, Sainsbury's*	1 Pizza/265g	729	275	11.8	29.3	12.3	3.5
Four Cheese, Thin Crust, Tesco*	1/2 Pizza/142g	386	272	14.5	31.8	9.6	1.8
Four Cheese, Weight Watchers*	1 Pizza/186g	400	215	10.8	34.9	3.8	1.6
French Bread, Blue Parrot Cafe, Sainsbury's*	1 Pizza/132g	271	205	10.7	30.8	4.3	1.3
Frutti Di Mare, Express, Pizza Express*	1 Pizza/373g	500	134	9.1	20.1	2.6	0.0
Funghi, Pizzaroma, Safeway*	1/2 Pizza/205g	506	247	10.8	29.3	9.6	2.9
Garlic & Mushroom, Asda*	1/2 Pizza/241g	696	289	10.0	24.0	17.0	1.6
Garlic & Mushroom, Thin & Crispy, Sainsbury's*	1 Pizza/260g	829	319	11.1	31.2	16.6	1.7
Garlic Bread, Stonebaked, Italiono, Tesco*	1 Serving/116.5g	405	346	7.8	43.6	15.6	1.5
Garlic Chicken & Spinach, Perfectly Balanced, Waitrose*	1/2 Pizza/172g	351	204	13.3	30.8	3.1	2.3
Garlic Chicken, Deep Pan, Sainsbury's*	1/2 Pizza/214g	464	217	11.2	28.3	6.5	3.3
Garlic Mushroom, BGTY, Sainsbury's*	1/2 Pizza/123g	262	213	11.6	37.2	2.0	2.7
Garlic Mushroom, Ciabatta Style, Stonebake, Goodfella's*	1/2 Pizza/186.6g	475	254	10.0	27.9	12.3	2.2
Garlic Mushroom, Classico, Tesco*	1/2 Pizza/207.5g	415	200	10.0	24.9	6.7	2.6
Garlic Mushroom, Tesco*	1 Pizza/425g	829	195	9.3	21.6	8.0	5.3
Garlic Mushroom, Thin Crust, Tesco*	1/2 Pizza/163g	340	209	11.0	21.1	9.0	3.6
Giardiniera, Pizza Express*	1 Pizza/300g	735	245	10.2	34.5	8.4	0.0
Grilled Pepper, Weight Watchers*	1 Pizza/220g	392	178	10.0	29.3	2.3	1.8
Ham & Cheese, Chunky, Asda*	1 Serving/90g	211	234	12.0	39.0	3.3	4.7
Ham & Cheese, Mini, Tesco*	1 Serving/92g	228	248	13.6	31.3	7.6	3.2
Ham & Cheese, Ultra Thin, Sodebo*	1 Pizza/200g	400	200	11.3	29.1	4.3	0.0
Ham & Mushroom Calzone, Waitrose*	1/2 Pizza/145g	363	250	10.0	31.6	9.3	1.6
Ham & Mushroom, COU, Marks & Spencer*	1 Pizza/245g	404	165	8.8	25.4	2.4	1.2
Ham & Mushroom, Deep & Crispy, Tesco*	1 Serving/210g	420	200	9.7	29.2	4.9	1.1
Ham & Mushroom, Deep Pan, Waitrose*	1/2 Pizza/219.9g	453	206	10.9	26.6	6.2	1.0
Ham & Mushroom, Finest, Tesco*	1/2 Pizza/240g	576	240	9.5	25.9	11.0	2.2
Ham & Mushroom, Healthy Eating, Tesco*	1 Pizza/252g	491	195	10.4	35.6	1.2	2.0
Ham & Mushroom, New, BGTY, Sainsbury's*	1 Pizza/248g	526	212	12.1	37.8	1.4	2.9
Ham & Mushroom, Stone Baked, Goodfella's*	1/2 Pizza/175g	439	251	9.6	27.6	11.4	1.2
Ham & Mushroom, Tesco*	1/6 /57g	132	232	11.2	29.2	7.8	1.9
Ham & Mushroom, Thin & Crispy, Asda*	1 Pizza/360g	760	211	11.0	26.0	7.0	2.4
Ham & Mushroom, Thin & Crispy, Tesco*	1 Serving/166g	349	210	13.0	23.9	6.9	2.4
Ham & Onion, Tesco*	1 Serving/181g	453	250	11.8	29.0	9.6	2.2
Ham & Pineapple, American Deep Pan, Sainsbury's*	1 Pizza/412g	1001	243	10.5	32.6	7.8	1.7
Ham & Pineapple, Chicago Town*	1 Pizza/435g	866	199	10.0	29.7	4.5	0.0
Ham & Pineapple, Deep Dish, Chicago Town*	1 Serving/170g	403	237	8.0	26.1	11.2	0.0
Ham & Pineapple, Deep Pan, Tesco*	1 Pizza/237g	437	184	9.8	29.8	2.9	1.9
Ham & Pineapple, Eat Smart, Safeway*	1 Serving/151g	279	185	13.6	27.2	2.4	2.5
Ham & Pineapple, Healthy Living, Tesco*	1/4 Pizza/105g	170	162	10.0	25.9	2.1	2.4
Ham & Pineapple, Loaded, Tesco*	1/2 Pizza/265g	557	210	11.3	28.7	5.5	1.4
Ham & Pineapple, Pizzerai, Simply Italian, Sainsbury's*	1/2 Pizza/178g	434	244	11.5	30.4	8.5	2.4
Ham & Pineapple, Stone Bake, Marks & Spencer*	1 Pizza/345g	690	200	10.1	28.3	5.7	1.6
Ham & Pineapple, Stonebaked, Tesco*	1 Pizza/161g	293	182	9.2	23.5	5.7	3.5
Ham & Pineapple, Tesco*	1/6 Pizza/56g	134	240	10.4	30.9	8.3	2.1
Ham & Pineapple, Thin & Crispy, 2 Pack, Sainsbury's*	1 Pizza/163g	417	256	13.8	32.0	8.1	1.7
Ham & Pineapple, Thin & Crispy, Goodfella's*	1 Serving/163g	333	204	10.6	22.8	7.8	2.4
Ham & Pineapple, Thin & Crispy, Sainsbury's*	1/2 Pizza/188g	441	235	12.3	29.9	7.4	2.8
Ham & Pineapple, Thin & Crispy, Somerfield*	1/2 Pizza/156g	348	223	12.3	28.2	6.8	3.0
Ham & Pineapple, Thin & Crispy, Waitrose*	1 Pizza/220g	616	280	12.8	33.3	9.6	2.2
Ham & Pineapple, Thin Base, Sainsbury's*	1/2 Pizza/150g	321	214	11.8	23.0	8.3	3.8

P

PIZZA

INFO/WEIGHT	Measure	per Measure KCAL	KCAL	PROT	CARB	FAT	FIBRE
Ham & Roast Onion, Classico, Italiano, Tesco*	1 Serving/181.5g	471	259	12.1	29.1	10.5	1.6
Ham, Mushroom & Gruyere, Sainsbury's*	1/4 Pizza/169.0g	404	239	10.2	31.3	8.1	3.7
Ham, Mushroom & Tomato, BGTY, Sainsbury's*	1/2 Pizza/150g	307	206	11.8	30.4	4.1	1.2
Ham, Pepperoni & Milano, Marks & Spencer*	1 Pizza/290g	696	240	14.0	23.3	9.8	1.1
Hawaiian, Healthy Living, Tesco*	1/2 Pizza/155g	293	189	12.5	29.6	2.3	3.0
Hawaiian, San Marco*	1/4 Pizza/90g	208	231	8.9	29.7	9.2	1.5
Hawaiian, Tesco*	1 Pizza/264g	649	246	12.1	32.4	7.6	1.5
Hawaiian, Thin Crust, Tesco*	1/2 Pizza/205g	387	189	12.5	29.6	2.3	3.0
Hickory Steak, Marks & Spencer*	1 Pizza/400g	820	205	9.9	25.7	6.7	1.4
Honey Roast Salmon & Broccoli, BGTY, Sainsbury's*	1 Serving/280g	613	219	10.2	34.4	4.5	3.5
Hot & Spicy Chicken, Deep Pan, Tesco*	1/2 Pizza/222g	423	191	10.5	30.0	3.3	2.1
Hot & Spicy, Deep Dish, Chicago Town*	1 Pizza/177g	434	245	8.6	30.4	9.9	0.9
Hot & Spicy, Deep Dish, Schwan's*	1 Pizza/170g	423	249	9.1	27.6	11.4	0.0
Hot & Spicy, Deep Pan, Tesco*	1 Serving/221g	423	191	10.5	30.0	3.3	2.1
Hot & Spicy, Pizzeria Style, Sainsbury's*	1 Pizza/376g	986	262	12.5	25.5	12.3	2.4
Hot Chicken, Stone Bake, Marks & Spencer*	1 Pizza/380g	798	210	11.5	25.1	6.8	1.3
Hot Dog, Kids, Tesco*	1 Pizza/95g	233	245	9.8	36.6	6.6	2.0
Italian Bacon, Mushroom & Parmesan, Marks & Spencer*	1 Pizza/315g	819	260	10.1	27.0	12.3	0.9
Italian Cheese & Ham, The Little Big Food Company*	1 Pizza/95g	236	248	11.0	36.3	6.6	1.0
Italian Meat Feast, Thin & Crispy, Waitrose*	1 Pizza/182g	477	262	10.7	26.5	12.6	1.8
Italian Meat, So Good, Somerfield*	1/2 Pizza/200g	468	234	14.0	32.4	5.4	2.4
Italian Meats, Finest, Tesco*	1/2 Pizza/217g	449	207	13.6	29.4	3.9	1.3
Italian Meats, TTD, Sainsbury's*	1/2 Pizza/223.7g	587	262	12.8	25.6	12.0	2.4
Italian Mozzarella & Black Forest Ham, Asda*	1/4 Pizza/110g	227	206	10.0	28.0	6.0	2.7
La Reine, Pizza Express, Sainsbury's*	1/2 Pizza/155g	361	233	12.3	29.8	7.2	1.9
Loaded Cheese, Goodfella's*	1 Pizza/410g	1115	272	11.4	29.4	12.1	1.7
Margherita Cheese & Tomato, San Marco*	1/2 Pizza/200g	454	227	10.7	29.8	7.2	1.2
Margherita Classico, Italiano, Tesco*	1/2 Pizza/191g	414	217	11.2	29.1	6.2	2.5
Margherita, 12", Finest, Tesco*	1/2 Pizza/254.5g	434	170	8.1	26.4	3.6	2.7
Margherita, BGTY, Sainsbury's*	1/2 Pizza/128.9g	254	197	11.8	32.5	2.2	2.0
Margherita, Finest, Tesco*	1 Serving/207g	441	213	11.0	30.5	5.2	1.2
Margherita, Healthy Living, Tesco*	1/2 Pizza/125g	222	178	10.8	29.3	2.0	2.5
Margherita, Italian Stone Baked, Somerfield*	1 Pizza/290g	554	191	10.0	22.0	7.0	0.0
Margherita, Italian Style, Somerfield*	1/2 Pizza/190g	424	223	10.0	32.0	6.0	0.0
Margherita, Italiano, Tesco*	1 Serving/172.5g	336	194	9.5	30.1	4.0	2.5
Margherita, Morrisons*	1/2 Pizza/163g	416	256	12.9	26.1	11.1	2.3
Margherita, Pizzeria, Sainsbury's*	1/2 Pizza/165g	450	273	13.9	34.5	8.8	2.9
Margherita, Stone Baked, GFY, Asda*	1/4 Pizza/73g	158	217	11.0	39.0	1.9	1.8
Margherita, Stone Baked, Goodfella's*	1 Slice/36g	95	263	10.9	31.9	11.4	7.6
Margherita, Stonebaked Ciabatta, Goodfella's*	1/2 Pizza/149.5g	405	270	11.3	32.8	11.5	2.6
Margherita, Thin Crust, Tesco*	1 Serving/170g	354	208	10.1	24.1	7.9	3.6
Marinated Tomato & Mascarpone, Piccadella, Tesco*	1 Pizza/260g	634	244	6.4	31.6	10.2	2.2
Massive On Meat, Deep Pan, Goodfella's*	1 Serving/106g	259	244	10.4	30.6	8.9	3.0
Meat Feast, American Style, Sainsbury's*	1/2 Pizza/263g	642	244	12.6	26.2	9.9	2.9
Meat Feast, Big Fill, Somerfield*	1 Pizza/455g	1019	224	11.0	26.0	8.0	0.0
Meat Feast, Deep & Loaded, Sainsbury's*	1/2 Pizza/297.5g	817	275	13.2	32.7	10.1	2.6
Meat Feast, Large, Tesco*	Per Pizza/735g	1904	259	10.9	32.6	9.4	2.0
Meat Feast, Loaded, Deep Pan, Large, Tesco*	1/2 Pizza/282g	776	275	12.0	26.1	13.6	1.9
Meat Feast, Thin & Crispy, Asda*	1/2 Pizza/183g	410	224	11.0	27.0	8.0	1.4
Meat Feast, Thin & Crispy, Somerfield*	1/2 Pizza/164.8g	413	250	12.4	25.7	10.8	3.2
Meat Feast, Thin Crust, Tesco*	1/2 Pizza/178g	430	242	13.6	21.3	11.4	2.3
Meat, Mediterranean Style, Pizzeria, Waitrose*	1/4 Pizza/174g	395	227	11.1	25.8	8.8	2.0
Mediterranean Madness, Goodfella's*	1/4 Pizza/108.8g	235	216	9.1	27.0	8.0	3.9

PIZZA

INFO/WEIGHT	Measure	per Measure KCAL	Nutrition Values per 100g / 100ml KCAL	PROT	CARB	FAT	FIBRE
Mediterranean Vegetable, Pizzeria, Sainsbury's*	1 Serving/211.3g	397	188	8.0	24.7	6.4	3.2
Mediterranean Vegetable, Stonebaked, Sainsbury's*	1/2 Pizza/260g	622	239	9.8	35.7	6.3	3.1
Mexican Chicken, COU, Marks & Spencer*	1 Pizza/248g	384	155	10.3	25.0	2.0	2.0
Micro, McCain*	1/2 Serving/133g	388	292	12.4	26.9	15.0	0.0
Mini, Party, Tesco*	1 Pizza/11g	26	248	11.4	28.6	10.5	1.9
Mozarella & Tomato, Gluten Free, Dietary Specials*	1 Pizza/320g	646	202	6.7	33.1	4.7	1.3
Mozarella E Provolone, La Bottega, Goodfella's*	1/2 Pizza/156g	372	238	10.1	27.9	9.6	2.4
Mozzarella & Cherry Tomato, Stonebaked, Safeway*	1/2 Pizza/262.5g	618	235	10.6	30.3	7.8	3.5
Mushroom & Roasted Onion, Waitrose*	1/2 Pizza/187.4g	402	215	9.8	28.9	6.7	1.3
Napoletana, Sainsbury's*	1/2 Pizza/186g	424	228	9.7	29.9	7.7	3.1
Napoletana, TTD, Sainsbury's*	1 Pizza/374g	1070	286	11.1	28.5	12.2	2.0
Napoli Ham & Mushroom, San Marco*	1/2 Pizza/219g	449	205	10.0	27.5	6.1	2.8
Napoli, Tesco*	1/2 Pizza/183.5g	432	235	11.9	32.6	6.3	1.4
Pasta, Ristorante, Dr Oetker*	1/2 Pizza/205.02g	449	219	8.0	26.6	8.9	0.0
Pepper Steak, Deep Dish, Chicago Town*	1 Pack/365g	372	102	6.1	13.4	2.7	0.0
Pepperonata, Delicata, Sainsbury's*	1 Pizza/330g	917	278	12.9	24.3	14.4	2.6
Pepperoni & Jalapeno Chill, Asda*	1 Pizza/277g	742	268	10.0	39.0	8.0	1.8
Pepperoni & Onion, 9", Sainsbury's*	1/2 Pizza/207g	615	297	13.4	31.7	13.0	1.9
Pepperoni Bacon, Primo*	1/2 Pizza/111g	360	324	10.5	42.5	13.1	0.0
Pepperoni Style, Italiano, Tesco*	1 Serving/215g	495	230	9.3	28.4	8.8	2.4
Pepperoni, American Style Deep Pan, Co-Op*	1 Pizza/395g	988	250	12.0	28.0	10.0	1.0
Pepperoni, Asda*	1/2 Pizza/150g	386	257	10.0	34.0	9.0	2.7
Pepperoni, Carb Control, Tesco*	1 Serving/118g	203	172	16.5	7.9	8.2	7.4
Pepperoni, Chicago Town*	1 Sm Pizza/170g	471	277	11.5	28.8	12.9	0.0
Pepperoni, Chilli & Vegetable, Fresh, Tesco*	1 Pizza/260g	660	254	9.5	35.1	8.4	1.7
Pepperoni, Classico, Tesco*	1/2 Pizza/205g	586	286	11.6	27.3	14.5	1.9
Pepperoni, Deep & Crispy, Tesco*	1 Pizza/375g	881	235	10.1	31.8	7.5	1.2
Pepperoni, Deep Crust, Big, Tesco*	1 Serving/208g	541	260	12.7	22.6	13.2	2.4
Pepperoni, Deep Filled, Chicago Town*	1 Serving/202.3g	620	307	11.5	28.0	16.6	1.3
Pepperoni, Deep Pan, Goodfella's*	1/4 Slice/109g	294	270	12.7	28.9	11.6	1.6
Pepperoni, Deep Pan, Sainsbury's*	1/2 Pizza/191g	478	250	9.9	28.3	10.8	3.2
Pepperoni, Deluxe, American Deep Pan, Sainsbury's*	1 Pizza/424g	1077	254	13.3	28.7	9.5	2.7
Pepperoni, Extra, Chicago Town*	1 Pizza/460g	994	216	9.6	27.7	7.4	0.0
Pepperoni, Feast, Deep Dish, Schwan's*	1 Pizza/435g	1188	273	9.9	26.3	14.2	0.0
Pepperoni, Freschetta, Schwan's*	1 Pizza/310g	846	273	10.8	31.6	11.5	0.0
Pepperoni, Goodfella's*	1 Pizza/337g	900	267	13.2	26.3	12.9	1.7
Pepperoni, Hot & Spicy, Stuffed Crust, Asda*	1 Pizza/245g	666	272	13.9	26.5	12.2	2.4
Pepperoni, Individual, Chicago Town*	1 Pizza/168g	496	295	9.9	30.9	14.6	0.8
Pepperoni, Italian Style, Somerfield*	1 Pizza/380g	920	242	11.0	32.0	8.0	0.0
Pepperoni, Italian, Thin & Crispy, Morrisons*	1 Pizza/365g	843	231	11.1	25.0	9.6	0.0
Pepperoni, Micro, McCain*	1 Serving/135g	405	300	12.1	26.5	16.2	0.0
Pepperoni, Mini, Tesco*	1 Serving/22g	71	323	11.8	30.5	16.8	2.7
Pepperoni, Oven Rising, Safeway*	1 Serving/95g	259	273	8.2	39.9	9.0	1.9
Pepperoni, Pizzeria Style, Sainsbury's*	1 Serving/183g	515	281	13.5	28.0	12.7	2.2
Pepperoni, Speciale, Sainsbury's*	1/2 Pizza/179g	448	250	11.9	26.6	10.9	2.3
Pepperoni, Stateside Foods*	1/2 Pizza/370g	988	267	12.2	32.3	9.8	1.4
Pepperoni, Stone Baked, Carlos*	1 Pizza/330g	832	252	13.0	23.0	12.0	0.0
Pepperoni, Stone Baked, Pizzaroma, Safeway*	1/2 Pizza/178.4g	479	269	12.9	30.6	10.6	2.2
Pepperoni, Stonebake, 10", Asda*	1/2 Pizza/170g	435	256	12.9	25.9	11.2	2.5
Pepperoni, Stonebaked Ciabatta, Goodfella's*	1/2 Pizza/181g	503	278	11.9	27.4	14.4	2.4
Pepperoni, Stonebaked, American Hot, Sainsbury's*	1/2 Pizza/276g	674	244	11.6	24.1	11.2	2.9
Pepperoni, Stonebaked, Tesco*	1 Serving/290g	771	266	11.7	25.9	12.8	2.7
Pepperoni, TTD, Sainsbury's*	1/3 Pizza/171g	461	270	14.2	29.3	10.7	2.3

P

PIZZA

INFO/WEIGHT	Measure per Measure KCAL	KCAL	PROT	CARB	FAT	FIBRE
Pepperoni, Thin & Crispy, Asda*	1/2 Pizza/180g 436	242	11.0	27.0	10.0	1.7
Pepperoni, Thin & Crispy, Goodfella's*	1 Pizza/593g 1595	269	13.8	26.9	11.8	2.3
Pepperoni, Thin & Crispy, Sainsbury's*	1/2 Pizza/132g 405	307	13.9	30.7	14.3	2.6
Pepperoni, Thin & Crispy, Tesco*	1/4 Pizza/132g 379	287	11.5	30.3	13.3	2.3
Pepperoni, Thin & Crispy, Waitrose*	1/2 Pizza/105g 359	342	12.9	35.1	15.8	1.9
Pepperoni, Thin Crust, Tesco*	1/2 Pizza/163g 460	283	14.0	23.0	15.0	2.5
Pepperoni, Zingy, Asda*	1 Serving/90g 255	283	12.0	43.0	7.0	4.0
Pleasure With Fire Roasted Vegetables, Heinz*	1/2 Pizza/200g 418	209	9.5	24.8	8.0	2.4
Pollo, Ristorante, Dr Oetker*	1/2 Pizza/177.55g 384	216	8.9	23.4	9.5	0.0
Pork, American Style Tennesse BBQ, Asda*	1 Pizza/248.7g 563	226	11.0	32.0	6.0	2.5
Prosciutto & Fresh Rocket, TTD, Sainsbury's*	1/2 Pizza/164.2g 541	330	11.9	39.9	13.6	2.5
Prosciutto & Mascarpone, Safeway*	1/2 Pizza/200g 522	261	12.3	29.8	10.3	2.2
Prosciutto Con Funghi, Lidl*	1/2 Pizza/200g 454	227	9.5	31.5	7.0	0.0
Prosciutto, Classico, Tesco*	1/2 Pizza/205g 461	225	11.7	33.6	4.9	2.5
Prosciutto, Pizzaria, Sainsbury's*	1 Pizza/325g 806	248	11.4	34.7	7.1	3.2
Prosciutto, Ristorante, Dr Oetker*	1 Pizza/330g 752	228	10.3	24.6	9.8	0.0
Quattro Formaggi, Ristorante, Dr Oetker*	1/2 Pizza/175g 473	270	11.4	23.9	14.3	0.0
Quattro Formaggio, Tesco*	1/2 Pizza/219.2g 583	266	13.3	25.1	12.5	1.8
Roasted Vegetable, For One, GFY, Asda*	1 Pizza/96.0g 190	198	9.0	32.0	3.8	1.5
Roasted Vegetable, Waitrose*	1 Pizza/300g 609	203	8.8	39.7	1.0	3.3
Roasted Vegetable, Wood Fired, Pizzaroma, Safeway*	1/2 Pizza/175g 350	200	7.9	27.0	6.3	5.1
Salame, Ristorante, Dr Oetker*	1/2 Pizza/159.82g 456	285	10.4	26.3	15.3	0.0
Salami & Ham, Pizzeria, Waitrose*	1/2 Pizza/205g 443	216	10.1	28.7	6.7	1.8
Salami & Pepperoni, Waitrose*	1/2 Pizza/190g 578	304	13.4	23.9	16.2	2.1
Salami Con Mozarella, Lidl*	1/2 Pizza/200g 534	267	9.9	31.5	11.2	0.0
Salami, Ultra Thin Italian, Tesco*	1 Serving/263g 692	263	12.0	31.9	9.7	1.0
Sicilian, Premium, Co-Op*	1 Pizza/600g 1320	220	9.0	27.0	8.0	2.0
Siciliana, Frozen, Finest, Tesco*	1 Serving/247.5g 432	174	8.5	21.9	5.8	3.2
Simply Cheese, Goodfella's*	1/4 Pizza/81.9g 226	276	16.3	22.5	13.4	1.9
Slice Selection, Marks & Spencer*	1 Serving/52g 120	230	9.4	30.3	7.8	1.9
Sloppy Giuseppe, Pizza Express, Sainsbury's*	1 Serving/362g 746	206	10.2	25.4	7.1	3.1
Smoked Ham & Mushroom, Thin & Crispy, Co-Op*	1 Pizza/400g 792	198	9.0	30.3	4.5	1.7
Smoked Ham & Peppers, Healthy Living, Tesco*	1 Serving/282g 386	137	8.7	21.1	2.0	1.8
Smoked Ham & Pineapple, Deep Pan, Co-Op*	1 Pizza/395g 1142	289	11.6	36.7	10.6	1.7
Smoked Ham & Pineapple, Weight Watchers*	1 Pizza/241g 429	178	10.3	27.6	2.9	1.5
Spicy Beef, Goodfella's*	1/2 Pizza/147.5g 392	265	12.4	26.5	12.1	2.2
Spicy Chicken, Foccacia, Sainsbury's*	1/2 Pizza/245g 581	237	12.0	30.3	7.6	2.5
Spicy Chicken, Healthy Living, Tesco*	1 Serving/252g 418	166	10.9	27.1	1.6	2.7
Spicy Chicken, Micro, McCain*	1 Pizza/133g 388	292	12.4	26.9	15.0	0.0
Spicy Chicken, Somerfield*	1 Serving/132.5g 305	229	13.4	29.7	6.3	0.0
Spicy Chorizo, Red Pepper & Chilli, Classico, Tesco*	1 Serving/218g 474	218	10.3	26.4	8.0	2.5
Spicy Pepperoni, Tesco*	1 Pizza/380g 756	199	8.9	27.7	5.8	2.6
Spicy Vegetable Nacho, GFY, Asda*	1 Pizza/282.7g 637	225	10.0	36.0	4.5	3.3
Spicy Vegetable, Low Fat, Bertorelli*	1 Pizza/180g 243	135	6.0	23.4	2.4	1.9
Spinach & Bacon, Thin & Crispy, Marks & Spencer*	1 Pizza/290g 740	255	10.6	26.8	12.1	1.0
Spinach & Goats Cheese, BGTY, Sainsbury's*	1/2 Pizza/160g 304	190	6.8	31.8	3.9	2.4
Spinach & Ricotta, BGTY, Sainsbury's*	1 Pizza/265g 535	202	10.4	34.4	2.5	2.6
Spinach & Ricotta, Classico, Tesco*	1/2 Pizza/215g 447	208	9.7	26.2	7.2	2.4
Spinach & Ricotta, Extra Special, Asda*	1 Pizza/400g 940	235	9.0	34.0	7.0	1.9
Spinach & Ricotta, GFY, Asda*	1 Pizza/160g 375	234	8.8	40.0	4.4	1.8
Spinach & Ricotta, Healthy Living, Tesco*	1 Pizza/304g 523	172	10.1	27.7	2.3	2.5
Spinach & Ricotta, Pizzaroma, Safeway*	1 Pizza/420g 1042	248	10.9	31.4	8.8	3.6
Spinach & Ricotta, Pizzeria, Sainsbury's*	1 Pizza/390g 897	230	9.5	29.2	8.4	2.6

PIZZA

INFO/WEIGHT	Measure per Measure KCAL	Nutrition Values per 100g / 100ml KCAL	PROT	CARB	FAT	FIBRE
Spinach With Bacon & Mushroom, GFY, Asda*	1 Serving/270g	618	229	13.0	34.0	4.5	2.6
Steak, Stone Bake, Marks & Spencer*	1 Pizza/400g	820	205	9.9	25.7	6.7	1.4
Sunblushed Tomato & Mascarpone, Pizzadella, Tesco*	1 Serving/275g	894	325	8.5	36.7	16.0	1.5
Super Supreme, Family, Chicago Town*	1/4 Pizza/225g	527	234	9.6	24.5	10.8	0.0
Supreme, Deep Dish, Individual, Chicago Town*	1 Pizza/170g	456	268	9.2	30.8	12.0	1.0
Supreme, Deep Pan, Safeway*	1 Serving/189g	450	238	10.8	27.0	9.6	4.7
Supreme, McCain*	1 Serving/125g	267	214	10.9	27.0	6.9	0.0
Supreme, Square To Share, Farmfoods*	1 Serving/93g	196	211	10.7	22.9	8.6	1.1
Sweet & Sour Chicken, Thin Crust, Tesco*	1/2 Pizza/186g	366	197	11.9	21.9	6.9	2.3
Sweet Chilli Chicken, BTGY, Sainsbury's*	1/2 Pizza/138g	276	200	13.0	33.2	1.7	2.1
Sweet Chilli Chicken, Stonebaked, Goodfella's*	1/2 Pizza/170g	423	249	12.9	22.3	12.1	3.0
The Big Cheese, Deep Pan, Goodfella's*	1/6 Pizza/118g	295	250	12.2	25.9	10.8	1.1
The Big Eat Meat X-Treme, Deep Pan, Goodfella's*	1/2 Pizza/352g	806	229	11.6	27.1	8.2	3.6
Three Cheese Calzone, Waitrose*	1 Calzone/265g	747	282	10.4	33.0	12.0	1.4
Three Cheese, Ultra Thin, Sodebo*	1 Pizza/180g	450	250	10.9	28.5	10.2	1.8
Three Cheeses & Tomato, Stonebaked, Co-Op*	1 Pizza/415g	888	214	10.0	25.2	8.1	1.5
Three Meat, Thin & Crispy, Sainsbury's*	1/2 Pizza/147g	344	234	12.5	23.4	10.7	1.3
Tomato	1oz/28g	54	193	3.3	22.6	10.6	1.4
Tomato & Cheese, Ross*	1 Pizza/81g	181	224	7.4	31.5	7.6	2.5
Tomato & Cheese, Savers, Safeway*	1 Pizza/140g	371	265	9.5	38.4	8.1	3.0
Tomato & Cheese, Stone Bake, Marks & Spencer*	1 Pizza/340g	782	230	10.8	30.1	8.4	1.6
Tomato & Cheese, Thin & Crispy, Marks & Spencer*	1 Pizza/300g	705	235	11.0	27.7	9.4	1.1
Tomato & Mascarpone Piccadella, Slow Roasted, Tesco*	1/2 Pizza/128g	281	220	8.4	29.8	7.6	1.5
Tomato & Pesto, Tesco*	1 Serving/176g	449	256	8.4	25.9	13.2	1.1
Tomato & Red Pepper, Perfectly Balanced, Waitrose*	1/2 Pizza/163g	313	192	6.6	38.1	1.5	1.9
Tomato & Ricotta, Waitrose*	1/2 Pizza/207.5g	443	214	7.8	25.7	8.9	2.2
Tomato, Aubergine & Spinach, Pizzeria, Waitrose*	1/2 Pizza/193g	403	209	7.8	35.4	4.0	3.6
Tomato, Basil & Garlic, Weight Watchers*	1 Serving/85g	169	199	12.3	29.8	3.4	1.6
Tomato, Mushroom & Bacon, Deep Pan, Co-Op*	1 Pizza/420g	882	210	9.0	25.0	8.0	2.0
Triple Cheese, Deep Dish, Chicago Town*	1 Serving/170g	418	246	9.9	27.6	10.7	0.0
Triple Cheese, Deep Pan, Morrisons*	1/6 Pizza/74.7g	199	265	10.4	28.2	12.3	1.9
Tuna & Caramelised Red Onion, COU, Marks & Spencer*	1 Pizza/245g	429	175	9.6	26.7	2.3	1.2
Tuna Sweetcorn, BGTY, Sainsbury's*	1 Pizza/304g	602	198	13.5	31.7	1.9	2.7
Tuscan Vegetable & Mozzarella, Way To Five, Sainsbury's*	1 Pizza/317g	552	174	5.7	26.6	5.0	2.3
Tuscana, Finest, Tesco*	1 Serving/255g	643	252	13.2	18.4	14.0	5.9
Ultimate Meat Feast, Sainsbury's*	1 Pizza/465g	1302	280	13.5	35.1	10.3	1.7
Vegetable Feast, Thin & Crispy, Iceland*	1 Slice/63g	148	237	7.8	26.5	11.1	1.8
Vegetable Supreme, Safeway*	1/4 Pizza/170g	352	207	10.4	25.9	6.9	2.9
Vegetable, COU, Marks & Spencer*	1 Pizza/294g	397	135	6.4	23.2	2.4	1.9
Vegetable, Deep & Crispy, Somerfield*	1/2 Pizza/212g	477	225	9.7	29.2	7.7	1.5
Vegetable, Frozen, Healthy Living, Tesco*	1 Pizza/400g	604	151	8.1	23.5	2.7	4.4
Vegetable, GFY, Asda*	1/4 Pizza/94g	141	150	7.0	24.0	2.9	3.7
Vegetable, Healthy Living, Tesco*	1 Serving/200g	302	151	8.1	23.5	2.7	4.4
Vegetable, Stone Bake, Marks & Spencer*	1 Serving/465g	837	180	7.8	25.0	5.6	1.5
Vegetale, Ristorante, Dr Oetker*	1/2 Pizza/184.93g	387	209	8.1	23.9	9.0	0.0
Verona, Frozen, Finest, Tesco*	1 Serving/237.5g	543	228	11.6	23.2	9.8	2.7

PIZZA BASE

INFO/WEIGHT	Measure per Measure KCAL	Nutrition Values per 100g / 100ml KCAL	PROT	CARB	FAT	FIBRE
Deep Pan, Italian, Sainsbury's*	1 Pizza/220g	684	311	7.0	59.5	5.0	1.4
Deep Pan, Napolina*	1 Base/260g	757	291	7.9	58.0	3.0	0.2
Deep, Standard Recipe, Pizza Two Four*	1oz/28g	63	225	7.0	48.7	0.2	0.0
Gluten & Wheat Free, Glutafin*	1 Base/110g	309	281	3.0	56.0	5.0	6.0
Gluten & Wheat Free, Sainsbury's*	1 Serving/75g	188	250	3.0	57.4	0.9	4.0
Gluten Free, Glutafin*	1 Base/110g	278	253	3.0	49.0	5.0	4.5

	Measure INFO/WEIGHT	per Measure KCAL	Nutrition Values per 100g / 100ml				
			KCAL	PROT	CARB	FAT	FIBRE
PIZZA BASE							
Italian, Sainsbury's*	1 Base/150g	452	301	7.6	57.0	4.8	1.5
Italian, The Pizza Compny*	1 Base/260g	624	240	7.6	46.5	2.6	0.0
Italiana, Parmalat*	1 Base/150g	450	300	9.0	55.0	4.9	0.0
Medium, Standard Recipe, Pizza Two Four*	1oz/28g	63	225	7.0	48.7	0.2	0.0
Mini, Napolina*	1 Base/75g	218	291	7.9	58.0	3.0	0.2
Thin & Crispy, 9", Sainsbury's*	1/2 Pizza/70.1g	176	251	8.4	47.3	3.1	4.4
Thin & Crispy, Napolina*	1 Base/150g	437	291	7.9	58.0	3.0	0.2
Thin & Crispy, Sainsbury's*	1 Base/135g	338	251	8.4	47.3	3.1	4.4
Thin & Crispy, Tesco*	1 Serving/110g	348	316	9.2	52.9	7.5	1.5
PIZZA BASE MIX							
Sainsbury's*	1 Pack/145g	486	335	12.8	62.3	3.8	2.9
Tesco*	1 Serving/36g	99	272	10.2	43.0	6.6	3.8
PIZZA POCKET							
Chargrilled Chicken & Veg, Healthy Eating, Tesco*	1 Pack/190g	304	160	11.4	23.1	2.4	2.8
PLAICE							
& Prawns, In Breadcrumbs, Aldi*	1 Serving/100g	212	212	8.6	25.4	8.4	0.0
Filled With Mushrooms, Somerfield*	1 Plaice/169.8g	338	199	10.2	15.7	10.6	1.2
Filled With Prawns & Garlic, Somerfield*	1 Plaice/171g	366	214	12.0	14.8	11.9	0.7
Fillets, In Breadcrumbs, Average	1 Serving/150g	331	221	12.8	15.5	11.9	0.8
Fillets, Lightly Dusted, Average	1 Fillet/113g	188	166	12.9	10.5	8.2	0.6
Fillets, Raw, Average	1oz/28g	24	87	18.3	0.0	1.5	0.0
Fillets, With Prawns, Asda*	1oz/28g	24	86	11.0	0.4	4.5	0.7
Goujons, Baked	1oz/28g	85	304	8.8	27.7	18.3	0.0
Goujons, Fried in Blended Oil	1oz/28g	119	426	8.5	27.0	32.3	0.0
In Batter, Fried in Blended Oil	1oz/28g	72	257	15.2	12.0	16.8	0.5
PLAICE WITH							
A Creamy Spinach Sauce, Morrisons*	1 Serving/170g	134	79	10.8	3.7	2.4	0.5
A Lightly Seasoned Coating, Whole, Filleted, Waitrose*	1 Fillet/88g	162	185	11.9	11.7	10.1	0.5
Mashed Potato, In Breadcrumbs, Apetito*	1 Serving/380g	420	111	6.6	13.6	3.4	1.7
Mushrooms & Prawns, Sainsbury's*	1 Serving/170g	354	208	12.0	15.9	10.7	1.7
Spinach & Cheddar Cheese, Fillets, Sainsbury's*	1 Serving/154g	222	144	13.6	3.1	8.6	0.8
Spinach & Ricotta Cheese, Whole, Sainsbury's*	1 Fillet/159g	334	210	11.6	17.2	10.5	0.8
PLANTAIN							
Boiled in Unsalted Water	1oz/28g	31	112	0.8	28.5	0.2	1.2
Raw	1oz/28g	33	117	1.1	29.4	0.3	1.3
Ripe, Fried in Vegetable Oil	1oz/28g	75	267	1.5	47.5	9.2	2.3
PLUMS							
Average	1oz/28g	10	36	0.6	8.6	0.1	1.6
Average, Stewed Without Sugar	1oz/28g	8	30	0.5	7.3	0.1	1.3
Soft Dried, Blue Parrot Cafe, Sainsbury's*	1 Pack/50g	119	237	2.6	55.6	0.5	7.1
Yellow, Waitrose*	1 Plum/50g	20	39	0.6	8.8	0.1	1.5
POLENTA							
Gourmet Merchant*	1 Serving/65g	232	357	7.4	78.8	1.4	1.3
Organic, Kallo*	1 Serving/150g	543	362	8.5	78.0	1.8	0.0
POLO							
Citrus Sharp, Nestle*	1 Tube/34g	134	393	0.0	96.6	1.0	0.0
Fruits, Nestle*	1 Tube/37g	142	383	0.0	96.0	0.0	0.0
Mints, Clear Ice, Nestle*	1 Polo/4g	16	390	0.0	97.5	0.0	0.0
Mints, Original, Nestle*	1 Mint/2g	8	404	0.0	98.9	1.1	0.0
Smoothies, Nestle*	1 Sweet/4g	16	408	0.1	86.9	6.8	0.0
Spearmint, Nestle*	1 Tube/35g	141	402	0.0	98.2	1.1	0.0
POMEGRANATE							
Raw, Fresh	1oz/28g	14	51	1.3	11.8	0.2	3.4

	Measure INFO/WEIGHT	per Measure KCAL	Nutrition Values per 100g / 100ml				
			KCAL	PROT	CARB	FAT	FIBRE
POMEGRANATE							
Weighed With Skin	1oz/28g	9	33	0.9	7.7	0.1	2.2
POP TARTS							
Chocolate, Kellogg's*	1 Pop Tart/50g	198	395	6.0	68.0	11.0	2.0
Cream Cheese & Cherry Swirl, Kellogg's*	1 Serving/62g	250	403	3.2	59.7	17.7	1.0
Frosted Brown Sugar Cinnamon, Kellogg's*	1 Serving/50g	210	420	6.0	68.0	14.0	2.0
Strawberry Sensation, Kellogg's*	1 Pop Tart/50g	198	395	4.0	70.0	11.0	2.0
POPCORN							
94% Fat Free, Orville, Redenbacher's*	1 Bag/76g	220	289	13.2	65.8	0.0	0.0
Air Popped, Plain	1 Av Sm/74g	282	382	12.0	77.7	4.2	0.0
Butter Flavour, Microwave, Popz*	1 Serving/100g	504	504	7.0	51.5	30.0	9.2
Butter Toffee, Asda*	1 Serving/100g	364	364	2.1	71.0	8.0	4.1
Butter Toffee, Marks & Spencer*	1 Serving/100g	495	495	5.7	59.0	26.3	2.3
Butter Toffee, Tesco*	1 Pack/350g	1418	405	2.2	81.7	7.7	4.3
Butter, Microwave, Act II*	1 Bag/90g	425	472	9.0	69.0	18.0	9.0
Chocolate Toffee, Mini Bites, Marks & Spencer*	1 Bite/9g	44	490	4.9	68.4	22.1	1.2
Plain, Oil Popped	1 Av Sm/74g	439	593	6.2	48.7	42.8	0.0
PlayTime Popcorn, Salt, Sold at Cinema	1 Av Sm/74g	384	519	8.3	45.9	33.6	0.0
Popping Corn, Organic, Evernat*	1oz/28g	165	588	6.2	44.4	42.8	6.6
Ready Salted, Microwave, Popz*	1 Serving/20g	101	504	7.0	51.5	30.0	9.2
Salted, Blockbuster*	1 Bowl/25g	99	397	10.6	62.2	11.7	8.6
Salted, Microwave, 93% Fat Free, Act II*	1 Pack/85g	345	406	10.0	76.0	7.0	13.0
Sea Salt, Sainsbury's*	1 Serving/10g	46	460	10.2	60.2	19.8	5.7
Super, Perri*	1 Packet/30g	139	464	8.4	55.5	23.2	8.5
Sweet, Blockbuster*	1 Serving/100g	431	431	6.9	67.3	14.9	8.6
Sweet, Cinema Style, Butterkist*	1 Serving/100g	391	391	4.9	76.2	7.4	0.0
Sweet, Microwave, Cinema, Popz*	1 Bag/85g	420	494	6.0	60.0	25.5	8.2
Toffee, 90% Fat Free, Butterkist*	1 Pack/35g	142	406	2.8	77.7	9.3	0.0
Toffee, Blockbuster*	1/4 Pack/50g	221	441	2.2	77.4	13.7	2.9
Toffee, Milk Chocolate Coated, Sainsbury's*	1/4 Bag/25g	130	520	6.5	64.1	26.4	1.3
Toffee, Sainsbury's*	1 Pack/100g	369	369	2.1	70.9	8.6	4.1
Vanilla, Cinema Sweet Microwave, Act II*	1/2 Pack/50g	234	468	9.0	71.0	16.0	12.0
POPCORN CAKES							
Caramel, Orville Redenbacher's*	1 Cake/12g	47	392	7.2	89.0	0.9	6.0
POPPADOM BITES							
Cool Yoghurt & Mint, Walkers*	1 Serving/35g	170	485	7.0	58.0	25.0	4.5
Mildly Spicy, Mini, Pataks, Red Mill*	1 Serving/30g	142	473	16.0	30.3	32.0	10.3
Spicy Tandoori Masala, Sensations, Walkers*	1 Sm Bag/18g	88	490	7.5	59.0	25.0	4.0
POPPADOMS							
Extra Large, Sharwood's*	1oz/28g	78	279	21.3	44.7	1.7	10.3
Fried in Vegetable Oil	1oz/28g	103	369	17.5	39.1	16.9	0.0
Garlic & Coriander, Sharwood's*	1oz/28g	130	464	17.7	37.9	26.8	7.7
Indian Spiced, Sharwood's*	1 Serving/12g	32	267	20.2	43.0	1.5	13.0
Madras Spiced, Sharwood's*	1oz/28g	79	281	20.4	45.6	1.9	10.3
Marks & Spencer*	1 Poppadom/9g	42	467	17.4	39.3	26.6	8.4
Mercifully Mild, Phileas Fogg*	1 Serving/30g	150	499	14.8	36.8	32.6	6.0
Mildly Spiced, Sharwood's*	1 Poppadom/13g	56	444	18.4	35.5	25.3	10.5
Mini, Sainsbury's*	1/2 Pack/50g	249	498	14.9	36.9	32.3	7.6
Patak's*	1 Serving/10g	28	275	21.5	43.2	1.9	0.0
Plain, Indian To Go, Sainsbury's*	1 Poppadom/8.4g	32	405	18.4	43.4	17.5	9.0
Plain, Sharwood's*	1oz/28g	77	274	20.7	44.7	1.4	10.1
Plain, Tesco*	1 Serving/9.4	41	439	17.8	44.4	21.1	4.6
Safeway*	1 Serving/35g	174	497	16.3	39.2	30.5	3.1
Sharwood's*	1 Serving/10g	41	408	21.0	39.3	18.6	9.1

P

	Measure INFO/WEIGHT	per Measure KCAL	Nutrition Values per 100g / 100ml KCAL	PROT	CARB	FAT	FIBRE
POPPADOMS							
Spicy, COU, Marks & Spencer*	1 Pack/26g	85	325	23.5	51.9	2.4	8.1
POPPETS*							
Chocolate Raisins	1 Box/100g	409	409	4.8	66.0	14.0	0.0
Mint Cream	1oz/28g	119	424	2.0	75.0	13.0	0.0
Peanut	1 Box/100g	544	544	16.4	37.0	37.0	0.0
Toffee, Milk Chocolate	1 Box/100g	491	491	5.3	68.0	23.0	0.0
PORK							
& Ham, Chopped, Tinned, BGTY, Sainsbury's*	1 Serving/50g	50	100	19.1	0.1	2.2	0.0
BBQ, Chunky, Tesco*	1 Pack/170g	226	133	23.3	4.6	2.4	0.2
Chop, Average	1oz/28g	67	240	29.2	0.0	13.7	0.0
Cooked, With Herbs, Italian, Finest, Tesco*	2 Slices/50g	117	234	18.0	1.0	17.5	0.0
Diced, Average	1oz/28g	31	109	22.1	0.0	1.8	0.0
Escalope, Average	1 Escalope/75g	108	145	31.1	0.0	2.3	0.0
Escalope, Lean, Healthy Range, Average	1 Escalope/75g	80	107	22.0	0.0	2.1	0.0
Joint, Ready To Roast, Average	1/2 Joint/254.2g	375	148	19.3	2.3	7.1	0.2
Joint, With Apricot & Orange Stuffing, Sainsbury's*	1/4 Joint/200g	566	283	29.0	0.9	18.1	1.4
Joint, With Crackling, Ready To Roast, Average	1 Joint/567g	1283	226	14.1	0.8	14.1	0.0
Leg, Joint, Healthy Range, Average	1 Serving/200g	206	103	20.1	0.6	2.2	0.0
Lemon & Thyme, TTD, Sainsbury's*	1 Serving/67g	159	238	19.8	5.6	15.2	0.3
Loin, Joint, Lean, Roast	1oz/28g	51	182	30.1	0.0	6.8	0.0
Loin, Oak Smoked, Sainsbury's*	1 Slice/13g	20	163	24.0	0.9	7.0	0.1
Loin, Roasted, With Rosemary, Arista, Sainsbury's*	1 Slice/17g	24	144	20.8	0.1	6.8	0.7
Loin, Smoked, Cured, Marks & Spencer*	1oz/28g	43	155	18.1	0.0	9.1	0.0
Loin, Steak, Fried, Lean	1oz/28g	53	191	31.5	0.0	7.2	0.0
Loin, Steak, Fried, Lean & Fat	1oz/28g	77	276	27.5	0.0	18.4	0.0
Loin, Steak, Lean, Raw, Average	1 Serving/175g	346	197	22.7	1.8	11.2	0.4
Loin, Steaks, With Bramley Apple Sauce, Tesco*	1 Serving/160g	232	145	15.5	9.1	5.2	0.5
Loin, Stuffed, Roast, Marks & Spencer*	1 Slice/12g	22	180	24.4	2.4	7.9	0.0
Medallions, Average	1 Pack/220g	179	163	35.1	0.1	2.5	0.5
Mince, Lean, Healthy Range, Average	1 Pack/400g	504	126	19.8	0.4	5.1	0.3
Mince, Raw	1oz/28g	46	164	19.2	0.0	9.7	0.0
Mince, Stewed	1oz/28g	53	191	24.4	0.0	10.4	0.0
Raw, Lean, Average	1oz/28g	42	151	28.6	0.0	4.1	0.0
Rib Roast, Outdoor Reared, TTD, Sainsbury's*	1 Serving/138g	206	150	27.6	1.2	3.8	1.2
Roast, Average	1oz/28g	34	121	22.7	0.3	3.3	0.0
Roast, Slices, Average	1 Slice/30g	40	134	22.7	0.5	4.5	0.0
Shoulder, Slices, Cured	1oz/28g	29	103	16.9	0.9	3.6	0.0
Shoulder, Steak, Hot & Spicy, Average	1 Steak/100g	219	219	22.3	2.5	13.3	0.5
Shoulder, Steaks, BBQ, Average	1 Steak/100g	234	234	26.8	2.8	13.0	0.5
Shoulder, Steaks, Chinese Style, Average	1 Steak/100g	277	277	26.7	3.9	17.1	0.6
Shoulder, With Leek & Bacon Stuffing, Roast, Sainsbury's*	1 Serving/150g	237	158	18.8	2.4	8.3	0.5
Sliced, Chinese, Marks & Spencer*	1 Serving/140g	224	160	26.4	6.1	3.1	0.0
Steak, Lean & Fat, Average	1oz/28g	61	219	23.8	0.0	13.7	0.1
Steak, Lean, Stewed	1oz/28g	49	176	33.6	0.0	4.6	0.0
Strips, For Stir Fry, Healthy Range, Average	1/4 Pack/113g	118	104	21.3	0.0	2.0	0.0
Tenderloin, Roulade, Waitrose*	1 Pack/171g	282	165	18.4	5.9	7.5	1.8
PORK &							
Apricots, Aromatic, Cafe Culture, Marks & Spencer*	1/2 Pack/420g	672	160	10.3	12.5	7.4	2.1
Chestnut Stuffing, Marks & Spencer*	1oz/28g	64	230	5.3	12.6	17.1	3.7
PORK CHAR SUI							
Chinese, Tesco*	1 Pack/400g	521	130	7.2	15.7	4.3	0.6
In Cantonese Sauce, Asda*	1 Pack/360g	623	173	9.8	28.4	2.2	0.5
Takeaway, Iceland*	1 Pack/400g	412	103	7.9	12.5	2.4	1.2

INFO/WEIGHT	Measure	per Measure KCAL	Nutrition Values per 100g / 100ml				
			KCAL	PROT	CARB	FAT	FIBRE
PORK CHAR SUI							
With Chicken, & Egg Fried Rice, Tesco*	1 Serving/450g	602	134	7.1	18.3	3.6	0.9
PORK CHINESE							
Style, GFY, Asda*	1 Serving/170g	286	168	18.8	15.3	3.5	0.4
With Noodles, Tesco*	1 Serving/450g	612	136	7.0	14.2	5.7	1.1
PORK DIJONNAISE							
Fillet, Finest, Tesco*	1 Pack/380g	536	141	16.5	1.8	7.5	0.5
PORK DINNER							
Roast, Birds Eye*	1 Pack/362g	348	96	7.4	11.2	2.4	1.3
PORK IN							
Mustard & Cream, Chops	1oz/28g	73	261	14.5	2.4	21.6	0.3
Rich Sage & Onion Gravy, Steaks, Tesco*	1 Serving/160g	218	136	16.0	3.2	6.5	1.5
PORK SCRATCHINGS							
KP*	1 Pack/20g	125	624	47.3	0.5	48.1	0.5
Mr Porkys*	1 Serving/20g	116	578	52.0	0.1	41.0	0.0
Pork Crunch, Low Carb, Top Notch, Freshers*	1 Bag/42g	211	502	66.2	0.9	26.0	0.6
Tavern Snacks*	1 Pack/30g	187	624	47.3	0.5	48.1	0.5
PORK WITH							
Bramley Apple, Medallions, Marks & Spencer*	1 Serving/380g	418	110	17.7	2.5	3.4	0.5
Cheese & Pineapple, Loin Steaks, Marks & Spencer*	1 Steak/141g	240	170	14.0	6.3	9.9	0.0
Herbes De Provence, Joint, Sainsbury's*	1/4 Joint/200g	302	151	19.2	0.1	8.2	0.6
Honey & Mustard Sauce, Steaks, Tesco*	1/2 Pack/160g	258	161	16.3	8.7	7.4	1.4
Honey & Soy, Sainsbury's*	1 Serving/260g	260	100	12.3	6.2	2.9	0.3
Leek & Cheese Stuffing, Joint, Sainsbury's*	1 Serving/100g	231	231	31.0	3.0	10.5	1.1
Maple & BBQ Sauce, Loin Steaks, Somerfield*	1/2 Pack/160g	336	210	20.4	9.2	10.0	0.0
Noodles, Chinese, Tesco*	1 Serving/450g	464	103	5.3	13.7	3.0	1.4
Peppers, Marinated, Tapas, Waitrose*	1 Serving/105g	181	172	26.3	2.2	6.4	0.3
Sage & Apple Crust, Asda*	1 Serving/100g	161	161	27.0	1.9	5.0	0.8
Sage & Onion Stuffing, Joint, Tesco*	1 Serving/200g	208	104	17.1	2.7	2.8	0.0
Thai Style Butter, Steaks, Asda*	4 Steaks/300g	810	270	26.0	1.0	18.0	0.0
PORT							
Average	1 Serving/50ml	79	157	0.1	12.0	0.0	0.0
POT NOODLE*							
Balti Curry, Made Up	1 Pot/301.1g	268	89	3.1	17.8	0.5	0.5
Beef & Tomato, Made Up	1 Pot/300g	378	126	3.1	18.1	4.7	1.1
Beef & Tomato, Mini	1 Pot/190g	254	134	3.5	18.7	5.0	1.7
Bombay Bad Boy, Hot, Made Up	1 Pot/300g	378	126	3.0	16.9	5.2	1.1
Chicken & Mushroom, King	1 Pack/401g	513	128	3.2	18.1	4.8	1.1
Chicken & Mushroom, Made Up	1 Pot/300g	384	128	3.2	18.0	4.7	1.1
Chicken & Mushroom, Mini, Made Up	1 Pot/189.8g	243	128	3.8	18.2	4.5	1.4
Chicken Curry, Hot, Made Up	1 Pot/300g	384	128	2.8	18.7	4.7	1.1
Chow Mein, Made Up	1 Pot/300g	381	127	3.0	18.0	4.8	1.1
Hot Dog & Ketchup, Fun Pots, Made Up	1 Pot/189.8g	243	128	3.6	18.3	4.5	1.5
Korma Curry, Made Up	1 Pot/300g	273	91	2.9	17.4	1.1	0.4
Nice & Spicy, Made Up	1 Pot/300g	381	127	2.8	18.3	4.7	1.1
Noodle, Hot, Made Up	1 Pot/300g	378	126	3.0	16.9	5.2	1.1
Seedy Sanchez, Made Up	1 Pot/300g	396	132	3.1	19.1	4.8	1.1
Spicy Chilli, Posh, Made Up	1 Pot/300.9g	337	112	1.8	15.6	4.7	0.5
Spicy Curry, Made Up	1 Pot/300g	393	131	2.9	19.1	4.8	1.1
Sweet & Sour, Dry	1 Pot/86g	376	437	12.1	60.9	16.1	3.1
Sweet & Sour, King, Dry	1 Serving/105g	473	450	8.8	60.0	19.1	4.8
Tikka Massala, Made Up	1 Pot/298.8g	245	82	3.1	17.5	0.8	0.3
POT RICE*							
Chicken & Sweetcorn, Dry	1 Pot/68g	243	357	13.1	65.8	4.6	4.0

P

	Measure INFO/WEIGHT	per Measure KCAL	Nutrition Values per 100g / 100ml				
			KCAL	PROT	CARB	FAT	FIBRE
POT RICE*							
Chicken Curry, Dry	1 Pot/74g	253	342	11.0	67.2	2.3	3.3
POTATO BAKED							
Chicken & Mushroom, Homepride*	1 Serving/105g	128	122	2.3	1.9	11.7	0.0
Leek & Cheese, Marks & Spencer*	1 Serving/206g	206	100	3.8	13.4	3.1	3.2
With Bacon, Finest, Tesco*	1 Pack/400g	484	121	3.7	15.1	5.2	0.9
With Cheddar Cheese, COU, Marks & Spencer*	1 Potato/164g	164	100	2.9	17.3	1.9	2.0
With Cheese & Bacon, Finest, Tesco*	1 Potato/245g	360	147	6.0	12.7	8.0	2.5
With Cheese & Vegetarian Bacon, Tesco*	1 Serving/225g	279	124	4.7	15.5	4.8	1.3
With Cheese, Healthy Living, Tesco*	1 Potato/200g	178	89	3.1	14.0	2.2	3.1
With Cheese, Tesco*	1 Pack/400g	448	112	2.7	18.7	2.9	1.0
With Chilli Con Carne, Eat Smart, Safeway*	1 Serving/300g	225	75	6.1	8.9	1.3	1.9
With Chilli, COU, Marks & Spencer*	1 Pack/300g	270	90	6.0	11.0	2.1	1.2
With Tuna & Sweetcorn, COU, Marks & Spencer*	1 Pack/300g	270	90	5.1	12.8	1.8	1.4
POTATO BITES							
Barbecue, Baked, COU, Marks & Spencer*	1 Pack/26g	92	355	7.1	76.7	2.4	4.2
Butter & Chive, Baked, COU, Marks & Spencer*	1 Serving/26g	92	355	7.6	77.2	2.0	4.7
Crispy, Safeway*	1 Serving/100g	209	209	3.5	32.6	7.2	2.2
POTATO BOMBAY							
Asda*	1/2 Can/196.0g	198	101	2.0	12.0	5.0	1.1
Average	1oz/28g	33	117	2.0	13.7	6.8	1.2
Canned, Sainsbury's*	1/2 Can/200g	160	80	2.4	13.3	1.9	1.8
Canned, Tesco*	1 Can/400g	296	74	1.6	11.9	2.2	0.7
Eat Smart, Safeway*	1 Serving/225g	124	55	1.3	7.3	1.9	2.3
Indian, Takeaway, Tesco*	1 Serving/200g	154	77	1.3	8.4	4.2	1.1
Indian, Tesco*	1 Pack/225g	187	83	1.8	12.4	3.0	2.8
Marks & Spencer*	1 Pack/300g	300	100	1.5	12.1	4.8	1.6
Meal Solutions, Co-Op*	1 Pack/300g	210	70	1.0	8.0	4.0	2.0
Mild, Flavour Of India, Sainsbury's*	1/2 Can/200g	166	83	2.0	13.0	2.5	1.4
Sainsbury's*	1 Pack/300g	303	101	1.8	11.8	5.2	1.7
Tesco*	1 Pack/350g	413	118	1.8	13.5	6.4	1.1
POTATO CAKES							
Average	1 Cake/70.4g	126	180	3.9	37.5	1.7	2.4
Fried, Average	1oz/28g	66	237	4.9	35.0	9.1	0.8
POTATO CHIPS							
Hand Fried Mature Cheddar, Burts*	1 Serving/40g	202	504	6.4	57.4	27.7	0.0
Lighly Salted, Organic, Kettle*	1 Serving/40g	189	472	6.2	53.6	25.8	5.1
Ready Salted, Sainsbury's*	1/4 Pack/33g	174	526	5.6	51.7	33.0	3.8
Reduced Fat, Cape Cod*	1 Bag/140g	664	474	7.9	53.5	25.4	6.4
Tyrells*	1 Pack/261g	1362	522	6.1	56.5	27.9	0.0
POTATO CREAMED							
With Cabbage, Asda*	1 Pack/350g	256	73	1.3	11.0	2.6	0.0
POTATO CRUNCHIES							
Oven Crunchies, Ross*	1 Serving/100g	240	240	3.6	30.0	11.7	2.4
POTATO FARLS							
Irish, Rankin*	1 Serving/60g	101	168	3.2	35.8	1.3	2.5
Marks & Spencer*	1 Farl/55g	79	144	4.2	33.8	0.4	4.7
Sunblest*	1 Slice/100g	156	156	3.8	33.2	0.9	1.9
POTATO FRIED							
Crispy, Marks & Spencer*	1 Pack/400g	660	165	2.0	22.6	7.1	1.4
POTATO FRITTERS							
Crispy, Birds Eye*	1 Fritter/20g	29	145	2.0	16.3	8.0	1.2
With Sweetcorn, Marks & Spencer*	1 Pack/135g	304	225	4.4	24.1	12.6	2.3

P

INFO/WEIGHT	Measure per Measure KCAL		Nutrition Values per 100g / 100ml				
			KCAL	PROT	CARB	FAT	FIBRE
POTATO INSTANT							
Made Up With Water, Average	1 Serving/180g	118	66	1.7	14.5	0.2	1.3
Mash, Dry, SmartPrice, Asda*	1/2 Pack/60g	209	349	8.0	78.0	0.5	7.0
Mashed, Dry, Tesco*	1 Serving/70g	225	321	7.7	72.0	0.2	7.1
Value, Tesco*	1 Serving/125g	400	320	8.0	71.0	0.5	6.7
POTATO JACKET							
Baked Bean & Sausage, Asda*	1 Pack/300g	447	149	5.0	25.0	3.2	2.7
Baked Bean Toppers, Safeway*	1 Topper/91.7g	166	180	5.0	22.1	7.8	4.5
Beef Chilli, Asda*	1 Pack/300g	381	127	5.0	21.0	2.6	2.0
Cheese & Beans, Somerfield*	1 Pack/338.9g	305	90	4.1	13.8	2.0	2.2
Cheese & Butter, Tesco*	1 Potato/200g	214	107	4.2	14.6	3.5	1.0
Cheesy, GFY, Asda*	1 Serving/155g	129	83	2.6	16.0	1.0	2.1
Chilli Con Carne, Somerfield*	1 Pack/340g	319	94	5.5	10.3	3.4	1.2
Creamy Mushroom, Asda*	1 Serving/100g	124	124	3.5	22.0	2.4	1.7
Halves, Marks & Spencer*	1 Serving/250g	188	75	2.0	14.2	1.1	1.7
Ham & Cheddar Cheese, Asda*	1 Pack/300g	435	145	7.0	21.0	3.7	1.6
Marfona, Marks & Spencer*	1 Serving/125g	106	85	2.6	16.8	1.0	2.9
Oven Baked, McCain*	1oz/28g	29	105	2.3	23.8	0.1	0.0
Spicy Chilli Con Carne, Spar*	1 Pack/340g	265	78	3.4	12.4	1.6	1.5
Stuffed With Garlic & Herb Butter, Mini, Tesco*	1 Pack/435g	570	131	1.3	14.6	7.5	1.0
Tuna & Sweetcorn, Deep Filled, Marks & Spencer*	1 Pack/300g	270	90	4.9	13.1	2.2	1.2
Tuna & Sweetcorn, Somerfield*	1 Pack/340g	333	98	3.2	12.5	3.9	1.0
With Baked Beans & Mozzarella, Eat Smart, Safeway*	1 Pack/283g	255	90	5.8	12.8	1.4	2.3
With Cheese Mash, GFY, Asda*	1 Potato/200g	192	96	4.8	13.0	2.8	2.2
With Cheese, Safeway*	1 Potato/200g	165	83	2.1	16.3	0.9	2.1
With Chicken Tikka, COU, Marks & Spencer*	1 Serving/300g	240	80	5.4	10.9	1.6	1.3
With Chilli Con Carne, COU, Marks & Spencer*	1 Potato/300g	270	90	6.0	11.0	2.1	1.2
With Chilli Con Carne, Eat Smart, Safeway*	1 Pack/300g	225	75	6.1	8.9	1.3	1.9
With Chilli, BGTY, Sainsbury's*	1 Pack/350g	319	91	5.3	14.3	1.4	1.2
With Garlic Butter, Mini, Safeway*	1 Pack/450g	495	110	1.8	14.6	4.6	2.4
With Garlic Mushrooms, BGTY, Sainsbury's*	1 Pack/350g	263	75	2.3	14.4	0.9	1.2
With Garlic Mushrooms, Eat Smart, Safeway*	1 Pack/300g	210	70	2.7	8.1	2.7	1.6
With Garlic, Mini, Asda*	1 Serving/65g	59	91	2.2	13.0	3.3	0.0
With Herb & Rock Salt Seasoning, Marks & Spencer*	1 Pack/500g	375	75	2.0	14.2	1.1	1.7
With Spicy Mushroom & Onion, Marks & Spencer*	1 Pack/300g	210	70	2.2	13.9	0.8	1.2
With Tuna & Sweetcorn, BGTY, Sainsbury's*	1 Pack/350g	361	103	6.5	13.2	2.7	1.3
With Tuna & Sweetcorn, COU, Marks & Spencer*	1 Pack/300g	270	90	5.1	12.8	1.8	1.4
POTATO MASH							
Bacon & Spring Onion, Finest, Tesco*	1/2 Pack/200g	214	107	4.3	10.8	5.2	1.6
Cabbage & Spring Onion, Sainsbury's*	1/2 Pack/225g	279	124	2.0	14.8	6.3	1.1
Carrot & Swede, Sainsbury's*	1/2 Pack/225g	230	102	1.9	11.7	5.3	1.5
Cheddar Cheese, Marks & Spencer*	1/2 Pack/225g	248	110	4.6	12.6	5.3	1.0
Cheddar, Irish, Finest, Tesco*	1 Serving/200g	312	156	7.4	9.4	9.9	1.6
Cheddar, Tesco*	1 Pack/500g	555	111	2.7	13.0	5.4	1.0
Cheese & Chive, Snack In A Pot, Tesco*	1 Pot/230g	304	132	2.2	9.6	9.4	0.9
Cheese & Onion, Tesco*	1 Serving/200g	210	105	3.2	12.6	4.7	1.0
Leek & Bacon, Tesco*	1 Serving/400g	356	89	3.0	11.1	3.6	1.9
Leek & Cheese, COU, Marks & Spencer*	1/2 Pack/225g	180	80	3.0	12.0	2.1	1.3
Mustard, With Caramelised Onions, Finest, Tesco*	1 Serving/200g	232	116	2.6	16.0	4.6	1.8
Olive Oil, Healthy Eating, Tesco*	1 Serving/100g	90	90	2.1	15.5	2.2	0.9
Onion & Thyme, Sainsbury's*	1 Serving/224g	195	87	1.9	18.1	0.8	1.5
Roast Onion, Snack In A Pot, Tesco*	1 Pot/218g	257	118	1.6	14.7	5.9	0.6
Savoy Cabbage & Spring Onion, Marks & Spencer*	1 Serving/225g	250	111	2.0	10.2	6.9	1.3
Sun Dried Tomato & Basil, COU, Marks & Spencer*	1 Serving/170g	128	75	1.0	14.4	1.5	1.2

P

	Measure INFO/WEIGHT	per Measure KCAL	Nutrition Values per 100g / 100ml				
			KCAL	PROT	CARB	FAT	FIBRE
POTATO MASH							
With Bacon & Cheese, Tesco*	1 Serving/200g	252	126	3.1	13.9	6.4	1.3
With Caramelised Onion, Taw Valley, Extra Special, Asda*	1/2 Pack/193g	361	187	5.0	17.0	11.0	2.3
With Carrot & Swede, Marks & Spencer*	1 Serving/225g	214	95	1.6	8.3	6.4	1.4
With Cracked Pepper & Sea Salt, Luxury, Sainsbury's*	1/2 Pack/225g	389	173	1.6	13.2	12.6	1.0
With Creme Fraiche, Waitrose*	1 Pack/450g	351	78	1.4	13.1	2.2	1.9
With Fried Onion, Smash*	1/2 Pack/269g	191	71	1.6	13.4	1.3	0.7
With Leeks, Creamy, Birds Eye*	1 Pack/300g	300	100	2.0	7.3	7.0	0.8
With Smoked Bacon, Smash*	1 Serving/169g	137	81	1.7	13.6	2.2	0.6
With Sweetcorn & Flaked Tuna, Quick, Sainsbury's*	1 Pot/224g	240	107	2.4	15.0	4.1	2.1
With Vegetables, Sainsbury's*	1/2 Pack/229.0g	142	62	1.8	11.4	1.0	3.1
POTATO RINGS							
Ready Salted, Marks & Spencer*	1 Serving/75g	375	500	3.5	58.9	28.1	2.6
Ready Salted, Sainsbury's*	1 Serving/50g	257	514	3.2	61.5	28.4	1.8
Salt Vinegar, Sainsbury's*	1 Pack/25g	114	456	3.6	65.6	19.6	2.8
POTATO ROAST							
& Caramelised Onions, Finest, Tesco*	1/2 Pack/200g	500	250	5.5	38.6	8.2	2.9
Pepper & Basil Layer, Safeway*	1 Pack/260g	195	75	1.7	8.8	3.4	1.9
POTATO SAUTE							
With Onion, & Bacon, Country Supper, Waitrose*	1/4 Pack/100g	112	112	1.9	16.4	4.3	1.3
POTATO SKINS							
1/4 Cut, Oven Baked, McCain*	1oz/28g	53	190	3.7	33.1	4.8	0.0
Cheese & Bacon, Sainsbury's*	1 Serving/140g	349	249	10.3	17.3	15.4	2.5
Cheese & Bacon, Tesco*	1 Serving/95g	241	254	9.2	19.5	15.5	3.0
Cheese & Chive, Sainsbury's*	2 Skins/150g	287	191	7.7	13.3	11.9	2.8
Loaded, American, Asda*	1 Serving/78.4g	293	375	15.0	27.0	23.0	2.4
Loaded, American, Tesco*	1 Serving/340g	388	114	6.8	16.3	2.4	3.3
Loaded, Cheese & Onion, Tesco*	1 Skin/60g	114	190	5.8	17.6	10.8	1.4
Loaded, Healthy Eating, Tesco*	1 Serving/340g	425	125	7.7	17.9	2.5	0.6
Loaded, New York Style, Tesco*	1 Burger/35g	89	254	9.2	19.5	15.5	3.0
Loaded, With Cheese & Bacon, Asda*	1 Serving/253.2g	314	124	6.0	16.0	4.0	2.3
Loaded, With Chilli & Cheese, Healthy Living, Tesco*	1 Pack/340g	388	114	6.8	16.3	2.4	3.3
Loaded, With Soured Cream & Chive Dip, Tesco*	1 Skin/59g	150	254	9.2	19.5	15.5	3.0
1/4 Cut, Deep Fried, McCain*	1oz/28g	52	186	3.0	30.1	6.0	0.0
POTATO SMILES							
McCain*	1 Piece/14g	27	192	3.2	29.2	6.9	0.0
Oven Baked, McCain*	1oz/28g	64	228	3.8	35.9	9.3	0.0
POTATO TWIRLS							
Sainsbury's*	1 Serving/50g	218	435	3.0	72.8	14.6	3.1
POTATO WAFFLES							
Bacon Flavour, Snacks, BGTY, Sainsbury's*	1 Bag/12g	41	345	6.4	79.9	1.4	2.9
Birds Eye*	1 Waffle/56g	94	167	2.0	20.7	8.5	1.5
Frozen, Cooked	1oz/28g	56	200	3.2	30.3	8.2	2.3
Frozen, Grilled, Asda*	1 Waffle/57g	104	183	2.0	21.0	10.1	1.7
Mini, Sainsbury's*	1 Waffle/11g	27	242	2.8	20.1	16.7	1.0
Oven Baked, Mini, McCain*	1oz/28g	62	221	3.9	32.0	8.6	0.0
Sainsbury's*	1 Waffle/55.7g	109	194	2.9	22.8	10.1	1.1
Southern Fried, Asda*	1 Waffle/51g	107	209	2.8	27.0	10.0	2.1
Tesco*	1 Waffle/56g	110	198	2.2	19.5	12.4	1.1
POTATO WEDGES							
& Dip, Marks & Spencer*	1 Pack/450g	698	155	2.5	20.4	7.4	1.8
Asda*	1 Wedge/40g	57	142	3.4	21.0	4.9	1.7
BBQ Chicken Spicy, Good Intentions, Somerfield*	1 Pack/400g	380	95	7.4	13.6	1.2	1.4
BBQ Flavour, Asda*	1 Serving/100g	185	185	2.9	23.0	9.0	1.7

	Measure INFO/WEIGHT	per Measure KCAL	Nutrition Values per 100g / 100ml				
			KCAL	PROT	CARB	FAT	FIBRE
POTATO WEDGES							
BGTY, Sainsbury's*	1/2 Pack/190g	179	94	3.0	16.4	1.8	3.4
Baked, GFY, Asda*	1 Pack/450g	617	137	3.4	25.0	2.6	3.4
Bombay, With Yoghurt & Mint Dip, Healthy Living, Tesco*	1 Serving/170g	139	82	1.3	14.5	2.1	0.9
Chunky, McCain*	10 Wedges/175g	242	138	2.4	23.3	4.7	0.0
Crispy, Marks & Spencer*	1 Serving/200g	340	170	1.3	25.3	7.1	1.7
Four Cheese & Red Onion, Chicago Town*	1 Serving/150g	210	140	2.1	21.0	5.3	2.4
Frozen, Tesco*	1 Serving/200g	262	131	2.0	22.4	3.7	1.8
Garlic & Herb Crusted, Chicago Town*	1 Serving/150g	216	144	1.9	24.4	4.3	2.2
Garlic & Herb, COU, Marks & Spencer*	1 Pack/300g	300	100	2.3	16.4	2.6	3.2
Hot & Spicy With Salsa Dip, Healthy Living, Tesco*	1 Serving/170g	112	66	1.1	12.4	1.3	1.4
Hot & Spicy, Frozen, Sainsbury's*	1 Serving/70g	98	140	2.8	23.7	3.8	2.0
In BBQ Sauce, Micro, McCain*	1 Box/200g	234	117	2.2	23.5	2.4	0.0
Jacket, Hot & Spicy, Sainsbury's*	12 Wedges/200g	280	140	2.8	23.7	3.8	2.0
Jacket, Sainsbury's*	1 Serving/100g	151	151	3.0	27.3	3.3	2.6
Micro, Tesco*	1 Pack/100g	170	170	2.6	24.5	6.8	2.3
New York Style, Healthy Eating, Tesco*	1/2 Pack/125g	124	99	2.3	16.4	2.7	1.3
Oven Baked, Waitrose*	1oz/28g	46	165	2.4	29.2	4.3	2.1
Perfectly Balanced, Waitrose*	1 Serving/275g	278	101	2.5	19.0	1.7	3.5
Savoury, McCain*	1 Serving/200g	300	150	2.9	22.7	6.2	0.0
Savoury, Waitrose*	1/3 Bag/250g	350	140	2.3	22.9	4.3	1.9
Sour Cream & Chives, McCain*	1 Serving/100g	132	132	2.4	24.0	4.1	0.0
Southern Fried Style, Tesco*	1 Serving/155g	233	150	3.0	14.1	9.1	2.0
Southern Fried, Asda*	1 Serving/188g	263	140	2.9	23.0	4.0	1.8
Spicy, & Garlic Dip, Linda McCartney*	1 Pack/300g	366	122	2.6	15.3	5.6	3.1
Spicy, American Style, Sainsbury's*	1/2 Pack/155.7g	190	122	3.0	20.1	3.3	3.5
Spicy, Deep Fried, McCain*	1oz/28g	52	187	3.6	27.3	8.1	0.0
Spicy, Marks & Spencer*	1/2 Pack/225g	349	155	2.4	21.8	6.5	1.3
Spicy, Occasions, Sainsbury's*	1 Serving/100g	144	144	2.5	23.7	4.3	0.4
Spicy, Oven Baked, McCain*	1oz/28g	61	219	4.2	34.8	8.4	0.0
Spicy, Simple Solutions, Tesco*	1 Serving/150g	141	94	4.6	12.2	3.0	1.4
Spicy, With Sour Cream & Chive Dip, Sainsbury's*	1/2 Pack/73g	284	387	5.5	27.0	28.5	3.7
Tesco*	1 Serving/110g	135	123	3.0	18.4	4.2	1.5
With Broccoli & Mozzerella Cheese, Weight Watchers*	1 Pack/320g	294	92	3.1	13.3	3.0	1.0
With Soured Cream & Chive Dip, Safeway*	1 Pack/450g	639	142	3.1	22.1	4.6	2.1
POTATOES							
Alphabites, Birds Eye*	9 Bites/56g	75	134	2.0	19.5	5.3	1.4
Anya, Sainsbury's*	1 Serving/100g	80	80	1.4	19.7	0.1	1.0
Baby, Garlic & Sea Salt Roasted, Finest, Tesco*	1 Serving/200g	192	96	3.1	13.5	3.3	1.0
Baby, New, With Mint Butter, The Best, Safeway*	1/2 Pack/190g	162	85	1.2	15.4	1.8	2.2
Baby, With Butter & Herbs, Sainsbury's*	1/4 Pack/141g	135	96	1.4	14.7	3.5	1.5
Baby, With Herb Butter, Safeway*	1 Serving/200g	158	79	1.4	15.6	1.2	1.4
Baked, Flesh & Skin, Average	1oz/28g	38	136	3.9	31.7	0.2	2.7
Baked, Flesh Only	1 Med/160g	123	77	2.2	18.0	0.1	1.4
Baked, Flesh Only, Weighed With Skin	1oz/28g	15	52	1.5	12.1	0.1	0.9
Baking, Average	1 Med Size/250g	193	77	2.0	16.8	0.2	1.4
Boiled, Average	1 Serving/120g	86	72	1.8	17.0	0.1	1.2
Boulangere, Marks & Spencer*	1/2 Pack/225g	180	80	2.8	15.9	0.9	0.9
Charlotte, Average	1 Serving/184g	139	76	1.6	17.4	0.3	3.3
Dauphinoise, Average	1 Serving/200g	335	168	2.2	12.8	12.0	1.5
Desiree, Average	1 Serving/200g	152	76	2.2	16.4	0.2	0.7
Garlic Roast, Sainsbury's*	1/2 Pack/225g	358	159	3.2	14.6	9.7	1.4
Garlic, Tapas Selection, Sainsbury's*	1 Serving/22g	49	224	2.6	10.4	19.1	0.7
Hasselback, Average	1 Serving/175g	182	104	1.9	22.0	0.9	2.9

POTATOES	Measure INFO/WEIGHT	per Measure KCAL	KCAL	PROT	CARB	FAT	FIBRE
Italian Style, & Vegetables, Waitrose*	1 Serving/126g	138	110	2.0	19.2	2.8	3.4
Jersey Royal, Canned, Average	1 Can/186g	116	62	1.4	14.0	0.1	1.2
Jersey Royal, New, Raw, Average	1oz/28g	21	75	1.7	17.2	0.2	1.5
Juliette, Sainsbury's*	1 Serving/250g	200	80	1.4	19.7	0.1	1.0
King Edward, Tesco*	1 Serving/100g	77	77	2.1	16.8	0.2	1.3
Lemon & Rosemary, Finest, Tesco*	1/2 Pack/200g	200	100	2.1	14.7	3.7	2.0
Maris Piper, In Salted Water, Asda*	1 Serving/95g	67	70	1.5	15.0	0.1	0.8
Maris Piper, New, Marks & Spencer*	1 Serving/100g	145	145	1.3	29.5	2.2	2.1
Maris Piper, Sainsbury's*	1 Serving/250g	180	72	1.8	17.0	0.1	1.2
Mashed, From Supermarket, Average	1/2 Pack/200g	197	98	1.8	13.3	4.1	1.5
Mashed, From Supermarket, Healthy Range, Average	1 Serving/200g	160	80	1.8	14.6	1.6	1.3
Mashed, From Supermarket, Premium, Average	1 Serving/225g	305	136	1.7	14.4	7.9	1.1
New, & Vegetables, Asda*	1 pack/230.6g	143	62	2.1	9.0	1.9	2.3
New, Baby, Average	1 Serving/180g	135	75	1.7	17.1	0.3	1.6
New, Baby, Canned, Average	1 Can/120g	70	59	1.4	13.2	0.2	1.4
New, Crushed, The Best, Safeway*	1 Pack/400g	440	110	2.2	12.6	5.2	1.3
New, Garlic, Herb & Parsley Butter, Co-Op*	1 Serving/100g	115	115	1.0	15.0	5.0	2.0
New, In A Herb Marinade, Tesco*	1/4 Pack/150g	152	101	1.3	13.0	4.9	1.5
New, In Herbs & Butter, Asda*	1 Pack/590g	637	108	1.6	17.0	3.3	1.2
New, With English Churned Butter, Marks & Spencer*	1 Pack/180g	261	145	1.3	29.5	2.2	2.1
New, With Herbs & Butter, Waitrose*	1 Serving/385g	443	115	1.7	13.8	5.9	1.2
New, With Parsley Butter, TTD, Sainsbury's*	1 Serving/150g	126	84	2.2	13.3	2.4	1.0
New, With Sunblush Tomato, Marks & Spencer*	1 Pack/385g	347	90	1.6	17.2	1.8	1.3
Parmentier, With Shallot Butter, Marks & Spencer*	1/4 Pack/125g	200	160	2.5	21.1	7.1	4.0
Red, Average	1 Serving/300g	218	73	2.0	16.4	0.2	1.3
Roast, Basted In Beef Dripping, Waitrose*	1 Serving/165g	213	129	2.2	18.0	5.4	1.9
Roast, Fresh Butter Basted, Tesco*	1 Serving/100g	134	134	2.3	19.3	5.4	1.4
Roast, Frozen, Average	1 Av Roastie/70g	105	149	2.6	23.5	5.0	1.4
Roast, Frozen, Healthy Range, Average	1 Av Roastie/70g	70	100	2.6	18.2	2.4	2.1
Roast, In Lard, Average	1oz/28g	42	149	2.9	25.9	4.5	1.8
Roast, In Oil, Average	1oz/28g	42	149	2.9	25.9	4.5	1.8
Roast, Old, Average	1 Av Potato/70g	104	149	2.9	25.9	4.5	1.8
Roasting, Average	1 Serving/150g	203	135	2.5	23.4	3.5	1.7
Rosemary & Garlic, Waitrose*	1 Serving/150g	237	158	3.8	30.7	2.2	2.9
Saute, Deep Fried, McCain*	1oz/28g	47	167	2.6	23.3	7.0	0.0
Saute, Oven Baked, McCain*	1oz/28g	56	199	4.4	36.9	3.8	0.0
Slices, Crispy, Marks & Spencer*	1oz/28g	55	195	3.2	20.2	11.3	2.8
Slices, Garlic & Herb, Heinz*	1oz/28g	23	82	1.7	10.2	3.9	0.7
Slices, Spicy Coated, Safeway*	1/2 Pack/150g	305	203	2.5	19.7	12.4	2.5
Spicy, With Chorizo, Tapas, Waitrose*	1 Serving/260g	512	197	6.7	11.8	13.7	1.1
Vivaldi, Boiled in Unsalted Water, Sainsbury's*	1 Serving/200g	160	80	1.4	19.7	0.1	1.0
White, Raw, Average	1oz/28g	21	75	2.0	16.8	0.2	1.3
With Garlic & Parsley Butter, Herb Oil Dressed, Co-Op*	1 Serving/178.3g	205	115	1.0	15.0	5.0	2.0
With Smoked Bacon, Oven Baked, Tesco*	1 Serving/200g	242	121	3.7	15.1	5.2	0.9
POUSSIN							
Raw, Meat & Skin	1oz/28g	57	202	19.1	0.0	13.9	0.0
Spatchcock, British, Waitrose*	1/2 Poussin/225g	365	162	19.0	1.2	9.0	0.0
Spatchcock, With Garlic & Herbs, Finest, Tesco*	1/2 Poussin/235g	348	148	19.7	1.0	7.3	0.5
POWERADE							
Citrus Charge, The Coca Cola Co*	1 Bottle/500ml	120	24	0.0	6.0	0.0	0.0
Ice Storm, The Coca Cola Co*	1 Bottle/500ml	120	24	0.0	6.0	0.0	0.0
Lemon & Grapefruit, The Coca Cola Co*	1 Bottle/500ml	120	24	0.0	6.0	0.0	0.0

P

	Measure	per Measure		Nutrition Values per 100g / 100ml				
	INFO/WEIGHT	KCAL		KCAL	PROT	CARB	FAT	FIBRE
PRAWN COCKTAIL								
20% More Prawns, Marks & Spencer*	1/2 Pack/100g	330		330	8.9	2.2	31.6	0.2
Asda*	1oz/28g	124		443	8.6	3.3	43.6	0.0
BFY, Morrisons*	1 Serving/100g	149		149	4.7	9.7	10.3	0.1
BGTY, Sainsbury's*	1oz/28g	45		160	7.5	2.3	13.4	0.5
Delicious, Boots*	1 Pack/250g	285		114	5.5	17.0	2.6	1.2
Half Fat, Safeway*	1 Serving/200g	362		181	8.0	6.4	13.8	0.6
Healthy Living, Tesco*	1 Serving/200g	276		138	6.8	2.3	11.3	0.6
Light, Asda*	1oz/28g	45		160	9.9	4.8	11.2	0.0
Marks & Spencer*	1oz/28g	97		345	8.7	3.0	33.1	1.2
Reduced Fat, Tesco*	1 Serving/200g	304		152	7.6	6.5	10.6	0.4
Reduced Fat, Waitrose*	1 Serving/200g	242		121	9.1	3.4	7.9	1.3
Safeway*	1/2 Pot/100g	373		373	7.6	3.4	36.5	0.2
Sainsbury's*	1 Serving/200g	706		353	7.9	2.7	34.5	0.5
Tesco*	1 Tub/200g	834		417	7.3	3.5	41.5	0.1
PRAWN CRACKERS								
Asda*	1 Serving/25g	134		535	2.0	53.0	35.0	0.0
Cooked In Sunflower Oil, Sharwood's*	5 Crackers/10g	48		479	0.7	68.3	22.6	0.8
Food To Go, Sainsbury's*	1 Bag/40g	214		534	2.9	60.2	31.3	0.4
Green Thai Curry, MS*	1 Packet/50g	250		500	3.2	62.2	25.8	1.6
Marks & Spencer*	1 Pack/15g	83		550	3.0	62.3	32.0	0.0
Ready To Eat, Sharwood's*	1 Bag/60g	316		527	0.5	62.0	30.8	1.2
Red Mill*	1 Bag/50g	282		563	2.8	53.1	37.7	0.7
Sainsbury's*	1 Cracker/3g	16		537	2.4	60.4	31.7	0.8
Tesco*	1/3 Pack/20g	114		568	3.7	44.0	41.9	0.5
Uncooked, Sharwood's*	1oz/28g	136		487	0.7	52.7	29.7	1.7
Waitrose*	1 Pack/50g	267		533	2.4	58.6	32.1	1.6
PRAWN CREOLE								
With Rice, Perfectly Balanced, Waitrose*	1 Serving/404g	275		68	4.2	10.3	1.1	2.9
PRAWN PINWHEEL								
Oriental Style, BGTY, Sainsbury's*	1 Pack/189.0g	274		145	6.0	26.7	1.1	0.0
PRAWN TOAST								
Chinese Snack Selection, Mini, Tesco*	1 Toast/11g	36		330	9.4	18.8	24.2	1.9
Dim Sum Selection, Sainsbury's*	1 Toast/8g	23		283	9.9	19.2	18.5	2.0
Marks & Spencer*	1oz/28g	78		280	11.5	18.4	18.1	2.2
Oriental Selection, Waitrose*	1 Toast/14g	38		272	11.1	18.3	17.2	2.1
Sesame, Marks & Spencer*	1 Toast/28g	84		300	10.6	15.3	21.5	3.2
Sesame, Occasions, Sainsbury's*	1 Toast/12g	34		283	9.9	19.2	18.5	2.0
Sesame, Oriental Snack Selection, Sainsbury's*	1 Toast/12g	40		335	9.3	23.0	22.9	5.1
Waitrose*	1 Toast/21g	47		223	9.7	7.4	17.2	5.8
PRAWNS								
Batter Crisp, Lyons*	1 Pack/160g	350		219	8.0	18.2	12.7	1.1
Boiled	1 Prawn/3g	3		99	22.6	0.0	0.9	0.0
Brine, John West*	1/2 Can/60g	58		97	21.0	1.0	1.0	0.0
Chilli & Coriander, Marks & Spencer*	1 Serving/70g	67		95	17.9	0.6	2.2	0.6
Chilli, Battered, Marks & Spencer*	1oz/28g	63		225	7.2	23.8	11.5	0.5
Chilli, Marks & Spencer*	1oz/28g	22		79	17.9	0.6	0.5	0.6
Cooked & Peeled, Average	1oz/28g	21		77	17.6	0.2	0.6	0.0
Dried	1oz/28g	79		281	62.4	0.0	3.5	0.0
Filo Wrapped & Breaded, Marks & Spencer*	1 Serving/19g	45		235	9.5	20.4	13.0	1.4
Hot & Spicy, Average	1 Serving/170g	461		271	9.4	22.9	15.8	2.2
Icelandic, Raw, Average	1oz/28g	30		106	22.7	0.0	1.6	0.0
King, Chilli & Coriander, Sainsbury's*	1 Pack/140g	133		95	13.8	0.5	4.2	0.5
King, Crevettes, Sainsbury's*	1 Pack/225g	205		91	21.8	0.1	0.5	0.3

P

PRAWNS	Measure INFO/WEIGHT	per Measure KCAL	Nutrition Values per 100g / 100ml				
			KCAL	PROT	CARB	FAT	FIBRE
King, In Filo, Finest, Tesco*	1 Prawn/20g	38	189	13.0	27.8	2.9	1.6
King, Raw, Average	1 Bag/200g	145	72	15.8	0.2	1.0	0.1
King, Tandoori, Average	6 Prawns/354g	195	55	5.7	5.9	1.1	0.7
King, Thai Sweet Chilli, Sainsbury's*	1 Serving/150g	177	118	6.4	13.9	4.1	1.9
King, With Garlic Butter, Marks & Spencer*	1 Serving/100g	165	165	12.5	9.1	9.0	0.5
Lemon & Pepper, Marks & Spencer*	1 Serving/70g	67	95	17.5	0.0	2.7	0.5
North Atlantic, Peeled, Cooked, Average	1oz/28g	22	80	17.5	0.0	1.1	0.0
North Atlantic, Raw, Average	1oz/28g	17	62	14.4	0.0	0.4	0.0
Raw, Average	1/4 Pack/112g	88	79	17.8	0.2	0.7	0.0
Thai, Marks & Spencer*	1oz/28g	29	103	5.2	13.6	3.1	1.3
Tiger, Cooked & Peeled, Average	1 Pack/180g	151	84	18.4	0.1	1.1	0.0
Tiger, Jumbo, Average	1 Serving/50g	39	78	18.3	0.3	0.5	0.0
Tiger, Raw, Average	1oz/28g	18	64	14.2	0.1	0.7	0.0
Tiger, Wrapped, Marks & Spencer*	1 Pack/190g	477	251	11.3	20.7	13.6	1.3
PRAWNS &							
Noodles in Sweet Chilli Sauce, COU, Marks & Spencer*	1 Pack/400g	300	75	5.4	11.7	0.4	2.1
PRAWNS BHUNA							
Tandoori, Indian, Sainsbury's*	1/2 Pack/200g	152	76	5.5	4.5	4.0	1.7
PRAWNS CHILLI							
With Spicy Chilli Dip, King, Sainsbury's*	1/2 Pack/150g	282	188	8.6	22.2	7.2	1.0
PRAWNS CHINESE							
Oriental Express*	1 Serving/320g	218	68	3.2	13.8	0.6	1.9
PRAWNS CREOLE							
GFY, Asda*	1 Serving/300g	222	74	3.2	13.0	1.0	1.4
Spicy, BGTY, Sainsbury's*	1 Pack/350g	357	102	4.8	15.6	2.4	0.4
With Vegetable Rice, King, COU, Marks & Spencer*	1 Pack/400g	300	75	4.5	13.3	0.6	0.7
PRAWNS GULNARI							
With Rice, COU, Marks & Spencer*	1 Pack/400g	400	100	4.0	18.7	0.8	1.6
PRAWNS IN							
Chilli, Coriander & Lime Marinade, King, Waitrose*	1/2 Pack/70g	71	102	19.9	0.5	2.3	0.6
Creamy Garlic Sauce, Young's*	1 Serving/158g	261	165	8.5	0.3	14.5	0.0
Sweet Chilli Sauce, Asda*	1 Pack/360g	500	139	4.1	15.0	6.9	0.3
PRAWNS JAPANESE							
King, Noodle Box, Marks & Spencer*	1 Pack/300g	330	110	5.8	16.0	2.7	1.6
PRAWNS ORIENTAL							
Marks & Spencer*	1 Pack/200g	440	220	11.9	16.9	11.7	0.9
PRAWNS SZECHUAN							
Spicy, COU, Marks & Spencer*	1 Pack/400g	380	95	4.5	16.9	0.9	1.5
PRAWNS WITH							
A Spicy Cajun Dip, King, Sainsbury's*	1 Pack/240g	254	106	14.8	9.1	1.8	1.4
A Sweet Chilli Sauce, Crispy, Marks & Spencer*	1 Pack/240g	444	185	6.6	23.1	7.4	1.6
Caribbean Style Sauce, GFY, Asda*	1 Serving/400g	408	102	4.7	17.0	1.7	2.1
Garlic & Herb Butter, King, Fresh, Marks & Spencer*	1 Serving/200g	330	165	12.5	9.1	9.0	0.5
Ginger & Spring Onion, Sainsbury's*	1 Pack/300g	198	66	4.7	4.7	3.1	0.3
Green Thai Sauce, Tiger, Waitrose*	1/2 Pack/117g	108	92	16.1	0.8	2.3	0.1
Noodles, King, Debenhams*	1 Serving/370g	537	145	5.4	20.2	4.8	0.0
Rice, Sweet Chilli, Tesco*	1 Pack/460g	488	106	2.4	19.2	2.2	0.5
With Creamy Lime Dip, King, Waitrose*	1 Pot/230g	518	225	15.8	0.8	17.7	0.2
PRETZELS							
American Style, Salted, Sainsbury's*	1 Serving/50g	191	381	9.6	81.8	4.0	5.2
Jumbo, Tesco*	1 Serving/50g	194	388	9.7	71.9	6.8	5.4
Lightly Salted, Tesco*	1 Serving/25g	99	395	9.3	73.4	7.1	5.5
Marks & Spencer*	1 Serving/100g	375	375	10.4	73.7	4.2	4.7

INFO/WEIGHT	Measure	per Measure KCAL	Nutrition Values per 100g / 100ml KCAL	PROT	CARB	FAT	FIBRE

PRETZELS

	INFO/WEIGHT	per Measure KCAL	KCAL	PROT	CARB	FAT	FIBRE
Mini, 99% Fat Free, Free Natural*	1 Serving/50g	188	376	10.1	81.7	1.0	0.0
Mini, Eat Smart, Safeway*	1 Bag/25g	90	360	9.6	79.7	2.5	5.5
New York Style, Salted, Mini, Shapers, Boots*	1 Bag/25g	94	375	10.0	79.0	2.1	4.2
New York Style, Shapers, Boots*	1 Bag/24g	94	391	11.0	81.0	2.5	3.8
Salt & Cracked Black Pepper, COU, Marks & Spencer*	1 Pack/25g	95	380	9.7	83.3	2.4	2.7
Salted, Sainsbury's*	1 Serving/50g	201	401	9.8	82.4	3.6	3.4
Salted, Stars, Tesco*	1oz/28g	104	371	8.2	73.7	4.8	3.1
Sea Salt & Black Pepper, Tesco*	1 Serving/50g	192	383	10.6	76.7	3.7	2.3
Sea Salt & Cracked Black Pepper, Sainsbury's*	1 Serving/50g	191	381	9.5	79.0	4.0	3.8
Selection Tray, Marks & Spencer*	1oz/28g	112	401	9.7	75.5	6.7	3.4
Snacks, Fabulous Bakin' Boys*	1 Pack/24g	96	401	9.0	79.5	4.9	2.5
Sour Cream & Chive Flavour, Penn State*	1 Serving/25g	114	454	12.7	70.3	14.4	0.8
Sour Cream & Chive, Sainsbury's*	1 Serving/25g	103	410	9.9	73.0	8.7	5.0
Sour Cream & Onion, Tesco*	1 Serving/25g	114	457	8.4	67.7	17.0	2.3
With Sea Salt, Giant, Marks & Spencer*	1 Pretzel/8g	31	390	9.7	77.3	6.8	5.4

PRINGLES*

	INFO/WEIGHT	per Measure KCAL	KCAL	PROT	CARB	FAT	FIBRE
Barbecue	1 Serving/50g	267	533	4.9	48.0	36.0	5.1
Cheese & Onion	1 Serving/50g	271	541	4.7	50.0	36.0	3.6
Curry	1 Serving/50g	266	531	5.2	46.0	36.0	3.4
Dippers, Original	1 Serving/100g	519	519	5.1	54.0	32.0	4.1
Dippers, Sour Cream & Onion	1 Tube/170g	886	521	5.5	52.0	33.0	3.9
Hot & Spicy	1 Serving/50g	273	546	5.0	49.0	37.0	3.3
Original	1 Serving/50g	274	547	4.7	47.0	38.0	5.1
Paprika	1 Serving/50g	273	545	5.1	49.0	36.0	3.4
Pizza	1 Serving/50g	268	536	5.1	43.0	37.0	4.8
Salt & Vinegar	1 Serving/50g	265	530	4.5	47.0	36.0	4.8
Sour Cream & Onion	1 Serving/50g	270	539	5.3	46.0	37.0	4.9
Sour Cream & Onion, Light	1 Serving/50g	233	466	5.4	56.0	25.0	4.6
Spanish Salsa	1 Serving/35g	193	550	5.0	48.0	37.0	3.5
Texas Barbecue Sauce	1 Serving/50g	272	544	4.4	50.0	36.0	3.4

PROBIOTIC DRINK

	INFO/WEIGHT	per Measure KCAL	KCAL	PROT	CARB	FAT	FIBRE
Cranberry & Raspberry, Dairy, Asda*	1 Bottle/100ml	64	64	2.3	12.0	0.8	2.4
Lidl*	1 Serving/125g	94	75	2.6	12.3	1.7	0.0
Orange, Health, Tesco*	1 Serving/100g	67	67	1.5	13.4	0.9	1.3
Orange, Pianola*	1 Serving/125ml	105	84	2.5	14.7	1.6	0.0
Peach, Dairy, Asda*	1 Bottle/100ml	68	68	2.3	13.0	0.8	2.3
Strawberry, Dairy, Asda*	1 Bottle/100ml	64	64	2.3	12.0	0.8	2.3
Yoghurt, Original, Tesco*	1 Bottle/100g	68	68	1.7	13.1	1.0	1.4

PROFITEROLES

	INFO/WEIGHT	per Measure KCAL	KCAL	PROT	CARB	FAT	FIBRE
Asda*	1 Serving/64g	218	343	5.0	20.0	27.0	0.0
Chocolate, 8 Pack, Co-Op*	1/4 Pack/112g	330	295	6.0	31.0	16.0	2.0
Choux & Chocolate Sauce, Tesco*	1 Serving/76.5g	297	386	5.1	26.9	28.7	0.5
Choux Fourres Nappes De Chocolat, Ed Marche*	1 Serving/90g	262	291	5.9	42.0	11.0	0.0
Classic French, Sainsbury's*	1 Serving/90g	284	316	6.6	33.7	17.2	0.1
Dairy Cream, Safeway*	1/4 Pack/67.1g	275	410	5.5	35.3	26.9	2.2
In A Pot, Waitrose*	1 Pot/80g	207	259	6.3	25.6	14.1	2.9
Stack, Sainsbury's*	1/4 Pack/74g	301	407	5.4	38.3	25.8	2.1
Waitrose*	4 Profiteroles/75g	269	359	4.8	31.1	23.9	0.7

PROVAMEL*

	INFO/WEIGHT	per Measure KCAL	KCAL	PROT	CARB	FAT	FIBRE
Soya Dessert, Caramel, Alpro Soya*	1 Pot/125g	103	82	3.0	13.7	1.7	0.3
Soya Dessert, Chocolate, Alpro Soya*	1 Pot/125g	110	88	3.0	13.8	2.3	0.9
Soya Dessert, Fruits Of The Forest, Alpro Soya*	1 Serving/125g	98	78	3.0	11.9	1.8	0.3
Soya Dessert, Hazelnut, Alpro Soya*	1 Pot/125g	126	101	3.0	16.0	2.8	1.2

P

	Measure INFO/WEIGHT	per Measure KCAL	Nutrition Values per 100g / 100ml				
			KCAL	PROT	CARB	FAT	FIBRE
PROVAMEL*							
Soya Dessert, Peach, Alpro Soya*	1 Pot/125g	109	87	3.8	12.4	2.2	0.3
Soya Dessert, Vanilla, Alpro Soya*	1 Pot/125g	108	86	3.0	14.4	1.8	1.0
Soya Dream, Alpro Soya*	1 Carton/250ml	445	178	3.0	1.7	17.7	1.1
Soya Milk, Banana Flavour, Alpro Soya*	1 Carton/250ml	188	75	3.6	10.5	2.1	1.2
Soya Milk, Chocolate, Alpro Soya*	1 Serving/100ml	82	82	3.8	10.7	2.4	1.2
Soya Milk, Rice, Alpro Soya*	1 Serving/100g	50	50	0.1	9.9	1.1	0.0
Soya Milk, Strawberry Flavour, Alpro Soya*	1 Carton/250ml	160	64	3.6	7.7	2.1	1.2
Soya Milk, Vanilla, Organic, Alpro Soya*	1 Serving/250ml	153	61	3.8	6.5	2.3	0.3
Yofu, Black Cherry, Alpro Soya*	1 Pot/125g	106	85	3.7	12.9	2.1	1.2
Yofu, Organic, Alpro Soya*	1oz/28g	15	53	4.5	2.8	2.6	1.5
Yofu, Peach & Mango, Organic, Alpro Soya*	1 Pot/125g	116	93	3.7	14.7	2.1	1.2
Yofu, Peach & Pear, Junior, Alpro Soya*	1 Pot/125g	105	84	3.8	12.4	2.2	0.0
Yofu, Peach, Alpro Soya*	1 Pot/125g	109	87	3.8	13.3	2.1	1.2
Yofu, Plain, Organic, Alpro Soya*	1 Serving/100g	59	59	4.7	3.2	2.7	0.2
Yofu, Red Cherry, Organic, Alpro Soya*	1 Pot/125g	116	93	3.7	14.8	2.1	1.2
Yofu, Strawberry & Banana, Junior, Alpro Soya*	1 Pot/125g	106	85	3.8	12.7	2.2	0.0
Yofu, Strawberry, Alpro Soya*	1 Pot/125g	106	85	3.8	12.6	2.1	1.3
Yofu, Vanilla, Alpro Soya*	1 Pot/125g	96	77	4.1	10.0	2.3	1.3
Yoghurt, Peach, Alpro Soya*	1 Pot/125g	109	87	3.8	12.4	2.2	0.3
Yoghurt, Plain, Organic, Alpro Soya*	1 Serving/125g	74	59	4.7	3.2	2.7	0.2
Yoghurt, Strawberry, Alpro Soya	1 Pot/125g	104	83	3.8	11.5	2.2	0.3
PROVENCALE							
Cabillaud à la, Weight Watchers*	1 Pack/380g	327	86	5.1	10.3	2.7	0.0
Chicken, Marks & Spencer*	1 Pack/430g	366	85	13.2	2.3	2.7	0.6
Chicken, Steam Cuisine, Marks & Spencer*	1oz/28g	34	120	9.6	12.7	3.8	1.4
Cod, Cote Table*	1 Serving/281g	185	66	8.6	3.4	2.0	0.0
King Prawn & Mushroom, Marks & Spencer*	1/2 Pack/185g	120	65	7.2	3.9	2.5	0.9
Mushroom, Fresh, COU, Marks & Spencer*	1/2 Pack/150g	60	40	2.6	4.1	1.5	1.8
Prawn & Mushroom With Pasta, COU, Marks & Spencer*	1 Pack/400g	360	90	5.9	15.7	0.5	0.0
Ratatouille, Tesco*	1/2 Can/195g	72	37	1.1	4.2	1.8	0.9
Ratatouille, Waitrose*	1/2 Can/195g	107	55	1.5	7.8	2.1	0.8
PRUNES							
Average	1 Serving/50g	79	158	2.5	36.4	0.4	5.8
In Apple Juice, Average	1 Serving/90g	76	84	0.8	19.8	0.1	1.4
In Fruit Juice, Average	1oz/28g	25	88	0.9	21.4	0.2	3.0
In Syrup, Average	1oz/28g	26	92	1.0	22.1	0.2	2.6
Stewed With Sugar	1oz/28g	29	103	1.3	25.5	0.2	3.1
Stewed Without Sugar	1oz/28g	23	81	1.4	19.5	0.3	3.3
PUDDING							
Apple & Blackberry Crumble, Custard Style, Somerfield*	1oz/28g	34	123	3.0	17.0	5.0	0.0
Apple & Custard, Sainsbury's*	1 Serving/115g	132	115	5.4	19.0	1.9	0.1
Apple Pie, Custard Style, Somerfield*	1oz/28g	34	123	3.0	17.0	5.0	0.0
Baklava Assortment, TTD, Sainsbury's*	1 Pastry/23.9g	105	439	10.6	33.4	29.2	4.2
Banana Fudge Crunch, Bird's*	1oz/28g	125	445	5.4	75.0	14.0	0.8
Blackberry & Bramley Apple, Marks & Spencer*	1/4 Pudding/152g	365	240	3.3	38.2	8.2	2.0
Bread	1oz/28g	83	297	5.9	49.7	9.6	1.2
Butterscotch, Instant, Fat Free, Jell-O*	1 Serving/7.5g	27	333	1.3	78.7	1.3	0.0
Cherry Cobbler, GFY, Asda*	1 Cobbler/100g	158	158	2.1	33.0	2.0	0.9
Chocolate, Marks & Spencer*	1 Serving/105g	401	382	6.2	40.7	21.6	1.1
Chocolate Sponge, Healthy Living, Tesco*	1 Serving/125g	239	191	4.4	34.7	3.8	0.9
Chocolate With Chocolate Sauce, BGTY, Sainsbury's*	1 Pudding/110.3g	161	146	3.5	28.6	1.9	2.3
Chocolate With Chocolate Sauce, Heinz*	1/4 Can/77g	221	287	3.1	47.7	9.3	1.4
Chocolate, BGTY, Sainsbury's*	1 Pot/110g	161	146	3.5	28.6	1.9	0.0

	INFO/WEIGHT	KCAL	KCAL	PROT	CARB	FAT	FIBRE
PUDDING							
Chocolate, Delice*	1 Pot/100g	136	136	2.5	18.9	5.4	0.0
Chocolate, Fat Free, Snacks, Jell-O*	1 Pudding/99g	90	91	2.0	20.2	0.0	0.0
Chocolate, For Two, Gu*	1 Pack/240g	780	325	3.9	51.8	11.4	1.6
Chocolate, Perfectly Balanced, Waitrose*	1 Pot/105g	196	187	3.8	36.0	3.1	0.8
Chocolate, Tesco*	1 Serving/110g	348	316	3.1	32.9	19.1	1.9
Creamed Sago, Ambrosia*	1 Serving/200g	158	79	2.5	13.6	1.6	0.2
Creamy Brioche With Apricot Compote, Co-Op*	1 Pack/230g	391	170	6.0	22.0	6.0	0.9
Creme aux Oeufs a la Vanille, Weight Watchers*	1 Pot/100g	116	116	4.8	17.0	3.2	0.0
Creme aux Oeufs au Chocolat, Weight Watchers*	1 Pot/100g	136	136	4.7	19.7	4.3	0.0
Diat, In Schoko-Creme, Onken*	1oz/28g	24	85	3.8	10.8	2.9	0.0
Eve's	1oz/28g	67	241	3.5	28.9	13.1	1.4
Eve's, 5% Fat, Marks & Spencer*	1 Pudding/223g	323	145	3.0	23.5	4.4	0.6
Eve's, BGTY, Sainsbury's*	1 Pudding/145g	164	113	2.2	23.4	1.2	0.7
Eve's, Marks & Spencer*	1 Serving/118g	254	215	2.7	32.3	8.3	0.4
Eve's, With Custard, Snack, Marks & Spencer*	1 Serving/230g	437	190	3.2	22.6	9.2	0.7
Forest Fruit Sponge, Eat Smart, Safeway*	1 Pot/88.2g	150	170	4.2	33.5	1.8	2.6
Jam Roly Poly & Custard, Co-Op*	1 Serving/105g	263	250	3.0	44.0	7.0	0.8
Lemon Crunch, Bird's*	1oz/28g	125	445	5.5	74.0	14.0	0.7
Lemon Sponge With Lemon Sauce, Eat Smart, Safeway*	1 Pudding/90g	135	150	2.2	29.0	2.6	1.4
Lemon, BGTY, Sainsbury's*	1 Serving/100g	151	151	2.9	31.0	1.9	0.5
Lemon, Marks & Spencer*	1 Pudding/105g	328	312	4.3	39.4	15.2	2.3
Low Fat Chocolate Pudding, Good Intentions, Somerfield*	1 Pudding/110g	200	182	3.0	37.6	2.2	2.4
Pear & Almond, Finest, Tesco*	1/6 Pudding/67g	181	270	4.8	25.6	16.5	1.9
Plum, Spiced, Safeway*	1 Pudding/125g	275	220	2.7	45.7	2.5	0.9
Queen of Puddings	1oz/28g	60	213	4.8	33.1	7.8	0.2
Rhubarb & Custard, BGTY, Sainsbury's*	1 Pudding/140g	137	98	2.0	18.4	2.0	1.4
Rhubarb Crumble, Custard Style, Somerfield*	1oz/28g	33	119	3.0	16.0	5.0	0.0
Rich Chocolate, Tryton Foods*	1oz/28g	76	273	4.7	41.7	9.5	1.8
Spotted Dick, Sainsbury's*	1/4 Pudding/82g	270	329	4.1	50.9	12.1	1.6
Spotted Dick, With Custard, Individual, Sainsbury's*	1 Pudding/205g	505	246	3.3	32.6	11.4	0.7
Sticky Toffee & Sticky Toffee Sauce, BGTY, Sainsbury's*	1 Serving/130g	319	245	5.0	49.3	4.1	2.2
Sticky Toffee, Bread, Marks & Spencer*	1oz/28g	83	295	4.1	46.3	10.6	2.2
Sticky Toffee, Healthy Living, Tesco*	1 Pack/125g	245	196	4.0	34.9	4.5	0.6
Sticky Toffee, Tesco*	1 Serving/110g	287	261	3.3	31.8	13.4	0.7
Sticky Toffee, With Custard, Somerfield*	1 Pack/245g	576	235	3.0	38.0	8.0	0.0
Strawberry Jam With Custard, Farmfoods*	1 Serving/145g	525	362	3.2	35.5	23.9	0.9
Summer Fruits, Healthy Eating, Tesco*	1 Serving/100g	72	72	1.3	16.3	0.2	2.9
Summer Fruits, Marks & Spencer*	1oz/28g	25	90	2.0	20.9	0.2	4.1
Summer Pudding, BGTY, Sainsbury's*	1 Pot/110g	223	203	3.2	40.9	4.6	2.4
Summer Pudding, Waitrose*	1 Pot/120g	125	104	2.0	23.1	0.4	1.4
Summer, Healthy Eating, Tesco*	1 Serving/100g	89	89	1.9	19.1	0.6	2.2
Syrup Sponge, Iceland*	1 Serving/72.8g	228	312	5.1	54.1	8.4	0.9
Syrup, Marks & Spencer*	1 Serving/105g	370	352	3.9	61.7	10.0	0.8
Treacle Sponge, Heinz*	1 Serving/160g	445	278	2.5	48.9	8.1	0.6
Truffle, Chocolate Amaretto, Gu*	1 Pot/80g	272	340	3.3	34.9	19.4	1.6
Truffle, Chocolate, With Rasberry Compote, Gu*	1 pot/80g	250	313	2.8	28.8	18.3	1.8
Truffle, Double Chocolate, Gu*	1 Pot/50g	220	440	3.5	25.9	25.0	2.7
PULSES							
Mixed, In Water, Sainsbury's*	1/2 Can/120g	131	109	8.7	13.6	2.2	4.6
PUMPKIN							
Boiled in Salted Water	1oz/28g	4	13	0.6	2.1	0.3	1.1
PUMPKIN							
Raw	1oz/28g	4	13	0.7	2.2	0.2	1.0

INFO/WEIGHT	Measure	per Measure KCAL	Nutrition Values per 100g / 100ml				
			KCAL	PROT	CARB	FAT	FIBRE

QUADRELLI

	Measure INFO/WEIGHT	per Measure KCAL	KCAL	PROT	CARB	FAT	FIBRE
Organic, Marks & Spencer*	1 Serving/75g	263	350	13.4	71.1	1.4	3.0

QUAVERS

Cheese, Walkers*	1 Bag/20g	103	515	3.0	61.0	29.0	1.2
Prawn Cocktail, Walkers*	1 Bag/16g	82	510	2.6	61.0	28.0	1.2
Salt & Vinegar, Walkers*	1 Bag/16g	80	500	2.3	58.0	29.0	1.1
Streaky Bacon, Walkers*	1 Pack/19.6g	103	515	2.2	62.0	29.0	1.3

QUICHE

Asparagus & Cheese, Safeway*	1/4 Quiche/100g	260	260	7.5	18.2	17.4	1.4
Asparagus & Mushroom, Tesco*	1/2 Quiche/200g	474	237	5.1	17.2	16.4	1.2
Baby Spinach & Gruyere, Sainsbury's*	1/4 Quiche/93g	228	245	7.4	15.1	17.2	1.0
Bacon & Cheese, Pork Farms*	1 Pack/120g	378	315	11.1	20.8	20.0	0.0
Bacon & Leek, Individual, Tesco*	1 Quiche/175g	485	277	8.3	19.4	18.5	0.9
Bacon & Leek, Tesco*	1 Serving/100g	251	251	6.8	21.5	15.3	1.2
Bacon & Tomato, Asda*	1 Serving/106.9g	201	188	8.0	21.0	8.0	1.1
Bacon & Tomato, Good Intentions, Somerfield*	1 Serving/145g	255	176	5.7	5.1	14.8	0.1
Bacon, Leek & Mushroom, Marks & Spencer*	1/4 Quiche/100g	250	250	8.7	14.2	17.9	2.1
Bacon, Mushroom & Tomato, Somerfield*	1/4 Quiche/100g	264	264	7.6	19.6	17.2	1.0
Bacon, Sausage & Tomato, Tesco*	1 Serving/130g	337	259	7.6	19.4	16.8	0.9
Brie & Smoked Bacon, Asda*	1/4 Quiche/90g	249	277	8.9	17.8	18.9	1.0
Broccoli & Cheddar Cheese, Safeway*	1 Pack/300g	813	271	7.7	19.8	17.9	1.9
Broccoli & Gruyere Cheese, Waitrose*	1 Serving/100g	241	241	7.3	13.0	17.8	2.9
Broccoli & Stilton, Mini, Sainsbury's*	1 Quiche/14g	52	369	8.8	35.2	21.4	3.3
Broccoli & Tomato, Marks & Spencer*	1oz/28g	59	210	6.7	14.7	13.8	1.6
Broccoli, Extra, Value, Tesco*	1 Serving/125g	341	273	10.0	15.1	19.2	0.8
Broccoli, Healthy Eating, Tesco*	1 Quiche/175g	308	176	6.7	21.5	7.0	1.4
Broccoli, Tesco*	1 Quiche/175g	340	194	7.0	20.9	9.2	1.4
Broccoli, Tomato & Cheese, BGTY, Sainsbury's*	1 Quiche/390g	632	162	6.4	15.7	8.2	1.3
Broccoli, Tomato & Cheese, Sainsbury's*	1 Serving/125g	279	223	6.3	17.9	14.0	0.9
Cheddar Cheese, & Onion, Safeway*	1/4 Quiche/100g	293	293	8.3	21.6	19.3	1.5
Cheese & Bacon, Healthy Eating, Tesco*	1 Serving/155g	307	198	9.1	19.9	9.1	1.4
Cheese & Bacon, SmartPrice, Asda*	1/4 Quiche/82g	208	257	6.0	20.0	17.0	0.7
Cheese & Bacon, Tesco*	1/4 Quiche/100g	324	324	10.5	16.4	24.0	1.7
Cheese & Broccoli, Good Intentions, Somerfield*	1 Quiche/145g	409	282	6.9	27.7	15.9	1.8
Cheese & Chive, Healthy Eating, Tesco*	1 Serving/86g	169	197	10.4	22.1	7.4	1.2
Cheese & Egg	1oz/28g	88	314	12.5	17.3	22.2	0.6
Cheese & Ham, Basics, Somerfield*	1/4 Quiche/81g	187	231	7.0	20.1	13.6	0.7
Cheese & Ham, Sainsbury's*	1 Serving/100g	266	266	9.3	14.4	19.0	1.2
Cheese & Mushroom, Budgens*	1/2 Quiche/170g	474	279	7.8	18.4	19.3	1.4
Cheese & Onion, BFY, Morrisons*	1 Serving/100g	212	212	10.1	20.2	10.2	1.4
Cheese & Onion, Finest, Tesco*	1 Serving/130g	346	266	9.1	15.3	18.7	2.5
Cheese & Onion, Marks & Spencer*	1 Slice/100g	250	250	8.2	16.1	17.2	1.5
Cheese & Onion, Mini, Somerfield*	1oz/28g	110	394	9.0	27.0	28.0	0.0
Cheese & Onion, Reduced Fat, Safeway*	1/4 Flan/100g	212	212	9.6	20.8	10.0	1.5
Cheese & Onion, Sainsbury's*	1/4 Quiche/100g	303	303	10.2	16.7	21.7	0.9
Cheese & Onion, Shell*	1 Slice/150g	362	241	7.9	16.1	15.4	0.0
Cheese & Onion, Small, Sainsbury's*	1/2 Quiche/90g	271	301	9.9	21.6	19.4	1.5
Cheese & Onion, Tesco*	1 Serving/90g	230	256	8.2	18.1	16.8	2.5
Cheese & Onion, Value, Tesco*	1/2 Quiche/200g	526	263	8.6	16.1	18.2	0.7
Cheese & Tomato, Asda*	1/4 Quiche/105g	274	261	8.0	19.0	17.0	0.9
Cheese & Tomato, Marks & Spencer*	1 Serving/100g	230	230	7.7	15.1	15.6	1.6
Cheese & Tomato, Tesco*	1 Serving/100g	274	274	7.5	18.3	19.0	1.4
Cheese Potato & Onion, Safeway*	1/3 Quiche/115g	361	314	8.8	24.1	20.3	1.5
Cheese, Broccoli & Tomato, Nisa Heritage*	1 Serving/85g	234	275	7.3	17.5	19.5	1.4

QUICHE	Measure INFO/WEIGHT	per Measure KCAL	Nutrition Values per 100g / 100ml KCAL	PROT	CARB	FAT	FIBRE
Cheese, Onion & Chive, Healthy Eating, Tesco*	1 Slice/100g	202	202	10.9	21.2	8.2	1.3
Cheese, Onion & Chive, SmartPrice, Asda*	1/4 Quiche/83g	213	257	6.0	20.0	17.0	0.7
Cheese, Onion & Chive, Tesco*	1oz/28g	90	320	10.6	15.5	24.0	0.6
Chicken & Basil, Finest, Tesco*	1 Serving/134g	381	284	9.3	19.8	18.6	1.3
Chicken & Mushroom, Somerfield*	1oz/28g	90	320	12.0	22.0	21.0	0.0
Chicken, Bacon & Mushroom, Asda*	1 Quiche/425g	1131	266	9.0	17.0	18.0	0.8
Chicken, Garlic & Herb, Asda*	1/8 Quiche/52g	137	264	10.0	20.0	16.0	1.2
Cumberland Sausage & Onion, Sainsbury's*	1 Serving/180g	486	270	7.0	18.8	18.5	1.3
Cumberland Sausage, Tesco*	1 Serving/100g	237	237	7.3	17.7	15.2	2.2
Davidstow Cheddar Cheese & Caramelised Onion, Asda*	1/3 Quiche/117g	367	315	7.0	20.0	23.0	1.0
Egg, Bacon & Cheese, Iceland*	1 Serving/90g	299	332	7.7	23.5	23.0	1.9
Gammon, Leek & Cheddar Cheese, Somerfield*	1/4 Quiche/95g	251	264	7.6	19.9	17.1	0.9
Garlic Mushroom, Asda*	1/4 Quiche/105g	273	260	7.0	22.0	16.0	0.7
Goats Cheese & Red Pepper, Tesco*	1 Serving/87g	271	312	5.8	19.2	23.6	0.9
Ham & Mustard, GFY, Asda*	1 Quiche/155g	327	211	9.0	19.0	11.0	3.9
Ham & Soft Cheese, Tesco*	1/4 Quiche/100g	280	280	7.4	17.5	20.1	1.9
Ham & Tomato, Marks & Spencer*	1/2 Pack/200g	440	220	8.1	12.4	15.5	2.9
Ham, Cheese & Chive, GFY, Asda*	1 Serving/78g	173	222	9.0	24.0	10.0	1.5
Leek & Sweet Potato, Waitrose*	1/2 Quiche/200g	440	220	5.3	17.0	14.5	2.3
Leek, Cheese & Chive, Sainsbury's*	1/3 Quiche/125g	293	234	7.1	14.9	16.2	1.3
Lincolnshire Sausage & Whole Grain Mustard, Somerfield*	1/4 Quiche/100g	282	282	6.7	17.7	20.5	0.8
Lorraine	1oz/28g	109	391	16.1	19.8	28.1	0.7
Lorraine, Asda*	1 Serving/106g	318	300	9.0	21.0	20.0	2.3
Lorraine, BGTY, Sainsbury's*	1 Serving/128g	273	213	10.9	17.7	10.9	0.7
Lorraine, Finest, Tesco*	1 Serving/100g	330	330	8.4	17.5	25.1	1.5
Lorraine, Improved Recipe, Marks & Spencer*	1oz/28g	78	280	12.5	14.9	18.9	0.9
Lorraine, Mini, Marks & Spencer*	1oz/28g	95	340	11.6	21.0	23.6	1.6
Lorraine, Reduced Fat, Waitrose*	1 Serving/120g	244	203	10.8	20.2	8.8	1.9
Lorraine, Sainsbury's*	1/3 Quiche/128g	341	265	9.3	14.4	19.0	0.9
Lorraine, Somerfield*	1/4 Quiche/87g	260	299	10.1	17.1	21.1	0.7
Lorraine, TTD, Sainsbury's*	1/3 Pie/158g	482	305	10.2	15.1	22.7	0.9
Lorraine, Tesco*	1 Serving/81g	220	272	9.1	18.7	17.9	1.2
Lorraine, With A Creamy Filling, Safeway*	1 Quiche/485g	1576	325	9.8	19.4	22.7	1.2
Mediterranean Pepper, Good Intentions, Somerfield*	1/3 Quiche/130g	264	203	7.9	22.2	9.2	1.3
Mediterranean Vegetable, BGTY, Sainsbury's*	1/2 Quiche/90g	160	178	7.3	19.2	8.0	1.7
Mediterranean Vegetable, Mini, Marks & Spencer*	1oz/28g	78	280	6.8	23.9	17.5	1.6
Mediterranean Vegetable, Sainsbury's*	1 Serving/200g	482	241	6.3	14.6	17.5	2.2
Mediterranean, GFY, Asda*	1 Serving/25g	54	217	9.0	25.0	9.0	2.4
Mediterranean, Marks & Spencer*	1oz/28g	64	230	6.6	16.6	15.3	0.9
Mushroom	1oz/28g	80	284	10.0	18.3	19.5	0.9
Mushroom Medley & Gruyere, TTD, Sainsbury's*	1/3 Quiche/158g	426	269	6.3	18.0	19.1	1.4
Mushroom Medley, Waitrose*	1/4 Quiche/100g	222	222	6.4	15.0	15.2	2.9
Mushroom, Bacon & Leek, Marks & Spencer*	1 Pack/170g	425	250	8.7	13.4	18.1	1.6
Mushroom, Marks & Spencer*	1/4 Quiche/100g	235	235	6.1	14.6	16.7	2.8
Mushroom, Somerfield*	1/4 Quiche/82g	212	258	9.0	20.0	16.0	0.0
Mushroom, Tesco*	1/4 Quiche/100g	250	250	5.6	17.4	17.5	1.0
Red Pepper, Goats Cheese & Spinach, Waitrose*	1 Serving/100g	218	218	6.5	15.8	14.3	2.6
Red Pepper, Rocket & Parmesan, Waitrose*	1 Serving/100g	236	236	6.1	14.8	16.9	1.9
Roast Sweet Potato, Carrot & Coriander, Asda*	1/2 Quiche/208g	523	252	7.0	20.0	16.0	1.0
Salmon & Asparagus, Healthy Eating, Tesco*	1 Quiche/345g	621	180	7.5	20.2	7.7	1.2
Salmon & Broccoli, Sainsbury's*	1 Serving	346	260	7.9	18.5	17.1	0.8
Salmon & Broccoli, Tesco*	1 Serving/133g	311	234	7.9	16.6	15.1	0.9
Salmon & Spinach, Sainsbury's*	1/3 Quiche/125g	318	254	8.2	15.9	17.5	1.0

Q

QUICHE	Measure INFO/WEIGHT	per Measure KCAL	KCAL	PROT	CARB	FAT	FIBRE
Sausage & Onion, Sainsbury's*	1 Serving/100g	287	287	7.1	19.7	20.0	1.2
Spinach & Gruyere, Mini, Somerfield*	1oz/28g	108	384	11.0	25.0	27.0	0.0
Spinach & Gruyere, Sainsbury's*	1/4 Quiche/100g	258	258	7.7	13.9	19.1	1.0
Spinach & Ricotta, Marks & Spencer*	1oz/28g	73	260	8.0	14.9	18.8	1.7
Spinach & Ricotta, Tesco*	1/4 Quiche/100g	237	237	5.8	19.9	14.9	1.0
Spinach Ricotta Cheese & Red Pepper, Safeway*	1 Serving/120g	304	253	6.2	20.2	16.4	1.2
Spinach, Ricotta & Gruyere Slice, Somerfield*	1 Slice/130g	348	268	7.0	15.0	20.0	0.0
Summer Vegetable, Marks & Spencer*	1/4 Quiche/100g	225	225	4.9	14.5	16.5	1.7
Sunblush Tomato, Basil & Mozzarella, Somerfield*	1/4 Quiche/88g	221	251	7.7	17.9	16.5	1.0
Sweet Cherry Pepper & Fontal Cheese, Finest, Tesco*	1/4 Slice/100g	293	293	6.7	16.9	22.1	0.9
Sweetfire Pepper, Feta & Olive, Waitrose*	1/4 Quiche/100g	238	238	5.7	15.7	16.9	1.4
Three Cheese & Onion, GFY, Asda*	1 Serving/73g	188	258	10.0	23.0	14.0	3.1
Tomato & Cheese, Sainsbury's*	1/3 Quiche/133g	374	281	7.9	20.9	18.4	1.5
Tomato Cheese & Courgette, GFY, Asda*	1 Serving/155g	333	215	7.0	22.0	11.0	3.3
Tomato, Broccoli & Cheese, Sainsbury's*	1 Serving/180g	437	243	6.7	19.6	15.3	1.5
Tomato, Cheese & Courgette, Asda*	1 Quiche/100g	333	333	11.0	34.0	17.0	5.0
Tomato, GFY, Asda*	1/4 Quiche/50g	94	188	8.0	21.0	8.0	0.8
Tomato, Mozzarella & Basil, Sainsbury's*	1/3 Quiche/133g	318	239	6.3	17.6	15.9	1.5
Tomato, Mushroom & Bacon, Sainsbury's*	1 Serving/187g	447	239	7.5	15.2	16.5	1.1
Tuna, Tomato & Basil, Asda*	1 Serving/125g	305	244	9.0	16.0	16.0	1.5
Vegetable, Tesco*	1 Serving/100g	257	257	6.9	17.5	17.7	1.5
QUICK SNACK							
Chicken & Mushroom Flavour, Value, Tesco*	1 Pot/80g	274	342	14.9	60.6	4.5	7.0
Mash, Roasted Onion, Sainsbury's*	1 Pot/58g	75	130	1.8	14.8	7.1	0.0
Rice, Chilli, Sainsbury's*	1 Pack/280g	241	86	2.5	18.6	0.2	0.0
QUINCE							
Average	1oz/28g	7	26	0.3	6.3	0.1	0.0
QUINOA							
Average	1oz/28g	87	309	13.8	55.7	5.0	8.9
QUORN*							
Bacon*	1 Rasher/30g	42	141	13.5	8.1	6.1	3.0
Balls, Al Forno	1 Serving/400g	348	87	4.7	13.1	1.8	1.8
Balls, Swedish Style	3 Balls/50g	72	144	22.0	5.4	3.8	3.2
Balls, Swedish Style, In Chunky Tomato & Basil Sauce	1 Pack/400g	296	74	8.2	5.0	2.3	2.0
Burgers	1 Burger/50g	69	137	17.8	8.8	3.4	3.7
Burgers, Original	1 Burger/50g	109	219	24.0	13.8	7.4	9.8
Burgers, Premium, Surprisingly Satisfying	1 Burger/82g	88	107	11.3	6.5	4.0	3.5
Burgers, Southern Style	1 Burger/63g	125	199	10.7	17.0	9.8	3.1
Casserole, With Dumplings	1oz/28g	36	127	4.5	14.2	5.8	1.7
Chicken Slices, Deli Style	3 Slices/33g	36	108	16.9	4.0	2.7	3.2
Chilli	1oz/28g	23	81	4.7	6.9	4.2	2.5
Curry, Red Thai	1 Pack/400g	464	116	4.6	15.5	3.9	4.0
Enchiladas	1 Pack/400g	384	96	5.3	11.7	3.1	1.9
Enchiladas, Marlow Foods*	1 Pack/401g	405	101	5.3	11.7	3.7	1.9
Escalopes, Garlic & Herb	1 Escalope/140g	293	209	8.9	16.9	11.8	3.8
Fajita, Ready Meal	1oz/28g	41	148	6.9	22.1	3.5	2.7
Fillets	2 Fillets/102g	92	90	12.6	5.9	1.8	4.7
Fillets, Cajun Spice	1 Serving/100g	176	176	10.9	14.7	8.2	3.4
Fillets, Chargrilled Tikka Style, Mini	1/2 Pack/85g	110	129	12.5	14.4	2.4	5.0
Fillets, Chinese Style Chargrilled, Mini	1 Serving/85g	115	135	12.1	15.6	2.7	4.7
Fillets, Garlic & Herb	1 Fillet/100g	198	198	10.7	16.7	9.8	4.1
Fillets, Hot & Spicy	1 Fillet/100g	176	176	10.9	14.7	8.2	6.4
Fillets, In A Mediterranean Marinade	1 Fillet/80g	90	112	12.5	8.8	3.0	4.0

Q

INFO/WEIGHT	Measure	per Measure KCAL	Nutrition Values per 100g / 100ml				
			KCAL	PROT	CARB	FAT	FIBRE
Fillets, In A White Wine Sauce With Mushrooms & Chives	1 Fillet/162.5g	142	87	6.2	4.4	5.0	1.5
Fillets, In Breadcrumbs	1 Fillet/94g	184	196	11.0	14.2	10.6	3.8
Fillets, In Mushroom & White Wine Sauce	1 Pack/325g	218	67	5.1	4.9	3.0	2.1
Fillets, Lemon & Black Pepper	1 Fillet/100g	195	195	11.6	17.2	8.9	3.3
Fillets, Mushroom & White Wine Sauce	1oz/28g	18	65	6.3	6.0	1.8	2.1
Fillets, Thai	1 Serving/79.4g	85	107	14.9	6.1	2.5	3.6
Fillets, With A Crispy Seasonal Coating	1 Fillet/100g	197	197	8.8	18.4	9.8	3.0
Florentine, Deli	1 Slice/15g	21	140	15.0	5.8	6.3	3.0
Goujons, With Chunky Salsa Dip	1oz/28g	57	204	10.4	17.0	10.5	3.0
Grills, Lamb Flavour	1 Grill/90g	104	116	11.4	10.4	3.2	4.2
Ham	1 Slice/12.5g	18	139	18.3	6.1	4.6	3.1
Ham, Wafer Thin, Deli	1 Serving/18g	23	130	19.3	6.1	3.1	3.1
Korma	1oz/28g	39	140	3.7	16.7	7.0	0.0
Lasagne	1 Pack/300g	249	83	4.1	9.9	3.0	1.3
Mince	1 Pack/350g	329	94	14.5	4.5	2.0	6.0
Moussaka	1 Pack/400g	364	91	3.6	9.8	4.1	1.2
Myco-Protein	1oz/28g	24	86	11.8	2.0	3.5	4.8
Noodles, Sweet Chilli	1 Pack/400g	352	88	4.2	12.7	2.3	1.5
Nuggets	1 nugget/20g	38	191	10.6	15.7	9.5	3.5
Nuggets, Southern Style	1 Nugget/20g	39	197	12.1	15.7	9.5	3.5
Pate, Brussels Style	1 Pack/130g	150	115	10.8	5.7	5.4	3.4
Pate, Country Style Coarse	1/2 Pot/65g	68	104	9.2	7.3	4.2	2.7
Pate, Deli	1oz/28g	32	115	10.8	5.7	5.4	3.4
Pie, Cottage	1 Pie/300g	177	59	2.5	9.0	1.4	2.6
Pie, Creamy Mushroom	1 Pie/134g	362	270	4.1	22.8	18.0	1.3
Pie, Mince & Onion	1 Pie/141g	368	261	5.3	27.1	14.6	1.5
Pie, Quorn & Vegetable	1oz/28g	52	186	6.9	14.7	11.5	2.0
Pieces	1 Pack/300g	309	103	14.0	5.8	2.6	6.0
Pork Ribsters	2 Ribsters/83.9g	99	118	15.9	4.8	3.9	2.8
Roast	2 Slices/90g	97	108	16.9	4.0	2.7	4.0
Roast, Chicken Style	1oz/28g	30	108	16.9	4.0	2.7	3.2
Sausage & Mash, Tesco*	1 Pack/400g	292	73	4.1	8.8	2.4	1.3
Sausage, Leek & Pork Style	1 Sausage/44g	56	127	15.1	5.5	4.9	4.3
Sausage, Spinach & Gruyere, Quorn*	1 Sausage/50g	64	128	15.2	6.6	4.6	2.8
Sausage, Vegetarian	1 Sausage/42g	46	109	14.3	4.5	3.7	3.7
Slices, Roast, With Sage & Onion Stuffing	1/4 Pack/70g	47	67	7.5	4.9	1.9	3.0
Spaghetti Bolognese	1 Pack/400g	240	60	3.7	9.2	0.9	1.6
Spaghetti Carbonara	1 Pack/400g	460	115	5.0	9.1	6.5	1.1
Steaks, Peppered	1 Steak/98.2g	107	109	11.4	7.4	3.8	4.0
Stir Fry, Spicy Chilli With Vegetables & Rice	1/2 Pack/170g	162	95	5.9	15.6	1.0	1.8
Tikka Masala, With Rice	1 Pack/400g	476	119	4.3	13.5	5.3	1.6
Turkey Flavour, With Stuffing, Deli	1 Slice/13g	15	114	15.1	8.3	2.3	4.7

Q

	Measure INFO/WEIGHT	per Measure KCAL	Nutrition Values per 100g / 100ml				
			KCAL	PROT	CARB	FAT	FIBRE
RABBIT							
Meat Only, Raw	1oz/28g	38	137	21.9	0.0	5.5	0.0
Meat Only, Stewed,	1oz/28g	32	114	21.2	0.0	3.2	0.0
Meat Only, Stewed, Weighed With Bone	1oz/28g	19	68	12.7	0.0	1.9	0.0
RADDICCIO							
Raw	1oz/28g	4	14	1.4	1.7	0.2	1.8
RADIATORE							
Dry, Average	1oz/28g	98	352	12.7	71.7	1.9	1.3
RADISH							
Red, Average	1oz/28g	3	12	0.7	1.9	0.2	0.9
White, Mooli, Raw	1oz/28g	4	15	0.8	2.9	0.1	0.0
RAISINS							
& Cranberries, Waitrose*	1 Serving/30g	94	312	1.5	75.7	0.3	3.4
& Sultanas, Jumbo, Marks & Spencer*	1 Pack/50g	133	265	2.4	62.4	0.5	2.6
Yoghurt Coated, Average	1 Bag/100g	424	424	2.7	66.3	17.8	1.0
Seedless, Average	1 Serving/75g	215	287	2.2	68.5	0.5	3.2
RAITA							
Cucumber & Mint, Patak's*	1oz/28g	33	117	3.9	12.9	5.5	0.1
Plain	1oz/28g	46	166	2.6	5.5	15.3	0.0
RASPBERRIES							
Average	1oz/28g	7	26	1.3	4.7	0.3	6.5
In Fruit Juice, Average	1oz/28g	9	32	0.9	6.7	0.2	1.7
In Syrup, Canned	1oz/28g	25	88	0.6	22.5	0.1	1.5
RATATOUILLE							
Average	1oz/28g	23	82	1.3	3.8	7.0	1.8
Chicken, Finest, Tesco*	1 Pack/550g	407	74	7.8	5.9	2.1	0.0
Princes*	1 Can/360g	86	24	1.0	4.2	0.4	0.0
Roasted Vegetable, Sainsbury's*	1 Pack/300g	134	45	1.4	7.5	1.0	2.3
Sainsbury's*	1 Pack/300g	99	33	1.5	5.5	0.6	1.6
Vegetable, Marks & Spencer*	1 Serving/100g	45	45	1.2	3.6	3.0	2.1
RAVIOLI							
Amatriciana, TTD, Sainsbury's*	1 Serving/125g	390	312	16.6	33.3	12.5	3.5
Asparagus & Ham, Healthy Eating, Tesco*	1/2 Pack/125g	203	162	8.2	26.5	2.6	0.6
Asparagus, Waitrose*	1 Serving/150g	303	202	10.5	26.4	6.0	2.0
Basil & Parmesan, Organic, Sainsbury's*	1/2 Pack/192g	290	151	7.4	21.1	5.2	2.1
Beef & Red Wine, Tesco*	1 Serving/125g	270	216	11.3	32.0	4.7	2.2
Beef & Shiraz, Finest, Tesco*	1/2 Pack/200g	358	179	8.4	26.1	4.5	1.8
Beef, Fresh, Safeway*	1 Serving/137g	352	257	10.0	39.4	6.6	3.0
Beef, In Tomato Sauce, Asda*	1 Serving/400g	352	88	3.6	14.0	2.0	3.0
Beef, Tesco*	1 Serving/194g	175	90	4.3	12.3	2.6	1.5
Blue Cheese & Bacon, Safeway*	1/2 Pack/125g	288	230	10.5	24.9	9.6	1.6
Cheese & Asparagus, Waitrose*	1 Serving/100g	242	242	12.6	31.7	7.2	2.4
Cheese & Sun Dried Tomato, Co-Op*	1/2 Pack/125g	356	285	12.0	38.0	9.0	2.0
Cheese & Tomato, Fresh, Organic, Tesco*	1 Serving/125g	343	274	12.5	30.8	11.2	1.1
Cheese & Tomato, Heinz*	1 Can/410g	332	81	2.7	14.1	1.5	0.6
Cheese, Garlic, & Herb, Fresh, Organic, Tesco*	1 Serving/125g	383	306	11.3	30.1	15.6	0.9
Cheese, Garlic, & Herb, Safeway*	1/2 Pack/125g	263	210	9.1	26.5	7.6	2.0
Cheese, Tomato & Basil, Italiano, Tesco*	1/2 Pack/125g	309	247	13.1	28.5	8.8	2.1
Cherry Tomato & Mushroom, Somerfield*	1 Pack/400g	436	109	3.5	9.8	6.2	1.2
Chicken & Mushroom, Finest, Tesco*	1/2 Pack/125g	268	214	11.6	25.8	7.1	1.1
Chicken & Rosemary, Perfectly Balanced, Waitrose*	1/2 Pack/125g	266	213	14.9	30.4	3.5	2.1
Chicken & Tomato, Perfectly Balanced, Waitrose*	1 Serving/125g	265	212	13.5	33.4	2.7	2.8
Chicken, Tomato & Basil, Finest, Tesco*	1 Serving/200g	358	179	9.6	21.7	6.0	1.0
Feta Cheese, Marks & Spencer*	1 Serving/100g	195	195	9.1	20.5	8.5	1.3

R

	Measure INFO/WEIGHT	per Measure KCAL	Nutrition Values per 100g / 100ml				
			KCAL	PROT	CARB	FAT	FIBRE
RAVIOLI							
Five Cheese, Weight Watchers*	1 Pack/330g	271	82	3.2	11.1	2.8	0.8
Florentine, Weight Watchers*	1 Serving/241g	220	91	3.7	14.1	2.1	1.2
Four Cheese, Good Intentions, Somerfield*	1 Pack/353g	367	104	4.1	14.0	3.5	1.7
Four Cheese, Italia, Marks & Spencer*	1 Pack/360g	432	120	6.7	13.1	4.6	1.0
Free Range Duck, TTD, Sainsbury's*	1/2 Pack/161g	314	195	11.5	21.0	7.3	2.3
Fresh, Bolognese, Safeway*	1 Serving/120g	200	167	8.8	22.6	4.6	2.0
Fresh, Pasta Reale*	1 Serving/150g	459	306	13.1	53.3	5.9	0.0
Garlic & Herb, Italiano, Tesco*	1 Serving/100g	318	318	11.1	39.1	13.0	2.6
Garlic Mushroom, Finest, Tesco*	1 Serving/250g	553	221	8.9	30.0	7.3	2.0
Goat's Cheese & Pesto, Asda*	1/2 Pack/150g	204	136	6.0	20.0	3.6	0.0
Goats Cheese & Roasted Red Pepper, Finest, Tesco*	1/2 Pack/125g	308	246	11.4	32.8	7.7	1.8
In Tomato Sauce, Bettabuy, Morrisons*	1oz/28g	21	75	2.7	14.0	0.9	1.3
In Tomato Sauce, Heinz*	1 Can/410g	299	73	2.6	13.0	1.1	0.6
In Tomato Sauce, Meat Free, Heinz*	1 Can/410g	308	75	2.4	14.4	0.8	0.5
In Tomato Sauce, Sainsbury's*	1oz/28g	23	83	3.1	15.5	1.0	0.5
In Tomato Sauce, Tesco*	1 Can/400g	272	68	2.4	12.1	1.1	1.3
Meat, Italian, Fresh, Asda*	1/2 Pack/150g	261	174	8.0	26.0	4.2	0.0
Meditteranean Vegetable, Healthy Eating, Tesco*	1 Serving/125g	199	159	6.7	27.2	2.6	0.9
Mozzarella Tomato & Basil, Tesco*	1 Serving/125g	304	243	13.6	24.1	10.2	0.5
Mushroom & Mascarpone, The Best, Safeway*	1 Pack/175g	466	266	9.9	31.8	11.0	1.0
Mushroom, Fresh, Sainsbury's*	1/2 Pack/125g	196	157	7.4	22.6	4.1	1.9
Mushroom, Italian, Fresh, Somerfield*	1/2 Pack/125g	336	269	10.8	34.4	9.8	1.8
Mushroom, Italiano, Tesco*	1 Serving/125g	333	266	10.4	27.0	12.9	3.0
Mushroom, Ready Meals, Marks & Spencer*	1oz/28g	38	135	8.1	22.0	1.9	2.2
Mushroom, Wild, Finest, Tesco*	1 Serving/200g	472	236	10.8	34.4	6.1	1.9
Mushroomi, Tesco*	1/2 Pack/125g	333	266	10.4	27.0	12.9	3.0
Pancetta & Mozzarella, Finest, Tesco*	1 Serving/125g	344	275	12.2	32.8	10.6	1.8
Prosciuttoi, Ready Meal, Marks & Spencer*	1 Pack/100g	195	195	13.3	17.0	8.1	1.0
Red Onion & Brunello Wine, TTD, Sainsbury's*	1 Serving/125g	235	188	7.5	23.0	7.3	2.5
Red Pepper, Basil & Chilli, Waitrose*	1/2 Pack/125g	313	250	11.6	32.0	8.4	1.7
Rich Beef & Red Wine, Morrisons*	1 Serving/150g	396	264	12.1	40.6	7.2	3.0
Roast Garlic & Herb, Tesco*	1/2 Pack/125g	343	274	12.8	31.1	10.9	1.1
Roasted Pepper, Marks & Spencer*	1 Pack/400g	540	135	5.4	11.0	7.7	1.1
Roasted Vegetable, Asda*	1/2 Pack/150g	218	145	6.0	29.0	0.5	0.0
Salmon, Open, Finest, Tesco*	1oz/28g	37	131	6.8	15.5	4.6	0.5
SmartPrice, Asda*	1 Can/400g	272	68	2.7	14.0	0.1	1.3
Smoked Ham, Bacon & Tomato, Italiano, Tesco*	1 Can/125g	303	242	10.8	32.3	7.7	2.9
Smoked Salmon & Dill, Sainsbury's*	1 Serving/125g	256	205	8.7	26.5	7.1	0.7
Spinach & Ricotta, Waitrose*	1 Serving/125g	309	247	10.5	35.0	7.2	1.9
Sweet Pepper & Chilli, Tesco*	1/2 Pack/125g	324	259	12.5	27.1	11.2	2.7
Tomato Cheese & Meat, Sainsbury's*	1 Serving/125g	314	251	12.4	21.4	12.9	2.2
Tomato, Cheese & Mortadell, Sainsbury's*	1 Serving/125g	273	218	10.3	20.3	10.6	2.4
Vegetable In Tomato Sauce, Italiana, Weight Watchers*	1 Can/385g	266	69	1.7	11.0	2.1	0.5
Vegetable, Sainsbury's*	1 Can/400g	328	82	2.6	16.3	0.7	0.7
Vegetable, Tesco*	1/2 Can/200g	164	82	2.6	16.3	0.7	0.7
Wild Mushroom, Al Forno, TTD, Sainsbury's*	1 Pack/300g	459	153	7.0	14.0	7.7	1.2
RAVIOLINI							
Gorgonzola & Walnut, Marks & Spencer*	1/2 Pack/125g	381	305	12.6	33.6	13.2	2.0
RED BULL*							
Regular	1 Can/250ml	113	45	0.0	11.3	0.0	0.0
REDCURRANT JELLY							
Average	1oz/28g	70	250	0.2	64.4	0.0	0.0

R

INFO/WEIGHT	Measure	per Measure KCAL	Nutrition Values per 100g / 100ml KCAL	PROT	CARB	FAT	FIBRE
REDCURRANTS							
Raw	1oz/28g	6	21	1.1	4.4	0.0	3.4
REEF*							
Orange & Passionfruit, Reef*	1 Bottle/275ml	179	65	0.0	9.5	0.0	0.0
REFRESHERS							
Bassett's*	1oz/28g	106	377	4.3	78.1	0.0	0.0
Lollipop, Bassett's*	1 Lolipop/6g	25	417	0.0	108.3	0.0	0.0
REHYDRATION DRINK							
Still Pink Grapefruit Sports, Shapers, Boots*	1 Bottle/500ml	10	2	0.1	0.2	0.1	0.0
RELISH							
Barbeque, Sainsbury's*	1 Serving/50g	50	100	1.0	19.3	2.1	1.1
Caramelised Onion & Chilli, Marks & Spencer*	1 Serving/20g	47	235	1.4	55.1	1.1	1.0
Caramelised Red Onion, Tesco*	1 Serving/10g	28	280	0.6	69.1	0.1	0.7
Hamburger, Bick's*	1oz/28g	27	96	1.3	22.3	0.2	0.0
Hot Chilli & Jalapeno, Branston*	1 Serving/10g	11	108	2.3	23.1	0.7	1.4
Onion & Garlic, Spicy, Waitrose*	1 Tbsp/15g	35	232	0.8	54.2	1.1	1.7
Onion, Marks & Spencer*	1oz/28g	46	165	1.0	32.1	3.0	1.1
Onion, Sainsbury's*	1 Serving/15g	23	151	0.9	36.0	0.4	0.7
Sweet Onion, Branston*	1 Serving/10g	15	145	1.0	34.2	0.4	0.6
Sweetcorn, Bick's*	1 Tbsp/22g	23	103	1.3	24.3	0.2	0.0
Tomato & Chilli Texan Style, Tesco*	1 Tbsp/14g	20	140	1.7	32.0	0.1	1.1
Tomato, Marks & Spencer*	1oz/28g	36	130	1.8	30.2	0.3	1.5
REVELS							
Mars*	1 Sm Bag/35g	166	475	5.0	67.7	20.4	1.2
RHUBARB							
Raw, Average	1 Serving/120g	8	7	0.9	0.8	0.1	1.4
Stewed With Sugar	1oz/28g	13	48	0.9	11.5	0.1	1.2
Stewed Without Sugar	1oz/28g	2	7	0.9	0.7	0.1	1.3
RIBENA*							
Apple Juice Drink	1 Carton/287ml	132	46	0.0	11.1	0.0	0.0
Blackcurrant Juice Drink	1 Carton/288ml	164	57	0.0	14.0	0.0	0.0
Blackcurrant, Diluted With Water	1 Serving/180ml	81	45	0.0	11.0	0.0	0.0
Light	1 Carton/288ml	26	9	0.1	2.1	0.0	0.0
Strawberry Juice Drink	1 Carton/288ml	156	54	0.0	13.2	0.0	0.0
RIBS							
Loin, BBQ, Sainsbury's*	1 Rib/42g	104	247	24.7	7.3	13.2	0.9
Pork, Barbecue, Average	1 Serving/100g	275	275	21.4	7.2	17.9	0.3
Pork, Chinese Style, Average	1 Serving/300g	736	245	17.9	10.0	14.9	0.7
Pork, Raw, Average	1oz/28g	47	169	18.6	1.8	9.9	0.2
Spare, Cantonese, Mini, Sainsbury's*	1 Rib/38g	97	259	17.2	17.3	13.4	1.0
Spare, Chinese Style, Summer Eating, Asda*	1 Serving/116g	334	288	32.0	4.1	16.0	0.8
Spare, Mini, Ready Meals, Marks & Spencer*	1oz/28g	57	205	16.6	8.6	11.5	0.2
Spare, Sticky, Glazed, Marks & Spencer*	1/2 Pack/150g	263	175	13.6	5.4	11.1	0.4
RIBSTEAKS							
Chinese Style, Dalepak*	1 Steak/75g	184	245	20.3	11.6	13.1	1.1
Smokey Barbecue Style, Dalepak*	1 Serving/75g	164	219	16.1	8.8	13.1	0.8
RICCOLI							
Egg, Fresh, Waitrose*	1oz/28g	81	289	11.4	53.1	3.4	2.1
RICE							
Arborio, Dry, Average	1 Serving/80g	279	348	7.1	78.3	0.8	0.8
BBQ & Spicy, Marks & Spencer*	1 Pack/250g	463	185	6.1	23.7	7.2	1.2
Balti Style, Quick, Sainsbury's*	1 Serving/228g	192	84	4.3	15.7	0.5	2.0
Balti, Break, Asda*	1 Serving/60g	209	348	13.3	70.0	1.7	0.0
Basmati, & Wild, Easy Cook, Tilda*	1oz/28g	98	349	9.4	77.0	0.4	0.9

R

RICE

INFO/WEIGHT	Measure	per Measure KCAL	Nutrition Values per 100g / 100ml KCAL	PROT	CARB	FAT	FIBRE
Basmati, & Wild, Sainsbury's* Cooked	1/2 Pack/125g	150	120	3.1	25.7	0.6	1.3
Basmati, Boil In The Bag, Dry, Average	1 Serving/50g	176	352	8.4	77.9	0.8	0.5
Basmati, Brown, Dry, Average	1 Serving/50g	177	353	9.5	71.8	3.0	2.2
Basmati, Cooked, Average	1 Serving/140g	189	135	3.6	26.0	1.8	0.7
Basmati, Dry Weight, Average	1 Serving/60g	212	353	8.1	77.9	1.0	0.6
Basmati, Easy Cook, Dry Weight, Average	1 Serving/40g	135	338	8.0	75.5	0.5	0.8
Basmati, Indian Takeaway, Tesco*	1 Serving/125g	219	175	4.5	37.6	0.7	0.4
Basmati, Indian, Dry, Average	1 Serving/75g	260	347	8.4	76.1	0.9	0.1
Basmati, Microwave, Cooked, Average	1 Serving/125g	182	146	2.7	30.1	1.9	0.0
Basmati, Pilau, Rizazz, Tilda* Cooked	1 Serving/125g	183	146	2.5	28.7	2.4	0.0
Basmati, Savory Mushroom, Tilda*	1 Pack/250g	353	141	2.6	27.5	2.3	0.0
Basmati, Spicy Mexican, Tilda*	1 Serving/125g	188	150	2.9	28.1	2.9	0.5
Basmati, Thai Lime & Coriander, Tilda*	1/2 Pack/125g	185	148	2.4	28.4	2.8	0.1
Basmati, White, Dry, Average	1 Serving/75g	262	349	8.1	77.1	0.6	2.2
Beef, Savoury, Batchelors*	1/2 Pack/62g	222	358	9.4	74.9	2.3	3.2
Brown, American, Easy Cook, Dry, Average	1 Serving/75g	262	350	7.4	75.3	2.2	1.5
Brown, Cooked, Average	1 Serving/140g	173	123	2.6	26.6	1.1	0.9
Brown, Dry, Average	1 Serving/75g	267	355	7.5	76.2	3.0	1.4
Brown, Long Grain, Dry, Average	1 Serving/50g	182	364	7.6	76.8	2.9	2.1
Brown, Whole Grain, Cooked, Average	1 Serving/170g	223	132	2.7	27.8	1.1	1.3
Brown, Whole Grain, Dry, Average	1 Serving/40g	138	344	7.4	71.6	2.9	3.0
Chicken & Sweetcorn, Savoury, Asda*	1/2 Pack/60g	195	325	10.0	65.0	2.8	10.0
Chicken, Savoury, Batchelors*	1 Pack/124g	455	367	8.9	79.4	1.5	2.6
Chicken, Savoury, Cooked, Safeway*	1 Serving/151g	213	141	3.6	28.3	1.5	2.2
Chicken, Savoury, Tesco*	1 Serving/87g	177	204	6.4	39.4	2.2	6.7
Chinese Five Spice, Special Recipe, Sainsbury's*	1oz/28g	37	133	2.9	29.9	0.3	0.9
Chinese Savoury, Batchelors*	1 Serving/50g	177	354	9.9	73.1	2.4	2.8
Chinese Style Savory Five Spice, Made Up, Tesco*	1 serving/141g	217	154	3.2	28.2	3.1	2.2
Chinese Style, Express, Uncle Ben's*	1 Pack/250g	338	135	3.1	27.3	1.5	0.0
Coconut & Lime, Asda*	1 Pack/360g	695	193	4.5	32.7	4.9	0.9
Coconut, Marks & Spencer*	1/2 Pack/124g	217	175	3.1	31.8	4.0	0.3
Coconut, Thai, Sainsbury's*	1/2 Pack/100g	178	178	2.6	21.3	9.1	1.9
Coriander & Herb, Packet, Cooked, Sainsbury's*	1/4 Pack/150g	204	136	2.5	30.4	0.5	1.5
Coriander & Herbs, Batchelors*	1/3 Pack/76g	280	369	7.9	79.6	3.5	5.0
Curry Style Savoury, Safeway*	1 Serving/100g	112	112	2.2	23.4	1.1	1.6
Curry, Savoury, Somerfield*	1/2 Pack/160g	194	121	2.2	26.0	0.9	1.3
Easy Cook, Cooked, Average	1 Serving/100g	139	139	2.8	29.3	1.2	0.2
Egg Fried	1oz/28g	58	208	4.2	25.7	10.6	0.4
Egg Fried, Asda*	1oz/28g	43	152	4.2	23.4	4.4	1.8
Egg Fried, Cantonese, Sainsbury's*	1/2 Pot/260g	456	175	4.5	28.4	5.1	0.6
Egg Fried, Chinese Style, Tesco*	1 Portion/250g	418	167	4.4	27.9	4.2	0.7
Egg Fried, Chinese Takeaway, Tesco*	1 Serving/200g	250	125	4.7	23.3	1.5	1.8
Egg Fried, Chinese, Sainsbury's*	1 Pack/200g	350	175	4.5	27.8	5.1	1.2
Egg Fried, Express, Uncle Ben's*	1 Pack/250g	440	176	4.1	30.5	4.2	0.0
Egg Fried, Healthy Living, Tesco*	1 Serving/250g	285	114	3.5	22.2	1.3	1.8
Egg Fried, Marks & Spencer*	1 Pack/200g	420	210	4.1	32.4	7.0	0.3
Egg Fried, Micro, Tesco*	1 Pack/250g	313	125	4.6	18.3	3.7	6.4
Egg Fried, Oriental Express*	1 Pack/425g	531	125	4.0	22.2	2.3	1.3
Egg Fried, Original, Asda*	1 Pack/250g	425	170	4.0	25.0	6.0	1.6
Egg Fried, Rizazz, Tilda*	1 Pack/250g	358	143	3.3	25.4	3.1	0.0
Egg Fried, Somerfield*	1 Pack/200g	298	149	7.2	25.0	2.2	1.1
Egg, Chinese Style, Morrisons*	1 Serving/250g	285	114	2.1	16.8	4.8	0.7
Fried, Chicken, Chinese Takeaway, Iceland*	1 Pack/340g	510	150	6.5	20.7	4.6	0.6

RICE

INFO/WEIGHT	Measure	per Measure KCAL	KCAL	PROT	CARB	FAT	FIBRE
Fried, Duck, Chicken & Pork Celebration, Sainsbury's*	1 Pack/450g	545	121	7.9	14.2	3.6	1.5
Garlic & Butter Flavoured, Batchelors*	1 Serving/50g	175	350	8.0	79.8	2.8	5.0
Garlic & Coriander Flavoured, Patak's*	1 Serving/125g	186	149	2.6	28.9	2.2	0.0
Garlic & Herb, Sainsbury's*	1/4 Pack/50g	66	132	2.3	28.8	0.8	1.1
Golden Savoury, Batchelors*	1/2 Pack/62g	226	364	10.1	74.7	2.8	2.4
Golden Savoury, New Improved Flavour, Batchelors*	1 Pack/120g	439	366	9.3	78.9	1.5	4.5
Golden Savoury, Nirvana, Aldi*	1 Pack/120g	142	118	2.5	25.4	0.7	2.9
Golden Savoury, Safeway*	1 Serving/205g	221	108	2.6	22.6	0.8	1.2
Golden Vegetable, Express, Uncle Ben's*	1 Pack/250g	350	140	2.9	28.2	1.8	0.0
Golden Vegetable, Savoury, Cooked, Value, Tesco*	1 Serving/145g	244	168	4.3	36.4	0.6	0.8
Golden Vegetable, Savoury, Sainsbury's*	1/4 Pack/100g	122	122	2.9	25.4	1.0	0.3
Golden Vegetable, Tesco*	1 Serving/125g	135	108	2.6	21.9	1.1	0.6
Golden, Savoury, 2 Minute, Batchelors*	1 Serving/130g	212	163	4.2	34.4	0.9	1.1
Golden, Savoury, Tesco* Cooked	1/2 Pack/159g	216	136	3.6	26.9	1.5	2.4
Imperial Red, Merchant Gourmet*	1oz/28g	85	305	8.6	61.2	2.5	8.6
Lemon Pepper Speciality, Asda*	1 Serving/52g	67	129	2.0	27.0	1.4	0.1
Lemon Pepper, In 5, Crosse & Blackwell*	1/2 Pack/163.4g	200	123	2.7	25.2	1.3	4.0
Long Grain, & Wild, Dry, Average	1 Serving/75g	254	338	7.6	72.6	2.0	1.7
Long Grain, American, Cooked, Average	1 Serving/160g	229	143	3.1	28.8	1.8	0.3
Long Grain, American, Dry, Average	1 Serving/50g	175	350	7.2	77.9	1.1	0.6
Long Grain, Dry, Average	1 Serving/50g	169	337	7.4	75.5	1.0	1.7
Long Grain, Microwavable, Cooked, Average	1 Serving/150g	180	120	2.7	25.8	0.6	0.7
Long Grain, Thai Fragrant, Tesco*	1 Serving/50g	175	349	7.3	79.1	0.4	0.8
Mediterranean Tomato, Rizazz, Tilda*	1/2 Pack/125g	194	155	2.7	28.6	3.3	0.0
Mexican Style, Old El Paso*	1 Serving/75g	268	357	9.0	78.0	1.0	0.0
Mexican, Ready Meals, Waitrose*	1 Pack/300g	432	144	2.6	27.8	2.5	0.5
Mild Curry, Savoury, Batchelors*	1/2 Pack/61g	217	355	8.4	76.0	1.9	1.8
Mild Curry, Tesco* Cooked	1 Serving/154g	217	141	3.1	29.7	1.1	2.1
Mixed Vegetable, Savoury, Tesco*	1 Serving/63g	219	347	8.8	71.1	3.0	6.4
Mushroom & Coconut, Organic, Waitrose*	1 Pack/300g	474	158	3.7	24.5	5.0	1.4
Mushroom & Pepper, Savoury, Safeway*	1/2 Pack/194g	227	117	2.7	25.4	0.5	0.7
Mushroom Pilau, Bombay Brasserie, Sainsbury's*	1 Pack/400g	672	168	3.7	28.6	4.3	0.7
Mushroom, Express, Uncle Ben's*	1 Pack/250g	380	152	3.1	30.9	1.8	0.0
Mushroom, Savoury, Batchelors*	1 Sachet/122g	439	360	10.9	74.3	2.1	2.5
Paella, Savoury, Tesco*	1 Serving/60g	220	367	8.4	72.7	4.7	4.5
Pilau, Cooked, Average	1 Serving/140g	244	174	3.5	30.3	4.4	0.8
Pilau, Dry, Average	1oz/28g	101	362	8.5	78.2	2.4	3.4
Pilau, Indian Mushroom, Sainsbury's*	1 Serving/100g	119	119	3.0	21.3	2.4	1.9
Pilau, Indian Take Away, Tesco*	1 Box/100g	135	135	2.7	23.7	3.3	2.2
Pilau, Spinach, Bombay Brasserie, Sainsbury's*	1 Pack/401g	642	160	3.5	26.9	4.3	0.8
Pudding, Tesco*	1 Serving/50g	175	349	7.3	77.3	1.2	0.2
Risotto, Dry, Average	1 Serving/50g	174	348	7.8	76.2	1.3	2.4
Saffron, Cooked, Average	1 Serving/150g	209	139	2.6	25.3	3.2	0.5
Spanish Style Savoury, Safeway*	1 Pack/394g	449	114	2.7	23.7	0.9	1.4
Special Fried, Asda*	1oz/28g	42	149	5.4	21.0	4.9	1.5
Special Fried, Chinese, Tesco*	1 Serving/300g	618	206	6.5	19.9	11.1	0.8
Special Fried, Marks & Spencer*	1 Pack/450g	923	205	6.2	27.2	7.8	0.5
Special Fried, Sainsbury's*	1 Serving/166g	272	164	5.1	25.5	4.6	0.7
Special Fried, Tesco*	1 Pack/250g	333	133	7.6	17.6	3.6	1.7
Spicy Mexican Style, Savoury, Tesco*	1 Serving/164g	584	356	9.0	69.9	4.5	6.0
Steamed, Asda*	1 Serving/200g	252	126	2.6	26.0	1.3	2.0
Sticky Thai, Safeway*	1 Pack/200g	260	130	2.5	25.6	1.8	1.4
Sweet & Sour Savoury, Cooked, Asda*	1/2 Pack/126g	154	122	2.5	26.0	0.9	3.0

R

RICE

Measure INFO/WEIGHT	per Measure KCAL	Nutrition Values per 100g / 100ml				
		KCAL	PROT	CARB	FAT	FIBRE
RICE						
Sweet & Sour, Rice Bowl, Uncle Ben's*	1 Pack/350g	364	104	5.2	19.5	0.6	0.0
Sweet & Sour, Savoury, Batchelors*	1 Serving/135g	419	310	9.4	75.6	2.1	3.1
Sweet & Sour, Savoury, Cooked, Tesco*	1/2 Pack/153g	214	140	2.7	29.1	1.4	2.3
Tandoori, Savoury, Batchelors*	1 Serving/120g	430	358	10.3	73.5	2.5	3.0
Thai Sticky, Tesco*	1 Serving/250g	358	143	2.5	27.6	2.5	0.4
Thai Style, Lemon Chicken, Savoury, Tesco*	1 Pack/105g	382	364	9.3	70.6	4.9	5.0
Thai, Chicken, Enjoy, Birds Eye*	1 Pack/500g	535	107	6.9	13.2	3.0	0.7
Thai, Cooked, Average	1 Serving/100g	136	136	2.5	27.4	1.8	0.3
Thai, Dry, Average	1 Serving/50g	174	348	7.1	78.9	0.5	0.9
Thai, Fragrant, Dry, Average	1 Serving/75g	272	363	7.2	82.0	0.7	0.3
Tomato & Basil, Express, Uncle Ben's*	1 Pack/250g	450	180	3.9	31.5	4.3	0.0
Valencia For Paella, Asda*	1 Serving/125g	435	348	6.0	79.0	0.8	0.0
Vegetable Pilau, Express, Uncle Ben's*	1 Pack/250g	445	178	3.4	33.8	3.2	0.0
Vegetable, Frozen, Tesco*	1 Serving/100g	105	105	4.0	20.8	0.6	1.1
Vegetable, Golden, Safeway*	1 Serving/125g	111	89	2.9	18.2	0.5	1.9
Vegetable, Original, Birds Eye*	1oz/28g	29	105	4.0	20.8	0.6	1.1
Vegetable, Savoury, Marks & Spencer*	1/2 Pack/250g	313	125	3.4	23.9	1.9	1.2
White, Cooked, Average	1 Serving/140g	182	130	2.6	28.7	0.8	0.2
White, Cooked, Frozen, Average	1 Serving/150g	168	112	2.9	23.9	0.6	1.2
White, Dry, Average	1 Serving/50g	181	362	7.1	79.1	1.9	0.4
White, Flaked, Raw	1oz/28g	97	346	6.6	77.5	1.2	0.0
White, Fried	1oz/28g	37	131	2.2	25.0	3.2	0.6
White, Microwave, Cooked, Average	1 Serving/150g	158	105	2.7	22.4	0.5	1.1
Whole Grain, Dry, Average	1 Serving/50g	171	342	8.2	72.0	2.3	4.1
Wild, Raw, Tilda*	1 Serving/40g	140	350	11.5	74.2	0.8	1.9
Yellow, Ready Cooked, Tesco*	1oz/28g	32	113	2.7	27.1	1.3	0.1
RICE &						
Red Kidney Beans, Average	1oz/28g	49	175	5.6	32.4	3.5	2.5
Vegetables, Marks & Spencer*	1 Serving/125g	125	100	3.1	18.8	1.6	1.9
RICE BITES						
Cheese & Onion Flavour, Asda*	1 Pack/30g	137	456	7.0	71.0	16.0	0.2
RICE BOWL						
Beef With Black Bean Sauce, Uncle Ben's*	1 Pack/350g	368	105	5.6	17.4	1.4	0.0
Chicken & Mushroom, Sharwood's*	1 Pack/350g	392	112	4.8	17.1	2.7	0.7
Chicken Tikka Masala, Uncle Ben's*	1 Pack/350g	382	109	5.9	15.9	2.4	0.0
Free From, Sainsbury's*	1 Serving/182g	146	80	1.6	17.1	0.6	1.4
Honey BBQ Chicken, Uncle Ben's*	1 Pack/350g	420	120	5.4	23.1	0.6	0.0
Sweet & Sour Chicken, Healthy Living, Tesco*	1 Serving/400g	376	94	6.3	14.3	1.3	0.6
Sweet N Sour, Sharwood's*	1 Serving/350g	438	125	4.8	18.6	3.5	0.8
Thai Green, Sharwood's*	1 Bowl/350g	550	157	4.8	17.3	7.6	0.9
Thai Red, Sharwood's*	1 Bowl/350g	487	139	4.7	18.1	5.3	1.0
RICE CAKES						
& Oats, High Fibre, Kallo*	1 Cake/8g	27	356	10.6	75.0	5.5	9.0
Apple & Cinnamon Flavour, Kallo*	1 Cake/11g	41	376	6.2	83.1	2.2	3.9
Bacon, Asda*	1 Cake/9g	42	462	8.0	67.0	18.0	0.0
Barbeque, Tesco*	1 Cake/9g	28	328	9.6	66.8	2.5	6.2
Black & White Sesame, Clearspring*	1 Cake/8g	31	385	7.4	82.2	2.9	0.0
Brink*	1 Cake/15g	56	370	8.8	78.8	2.2	0.0
Caramel Flavour, Kallo*	1 Cake/9.9g	38	383	6.2	78.9	4.8	3.9
Caramel, Jumbo, Tesco*	1 Cake/10g	36	364	6.5	73.9	2.5	5.1
Caramel, Less Than 3% Fat, Sainsbury's*	1 Pack/35g	134	382	5.6	86.4	1.6	1.8
Caramel, Snack Size, Tesco*	1 Bag/35g	133	379	5.5	82.7	2.9	0.9
Caramel, Tesco*	1 Serving/2.3g	8	379	5.5	98.2	2.9	0.9

RICE CAKES

INFO/WEIGHT	Measure per Measure KCAL	KCAL	PROT	CARB	FAT	FIBRE
Cheese & Onion, Namchow*	1 Serving/38g	141	377	7.2	79.5	3.3	0.0
Cheese, Jumbo, Free From, Tesco*	1 Serving/10g	44	439	8.1	62.1	17.6	3.8
Chocolate, Fabulous Bakin' Boys*	1 Biscuit/17g	83	490	6.4	66.7	22.0	1.6
Crispy, Somerfield*	1oz/28g	134	479	5.0	77.0	17.0	0.0
Dark Chocolate, Organic, Kallo*	1 Cake/12g	57	471	6.8	57.2	24.1	7.4
Five Grain, Finn Crisp*	1 Piece/10g	36	356	9.8	73.9	1.7	9.7
Honey, Puffed, Kallo*	1 Serving/50g	182	364	7.0	80.0	2.0	6.7
Kallo*	1 Cake/7g	27	386	8.2	81.1	3.2	3.2
Lightly Salted, Perfectly Balanced, Waitrose*	1 Cake/8g	31	387	8.3	82.4	2.7	2.1
Lightly Salted, Thick Slice, Low Fat, Kallo*	1 Cake/8g	30	372	8.0	78.7	2.8	5.1
Low Fat, Kallo*	1 Cake/10g	38	375	6.2	83.1	2.2	3.9
Milk Chocolate, Organic, Kallo*	1 Cake/15g	77	511	6.5	56.2	28.7	3.5
Oat, Kallo*	1 Slice/7.7g	28	351	10.6	75.3	5.5	9.1
Oat, Lightly Salted, Thick Slice, Kallo*	1 Cake/7.6g	28	356	10.6	75.0	5.5	9.0
Organic, Organix*	3 Cakes/5.9g	22	370	6.5	83.0	1.4	3.2
Rice Bites, Asda*	1 Cake/8.8g	42	466	8.0	68.0	18.0	0.0
Rice Crunchies, Safeway*	1 Small Pack/25g	95	378	7.4	84.2	1.3	1.5
Rikarikas, The Positive Food Co*	1 Bag/25g	92	366	7.5	83.0	0.6	1.6
Ryvita*	1 Cake/7g	28	394	8.1	83.1	3.2	1.2
Salt & Vinegar, Sainsbury's*	1 Bag/30g	121	403	8.3	73.3	8.3	2.7
Salt & Vinegar, Snack, Tesco*	1 Pack/35g	116	332	7.5	71.5	1.8	1.1
Salt 'n' Vinegar, Jumbo, Tesco*	1 Cake/8.8g	28	306	8.4	62.5	7.5	6.0
Savoury With Yeast Extract, Kallo*	1 Slice/11g	40	364	12.7	72.0	2.8	4.7
Savoury, Kallo*	1 Cake/8g	28	355	14.2	67.5	3.2	4.4
Savoury, Thick Slice, Organic, Kallo*	1 Slice/9g	31	364	12.7	72.0	2.8	4.5
Sesame Garlic, Clearspring*	1 Serving/8g	29	382	7.8	82.3	2.4	0.0
Sesame Teriyaki, Clearspring*	1 Cake/8g	28	377	6.5	82.8	2.2	0.0
Sesame, Ryvita*	1 Slice/7.3g	28	396	8.2	82.3	3.8	1.3
Slightly Salted, Thick Slice, Organic, Kallo*	1 Cake/8g	30	372	8.0	78.7	2.8	5.1
Slightly Salted, With Cracked Pepper, Snack Size, Kallo*	1 Rice Cake/2g	8	372	8.0	78.7	2.8	5.1
Thin Slice, Organic, Kallo*	1 Cake/5g	19	372	8.0	78.7	2.8	5.1
Thin Slice, Organic, Waitrose*	1 Serving/5g	17	340	8.0	70.0	2.0	4.0
Thin Slice, Organic, Waitrose*	1 Cake/6g	23	391	9.0	81.3	3.3	3.8
Whole Grain, No Added Salt, Thick Slice, Organic, Kallo*	1 Cake/9g	33	365	7.6	80.0	3.1	3.4
With Sesame, Organic, Evernat*	1 Cake/4g	15	368	8.5	74.5	4.0	0.0
With Sesame, Organic, Kallo*	1 Cake/7.5g	30	373	8.0	78.0	3.2	5.4
With Sesame, Thick Sliced, No Added Salt, Kallo*	1 Cake/10g	37	373	8.0	78.0	3.2	5.4
With Yeast Extract, Snack Size, Kallo*	1 Cake/2g	7	364	12.6	71.1	2.8	4.7

RICE CRACKERS

INFO/WEIGHT	Measure per Measure KCAL	KCAL	PROT	CARB	FAT	FIBRE
Barbecue Flavour, Tesco*	1 Bag/25g	102	409	6.7	78.8	7.4	1.7
Brown, Wakama*	1 Cracker/5g	19	375	8.0	84.8	0.4	0.0
Cheese, Tesco*	1 Serving/25g	104	416	7.9	78.1	8.0	1.8
Chilli, Temptations, Tesco*	1 Serving/25g	128	512	4.4	58.0	28.8	0.0
Choco Noir, Bonvita*	1 Cracker/18g	79	440	6.8	64.0	18.5	0.0
Cracked Pepper, Sakata*	1/2 Pack/50g	200	400	7.3	84.4	3.0	2.0
Crispy, Chilli & Lime, Go Ahead, McVitie's*	1 Serving/25g	101	405	7.1	83.6	3.6	2.1
Crispy, Sea Salt & Vinegar, Go Ahead, McVitie's*	1 Serving/25g	102	408	6.6	80.6	5.4	1.8
Crispy, Sour Cream & Herbs, Go Ahead, McVitie's*	1 Serving/25g	106	422	7.1	78.2	8.0	1.8
Japanese, Hider*	1 Bag/70g	303	433	11.3	61.7	17.3	0.0
Japanese, Holland & Barratt*	1oz/28g	111	397	9.0	79.7	4.7	0.3
Japanese, Mini, Sunrise*	1 Serving/50g	180	360	7.0	83.0	0.0	7.0
Mix, Marks & Spencer*	1/2 Pack/62.5g	227	360	6.5	82.9	0.1	1.6
Paprika Flavour, Namchow*	1 Serving/38g	141	375	7.5	78.9	3.3	0.0

R

	INFO/WEIGHT	KCAL	KCAL	PROT	CARB	FAT	FIBRE
RICE CRACKERS							
Sainsbury's*	1 Serving/20g	87	433	11.2	74.3	9.4	1.0
Salt & Vinegar, Namchow*	1 Serving/38g	139	370	6.7	77.5	3.7	0.0
Thai Chilli, Nature's Harvest*	1 Pack/75g	401	535	4.6	61.5	29.7	4.2
Thai, Marks & Spencer*	1 Serving/55g	209	380	7.0	80.2	3.3	1.2
Thai, Sesame & Soy Sauce, Marks & Spencer*	1 Pack/54.5g	212	385	7.6	77.8	4.8	1.4
Thai, Wakama*	1 Cracker/2g	8	400	6.9	86.9	2.7	0.5
Thin, Blue Dragon*	3 Crackers/5g	20	395	6.1	84.4	3.7	0.0
Tomato Salsa Flavour, Tesco*	1 Pack/25g	103	412	6.8	79.6	7.2	1.6
With Tamari, Clearspring*	1 Bag/50g	190	380	8.2	83.4	1.5	0.3
RICE PUDDING							
& Conserve, Marks & Spencer*	1oz/28g	53	190	2.3	17.4	12.5	0.3
50% Less Fat, Asda*	1/2 Can/212g	170	85	3.3	16.2	0.8	0.2
Apple, 99% Fat Free, Mullerice, Muller*	1 Pot/150g	125	83	3.5	15.3	0.9	0.0
Apple, Mullerice, Muller*	1 Pot/200g	244	122	3.3	21.7	2.4	0.0
BGTY, Sainsbury's*	1/2 Can/212g	180	85	3.3	16.2	0.8	0.2
Banana, Ambrosia*	1 Pot/150g	153	102	3.2	16.6	2.5	0.0
Canned	1oz/28g	25	89	3.4	14.0	2.5	0.2
Caramel, Ambrosia*	1 Pot/150g	149	99	3.1	16.1	2.5	0.0
Caramel, Mullerice, Muller*	1 Pot/200g	210	105	3.5	17.4	2.4	0.0
Chocolate, Mullerice, Muller*	1 Pot/200g	246	123	3.4	21.5	2.6	0.0
Clotted Cream, Cornish, Waitrose*	1 Serving/150g	305	203	3.0	17.6	13.4	0.5
Clotted Cream, Tesco*	1/2 Pack/250g	473	189	2.4	17.9	12.0	0.1
Creamed With Sultanas & Nutmeg, Ambrosia*	1/2 Can/200g	210	105	3.2	16.6	2.9	0.1
Creamed, Canned, Ambrosia*	1 Can/425g	383	90	3.1	15.2	1.9	0.0
Creamed, Healthy Living, Tesco*	1 Serving/213g	142	67	3.0	12.0	0.8	0.2
Creamed, Low Fat, Ambrosia*	1 Serving/150g	129	86	3.3	16.1	0.9	0.0
Creamed, Luxury, Sainsbury's*	1 Can/425g	544	128	3.3	15.9	5.7	0.0
Creamed, Pot, Ambrosia*	1 Pot/150g	152	101	3.2	16.5	2.5	0.0
Creamed, Sainsbury's*	1 Serving/213g	202	95	3.2	16.2	1.5	0.1
Creamed, Weight Watchers*	1 Pot/130.1g	108	83	3.2	16.0	0.7	0.3
Creamy Rice With Tropical Crunch, Ambrosia*	1 Pack/210g	307	146	3.6	23.4	4.2	0.6
Creamy Rice, Shape*	1 Serving/175g	149	85	3.5	15.4	1.0	0.4
Creamy With Strawberry Crunch, Ambrosia*	1 Pack/205g	297	145	3.9	23.0	4.2	0.7
Eat Smart, Safeway*	1 Serving/212g	138	65	3.4	10.3	0.8	0.0
Everyday, Co-Op*	1 Can/396	333	84	3.4	15.5	0.9	0.1
GFY, Asda*	1 Pudding/119g	115	97	4.2	17.0	1.4	0.5
Libby's*	1 Serving/200g	180	90	3.3	16.2	1.6	0.2
Light, Mullerice, Muller*	1 Pot/100g	72	72	3.5	12.2	0.9	0.0
Low Fat, Ambrosia*	1 Pot/150g	121	81	3.2	15.2	0.8	0.0
Low Fat, Good Intentions, Somerfield*	1/2 Can/212g	164	77	3.0	15.1	0.6	0.2
Low Fat, Healthy Selection, Somerfield*	1 Pot/213g	173	81	4.0	15.0	1.0	0.0
Low Fat, No Added Sugar, Weight Watchers*	1/2 Can/212g	155	73	3.7	11.4	1.5	0.0
Luxury Rice, Llangadog Creamery*	1 Serving/220g	310	141	3.1	15.2	7.7	0.0
Milk, Economy, Sainsbury's*	1/2 Can/198g	139	70	3.2	12.6	0.8	0.2
Organic, Ambrosia*	1 Can/425g	455	107	3.4	15.1	3.7	0.0
Organic, Evernat*	1oz/28g	39	141	5.5	22.9	3.0	0.0
Original, 99% Fat Free, Mullerice, Muller*	1 Pot/150g	108	72	3.9	11.8	1.0	0.0
Original, Mullerice, Muller*	1 Pot/200g	232	116	3.7	19.1	2.7	0.0
Perfectly Balanced, Waitrose*	1 Serving/154g	140	91	3.4	15.7	1.6	1.2
Raisin & Nutmeg, Muller*	1 Pot/200g	244	122	3.3	22.0	2.3	0.0
Rasberry, BGTY, Sainsbury's*	1 Pot/135g	126	93	3.2	17.2	1.2	1.3
Raspberry, Mullerice, Muller*	1 Pot/200g	228	114	3.4	20.0	2.3	0.0
Sainsbury's*	1 Serving/100g	102	102	3.8	14.5	3.2	0.2

R

	Measure INFO/WEIGHT	per Measure KCAL	Nutrition Values per 100g / 100ml				
			KCAL	PROT	CARB	FAT	FIBRE
RICE PUDDING							
Strawberry, 99% Fat Free, Muller*	1 Serving/150g	116	77	3.5	13.6	0.9	0.0
Strawberry, Mullerice, Muller*	1 Pot/200g	230	115	3.4	20.0	2.4	0.0
Thick & Creamy, Co-Op*	1 Can/425g	531	125	3.0	16.0	6.0	0.0
Thick & Creamy, Nestle*	1 Can/425g	527	124	3.1	15.4	5.6	0.2
Toffee, 99% Fat Free, Mullerice, Muller*	1 Pot/150g	119	79	3.3	14.3	1.0	0.0
Value, Tesco*	1/2 Can/212g	178	84	3.3	15.5	0.9	0.2
Vanilla Custard, Mullerice, Muller*	1 Pot/200g	250	125	3.3	22.1	2.6	0.0
Venetian, Cafe Culture, Marks & Spencer*	1 Serving/120g	300	250	3.4	21.8	16.4	0.2
With Cream, Sainsbury's*	1 Can/229.5g	242	105	3.1	9.8	5.9	0.0
With Jam, Kosy Shack, Costcutters*	1 Serving/150g	173	115	3.5	19.8	2.5	0.9
With Sultanas & Nutmeg, Ambrosia*	1 Pack/425g	446	105	3.2	16.6	2.9	0.1
RICE STICKS							
Mediterranean Tomato, Weight Watchers*	1 Bag/20g	72	360	7.3	77.7	2.2	2.8
Salt & Vinegar, Weight Watchers*	1 Serving/20g	73	365	7.7	79.7	1.7	2.4
Thai Sweet Chilli Flavour, Weight Watchers*	1 Serving/20g	73	363	7.6	79.5	1.6	2.2
Weight Watchers*	1 Serving/20g	15	73	1.5	15.9	0.3	0.4
RIGATONI							
Carbonara, Tesco*	1 Serving/205g	236	115	5.2	10.6	5.8	1.2
Dry, Average	1 Serving/80g	272	340	11.4	68.5	1.5	2.7
Tomato & Cheese, Perfectly Balanced, Waitrose*	1 Pack/400g	664	166	7.6	28.6	2.3	2.3
RISOTTO							
Balls, Mushroom, Occasions, Sainsbury's*	1 Ball/25g	76	304	3.8	41.2	13.8	1.7
Balls, Sun Dried Tomato, Occasions, Sainsbury's*	1 Ball/25g	71	285	6.8	30.8	15.0	2.9
Beef, Vesta*	1 Serving/100g	346	346	15.3	57.8	5.9	5.6
Caramelised Onion & Gruyere Cheese, Marks & Spencer*	1 Pack/200g	350	175	3.0	17.8	10.3	1.7
Chargrilled Chicken, Ready Meal, Marks & Spencer*	1 Pack/365g	493	135	6.4	11.6	6.9	0.7
Chicken & Asparagus, Eat Smart, Safeway*	1 Pack/380g	418	110	6.2	16.8	1.5	0.6
Chicken & Bacon, Italiano, Tesco*	1 Pack/450g	653	145	5.9	20.2	4.5	1.5
Chicken & Lemon, Weight Watchers*	1 Pack/330g	323	98	5.9	12.5	2.8	0.5
Chicken & Mushroom, Finest, Tesco*	1 Pack/400g	496	124	7.4	17.2	2.8	0.5
Chicken & Mushroom, Good Intentions, Somerfield*	1 Pack/300g	345	115	5.7	19.0	1.8	0.3
Chicken & Sun Dried Tomato, Waitrose*	1 Pack/350g	385	110	6.0	7.2	6.3	0.3
Chicken, BGTY, Sainsbury's*	1 Pack/327g	356	109	7.5	15.5	1.9	1.0
Chicken, Enjoy, Birds Eye*	1 Pack/500g	735	147	8.5	14.0	6.3	0.5
Chicken, Lemon & Wild Rocket, Sainsbury's*	1 Pack/360g	683	190	16.2	5.6	11.4	0.1
Chicken, Ready Meal, Marks & Spencer*	1 Pack/360g	450	125	6.7	14.4	4.4	0.9
Haddock & Mushroom, COU, Marks & Spencer*	1 Pack/400g	320	80	6.4	12.1	0.8	2.0
Hot Smoked Salmon & Spinach, Marks & Spencer*	1/2 Pack/300g	420	140	6.4	11.0	8.0	0.6
Italian Red Wine With Creamed Spinach, Sainsbury's*	1 Pack/400g	596	149	2.4	19.3	6.9	0.4
King Prawn & Snow Crab, Marks & Spencer*	1 Pack/365g	402	110	4.1	12.7	4.5	0.5
King Prawn, Pea & Mint, Marks & Spencer*	1/2 Pack/300g	405	135	3.8	15.9	6.2	0.9
Lemon & Mint, Perfectly Balanced, Waitrose*	1 Pack/350g	462	132	3.9	20.7	3.7	1.0
Mushroom, BGTY, Sainsbury's*	1 Pack/400g	320	80	2.6	15.6	0.8	0.6
Mushroom, COU, Marks & Spencer*	1 Pack/330g	347	105	4.4	15.2	2.7	1.5
Mushroom, Finest, Tesco*	1 Pack/350g	550	157	3.1	16.4	8.8	1.2
Mushroom, Healthy Living, Tesco*	1 Pack/400g	320	80	2.6	15.6	0.8	0.6
Mushroom, Italiano, Tesco*	1 Pack/340g	367	108	2.4	20.0	2.0	4.6
Mushroom, Ready Meals, Marks & Spencer*	1 Pack/360g	450	125	2.8	16.9	4.9	1.0
Mushroom, Waitrose*	1 Pack/350g	277	79	1.9	6.9	4.9	0.5
Roasted Vegetable & Sunblush Tomato, Finest, Tesco*	1/2 Pack/200g	306	153	3.7	14.5	9.0	1.4
Roasted Vegetables, Stir-in, Uncle Ben's*	1/2 Pack/75g	86	115	1.7	5.0	9.7	0.0
Seafood, Young's*	1 Pack/350g	424	121	4.5	17.4	3.7	0.1
Spring Vegetable, Marks & Spencer*	1 Serving/330g	330	100	2.0	14.2	4.0	0.9

R

	Measure INFO/WEIGHT	per Measure KCAL	Nutrition Values per 100g / 100ml KCAL	PROT	CARB	FAT	FIBRE
RISOTTO							
Tomato & Cheese, GFY, Asda*	1 Pack/400g	428	107	3.1	17.0	3.0	0.7
Tomato & Mascarpone, Marks & Spencer*	1 Pack/360g	468	130	2.7	17.5	5.3	0.9
Vegetable	1oz/28g	41	147	4.2	19.2	6.5	2.2
Vegetable, Brown Rice	1oz/28g	40	143	4.1	18.6	6.4	2.4
Wild Mushroom & Garlic, Tesco*	1 Pack/320g	522	163	3.6	27.2	4.4	1.6
RISPINOS							
Apple & Cinnamon, Uncle Ben's*	1 Bag/60g	230	383	4.7	90.0	0.5	0.0
Barbecue, Uncle Ben's*	1 Pack/50g	182	363	8.4	82.0	0.2	0.0
Caramel, Uncle Ben's*	1 Pack/60g	229	382	5.1	89.0	0.7	0.0
Cheese & Onion, Uncle Ben's*	1 Pack/50g	181	361	8.4	81.0	0.4	0.0
Chocolate, Uncle Ben's*	1oz/28g	108	385	5.3	89.0	1.1	0.0
Coconut, Uncle Ben's*	1oz/28g	111	396	6.7	86.0	2.8	0.0
Hot & Spicy, Uncle Ben's*	1 Bag/50g	183	366	7.5	83.0	0.6	0.0
Pizza, Uncle Ben's*	1 Pack/50g	182	363	8.4	82.0	0.2	0.0
Vanilla, Uncle Ben's	1oz/28g	107	383	7.7	87.0	0.5	0.0
RISSOLES							
Lentil, Fried in Vegetable Oil	1oz/28g	59	211	8.9	22.0	10.5	3.6
RIVELLA*							
Blue	1 Can/330ml	17	5	0.0	1.3	0.0	0.0
ROAST							
Vegetarian, Chicken Style, Tesco*	1 Serving/113g	214	189	22.1	4.8	9.0	1.7
Veggie, Chicken Style, Realeat*	1 Pack/454g	844	186	23.0	3.2	9.0	0.0
ROCK SALMON							
Raw, Meat Only, Average	1oz/28g	43	154	16.6	0.0	9.7	0.0
ROCKET							
Fresh, Average	1 Serving/50g	10	21	2.6	1.7	0.4	0.8
ROE							
Cod, Average	1 Can/100g	96	96	17.1	0.5	2.8	0.0
Cod, Hard, Coated in Batter, Fried	1oz/28g	53	189	12.4	8.9	11.8	0.2
Cod, Hard, Fried in Blended Oil	1oz/28g	57	202	20.9	3.0	11.9	0.1
Herring, Soft, Fried in Blended Oil	1oz/28g	74	265	26.3	4.7	15.8	0.2
Herring, Soft, Raw	1oz/28g	25	91	16.8	0.0	2.6	0.0
ROGAN JOSH							
Chicken & Rice, Sainsbury's*	1 Pack/500g	675	135	6.7	14.1	5.4	2.4
Chicken, Breast, Chunks, Hot, Sainsbury's*	1/2 Pack/114g	143	126	23.6	3.9	1.8	1.0
Chicken, Patak's*	1oz/28g	34	123	8.1	17.2	2.4	0.7
Chicken, With Pilau Rice, Farmfoods*	1 Pack/325g	354	109	5.3	17.1	2.1	0.4
Lamb With Basmati Rice, Eat Smart, Safeway*	1 Pack/380g	380	100	6.9	14.0	1.5	1.9
Lamb, Indian Takeaway, Tesco*	1 Serving/350g	494	141	9.0	7.5	8.3	1.3
Lamb, Marks & Spencer*	1 Pack/300g	360	120	14.4	3.9	5.1	1.2
Lamb, Sainsbury's*	1 Pack/400g	660	165	11.3	4.9	11.1	1.9
Lamb, Tesco*	1 Pack/350g	340	97	4.8	9.6	4.4	1.5
Lamb, With Pilau Rice, Eastern Classics, Aldi*	1 Pack/400g	604	151	5.6	19.9	5.4	1.0
Prawn & Pilau Rice, BGTY, Sainsbury's*	1 Pack/401g	353	88	4.8	15.3	0.8	1.9
Prawn, COU, Marks & Spencer*	1 Pack/400g	360	90	4.9	16.2	0.6	0.8
ROLL							
All Day Breakfast, Asda*	1 Roll/220g	581	264	10.0	29.0	12.0	0.0
Bacon & Sausage, Marks & Spencer*	1oz/28g	88	315	13.3	3.4	27.7	0.7
Bacon, Marks & Spencer*	2 Rolls/18g	40	220	14.2	0.4	18.3	0.0
Beef, Weight Watchers*	1 Roll/174g	276	159	10.8	23.1	2.5	1.0
Brie & Grapes, Marks & Spencer*	1 Roll/57g	174	306	11.1	24.5	18.2	1.4
Cheese & Chutney, Marks & Spencer*	1 Roll/165g	256	155	13.9	23.1	0.7	1.2
Cheese & Onion, Asda*	1 Serving/66.8g	200	298	7.0	27.0	18.0	2.0

ROLL

	Measure INFO/WEIGHT	per Measure KCAL	KCAL	PROT	CARB	FAT	FIBRE
Cheese & Onion, King Size, Pork Farms*	1 Serving/130g	443	341	7.4	28.4	22.0	0.0
Cheese & Onion, Marks & Spencer*	1 Roll/25g	80	320	9.6	24.7	20.5	1.3
Cheese & Onion, Sainsbury's*	1 Roll/67g	205	306	8.0	22.9	20.3	1.9
Cheese & Onion, Tesco*	1 Roll/66.6g	212	317	7.5	27.9	19.4	2.3
Cheese & Pickle, Sainsbury's*	1 Roll/136g	359	264	10.6	35.1	10.0	0.0
Cheese Ploughman's, Malted Wheat, BGTY, Sainsbury's*	1 Roll/171.7g	310	180	10.9	29.3	2.1	3.8
Cheese, Tomato & Onion, Sainsbury's*	1 Pack/100g	518	518	18.4	47.9	28.1	0.0
Chicken & Beef Duo, Marks & Spencer*	1 Serving/146.9g	235	160	12.0	22.1	2.6	2.7
Chicken & Herb, Shapers, Boots*	1 Roll/167.6g	291	173	12.0	25.0	2.8	1.7
Chicken & Stuffing, Tesco*	1 Roll/323g	1043	323	10.4	29.4	18.2	1.0
Chicken & Sun Dried Tomato, Weight Watchers*	1 Pack/170g	272	160	12.9	22.7	1.9	1.2
Chicken & Sweetcorn, Sainsbury's*	1 Serving/170g	462	272	12.5	24.2	13.9	0.0
Chicken Salad, Healthy Living, Tesco*	1 Serving/100g	149	149	10.6	22.3	2.0	1.2
Chicken Salsa, BGTY, Sainsbury's*	1 Pack/197g	323	164	11.1	24.8	2.3	0.0
Chunky Cheese & Mustard, Finest, Tesco*	1 Roll/88g	260	295	10.9	40.0	10.2	2.4
Chunky Herbes de Provence, Finest, Tesco*	1 Roll/82g	196	239	7.4	45.2	3.2	2.6
Cornish, In Pastry, Pork Farms*	1 Roll/75.1g	226	301	6.6	24.5	20.1	0.0
Egg & Bacon, Sub, Shapers, Boots*	1 Serving/169.3g	319	189	11.0	27.0	4.3	1.3
Egg & Cress, Healthy Living, Tesco*	1 Pack/175g	322	184	9.6	27.7	3.9	1.2
Egg & Tomato, Shapers, Boots*	1 Roll/166.3g	300	181	8.0	30.0	3.2	2.6
Egg Mayo & Cress, Fullfillers*	1 Roll/125g	266	213	10.0	25.7	9.4	0.0
Egg Mayonnaise & Cress, Sub, Shapers, Boots*	1 Pack/156.9g	306	195	9.5	30.0	4.0	1.7
Egg Mayonnaise, & Cress, White, Soft, Somerfield*	1 Serving/211g	475	225	9.4	28.2	8.2	2.1
Ham & Cheese, In Pastry, Pork Farms*	1 Roll/70.1g	216	308	8.0	28.8	17.9	0.0
Ham & Pineapple, Eat Smart, Safeway*	1 Serving/180g	225	125	11.2	17.2	1.1	2.6
Ham & Tomato, Taste!*	1 Serving/112.2g	211	188	10.4	27.0	4.3	0.0
Ham Salad, BGTY, Sainsbury's*	1 Roll/178g	292	164	10.8	25.9	1.9	0.0
Ham Salad, Healthy Living, Tesco*	1 Roll/203g	284	140	9.8	19.3	2.6	0.0
Ham, Darwins Deli*	1 Serving/125g	298	238	11.0	37.4	6.0	0.0
Leicester Ham & Cheese, Sub, Waitrose*	1 Pack/206.4ml	581	282	12.6	24.0	15.1	13.0
Mushroom & Bacon, Crusty, Marks & Spencer*	1 Roll/160g	424	265	8.7	29.0	12.6	2.3
Oak Smoked Salmon, Marks & Spencer*	1 Roll/55g	139	252	14.6	23.1	11.3	1.2
Roast Chicken & Mayonnaise, Big, Sainsbury's*	1 Pack/185g	479	259	9.6	21.8	14.8	0.0
Roast Chicken & Sweetcure Bacon, Boots*	1 Pack/244.7g	691	282	13.0	26.0	14.0	1.6
Roast Chicken Salad, Improved, Shapers, Boots*	1 Pack/187.6g	303	161	11.0	25.0	1.9	1.6
Roast Pork, Stuffing & Apple Sauce, Boots*	1 Roll/218.1g	602	276	10.0	32.0	12.0	1.8
Smoked Ham & Free Range Egg, Marks & Spencer*	1 Serving/208.3g	499	240	11.1	20.5	12.4	1.0
Spicy Chicken, Crusty, Marks & Spencer*	1 Roll/150g	383	255	12.8	25.8	11.1	2.0
Steak & Onion, Marks & Spencer*	1 Serving/150g	308	205	11.0	24.5	7.0	3.8
Taiko California, Waitrose*	4 Pieces/120g	196	163	4.4	26.8	4.1	1.5
Tomato & Basil, Sub, COU, Marks & Spencer*	1 Roll/35g	93	265	11.0	48.7	2.7	2.4
Tuna & Sweetcorn With Mayonnaise, Shell*	1 Pack/180g	536	298	13.1	28.6	14.6	0.0
Tuna Cheese Melt, Boots*	1 Roll/198.7g	613	308	13.0	23.0	18.0	1.2
Tuna Mayo & Cucumber, Taste!*	1 Serving/110.9g	274	247	9.0	27.3	11.3	0.0
Tuna Mayonnaise, With Cucumber, Yummies*	1 Serving/132.3g	339	257	10.4	22.5	14.0	0.0
Turkey Salad, Northern Bites*	1 Roll/230.7g	323	140	8.6	19.6	3.6	3.0
Turkey, Stuffed, GFY, Asda*	1/2 Pack/225g	320	142	14.0	12.0	4.2	0.8
White, Cheese & Onion, Shell*	1 Roll/178g	554	311	14.5	30.2	14.8	0.0

ROLLMOPS

	Measure INFO/WEIGHT	per Measure KCAL	KCAL	PROT	CARB	FAT	FIBRE
Tesco*	1 Serving/130g	181	139	7.8	8.6	8.2	0.4

ROLO

	Measure INFO/WEIGHT	per Measure KCAL	KCAL	PROT	CARB	FAT	FIBRE
Giant, Nestle*	1 Rolo/9g	42	471	3.2	68.5	20.5	0.3
Minis, Nestle*	1 Pack/26g	123	471	3.2	68.5	20.5	0.3

	Measure	per Measure	Nutrition Values per 100g / 100ml				
	INFO/WEIGHT	KCAL	KCAL	PROT	CARB	FAT	FIBRE
ROLO							
Nestle*	1 Rolo/5g	24	471	3.2	68.5	20.5	0.3
ROLY POLY							
Frozen, Tesco*	1 Serving/81g	287	354	4.4	52.7	14.0	0.5
Jam & Custard, Sainsbury's*	1 Pack/205g	521	254	3.3	34.1	11.6	0.5
Jam, Sainsbury's*	1/4 Pack/81g	291	359	4.4	53.3	14.2	0.5
Jam, Tesco*	1 Serving/82g	308	375	4.7	51.5	16.7	1.2
ROOT BEER							
Average	1 Can/330ml	135	41	0.0	10.6	0.0	0.0
ROSEMARY							
Dried	1 Tsp/1g	3	331	4.9	46.4	15.2	0.0
Fresh	1oz/28g	28	99	1.4	13.5	4.4	0.0
ROSTI							
Garlic & Mushroom, Finest, Tesco*	1 Serving/200g	346	173	5.7	15.4	9.8	1.7
Oven Baked, McCain*	1 Rosti/95g	234	246	3.7	29.7	12.8	0.0
Peppered Steak, British Classics, Tesco*	1 Pack/450g	599	133	9.0	10.7	6.2	1.7
Potato & Leek, Sainsbury's*	1/2 Pack/190g	296	156	4.5	9.8	11.0	0.3
Potato & Root Vegetable, COU, Marks & Spencer*	1 Cake/100g	85	85	1.6	13.3	2.7	1.5
Potato Cakes, Baby, Marks & Spencer*	1 Rosti/22.9g	40	175	3.5	25.1	6.7	1.6
Potato Cakes, Marks & Spencer*	1 Serving/100g	140	140	1.5	16.8	7.5	1.8
Potato, Waitrose*	1 Rosti/45g	112	248	3.8	22.5	15.9	2.7
Potato, Chicken & Sweetcorn Bake, Asda*	1 Serving/400g	440	110	7.0	10.0	4.7	0.6
Potato, Fresh, Safeway*	1 Rost/100g	138	138	2.8	19.2	5.5	2.8
Potato, McCain*	1 Rosti/95g	161	169	2.2	19.6	9.1	0.0
Potato, Mini, Party Bites, Sainsbury's*	1 serving/100g	218	218	2.5	26.2	11.5	3.0
Potato, Mini, Party Range, Tesco*	1 Rosti/16.7g	33	193	2.1	20.6	11.4	3.3
Potato, Onion & Gruyere, Finest, Tesco*	1 Pack/350g	403	115	3.5	11.9	5.9	1.4
Potato, Spinach & Mozzarella, Tesco*	1 Serving/140g	228	163	3.8	24.5	5.5	2.0
Vegetable, Waitrose*	1 Pack/400g	248	62	1.4	8.8	2.3	1.3
ROUGHY							
Orange, Raw	1oz/28g	35	126	14.7	0.0	7.0	0.0
ROULADE							
Chocolate, Finest, Tesco*	1 Serving/80g	222	277	3.4	53.2	5.6	2.3
Chocolate, TTD, Sainsbury's*	1/4 Roulade/119g	420	354	5.4	47.3	16.0	2.5
Lemon Meringue, Marks & Spencer*	1 Serving/74g	230	311	3.2	46.6	12.5	0.3
Lemon Meringue, TTD, Sainsbury's*	1 Serving/100g	277	277	2.4	44.7	9.8	0.5
Lemon, Asda*	1 Serving/100g	343	343	2.7	56.0	12.0	0.0
Mini, Marks & Spencer*	1 Serving/62.5g	202	321	8.5	3.0	30.5	0.0
Orange & Lemon Meringue, Co-Op*	1 Serving/82g	287	350	3.0	57.0	12.0	0.3
Passion Fruit, Marks & Spencer*	1oz/28g	83	295	2.8	50.0	9.2	0.2
Raspberry & Vanilla, Somerfield*	1oz/28g	118	420	3.0	56.0	20.0	0.0
Raspberry, Finest, Tesco*	1 Slice/67g	203	303	3.3	33.2	17.4	1.7
Raspberry, Marks & Spencer*	1oz/28g	88	315	3.3	50.3	11.0	0.1
Salmon, Smoked, Waitrose*	1 Roulade/10g	23	228	13.1	1.6	18.8	0.7
Smoked Salmon & Asparagus, Sainsbury's*	1 Serving/60g	122	204	13.0	2.2	16.0	0.3
Smoked Salmon & Spinach, Finest, Tesco*	1 Serving/60g	91	152	11.5	3.6	10.2	0.6
Toffee & Walnut, Somerfield*	1oz/28g	130	465	4.0	50.0	28.0	0.0
Toffee Pecan, Finest, Tesco*	1 Serving/60g	218	363	3.6	53.8	14.8	0.5
Toffee, Marks & Spencer*	1oz/28g	104	371	4.1	56.0	14.5	0.3
RUM							
37.5% Volume	1 Shot/25ml	52	207	0.0	0.0	0.0	0.0
40% Volume	1 Shot/25ml	56	222	0.0	0.0	0.0	0.0
Southern Comfort*, 37.5% Volume	1 Shot/25ml	52	207	0.0	0.0	0.0	0.0
White	1 Shot/25ml	52	207	0.0	0.0	0.0	0.0

R

	Measure INFO/WEIGHT	per Measure KCAL	Nutrition Values per 100g / 100ml				
			KCAL	PROT	CARB	FAT	FIBRE
RUSKS							
Banana, Farleys*	1 Serving/17.1g	70	409	7.3	75.1	8.8	2.9
Mini, Farleys*	1 Serving/30g	122	405	7.0	77.7	7.3	2.1
RYVITA BREAKS							
Ryvita*	1 Slice/14.4g	47	333	8.0	69.5	2.5	12.0

R

INFO/WEIGHT	Measure	per Measure KCAL	Nutrition Values per 100g / 100ml				
			KCAL	PROT	CARB	FAT	FIBRE

SAAG
Aloo Gobi, Waitrose*	1 Pack/300g	336	112	2.4	5.4	9.0	2.2
Aloo, Canned, Tesco*	1/2 Can/200g	124	62	1.8	9.3	1.9	2.0
Aloo, Fresh, Sainsbury's*	1 Pack/400g	388	97	2.0	14.7	3.3	4.8
Aloo, Jar, Sainsbury's*	1/2 Jar/135g	122	90	1.6	11.0	4.3	1.7
Aloo, North Indian, Sainsbury's*	1 Pack/300g	354	118	2.4	9.0	8.0	1.6
Aloo, Packet, Sainsbury's*	1/2 Pack/150g	185	123	2.1	9.9	8.3	2.7
Aloo, Tesco*	1 Serving/200g	144	72	2.1	8.0	3.5	2.0
Chicken, Marks & Spencer*	1/2 Pack/175g	192	110	11.3	4.1	5.2	1.2
Chicken, Masala, Sainsbury's*	1oz/28g	36	127	13.2	2.4	7.2	2.3
Chicken, Safeway*	1 Pack/350g	504	144	11.6	5.4	8.4	1.4
Gobi Aloo, Indian Takeaway, Sainsbury's*	1 Pack/334g	164	49	1.7	8.0	1.1	1.5
Gobi Aloo, Indian, Tesco*	1 Pack/225g	225	100	2.1	6.5	7.3	1.8
Gobi Aloo, Tesco*	1 Serving/175g	179	102	1.7	6.8	7.6	2.2
Paneer, Sainsbury's*	1/2 Pack/200g	342	171	7.7	4.5	13.6	2.4

SAFFRON
Average	1 Tsp/0.7g	3	310	11.4	61.5	5.9	0.0

SAGE
Dried, Ground	1 Tsp/1g	3	315	10.6	42.7	12.7	0.0
Fresh	1oz/28g	33	119	3.9	15.6	4.6	0.0

SAGO
Raw	1oz/28g	99	355	0.2	94.0	0.2	0.5

SALAD
Alfresco Style, Tesco*	1 Serving/200g	40	20	0.9	3.3	0.3	1.4
All Seasons, Sainsbury's*	1oz/28g	3	12	1.0	1.5	0.2	1.2
American Ranch, Asda*	1 Serving/220g	253	115	2.5	6.0	9.0	2.0
American Style, Morrisons*	1 Serving/25g	5	22	1.1	3.9	0.3	2.3
Aromatic Herb, Waitrose*	1/4 Pack/27g	4	15	0.9	1.7	0.5	1.0
Assorted, Asda*	1 Serving/100g	22	22	2.4	1.7	0.6	0.0
Baby Leaf & Herb, Asda*	1 Serving/50g	7	14	2.3	0.7	0.2	2.4
Baby Leaf With Watercress, Tesco*	1/4 Bag/25g	5	19	2.0	1.3	0.7	1.4
Baby Leaf, Fully Prepared, Sainsbury's*	1/2 Bag/63g	10	16	1.3	1.9	0.4	1.5
Baby Leaf, Italian Style, Marks & Spencer*	1 Serving/55g	74	135	1.6	2.7	13.1	1.4
Baby Leaf, Organic, Sainsbury's*	1 Serving/20g	3	14	1.5	1.4	0.3	1.1
Baby Leaf, Sainsbury's*	1 Serving/60g	13	21	1.3	1.7	1.0	3.3
Baby Plum & Sundried Tomato Salad, Waitrose*	1 Serving/200g	226	113	1.3	6.8	8.9	0.8
Baby Spinach & Red Mustard, Marks & Spencer*	1 Pack/170g	264	155	1.7	1.1	15.7	0.1
Baby Tomato, Tesco*	1 Pack/205g	35	17	0.8	2.8	0.3	0.9
Bacon Caesar, Marks & Spencer*	1oz/28g	48	170	5.5	5.7	14.0	1.2
Bacon Caesar, Sainsbury's*	1 Pack/256g	415	162	4.7	12.0	12.7	1.4
Bacon, Pasta, Budgens*	1 Salad/200g	570	285	5.1	12.6	23.9	0.7
Bean & Chorizo, Tapas Selection, Sainsbury's*	1 Serving/22g	29	132	8.1	10.7	6.3	1.9
Bean & Sweetcorn, Side, Marks & Spencer*	1 Serving/125g	131	105	2.5	7.0	7.2	1.3
Bean, & Mexican Rice, COU, Marks & Spencer*	1 Serving/250g	250	100	6.0	15.6	1.4	1.2
Bean, Marks & Spencer*	1 Serving/80g	72	90	6.4	14.3	0.9	3.9
Bean, Mint & Coriander, Somerfield*	1 Pack/250g	288	115	7.0	19.4	1.1	4.7
Bean, Retail	1oz/28g	41	147	4.2	12.8	9.3	3.0
Bean, Three, Marks & Spencer*	1 Pack/225g	225	100	5.8	16.7	1.3	3.9
Bean, Vinaigrette Mixed, Tesco*	1 Can/400g	280	70	3.2	13.1	0.5	1.9
Beetroot	1oz/28g	28	100	2.0	8.4	6.8	1.7
Beetroot & Carrot, Continental, Iceland*	1 Serving/100g	24	24	1.2	4.3	0.2	2.1
Beetroot & Lettuce, Asda*	1 Serving/30g	5	16	1.4	2.7	0.0	2.5
Beetroot, 1% Fat, Marks & Spencer*	1 Serving/225g	131	58	1.1	7.7	2.7	1.7
Beetroot, GFY, Asda*	1 Serving/84g	46	55	1.0	12.0	0.3	1.8

S

SALAD

INFO/WEIGHT	Measure	per Measure KCAL	KCAL	PROT	CARB	FAT	FIBRE
Beetroot, Healthy Living, Tesco*	1 Serving/200g	116	58	0.9	11.3	1.0	2.0
Beetroot, Marks & Spencer*	1 Serving/225g	124	55	1.0	12.0	0.3	3.0
Beetroot, Organic, Marks & Spencer*	1oz/28g	20	73	1.5	9.1	3.4	1.9
Beetroot, Pots, Healthy Living, Tesco*	1 Serving/200g	110	55	1.7	11.5	0.2	1.3
Beetroot, Sainsbury's*	1 Tub/200g	160	80	0.9	11.7	3.3	2.1
Bistro, Asda*	1 Serving/180g	29	16	1.4	2.7	0.0	2.5
Bistro, Sainsbury's*	1 Pack/150g	33	22	1.1	3.6	0.4	1.3
Bistro, Washed Ready To Eat, Tesco*	1 Pack/140g	22	16	1.1	1.7	0.5	1.0
Bowl, French Style, Way to Five, Sainsbury's*	1 Pack/264g	103	39	0.7	4.2	2.2	2.2
Bowl, Large, Sainsbury's*	1 Pack/300g	51	17	1.1	2.9	0.2	2.3
Cabbage & Leek, Crunchy Mix, Sainsbury's*	1/2 Pack/126.3g	24	19	1.2	2.1	0.6	1.9
Caesar, BGTY, Sainsbury's*	1/3 Pack/75g	78	104	3.6	9.8	5.6	1.7
Caesar, Bacon, Marks & Spencer*	1 Serving/250g	400	160	7.1	4.1	12.5	1.3
Caesar, Bistro, Waitrose*	1/2 Pack/112.5g	172	152	6.4	6.3	11.2	7.6
Caesar, Finest, Tesco*	1 Bowl/220g	532	242	5.2	4.7	22.5	0.9
Caesar, GFY, Asda*	1/2 Pack/87.4g	76	87	8.0	7.0	3.0	1.5
Caesar, Healthy Eating, Tesco*	1 Serving/100g	101	101	3.2	8.0	6.2	0.7
Caesar, Improved Recipe, Marks & Spencer*	1 Pack/290g	551	190	5.0	1.3	18.1	1.3
Caesar, Sainsbury's*	1/2 Bag/128g	227	177	3.6	6.7	15.1	1.0
Caesar, Somerfield*	1 Pack/255g	339	133	4.6	5.1	10.5	1.3
Caesar, Waitrose*	1 Serving/115g	175	152	6.4	6.3	11.2	0.8
Caesar, Washed & Ready to Eat, Somerfield*	1/2 Bag/125g	155	124	5.0	6.5	8.7	0.8
Caesar, With Parmigiano Reggiano, Tesco*	1 Bag/275g	552	201	4.1	5.8	17.8	1.3
Cajun Chicken, David lloyd leisure*	1 Pack/300g	429	143	11.7	17.7	3.3	1.0
Californian Crunch, GFY, Asda*	1 Pack/160g	75	47	0.9	8.0	1.3	1.8
Cannellini Bean & Chicken, Marks & Spencer*	1 Serving/225g	250	111	5.9	7.4	6.5	3.1
Cannellini Bean & Tuna, Marks & Spencer*	1 Serving/255g	215	84	5.3	5.4	4.5	2.1
Caribbean Chicken, Shapers, Boots*	1 Pack/220g	222	101	5.8	14.0	2.3	1.2
Carrot & Nut With Dressing, Retail, French's*	1oz/28g	61	218	2.1	13.7	17.6	2.4
Carrot & Sultana, BGTY, Sainsbury's*	1/2 Pack/100g	55	55	0.6	12.4	0.3	0.0
Carrot & Sultana, Healthy Living, Tesco*	1 Tub/225g	142	63	1.2	13.2	0.6	2.5
Carrot, Marks & Spencer*	1 Pack/215.4g	280	130	3.1	22.4	3.4	2.7
Carrot, Orange & Ginger, Good Intentions, Somerfield*	1 Serving/250g	275	110	2.0	22.4	1.4	1.4
Carrot, Peanut & Sultana, Asda*	1 Serving/20g	54	272	8.0	15.0	20.0	4.5
Celery, Nut & Sultana, Asda*	1oz/28g	76	272	2.9	11.2	23.9	1.9
Chargrilled Chicken & Bacon, Tesco*	1 Pack/300g	657	219	7.8	18.7	12.6	0.9
Chargrilled Chicken & Pesto, Sainsbury's*	1 Pack/250g	375	150	7.9	15.8	6.1	1.3
Chargrilled Chicken Wholefood, Marks & Spencer*	1 Pot/219g	230	105	10.1	11.6	1.9	4.8
Chargrilled Chicken, Tesco*	1 Serving/300g	384	128	6.1	15.0	4.8	2.4
Chargrilled Pepper With Cous Cous, Asda*	1 Pack/325.2g	426	131	4.3	21.0	3.3	0.0
Cheddar Cheese & Pasta, Tesco*	1 Pot/215g	546	254	5.7	12.0	20.4	0.8
Cheese & Coleslaw, Tesco*	1 Pack/250g	265	106	3.4	3.5	8.7	1.4
Cheese Coleslaw, Sainsbury's*	1oz/28g	61	218	5.1	6.0	19.3	0.1
Cheese Layered, Marks & Spencer*	1 Pack/450g	923	205	4.3	9.0	17.0	0.7
Cheese Potato, Sainsbury's*	1 Serving/125g	200	160	2.7	7.9	13.1	3.4
Cheese, Carb Control, Tesco*	1 Serving/195g	294	151	10.1	2.5	11.2	0.6
Cheese, Layered, Tesco*	1 Serving/225g	437	194	5.8	10.8	14.2	0.8
Cherry Tomato, All Good Things*	1 Pack/185g	31	17	0.8	2.8	0.3	1.4
Cherry Tomato, Fresh, Safeway*	1 Pack/170g	31	18	0.8	2.9	0.3	0.9
Cherry Tomato, Large, Fresh, Safeway*	1 Serving/245g	49	20	1.0	3.1	0.4	1.9
Chick Pea & Cous Cous, Tesco*	1 Serving/250g	245	98	3.2	15.5	2.6	0.0
Chick Pea & Spinach, Marks & Spencer*	1 Serving/260g	299	115	7.3	12.5	4.1	2.7
Chicken & Bacon, Caesar, Marks & Spencer*	1 Salad/380g	798	210	8.8	14.1	12.9	3.9

SALAD

INFO/WEIGHT	per Measure KCAL	KCAL	PROT	CARB	FAT	FIBRE
Chicken & Bacon, Carb Control, Tesco*	1 serving/188g	244	130	13.2	1.7	7.8	0.5
Chicken & Bacon, Layered, Asda*	1 Serving/375g	473	126	7.0	11.0	6.0	0.0
Chicken & Caesar, Boots*	1 Serving/200g	144	72	4.9	2.8	4.6	1.4
Chicken & Rice, Safeway*	1 Serving/200g	220	110	6.4	17.6	1.3	1.4
Chicken Caesar Bistro, Marks & Spencer*	1/2 Pack/135g	189	140	5.0	6.5	10.6	0.6
Chicken Caesar, Fresh, Sainsbury's*	1 Serving/200g	278	139	6.0	6.2	10.0	1.2
Chicken Caesar, Marks & Spencer*	1/2 Pack/140g	266	190	6.7	8.7	14.3	0.8
Chicken Caesar, Menu, Boots*	1 Serving/171g	139	81	7.8	6.3	2.7	1.9
Chicken Caesar, Shapers, Boots*	1 Serving/203g	164	81	7.8	6.3	2.7	1.9
Chicken Caesar, Simply, Boots*	1 Pack/162g	196	121	12.0	4.8	6.0	1.3
Chicken Caesar, TTD, Sainsbury's*	1 Serving/190g	308	162	11.1	1.6	12.3	1.5
Chicken Caesar, Tesco*	1 Pack/300g	330	110	6.8	10.6	4.5	0.8
Chicken Noodle & Sweet Chilli, Shapers, Boots*	1 Pack/197g	266	135	12.0	16.0	2.6	0.9
Chicken Noodle, Thai Style, Sainsbury's*	1 Pack/260g	283	109	6.6	14.2	2.9	1.3
Chicken Tikka & Rice, COU, Marks & Spencer*	1 Pack/390g	410	105	5.1	18.7	1.0	0.6
Chicken With Mayonnaise, Waitrose*	1 Pack/208g	406	195	10.3	17.1	9.5	2.5
Chicken, Avacado & Bacon, Marks & Spencer*	1 Serving/235g	235	100	8.5	2.8	5.8	2.8
Chicken, Healthy Eating, Tesco*	1 Salad/216g	296	137	8.4	22.6	1.4	1.2
Chicken, Healthy Option, Mattessons*	1 Pack/200g	344	172	11.1	20.0	5.3	2.9
Chicken, Italian Style, Snack Pot, Carb Check, Heinz*	1 Pot/218g	131	60	5.9	4.3	2.0	1.0
Chicken, Sweet Chilli, BGTY, Sainsbury's*	1 Serving/200g	206	103	6.0	18.7	0.4	0.0
Chicken, Sweetcorn & Pasta, Safeway*	1 Serving/200g	230	115	7.5	16.3	1.8	1.0
Chicken, Tesco*	1 Serving/300g	348	116	5.3	7.0	7.4	1.0
Chicken, Tomato, & Basil, Safeway*	1 Serving/200g	330	165	6.9	14.2	8.9	0.6
Chilli Chicken & Spicy Cous Cous, Healthy Eating, Tesco*	1 Serving/190g	251	132	6.5	21.1	2.4	1.5
Chilli, Tomato, Chick Pea & Butterbean, Tesco*	1 Pack/130g	146	112	3.4	14.3	4.6	0.5
Chunky, Somerfield*	1 Serving/250g	40	16	1.0	3.0	0.0	0.9
Citrus, Tesco*	1 Serving/142g	57	40	0.3	9.6	0.0	0.4
Classic Caesar, Reduced Fat, Marks & Spencer*	1 Serving/115g	132	115	4.8	12.7	4.9	0.5
Classic With Green Herb Dressing, Co-Op*	1 Serving/90g	86	95	1.0	2.0	9.0	1.0
Classic, Marks & Spencer*	1 pack/255g	38	15	0.8	2.1	0.4	1.2
Club, Safeway*	1 Serving/215g	226	105	1.3	6.0	8.4	1.3
Coleslaw & Potato, 3% Fat, Marks & Spencer*	1oz/28g	20	72	2.7	7.7	3.4	1.5
Coleslaw Layered, Fresh, Asda*	1 Tub/197g	209	106	1.2	5.0	9.0	1.5
Coleslaw, Deli Style, Marks & Spencer*	1 Serving/320g	336	105	3.5	1.5	9.7	1.4
Coleslaw, Sainsbury's*	1 Serving/150g	191	127	0.9	6.8	10.7	1.9
Complete Hot Greek, Sainsbury's*	1 Pack/299g	287	96	4.3	2.9	7.5	1.7
Continental Four Leaf, Sainsbury's*	1oz/28g	5	18	1.6	2.1	0.3	0.8
Continental Leaf, Asda*	1oz/28g	4	16	1.4	1.4	0.5	1.4
Coronation Chicken & Rice, Asda*	1oz/28g	67	241	6.7	15.2	17.0	0.4
Coronation Chicken, Sainsbury's*	1 Serving/62.4g	180	290	6.3	14.4	23.0	1.4
Coronation Chicken, Salad Bar, Asda*	1oz/28g	82	293	5.7	16.4	22.7	0.7
Coronation Rice, Tesco*	1 Serving/50g	104	207	2.0	15.9	15.1	0.8
Cosmopolitan, Fresh, Sainsbury's*	1 Serving/10g	2	21	2.2	0.3	1.2	1.6
Country Style, Co-Op*	1/2 Pack/100g	20	20	1.0	3.0	0.4	2.0
Cous Cous & Roast Vegetable, GFY, Asda*	1 Serving/100g	120	120	3.5	23.0	1.6	2.7
Cous Cous With Chargrilled Chicken, Sainsbury's*	1 Pack/240g	446	186	7.4	19.6	8.7	0.0
Cous Cous, BFY, Morrisons*	1/2 Pot/113g	164	145	4.6	23.8	3.5	0.5
Cous Cous, Tesco*	1 Serving/25g	35	141	4.8	26.9	1.6	0.6
Cous Cous, With Mixed Peppers & Cucumber, GFY, Asda*	1/4 Pot/56g	66	117	3.9	25.0	0.2	1.5
Creamy Potato With Onion & Chives, Sainsbury's*	1/4 Pot/62.5g	96	153	1.3	9.0	12.4	2.7
Crisp & Crunchy, Asda*	1 Pack/250g	55	22	0.8	3.3	0.6	1.4
Crisp & Cruncy With French Dressing, GFY, Asda*	1/3 Pack/116g	26	22	0.8	3.3	0.6	1.4

SALAD

INFO/WEIGHT	per Measure KCAL	KCAL	PROT	CARB	FAT	FIBRE
SALAD						
Crisp & Light, Marks & Spencer*	1 Serving/170g	51	30	0.5	5.4	0.8	1.0
Crisp & Sweet, Asda*	1 Serving/100g	19	19	0.9	3.1	0.3	1.7
Crisp Mixed, Tesco*	1 Pack/200g	38	19	1.1	2.8	0.3	1.5
Crispy Duck & Herb, Marks & Spencer*	1/2 Pack/140g	378	270	20.7	3.7	18.3	1.4
Crispy Green, Sainsbury's*	1 Serving/70g	8	12	0.9	1.6	0.2	0.8
Crispy Leaf, Asda*	1oz/28g	4	14	0.8	1.6	0.5	0.9
Crispy Leaf, Sainsbury's*	1/2 Pack/75g	9	12	1.0	1.2	0.4	1.5
Crispy Medley, Waitrose*	1 Serving/50g	8	15	0.8	1.7	0.5	0.9
Crispy, Tesco*	1oz/28g	6	20	1.2	3.0	0.3	1.6
Crunchy Coleslaw Bowl, Marks & Spencer*	1 Pack/325g	455	140	1.0	2.5	13.8	2.0
Crunchy Layered, Tesco*	1 Serving/54g	15	27	1.1	4.9	0.3	1.7
Crunchy Shredded, Safeway*	1 Serving/50g	10	19	1.2	2.9	0.3	1.5
Crunchy Spring, Side, Marks & Spencer*	1 Serving/160g	32	20	0.9	4.1	0.2	1.3
Crunchy, Basics, Sainsbury's*	1 Pack/200g	40	20	1.3	3.4	0.2	2.2
Crunchy, Fully Prepared, Sainsbury's*	1/2 Pack/150g	24	16	1.1	3.0	0.1	1.7
Crunchy, Tesco*	1 serving/56.3g	11	19	1.2	2.8	0.3	2.1
Crunchy, Value, Tesco*	1 Serving/56g	11	19	1.2	2.8	0.3	2.1
Eat Me Keep Me, Tesco*	1 Serving/80g	14	18	0.8	3.0	0.3	1.7
Egg & Baby Spinach, Waitrose*	1 Pack/215g	167	78	3.5	1.8	6.3	1.0
Egg & Coleslaw, Boots*	1 Pot/233g	405	174	3.0	4.6	16.0	1.0
Egg & Potato, Fresh, Marks & Spencer*	1 Serving/250g	150	60	3.0	4.6	2.9	0.9
Egg & Potato, GFY, Asda*	1 Serving/290g	160	55	2.4	5.2	2.8	1.2
Egg Layered Bowl, Tesco*	1 Pack/410g	726	177	4.2	8.4	14.1	1.3
Endive & Radicchio, Somerfield*	1 Pack/150g	20	13	2.0	1.0	0.0	0.0
English Garden, Tesco*	1 Serving/180g	22	12	0.7	1.8	0.2	0.7
Family, Florette*	1 Serving/50g	11	21	1.1	3.6	0.3	0.0
Family, Somerfield*	1 Serving/67g	12	18	0.8	2.9	0.4	1.3
Feta Cheese & Sunblushed Tomato, Marks & Spencer*	1 Serving/190g	361	190	5.5	17.2	11.1	2.1
Fine Cut, Asda*	1oz/28g	7	24	1.2	4.1	0.3	2.1
Fine Noodle With Duck Breast, COU, Marks & Spencer*	1 Pack/280g	294	105	5.5	18.9	1.1	1.1
Florida, Retail	1oz/28g	63	224	0.9	9.7	20.5	1.0
Four Bean, Finest, Tesco*	1 Pack/225g	259	115	5.0	14.2	4.2	4.6
Four Leaf, Tesco*	1oz/28g	4	15	0.8	1.8	0.5	0.9
French Goat's Cheese, Extra Fine, Asda*	1 Pack/185g	463	250	8.4	11.4	19.0	0.8
French Style, Marks & Spencer*	1 Pack/140g	140	100	1.0	2.5	9.7	0.9
French Style, Waitrose*	1/2 Pack/82g	149	182	5.1	7.2	14.8	1.8
Fusion, Fully Prepared, Sainsbury's*	1/2 Pack/62.5g	15	24	3.7	0.3	0.8	3.4
Garden With Watercress, Marks & Spencer*	1 Salad/80g	10	12	1.5	1.4	0.1	1.4
Garden With Yoghurt & Mint Dressing, GFY, Asda*	1 Serving/195g	51	26	1.1	3.2	1.0	0.0
Garden, Fresh, Safeway*	1/2 Pack/105g	27	26	1.1	4.8	0.3	1.1
Garden, Shapers, Boots*	1 Pack/237.3g	159	67	1.5	8.8	2.9	1.5
Garden, Sweet And Crispy, Tesco*	1 Bag/225g	54	24	1.0	4.2	0.4	1.4
Garden, Tesco*	1 Serving/225g	34	15	1.0	2.0	0.3	0.9
Gourmet Nicoise, Marks & Spencer*	1 Serving/500g	575	115	4.8	3.9	8.9	0.0
Gourmet Caesar, Marks & Spencer*	1 Serving/100g	155	155	4.1	7.1	12.1	0.8
Gourmet Chargrilled Chicken & Bacon, Atkins*	1 Pack/245g	311	127	12.0	2.5	8.2	1.0
Gourmet Continental, Waitrose*	1 Serving/150g	23	15	0.8	1.7	0.5	0.9
Greek	1oz/28g	36	130	2.7	1.9	12.5	0.8
Greek Style Collection, Marks & Spencer*	1 Pack/328.6g	461	140	4.4	8.8	9.9	1.2
Greek Style Feta, Marks & Spencer*	1 Serving/255g	268	105	3.5	1.5	9.7	1.4
Greek Style Feta, Tip & Mix, Marks & Spencer*	1 Pack/195g	215	110	4.0	2.5	9.4	1.6
Greek Style Layered, Perfectly Balanced, Waitrose*	1 Pack/280g	134	48	2.4	3.2	2.8	0.7
Greek Style, Fresh, Food Counter, Sainsbury's*	1 Serving/166g	247	149	1.9	2.7	14.0	0.0

SALAD

INFO/WEIGHT	Measure	per Measure KCAL	Nutrition Values per 100g / 100ml KCAL	PROT	CARB	FAT	FIBRE
Greek Style, Marks & Spencer*	1/2 Pack/120.8g	145	120	3.7	3.7	11.3	0.7
Greek Style, Waitrose*	1/2 Pack/125g	54	43	1.9	4.0	2.2	1.2
Greek Style, With Herb Dressing, Tesco*	1 Pack/240g	305	127	3.2	2.0	11.8	1.0
Greek Style, With Houmous Dip, & Pitta, Sainsbury's*	1 Bowl/195g	296	152	5.4	12.5	8.9	2.6
Greek Style, With White Wine Vinaigrette, Tesco*	1 Pack/235g	256	109	3.5	2.3	9.5	1.5
Greek, BGTY, Sainsbury's*	1 Serving/198.5g	133	67	2.0	9.0	2.5	0.8
Greek, Marks & Spencer*	1 Serving/125g	119	95	2.5	2.4	8.2	0.7
Greek, Waitrose*	1 Serving/200g	206	103	3.3	5.0	7.8	1.0
Green	1oz/28g	3	12	0.7	1.8	0.3	1.0
Green Side, Sainsbury's*	1 Pack/200g	28	14	1.2	2.1	0.1	1.4
Green Side, Tesco*	1 Serving/100g	12	12	0.7	1.6	0.3	1.3
Green With Chives, Tesco*	1/2 Pack/90g	13	14	1.0	1.6	0.4	1.7
Green With Honey & Mustard Dressing, Marks & Spencer*	1 Pack/200g	120	60	0.9	2.7	4.8	0.8
Green With Sweetcorn & Radish, Fresh, Safeway*	1 Pack/210g	55	26	1.1	4.8	0.3	1.1
Green, Crispy, Fresh, Sainsbury's*	1 serving/40g	5	12	0.9	1.6	0.2	0.8
Green, Marks & Spencer*	1oz/28g	4	13	0.8	1.7	0.3	0.9
Herb Garden, Morrisons*	1 Serving/28g	4	14	0.9	1.7	0.5	0.0
Herb, Marks & Spencer*	1 Pack/100g	20	20	2.9	1.4	0.4	1.9
Herb, Organic, Sainsbury's*	1 Serving/100g	17	17	1.8	1.3	0.5	1.8
Herb, Sainsbury's*	1 Serving/40g	10	26	1.9	2.0	1.1	1.7
Herb, Tesco*	1oz/28g	4	16	1.1	1.8	0.5	0.9
Honey Smoked Salmon & New Potato, Marks & Spencer*	1 Pack/270g	270	100	5.5	7.5	5.3	1.5
Hot Smoked Salmon & Rice, Deli Meal, Marks & Spencer*	1 Pack/380g	570	150	6.5	15.1	6.9	0.2
Iceberg & Cabbage, Asda*	1/2 Pack/125g	24	19	1.0	3.1	0.3	1.5
Italian Style Side, Waitrose*	1 Serving/160g	32	20	1.1	3.1	0.3	2.6
Italian Style, Marks & Spencer*	1 Bag/100g	18	18	1.3	1.8	0.5	1.4
Italian Style, Sainsbury's*	1/3 Pack/60g	80	134	2.1	8.0	10.9	1.1
Italian Style, Tesco*	1/3 Pack/40g	6	16	1.0	1.9	0.5	1.2
Italian Wild Rocket & Parmesan, Sainsbury's*	1 Serving/50g	89	177	7.5	3.4	14.8	0.5
Italian, Complete, Sainsbury's*	1 Pack/160g	203	127	3.6	9.0	8.5	1.5
Jardin, Tesco*	1 Serving/25g	4	14	0.8	1.7	0.5	0.9
King Prawn & Pasta, COU, Marks & Spencer*	1 Pack/270g	284	105	5.9	15.1	2.4	2.7
King Prawn, Thai Style, Marks & Spencer*	1 Pack/295g	266	90	4.4	12.6	2.5	1.3
Layered With Egg, Somerfield*	1 Pot/300g	543	181	3.0	3.0	18.0	0.0
Layered With Tuna, Somerfield*	1 Pot/255g	599	235	5.0	5.0	22.0	0.0
Leafy Mixed, Safeway*	1oz/28g	4	14	0.9	1.5	0.5	1.0
Leafy, Organic, Sainsbury's*	1/2 Pack/50g	8	15	1.7	1.3	0.3	1.8
Leafy, Tesco*	1oz/28g	4	14	1.2	1.5	0.4	1.9
Leafy, With Tatsoi, Tesco*	1 Serving/42g	6	14	1.2	1.5	0.4	1.9
Lemonss & Roasted Pepper, COU, Marks & Spencer*	1 Pack/340g	306	90	3.2	14.6	2.3	1.8
Luxury Potato, Asda*	1 Serving/50g	119	237	1.0	11.0	21.0	0.0
Marinated Seafood, Waitrose*	1 Tub/160g	331	207	15.7	3.1	14.6	0.0
Mediterranean Style Side, Way to Five, Sainsbury's*	1 Serving/245g	64	26	1.2	3.0	1.0	2.7
Mediterranean Style, Asda*	1/2 Pack/135g	22	16	1.0	3.0	0.0	0.0
Mediterranean Style, Tesco*	1/2 Pack/100g	123	123	3.5	1.9	11.3	1.3
Mediterranean Tuna, John West*	1oz/28g	30	106	8.0	5.0	6.0	2.0
Mexican Style Bean & Cheese, Marks & Spencer*	1/2 Pot/150g	150	100	6.1	11.2	3.5	4.8
Mixed Bean With Onions & Peppers, Safeway*	1/2 Can/210g	141	67	4.0	11.4	0.6	2.7
Mixed Bean, Tesco*	1 Serving/70g	49	70	3.2	13.1	0.5	1.9
Mixed Bean, Waitrose*	1 Serving/210g	229	109	8.7	13.6	2.2	4.6
Mixed Bean, Way To Five, Sainsbury's*	1/2 Can/205g	172	84	5.4	13.5	0.9	3.8
Mixed Leaf Medley, Waitrose*	1 Serving/25g	4	15	0.8	1.7	0.5	0.9
Mixed Leaf Tomato & Olive, Tesco*	1 Serving/170g	150	88	1.0	3.4	7.8	2.0

SALAD

INFO/WEIGHT	Measure	per Measure KCAL	Nutrition Values per 100g / 100ml KCAL	PROT	CARB	FAT	FIBRE
Mixed Leaf With Olive Oil Dressing, Pizza Express*	1 Pack/240g	326	136	0.9	2.1	14.1	0.7
Mixed Leaf, Tomato & Olive, Tesco*	1 Serving/170g	150	88	1.0	3.4	7.8	0.0
Mixed Leaf, Tomato, Feta, Boots*	1 Pack/179g	218	122	3.7	5.4	9.5	1.0
Mixed Leaves, Bondelle*	1 serving/50g	11	21	1.4	3.3	0.2	0.0
Mixed Leaves, Tesco*	1 Serving/20g	3	14	0.9	1.6	0.4	0.9
Mixed Pepper, Asda*	1/2 Pack/100g	24	24	1.0	4.3	0.3	1.7
Mixed With Peppers & Iceberg Lettuce, Somerfield*	1 Pack/200g	50	25	1.0	5.0	0.0	0.0
Mixed With Tatsoi, Safeway*	1 Serving/34g	5	15	1.1	1.5	0.4	1.2
Mixed, Florette*	1 Serving/100g	18	18	1.3	3.6	0.0	0.0
Mixed, Sainsbury's*	1 Serving/100g	21	21	1.4	3.4	0.2	2.1
Mixed, Sweet & Crispy, Tesco*	1 Serving/200g	48	24	1.0	4.2	0.3	2.0
Mixed, Tesco*	1 serving/100g	24	24	1.0	4.2	0.3	2.0
Moroccan Styles, COU, Marks & Spencer*	1/2 Pack/100g	160	160	5.0	32.8	1.2	4.8
Mozzarella & Cherry Tomato, Shapers, Boots*	1 Bowl/194g	184	95	4.1	3.3	7.3	0.9
Mozerella & Tomato, Marks & Spencer*	1 Serving/310g	400	129	5.5	15.5	4.8	0.9
Mozzarella & Sunkissed Tomato, Tesco*	1 Bag/160g	270	169	4.6	4.3	14.3	2.1
Mozzarella, With Sun Ripened Tomato, Marks & Spencer*	1 Serving/100g	250	250	9.8	4.9	21.4	2.0
Nantaise, Waitrose*	1 Pack/160g	34	21	1.5	2.9	0.4	2.0
New Potato & Free Range Egg, Side, Sainsbury's*	1 Pack/315g	189	60	2.5	3.1	4.2	1.4
New Potato & King Prawn, Marks & Spencer*	1 Pack/210g	221	105	5.6	10.2	4.5	1.7
New Potato & Sweet Chilli Prawn, Marks & Spencer*	1 Pack/210g	147	70	2.8	14.0	0.5	0.7
New Potato, Less Than 3% Fat, Marks & Spencer*	1 Pot/190g	143	75	1.7	14.4	1.3	1.2
New Potato, Marks & Spencer*	1 Serving/60g	63	105	1.6	15.0	4.5	1.0
New World, Finest, Tesco*	1 Bag/125g	24	19	1.7	1.9	0.5	1.1
Nicoise Style, Layered, Waitrose*	1 Bowl/275g	129	47	2.7	5.8	1.4	1.0
Nicoise, Food To Go, Marks & Spencer*	1 Pack/350g	473	135	5.9	7.5	9.0	0.5
Nicoise, Lunch Pot, Marks & Spencer*	1 Pot/330g	330	100	5.6	4.9	6.7	1.0
Noodle & King Prawn, Perfectly Balanced, Waitrose*	1 Pack/225g	223	99	5.0	17.4	1.0	1.0
Noodle With Thai Style Chicken, Marks & Spencer*	1/2 Pot/145g	160	110	5.2	11.6	4.9	1.4
Noodle, Sweet Chilli Chicken, Shapers, Boots*	1 Serving/197g	256	130	11.0	17.0	2.1	1.1
Noodle, Thai Style, BGTY, Sainsbury's*	1 Pack/185g	150	81	2.7	13.5	1.9	0.0
Pancetta, Express, Pizza Express*	1 Salad/90g	200	223	7.4	3.3	20.0	0.0
Pasta & Cheese, Asda*	1 Serving/125g	319	255	6.0	15.0	19.0	1.2
Pasta & Cheese, Somerfield*	1/2 Pack/225g	342	152	3.6	11.8	10.4	1.5
Pasta & Garlic, Iceland*	1 Serving/75g	149	199	2.2	15.4	14.3	1.6
Pasta & Ham, Safeway*	1 Pot/225g	284	126	4.5	16.9	4.5	0.3
Pasta & Mushroom, Waitrose*	1 Pack/200g	320	160	4.1	14.0	9.7	0.6
Pasta & Pepper Side, Tesco*	1 Pack/230g	278	121	2.4	13.0	6.6	1.3
Pasta & Sweetcorn, Less Than 3% Fat, Marks & Spencer*	1/2 Pack/100g	85	85	2.8	14.7	1.4	1.5
Pasta & Tomato, GFY, Asda*	1 Pack/300g	348	116	3.0	19.0	3.1	1.6
Pasta, Spinach & Pinenut, Safeway*	1 Serving/200g	295	148	5.3	15.2	7.2	1.7
Pea Leaf, With Baby Mint, TTD, Sainsbury's*	1 Serving/80g	11	14	1.5	1.8	0.1	1.7
Potato & Cheese, Pasta & Mixed Leaf, Waitrose*	1 Serving/205g	267	130	3.2	10.1	8.5	1.1
Potato & Egg Side, Tesco*	1 Pack/300g	192	64	2.5	4.2	4.1	1.1
Potato & Egg, Fresh, Safeway*	1 Serving/105g	84	80	8.4	3.0	3.6	1.6
Potato & Egg, With Mayo, Side, Tesco*	1 Serving/300g	225	75	2.9	3.1	5.7	1.2
Potato Baby, With Mint, TTD, Sainsbury's*	1 Serving/100g	204	204	2.0	10.8	17.0	0.7
Potato Layered, Tesco*	1 Pack/350g	284	81	1.3	7.8	4.9	1.3
Potato With Mayonnaise	1oz/28g	67	239	1.6	12.2	20.8	0.9
Potato With Mayonnaise, Retail	1oz/28g	80	287	1.5	11.4	26.5	0.8
Potato With Reduced Calorie Dressing, Retail	1oz/28g	27	97	1.3	14.8	4.1	0.8
Potato, 30% Less Fat, Sainsbury's*	1/2 Pot/150g	159	106	1.7	11.1	6.1	1.1
Potato, 50% Less Fat, Asda*	1/2 Pot/62g	47	76	1.6	11.2	2.7	1.5

S

SALAD

	Measure INFO/WEIGHT	per Measure KCAL	Nutrition Values per 100g / 100ml				
			KCAL	PROT	CARB	FAT	FIBRE
Potato, 60% Less Fat, Asda*	1 Serving/100g	101	101	1.7	10.0	6.0	0.0
Potato, Asda*	1/4 Pot/57g	67	117	0.9	12.5	7.0	1.1
Potato, Chunky, Somerfield*	1oz/28g	59	212	1.0	3.0	22.0	0.0
Potato, Creamy, Asda*	1oz/28g	61	219	1.0	11.9	18.6	0.7
Potato, Eat Smart, Safeway*	1/2 Pack/121g	85	70	1.7	10.2	2.0	1.9
Potato, Finest, Tesco*	1 Serving/25g	51	204	1.8	10.1	17.4	0.8
Potato, From Salad Selection, Sainsbury's*	1 Serving/50g	102	204	1.0	10.5	17.5	1.3
Potato, GFY, Asda*	1/2 Pack/125g	145	116	1.3	12.0	7.0	0.0
Potato, Good Intentions, Somerfield*	1 Serving/50g	50	100	1.2	14.0	4.4	1.0
Potato, Healthy Living, Tesco*	1 Sm Serving/25g	28	112	1.7	15.4	4.8	1.2
Potato, Heinz*	1/2 Can/97g	137	141	1.4	14.8	8.5	0.8
Potato, Less Than 4% Fat, Safeway*	1 Serving/250g	213	85	2.1	13.1	2.7	0.9
Potato, Less Than 5% Fat, Somerfield*	1oz/28g	24	86	2.0	11.0	4.0	0.0
Potato, Marks & Spencer*	1oz/28g	55	195	1.2	8.5	17.3	1.3
Potato, Perfectly Balanced, Waitrose*	1/2 Pot/125g	99	79	2.4	10.5	3.0	1.0
Potato, Reduced Fat, Sainsbury's*	1oz/28g	45	162	1.0	12.0	12.3	0.7
Potato, Sainsbury's*	1 Serving/30g	43	143	0.9	10.0	11.0	0.9
Potato, Salad Bar, Asda*	1oz/28g	52	187	0.6	11.6	15.4	1.1
Potato, Tesco*	1 Pot/125g	219	175	1.5	12.2	13.3	0.9
Potato, Value, Tesco*	1/2 Pack/125g	138	110	1.0	12.0	6.5	0.4
Potato, With Onions & Chives, Sainsbury's*	1/4 Pot/63g	88	140	0.9	10.0	11.0	0.9
Potato, With Salad Cream, Tesco*	1/2 Tub/125g	143	114	1.1	11.0	7.3	2.6
Prawn & Avacado, Marks & Spencer*	1 Serving/220g	176	80	3.0	2.0	6.8	3.1
Prawn & Egg, Leaf, Shapers, Boots*	1 Pack/182g	193	106	6.7	2.1	7.9	1.0
Prawn Cocktail, Boots*	1 Pack/202g	234	116	4.4	2.1	10.0	1.2
Prawn Cocktail, Healthy Living, Tesco*	1 Serving/300g	279	93	5.7	15.3	1.0	2.0
Prawn Cocktail, Tesco*	1 Pack/300g	360	120	5.7	10.9	6.0	0.8
Prawn Layered, Food To Go, Marks & Spencer*	1 Pack/220g	176	80	4.8	9.6	2.4	1.1
Prawn Layered, Marks & Spencer*	1 Pack/450g	358	80	4.8	9.6	2.4	1.1
Prawn Satay & Noodle, Tesco*	1 Serving/250g	320	128	7.1	9.5	6.8	1.2
Prawn, Layered, Sainsbury's*	1 Pack/275g	355	129	3.6	11.2	7.7	1.1
Prawn, Tesco*	1 Pack/280g	314	112	4.7	12.0	5.0	0.9
Primavera, Finest, Tesco*	1 Pack/100g	25	25	2.4	2.4	0.6	2.6
Rainbow Rice, Marks & Spencer*	1 Serving/261.5g	341	130	2.5	23.3	3.2	1.5
Red Hot, Very Special, Asda*	1 Serving/85g	9	11	1.9	0.9	0.0	1.4
Red Leaf & Rocket, Sainsbury's*	1 Serving/50g	11	21	3.5	1.6	0.1	1.1
Red Rice & Feta, Marks & Spencer*	1 Pack/244.4g	439	180	4.8	21.0	8.5	1.3
Red Thai Chicken With Noodles, Tesco*	1 Pack/300g	342	114	7.2	20.2	0.5	1.4
Ribbon, Marks & Spencer*	1oz/28g	5	17	0.8	3.2	0.2	1.7
Rice, Courgette & Pine Nut, BGTY, Sainsbury's*	1/3rd Pot/65g	68	105	2.7	20.0	1.6	1.5
Roast Chicken & Coleslaw, Boots*	1 Serving/245g	392	160	4.5	3.9	14.0	1.3
Roast Chicken, Layered, Healthy Living, Tesco*	1 Salad/400g	268	67	5.8	8.4	1.1	2.1
Roast Chicken, Tesco*	1 Salad/300g	348	116	5.3	7.0	7.4	1.0
Roasted Artichoke & Pepper, Marks & Spencer*	1 Serving/220g	638	290	4.1	12.8	24.5	5.1
Roasted Vegetable, Feta & Cous Cous, Somerfield*	1 Pack/299.4g	490	164	5.0	22.9	5.8	1.6
Roasted Vegetables & Cous Cous, Sainsbury's*	1 Pot/225g	378	168	5.3	12.6	10.7	1.9
Rocket, Leafy, Asda*	1 Serving/75g	10	13	1.5	1.4	0.1	1.8
Rocket, Organic, Sainsbury's*	1 Serving/25g	6	25	3.3	2.3	0.3	1.7
Rocket, Tesco*	1oz/28g	4	14	0.8	1.7	0.5	0.9
Rocket, Washed & Ready To Serve, Sainsbury's*	1/4 Pack/4g	1	16	2.6	0.2	0.5	2.3
Rocket, Wild, Fully Prepared, Sainsbury's*	1/2 Pack/25g	7	28	3.9	2.6	0.2	0.6
Rocket, Wild, Safeway*	1 Serving/25g	6	25	3.3	2.3	0.3	1.7
Ruby, Tesco*	1 Serving/48g	12	25	1.4	4.1	0.4	2.2

S

SALAD

INFO/WEIGHT	Measure per Measure KCAL	KCAL	PROT	CARB	FAT	FIBRE
Salad, Bistro, Somerfield*	1/2 pack/50g	7	14	0.8	1.6	0.5	1.4
Salmon & Roquette, Marks & Spencer*	1 Serving/255g	306	120	3.9	8.5	8.0	1.0
Santa Plum Tomato & Avocado, Marks & Spencer*	1 Pack/240g	348	145	1.7	4.1	13.4	0.2
Santa Plum Tomato With Dressing, Marks & Spencer*	1 Pack/225g	135	60	0.9	3.1	4.8	0.9
Santa Tomato, Side, Marks & Spencer*	1 Pack/225g	146	65	0.8	3.3	5.5	0.9
Sea Food, Family Mart*	1 Serving/100g	29	29	1.6	4.1	0.6	0.0
Seafood, Marinated, Marks & Spencer*	1 Serving/90g	108	120	13.4	2.3	6.4	0.8
Seafood, Sunkis*	1 Tub/100g	83	83	4.6	7.4	3.9	0.0
Seasonal, Organic, Waitrose*	1/4 Pack/25g	4	15	0.8	1.7	0.5	0.9
Selection, Fresh, Marks & Spencer*	1 Pack/230g	32	14	0.7	2.1	0.3	0.9
Selection, Side, Marks & Spencer*	1 Serving/255g	153	60	1.1	2.5	5.0	1.3
Shredded Beetroot, Asda*	1 Serving/140g	29	21	1.1	3.5	0.3	1.5
Side, Fresh & Crispy, Tesco*	1 Salad/230g	30	13	0.7	1.9	0.3	1.3
Side, Garden, With Cherry Tomatoes, Waitrose*	1 Pack/170g	25	15	0.8	2.0	0.4	1.3
Simply Chicken, Ginsters*	1 Pack/186.5g	316	170	11.4	22.7	3.7	0.0
Skipjack Tuna, John West*	1 Can/192g	190	99	7.3	3.7	6.1	0.0
Smoked Ham, Weight Watchers*	1 Pack/181g	233	129	11.0	16.6	2.0	3.0
Spanish Style Rice, Marks & Spencer*	1 Serving/220g	319	145	5.8	17.4	5.8	0.5
Spicy Bean, Tesco*	1 Serving/125g	111	89	4.9	12.1	2.3	2.5
Spicy Rice, Waitrose*	1 Serving/200g	318	159	3.2	21.7	6.6	0.9
Spinach, Rocket, & Watercress, Asda*	1 serving/100g	21	21	2.8	1.2	0.6	1.9
Spinach, Waitrose*	1 Pack/100g	25	25	2.8	1.6	0.8	2.1
Spinach, Watercress & Rocket, Safeway*	1 Serving/60g	14	24	3.0	1.5	0.7	1.8
Spring, American Style, Marks & Spencer*	1 Serving/60g	9	15	1.9	1.4	0.2	1.3
Sugar Plum Tomato, Fresh, Safeway*	1 Serving/160g	46	29	1.1	3.2	1.3	1.2
Summer, Marks & Spencer*	1oz/28g	6	20	0.8	3.6	0.4	1.2
Sweet & Crispy, Marks & Spencer*	1 Serving/140g	49	35	1.7	4.7	1.0	1.6
Sweet & Crispy, Side, Sainsbury's*	1/4 Bag/93g	23	25	1.3	4.4	0.2	2.2
Sweet & Crunchy, Eat One Keep One, Somerfield*	1 Serving/150g	33	22	0.8	3.9	0.3	2.0
Sweet & Crunchy, Sainsbury's*	1 Serving/125g	21	17	0.8	2.9	0.2	1.3
Sweet & Crunchy, Tesco*	1 Pack/285g	51	18	0.8	3.0	0.3	1.7
Sweet & Sour Prawn Noodle, Healthy Eating, Tesco*	1 Pack/190g	122	64	5.0	9.4	0.7	0.4
Sweet Carrot & Sultana, Marks & Spencer*	1 Serving/100g	55	55	0.8	11.4	0.7	2.6
Sweet Carrot, 3% Fat, Marks & Spencer*	1oz/28g	21	75	1.3	16.7	1.2	1.4
Sweet Chilli Chicken Noodle, COU, Marks & Spencer*	1 Pack/340g	408	120	6.8	17.4	2.3	1.2
Sweet Crispy, Eat Smart, Safeway*	1 Serving/220g	59	27	1.0	4.9	0.4	1.3
Sweet Crispy, Safeway*	1 Serving/220g	132	60	2.2	10.8	0.9	2.9
Sweet Green, Marks & Spencer*	1 Serving/150g	23	15	1.5	1.3	0.3	2.0
Sweet Leaf & Carrot, Asda*	1/2 Pack/164g	34	21	0.9	3.6	0.3	1.4
Sweet Leaf, Fully Prepared, Fresh, Sainsbury's*	1/4 Pack/75g	12	16	0.8	3.0	0.1	2.1
Sweet Leafy, Organic, Tesco*	1 Serving/250g	45	18	0.8	2.7	0.4	1.9
Sweet Pepper Side, Tesco*	1 Serving/54g	22	41	1.3	8.0	0.4	2.1
Sweet Pepper With Corn, Tesco*	1 Pack/270g	103	38	1.3	7.2	0.5	1.5
Sweet Pepper, Medley, Waitrose*	1/2 Pack/100g	22	22	0.9	3.8	0.4	1.5
Sweet, Baby Leaf Mix, Co-Op*	1 Serving/50g	8	15	0.8	2.0	0.5	2.0
Sweet, Crunchy, Mixed, Co-Op*	1 Serving/100g	30	30	1.0	6.0	0.2	2.0
Sweet, Layered, Tesco*	1 Serving/285g	80	28	1.1	5.0	0.4	1.6
Sweet, Shredded, Tesco*	1 Serving/100g	20	20	1.1	2.9	0.4	1.9
Sweet, Waitrose*	1 Serving/160g	27	17	0.7	2.8	0.3	1.7
Tabbouleh & Feta, Tesco*	1 Pack/225g	302	134	5.4	16.7	5.0	0.6
Tabbouleh Feta, Finest, Tesco*	1 Pack/225g	266	118	4.2	13.7	5.2	0.6
Tabbouleh Style, Perfectly Balanced, Waitrose*	1 Pack/225g	234	104	2.8	14.3	3.9	2.6
Tabbouleh, Healthy Living, Tesco*	1 Serving/200g	194	97	3.5	16.8	1.8	1.3

S

INFO/WEIGHT	Measure per Measure	KCAL	Nutrition Values per 100g / 100ml				
			KCAL	PROT	CARB	FAT	FIBRE

SALAD
Tatsoi, Fully Prepared, Sainsbury's*	1 Pack/115g	21	18	1.7	2.2	0.3	1.3
Tenderleaf, Waitrose*	1 Serving/200g	30	15	0.9	1.6	0.5	1.1
Tenderleaf, With Mizuna, Sainsbury's*	1 Serving/50g	10	20	3.6	0.2	0.6	2.2
Thai Style Chicken, Marks & Spencer*	1 Serving/195g	205	105	6.7	15.1	1.9	1.9
Thai Style Noodle With King Prawns, Marks & Spencer*	1 Serving/425g	425	100	5.2	17.5	1.0	1.8
Three Bean & Pesto, Italian Style, Boots*	1 Serving/290g	374	129	8.3	14.0	4.3	1.8
Three Bean, Pot, Tesco*	1 Pot/210g	204	97	4.1	10.2	4.4	2.3
Three Bean, Sainsbury's*	1 Serving/125g	108	86	4.2	6.0	5.0	0.0
Three Bean, Tinned, Tesco*	1 Tin/160g	176	110	7.7	17.6	1.0	5.3
Three Leaf Blend, Sainsbury's*	1 Pack/50g	10	19	1.7	1.8	0.6	1.2
Tiger Prawn & Pasta, GFY, Asda*	1 Serving/200g	250	125	4.6	20.0	2.9	2.0
Tomato & Mozarella Cheese, Marks & Spencer*	1/2 Pack/110g	155	141	10.0	3.2	9.6	0.5
Tomato & Onion	1oz/28g	20	72	0.8	4.0	6.1	1.0
Tomato, Avocado & Rocket, Marks & Spencer*	1 Pack/350g	508	145	1.7	4.1	13.4	0.2
Tomato, Pasta & Mozarella, Waitrose*	1 Serving/100g	169	169	4.3	10.0	12.4	0.6
Tuna & Tomato, Boots*	1 Pack/171g	150	88	6.5	2.0	6.0	1.0
Tuna In a Tomato & Herb Dressing, John West*	1 Can/192g	190	99	7.3	3.7	6.1	0.0
Tuna Layered, COU, Marks & Spencer*	1 Tub/450g	338	75	6.8	7.2	2.2	2.2
Tuna Layered, Waitrose*	1 Bowl/300g	636	212	4.0	4.8	19.6	1.0
Tuna Nicoise, BGTY, Sainsbury's*	1 Pack/300g	315	105	6.3	15.5	2.0	2.5
Tuna Nicoise, Finest, Tesco*	1 Serving/250g	430	172	8.5	13.3	9.4	0.8
Tuna Nicoise, Marks & Spencer*	1/2 Pack/255g	306	120	6.0	3.7	8.8	0.2
Tuna Nicoise, No Mayonnaise, Shapers, Boots*	1 Pack/276.4g	132	48	4.0	5.0	1.3	0.8
Tuna Nicoise, Sainsbury's*	1 Pack/183g	234	128	11.3	1.8	8.4	0.0
Tuna Nicoise, Shapers, Boots*	1 Serving/290g	138	48	4.1	4.8	1.3	0.8
Tuna, Breton Style, Snack Pot, Carb Check, Heinz*	1 Pot/219g	239	109	8.4	4.6	6.3	1.5
Tuna, Healthy Eating, Tesco*	1 Serving/300g	399	133	6.2	10.5	7.3	0.9
Tuna, Layered, Tesco*	1 Serving/370g	466	126	4.4	9.4	7.9	1.0
Tuna, With Lemon Dressing, Tesco*	1 Serving/300g	282	94	4.2	1.4	8.0	1.0
Tuscan Style Bean & Sunblush Tomato, Waitrose*	1 Pot/225g	308	137	5.6	17.9	4.8	1.0
Vegetable, Canned	1oz/28g	40	143	1.6	13.0	9.8	1.2
Vegetable, Heinz*	1 Can/195g	259	133	1.5	12.6	8.5	1.3
Waldorf	1oz/28g	54	193	1.4	7.5	17.7	1.3
Waldorf, Side, Waitrose*	1 Pack/160g	32	20	1.1	3.1	0.3	2.6
Waldorf, Waitrose*	1 Serving/50g	161	321	2.6	7.6	31.1	1.3
Watercress & Spinach, Asda*	1 Serving/50g	11	21	2.8	1.2	0.6	1.9
Watercress, Baby Spinach & Rocket, Somerfield*	1 Serving/100g	25	25	3.0	1.2	0.9	1.7
Watercress, Mustard Leaf & Mizuna, Marks & Spencer*	1/2 Pack/60g	9	15	2.4	0.4	0.3	3.0
Watercress, Spinach & Rocket, Tesco*	1 Serving/30g	7	22	3.0	0.8	0.8	1.9
Watercress, Spinach & Rocket, Waitrose*	1 Bag/135g	28	21	2.2	1.2	0.8	1.5
Wheat With Roasted Vegetables, Sainsbury's*	1 Pack/220g	339	154	3.3	17.0	8.3	4.5
Wild Rocket, Spinach & Watercress, Asda*	1 Serving/100g	21	21	2.8	1.2	0.6	1.9
With Sweetcorn, Side, Tesco*	1 Serving/135g	51	38	1.3	7.2	0.5	1.5
World Fusion, Somerfield*	1 Serving/100g	17	17	1.3	1.6	0.6	1.7

SALAD BOWL
Avocado & Tomato, Sainsbury's*	1 Pack/180g	97	54	1.0	6.7	2.6	1.3
Coleslaw, Marks & Spencer*	1 Pack/325g	293	90	1.3	4.9	7.4	1.3
Coleslaw, Tesco*	1 Bowl/300g	327	109	1.0	3.4	10.1	1.3
Crispy, Marks & Spencer*	1 Serving/250g	88	35	1.3	6.6	0.5	1.2
French Style, Sainsbury's*	1oz/28g	15	55	1.0	4.8	3.5	1.5
Fruit Crunch, Marks & Spencer*	1/2 Pack/120g	174	145	3.1	25.5	3.4	0.6
Goats Cheese, Sainsbury's*	1 Serving/100g	161	161	5.8	7.6	11.9	1.3
Greek Style, Marks & Spencer*	1 Bowl/255g	242	95	2.5	2.4	8.2	0.7

SALAD BOWL	Measure INFO/WEIGHT	per Measure KCAL	KCAL	PROT	CARB	FAT	FIBRE
Greek Style, Somerfield*	1 Bowl/225g	178	79	2.2	3.5	6.2	1.1
Honey & Mustard Chicken, Fresh, Sainsbury's*	1 Serving/300g	408	136	5.9	10.3	7.9	1.7
Italian Avocado & Tomato, Sainsbury's*	1 Bowl/180g	97	54	1.0	6.7	2.6	1.3
Large, Sainsbury's*	1/6 Pack/52g	12	23	0.9	4.3	0.3	1.1
Mixed, Medley, Waitrose*	1/4 Pack/60g	9	15	0.9	1.7	0.5	1.0
Mixed, Waitrose*	1/4 pack/64.3g	9	14	0.8	1.6	0.5	1.4
Mushrooms in Tomato Sauce, Sainsbury's*	1 Serving/100g	72	72	2.5	3.3	4.8	0.5
New Potato, Tuna & Egg, Marks & Spencer*	1 Pack/340g	255	75	3.8	6.7	3.8	0.7
Pasta With Sun Dried Tomato Dressing, WTF, Sainsbury's*	1 Bowl/320g	470	147	3.2	20.0	6.0	1.5
Pasta, Somerfield*	1 Pack/320g	541	169	3.3	20.8	8.1	1.5
Prawn, Sainsbury's*	1 Bowl/400g	632	158	3.7	9.4	11.7	1.2
Red Cheddar & Edam, Way to Five, Sainsbury's*	1/2 Pack/224g	240	107	4.4	12.8	4.2	1.1
Roast Chicken, Layered, Healthy Eating, Tesco*	1 Bowl/400g	268	67	5.8	8.4	1.1	2.1
Tomato & Basil, Marks & Spencer*	1 Serving/225g	225	100	0.8	3.7	10.1	1.1
Tomato, Sainsbury's*	1/2 Bowl/150g	93	62	0.9	4.4	4.5	1.6
Tomato, WTF, Sainsbury's*	1 Bowl/300g	174	58	0.8	4.5	4.1	2.8
Tuna, Fresh, Asda*	1 Serving/160g	184	115	8.0	5.0	7.0	0.0
Tuna, Layered, Tesco*	1 Serving/185g	313	169	6.3	8.3	12.3	1.3
Tuna, Sainsbury's*	1 Serving/200g	336	168	6.1	11.7	10.7	1.5
Tuscan, Tesco*	1 Pack/175g	166	95	0.9	3.5	8.6	1.2
SALAD CREAM							
Average	1 Tsp/5g	17	335	1.7	18.6	27.9	0.1
Reduced Calorie, Average	1 Tsp/5g	6	130	1.0	12.9	7.9	0.2
SALAD KIT							
Caesar, Asda*	1/2 Pack/113g	154	136	5.0	11.0	8.0	1.4
Caesar, BGTY, Sainsbury's*	1/2 Pack/130g	135	104	3.6	9.8	5.6	1.7
Caesar, Healthy Living, Tesco*	1/2 Pack/132.5g	149	112	3.3	5.9	8.3	1.4
Caesar, New Improved, Tesco*	1/2 Pack/138g	279	202	4.7	4.5	18.3	1.3
Ranch, Healthy Living, Tesco*	1 Serving/115g	69	60	4.4	5.0	2.5	1.8
SALAD SNACK							
Chargrilled Chicken & Pesto Pasta, Sainsbury's*	1 Pack/240g	454	189	7.2	19.4	9.2	0.0
Chargrilled Chicken, Tesco*	1 Pot/300g	384	128	6.1	15.0	4.8	2.4
Chargrilled Vegetable Tortellini, Tesco*	1 Serving/300g	492	164	5.1	18.7	7.7	1.7
Cheese & Tomato, Tesco*	1 Pot/300g	519	173	6.3	21.7	6.8	2.2
Cheese Layered, Sainsbury's*	1 Pack/190g	397	209	5.4	12.4	15.3	0.0
Chicken & Bacon, Tesco*	1 Pack/300g	501	167	7.2	10.9	10.5	3.2
Chicken Caesar, Sainsbury's*	1 Pack/182.2g	164	90	5.9	5.3	5.0	1.0
Chicken Caesar, Tesco*	1 Serving/300g	420	140	8.2	11.4	6.8	1.7
Chicken Noodle, Sainsbury's*	1 Snack/240g	278	116	5.2	12.4	5.1	1.4
Greek Style, BGTY, Sainsbury's*	1 Pack/198.5g	133	67	2.0	9.0	2.5	0.8
Ham & Mushroom, Tesco*	1 Pot/300g	600	200	4.7	21.2	10.7	1.4
Hoi Sin Chicken & Noodle, TTD, Sainsbury's*	1 Pack/230g	214	93	4.7	15.2	1.5	1.8
Honey & Mustard Chicken Pasta, Sainsbury's*	1 Pack/190.1g	344	181	7.1	18.0	8.9	0.0
Honey & Mustard Chicken, Tesco*	1 Pot/300g	585	195	8.4	20.4	8.9	1.1
Pasta & Tuna, BGTY, Sainsbury's*	1 Pack/260g	218	84	6.0	11.5	1.6	2.3
Pasta & Tuna, Healthy Selection, Somerfield*	1 Pot/190g	194	102	6.5	13.0	2.7	1.1
Pasta, Cheese, Somerfield*	1 Salad/200g	422	211	8.0	14.0	14.0	0.0
Pasta, Egg Mayo, Asda*	1 Serving/180g	364	202	4.0	12.8	15.0	0.3
Pasta, Tuna, Asda*	1 Serving/180g	196	109	5.5	13.2	3.8	0.9
Pasta, Tuna, Sainsbury's*	1 Pot/260g	218	84	6.0	11.5	1.6	2.3
Roast Chicken, Tesco*	1 Pack/300g	324	108	6.0	4.8	7.2	1.9
Salmon & Dill, Tesco*	1 Pack/300g	600	200	7.7	13.4	12.8	0.8
Sausage & Tomato, Tesco*	1 Serving/300g	529	176	4.5	19.1	9.1	4.0

S

	Measure INFO/WEIGHT	per Measure KCAL	Nutrition Values per 100g / 100ml				
			KCAL	PROT	CARB	FAT	FIBRE
SALAD SNACK							
Thai Prawn, Good Intentions, Somerfield*	1 Serving/215g	230	107	5.0	17.9	1.7	1.1
Tuna & Pasta, BGTY, Sainsbury's*	1 Pack/260g	255	98	5.7	13.9	2.2	1.3
Tuna & Sweetcorn, Good Intentions, Somerfield*	1 Pot/215g	219	102	6.6	12.7	2.8	0.9
Tuna & Sweetcorn, Tesco*	1 Pack/300g	540	180	7.3	23.9	6.1	0.7
Tuna Pasta With Balsamic Dressing, GFY, Asda*	1 Pack/199.2g	263	132	5.0	20.0	3.6	1.5
Tuna, Healthy Living, Tesco*	1 Serving/300g	252	84	7.6	11.5	0.9	0.9
SALAMI							
Ardennes Pepper, Waitrose*	2 Slices/14g	60	429	18.6	1.9	38.5	1.1
Average	1 Slice/5g	18	360	28.4	1.9	26.2	0.0
Danish, Average	1 Serving/17g	89	524	13.2	1.3	51.7	0.0
Emiliano, Sainsbury's*	1 Serving/70g	209	298	28.8	0.1	20.3	0.0
German, Average	1 Serving/60g	200	333	20.3	1.6	27.3	0.1
German, Peppered, Average	3 Slices/25g	86	342	22.2	2.5	27.1	0.2
Healthy Range, Average	4 Slices/25g	55	221	22.4	0.7	14.3	0.0
Milano, Average	1 Serving/70g	278	397	25.9	0.9	32.2	0.0
Napoli, Average	1 Slice/5g	17	342	27.1	0.8	25.5	0.1
Spanish, Wafer Thin, Tesco*	1 Pack/80g	273	341	25.5	6.8	23.5	0.0
Ungherese, Tesco*	1 Serving/35g	136	388	24.5	0.5	32.0	0.0
SALMON							
Appetisers, Smoked, Tesco*	1 Pack/100g	224	224	15.1	0.7	17.9	1.7
Blinis, Smoked, Marks & Spencer*	1oz/28g	67	240	11.9	18.9	13.0	1.8
Crunchies, Tesco*	1 Serving/112g	211	188	9.0	15.9	9.8	1.3
Crusted, Mediterranean Style, Sainsbury's*	1 Serving/166g	322	194	18.0	5.3	11.5	0.8
Fillets, & Butter, Marks & Spencer*	1oz/28g	64	230	16.7	0.0	18.0	0.0
Fillets, Cajun, Waitrose*	1 Serving/150g	215	143	20.6	0.4	6.5	0.0
Fillets, Chargrilled, Sainsbury's*	1 Serving/270 g	270	243	20.9	0.2	17.6	0.0
Fillets, In White Wine & Parsley Dressing, Tesco*	1 Fillet/150g	291	194	17.5	0.3	13.6	0.6
Fillets, Lime & Coriander Marinade, Pacific, Sainsbury's*	1 Serving/100g	139	139	24.4	1.3	4.1	0.9
Fillets, Lime & Coriander, Tesco*	1 Pack/250g	283	113	18.2	5.4	2.1	0.0
Fillets, Raw, Average	1 Fillet/79g	149	189	20.9	0.1	11.7	0.1
Fillets, With Lemon & Herb Butter, Asda*	1 Fillet/125g	305	244	20.0	0.4	18.0	0.0
Fillets, With Orange & Dill Dressing, Tesco*	1 Serving/300g	540	180	17.7	4.1	10.3	0.7
Fillets, With Sea Salt & Black Pepper Butter, Safeway*	1 Fillet/115g	288	250	20.4	0.1	18.7	0.0
Fillets, With Sicilian Citrus Glaze, Sainsbury's*	1 Fillet/144.9g	371	256	21.9	2.3	17.8	0.0
Flakes, Honey Roast, Average	1oz/28g	56	198	24.0	1.9	10.7	0.2
Goan, Limited Edition, Sainsbury's*	1 Pack/351g	358	102	11.1	2.3	5.4	2.4
Goujons, Average	1 Pack/150g	321	214	16.4	12.4	11.0	1.1
Hot Smoked, Average	1 Serving/62g	103	166	24.0	0.9	7.2	0.1
In Crust, Wild Alaska, Young's*	1 Serving/160g	224	140	19.5	7.2	3.6	0.2
Lime & Coriander, Tesco*	1 Serving/120g	176	147	21.4	7.0	3.7	0.7
Mild Oak Smoked, Average	1 Slice/25g	46	182	22.6	0.1	10.2	0.0
Pink, Average	1 Serving/125g	162	130	19.5	0.1	5.8	0.1
Pink, In Brine, Average	1oz/28g	43	153	23.5	0.0	6.6	0.0
Poached, Average	1 Serving/90g	176	195	22.5	0.2	11.7	0.3
Potted, Marks & Spencer*	1 Serving/75g	184	245	17.1	0.5	19.4	1.2
Red, Average	1/2 Can/90g	141	156	20.5	0.1	8.2	0.1
Red, In Brine, Average	1oz/28g	47	169	22.4	0.0	8.9	0.0
Rillettes, John West*	1/2 Can/62g	169	272	14.9	0.1	23.5	0.0
Smoked, Average	1 Serving/70g	126	179	21.9	0.5	10.0	0.1
Smoked, Birch & Juniper, Sainsbury's*	1/2 Pack/30g	47	156	24.7	0.3	6.4	0.0
Smoked, Oak & Beech, Shetland Isles, Finest, Tesco*	1 Serving/65g	116	179	22.0	0.2	10.0	0.0
Smoked, Trimmings, Average	1 Serving/55g	101	184	22.9	0.2	10.3	0.0
Steak, Chunky, Sainsbury's*	1 Serving/175g	376	215	24.2	0.1	13.1	0.1

S

	Measure INFO/WEIGHT	per Measure KCAL	Nutrition Values per 100g / 100ml				
			KCAL	PROT	CARB	FAT	FIBRE
SALMON							
Tail Joint, Lemon & Herb Butter, Marks & Spencer*	1 Pack/480g	864	180	18.8	0.8	11.4	0.2
SALMON &							
Dill Sauce, Young's*	1 Pack/435g	265	61	6.1	4.2	2.3	0.1
Pasta, Young's*	1 Pack/300g	411	137	7.8	16.6	4.4	1.2
Spinach, Roulade, Tesco*	1 Serving/60g	155	258	9.5	1.7	23.7	0.2
Thai Noodles, Healthy Eating, Tesco*	1 Pack/350g	231	66	6.7	7.1	1.2	1.5
Vegetables, Marks & Spencer*	1 Serving/200g	220	110	6.0	5.2	6.9	0.8
SALMON EN CROUTE							
Iceland*	1 Serving/170g	476	280	8.5	20.1	18.4	1.0
Luxury, Marks & Spencer*	1oz/28g	59	210	11.9	9.4	13.7	2.2
Marks & Spencer*	1/2 Pack/185g	574	310	10.4	17.3	21.9	0.6
Retail	1oz/28g	81	288	11.8	18.0	19.1	0.0
Sainsbury's*	1 Serving/179g	553	309	10.9	17.3	21.8	0.7
Tesco*	1 Serving/205g	568	277	9.7	15.4	19.6	0.6
Young's*	1 Serving/200g	330	165	5.3	9.2	11.9	0.4
SALMON FLORENTINE							
Asda*	1 Serving/190g	306	161	16.0	1.8	10.0	0.0
SALMON IN							
A Creamy Horseradish Sauce, Fillets, Wonnemeyer*	1 Serving/300g	459	153	9.4	5.3	10.5	0.0
A Watercress Sauce, Marks & Spencer*	1 Pack/400g	480	120	7.1	8.1	6.8	1.7
Creamy Watercress Sauce, Fillets, Sainsbury's*	1 Serving/180g	292	162	13.0	2.2	11.3	0.4
Creamy Watercress Sauce, Fillets, Scottish, Seafresh*	1 Pack 300g	528	176	13.7	1.2	12.9	0.1
Dill Sauce, Fillets, Steamfresh, Birds Eye*	1 Pack/340g	357	105	13.0	2.9	4.2	0.1
Lemon Mayonnaise, Weight Watchers*	1 Can/80g	130	163	10.2	6.4	10.6	0.1
Lime & Coriander, Fillets, Good Choice, Iceland*	1/2 Pack/150g	189	126	19.8	5.1	2.9	0.8
Pancetta, Wrapped, Finest, Tesco*	1 Serving/150g	328	219	14.9	1.0	17.2	0.1
Tomato & Mascarpone Sauce, Fillets, Asda*	1/2 Pack/181.0g	279	154	13.0	0.8	11.0	0.6
Watercress Sauce, Fillet, Finest, Tesco*	1 Serving/500g	690	138	7.4	5.1	9.8	2.6
Watercress Sauce, Somerfield*	1 Pack/210g	386	184	12.9	1.2	14.2	1.1
Watercress Sauce, Waitrose*	1/2 Pack/150g	264	176	13.7	1.2	12.9	0.1
SALMON LUNCHBOX							
COU, Marks & Spencer*	1 Pack/235g	200	85	5.1	13.1	1.4	0.9
SALMON MOROCCAN							
Style, Fillets, Asda*	1 Serving/240g	454	189	19.0	1.3	12.0	0.0
SALMON PARCELS							
& Garlic Butter, Finest, Tesco*	1 Serving/164g	321	196	16.8	0.6	14.1	0.5
In Lemon Sauce, Marks & Spencer*	1 Serving/185g	350	189	12.1	1.4	15.1	0.5
Smoked, Scottish, Marks & Spencer*	1 Parcel/58g	130	226	16.7	1.2	17.6	0.0
Smoked, Tesco*	1 Serving/50g	147	293	16.4	0.0	25.3	0.2
Smoked, Waitrose*	1 Serving/57g	140	246	14.6	1.2	20.2	0.0
With Light Creamy Mousse Filling, Smoked, Tesco*	1 Parcel/56.5g	99	177	17.5	1.7	11.1	0.1
SALMON PEPPERONATA							
BGTY, Sainsbury's*	1 Pack/380g	300	79	5.8	8.8	2.3	0.9
SALMON PLATTER							
GFY, Asda*	1 Pack/400g	376	94	7.0	8.0	3.8	1.4
SALMON WITH							
A Cream Sauce, Scottish Fillets, Marks & Spencer*	1 Serving/200g	360	180	13.8	1.0	13.0	0.1
Asparagus & Rice, Fillets, Perfectly Balanced, Waitrose*	1 Serving/400g	348	87	8.2	11.4	1.0	0.9
Coriander & Lime, Pacific, Asda*	1 serving/113g	154	137	27.0	0.5	3.0	0.0
Herb Vegetables, Healthy Eating, Tesco*	1 Pack/350g	228	65	6.6	3.8	2.6	0.9
Mozzarella & Tomato Crust, Just Cook, Sainsbury's*	1/2 Pack/171g	208	122	15.8	3.8	4.8	0.3
Potatoes & Vegetables, Scottish, Marks & Spencer*	1 Pack/400g	460	115	7.9	5.8	6.9	0.9
Spinach & Cheese, Atlantic, Birds Eye*	1 Serving/241g	415	172	9.8	4.2	12.9	0.1

S

	Measure	per Measure		Nutrition Values per 100g / 100ml				
	INFO/WEIGHT	KCAL		KCAL	PROT	CARB	FAT	FIBRE

SALSA

Chunky Tomato & Avocado, COU, Marks & Spencer*	1/2 Pot/85g	30		35	0.8	5.4	1.4	1.4
Chunky, Sainsbury's*	0.5 pot/84.3g	43		51	1.1	7.8	1.7	1.2
Cool, Sainsbury's*	1 Serving/100g	31		31	1.0	6.1	0.3	1.2
Cool, Tesco*	1oz/28g	11		38	0.9	7.1	0.3	0.8
Extra Hot, Fresh, Somerfield*	1oz/28g	13		47	1.0	8.0	1.0	0.0
Fire Roasted Pepper, Somerfield*	1 Pot/120g	50		42	1.2	8.1	0.5	1.3
Fresh, Asda*	1oz/28g	10		35	1.2	6.2	0.6	2.0
Fresh, Sainsbury's*	1oz/28g	15		54	1.7	7.0	2.1	0.9
GFY, Asda*	1/2 Pot/236g	85		36	1.1	7.0	0.4	0.7
Hot, Fresh, Tesco*	1oz/28g	16		57	1.4	7.5	2.4	1.2
Hot, Primula*	1oz/28g	10		35	1.8	6.6	0.2	0.0
Hot, Tesco*	1/2 Jar/150g	38		25	1.2	4.7	0.2	1.1
Marks & Spencer*	1/2 Jar/136g	95		70	1.2	12.0	2.4	1.5
Medium Hot, Discovery*	1oz/28g	16		58	1.1	8.1	2.4	2.1
Prawn & Tomato, Fresh, Anti Pasti, Asda*	1 Pot/150g	101		67	8.0	3.1	2.5	1.3
Red Onion & Tomato, Tapas Selection, Sainsbury's*	1 Serving/22g	17		77	3.0	6.0	4.5	0.9
Red Pepper, Sainsbury's*	1 Serving/85g	31		37	1.7	3.8	1.7	1.5
Smokey BBQ, Weight Watchers*	1 Serving/56g	20		36	1.1	7.6	0.1	2.3
Spiced Mango, Ginger & Chilli, Weight Watchers*	1/2 Pot/50g	43		85	1.0	19.9	0.2	2.6
Spicy Mango & Lime, Morrisons*	1/2 Pot/85g	62		73	1.0	15.9	0.4	1.3
Spicy Red Pepper, Sainsbury's*	1 Pot/170g	54		32	1.4	3.2	1.4	1.3
Spicy, Less Than 3% Fat, Marks & Spencer*	1/2 Pot/85g	30		35	1.3	5.6	0.8	0.8
Spicy, Marks & Spencer*	1oz/28g	17		60	1.3	7.2	2.7	1.2
Sweetcorn, Fresh, Sainsbury's*	1/4 Pot/51g	32		63	1.1	10.5	1.8	1.3
Taco, Old El Paso*	1/4 Pack/29g	13		46	1.5	10.0	0.0	0.0
Tomato & Avocado, Marks & Spencer*	1/2 Pack/85.7g	30		35	0.8	5.4	1.4	1.4
Tomato, Chunky, Tesco*	1 Pot/170g	68		40	1.1	5.9	1.3	1.1
Tomato, Chunky, Tex Mex, Tesco*	1 Serving/50g	26		52	1.0	6.4	2.5	1.0
Tomato, Marks & Spencer*	1 Tbsp/25g	9		35	1.0	4.7	1.2	0.9
Tomato, Reduced Fat, Waitrose*	1 Serving/1g	0		27	1.5	4.7	0.2	1.4
Tomato, Vine Ripened, Tesco*	1/2 Pack/95g	45		47	1.0	6.7	1.8	1.1
Tomato, Waitrose*	1 Serving/50g	24		47	1.5	5.0	2.3	1.7

SALT

Cooking, Sainsbury's*	1oz/28g	0		0	0.0	0.0	0.0	0.0
Table	1 Tsp/5g	0		0	0.0	0.0	0.0	0.0

SAMOSAS

Chicken Tikka, Sainsbury's*	2 Samosas/100g	239		239	8.3	22.5	12.9	3.1
Chicken, Mumtaz*	1 Serving/105g	177		169	19.6	4.9	7.9	0.0
Dim Sum Selection, Sainsbury's*	1 Samosas/12g	24		196	3.4	28.6	7.6	2.8
Indian Style Selection, Co-Op*	1 Samosa/20.8g	50		240	5.0	27.0	13.0	3.0
Lamb, Waitrose*	1oz/28g	87		310	8.5	18.1	22.6	0.8
Mini, Sainsbury's*	1 Serving/28g	82		294	6.9	33.2	14.8	2.7
Vegetable, Delicately Spiced, Sainsbury's*	1 Samosa/50g	90		180	3.6	20.2	9.4	2.9
Vegetable, Marks & Spencer*	1 Samosa/45g	115		255	5.1	24.8	15.3	2.8
Vegetable, Mini Indian Selection, Tesco*	1 Samosa/32g	66		207	4.8	25.6	9.5	3.4
Vegetable, Mini, Waitrose*	2 Samosas/59.8g	146		244	4.5	28.7	12.4	2.8
Vegetable, Northern Indian, Sainsbury's*	1 Samosa/50g	126		252	5.8	30.6	11.8	2.6
Vegetable, Retail	1oz/28g	61		217	5.1	30.0	9.3	2.5
Vegetable, Sainsbury's*	1 Samosa/50g	90		180	3.6	20.2	9.4	3.0
Vegetable, Tesco*	1 Samosa/50g	126		252	5.0	28.4	13.2	2.7
Vegetable, Waitrose*	1 Samosas/50g	107		214	3.3	26.3	10.6	0.8

SANDWICH

All Day Breakfast, BGTY, Sainsbury's*	1 Pack/188g	294		156	9.6	22.7	2.4	0.0

S

SANDWICH

INFO/WEIGHT	Measure per Measure KCAL	Nutrition Values per 100g / 100ml KCAL	PROT	CARB	FAT	FIBRE
All Day Breakfast, Eat Smart, Safeway*	1 Pack/157g	236	150	10.0	21.6	2.1	2.2
All Day Breakfast, Finest, Tesco*	1 Pack/275g	660	240	9.7	16.4	15.1	1.6
All Day Breakfast, Ginsters*	1 Pack/241.3g	537	223	10.8	20.3	11.0	0.0
All Day Breakfast, Healthy Living, Tesco*	1 Pack/223.1g	328	147	11.9	16.8	3.6	2.7
All Day Breakfast, Shapers, Boots*	1 Pack/207.1g	323	156	11.0	23.0	2.5	2.2
All Day Breakfast, The Big Eat Street, Safeway*	1 Pack/213.1g	584	274	12.1	23.1	14.8	2.1
All Day Breakfast, Wall's*	1 Pack/225.1g	610	271	9.2	24.3	15.4	1.4
All Day Breakfast, Weight Watchers*	1 Pack/157.7g	299	189	11.0	30.2	2.7	1.9
Avocado, & Spinach, Marks & Spencer*	1 Pack/241.7g	581	240	4.5	24.7	13.6	2.2
Avocado, Mozzarella & Tomato, Marks & Spencer*	1 Pack/272.9g	655	240	8.8	21.7	13.2	2.3
BLT, & Chicken Salad, Co-Op*	1 Pack/230g	472	205	10.0	21.0	9.0	2.0
BLT, Asda*	1 Pack/262g	618	236	12.2	20.3	12.0	3.0
BLT, BGTY, Sainsbury's*	1 Pack/196g	331	169	10.4	27.0	2.2	0.0
BLT, COU, Marks & Spencer*	1 Pack/174g	278	160	9.5	25.6	2.7	2.5
BLT, Classic, Taste!*	1 Serving/150g	345	230	9.3	25.2	9.9	0.0
BLT, Deep Fill, Safeway*	1 Pack/202g	565	280	14.0	29.2	12.0	2.2
BLT, Deep Fill, Tesco*	1 Pack/231g	635	275	11.8	19.8	16.5	1.2
BLT, Deep Filled, Asda*	1 Pack/206g	606	294	13.3	21.8	17.0	3.0
BLT, Eat Smart, Safeway*	1 Pack/165g	231	140	9.8	21.8	1.4	2.4
BLT, GFY, Asda*	1 Pack/171g	294	172	9.0	26.0	3.5	1.6
BLT, Ginsters*	1 Pack/192g	516	269	15.6	21.2	15.6	0.0
BLT, Healthy Living, Tesco*	1 Pack/190g	287	151	10.1	24.5	1.4	1.6
BLT, Healthy Selection, Budgens*	1 Pack/183g	361	197	10.0	22.9	7.3	2.5
BLT, Marks & Spencer*	1 Serving/181g	534	295	10.3	22.4	18.2	1.9
BLT, Max, Shell*	1 Pack/249.1g	665	267	10.8	24.1	14.1	0.0
BLT, Platter, Marks & Spencer*	1/4 Sandwich/49.2g	159	325	11.7	21.2	21.4	1.3
BLT, Safeway*	1 Pack/230g	529	230	15.9	35.4	2.3	3.9
BLT, Salt Controlled, Shapers, Boots*	1 Pack/180.1g	290	161	9.3	23.0	3.4	3.0
BLT, Shapers, Boots*	1 Pack/171g	328	192	10.0	22.0	7.1	2.3
BLT, Somerfield*	1 Pack/157g	425	270	10.3	23.8	14.7	2.3
BLT, Sutherland*	1 Pack/216g	624	289	9.1	23.8	17.5	0.0
BLT, Taste!*	1 Pack/168.9g	353	209	8.5	22.4	9.5	0.0
BLT, Tesco*	1 Pack/203g	520	256	11.9	19.5	14.4	1.5
BLT, Waitrose*	1 Pack/210g	578	275	9.3	25.6	15.0	2.3
BLT, Weight Watchers*	1 Pack/171g	267	156	9.8	23.5	2.5	2.4
BLT, With Mayo, Safeway*	1 Pack/168g	462	275	10.4	20.7	16.7	2.3
Bacon, & Brie, Asda*	1 Pack/181g	603	333	13.3	22.9	21.1	1.3
Bacon, & Brie, Finest, Tesco*	1 Pack/201.1g	571	284	14.1	19.4	16.7	2.1
Bacon, & Egg, Boots*	1 Pack/179g	480	268	12.0	19.0	16.0	1.4
Bacon, & Egg, Co-Op*	1 Pack/188g	536	285	13.0	20.0	17.0	2.0
Bacon, & Egg, Deep Fill, Ginsters*	1 Pack/210g	590	281	11.5	18.8	18.2	0.0
Bacon, & Egg, Felix Van Den Berghe*	1 Pack/137.9g	382	277	8.9	22.2	17.0	0.0
Bacon, & Egg, Ginsters*	1 Pack/210g	523	249	13.2	22.0	11.6	0.0
Bacon, & Egg, Healthy Living, Tesco*	1 Serving/178.3g	328	184	11.5	22.7	5.2	1.7
Bacon, & Egg, Marks & Spencer*	1 Pack/215g	525	244	13.4	15.8	14.2	2.1
Bacon, & Egg, On Malted Whole Grain Bread, Budgens*	1 Pack/174.9g	593	339	12.3	21.4	21.4	1.6
Bacon, & Egg, Sainsbury's*	1 Pack/215g	535	249	12.3	23.2	11.9	0.0
Bacon, & Egg, Shell*	1 Pack/191g	579	303	12.2	18.7	19.9	0.0
Bacon, & Egg, Taste!*	1 Pack/186.8g	496	265	12.8	19.1	15.3	0.0
Bacon, & Egg, Tesco*	1 Pack/188g	481	256	14.1	21.0	12.9	1.9
Bacon, & Tomato, COU, Marks & Spencer*	1 Pack/168.8g	270	160	9.5	25.6	2.7	2.5
Bacon, Brie, & Mango Chutney, Daily Bread*	1 Serving/212.6g	556	261	12.7	28.6	10.7	0.0
Bap, Chicken, & Sweetcorn, Sainsbury's*	1 Serving/169.9g	462	272	12.5	24.2	13.9	0.0

SANDWICH

INFO/WEIGHT	Measure	per Measure KCAL	KCAL	PROT	CARB	FAT	FIBRE
Bap, Chicken, Chargrilled, Malted, Co-Op*	1 Bap/201g	492	245	9.0	23.0	13.0	2.0
Bap, Corned Beef, & Onion, White, Open Choice Foods*	1 Roll/144g	331	230	12.7	30.7	6.1	0.0
Bap, Ham, & Salad, Co-Op*	1 Bap/163.9g	295	180	8.0	30.0	3.0	2.0
Bap, Tuna, & Sweetcorn, Malted, Co-Op*	1 Bap/212g	530	250	9.0	24.0	13.0	2.0
Beef, & English Mustard Mayonnaise, Roast, Oldfields*	1 Pack/150g	405	270	16.0	29.0	11.9	0.0
Beef, & Horseradish Mayonnaise, Roast, Finest, Tesco*	1 Pack/222.8g	439	197	12.5	20.7	7.1	1.6
Beef, & Horseradish Mayonnaise, Roast, Rare, Waitrose*	1 Pack/197g	415	211	12.2	23.1	7.8	2.0
Beef, & Horseradish Mayonnaise, Shapers, Boots*	1 Pack/159.3g	266	167	12.0	25.0	2.1	2.6
Beef, & Horseradish, Deep Filled, BGTY, Sainsbury's*	1 Pack/202g	313	155	11.4	22.0	2.4	2.4
Beef, & Horseradish, Rare Roast, Marks & Spencer*	1 Pack/168g	311	185	14.8	21.1	4.3	2.4
Beef, & Horseradish, Roast, So Good, Somerfield*	1 Pack/188g	404	215	12.4	27.6	6.1	1.8
Beef, & Horseradish, Sainsbury's*	1 Pack/187g	389	208	12.0	24.1	7.1	0.0
Beef, & Horseradish, Shapers, Boots*	1 Sandwich/155.9g	276	177	12.0	28.0	1.7	1.8
Beef, & Onion, Roast, Deep Filled, Asda*	1 Pack/258g	550	213	11.3	22.6	10.8	1.1
Beef, & Onion, Roast, Healthy Living, Tesco*	1 Pack/185.3g	278	150	13.3	20.0	1.9	2.7
Beef, & Pate, Marks & Spencer*	1 Pack/187.9g	310	165	11.2	21.6	3.9	2.4
Beef, & Salad, Gibsons*	1 Pack/185g	348	188	10.6	23.5	5.7	0.0
Beef, & Salad, Roast, Daily Bread*	1 Pack/202g	319	158	9.0	21.4	4.1	0.0
Beef, Peppered, Shell*	1 Pack/181.0g	400	221	7.3	29.0	8.4	1.3
Beef, Roast, Feel Good, Shell*	1 Pack/153g	390	255	17.6	24.2	9.7	0.0
Beef, Roast, Handmade, Tesco*	1 Pack/223g	439	197	12.5	20.7	7.1	1.6
Beef, Roast, Sainsbury's*	1 Pack/173.9g	426	245	9.4	29.3	10.0	0.0
Beef, Salt, With Gherkins, & Mustard Mayo, Sainsbury's*	1 Pack/242g	486	201	9.3	24.1	7.5	3.1
Beef, Tomato & Horseradish, Asda*	1 Pack/168.9g	255	151	10.0	22.0	2.6	2.7
Beef, Topside, Deli*	1 Serving/191g	447	234	15.4	18.3	11.0	0.0
Big Three, Iceland*	1 Pack/246.3g	637	259	10.6	20.8	14.9	1.7
Breakfast Special, Fulfilled*	1 Pack/218g	483	222	10.0	18.6	11.5	0.0
Breakfast, Big, Gourmet, Felix Van Den Berghe*	1 Serving/235.4g	691	294	10.6	23.2	16.0	0.0
Breakfast, Mega Triple, Co-Op*	1 Pack/267g	750	281	11.6	25.5	15.0	3.4
Brie, & Grape, Finest, Tesco*	1 Pack/209g	527	252	8.5	20.6	15.1	1.5
Brie, With Apple & Grapes, Sainsbury's*	1 Pack/220g	473	215	8.2	20.8	11.0	0.0
Brunch, Eat Smart, Safeway*	1 Pack/250g	363	145	9.4	21.6	1.9	2.9
Brunch, St Ivel*	1 Pack/225g	581	258	10.2	26.0	12.6	0.0
Brunch, Triple, Sainsbury's*	1 Serving/241g	567	235	10.5	25.6	10.2	0.0
Cheddar, & Celery, Marks & Spencer*	1 Pack/200g	540	270	9.7	22.4	15.9	1.5
Cheddar, & Coleslaw, Simply, Boots*	1 Pack/185g	538	291	9.2	23.0	18.0	1.8
Cheddar, & Ham, British, Marks & Spencer*	1 Serving/164.6g	396	240	15.1	20.0	11.3	1.7
Cheddar, & Ham, Oldfields*	1 Pack/246.0g	674	274	11.7	20.5	16.1	2.0
Cheddar, & Ham, Platter, Marks & Spencer*	1/4 Sandwich/41.7g	101	240	15.1	20.0	11.3	1.7
Cheddar, & Ham, Smoked, Deep Filled, Tesco*	1 Serving/203.2g	572	282	14.3	19.5	16.3	1.2
Cheddar, & Ham, With Pickle, Smoked, Finest, Tesco*	1 Pack/217.1g	532	245	11.9	23.7	11.4	3.9
Cheddar, & Pickle, Mature, Sainsbury's*	1 Pack/171g	588	344	14.3	38.7	15.8	7.0
Cheddar, & Salad, Mature, Upper Crust*	1 Pack/225.1g	466	207	9.5	20.3	9.8	0.0
Cheddar, & Tomato, Mature, Big, Sainsbury's*	1 Pack/233g	596	256	12.9	26.3	11.0	0.0
Cheddar, & Tomato, Red, Tesco*	1 Pack/182g	526	289	9.2	24.0	17.4	1.1
Cheddar, Oldfields*	1 Pack/121.1g	384	317	12.8	33.2	14.3	1.5
Cheddar, Red Leicester, & Onion, Tesco*	1 Pack/182g	604	332	11.0	23.8	21.4	2.5
Cheese, & Apple & Grape, COU, Marks & Spencer*	1 Pack/186.2g	270	145	8.5	24.9	1.2	2.0
Cheese, & Apple, & Celery, Asda*	1 Pack/173.0g	244	141	8.0	21.0	2.8	2.7
Cheese, & Celery, Marks & Spencer*	1 Pack/180g	466	259	10.8	14.7	17.4	2.9
Cheese, & Celery, Shapers, Boots*	1 Pack/181g	288	159	11.0	24.0	2.3	3.0
Cheese, & Coleslaw, Asda*	1 Pack/262g	799	305	10.1	22.1	19.6	3.3
Cheese, & Coleslaw, Eat Smart, Safeway*	1 Pack/169.0g	245	145	10.1	20.7	2.2	4.0

S

SANDWICH

INFO/WEIGHT	Measure	per Measure KCAL	Nutrition Values per 100g / 100ml KCAL	PROT	CARB	FAT	FIBRE
Cheese, & Coleslaw, Marks & Spencer*	1 Pack/186g	498	268	10.2	17.6	17.4	3.2
Cheese, & Coleslaw, Shapers, Boots*	1 Pack/224g	338	151	11.0	22.0	2.1	3.2
Cheese, & Coleslaw, Sutherland*	1 Pack/185g	376	203	10.7	29.9	4.5	0.0
Cheese, & Ham, & Pickle, Healthy Living, Tesco*	1 Pack/201.3g	312	155	13.1	21.0	2.1	1.7
Cheese, & Ham, & Pickle, Simply, Boots*	1 Pack/225g	551	245	11.0	21.0	13.0	2.4
Cheese, & Ham, & Pickle, Tesco*	1 Serving/215g	497	231	11.7	20.3	11.5	1.8
Cheese, & Ham, Eat Smart, Safeway*	1 Pack/170g	254	149	12.5	19.2	2.5	4.1
Cheese, & Ham, Smoked, Tesco*	1 Pack/204g	620	304	14.1	19.7	18.7	1.6
Cheese, & Marmite, No Mayonnaise, Boots*	1 Pack/156g	420	269	12.2	26.3	12.8	1.7
Cheese, & Onion, Deep Fill, Tesco*	1 Pack/212g	742	350	12.3	20.2	24.5	1.3
Cheese, & Onion, GFY, Asda*	1 Pack/156g	253	162	13.0	23.0	2.0	0.0
Cheese, & Onion, Good Intentions, Somerfield*	1 Pack/171.9g	294	171	10.8	24.8	3.2	2.1
Cheese, & Onion, Healthy Living, Tesco	1 Pack/168g	314	187	10.3	23.2	5.9	1.7
Cheese, & Onion, Heinz*	1 Pack/197g	563	286	11.2	24.0	16.1	3.2
Cheese, & Onion, Tesco*	1 Pack/178g	621	349	11.5	17.1	26.1	2.2
Cheese, & Onion, Triple, Tesco*	1 Pack/273g	906	332	11.0	23.8	21.4	2.5
Cheese, & Onion, Waitrose*	1 Pack/176g	579	329	12.5	20.2	22.0	2.8
Cheese, & Pickle, & Tomato, Somerfield*	1 Pack/166.5g	317	191	12.5	25.6	4.3	3.5
Cheese, & Pickle, BHS*	1 Pack/177.7g	504	283	12.5	29.6	12.7	1.8
Cheese, & Pickle, Heinz*	1 Pack/178g	543	305	13.8	28.4	15.1	3.8
Cheese, & Pickle, Shapers, Boots*	1 Pack/165g	342	207	9.8	31.0	4.9	2.3
Cheese, & Pickle, Tesco*	1 Pack/140g	400	286	12.7	27.8	13.8	1.4
Cheese, & Pickle, Virgin Trains*	1 Sandwich/158g	444	281	11.5	31.1	12.4	0.0
Cheese, & Salad, & Reduced Fat Mayonnaise, Waitrose*	1 Pack/180g	301	167	9.8	20.8	5.0	3.1
Cheese, & Salad, Budgens*	1 Pack/168.9g	250	148	10.9	21.9	1.8	1.6
Cheese, & Salad, COU, Marks & Spencer*	1 Pack/188g	244	130	12.1	17.0	1.6	2.4
Cheese, & Salad, Shapers, Boots*	1 Pack/205g	308	150	9.7	22.0	2.5	2.2
Cheese, & Salad, Tesco*	1 Serving/188g	429	228	10.1	20.2	11.9	2.1
Cheese, & Spring Onion, Asda*	1 Pack/159.6g	578	361	13.0	21.0	25.0	1.9
Cheese, & Spring Onion, Mixed, Scottish Slimmers*	1 Pack/139.3g	297	214	12.4	26.5	6.5	2.1
Cheese, & Spring Onion, Sainsbury's*	1 Serving/177g	605	342	11.4	24.0	22.3	1.1
Cheese, & Tomato, Asda*	1 Pack/154g	388	252	11.0	23.2	12.8	3.7
Cheese, & Tomato, Freshmans*	1 Pack/111g	248	223	11.0	8.0	16.8	0.0
Cheese, & Tomato, Ginsters*	1 Serving/176.2g	451	256	8.8	27.3	12.4	0.0
Cheese, & Tomato, Organic, Marks & Spencer*	1 Pack/165g	559	339	11.8	24.8	21.4	1.9
Cheese, & Tomato, Sainsbury's*	1 Pack/215.9g	542	251	12.9	22.8	12.2	0.0
Cheese, & Tomato, Tesco*	1 Pack/182g	582	320	9.2	22.6	21.4	1.1
Cheese, Asda*	1 Pack/262g	618	236	12.2	20.3	12.0	3.0
Cheese, Crunch, Scottish Slimmers*	1 Pack/137.1g	292	213	11.0	27.6	6.6	2.3
Cheese, Ham, BLT, Triple Pack, Asda*	1 Pack/260g	614	236	12.2	20.3	12.0	3.0
Cheese, Savoury, Northern Bites*	1 Serving/210g	212	101	3.6	18.5	1.9	0.0
Cheese, Savoury, Sandwich King*	1 Pack/135.2g	328	243	11.6	30.2	8.3	0.0
Cheese, Smoked, Folded Focaccia, TTD, Sainsbury's*	1/4 Focaccia/220g	607	276	13.1	34.6	9.4	2.9
Cheese, Three, & Onion, Boots*	1 Pack/169g	566	335	11.0	28.0	20.0	1.9
Cheese, Three, & Onion, New Style, Weight Watchers*	1 Pack/148g	275	186	14.8	26.2	2.4	1.4
Cheese, Three, & Spring Onion, Shell*	1 Pack/168g	672	400	11.1	20.8	30.3	0.0
Chicken & Salad, Ham & Cheese, Twin, Tesco*	1 Pack/189g	434	230	10.8	21.1	11.4	2.3
Chicken, & Avocado, Tesco*	1 Serving/219.2g	558	255	11.9	19.5	14.4	2.4
Chicken, & Bacon & Tomato, Paprika, Shapers, Boots*	1 Pack/184g	296	161	11.0	19.0	4.6	2.3
Chicken, & Bacon, & Lettuce, Tesco*	1 Pack/195g	515	264	15.4	16.0	15.4	1.6
Chicken, & Bacon, & Salad, Big, Sainsbury's*	1 Pack/249g	610	245	11.1	21.7	12.7	0.0
Chicken, & Bacon, BGTY, Sainsbury's*	1 Pack/211.4g	314	149	11.7	20.8	2.3	0.0
Chicken, & Bacon, Baton, Tesco*	1 Pack/201g	511	254	9.4	24.7	13.1	1.7

SANDWICH

	INFO/WEIGHT	KCAL	KCAL	PROT	CARB	FAT	FIBRE
Chicken, & Bacon, Big Fill, Somerfield*	1 Pack/209.6g	567	270	12.0	25.0	13.5	2.3
Chicken, & Bacon, COU, Marks & Spencer*	1 Pack/178g	276	155	13.0	21.6	1.5	1.9
Chicken, & Bacon, Chunky, Heinz*	1 Pack/168.1g	506	301	12.7	26.8	15.9	4.7
Chicken, & Bacon, Deep Filled, Eat Street, Safeway*	1 Pack/206.5g	476	230	14.6	23.6	8.5	1.9
Chicken, & Bacon, Deep Filled, Ginsters*	1 Pack/200g	540	270	13.1	18.3	16.1	0.0
Chicken, & Bacon, Good Intentions, Somerfield*	1 Pack/209g	335	160	11.9	19.9	3.4	2.7
Chicken, & Bacon, Healthy Living, Tesco*	1 Sandwich/193g	301	156	13.9	20.8	2.0	1.3
Chicken, & Bacon, Marks & Spencer*	1 Pack/173g	400	231	17.7	6.4	14.9	5.5
Chicken, & Bacon, Mattessons*	1 Pack/190g	604	318	13.3	26.0	17.9	1.1
Chicken, & Bacon, Roast, Boots*	1 Pack/250g	599	240	11.6	16.8	14.0	1.4
Chicken, & Bacon, Roast, Marks & Spencer*	1 Pack/173.1g	450	260	14.1	23.8	12.1	3.4
Chicken, & Bacon, Roast, Sainsbury's*	1 Pack/167g	433	259	14.1	18.6	14.2	0.0
Chicken, & Bacon, Sainsbury's*	1 Pack/214.9g	574	267	12.6	25.0	13.0	1.3
Chicken, & Bacon, Shapers, Boots*	1 Pack/179g	317	177	14.0	19.0	5.0	3.1
Chicken, & Bacon, Sutherland*	1 Pack/170.9g	535	313	15.3	21.4	18.4	0.0
Chicken, & Bacon, Tesco*	1 Pack/195g	493	253	14.3	21.0	12.4	1.7
Chicken, & Bcaon, On Pepper Bread, Marks & Spencer*	1 Serving/176.7g	266	150	13.2	22.7	0.9	2.1
Chicken, & Chorizo, Sainsbury's*	1 Serving/215g	432	201	10.9	17.0	9.9	3.4
Chicken, & Coleslaw, Roast, Sainsbury's*	1 Pack/186g	348	187	11.4	21.0	7.9	0.0
Chicken, & Coriander, Taste!*	1 Serving/159.4g	227	143	5.6	23.3	2.9	0.0
Chicken, & Coriander, With Lime, BGTY, Sainsbury's*	1 Pack/168g	282	168	10.6	23.5	3.5	0.0
Chicken, & Ham, Healthy Living, Tesco*	1 Serving/244g	327	134	13.2	17.9	1.1	1.3
Chicken, & Ham, Oak Smoked, Big, Sainsbury's*	1 Pack/244g	461	189	12.3	18.8	7.2	0.0
Chicken, & Ham, Roast, Ginsters*	1 Pack/180g	425	236	11.2	18.5	13.6	0.0
Chicken, & Ham, Roast, Tesco*	1 Pack/228g	561	246	13.3	16.6	14.0	1.2
Chicken, & Mayo, The Sandwich Company*	1 Pack/72g	251	348	17.8	35.9	14.8	0.0
Chicken, & Mayonnaise, Simply, Oldfields*	1 Pack/128g	357	279	12.8	30.2	12.8	2.1
Chicken, & Pepperonata, COU, Marks & Spencer*	1 Pack/171.4g	239	140	10.4	20.9	1.7	1.3
Chicken, & Pesto, Shapers, Boots*	1 Pack/181g	311	172	12.0	26.0	2.3	1.7
Chicken, & Pesto, With Rocket, Woolworths*	1 Pack/195g	326	167	5.0	16.9	8.8	0.0
Chicken, & Roasted Peppers, Chargrilled, BHS*	1 Pack/183.2g	295	161	11.5	22.0	3.1	3.1
Chicken, & Salad With Mayo, Roast, Big, Sainsbury's*	1 Pack/268.8g	560	208	11.0	20.9	8.9	9.0
Chicken, & Salad, BGTY, Sainsbury's*	1 Pack/197g	278	141	10.3	18.6	3.0	0.0
Chicken, & Salad, Bernard Matthews*	1 Pack/162g	269	166	7.0	22.7	5.2	0.0
Chicken, & Salad, Best For You, BHS*	1 Pack/315g	992	315	23.2	43.1	5.3	3.3
Chicken, & Salad, Big Fill, Somerfield*	1 Pack/247.8g	513	207	11.5	20.4	8.8	2.0
Chicken, & Salad, Big, Marks & Spencer*	1 Pack/283g	509	180	9.8	19.4	7.3	1.5
Chicken, & Salad, COU, Marks & Spencer*	1 Pack/194g	262	135	9.8	19.0	1.9	1.6
Chicken, & Salad, Co-Op*	1 Pack/195g	449	230	10.0	24.0	11.0	2.0
Chicken, & Salad, Daily Bread*	1 Serving/187g	322	172	8.9	19.5	6.9	0.0
Chicken, & Salad, Deep Filled, Safeway*	1 Pack/211.9g	445	210	11.0	21.1	8.8	3.7
Chicken, & Salad, Deep Filled, Tesco*	1 Pack/237.8g	440	185	13.1	14.6	8.2	2.8
Chicken, & Salad, Deli-Lite, Brambles*	1 Pack/175.2g	268	153	11.7	23.7	1.3	2.0
Chicken, & Salad, Eat Smart, Safeway*	1 Pack/183g	265	145	13.7	17.1	2.3	0.8
Chicken, & Salad, Eat Street, Safeway*	1 Pack/200g	330	165	10.3	22.2	3.4	1.8
Chicken, & Salad, GFY, Asda*	1 Pack/194g	239	123	11.0	19.0	0.9	2.8
Chicken, & Salad, Good Intentions, Somerfield*	1 Pack/186g	294	158	10.4	23.5	2.5	1.5
Chicken, & Salad, Healthy Choice, Safeway*	1 Pack/185g	287	155	10.7	20.5	3.4	1.9
Chicken, & Salad, Healthy Eating, Tesco*	1 serving/200g	510	255	20.7	32.4	4.8	7.7
Chicken, & Salad, Healthy Living, Tesco*	1 Pack/195g	257	132	10.7	16.8	2.5	4.0
Chicken, & Salad, Heinz*	1 Pack/165.5g	332	200	8.6	19.9	9.6	2.0
Chicken, & Salad, Low Fat, Heinz*	1 Pack/166g	246	148	11.8	22.3	1.3	5.3
Chicken, & Salad, Low Fat, Waitrose*	1 Pack/188g	291	155	10.4	18.6	4.3	2.1

S

SANDWICH

INFO/WEIGHT	Measure	per Measure KCAL	KCAL	PROT	CARB	FAT	FIBRE
Chicken, & Salad, Marks & Spencer*	1 Pack/200g	408	204	9.2	17.6	10.8	1.5
Chicken, & Salad, Mattessons*	1 Pack/193g	313	162	11.2	18.8	4.7	2.8
Chicken, & Salad, Millers*	1 Pack/200g	310	155	11.3	16.3	4.9	0.0
Chicken, & Salad, Montagu's*	1 Pack/162g	275	170	10.5	20.9	5.3	0.0
Chicken, & Salad, On Malted Bread With Mayo, Safeway*	1 Pack/195g	392	201	10.9	18.7	9.2	2.1
Chicken, & Salad, Roast, BGTY, Sainsbury's*	1 Pack/204g	298	146	10.4	21.0	2.3	2.0
Chicken, & Salad, Roast, COU, Marks & Spencer*	1 Pack/196g	265	135	8.9	19.6	2.3	2.2
Chicken, & Salad, Roast, Feel Good, Shell*	1 Pack/190.6g	327	171	9.8	22.4	4.7	0.0
Chicken, & Salad, Roast, Finest, Tesco*	1 Pack/237g	593	250	11.0	22.7	12.8	1.7
Chicken, & Salad, Roast, Marks & Spencer*	1 Pack/200g	430	215	8.5	19.5	9.5	2.6
Chicken, & Salad, Roast, Shapers, Boots*	1 Pack/230g	308	134	11.0	17.0	2.5	3.7
Chicken, & Salad, Roast, Waitrose*	1 Pack/217g	482	222	9.4	21.1	11.1	2.0
Chicken, & Salad, Roast, Weight Watchers*	1 Pack/186g	266	143	10.3	15.8	4.3	2.8
Chicken, & Salad, Sainsbury's*	1 Pack/240.1g	425	177	12.1	18.8	5.9	0.0
Chicken, & Salad, Sandwich King*	1 Pack/228g	534	234	11.9	26.8	8.6	0.0
Chicken, & Salad, Shell*	1 Pack/201.0g	404	201	8.7	19.4	9.8	0.0
Chicken, & Salad, Tesco*	1 Pack/193g	386	200	11.9	17.6	9.1	1.5
Chicken, & Salad, Waitrose*	1 Pack/208g	406	195	10.3	17.1	9.5	2.5
Chicken, & Salad, Wild Bean Cafe*	1 Pack/210g	273	130	12.4	18.9	0.5	2.8
Chicken, & Salad, With Mayo, Yummies*	1 Packet/154.5g	274	178	11.9	17.8	6.6	0.0
Chicken, & Salad, With Mayo. BGTY, Sainsbury's*	1 Serving/200g	314	157	12.0	21.9	2.4	0.0
Chicken, & Stuffing, Co-Op*	1 Pack/201g	503	250	12.0	22.0	13.0	3.0
Chicken, & Stuffing, Roast, Boots*	1 Pack/234.7g	670	285	12.0	22.0	17.0	1.9
Chicken, & Stuffing, Roast, Deep Fill, Tesco*	1 Serving/220g	532	242	14.0	19.0	12.2	1.3
Chicken, & Stuffing, Roast, Marks & Spencer*	1 Pack/182g	557	306	14.3	25.4	16.6	3.2
Chicken, & Stuffing, Roast, Tesco*	1 Pack/164g	313	191	14.6	20.3	5.7	1.7
Chicken, & Stuffing, Shapers, Boots*	1 Serving/184.7g	327	177	13.0	25.0	2.8	2.2
Chicken, & Stuffing, Tesco*	1 Pack/323g	1043	323	10.4	29.4	18.2	1.0
Chicken, & Sweetcorn, Marks & Spencer*	1 Pack/186g	363	195	12.7	22.8	5.7	4.0
Chicken, & Sweetcorn, Shapers, Boots*	1 Pack/180g	324	180	12.0	25.0	3.5	2.0
Chicken, & Sweetcorn, Tesco*	1 Pack/194g	411	212	13.2	20.1	8.7	3.0
Chicken, & Sweetcorn, With Mayo, Benedicts*	1 Pack/185g	437	236	12.2	20.6	10.7	0.0
Chicken, & Tomato Relish, Chargrilled, Shapers, Boots*	1 Pack/190g	295	155	12.0	20.0	3.0	3.1
Chicken, & Tomato Salsa, Chargrilled, BGTY, Sainsbury's*	1 Pack/225g	218	97	1.5	15.9	1.8	2.9
Chicken, & Tomatoes, Roast, COU, Marks & Spencer*	1 Pack/195g	273	140	12.0	21.7	2.1	4.2
Chicken, & Watercress, BGTY, Sainsbury's*	1 Pack/170g	284	167	14.2	22.9	2.1	2.0
Chicken, & Watercress, COU, Marks & Spencer*	1 Pack/164g	266	162	12.8	23.9	1.7	2.1
Chicken, & Watercress, Chargrilled, BGTY, Sainsbury's*	1 Pack/172g	318	185	14.5	24.1	3.4	0.0
Chicken, & Watercress, Healthy Eating, Tesco*	1 Pack/160g	253	158	13.8	21.7	1.8	1.7
Chicken, Asian, Shapers, Boots*	1 Pack/189.6g	274	144	12.0	19.0	2.4	2.9
Chicken, BBQ, & Ranch Coleslaw, Big, Sainsbury's*	1 Pack/276.6g	474	171	9.2	22.7	4.8	0.0
Chicken, BBQ, On Malted Bread, Fresh Bite*	1 Pack/225.8g	341	151	9.0	23.4	2.4	0.0
Chicken, BLT, Daily Bread*	1 Pack/187.2g	322	172	9.0	19.5	7.0	0.0
Chicken, BLT, Taste!*	1 Pack/238.5g	459	192	10.3	19.0	8.3	0.0
Chicken, Bacon & Avocado, Finest, Tesco*	1 Pack/208g	516	248	12.2	19.3	13.5	1.9
Chicken, Bacon & Sweet Chilli, Feel Good, Shell*	1 Pack/173.5g	365	211	14.1	29.2	5.0	0.0
Chicken, Bacon & Tomato, BGTY, Sainsbury's*	1 Pack/190g	270	142	11.4	19.0	2.3	0.0
Chicken, Bacon, & Avocado, Ultimate, Marks & Spencer*	1 Pack/241g	552	229	10.7	17.9	12.7	2.8
Chicken, Basil & Sunblush Tomato, Harry Mason*	1 Pack/163.9g	272	166	13.0	21.8	3.2	0.6
Chicken, Bechamel & Leek, Daily Bread*	1 Pack/210.4g	382	182	11.0	26.8	3.4	0.0
Chicken, Beef, & Ham, Triple Pack, Tesco*	1 Serving/272g	583	214	12.1	24.3	7.6	2.0
Chicken, Breast, BGTY, Sainsbury's*	1 Pack/165g	251	152	12.2	24.7	0.5	0.0
Chicken, Caesar, & Bacon, Club, TTD, Sainsbury's*	1 Pack/246.6g	662	268	14.0	21.2	14.1	0.0

S

SANDWICH

INFO/WEIGHT	Measure	per Measure KCAL	Nutrition Values per 100g / 100ml				
			KCAL	PROT	CARB	FAT	FIBRE
Chicken, Caesar, & Salad, GFY, Asda*	1 Pack/163g	289	177	11.0	27.0	2.8	2.1
Chicken, Caesar, & Salad, Sainsbury's*	1 Pack/186g	299	161	11.2	20.4	3.8	0.0
Chicken, Caesar, Boots*	1 Pack/226.0g	531	235	9.8	22.0	12.0	1.7
Chicken, Caesar, COU, Marks & Spencer*	1 Pack/181g	244	135	12.2	19.9	2.4	4.3
Chicken, Caesar, Chargrilled, Big, Sainsbury's*	1 Pack/216g	657	304	12.2	25.3	17.1	0.0
Chicken, Caesar, Finest, Tesco*	1 Pack/199g	454	228	15.4	19.2	10.0	1.4
Chicken, Caesar, The Best, Safeway*	1 Pack/198g	505	255	14.3	20.8	12.3	2.6
Chicken, Chargrilled, Ginsters*	1 Pack/209g	431	206	11.3	21.6	8.3	0.0
Chicken, Chargrilled, Go Foods Ltd*	1 Pack/331g	695	210	14.5	29.0	4.1	0.0
Chicken, Chargrilled, No Mayo, Rustlers*	1 Pack/150g	228	152	16.0	20.1	0.8	0.0
Chicken, Chargrilled, Pitta Pocket, Marks & Spencer*	1 Pack/208g	279	134	11.2	14.5	3.5	1.6
Chicken, Cheese, Bacon, Big, Sainsbury's*	1 Pack/254g	734	289	11.7	18.0	17.9	0.0
Chicken, Cheese, Bacon, Triple, BGTY, Sainsbury's*	1 Pack/263g	534	203	11.7	19.4	7.6	4.4
Chicken, Chilli, Fresh, Taste!*	1 Pack/154.5g	223	145	5.6	23.4	3.2	0.0
Chicken, Chinese, Esso*	1 Pack/177.8g	409	230	13.0	22.8	9.0	4.0
Chicken, Chinese, Low Calorie, Tesco*	1 Pack/169g	270	160	11.8	22.6	2.5	2.0
Chicken, Chinese, Malted Brown Bread, Waitrose*	1 Pack/164g	333	203	13.5	21.9	6.8	3.3
Chicken, Chinese, Treat Yourself, Shell*	1 Pack/178g	409	230	13.0	22.8	9.6	0.0
Chicken, Coronation, Marks & Spencer*	1 Pack/210g	420	200	11.2	20.2	9.7	3.1
Chicken, Coronation, Indulgence, Taste*	1 Pack/159.0g	396	249	9.1	26.5	11.8	0.0
Chicken, Coronation, Taste*	1 Pack/178.2g	367	206	10.6	24.0	7.5	0.0
Chicken, Coronation, Woolworths*	1 Serving/159g	396	249	9.1	26.5	11.8	0.0
Chicken, Creole, & Italian Leaves, Northern Bites*	1 Pack/189.8g	298	157	13.1	22.1	2.4	2.4
Chicken, Curry, Lifestyle*	1 Serving/160g	211	132	13.0	6.0	6.0	0.0
Chicken, Eat Smart, Safeway*	1 Pack/141g	240	170	14.9	22.2	2.0	0.6
Chicken, Flame Grilled, Rustlers*	1 Pack/150g	347	231	16.3	20.1	9.5	0.0
Chicken, Ham, Prawn, Triple Pack, Healthy Living, Tesco*	1 Pack/246.5g	349	142	10.7	20.2	2.1	2.2
Chicken, Harvester, Taste!*	1 Pack/200g	295	148	7.7	20.3	4.0	0.0
Chicken, Healthier Choice, Ginsters*	1 Pack/183g	247	135	10.2	20.5	1.4	0.0
Chicken, Healthy, BHS*	1 Pack/250g	393	157	10.9	20.5	3.5	3.1
Chicken, Honey & Mustard, BGTY, Sainsbury's*	1 Pack/171g	296	173	13.1	24.0	2.7	0.0
Chicken, Honey & Mustard, On Softgrain Bread, Tasties*	1 Pack/152g	304	200	14.4	28.5	3.3	0.0
Chicken, Honey & Mustard, Safeway*	1 Pack/167g	399	239	12.7	23.6	10.4	2.5
Chicken, Jalfrezi, Naan, Ready To Go, Marks & Spencer*	1 Pack/288g	576	200	9.8	26.3	6.3	2.9
Chicken, Kashmir, French Cuisiniers*	1 Pack/145g	204	141	12.9	20.3	1.6	2.9
Chicken, Lemon, & Relish, Perfectly Balanced, Waitrose*	1 Pack/151g	243	161	12.3	21.4	2.9	3.5
Chicken, Lemon, &With Mint, Brambles*	1 Pack/161.0g	338	210	13.4	24.6	5.4	3.2
Chicken, Lime & Coriander, BP*	1 Pack/154.5g	291	189	12.5	25.2	4.2	0.0
Chicken, Low Fat, BHS*	1 Pack/200g	336	168	11.0	20.7	4.6	3.0
Chicken, Mexican, Healthy Choices, Shell*	1 Serving/167.9g	376	224	12.2	28.1	7.0	0.0
Chicken, Moroccan, Sainsbury's*	1/2 Pack/99.5g	184	186	10.6	27.9	3.6	0.0
Chicken, No Mayo, Cafe Revive, Marks & Spencer*	1 Pack/153g	230	150	14.1	17.9	2.4	3.1
Chicken, No Mayo, Daily Bread*	1 Pack/160.3g	278	174	8.6	23.8	4.4	0.0
Chicken, No Mayo, Marks & Spencer*	1 Pack/142g	220	155	15.0	17.5	3.0	3.1
Chicken, No Mayo, Roast, COU, Marks & Spencer*	1 Serving/147g	250	170	14.5	21.1	2.6	1.4
Chicken, No Mayonnaise, Waitrose*	1 Pack/173g	332	192	11.6	24.0	5.5	2.1
Chicken, Oriental, Triple, Shapers, Boots*	1 Pack/215g	398	185	12.0	22.0	5.4	2.6
Chicken, Pesano Pesto, Brambles*	1 Pack/417g	826	198	10.8	24.0	6.3	1.5
Chicken, Prawn Mayo, Mixed, Shapers, Boots*	1 Pack/220g	416	189	12.0	20.0	6.8	2.8
Chicken, Red Thai, BGTY, Sainsbury's*	1 pack/195g	326	167	11.3	26.4	1.9	0.0
Chicken, Red Thai, Taste!*	1 Pack/164g	335	204	11.5	26.1	6.0	0.0
Chicken, Roast, Breast, BGTY, Sainsbury's*	1 Pack/174g	275	158	14.8	20.9	2.5	1.8
Chicken, Roast, Healthy Living, Tesco*	1 Pack/155.1g	288	186	13.5	25.4	3.4	1.4

S

SANDWICH

	Measure INFO/WEIGHT	per Measure KCAL	KCAL	PROT	CARB	FAT	FIBRE
Chicken, Roast, No Mayo, COU, Marks & Spencer*	1 Pack/160.6g	244	151	14.2	18.6	2.3	1.8
Chicken, Roast, Shapers, Boots*	1 Pack/163g	259	159	16.0	21.0	1.3	2.5
Chicken, Roast, Tesco*	1 Pack/158g	412	261	13.1	23.9	12.5	1.5
Chicken, Roast, Triple, Perfectly Balanced, Waitrose*	1 Pack/254g	356	140	8.7	19.2	3.2	2.8
Chicken, Rustlers*	1 Pack/150g	347	231	16.3	20.1	9.5	0.0
Chicken, Safeway*	1 Serving/200g	350	175	10.7	20.6	5.6	2.5
Chicken, Salad, Chargrilled, Weight Watchers*	1 Pack/186g	296	159	9.9	20.4	4.2	1.9
Chicken, Sesame, Sainsbury's*	1 Pack/191g	397	208	9.8	23.7	8.2	2.4
Chicken, Shell*	1 Pack/121g	334	276	13.9	25.9	13.0	0.0
Chicken, Simply, Eat Smart, Safeway*	1 Pack/147g	250	170	14.5	23.0	2.2	1.4
Chicken, Simply, Healthy Selection, Budgens*	1 Pack/148.2g	286	193	14.3	28.4	2.5	2.1
Chicken, Smokey, BGTY, Sainsbury's*	1 Pack/178g	276	155	11.1	25.6	1.0	0.0
Chicken, Southern Fried Breast, Microwave, Tesco*	1 Burger/135g	381	282	13.0	28.9	12.7	1.6
Chicken, Southern Fried, Rustlers*	1 Serving/145g	436	301	11.7	30.6	14.7	0.0
Chicken, Southern Spiced, Marks & Spencer*	1 Pack/179g	421	235	11.2	21.7	13.0	3.1
Chicken, Spicy, Deep Filled, Co-Op*	1 Pack/216g	421	195	10.0	24.0	7.0	3.0
Chicken, Sundried Tomato & Herb, Bells*	1 Pack/198g	400	202	10.2	18.9	9.5	0.0
Chicken, Sutherland*	1 Pack/220g	465	211	10.4	22.9	8.7	0.0
Chicken, Tandoori, Finest, Tesco*	1 Pack/224g	421	188	10.8	19.2	7.5	1.4
Chicken, Tangy Lime & Ginger, Shapers, Boots*	1 Pack/168g	319	190	12.0	21.0	6.4	5.1
Chicken, Thai, BGTY, Sainsbury's*	1 Pack/195.8g	280	143	10.2	19.6	2.6	0.6
Chicken, Thai, Tesco*	1 Pack/244g	634	260	8.5	21.1	15.7	1.5
Chicken, Tikka Masala, Go Foods Ltd*	1 Pack/136g	343	252	11.4	23.5	12.8	0.0
Chicken, Tikka, & Yoghurt, Taste!*	1 Pack/215.3g	436	203	8.2	20.4	9.8	0.0
Chicken, Tikka, Asda*	1 Pack/186g	316	170	11.0	21.0	4.7	1.5
Chicken, Tikka, COU, Marks & Spencer*	1 Pack/185g	268	145	12.1	20.5	1.8	3.2
Chicken, Tikka, Eat Smart, Safeway*	1 Pack/159g	240	151	11.8	21.6	1.9	2.5
Chicken, Tikka, Garlic & Herb Bread Pocket, Somerfield*	1 Pack/168g	341	203	11.0	30.0	4.3	2.0
Chicken, Tikka, Healthy Eating, Tesco*	1 Pack/159g	270	170	14.5	21.9	2.7	1.8
Chicken, Tikka, Marks & Spencer*	1 Pack/180g	391	217	10.4	19.5	10.9	2.0
Chicken, Tikka, Naan, Ready To Go, Marks & Spencer*	1 Pack/298g	641	215	9.9	26.5	7.8	4.0
Chicken, Tikka, On Pepper Chilli Bread, Shapers, Boots*	1 Pack/172.1g	296	172	13.0	25.0	2.6	2.5
Chicken, Tikka, Open, COU, Marks & Spencer*	1 Pack/190g	260	137	9.6	21.8	1.2	2.2
Chicken, Tikka, Thai Style, Korma, Big, Sainsbury's*	1 Pack/268g	581	217	11.9	20.5	9.7	0.0
Chicken, Tikka, Weight Watchers*	1 Pack/158g	289	183	12.8	23.4	4.3	1.6
Chicken, Tomato & Basil, Healthy Eating, Tesco*	1 Pack/176g	266	151	11.5	21.1	2.3	2.0
Chicken, Triple, GFY, Asda*	1 Pack/230g	453	197	13.0	25.0	5.0	1.6
Chicken, Triple, Shapers, Boots*	1 Serving/228g	440	193	13.0	23.0	5.4	2.3
Chicken, Tzatziki, Perfectly Balanced, Waitrose*	1 Pack/189g	270	143	12.4	19.4	1.7	1.7
Chicken, With Fresh Herb Salad, Roast, British, Asda*	1 Pack/213.9g	447	209	11.0	21.0	9.0	2.0
Chicken, With Honey Mustard Mayo, Chargrilled, Spar*	1 Pack/168g	428	255	13.1	25.0	11.4	0.0
Chicken, With Mango, Chargrilled, TTD, Sainsbury's*	1 Pack/217g	352	162	11.0	22.2	3.2	0.0
Chicken, With Mayo, On Thick Softgrain, Tasties*	1 Pack/192g	338	176	9.5	16.1	7.9	0.0
Chicken, With Salad, Chargrilled, Debenhams*	1 Pack/250g	325	130	7.6	18.0	3.6	0.0
Christmas Special, Ginsters*	1 Pack/220g	583	265	9.5	23.2	15.6	0.0
Christmas, BGTY, Sainsbury's*	1 Pack/186.4g	370	199	14.6	27.3	3.5	0.0
Christmas, Shell*	1 Pack/182.7g	414	226	11.1	25.5	8.2	2.1
Christmas, Weight Watchers*	1 Pack/173.1g	296	171	12.2	28.8	2.8	2.1
Classic Feast, Marks & Spencer*	1 Serving/295g	841	285	10.6	21.3	17.5	4.7
Classic, Triple Pack, Somerfield*	1 Serving/250g	653	261	10.2	22.1	14.6	2.5
Club, New York Style, Sainsbury's*	1 Serving/212g	608	287	13.3	22.8	15.8	2.7
Corned Beef, & Tomato, & Onion, The Salad Garden*	1 Pack/137g	338	247	14.2	23.0	10.8	0.0
Corned Beef, On White, Simply, Brambles*	1 Pack/126g	325	258	14.2	30.8	8.6	1.4

SANDWICH

	INFO/WEIGHT	KCAL	KCAL	PROT	CARB	FAT	FIBRE
Cottage Cheese, & Tomato, Shapers, Boots*	1 Pack/150g	219	146	7.8	18.0	4.8	2.4
Crab, Marie Rose, Brown Bread, Royal London Hospital*	1 Pack/158g	293	185	9.7	22.0	7.1	0.0
Crayfish, & Lemon Mayonnaise, Daily Bread*	1 Pack/173.0g	391	226	9.5	31.0	6.6	0.0
Crayfish, & Rocket, Bistro, Waitrose*	1 Pack/192.7g	423	219	11.5	20.4	10.1	2.4
Crayfish, & Rocket, Go Eat*	1 Pack/163g	289	177	10.6	24.6	4.3	1.9
Crayfish, & Rocket, Shapers, Boots*	1 Pack/172.2g	291	169	11.0	26.0	2.2	2.5
Crayfish, & Rocket, So Good, Somerfield*	1 Pack/205.5g	486	237	9.5	25.8	10.6	1.0
Crayfish, With Lime & Chilli, Healthy Choice!, Shell*	1 Pack/162.6g	336	206	10.7	26.5	6.4	0.0
Cream Cheese, & Cucumber, Gourmet Express*	1 Pack/104g	267	257	8.9	39.5	7.0	0.0
Cream Cheese, & Ham, Tesco*	1 Pack/212g	655	309	11.0	27.2	17.3	1.2
Cream Cheese, & Peppers, Taste!*	1 Pack/154.2g	296	192	7.3	25.5	6.8	0.0
Cream Cheese, & Salad, The Sandwich Box*	1 Pack/138g	250	181	5.6	26.3	5.8	0.0
Cream Cheese, Red Pepper & Spinach, Daily Bread*	1 Pack/156g	273	175	7.4	24.0	5.2	0.0
Duck, Aromatic, Marks & Spencer*	1 Serving/186.8g	496	265	13.1	21.0	14.5	2.1
Duck, Peking, No Mayo, Boots*	1 Pack/221.7g	400	180	7.7	27.0	4.6	1.7
Edam, & Tomato, & Spring Onion, BHS*	1 Serving/184.1g	313	170	8.6	22.5	5.1	3.2
Edam, & Tomato, Low Fat, Oldfields*	1 Pack/172.9g	306	177	9.6	26.3	3.7	2.7
Edam, Oldfields*	1 Pack/175g	326	186	9.8	23.9	5.7	0.0
Egg Mayonaise, & Iceburg Lettuce, Northern Bites*	1 Serving/152.1g	333	219	7.7	20.9	11.3	0.0
Egg Mayonnaise, & Bacon, Boots*	1 Serving/200g	426	213	13.5	23.5	7.0	2.8
Egg Mayonnaise, & Cress, BHS*	1 Serving/187.8g	462	246	10.0	24.7	12.7	1.9
Egg Mayonnaise, & Cress, Go Simple, Asda*	1 Pack/169g	370	219	10.0	20.0	11.0	1.7
Egg Mayonnaise, & Cress, Millers*	1 Pack/166g	369	222	9.4	18.8	12.2	0.0
Egg Mayonnaise, & Cress, Reduced Fat, Waitrose*	1 Pack/162g	300	185	10.4	18.1	7.9	3.4
Egg Mayonnaise, & Cress, Shapers, Boots*	1 Pack/161g	296	184	11.0	26.0	4.4	1.9
Egg Mayonnaise, & Cress, Wheatgerm Bread, Asda*	1 Pack/158g	371	235	9.7	21.3	12.4	1.9
Egg Mayonnaise, & Cress, Wheatgerm, Tesco*	1 Pack/146g	368	252	9.8	18.4	15.5	1.3
Egg Mayonnaise, & Cress, Wholemeal Bread, Oldfields*	1 Pack/128g	301	235	9.7	24.0	11.2	3.6
Egg Mayonnaise, & Cress, Yummies*	1 Serving/149.8g	428	285	8.4	17.8	20.0	0.0
Egg Mayonnaise, & Gammon Ham, Strollers*	1 Pack/169.5g	399	236	13.0	20.5	11.4	0.0
Egg Mayonnaise, & Salad, Superdrug*	1 Pack/169g	286	169	7.6	18.3	7.3	2.4
Egg Mayonnaise, Boots*	1 Pack/183.6g	449	244	9.7	22.0	13.0	2.3
Egg Mayonnaise, Deep Fill, Benedicts*	1 Pack/195g	560	287	9.6	36.3	11.1	0.0
Egg Mayonnaise, Free Range, Finest, Tesco*	1 Pack/217g	412	190	10.9	16.8	8.8	2.3
Egg Mayonnaise, Good Intentions, Somerfield*	1 Pack/150.3g	263	175	10.8	23.7	4.1	3.0
Egg Mayonnaise, Healthy Living, Tesco*	1 Pack/162.2g	253	156	9.3	21.4	3.7	2.8
Egg Mayonnaise, On Hi Bran Bread, Ginsters*	1 Pack/143g	343	240	10.7	17.6	15.2	0.0
Egg Mayonnaise, On Malted Wheatgrain, Taste!*	1 Serving/169g	394	233	10.6	20.0	12.3	0.0
Egg Mayonnaise, Shell*	1 Pack/189g	522	276	9.8	24.7	15.4	0.0
Egg Mayonnaise, Simply, Boots*	1 Pack/181g	449	248	9.2	19.0	15.0	2.9
Egg Mayonnaise, Simply, Ginsters*	1 Pack/161g	309	192	8.5	24.1	6.8	0.0
Egg Mayonnaise, Snack & Shop, Esso*	1 Pack/240g	624	260	9.4	25.5	13.4	0.0
Egg Mayonnaise, Waitrose*	1 Pack/180g	396	220	10.1	19.1	11.4	3.4
Egg, & Bacon, & Lincolnshire Sausage, Waitrose*	1 Pack/249g	655	263	11.3	24.7	13.2	0.9
Egg, & Cress, BGTY, Sainsbury's*	1 Pack/166g	281	169	9.7	23.1	4.2	3.8
Egg, & Cress, COU, Marks & Spencer*	1 Pack/192g	240	125	9.8	15.5	2.7	2.8
Egg, & Cress, Deep Fill, Tesco*	1 Pack/218g	521	239	11.1	17.0	14.1	1.1
Egg, & Cress, Free Range, Marks & Spencer*	1 Pack/192g	307	160	10.7	17.8	4.7	3.0
Egg, & Cress, Free Range, Sainsbury's*	1 Pack/204g	404	198	10.5	20.3	8.3	3.3
Egg, & Cress, Free Range, Tesco*	1 Pack/195g	402	206	10.4	12.9	12.5	3.0
Egg, & Cress, Heinz*	1 Pack/162g	241	149	9.6	22.7	2.2	5.4
Egg, & Cress, Marks & Spencer*	1 Pack/182g	331	182	10.1	13.6	9.7	3.2
Egg, & Cress, Organic, Marks & Spencer*	1 Pack/185g	444	240	9.6	18.0	14.2	3.6

S

SANDWICH

INFO/WEIGHT	Measure	per Measure KCAL	KCAL	PROT	CARB	FAT	FIBRE
Egg, & Cress, Reduced Fat, Waitrose*	1 Pack/162g	262	162	9.7	16.5	6.4	6.4
Egg, & Cress, Sainsbury's*	1 Pack/170g	384	226	10.6	19.8	11.6	0.0
Egg, & Cress, Tesco*	1 Pack/174g	445	256	10.0	20.3	15.0	1.7
Egg, & Cress, White Batton, Sandwich King*	1 Sandwich/155g	387	250	8.1	25.3	13.7	0.0
Egg, & Gammon, Safeway*	1 Pack/233.3g	489	210	12.9	20.4	8.0	0.0
Egg, & Ham, Asda*	1 Pack/262g	590	225	10.4	16.8	12.8	2.1
Egg, & Salad, Deep Filled, Asda*	1 Pack/231g	395	171	8.0	19.0	7.0	1.0
Egg, & Salad, Free Range, Good Intentions, Somerfield*	1 Pack/173g	260	150	7.2	21.6	3.9	2.9
Egg, & Salad, Free Range, Sainsbury's*	1 Pack/224.5g	450	200	8.5	24.5	7.5	0.0
Egg, & Salad, GFY, Asda*	1 Pack/156.8g	229	146	8.0	22.0	2.9	2.9
Egg, & Salad, Healthy Living, Tesco*	1 Pack/182g	264	145	7.2	18.6	4.2	1.8
Egg, & Salad, Shapers, Boots*	1 Pack/184g	304	165	6.9	24.0	4.6	1.1
Egg, & Salad, Weight Watchers*	1 Pack/171.6g	255	148	7.5	22.8	3.0	1.4
Egg, & Salad, With Mayonnaise, Wholemeal, Waitrose*	1 Pack/180g	257	143	8.3	16.5	4.9	3.6
Egg, & Tomato, Deep Fill, Spar*	1 Serving/183.2g	348	190	8.2	22.8	7.4	0.0
Egg, & Tomato, On Softgrain Bread, Daily Bread*	1 Pack/160.3g	278	174	8.6	23.8	4.4	0.0
Egg, & Tomato, Organic, Waitrose*	1 Pack/192g	359	187	9.7	15.3	9.7	4.0
Egg, & Tomato, Tesco*	1 Pack/172g	311	181	8.5	22.6	6.3	2.3
Egg, & Tomato, With Salad Cream, Big, Sainsbury's*	1 Pack/266g	463	174	9.1	21.3	5.8	0.0
Egg, & Watercress, Free Range, Marks & Spencer*	1 Pack/191.9g	355	185	9.2	18.1	8.2	2.9
Egg, Co-Op*	1 Pack/190g	285	150	6.8	22.1	3.7	3.7
Egg, Old Fashioned, Brambles*	1 Pack/172.7g	247	143	6.9	26.1	1.2	1.9
Feta Cheese, & Salad, Taste*	1 Pack/178.2g	367	206	10.6	24.0	7.5	0.0
Feta Cheese, Bells*	1 Pack/222.9g	468	210	7.1	18.8	11.8	0.0
Gammon, & Salad, Tasties*	1 Pack/172g	261	152	9.6	20.6	3.5	0.0
Goat's Cheese, & Cranberry, Shapers, Boots*	1 Pack/149.7g	324	216	8.4	36.0	4.2	2.6
Goat's Cheese, & Sunblush Tomato, Pesto Mayo, Deli*	1 Pack/179.1g	480	268	9.5	20.5	16.4	0.0
Greek Salad, Classic, Cafe Primo*	1 Serving/215.5g	514	238	8.6	23.1	12.5	1.8
Greek Salad, Waitrose*	1 Serving/225.1g	376	167	6.2	17.2	8.1	2.2
Ham, & Coleslaw, Smoked, Brambles*	1 Pack/165.5g	282	171	8.2	28.8	2.5	1.8
Ham, & Dijon Mustard, Healthy Selection, Budgens*	1 Pack/120g	190	158	9.7	21.9	2.5	2.0
Ham, & Edam, Smoked, Shapers, Boots*	1 Pack/183g	315	172	9.3	19.0	6.5	2.7
Ham, & Mustard, Eat Smart, Safeway*	1 Pack/139g	250	180	13.7	26.3	2.2	2.0
Ham, & Mustard, Eat Street, Safeway*	1 Pack/150g	285	190	12.3	25.2	4.2	1.0
Ham, & Mustard, Heinz*	1 Pack/180.4g	459	255	11.8	25.6	11.5	5.0
Ham, & Mustard, Simply, Ginsters*	1 Pack/157.1g	399	254	11.7	23.5	12.6	0.0
Ham, & Mustard, Smoked, Sainsbury's*	1 Serving/160g	344	215	11.2	21.9	8.5	0.0
Ham, & Mustard, Smoked, Tesco*	1 Pack/156g	385	247	11.1	22.4	12.5	1.0
Ham, & Mustard, Tesco*	1 Pack/147g	437	297	10.6	20.8	19.0	1.2
Ham, & Pineapple Salsa, Maple Flavoured, Waitrose*	1 Pack/193.5g	330	170	8.4	23.8	4.6	3.1
Ham, & Salad, & Mustard, Darwins Deli*	1 Serving/180g	574	319	14.0	48.5	7.6	0.0
Ham, & Salad, Big Fill, Somerfield*	1 Pack/222g	515	232	9.4	22.9	11.4	2.3
Ham, & Salad, Brambles*	1 Serving/173g	289	167	10.1	23.2	3.9	1.2
Ham, & Salad, British, COU, Marks & Spencer*	1 Pack/183g	265	145	10.5	19.9	2.6	1.8
Ham, & Salad, British, Marks & Spencer*	1 Serving/182.8g	265	145	10.5	19.9	2.6	1.8
Ham, & Salad, Danish, COU, Marks & Spencer*	1 Pack/138g	181	131	9.3	17.4	2.7	1.9
Ham, & Salad, Danish, Lean, COU, Marks & Spencer*	1 Pack/182g	237	130	10.6	19.5	0.9	1.4
Ham, & Salad, Food Go*	1 Pack/177.8g	297	167	9.8	22.9	4.0	0.0
Ham, & Salad, Ginsters*	1 Pack/179g	287	161	8.9	23.6	3.5	0.0
Ham, & Salad, Good Intentions, Somerfield*	1 Pack/178g	287	161	9.5	23.8	3.1	1.1
Ham, & Salad, Healthy Living, Tesco*	1 pack/183.8g	272	148	9.7	23.3	1.7	1.4
Ham, & Salad, Healthy Options, Oldfields*	1 Pack/156g	229	147	8.7	24.0	1.9	0.0
Ham, & Salad, Healthy, Spar*	1 Serving/181g	286	158	8.4	22.7	3.7	0.0

S

SANDWICH

	Measure	per Measure KCAL		KCAL	PROT	CARB	FAT	FIBRE
Ham, & Salad, Leicester, Waitrose*	1 Serving/186.8g	325		174	8.6	24.0	4.8	1.6
Ham, & Salad, Select*	1 Serving/180g	266		148	8.0	23.2	2.6	0.0
Ham, & Salad, Shapers, Boots*	1 Pack/195g	269		138	9.4	22.0	1.4	1.8
Ham, & Salad, Smoked, Ainsley Harriott*	1 Pack/217.7g	307		141	8.9	19.9	2.9	0.0
Ham, & Salad, Smoked, Taste*	1 Serving/188g	309		164	9.8	19.8	5.2	0.0
Ham, & Salad, Smoked, Weight Watchers*	1 Pack/190.9g	252		132	10.2	19.1	1.6	3.5
Ham, & Salad, Snack & Shop, Esso*	1 Pack/191.2g	304		159	9.2	22.9	3.4	5.0
Ham, & Salad, Tesco*	1 Pack/183.8g	272		148	9.7	23.3	1.7	1.4
Ham, & Salad, Wild Bean Cafe*	1 Pack/212.0g	301		142	10.7	18.8	2.6	2.0
Ham, & Salad, With Mustard, Finest, Tesco*	1 Pack/200g	466		233	15.3	19.3	10.5	1.3
Ham, & Soft Cheese, Tesco*	1 Serving/164g	333		203	11.6	22.5	7.4	2.2
Ham, & Swiss Cheese, BIG, Sainsbury's*	1 Pack/218g	652		299	11.6	25.4	16.7	0.5
Ham, & Swiss Cheese, Marks & Spencer*	1 Pack/159g	393		247	14.7	18.9	12.6	3.3
Ham, & Swiss Cheese, Safeway*	1 Pack/201.1g	533		265	14.5	19.7	14.3	1.5
Ham, & Tomato, Brambles*	1 Pack/159.1g	288		181	11.1	24.1	4.6	3.3
Ham, & Tomato, GFY, Asda*	1 Pack/173g	254		147	10.0	23.0	1.7	1.4
Ham, & Tomato, Honey Roast, Feel Good, Shell*	1 Pack/170.9g	388		227	9.8	22.1	11.0	0.0
Ham, & Turkey, & Salad, Sutherland*	1 Pack/185g	303		164	9.8	25.2	2.6	0.0
Ham, & Turkey, Asda*	1 Pack/190g	393		207	12.9	15.8	10.2	2.3
Ham, & Turkey, Healthy, Felix Van Den Berghe*	1 Pack/148.6g	264		177	9.4	26.2	4.0	0.0
Ham, & Turkey, With Salad, Healthy Living, Co-Op*	1 Serving/181.3g	290		160	10.0	24.0	3.0	3.0
Ham, Asda*	1 Pack/262g	618		236	12.2	20.3	12.0	3.0
Ham, Beef, Chicken, Triple, Tesco*	1 Pack/272g	582		214	12.1	24.3	7.6	2.0
Ham, Cheese, & Pickle, BGTY, Sainsbury's*	1 Sandwich/198g	325		164	14.0	21.3	2.5	2.1
Ham, Cheese, & Pickle, Healthy Choice, Sutherland*	1 Pack/185g	368		199	13.4	27.4	4.0	0.0
Ham, Cheese, & Pickle, Healthy Living, Co-Op*	1 Pack/185g	370		200	13.0	27.0	4.0	3.0
Ham, Cheese, & Pickle, Heinz*	1 Pack/187.9g	466		248	11.3	21.7	12.9	4.8
Ham, Cheese, & Pickle, Leicester, Waitrose*	1 Pack/205g	513		250	11.9	23.7	11.9	2.1
Ham, Cheese, & Pickle, Marks & Spencer*	1 Pack/197g	459		233	13.0	15.9	13.1	2.4
Ham, Cheese, & Pickle, Platter, Marks & Spencer*	1/4 Sandwich/55.8g	146		260	11.9	19.3	14.9	5.3
Ham, Cheese, & Pickle, Taste!*	1 Pack/173.9g	414		238	11.1	20.3	12.5	0.0
Ham, Marks & Spencer*	1 Pack/200g	220		110	17.2	3.2	2.6	0.0
Ham, Smoked, Fresh, Taste!*	1 Pack/186.9g	286		153	9.1	18.4	4.8	0.0
Ham, Tomato, & Lettuce, Oldfields*	1 Pack/215.9g	393		182	12.3	19.0	8.1	3.5
Houmous, & Crunchy Salad, Oldfields*	1 Pack/180g	256		142	6.3	20.0	4.2	0.0
Houmous, Tomato, & Red Onion, Daily Bread*	1 Serving/184g	367		199	6.9	22.7	9.6	0.0
Indian Triple, Sainsbury's*	1 Serving/265.2g	549		207	12.8	25.2	6.1	0.0
King Prawn, & Wild Rocket, Honduran, Marks & Spencer*	1 Serving/195.7g	451		230	9.4	20.3	12.2	1.4
King Prawn, Sainsbury's*	1 Pack/203.8g	424		208	11.6	22.3	8.0	0.0
Lovely Stuff, Cranks*	1 Pack/209.5g	353		169	5.2	26.1	4.9	2.7
Lunch Triple, Sainsbury's*	1 Serving/238g	635		267	11.3	22.0	14.9	0.0
Mediterranean Style, Triple, GFY, Asda*	1 Pack/211g	352		167	11.0	26.0	2.1	2.3
Mozzarella, & Pepperoni, Sainsbury's*	1 Pack/171.2g	380		222	10.5	29.0	7.1	0.0
Mozzarella, & Roast Vegetables, Felix Van Den Berghe*	1 Pack/157.9g	330		209	9.5	23.8	8.4	0.0
Mozzarella, & Tomato, & Basil, Debenhams*	1 Pack/152.5g	339		223	10.0	25.0	9.2	0.0
Mozzarella, & Tomato, Waitrose*	1 Pack/193.0g	359		186	9.7	15.7	9.4	0.3
Mozzarella, Italian Style, Taste!*	1 Pack/183.1g	390		213	9.2	20.1	10.6	2.0
Mozzarella, Pesto & Pine Nuts, Sainsbury's*	1 Pack/180g	423		235	10.2	26.8	9.7	2.8
Mozzarella, Tomato, & Basil, Healthy Options, Oldfields*	1 Pack/175g	285		163	8.1	22.1	4.8	3.3
Mozzarrella, & Tomato Calzone, Waitrose*	1 Pack/175g	410		234	10.8	22.7	11.1	2.2
New York Deli, Boots*	1 Pack/245g	397		162	10.0	19.0	5.1	1.7
Old Smokey, Gourmet Organics*	1 Sandwich/191.7g	278		145	6.9	22.3	3.1	0.0
Pastrami, & Gherkin, BGTY, Sainsbury's*	1 Pack/230g	357		155	9.8	23.1	2.6	3.0

S

SANDWICH

INFO/WEIGHT	Measure	per Measure KCAL	KCAL	PROT	CARB	FAT	FIBRE
Philadelphia Salad, The Classic Sandwich Co*	1 Pack/135g	264	196	6.2	22.1	9.1	0.0
Ploughman's, Cheddar Cheese, Deep Fill, Asda*	1 Pack/228.6g	472	206	9.0	20.0	10.0	4.3
Ploughman's, Cheddar Cheese, Marks & Spencer*	1 Pack/185g	435	235	9.6	23.7	12.4	2.5
Ploughman's, Cheddar, Heinz*	1 Pack/208.3g	551	265	9.3	27.1	13.3	2.4
Ploughman's, Cheddar, Mature Vintage, Sainsbury's*	1 Pack/204.2g	439	215	9.3	22.3	9.9	0.0
Ploughman's, Cheese, 50% Less Fat, BGTY, Sainsbury's*	1 Pack/204g	335	164	10.7	23.3	3.1	3.1
Ploughman's, Cheese, BGTY, Sainsbury's*	1 Pack/216.7g	373	172	12.5	20.5	4.4	0.0
Ploughman's, Cheese, Boots*	1 Pack/260g	640	246	7.8	20.0	15.0	1.9
Ploughman's, Cheese, Healthy Living, Tesco*	1 Pack/186g	279	150	11.2	22.3	1.8	0.9
Ploughman's, Cheese, Marks & Spencer*	1 Pack/192g	499	260	9.1	25.1	13.4	3.0
Ploughman's, Cheese, Simply, Boots*	1 Pack/260g	640	246	7.8	20.0	15.0	1.9
Ploughman's, Deep Fill, Ginsters*	1 Pack/232g	636	274	9.6	20.8	17.6	0.0
Ploughman's, Deep Fill, Tesco*	1 Pack/245g	551	225	10.9	20.2	11.2	1.4
Ploughman's, Deep Filled, Asda*	1 Pack/254g	650	256	10.3	21.3	14.5	2.9
Ploughman's, Healthy Living, Tesco*	1 Serving/197g	331	168	10.8	20.7	4.7	1.5
Ploughman's, On Malted Bread, Tesco*	1 Serving/246g	595	242	10.6	21.3	12.8	1.1
Ploughman's, Shell*	1 Pack/225.9g	540	239	9.0	19.4	13.9	1.0
Ploughman's, Taste!*	1 Pack/205g	492	240	9.5	20.6	13.3	0.0
Pork, & Applesauce, Bells*	1 Pack/179.5g	340	190	11.5	26.1	4.5	0.0
Prawn Cocktail, & Salad, Shapers, Boots*	1 Pack/167g	296	177	10.0	18.0	7.2	2.9
Prawn Cocktail, Classic, Heinz*	1 Pack/193g	409	212	8.4	25.0	8.7	2.5
Prawn Cocktail, Healthy Eating, Tesco*	1 Pack/154g	245	159	11.0	22.0	2.7	1.8
Prawn Cocktail, Jumbo Tiger, Benedicts*	1 Serving/225g	349	155	7.4	20.4	4.8	0.0
Prawn Cocktail, Platter, Marks & Spencer*	1/4 Sandwich/50g	115	230	8.1	22.3	12.8	2.2
Prawn Cocktail, Weight Watchers*	1 Pack/168g	252	150	8.9	18.1	4.6	2.8
Prawn Mayo, BLT, Smoked Ham & Cheese, Triple, Tesco*	1 Pack/265g	708	267	11.8	20.3	15.4	1.0
Prawn Mayo, Ham Salad Triple Pack, Sutherland*	1 Pack/253g	620	245	9.8	24.8	11.9	0.3
Prawn Mayonnaise, BGTY, Sainsbury's*	1 Serving/170.5g	250	146	8.9	24.6	1.3	0.0
Prawn Mayonnaise, COU, Marks & Spencer*	1 Pack/155g	240	155	10.2	22.9	2.3	2.8
Prawn Mayonnaise, Daily Bread*	1 Pack/156.5g	373	239	11.9	23.0	11.0	0.0
Prawn Mayonnaise, Deep Filled, Eat Street, Safeway*	1 Pack/225g	450	200	10.7	23.6	6.5	2.1
Prawn Mayonnaise, Eat Smart, Safeway*	1 Pack/165g	256	155	10.4	23.0	2.3	2.0
Prawn Mayonnaise, GFY, Asda*	1 Pack/160g	251	157	10.0	23.0	2.8	2.8
Prawn Mayonnaise, Ginsters*	1 Pack/152g	415	273	12.4	17.8	17.8	0.0
Prawn Mayonnaise, Healthy Living, Tesco*	1 Pack/157g	245	156	10.2	21.8	3.1	0.5
Prawn Mayonnaise, Heinz*	1 Pack/180g	493	274	8.9	24.0	15.8	2.5
Prawn Mayonnaise, Marks & Spencer*	1 Pack/156g	382	245	10.5	20.2	13.5	2.7
Prawn Mayonnaise, Oatmeal Bread, Co-Op*	1 Pack/159g	445	280	11.0	28.0	14.0	2.0
Prawn Mayonnaise, Oatmeal Bread, Waitrose*	1 Pack/180g	463	257	10.2	20.4	15.0	3.2
Prawn Mayonnaise, On Oatmeal Bread, Big, Sainsbury's*	1 Pack/259g	686	265	10.1	21.1	15.6	0.0
Prawn Mayonnaise, On Oatmeal Bread, Fulfilled*	1 Pack/144.0g	393	273	12.7	24.3	13.8	0.0
Prawn Mayonnaise, On Oatmeal Bread, Taste*	1 Pack/144.1g	320	222	12.6	24.3	8.3	1.5
Prawn Mayonnaise, On Oatmeal Bread, Weight Watchers*	1 Pack/158g	254	161	10.4	23.7	2.7	2.3
Prawn Mayonnaise, Reduced Fat, Waitrose*	1 Pack/155g	284	183	8.9	20.0	7.5	2.8
Prawn Mayonnaise, Sainsbury's*	1 Pack/150.9g	323	214	11.6	20.9	9.3	0.0
Prawn Mayonnaise, Shapers, Boots*	1 Pack/161g	245	152	10.0	22.0	2.4	2.7
Prawn Mayonnaise, Simply, Boots*	1 Pack/261g	736	282	11.0	19.0	18.0	2.2
Prawn Mayonnaise, Tesco*	1 Pack/154g	402	261	9.5	23.5	14.3	1.6
Prawn Mayonnaise, Triple, Asda*	1 Pack/248.0g	635	256	9.0	19.0	16.0	3.4
Prawn Mayonnaise, Triple, Tesco*	1 Pack/231g	603	261	9.5	23.5	14.3	1.6
Prawn Mayonnaise, Upper Crust*	1 Pack/207.9g	343	165	9.2	20.9	5.0	0.0
Prawn Mayonnaise, Waitrose*	1 Pack/178g	309	174	9.3	20.1	6.2	2.2
Prawn, & Citrus Mango, Healthy Options, Oldfields*	1 Pack/220g	275	125	9.0	18.5	1.8	0.0

S

	Measure INFO/WEIGHT	per Measure KCAL	Nutrition Values per 100g / 100ml KCAL	PROT	CARB	FAT	FIBRE

SANDWICH

	Measure/INFO/WEIGHT	per Measure/KCAL	KCAL	PROT	CARB	FAT	FIBRE
Prawn, & Coriander, Marks & Spencer*	1 Serving/213.0g	575	270	9.5	20.6	16.6	3.7
Prawn, & Egg, Deep Filled, Asda*	1 Pack/250g	570	228	12.0	17.0	12.0	2.3
Prawn, & Egg, Safeway*	1 Pack/216g	400	185	9.4	18.8	8.0	1.0
Prawn, & Rocket, Jumbo, TTD, Sainsbury's*	1 Sandwich/224g	459	205	10.9	19.8	9.1	0.0
Prawn, & Salmon, Waitrose*	1 Pack/154g	345	224	12.5	22.0	9.5	2.8
Prawn, & Smoked Salmon, Marks & Spencer*	1 Pack/445g	1135	255	11.7	19.3	14.3	1.4
Prawn, & Thai Dressing, Tiger, Waitrose*	1 Pack/200g	342	171	9.6	23.6	4.3	2.2
Prawn, Bells, Lighter Eating, Ready To Go, Bells*	1 Serving/154.5g	257	167	12.5	24.0	2.3	0.0
Prawn, Marie Rose, Fulfilled*	1 Pack/149g	292	196	13.4	26.3	4.1	0.0
Prawn, Marie Rose, Waitrose*	1 Pack/164g	303	185	9.4	17.3	8.7	2.7
Prawn, Mayo, Tomato & Lettuce, Deep Fill, Benedicts*	1 Pack/200g	330	165	10.2	21.9	3.9	0.0
Prawn, Roast Chicken, BLT, Triple, Waitrose*	1 Pack/241g	653	271	9.2	18.8	17.7	1.6
Prawn, Shell*	1 Serving/209.2g	523	250	9.4	23.7	13.1	0.0
Prawn, Thai Style, Ginsters*	1 Pack/183.0g	313	171	9.2	22.5	4.9	0.0
Rib, BBQ, Rustlers*	1 Pack/170g	444	261	14.6	23.8	11.9	0.0
Ribsteak, BBQ, Snack Express*	1 Serving/145g	410	283	14.6	26.2	13.3	0.0
Salad, & Pepper Salsa, Hackens*	1 Pack/157.0g	197	126	5.1	21.8	2.0	0.0
Salad, & Salad Cream, Fulfilled*	1 Pack/172g	244	142	4.9	21.5	4.1	0.0
Salad, Healthy, Cambridge University Catering*	1 Pack/155.7g	246	158	5.9	27.4	2.8	0.0
Salad, Mixed, Good Food*	1 Pack/155.7g	246	158	5.9	27.4	2.8	10.0
Salad, Northern Bites*	1 Pack/210g	193	92	4.1	15.3	2.0	3.0
Salad, Serious About Sandwiches*	1 Pack/236.8g	322	136	5.8	17.1	4.9	0.8
Salad, Simply, Brambles*	1 Serving/151.3g	242	160	5.8	25.2	4.0	3.6
Salad, Simply, Shapers, Boots*	1 Pack/216g	300	139	5.2	23.0	2.9	1.8
Salad, Taste!*	1 Serving/200g	246	123	4.4	18.9	3.3	0.0
Salmon, & Black Pepper, Smoked, Fulfilled*	1 Pack/120g	293	244	13.8	29.0	8.6	0.0
Salmon, & Cream Cheese, Smoked, Marks & Spencer*	1 Pack/162g	437	270	11.7	19.3	16.2	2.5
Salmon, & Creme Fraiche, Smomked, Safeway*	1 Pack/171.4g	359	210	11.0	23.6	7.8	2.5
Salmon, & Cucumber, BGTY, Sainsbury's*	1 Pack/161g	266	165	9.7	21.0	3.0	3.5
Salmon, & Cucumber, Brown Bread, Waitrose*	1 Pack/150g	296	197	10.5	22.7	7.1	1.4
Salmon, & Cucumber, Heallthy Choice, Sutherland*	1 Pack/164g	321	196	9.8	26.6	5.6	0.0
Salmon, & Cucumber, Healthy Living, Tesco*	1 Serving/155g	256	165	11.3	24.8	2.3	1.6
Salmon, & Cucumber, Marks & Spencer*	1 Pack/168g	329	196	11.0	19.5	8.3	2.6
Salmon, & Cucumber, Red, BGTY, Sainsbury's*	1 Pack/192g	278	145	9.4	21.7	2.3	2.4
Salmon, & Cucumber, Red, Marks & Spencer*	1 Pack/183g	375	205	11.1	18.5	9.3	1.4
Salmon, & Cucumber, Red, Tesco*	1 Pack/144g	284	197	11.1	23.8	6.4	1.9
Salmon, & Cucumber, Shapers, Boots*	1 Pack/181.3g	272	150	10.0	19.0	3.8	2.9
Salmon, & Cucumber, Tesco*	1 Pack/143.8g	266	185	12.9	21.0	5.5	4.4
Salmon, & Lemon, & Black Pepper, Smoked, Deli*	1 Pack/115.6g	283	244	12.9	29.5	8.3	0.0
Salmon, & Rocket, Poached, Marks & Spencer*	1 Pack/180g	495	275	13.5	21.2	14.9	2.1
Salmon, & Soft Cheese, Feel Good, Shell*	1 Pack/174.1g	404	232	13.5	28.0	7.4	1.0
Salmon, & Soft Cheese, Smoked, Waitrose*	1 Pack/154g	300	195	14.8	19.2	6.5	4.2
Salmon, & Spinach, Poached, Shapers, Boots*	1 Pack/168.0g	284	169	9.2	23.0	4.5	3.1
Salmon, Poached, Marks & Spencer*	1 Pack/180g	495	275	13.5	21.2	14.9	2.1
Salmon, Poached, Prawn & Rocket, Waitrose*	1 Pack/165.6g	309	186	11.2	23.5	5.2	2.1
Salmon, Smoked, Daily Bread*	1 Pack/121.8g	296	243	13.5	28.0	8.7	0.0
Salmon, Smoked, Luxury, Marks & Spencer*	1 Pack/137g	333	243	15.0	19.0	11.9	1.8
Sausage, Egg & Bacon, Boots*	1 Pack/325g	887	273	9.3	23.0	16.0	2.2
Sausage, Triple Pack, GFY, Asda*	1 Pack/215g	424	197	9.0	30.0	4.5	2.3
Seafood Cocktail, Asda*	1 Pack/190g	486	256	6.7	21.3	15.8	1.6
Seafood Cocktail, Marks & Spencer*	1 Pack/226g	463	205	7.2	16.3	12.4	3.5
Seafood Cocktail, Waitrose*	1 Pack/210.2g	267	127	7.3	17.6	3.0	8.1
Seafood Medley, Marks & Spencer*	1 Pack/227g	468	206	7.2	16.3	12.4	3.5

S

SANDWICH

	Measure INFO/WEIGHT	per Measure KCAL	KCAL	PROT	CARB	FAT	FIBRE
Seafood, Mixed, Tesco*	1 Pack/184g	502	273	7.3	23.2	16.8	0.8
Soft Cheese, & Roasted Pepper, Weight Watchers*	1 Pack/158g	289	183	9.4	27.7	3.8	1.5
Southern Amercian Style, Boots*	1 Pack/270.0g	548	203	9.9	24.0	7.5	1.3
Sub, Beef, & Onion, Marks & Spencer*	1 Pack/207g	611	295	13.3	25.6	15.3	1.5
Sub, Beef, & Onion, Roast, Sainsbury's*	1 Serving/174g	426	245	9.4	29.3	10.0	0.0
Sub, Chicken & Bacon, Sainsbury's*	1 Pack/190g	554	291	13.4	27.4	14.2	0.8
Sub, Chicken, & Bacon, Compass Foods*	1 Pack/165g	450	273	12.2	28.7	12.2	0.0
Sub, Chicken, & Bacon, The Big, Marks & Spencer*	1 Pack/218g	545	250	15.6	24.9	10.0	1.4
Sub, Chicken, & Salad, Asda*	1 Sub/200g	460	230	9.4	17.4	13.6	0.9
Sub, Chicken, & Stuffing, Safeway*	1 Roll/275g	605	220	10.3	21.3	10.4	4.2
Sub, Chicken, & Stuffing, Shell*	1 Serving/182.8g	437	239	13.3	32.0	6.4	0.0
Sub, Chicken, Caesar, Chargrilled, Sainsbury's*	1 Pack/216g	611	283	13.4	25.6	14.1	0.0
Sub, Chicken, Nacho Style, Global, Somerfield*	1 Roll/226g	513	227	7.4	30.8	8.3	4.2
Sub, Egg Mayonnaise, Daily Bread*	1 Pack/165.2g	441	267	9.6	29.6	13.5	0.0
Sub, Ham, & Tomato Salad, Shapers, Boots*	1 Pack/170.2g	286	168	9.2	28.0	2.3	1.4
Tuna Mayonnaise, & Cucumber, Daily Bread*	1 Pack/190.3g	391	206	12.1	19.8	8.7	0.0
Tuna Mayonnaise, & Cucumber, Simply, Boots*	1 Pack/200g	498	249	12.0	21.0	13.0	2.4
Tuna Mayonnaise, & Salad, Cafe Nero*	1 Serving/176g	359	204	9.5	20.1	9.5	0.0
Tuna Mayonnaise, & Salad, Serious About Sandwiches*	1 Pack/191.8g	305	159	8.6	20.5	4.7	2.9
Tuna Mayonnaise, & Sweetcorn, Whistlestop*	1 Pack/139.5g	377	271	13.6	25.5	12.7	0.0
Tuna Mayonnaise, Menu, Boots*	1 Pack/181.9g	451	248	13.0	23.0	11.0	1.1
Tuna Mayonnaise, On White Bread, Oldfields*	1 Pack/141.7g	395	278	15.2	27.4	12.8	2.0
Tuna Mayonnaise, White Bread, Open Choice Foods*	1 Pack/120g	298	248	12.0	29.6	8.4	0.0
Tuna, & Celery, Perfectly Balanced, Waitrose*	1 Pack/172g	272	158	11.7	20.5	3.2	3.9
Tuna, & Celery, Waitrose*	1 Pack/168.2g	254	151	10.2	19.5	3.6	3.0
Tuna, & Chargrilled Vegetables, BGTY, Sainsbury's*	1 Pack/196g	329	168	10.7	21.5	4.4	0.0
Tuna, & Cucumber, & Red Onion, Brambles*	1 Pack/161.0g	264	164	11.3	24.3	2.4	1.6
Tuna, & Cucumber, BGTY, Sainsbury's*	1 Pack/178g	268	151	11.3	22.3	1.8	3.1
Tuna, & Cucumber, BHS*	1 Pack/210g	479	228	10.8	24.2	11.5	1.2
Tuna, & Cucumber, Feel Good, Shell*	1 Pack/214.0g	518	242	12.6	31.2	7.5	0.0
Tuna, & Cucumber, Fulfilled*	1 Sandwich/183.5g	368	200	11.0	20.4	8.4	0.0
Tuna, & Cucumber, GFY, Asda*	1 Pack/169.3g	275	163	12.0	24.0	2.1	2.7
Tuna, & Cucumber, Healthy Choice, Asda*	1 Pack/164g	315	192	10.9	22.3	6.6	1.1
Tuna, & Cucumber, Healthy Choice, Sutherland*	1 Pack/179g	344	192	12.2	22.0	6.2	0.0
Tuna, & Cucumber, Less Than 350 Cals, Ginsters*	1 Serving/193g	298	154	10.8	19.0	3.9	3.1
Tuna, & Cucumber, Low Fat, Heinz*	1 Serving/183.4g	276	151	12.3	21.6	1.6	6.8
Tuna, & Cucumber, Marks & Spencer*	1 Pack/170g	430	253	12.0	18.0	14.8	2.4
Tuna, & Cucumber, On Malted Wheatgrain, Ginsters*	1 Pack/175g	319	182	14.1	21.8	4.3	0.0
Tuna, & Cucumber, Shapers, Boots*	1 Pack/179g	322	180	11.0	24.0	4.4	1.7
Tuna, & Cucumber, Shell*	1 Pack/188g	431	229	12.3	21.9	10.2	0.0
Tuna, & Cucumber, Waitrose*	1 Serving/175g	236	135	11.0	18.3	2.0	3.6
Tuna, & Cucumber, Weight Watchers*	1 Pack/173.3g	279	161	11.4	25.1	1.7	1.4
Tuna, & Green Pesto, BGTY, Sainsbury's*	1 Pack/211.4g	279	132	11.0	17.0	2.2	0.0
Tuna, & Lemon Mayo, Shapers, Boots*	1 Pack/206g	318	154	10.0	18.0	4.7	1.7
Tuna, & Pepper & Sweetcorn Salad, Shapers, Boots*	1 Pack/204g	345	169	9.2	24.0	4.0	1.9
Tuna, & Peppers, Virgin Trains*	1 Pack/177.5g	338	191	9.9	26.5	5.0	0.0
Tuna, & Salad, Bloomer, Marks & Spencer*	1 Pack/230.8g	601	260	11.8	17.8	16.0	2.6
Tuna, & Salad, Cafe Primo*	1 Pack/230.3g	449	195	8.7	27.3	6.9	2.1
Tuna, & Salad, Debenhams*	1 Pack/249g	309	124	7.7	16.9	3.4	0.0
Tuna, & Salad, Marks & Spencer*	1 Pack/250g	575	230	12.5	16.8	12.6	2.1
Tuna, & Salad, Maxi, Greenhalgh's, Booths*	1 Serving/215.5g	389	181	8.3	17.4	8.8	1.0
Tuna, & Salad, Mediterranean, Waitrose*	1 Pack/207g	253	122	7.2	17.1	2.8	2.6
Tuna, & Salad, On White, Tesco*	1 Pack/190g	352	185	9.8	20.8	7.0	1.1

SANDWICH

INFO/WEIGHT	Measure per Measure KCAL		Nutrition Values per 100g / 100ml				
			KCAL	PROT	CARB	FAT	FIBRE
Tuna, & Salad, Tesco*	1 Pack/197g	339	172	9.9	16.5	7.4	2.8
Tuna, & Salad, Weight Watchers*	1 Pack/191g	248	130	10.6	15.8	2.7	2.6
Tuna, & Sweetcorn, & Red Onion, Co-Op*	1 Pack/256g	614	240	11.0	23.0	11.0	4.0
Tuna, & Sweetcorn, Asda*	1 Pack/205g	592	289	11.5	21.8	17.2	2.7
Tuna, & Sweetcorn, BGTY, Sainsbury's*	1 Packet/187.3g	309	165	10.8	24.7	2.7	2.8
Tuna, & Sweetcorn, COU, Marks & Spencer*	1 Pack/180g	270	150	12.6	19.0	2.4	3.8
Tuna, & Sweetcorn, Eat Smart, Safeway*	1 Pack/204.2g	337	165	12.8	23.2	1.8	1.7
Tuna, & Sweetcorn, Felix Van Den Berghe*	1 Pack/128.7g	373	289	10.4	29.3	12.4	0.0
Tuna, & Sweetcorn, Healthy Living, Tesco*	1 Pack/184g	289	157	13.0	22.5	1.7	2.3
Tuna, & Sweetcorn, Heinz*	1 Pack/208g	528	254	10.4	23.5	13.2	1.6
Tuna, & Sweetcorn, Marks & Spencer*	1 Pack/185g	426	230	11.4	23.0	10.2	4.0
Tuna, & Sweetcorn, Sainsbury's*	1 Pack/183g	392	214	12.1	22.3	8.5	0.0
Tuna, & Sweetcorn, Shapers, Boots*	1 Pack/170g	295	174	12.4	25.3	2.6	2.0
Tuna, & Sweetcorn, Tesco*	1 Pack/174g	432	248	11.3	24.4	11.7	1.8
Tuna, & Tomato, & Onion, COU, Marks & Spencer*	1 Pack/177g	250	141	11.1	18.8	2.4	2.2
Tuna, Crunch, Healthy Living, Tesco*	1 Pack/180g	261	145	11.0	19.9	2.4	0.5
Tuna, Crunch, Shapers, Boots*	1 Pack/200g	290	145	9.1	20.0	3.2	3.2
Tuna, Healthy Options, Spar*	1 Pack/150g	269	179	14.3	24.9	2.4	0.0
Tuna, Heinz*	1 Serving/183.4g	276	151	12.3	21.6	1.6	6.8
Tuna, Mediterranean, COU, Marks & Spencer*	1 Pack/260g	364	140	10.3	19.6	2.2	1.6
Tuna, Melt, Swedish Bread, Shapers, Boots*	1 Pack/163g	254	156	14.0	20.0	2.2	2.1
Tuna, Nicoise, Taste!*	1 Pack/218.4g	403	185	11.3	20.1	6.6	0.0
Tuna, Simply, Ginsters*	1 Pack/167.0g	466	279	12.8	22.9	15.1	0.0
Turkey, & Bacon, COU, Marks & Spencer*	1 Pack/165g	256	155	12.0	21.0	2.4	1.7
Turkey, & Cheese, & Bacon, Bernard Matthews*	1 Serving/192.0g	482	251	9.2	28.3	11.2	0.0
Turkey, & Cranberry Salad, Fullfillers*	1 Serving/180g	319	177	13.0	23.3	3.2	0.0
Turkey, & Cranberry, COU, Marks & Spencer*	1 Pack/180g	279	155	12.1	22.8	1.7	2.9
Turkey, & Lettuce & Tomato, Shapers, Boots*	1 Pack/217g	310	143	9.8	21.0	2.2	2.9
Turkey, & Sage, & Mayonnaise, Bells*	1 Pack/163.6g	415	253	11.6	21.2	13.5	0.0
Turkey, & Salad, Healthy Eating, Wild Bean Cafe*	1 Serving/230g	315	137	10.0	21.5	1.1	1.8
Turkey, & Stuffing, & Cranberry Sauce, Shapers, Boots*	1 Pack/167g	316	189	10.0	26.0	5.0	1.5
Turkey, & Stuffing, Marks & Spencer*	1 Pack/190g	352	185	12.3	23.1	4.9	1.9
Turkey, & Sun Dried Tomato, Festive Feast, Taste!*	1 Pack/159.1g	401	252	8.8	23.0	13.9	0.0
Turkey, Northern Bites*	1 Pack/200g	354	177	11.9	22.8	4.3	0.0
Turkey, Smoked, On Wholemeal, Sodhexo*	1 Pack/128g	259	202	16.1	23.8	4.8	3.6
Vegetable, & Chilli Bean, Roasted, Marks & Spencer*	1 Pack/200g	340	170	5.2	24.5	5.7	2.1
Vegetable, Marks & Spencer*	1 Serving/180g	252	140	6.1	23.5	2.3	2.1
Vegetable, Roasted, Open, COU, Marks & Spencer*	1 Pack/150g	260	173	8.4	31.3	1.5	4.4
Vegetable, Spicy Cajun, Sandwich King*	1 Pack/140.5g	287	205	6.0	30.3	6.7	0.0
Wedge, Chicken, & Salad, Tesco*	1 Pack/220g	458	208	9.4	18.2	10.8	1.2
Wedge, Chicken, BBQ, Tesco*	1 Pack/195g	321	165	10.2	27.4	1.6	1.0
Wedge, Ham, & Salad, Healthy Eating, Tesco*	1 Pack/198g	269	136	7.1	23.0	1.7	1.0
Wedge, Ploughman's, Tesco*	1 Pack/269.1g	705	262	10.5	26.9	12.5	1.4
Wedge, Sausage, & Egg, Tesco*	1 Pack/269g	699	260	9.1	23.6	14.4	1.1
Wedge, Tuna, & Salad, Tesco*	1 Pack/204.9g	291	142	8.1	23.9	1.5	0.8
Wensleydale, & Carmelised Carrot Chutney, Brambles*	1 Pack/180.9g	445	246	10.8	24.4	11.9	1.9
Wensleydale, & Carrot, Marks & Spencer*	1 Pack/183g	430	235	9.9	21.4	12.3	2.8

SANDWICH FILLER

Beef & Onion, Deli, Asda*	1 Serving/50g	79	157	10.0	0.1	13.0	1.1
Big Breakfast, Deli, Asda*	1 Serving/100g	251	251	12.0	3.5	21.0	0.5
Chargrilled Vegetable, Sainsbury's*	1/2 Pot/85g	192	226	3.4	2.2	22.7	0.6
Cheese & Bacon, Tesco*	1 Serving/50g	199	398	12.2	2.6	37.6	1.2
Cheese & Ham, Sainsbury's*	1 Serving/25g	124	497	12.4	0.8	49.3	0.3

SANDWICH FILLER

INFO/WEIGHT	Measure	per Measure KCAL	Nutrition Values per 100g / 100ml KCAL	PROT	CARB	FAT	FIBRE
Cheese & Onion, Sainsbury's*	1 Serving/85g	463	545	10.8	1.1	55.3	0.4
Cheese & Spring Onion, Healthy Eating, Tesco*	1 Serving/85g	185	218	13.2	6.8	15.4	0.6
Cheese & Spring Onion, Marks & Spencer*	1 Serving/56g	199	355	8.5	5.0	33.6	0.2
Chicken & Bacon With Sweetcorn, Sainsbury's*	1 Serving/60g	187	312	13.2	2.6	27.6	1.1
Chicken & Sweetcorn, Deli, Marks & Spencer*	1 Pot/170g	306	180	11.6	4.2	12.9	1.5
Chicken & Sweetcorn, Tesco*	1/2 Tub/125g	285	228	10.9	3.7	18.8	0.9
Chicken Caesar, BGTY, Sainsbury's*	1/2 Jar/85.4g	116	137	15.6	2.5	7.2	2.2
Chicken Tikka & Citrus Raita, COU, Marks & Spencer*	1/2 Pot/85g	77	90	12.6	4.9	2.0	0.9
Chicken Tikka, BGTY, Sainsbury's*	1/2 Pot/85g	99	117	16.5	6.0	3.0	1.0
Chicken Tikka, Healthy Eating, Tesco*	1 Serving/100g	110	110	7.1	12.4	3.6	1.0
Chicken Tikka, Mild, Heinz*	1 Serving/52g	102	196	5.2	12.3	14.0	0.7
Chicken With Salad Vegetables, Heinz*	1 Filling/56g	114	203	5.1	11.7	15.1	0.5
Chicken, Coronation, Deli, Asda*	1 Serving/56.1g	171	305	13.0	7.0	25.0	0.8
Chicken, Stuffing & Bacon, COU, Marks & Spencer*	1 Pack/170g	170	100	13.1	6.2	2.2	1.3
Chicken, Sweetcorn & Bacon, Tesco*	1 Serving/50g	167	334	12.3	4.3	29.7	1.6
Chicken, Sweetcorn & Sage, Healthy Eating, Tesco*	1 Serving/125g	105	84	9.4	8.8	1.3	1.3
Chicken, Tikka, Deli, Asda*	1 Serving/40g	114	284	13.0	13.0	20.0	0.7
Chicken, Tomato & Sweetcure Bacon, Marks & Spencer*	1 Pot/170g	502	295	11.4	2.8	26.4	0.7
Chunky Egg & Smoked Ham, Tesco*	1 Serving/100g	234	234	11.8	0.2	20.7	0.3
Chunky Seafood Cocktail, Tesco*	1 Serving/100g	347	347	5.6	3.3	34.6	1.7
Corned Beef & Onion, Deli, Asda*	1 Serving/50g	170	340	12.0	3.3	31.0	0.7
Coronation Chicken, Sainsbury's*	1 Serving/75g	229	305	12.1	8.9	24.6	1.2
Coronation Chicken, Tesco*	1 Tbsp/30g	84	279	14.7	6.1	21.8	0.7
Coronation Chicken, Waitrose*	1 Pack/170g	554	326	11.1	13.2	25.4	2.0
Creamy Chicken Tikka, Sainsbury's*	1 Serving/85g	184	217	14.6	1.1	17.1	1.4
Egg & Bacon, Fresh, Tesco*	1 Serving/45g	112	248	12.7	4.2	20.1	0.6
Egg & Bacon, Safeway*	1 Serving/85g	302	355	12.2	1.0	33.5	0.0
Egg Mayonaise, BFY, Morrisons*	1 Spread/50g	71	142	10.0	1.7	10.6	0.0
Egg Mayonnaise & Bacon, Free Range, Co-Op*	1 Pot/200g	500	250	13.0	0.9	22.0	0.6
Egg Mayonnaise, BGTY, Sainsbury's*	1 Serving/85g	102	120	10.9	0.9	7.1	1.2
Egg Mayonnaise, Chunky Free Range, Tesco*	1 Serving/50g	104	208	12.3	0.2	17.6	0.3
Egg Mayonnaise, Deli, Asda*	1 Serving/50g	114	227	11.0	0.8	20.0	0.3
Egg Mayonnaise, Sainsbury's*	1 Serving/50g	127	254	10.8	0.6	23.2	0.7
Egg Mayonnaise, Tesco*	1 Serving/50g	134	267	10.8	0.2	24.8	0.6
Ham & Salad Vegetables, Heinz*	1oz/28g	57	204	5.3	10.0	15.9	0.4
Poached Salmon & Cucumber, Deli, Marks & Spencer*	1 Pot/170g	349	205	14.0	1.0	16.3	0.5
Prawn Mayonaise, Deli, Asda*	1 Serving/50g	170	339	9.0	1.6	33.0	0.4
Prawn Mayonnaise, Marks & Spencer*	1/2 Pack/170g	502	295	10.6	0.6	28.0	0.3
Prawn Mayonnaise, Waitrose*	1 Pot/170g	537	316	8.9	0.2	31.1	0.0
Red Leicester & Bacon, Tesco*	1 Serving/125g	518	414	13.1	8.0	36.6	1.1
Roast Beef, Onion & Horseradish, Sainsbury's*	1 Serving/100g	372	372	6.4	3.7	36.8	1.2
Roast Chicken & Stuffing, Sainsbury's*	1 Serving/100g	424	424	10.8	1.9	41.5	1.2
Seafood Cocktail, Marks & Spencer*	1oz/28g	76	272	6.4	8.2	23.8	0.2
Seafood Cocktail, Sainsbury's*	1 Serving/50g	138	275	10.1	1.1	25.6	0.5
Seafood, BGTY, Sainsbury's*	1oz/28g	36	128	8.7	7.6	7.0	0.5
Smoked Ham, Roasted Onion & Mustard, Sainsbury's*	1 Serving/100g	343	343	7.3	3.4	33.4	0.0
Smoked Salmon & Soft Cheese, Marks & Spencer*	1 Pack/170g	451	265	11.1	4.9	23.9	0.0
Tex-Mex Chicken, Tesco*	1 Pack/250g	255	102	12.3	11.2	0.9	1.2
Three Cheese & Onion, Premier Deli*	1 Serving/100g	540	540	10.8	1.0	54.8	2.0
Tuna & Sweetcorn With Salad Vegetables, Heinz*	1oz/28g	53	191	5.8	12.1	13.2	0.7
Tuna & Sweetcorn, COU, Marks & Spencer*	1/2 Pot/85g	77	90	11.6	5.7	2.0	1.3
Tuna & Sweetcorn, Deli, Asda*	1 Serving/50g	148	296	12.0	3.4	26.0	1.4
Tuna & Sweetcorn, Marks & Spencer*	1oz/28g	70	250	14.2	2.3	20.7	1.3

	Measure INFO/WEIGHT	per Measure KCAL	Nutrition Values per 100g / 100ml				
			KCAL	PROT	CARB	FAT	FIBRE
SANDWICH FILLER							
Tuna Crunch, Tesco*	1 Serving/100g	336	336	12.1	2.6	30.8	0.4
Tuna Mayonnaise & Sweetcorn, BGTY, Sainsbury's*	1 Serving/100g	92	92	13.8	5.9	1.5	1.1
Tuna Mayonnaise, & Cucumber, Choice, Tesco*	1 Serving/200g	463	232	12.9	23.3	11.4	1.6
Tuna Mayonnaise, BGTY, Sainsbury's*	1 Serving/100g	114	114	17.6	3.5	3.4	0.1
Tuna, Carb Check, Heinz*	1 Serving/52g	84	161	6.6	6.3	12.0	0.7
Tuna, Tomato & Black Olive, BGTY, Sainsbury's*	1 Pack/100g	88	88	12.6	5.9	1.6	1.2
SANDWICH FILLING							
Big Breakfast, Asda*	1 Serving/125g	314	251	12.0	3.5	21.0	0.5
Cheese & Onion, Asda*	1 Serving/56g	288	515	9.8	4.4	50.9	0.3
Cheese & Onion, GFY, Asda*	1 Serving/80g	206	257	11.0	6.0	21.0	0.8
Cheese & Spring Onion, BFY, Morrisons*	1/2 Pot/85g	216	254	10.4	7.0	20.0	2.2
Chicken & Bacon, Asda*	1 Serving/100g	341	341	17.0	3.0	29.0	0.5
Chicken & Sweetcorn, Asda*	1 Serving/60g	187	312	11.0	4.0	28.0	2.0
Chicken & Sweetcorn, Low Fat, Morrisons*	1 Serving/56g	101	180	8.8	8.5	12.3	1.6
Chicken Tikka, Asda*	1 Serving/28g	80	284	13.0	13.0	20.0	0.7
Chicken Tikka, Less Than 5% Fat, Asda*	1 Serving/56g	65	116	11.0	7.3	4.7	1.2
Crab, BGTY, Sainsbury's*	1oz/28g	36	128	8.7	7.6	7.0	0.5
Egg Mayonnaise With Chives, Asda*	1oz/28g	92	327	9.1	1.1	31.8	0.0
Egg Mayonnaise, Asda*	1oz/28g	72	258	10.3	1.9	23.3	0.7
Houmous & Vegetable, Asda*	1/3 tub/57g	133	233	8.0	12.0	17.0	3.5
Prawn Mayonnaise, GFY, Asda*	1 Serving/57g	101	177	12.0	3.0	13.0	0.1
Prawns With Seafood Sauce, Asda*	1oz/28g	107	382	11.7	1.4	36.8	0.0
Tuna & Sweetcorn With Mayonnaise, Morrisons*	1 Serving/25g	72	289	13.1	5.9	23.7	0.6
Tuna & Sweetcorn, Asda*	1oz/28g	83	295	8.2	6.0	26.5	0.6
Tuna & Sweetcorn, GFY, Asda*	1/3 Pot/57g	71	125	12.0	10.0	4.1	0.8
Tuna & Sweetcorn, Reduced Fat, Co-Op*	1 Serving/50g	103	205	13.0	7.0	14.0	0.9
SANDWICH SPREAD							
Chicken & Bacon, Asda*	1 Jar/170g	610	359	18.0	2.0	31.0	1.0
Chicken Tikka, Asda*	1 Serving/50g	77	154	7.0	9.0	10.0	0.2
Cucumber, Heinz*	1oz/28g	46	164	1.7	12.7	11.6	0.6
Original, Heinz*	1oz/28g	66	237	1.7	15.2	18.6	0.7
Somerfield*	1oz/28g	59	212	1.0	26.0	11.0	0.0
SARDINES							
Cook!, Marks & Spencer*	1 Serving/128g	262	205	16.4	1.2	14.1	0.1
Grilled	1oz/28g	55	195	25.3	0.0	10.4	0.0
In Barbecue Sauce, Princes*	1 Can/120g	182	152	15.1	5.0	8.0	0.0
In Brine, Canned, Drained	1oz/28g	48	172	21.5	0.0	9.6	0.0
In Oil, Canned, Drained	1oz/28g	62	220	23.3	0.0	14.1	0.0
In Salsa, Norwegian, Canned, Finest, King Oscar*	1 Can/106g	180	170	13.2	2.8	11.3	0.0
In Smoky Barbecue Sauce, Princes*	1 Can/120g	182	152	15.1	5.0	8.0	0.0
In Spring Water, Portuguese, Sainsbury's*	1 Can/90g	165	183	22.4	0.0	10.3	0.0
In Sunflower Oil, Drained, Princes*	1 Can/90g	189	210	22.0	0.0	13.9	0.0
In Sunflower Oil, John West*	1 Can/96g	209	218	23.0	0.0	14.0	0.0
In Sunflower Oil, Portuguese, Sainsbury's*	1 Can/90g	167	186	25.1	0.1	10.3	0.1
In Tomato Sauce, Canned	1oz/28g	45	162	17.0	1.4	9.9	0.0
Picante, Waitrose*	1 Serving/88g	265	301	17.9	0.3	25.4	0.0
Raw	1oz/28g	46	165	20.6	0.0	9.2	0.0
SATAY							
Chicken & Turkey, Sainsbury's*	1 Stick/20g	44	222	20.0	4.0	14.0	1.9
Chicken Tikka, Cocktail Selection, Somerfield*	1oz/28g	48	171	24.0	4.0	7.0	0.0
Chicken, GFY, Asda*	1 Serving/168.1g	242	144	22.0	6.0	3.6	0.8
Chicken, Indonesian, Mini, Sainsbury's*	1 Stick/10g	17	171	23.0	4.0	7.0	0.7
Chicken, Marks & Spencer*	1 Satay/43g	90	210	19.1	4.4	12.7	0.7

	INFO/WEIGHT	KCAL	KCAL	PROT	CARB	FAT	FIBRE
SATAY							
Chicken, Occasions, Sainsbury's*	1 Satay/10g	15	150	22.0	2.0	6.0	0.7
Chicken, Sainsbury's*	1 Pack/350g	301	86	7.6	7.8	2.7	0.4
Chicken, Sticks, Asda*	1 Stick/20g	43	216	18.0	4.5	14.0	0.0
Chicken, Tesco*	1 Serving/350g	483	138	13.4	5.1	7.1	0.7
Chicken, Thai Cocktail Sel & Peanut Sauce, Somerfield*	1oz/28g	43	152	23.0	2.0	6.0	0.0
Chicken, Waitrose*	1 Serving/350g	679	194	17.1	6.7	11.0	1.3
Chicken, With Jasmin Rice, Eat Smart, Safeway*	1 Pack/400g	380	95	5.3	14.3	1.5	0.7
Selection, Safeway*	1 Satay/10g	20	200	26.0	9.0	8.0	3.0
Szechuan Style, Occasions, Sainsbury's*	1 Satay/10g	20	196	22.8	6.4	8.8	0.5
SATSUMAS							
Fresh, Raw	1oz/28g	10	36	0.9	8.5	0.1	1.3
Weighed With Peel	1 Med/80g	21	26	0.6	6.0	0.1	0.9
SAUCE							
Amatrician, Sainsbury's*	1 Serving/100g	52	52	3.8	4.3	2.2	1.4
Apple & Brandy, Asda*	1 Serving/125g	56	45	0.2	11.0	0.0	0.0
Apple, Baxters*	1 Tsp/15g	7	49	0.1	11.1	0.4	0.7
Apple, Bramley, Colman's*	1 Tsp/15ml	16	108	0.2	26.0	0.0	0.0
Apple, Bramley, Marks & Spencer*	1 Serving/50g	53	106	0.3	25.0	0.1	0.8
Apple, Bramley, Safeway*	1 Serving/50g	61	121	0.2	29.9	0.1	1.0
Apple, Bramley, Sainsbury's*	1 Tsp/15g	17	111	0.2	27.2	0.1	1.8
Apple, Bramley, Tesco*	1 Serving/50g	70	140	0.3	33.7	0.1	1.1
Apple, Heinz*	1 Tsp/15g	8	56	0.3	13.4	0.2	1.5
Apple, Value, Tesco*	1 Serving/50g	29	58	0.1	14.4	0.0	0.5
Apricot & Almond Tagine, Sainsbury's*	1/3 Jar/120g	98	82	2.0	17.9	1.6	2.5
Aromatic Cantonese, Express, Uncle Ben's*	1 Serving/170g	172	101	0.6	24.6	0.1	0.0
Arrabbiata, Asda*	1/2 Tub/150g	72	48	1.2	7.0	1.7	0.7
Arrabbiata, Lazio, Sainsbury's*	1/3 Jar/113g	154	136	2.2	7.2	10.9	0.0
Arrabbiata, Red Pepper, Sainsbury's*	1 Serving/75g	34	45	1.3	4.3	2.5	2.1
Arrabiata, Italiano, Fresh, Tesco*	1 Pot/350g	126	36	1.4	7.1	0.2	1.1
Arrabiata, Safeway*	1/2 Pot/175g	250	143	2.9	14.1	8.3	2.9
Au Poivre, TTD, Sainsbury's*	1 Serving/150g	300	200	2.5	6.2	18.4	0.6
BBQ Original, Heinz*	1 Serving/9.5g	12	137	1.3	31.0	0.3	0.3
BBQ, HP*	1 Serving/20ml	29	143	0.8	33.1	0.2	0.0
BBQ, Smokey Tomato, HP*	1oz/28g	40	143	0.8	33.1	0.2	0.0
BBQ, Spicy Mayhem, HP*	1 Serving/2g	3	156	0.9	36.7	0.1	0.0
Balti Curry, Tesco*	1 Serving/200g	126	63	1.7	4.3	4.6	1.7
Balti Indian, Marks & Spencer*	1oz/28g	25	90	1.6	5.6	6.7	1.8
Balti, 97% Fat Free, Homepride*	1 Serving/230g	133	58	1.1	9.1	1.9	1.8
Balti, Cooking, BGTY, Sainsbury's*	1/4 Jar/129g	98	76	1.1	10.9	3.1	0.6
Balti, Cooking, Organic, Perfectly Balanced, Waitrose*	1 Jar/450g	302	67	1.6	12.1	1.3	3.1
Balti, Cooking, Organic, Sainsbury's*	1 Serving/225g	158	70	2.2	10.0	2.3	0.5
Balti, Cooking, Sharwood's*	1 Jar/420g	370	88	1.1	9.1	5.2	0.5
Balti, Cooking, Tesco*	1 Serving/500g	575	115	2.3	8.6	7.8	1.6
Balti, Curry, Asda*	1/4 Jar/125g	155	124	1.6	7.0	10.0	1.7
Balti, Curry, Loyd Grossman*	1 Serving/212g	346	163	1.7	8.8	13.4	1.4
Balti, Curry, Sharwood's*	1 Serving/140g	123	88	1.1	9.1	5.2	0.5
Balti, Deliciously Good, Homepride*	1/3 Jar/153g	89	58	1.1	9.1	1.9	0.6
Balti, Indian Style, Iceland*	1 Serving/220g	154	70	1.6	10.1	2.6	0.5
Balti, Sizzle & Stir, Chicken Tonight*	1/3 Jar/168g	195	116	1.3	6.3	9.5	2.9
Balti, Tomato & Coriander, Patak's*	1 Serving/70g	58	83	0.8	6.5	6.0	1.2
Barbecue, Asda*	1 Serving/135g	128	95	1.2	22.0	0.2	0.6
Barbecue, Chicken Tonight*	1/4 Jar/125g	76	61	2.0	12.4	0.4	0.9
Barbecue, Cooking, BGTY, Sainsbury's*	1/4 Jar/124g	46	37	0.4	8.4	0.2	0.7

SAUCE	Measure INFO/WEIGHT	per Measure KCAL	Nutrition Values per 100g / 100ml				
			KCAL	PROT	CARB	FAT	FIBRE
Barbecue, Original, Sainsbury's*	1 Tbsp/15g	19	127	0.9	29.6	0.1	0.3
Barbeque, Cook In, Homepride*	1 Serving/130g	96	74	0.8	14.0	1.6	0.0
Barbeque, Simply Sausages Ranch, Colman's*	1 Serving/130g	96	74	1.8	16.6	0.1	1.1
Bearnaise, Sainsbury's*	1 Tbsp/15.0g	59	393	0.6	5.0	41.0	0.0
Beef In Ale, Cooking, Asda*	1 Jar/500g	160	32	1.6	6.0	0.2	0.0
Bhuna Cooking, Shere Khan*	1 Jar/425g	244	57	1.3	4.5	3.8	0.0
Bhuna, Sharwood's*	1 Jar/420g	361	86	0.8	8.4	5.4	0.6
Black Bean & Chillli, Stir Fry, Asda*	1/2 Jar/97g	158	163	3.7	10.0	12.0	0.8
Black Bean & Green Pepper, Stir Fry, Sharwood's*	1 Serving/150g	83	55	2.0	11.0	0.3	0.5
Black Bean, Amoy*	1oz/28g	42	150	10.0	23.0	2.0	0.0
Black Bean, Aromatic, Stir Fry, Amoy*	1 Serving/150g	228	152	3.8	33.7	0.2	0.0
Black Bean, Asda*	1 Serving/55g	55	100	2.9	19.0	1.4	0.0
Black Bean, Canton, Stir Fry, Blue Dragon*	1/2 Pack/60g	53	88	2.8	14.8	2.0	1.5
Black Bean, Cantonese, Stir Fry, Sainsbury's*	1 Serving/70ml	116	166	2.6	33.4	2.4	2.6
Black Bean, Cook In, Co-Op*	1 Serving/100g	80	80	1.0	18.0	0.6	0.8
Black Bean, Finest, Tesco*	1 Jar/350g	252	72	0.8	16.1	0.5	0.8
Black Bean, Fresh, Sainsbury's*	1 Sachet/50ml	78	156	6.7	27.5	2.6	1.7
Black Bean, Lloyd Grossman*	1 Serving/175g	177	101	2.4	12.6	4.5	0.7
Black Bean, Sharwood's*	1 Serving/97.5g	96	98	2.2	18.8	1.5	0.6
Black Bean, Stir Fry Additions, Tesco*	1 Sachet/50g	69	138	4.1	23.6	3.0	0.0
Black Bean, Stir Fry, Amoy*	1oz/28g	29	104	1.8	12.0	5.6	0.0
Black Bean, Stir Fry, Fresh Ideas, Tesco*	1/2 Sachet/25g	33	132	4.2	22.6	2.8	0.8
Black Bean, Stir Fry, Marks & Spencer*	1 Serving/60g	108	180	6.3	20.0	8.0	2.0
Black Bean, Stir Fry, Morrisons*	1/2 Jar/237g	135	57	1.7	11.2	0.6	0.0
Black Bean, Stir Fry, Safeway*	1/3 Pack/33g	43	129	3.7	20.2	3.7	0.9
Black Bean, Stir Fry, Sharwood's*	1 Jar/160g	149	93	0.3	19.9	1.3	1.2
Black Bean, Stir Fry, Straight To Wok, Amoy*	1 Pack/220g	411	187	2.7	42.7	0.6	0.0
Black Bean, Stir Fry, Tesco*	1/2 Jar/220g	216	98	2.3	17.9	1.6	0.7
Black Bean, Uncle Ben's*	1 Serving/125g	89	71	2.0	12.8	1.3	0.0
Black Pepper, Hong Kong, Straight To Wok*	1oz/28g	40	142	2.2	20.5	5.7	0.0
Black Pepper, Lee Kum Kee*	1 Serving/90g	107	119	3.2	19.0	3.3	1.3
Black Pepper, Stir Fry, Blue Dragon*	1/2 Sachet/60g	47	79	1.6	8.4	4.4	0.1
Bolognese, Emilia Romagna, Fresh, Sainsbury's*	1/2 Pot/150g	99	66	5.9	3.4	3.2	1.7
Bolognese, Fresh, Safeway*	1/2 Pot/153g	182	119	7.3	6.3	7.2	1.6
Bolognese, Italiano, Tesco*	1 Serving/175g	194	111	5.9	4.8	7.5	0.8
Bolognese, Lloyd Grossman*	1/4 Jar/106g	80	75	2.0	10.2	2.9	1.4
Bolognese, Original, Deliciously Good, Homepride*	1/4 Jar/112g	39	35	1.3	7.1	0.2	0.8
Bolognese, Original, Dolmio*	1 Serving/250g	130	52	1.7	8.7	1.2	0.0
Bolognese, Tinned, Sainsbury's*	1/3 Can/141g	86	61	4.5	5.7	2.2	1.0
Bolognese, Waitrose*	1 Serving/175g	151	86	5.4	5.3	4.9	2.0
Branston Smooth, Crosse & Blackwell*	1 Serving/25g	35	139	0.6	34.0	0.1	1.4
Brazilian Chicken, Chicken Tonight*	1 Serving/125g	49	39	1.2	7.0	0.7	1.3
Bread, Christmas, Tesco*	1 Serving/60g	64	107	3.3	11.8	5.3	0.5
Bread, Luxury, Marks & Spencer*	1 Serving/115g	196	170	3.2	8.1	14.1	2.2
Bread, Made With Semi-Skimmed Milk	1 Serving/45g	42	93	4.3	12.8	3.1	0.3
Bread, Marks & Spencer*	1 Serving/85g	153	180	3.1	8.7	14.6	0.2
Brown, Daddies Favourite, HP*	1 Tsp/6g	6	102	0.9	24.3	0.1	0.0
Brown, Tesco*	1 Tsp/10g	10	104	0.7	25.1	0.1	0.6
Burger, Hellmann's*	1 Tbsp/15g	36	240	1.1	12.0	21.0	0.0
Butter & Tarragon, Chicken Tonight*	1oz/28g	30	106	1.0	2.1	10.4	0.7
Buttermilch Banane, Lifestyle, Co-Op*	1 Serving/250ml	65	26	2.1	4.0	0.2	0.0
Cajun, Sizzle & Stir, Chicken Tonight*	1/3 Jar/150g	189	126	0.8	12.0	8.3	0.0
Cantonese Chow Mein Stir Fry, Sainsbury's*	1/2 Jar/100g	67	67	0.4	12.1	1.9	0.8

S

	Measure INFO/WEIGHT	per Measure KCAL	KCAL	PROT	CARB	FAT	FIBRE
SAUCE							
Cantonese, Sizzling, Uncle Ben's*	1/2 Jar/270g	416	154	0.7	24.0	6.1	0.0
Carbonara, BGTY, Sainsbury's*	1 Serving/150g	138	92	5.5	10.1	3.3	1.5
Carbonara, Creamy, Loyd Grossman*	1oz/28g	52	186	3.8	8.9	15.0	0.3
Carbonara, Creamy, Microwaveable, Dolmio*	1 Serving/75g	116	155	3.3	4.0	13.5	0.0
Carbonara, Finest, Tesco*	1 Serving/175g	194	111	6.2	5.6	7.1	0.5
Carbonara, Fresh, Sainsbury's*	1/2 Pot/150g	333	222	5.9	2.2	21.1	0.8
Carbonara, GFY, Asda,*	1 Serving/170g	167	98	5.0	6.0	6.0	0.0
Carbonara, Healthy Eating, Tesco*	1 Serving/175g	121	69	5.2	6.2	2.6	0.0
Carbonara, Less Than 5% Fat, Safeway*	1 Serving/175g	130	74	4.1	4.8	4.2	0.2
Carbonara, Stir In, Dolmio*	1 Serving/75g	140	186	6.5	3.7	15.8	0.0
Carbonara, With Cheese & Bacon, Sainsbury's*	1/2 Pot/150g	177	118	6.3	4.1	8.5	1.2
Carmelised Onion & Red Wine, Marks & Spencer*	1 Serving/52g	31	60	1.9	6.7	3.1	0.6
Casserole, Sausage, Cook In, Homepride*	1 Jar/720g	504	70	0.8	16.0	0.2	0.0
Chasseur, Cook In, Homepride*	1 Can/390g	156	40	0.7	9.2	0.1	0.0
Chausseur, Classic, Chicken Tonight*	1 Serving/100g	45	45	0.7	3.9	2.9	1.3
Cheese, Dry, Asda*	1 Serving/27g	101	373	4.4	64.0	11.0	7.0
Cheese, For Broccoli, Creamy, Dry, Schwartz*	1 Pack/40g	144	361	8.1	66.5	6.9	1.4
Cheese, Fresh, Italiano, Tesco*	1/2 Tub/175g	236	135	6.8	6.2	9.2	0.0
Cheese, Fresh, Waitrose*	1 Pot/350g	459	131	5.1	5.7	9.8	0.0
Cheese, Granules, Bisto*	1 Serving/200ml	168	84	1.2	7.4	5.4	0.2
Cheese, Instant, Morrisons*	1 Serving/14g	38	272	7.9	14.3	20.3	0.0
Cheese, Italian Style, Finest, Tesco*	1/2 Pot/175g	355	203	10.1	14.0	11.9	0.0
Cheese, Italiano, Tesco*	1 Pot/350g	368	105	5.3	8.0	5.7	0.0
Cheese, Made With Semi-Skimmed Milk	1 Serving/60g	107	179	8.1	9.1	12.6	0.2
Cheese, Made With Whole Milk	1 Serving/60g	118	197	8.0	9.0	14.6	0.2
Cheese, Sainsbury's*	1 Serving/125g	140	112	5.0	6.1	7.5	1.2
Cherry Tomato & Fresh Basil, Marks & Spencer*	1 Serving/175g	131	75	1.2	5.5	5.3	1.1
Chicken Jalfrezi, Knorr, Sizzle & Stir*	1 Jar/455g	514	113	1.1	4.4	10.1	2.4
Chicken, Sizzling, Dolmio*	1 Serving/100g	102	102	1.2	7.5	7.5	0.0
Chicken, Spanish, Chicken Tonight*	1 Serving/250g	123	49	1.7	8.0	1.3	1.0
Chilli & Garlic, Lea & Perrins*	1 Tsp/6g	4	60	1.0	14.9	0.0	0.0
Chilli & Garlic, Stir Fry, Marks & Spencer*	1 Serving/82.5g	120	145	0.7	32.4	1.2	1.1
Chilli Con Carne, 2 Step Season, Discovery*	1/2 Jar/185g	176	95	3.8	17.6	1.2	3.1
Chilli Con Carne, Asda*	1 Large Jar/570g	371	65	2.6	12.0	0.7	0.0
Chilli Con Carne, Cook In, Homepride*	1 Can/390g	234	60	2.5	11.2	0.6	0.0
Chilli Con Carne, Cooking, BGTY, Sainsbury's*	1 Jar/500g	190	38	0.8	8.2	0.2	0.6
Chilli Con Carne, Hot, Sainsbury's*	1 Serving/116g	66	57	2.4	11.3	0.2	1.6
Chilli Soy, Amoy*	1 Tbsp/15g	8	54	4.2	9.2	0.0	0.0
Chilli With Kidney Beans, Old El Paso*	1 Serving/115g	92	80	4.3	14.8	0.4	0.0
Chilli, Amoy*	1 Tsp/6g	2	25	1.0	5.2	0.0	1.0
Chilli, Cooking, SmartPrice, Asda*	1 Serving/140g	80	57	2.5	11.0	0.3	1.1
Chilli, HP*	1 Tsp/6g	8	134	1.2	32.3	0.1	0.0
Chilli, Hot, Co-Op*	1 Jar/440g	242	55	2.0	10.0	0.5	2.0
Chilli, Hot, Mexican, Morrisons*	1/4 Jar/125g	73	58	2.2	11.2	0.5	2.0
Chilli, Medium, Deliciously Good, Homepride*	1 Jar/460g	258	56	2.3	10.4	0.5	1.2
Chilli, Mild, Dry, Colman's*	1 Pack/35g	113	322	9.2	60.0	3.9	0.0
Chilli, Mild, Healthy Eating, Asda*	1/2 Jar/250g	173	69	2.1	10.0	2.3	1.7
Chilli, Mild, Safeway*	1 Serving/250g	188	75	2.4	11.3	2.2	1.2
Chilli, Seeds Of Change*	1 Jar/400g	408	102	4.0	18.2	1.5	2.2
Chinese 5 Spice, Stir It Up, Chicken Tonight*	1 Jar/80g	478	597	2.4	34.1	50.1	6.6
Chinese Orange, Honey & Ginger, Cooking, Sainsbury's*	1 Serving/125g	91	73	0.3	17.2	0.3	0.3
Chinese Style, Stir Fry, Fresh, Asda*	1/2 Sachet/50ml	93	186	1.5	18.0	12.0	0.0
Chinese Sweet & Sour Stir Fry, Sainsbury's*	1 Serving/200g	248	124	0.2	30.0	0.3	0.5

Nutrition Values per 100g / 100ml apply to the KCAL, PROT, CARB, FAT, FIBRE columns.

SAUCE

INFO/WEIGHT	Measure	per Measure KCAL	Nutrition Values per 100g / 100ml KCAL	PROT	CARB	FAT	FIBRE
Chinese Sweet & Sour, Cooking, Sainsbury's*	1/4 Jar/125g	109	87	0.7	20.1	0.1	0.7
Chinese, Curry, Farmfoods*	1 Sachet/200g	220	110	0.6	7.1	8.8	0.7
Chinese, Stir Fry, Dry, Tesco*	1 Pack/50g	170	340	0.8	17.3	29.7	0.0
Chinese, Stir Fry, Sachet, Fresh, Sainsbury's*	1/2 Sachet/51ml	83	163	1.7	14.1	11.1	1.8
Chip Shop Curry, Dry, Bisto*	1 Serving/10.7g	51	468	4.3	72.6	17.8	2.7
Chocolate Flavour, Dry, Lyle's*	1 Serving/10g	31	305	1.0	74.0	0.5	0.0
Chocolate, Dry, Sainsbury's*	1 Serving/30g	108	360	1.3	62.8	11.6	0.9
Chop Suey, Blue Dragon*	1/2 Sachet/60g	34	57	0.5	8.3	2.4	0.5
Chop Suey, Cantonese, Sharwood's*	1 Serving/200g	146	73	0.6	14.4	1.4	0.4
Chop Suey, Cooking, Asda*	1 Serving/240g	214	89	0.6	17.0	2.1	0.2
Chop Suey, Stir Fry, Sharwood's*	1 Jar/160g	120	75	0.7	14.6	1.5	0.2
Chow Mein, Sainsbury's*	1 Serving/50g	36	71	1.8	10.5	2.4	0.0
Chow Mein, Stir Fry, Asda*	1/2 Jar/97.5g	97	99	1.6	21.0	1.0	0.1
Chow Mein, Stir Fry, Blue Dragon*	1 Sachet/120g	110	92	1.1	15.4	2.9	0.4
Chow Mein, Stir Fry, Safeway*	1 Serving/75ml	128	170	1.3	29.0	5.1	0.7
Chunky Onions & Garlic, Ragu*	1/4 Jar/129g	66	51	1.9	7.6	1.4	2.0
Classic Sweet & Sour Stir-Fry, Amoy*	.5 Pack/75g	166	221	0.5	54.4	0.2	0.0
Coconut, Chilli & Lime, Cook-In, Homepride*	1 Serving/115g	110	96	1.1	5.9	7.5	0.0
Coconut, Lime & Coriander, Cooking, Nando's*	1 Serving/65g	88	135	1.5	12.2	10.0	1.2
Coconut, Thai Style, Stir Fry, Waitrose*	1/2 Pack/50ml	53	105	1.5	5.5	8.6	1.8
Cooking, Balti, Asda*	1/4 Jar/145g	155	107	1.9	9.0	7.0	1.1
Coronation Chicken, Cook In, Homepride*	1 Serving/250g	233	93	0.8	13.2	4.2	0.0
Coronation, Heinz*	1 Tbsp/10g	33	334	0.8	13.1	31.0	0.9
Country French, Chicken Tonight*	1/4 Jar/125g	123	98	0.7	3.3	9.1	0.7
Country French, Low Fat, Chicken Tonight*	1 Serving/125g	58	46	0.9	4.2	2.8	0.7
Country Mushroom, Ragu*	1/4 Jar/129g	88	68	2.0	9.5	2.1	1.2
Cowboy Joe BBQ, Eazy Squirt, Heinz*	1 Serving/10ml	11	114	0.5	27.4	0.2	0.2
Cracked Black Pepper Stir-Fry, Amoy*	.5 Pack/75g	192	256	1.8	51.0	5.0	0.0
Cracked Black Pepper, Marks & Spencer*	1 Jar/300g	345	115	2.7	6.7	8.9	0.4
Cracked Black Pepper, Stir Fry, Amoy*	1 Serving/60g	151	251	1.9	49.4	5.1	0.0
Cranberry & Port, Marks & Spencer*	1 Serving/75g	71	95	2.3	20.2	0.4	2.1
Cranberry & Red Onion, Sizzling, Homepride*	1 Serving/100g	83	83	0.5	17.7	1.0	0.0
Cranberry Jelly, Baxters*	1 Tsp/15g	40	268	0.0	67.0	0.0	0.0
Cranberry, Sainsbury's*	1 Tsp/15g	23	154	0.8	37.1	0.3	1.3
Cranberry, Tesco*	1 Tsp/15g	23	156	0.1	38.8	0.0	0.9
Cranberry, With Brandy & Orange Zest, Finest, Tesco*	1 Serving/10g	24	235	0.3	57.2	0.6	1.3
Cream, Graddsås, Ikea*	1 Serving/60ml	72	120	1.0	4.0	11.0	0.0
Creamy Garlic & Herb, Schwartz*	1 Serving/75g	83	110	3.6	11.6	5.5	0.4
Creamy Ham, Knorr*	1 Pouch/100ml	163	163	0.3	4.0	16.0	0.3
Creamy Horseradish With Garlic, So Good, Somerfield*	1 Tsp/6g	19	317	4.1	25.0	22.3	0.0
Creamy Lemon & Dill, Fresh, Sainsbury's*	1/2 Pot/150g	242	161	1.6	4.2	15.3	1.5
Creamy Mushroom Stroganoff, Marks & Spencer*	1 Serving/75g	86	115	3.3	4.8	9.2	0.6
Creamy Mushroom, Cooking, Marks & Spencer*	1 Jar/510g	663	130	1.3	5.4	11.3	0.5
Creamy Mushroom, Knorr*	1 Serving/125g	111	89	0.4	4.5	7.7	0.4
Creamy Mushroom, Low Fat, Chicken Tonight*	1 Serving/250g	108	43	1.3	2.9	2.9	1.0
Creamy Peppercorn & Whisky, Baxters*	1 Pack/320g	422	132	1.9	6.7	10.8	0.2
Creamy Peppercorn, Chicken Tonight*	1/4 Jar/125g	114	91	0.3	5.3	7.6	1.0
Creamy, Curry, BGTY, Sainsbury's*	1/4 Jar/125g	84	67	1.4	6.8	3.8	0.5
Creamy, Curry, Chicken Tonight*	1/4 Jar/125g	106	85	1.5	4.6	6.7	0.8
Creole Recipe, Discovery*	1/4 Jar/66g	62	94	0.9	17.9	1.8	0.7
Creole Style, Aldi*	1 Serving/160g	158	99	1.3	18.6	2.2	0.0
Cumberland Sausage, Colman's*	1/4 Jar/126g	43	34	0.7	7.4	0.2	0.8
Curry Moglai Passanda, Asda*	1/2 Jar/170g	277	163	2.9	10.0	12.4	1.1

S

SAUCE

INFO/WEIGHT	Measure	per Measure KCAL	KCAL	PROT	CARB	FAT	FIBRE
Curry, 98% Fat Free, Homepride*	1oz/28g	16	56	1.1	8.6	1.9	0.5
Curry, Chinese Style, Asda*	1 Serving/184.2g	140	76	1.6	7.0	4.6	2.5
Curry, Cook In, Homepride*	1/2 Can/250g	175	70	0.8	10.7	2.7	0.9
Curry, Cooking, Savers, Safeway*	1 Jar/440g	295	67	1.4	7.4	3.5	0.9
Curry, Creamy, Cooking, BGTY, Sainsbury's*	1/4 Jar/125g	94	75	1.8	10.1	3.0	1.0
Curry, Deliciously Good, Homepride*	1/3 Jar/149g	91	61	1.1	10.0	1.8	0.5
Curry, Green Thai, Asda*	1 Jar/340g	309	91	0.5	4.3	8.0	0.2
Curry, Green Thai, BGTY, Sainsbury's*	1/4 Jar/125g	61	49	0.6	5.7	2.6	1.4
Curry, Green Thai, Express, Uncle Ben's*	1 Pack/170g	131	77	1.1	5.4	5.8	0.0
Curry, Green Thai, Finest, Tesco*	1 Serving/350g	420	120	1.4	4.8	10.6	0.7
Curry, Green Thai, Sharwood's*	1 Serving/403g	431	107	1.1	8.4	7.6	0.1
Curry, Green Thai, Stir Fry, Blue Dragon*	1 Sachet/120g	74	62	0.9	5.7	4.0	0.5
Curry, Hot & Spicy, Concentrate, Keejays*	1oz/28g	151	538	7.3	30.4	43.0	4.5
Curry, Madras, Tesco*	1/2 Jar/200g	168	84	1.1	5.2	6.5	1.3
Curry, Medium, Uncle Ben's*	1 Serving/100g	66	66	0.9	11.1	2.0	0.0
Curry, Mild, Tesco*	1 Jar/500g	420	84	1.1	13.4	2.8	0.8
Curry, Red Thai, Asda*	1/2 Jar/158g	248	157	2.0	8.0	13.0	2.5
Curry, Red Thai, BGTY, Sainsbury's*	1 Serving/124g	77	62	0.6	6.0	3.9	1.4
Curry, Red Thai, Finest, Tesco*	1 Jar/350g	389	111	1.3	6.2	9.0	0.9
Curry, Red Thai, Sainsbury's*	1/2 Pouch/250g	390	156	1.7	5.0	14.3	1.5
Curry, Red Thai, Sharwood's*	1 Serving/138g	150	109	1.2	7.9	8.0	0.2
Curry, Red Thai, Sizzle & Stir, Chicken Tonight*	1 Jar/485g	873	180	1.5	4.5	17.3	1.7
Curry, Red Thai, Stir Fry, Blue Dragon*	1 Serving/60g	55	91	1.0	7.3	6.4	1.2
Curry, SmartPrice, Asda*	1/4 Jar/110g	73	66	1.4	11.0	1.8	0.6
Curry, Sweet	1 Serving/115g	105	91	1.2	9.6	5.6	1.4
Curry, Thai Coconut, Uncle Ben's*	1 Serving/125g	128	102	1.4	13.2	4.8	0.0
Curry, Value, Tesco*	1 Can/390g	355	91	1.6	11.0	4.5	1.3
Curry, Yellow Thai, Cooking, Sainsbury's*	1 Jar/500g	785	157	2.3	5.4	14.0	2.3
Dark Soya, Amoy*	1 Serving/10g	9	87	1.7	20.0	0.0	0.0
Dhansak, Medium, Sharwood's*	1 Jar/420g	370	88	3.6	11.1	3.2	1.0
Dhansak, Sharwood's*	1 Jar/445g	668	150	4.7	15.2	7.8	1.4
Diane, Safeway*	1/2 Pot/85g	40	47	0.8	3.3	3.5	0.3
Dipping For Dim Sum, Amoy*	1 Tbsp/15ml	29	190	0.0	48.0	0.0	0.0
Dopiaza, Cooking, Tesco*	1 Serving/166g	176	106	2.2	9.4	6.6	1.9
Dopiaza, Patak's*	1 Serving/212g	237	112	1.6	9.8	7.3	1.2
Dopiaza,Medium, Cook In, Sharwood's*	1/2 Bottle/210g	193	92	1.4	10.2	5.1	0.6
Enchilada, Medium, Old El Paso*	1 Can/270g	92	34	0.0	5.0	1.7	0.0
Exotic Curry, Heinz*	1 Serving/15ml	41	271	0.7	15.3	22.8	0.6
Extra Creamy Mushroom, Chicken Tonight*	1 Serving/250g	218	87	0.4	5.5	7.0	0.5
Fajita, Asda*	1/4 Jar/125g	79	63	1.0	5.0	4.3	1.0
Fajita, Marks & Spencer*	1oz/28g	24	85	1.3	6.4	6.1	2.2
Fish, Nam Plam, Blue Dragon*	1 Tbsp/15ml	12	80	13.4	6.7	0.0	0.0
Florentina, Italiano, Tesco*	1/2 Tub/175g	128	73	2.1	3.8	5.5	0.6
Flour, Dry, Sainsbury's*	1 Serving/20g	69	343	9.8	73.0	1.3	3.0
For Bolognese, Extra Onion & Garlic, Dolmio*	1 Serving/125g	66	53	1.7	9.0	1.0	0.0
For Bolognese, Light, Original, Ragu*	1 Jar/515g	196	38	1.4	8.2	0.1	1.2
For Bolognese, Original, Ragu*	1 Jar/515g	242	47	1.4	8.2	0.9	1.2
For Lasagne, Tomato, Ragu*	1 Jar/515g	191	37	1.5	7.4	0.2	1.0
For Lasagne, White, Dolmio*	1 Serving/140g	154	110	2.1	3.7	9.6	0.0
For Lasagne, White, Light, Ragu*	1/4 Jar/122g	88	72	0.5	6.3	5.0	0.2
For Lasagne, White, Ragu	1/4 Jar/123g	205	167	0.5	4.7	16.3	0.3
Four Cheese, Asda*	1/2 Jar/155g	242	156	3.5	3.9	14.0	0.1
Four Cheese, Dry, Colman's*	1 Serving/100g	357	357	18.1	46.3	11.1	1.7

SAUCE

	Measure INFO/WEIGHT	per Measure KCAL	Nutrition Values per 100g / 100ml				
			KCAL	PROT	CARB	FAT	FIBRE
Four Cheese, Less Than 5% Fat, Safeway*	1/2 Pot/175g	140	80	4.9	5.8	4.1	0.2
Fruity, HP*	1 Tsp/6g	8	141	1.2	35.1	0.1	0.0
Garlic, Heinz*	1 Serving/10ml	32	323	1.0	12.1	29.9	1.2
Garlic, Lea & Perrins*	1 Tsp/6g	20	337	1.8	17.8	29.0	0.0
Granules, White, Dry, Bisto*	1 Serving/10g	50	499	3.3	58.6	28.0	1.0
Gravadlax, Dill, & Mustard, Dry, Waitrose*	1 Sachet/35g	123	352	2.5	27.8	25.7	0.6
Green Peppercorn, Dry, Sainsbury's*	1 Tbsp/15ml	68	455	0.4	3.8	48.5	0.1
Green Pesto, Barto's*	1 Serving/20g	92	460	5.0	4.5	47.0	0.0
Green Tandoori, Marks & Spencer*	1 Jar/385g	501	130	3.6	6.8	9.9	1.5
Green Thai, Cooking, Perfectly Balanced, Waitrose*	1/2 Jar/215g	112	52	0.8	4.9	3.2	1.5
Green Thai, Loyd Grossman*	1/2 Jar/175g	182	104	1.6	10.0	6.4	0.8
Green Thai, So Good, Somerfield*	1 Jar/350g	413	118	1.2	7.0	9.5	0.5
Green Thai, Stir Fry, Fresh Ideas, Tesco*	1 Pack/50g	91	182	2.1	6.2	16.6	0.1
Green Thai, Stir Fry, Safeway*	1 Serving/75ml	259	345	1.2	12.2	32.0	2.1
Gujarati Ras, TTD, Sainsbury's*	1/2 Jar/175g	165	94	0.7	11.9	4.8	1.6
HP*	1oz/28g	33	119	1.1	27.1	0.2	0.0
Ham & Mushroom For Pasta, Stir & Serve, Homepride*	1 Serving/100g	95	95	1.5	1.3	9.3	0.0
Ham & Mushroom, Safeway*	1/2 Pot/154g	149	97	6.5	6.5	5.0	0.7
Hoi Sin & Garlic, Blue Dragon*	1 Serving/60g	80	133	1.2	26.1	2.6	0.0
Hoi Sin & Plum, Chinatown, Knorr*	1/4 Jar/131g	96	73	0.8	15.8	0.7	1.2
Hoi Sin & Plum, Sweet & Fruity Stir Fry, Sharwood's*	1 Serving/136g	128	94	0.7	19.9	1.3	0.9
Hoi Sin & Spring Onion, Stir Fry, Sharwood's*	1 Jar/165g	196	119	1.3	26.5	0.8	0.8
Hoi Sin, Marks & Spencer*	1/2 Pot/50ml	80	160	3.2	31.8	2.0	2.2
Hoi Sin, Sharwood's*	1 Tbsp/20g	42	211	2.7	49.5	0.3	0.6
Hoisin & Plum, Dipping, Finest, Tesco*	1 Serving/50g	78	156	2.3	35.3	0.6	1.4
Hoisin & Plum, Stir Fry, Healthy Living, Tesco*	1 Serving/250g	148	59	2.1	9.7	1.3	1.3
Hollandaise, Dry, Colman's*	1 Pack/27g	100	372	6.4	61.6	11.1	1.8
Hollandaise, Dry, Marks & Spencer*	1oz/28g	115	410	0.9	3.6	43.6	0.5
Hollandaise, Dry, Sainsbury's*	1 Tbsp/15ml	77	515	0.5	4.2	55.0	0.0
Hollandaise, Dry, Schwartz*	1 Pack/25g	98	392	11.3	61.5	11.2	0.0
Hollandaise, Finest, Dry, Tesco*	1 Serving/98g	473	485	1.4	17.2	45.6	0.3
Hollandaise, Full Fat, Dry, Marks & Spencer*	1 Tbsp/20g	67	336	1.1	4.5	34.9	0.1
Hollandaise, Homemade	1oz/28g	198	707	4.8	0.0	76.2	0.0
Hollandaise, Pour Over, Knorr*	1oz/28g	44	158	0.0	7.0	14.0	0.0
Honey & Coriander, Stir Fry, Blue Dragon*	1 Pack/120g	115	96	0.5	22.1	0.6	0.3
Honey & Mustard, COU, Marks & Spencer*	1/2 Jar/160g	112	70	2.3	9.2	2.9	0.7
Honey & Mustard, Chicken Tonight*	1/4 Jar/130g	139	107	1.6	13.5	5.2	1.3
Honey & Mustard, For Cooking, Asda*	1 Serving/200g	234	117	0.6	13.0	7.0	0.0
Honey n Chilli, Stir Fry, Discovery*	1/2 Pack/75g	123	164	1.1	37.3	1.1	1.9
Hong Kong Curry, Loyd Grossman*	1 Jar/350g	371	106	1.3	7.8	7.7	0.8
Horseradish, Creamed, Colman's*	1 Tsp/16g	37	229	4.3	21.4	13.3	0.0
Horseradish, Creamed, Marks & Spencer*	1 Tsp/5g	16	325	2.4	12.1	29.3	2.5
Horseradish, Creamed, Tesco*	1 Serving/15g	30	202	2.4	23.0	10.3	1.9
Horseradish, Creamed, Waitrose*	1 Tbsp/16g	30	185	2.4	19.6	9.9	2.3
Horseradish, Creamy, Sainsbury's*	1 Tsp/5g	9	185	2.4	19.6	9.9	2.3
Horseradish, Hot, Colman's*	1 Tbsp/15ml	16	105	1.8	9.7	5.7	0.0
Horseradish, Hot, Tesco*	1 Serving/10g	11	110	2.0	12.0	6.0	2.0
Horseradish, Mustard, Sainsbury's*	1 Tsp/5g	8	163	7.9	18.2	6.6	3.5
Horseradish, Sainsbury's*	1 Dtsp/10g	15	145	1.5	17.8	6.6	2.4
Hot Chilli, Asda*	1/4 Jar/126g	82	65	2.0	8.0	2.8	1.2
Hot Chilli, Deliciously Good, Homepride*	1 Serving/120g	62	52	1.3	10.6	0.5	1.1
Hot Chilli, Sharwood's*	1fl oz/30ml	36	120	0.5	29.4	0.6	1.3
Hot Chilli, Uncle Ben's*	1 Jar/500g	250	50	2.0	9.6	0.4	0.0

S

SAUCE

INFO/WEIGHT	Measure per Measure KCAL		KCAL	PROT	CARB	FAT	FIBRE
Hot Onion, TTD, Sainsbury's*	1 Serving/10g	17	167	0.2	41.0	0.1	0.1
Hot Pepper	1oz/28g	7	26	1.6	1.7	1.5	0.0
Indian Tikka, Chicken Tonight*	1 Serving/250g	320	128	1.3	10.0	9.2	1.2
Italian Hot Chilli, Dolmio*	1/2 Pack/150g	104	69	1.3	7.1	3.9	0.0
Italian Onion & Garlic, Sainsbury's*	1 Jar/500g	375	75	2.2	12.1	2.0	1.7
Italian Tomato & Herb, For Pasta, BGTY, Sainsbury's*	1/2 Jar/250g	138	55	2.1	10.9	0.3	0.0
Italian Tomato & Herb, Sainsbury's*	1/4 Jar/126g	88	70	2.0	11.1	2.0	1.4
Italian Tomato & Sweet Basil, Go Organic*	1 Serving/80g	51	64	1.2	4.3	4.7	0.9
Italian With Onion, Garlic & Herb, Safeway*	1 Serving/210g	143	68	2.1	11.5	1.6	1.8
Jalfrezi, Cooking, Asda*	1 Jar/500g	470	94	1.0	9.0	6.0	0.7
Jalfrezi, Cooking, Sainsbury's*	1 Serving/250g	160	64	1.0	9.6	2.4	1.7
Jalfrezi, Cooking, Shere Khan*	1 Jar/425g	202	48	0.8	3.9	3.2	0.0
Jalfrezi, Cooking, Tesco*	1/4 Jar/125g	144	115	2.6	11.4	6.5	1.6
Jalfrezi, Curry, Loyd Grossman*	1 Jar/425g	540	127	2.1	8.2	9.5	1.2
Jalfrezi, Curry, Patak's*	1 Serving/135g	157	116	1.7	11.3	7.0	1.4
Jalfrezi, Hot, Cooking, Sharwood's*	1 Jar/440g	264	60	1.4	7.8	2.6	1.5
Jalfrezi, Hot, Tesco*	1 Serving/220g	125	57	1.1	8.3	2.1	0.8
Jalfrezi, Marks & Spencer*	1 Jar/385g	308	80	1.7	6.6	5.2	1.9
Jalfrezi, Mild, Sharwood's*	1 Jar/420g	315	75	1.1	8.1	4.2	1.2
Jalfrezi, Piri Piri, Finest, Tesco*	1 Serving/175g	145	83	1.2	5.7	6.2	1.5
Jalfrezi, Stir Fry, Patak's*	1 Jar/250g	260	104	1.4	7.6	7.5	1.4
Kaffir Lime Chilli & Basil, Stir Fry, Sainsbury's*	1 Serving/150g	158	105	1.2	10.6	6.4	1.0
Karai Tomato & Coriander, Patak's*	1 Serving/135g	170	126	4.0	15.7	5.2	1.1
Kashmiri Moglai, TTD, Sainsbury's*	1/2 Jar/175g	184	105	1.7	8.1	7.3	1.6
Kashmiri, Butter, Patak's*	1 Jar/420g	496	118	0.8	11.2	7.8	1.0
Kashmiri, Sharwood's*	1/2 Bottle/210g	231	110	3.0	13.0	5.1	1.5
Korma, Asda*	1 Serving/225g	434	193	2.5	12.0	15.0	2.2
Korma, Coconut & Cream, Mild, Patak's*	1 Serving/135g	235	174	1.3	9.1	14.7	0.8
Korma, Cooking, BGTY, Sainsbury's*	1/4 Jar/129g	119	92	1.1	10.8	4.9	1.4
Korma, Cooking, Healthy Eating, Tesco*	1/4 Jar/125g	120	96	1.9	7.4	6.4	0.6
Korma, Cooking, Sainsbury's*	1/4 Jar/125g	159	127	1.4	8.0	9.9	1.0
Korma, Deliciously Good, Homepride*	1 Jar/450g	396	88	1.4	10.6	4.4	1.4
Korma, Free From, Sainsbury's*	1/2 Jar/175g	191	109	1.9	7.6	7.9	1.2
Korma, GFY, Asda*	1 Serving/240g	312	130	3.0	7.0	10.0	1.6
Korma, Homepride*	1 Serving/160g	110	69	1.3	11.6	2.0	0.0
Korma, Indian, Marks & Spencer*	1oz/28g	60	215	3.8	11.7	17.3	0.9
Korma, Loyd Grossman*	1/2 Jar/222g	542	244	3.6	19.1	17.0	0.6
Korma, Organic, Patak's*	1/4 Jar/106g	148	140	1.9	5.9	12.0	0.9
Korma, Patak's*	1 Jar/540g	913	169	3.6	8.5	13.4	2.3
Korma, Seeds Of Change*	1/2 Jar/175g	231	132	1.2	12.8	8.4	1.3
Korma, Sharwood's*	1 Serving/105g	150	143	1.4	12.2	9.8	1.8
Korma, Sizzle & Stir, Knorr*	1 Serving/152g	365	240	1.2	11.2	21.2	2.7
Korma, Tesco*	1/4 Jar/125g	193	154	2.4	9.9	11.7	1.3
Korma, Tin, Patak's*	1 Can/283g	478	169	3.6	8.5	13.4	2.3
Korma, Uncle Ben's*	1 Jar/500g	625	125	1.2	11.4	7.8	0.0
Lamb Hot Pot, For Cooking, Dry, Asda*	1 Pack/42g	147	351	7.0	65.0	7.0	3.3
Lemon & Ginger, Stir Fry, Finest, Tesco*	1/4 Jar/85g	144	169	0.2	41.7	0.2	0.2
Lemon & Sesame, Sharwood's*	1 Serving/100g	118	118	0.2	28.9	0.2	0.1
Lemon Butter, Dry, Schwartz*	1 Serving/9g	35	388	10.2	61.4	11.3	0.0
Lemon, Amoy*	1 Tsp/5ml	5	104	0.0	26.0	0.0	0.0
Lemon, Stir Fry, Straight to Wok, Amoy*	1/2 Sachet/50g	81	162	0.3	40.0	0.2	0.0
Lemon, Stir Fry, Tesco*	1 Jar/450g	369	82	0.1	19.3	0.2	0.1
Lime Honey & Ginger, Stir Fry, Sharwood's*	1 Serving/50g	35	69	0.3	16.6	0.1	0.2

SAUCE	Measure INFO/WEIGHT	per Measure KCAL	KCAL	PROT	CARB	FAT	FIBRE
				Nutrition Values per 100g / 100ml			
Madras Cumin & Chilli, Patak's*	1/4 Jar/135g	162	120	2.1	11.9	7.1	1.8
Madras, Cooking, Asda*	1/4 Jar/141.6g	109	77	1.3	8.0	4.4	1.0
Madras, Cooking, Sharwood's*	1 Tsp/2g	2	86	1.5	6.9	5.8	1.3
Madras, Curry, Sharwood's*	1 Jar/420g	521	124	1.7	8.9	9.1	1.4
Madras, Indian, Sharwood's*	1 Jar/420g	433	103	1.8	9.7	6.3	1.9
Madras, Patak's	1 Jar/283g	631	223	2.7	11.0	18.7	2.8
Makhani, Sharwood's*	1 Jar/420g	399	95	0.9	7.2	6.9	0.4
Mango, Kashmiri Style, Finest, Tesco*	1/2 Jar/175g	285	163	2.4	7.7	13.6	0.9
Mediterranean Vegetable, Roasted, Sainsbury's*	1/2 Pot/150g	102	68	1.6	6.7	3.9	0.4
Mediterranean Vegetable, Waitrose*	1/3 Pot/120g	60	50	1.3	4.5	3.0	1.6
Mediterranean Vegetables, Stir In, BGTY, Sainsbury's*	1 Jar/150g	123	82	1.9	9.0	4.3	1.4
Mexican Recipe, Discovery*	1 Jar/265g	355	134	1.5	18.2	5.5	1.4
Mexican Style, Cooking, Eat Smart, Safeway*	1 Serving/178g	134	75	1.3	15.8	0.6	1.2
Mexican, Cooking, BGTY, Sainsbury's*	1/4 Jar/124.4g	51	41	0.7	9.2	0.2	0.8
Mint Garden, Fresh, Tesco*	1 Tsp/5g	2	40	2.6	3.6	0.4	1.5
Mint Jelly, Average	1 Serving/14ml	37	261	0.1	64.5	0.1	0.1
Mint Raita, Patak's*	1 Jar/270g	340	126	3.9	13.6	5.5	0.1
Mint, Baxters*	1oz/28g	17	62	1.7	13.2	0.3	0.0
Mint, Sainsbury's*	1 Dtsp/10g	13	126	2.5	28.7	0.1	4.0
Moglai, Tomato & Fennel, Cooking, Patak's*	1 Jar/283g	374	132	3.1	9.7	8.9	1.8
Mornay, Cheese, Asda*	1/4 Pot/71g	114	161	6.8	6.6	12.7	0.4
Moroccan Seven Vegetable Cous Cous, Sainsbury's*	1 Serving/50g	89	178	2.6	5.9	16.0	0.0
Moroccan Tagine, Pan Fry, Loyd Grossman*	1oz/28g	15	53	0.9	5.4	3.1	0.4
Morrocan Chicken, Chicken Tonight*	1 Jar/500g	365	73	0.4	14.7	1.3	1.4
Mushroom & Garlic, 95% Fat Free, Homepride*	1 Serving/220g	154	70	0.9	7.0	4.2	0.3
Mushroom & Herb, Cooking, BGTY, Sainsbury's*	1/4 Jar/125g	68	54	1.8	6.6	2.3	0.5
Mushroom & White Wine, Knorr*	1 Serving/100ml	99	99	1.0	4.0	8.0	0.6
Mushroom, Creamy, Asda*	1 Serving/125g	76	61	0.8	6.0	3.7	0.5
Mushroom, Creamy, Tesco*	1/2 Pot/175g	142	81	1.5	5.6	5.8	0.4
Mushroom, For Pasta, Organic, Safeway*	1 Serving/220g	130	59	1.4	7.8	2.5	1.2
Mushroom, Not Just For Pasta, Sainsbury's*	1/2 Pot/150g	92	61	1.7	3.6	4.4	0.9
Mushroom, TTD, Sainsbury's*	1 Serving/150g	251	167	2.6	3.5	15.8	1.4
Napoletana, Fresh, Sainsbury's*	1/2 Pot/150g	95	63	1.7	7.3	3.0	2.3
Napoletana, Italiano, New Improved Recipe, Tesco*	1/2 Pot/175g	126	72	1.6	8.7	3.4	1.1
Napoletana, Safeway*	1 Serving/175g	107	61	1.3	6.1	3.5	1.4
Napoletana, Waitrose*	1 Pot/600g	252	42	1.8	5.5	1.4	1.7
Nasi Goreng, Indonesion, Sainsbury's*	1 Tbsp/15g	24	162	3.3	11.8	11.3	2.1
Olive & Tomato, Stir Through, Sacla*	1/2 Jar/95g	189	199	2.1	4.1	19.4	0.0
Onion, Made With Semi-Skimmed Milk	1 Serving/60g	52	86	2.9	8.4	5.0	0.4
Onion, Made With Skimmed Milk	1 Serving/60g	46	77	2.9	8.4	4.0	0.4
Orange & Green Ginger, Blue Dragon*	1 Pack/120g	118	98	0.5	20.4	1.6	0.5
Oriental Orange & Ginger, Homepride*	1 Serving/100g	68	68	0.7	15.9	0.1	0.0
Oriental Sweet & Sour, Express, Uncle Ben's*	1 Serving/170g	221	130	0.8	27.5	1.9	0.0
Oyster & Garlic, Stir Fry, Straight To Wok, Amoy*	1/2 Pack/50g	98	195	4.9	37.0	3.0	0.0
Oyster & Spring Onion, Stir Fry, Blue Dragon*	1 Serving/80g	74	92	1.6	19.9	0.7	1.1
Oyster Flavoured, Amoy*	1 Tsp/5ml	5	108	2.0	25.0	0.0	0.0
Oyster, Stir Fry, Sainsbury's	1 Tbsp/15g	9	61	1.6	13.3	0.1	0.2
Pad Thai, Blue Dragon*	1 Serving/50g	117	234	1.0	44.0	6.0	0.0
Paprika Chicken, Chicken Tonight*	1 Serving/250g	240	96	0.9	3.5	8.7	1.4
Parsley & Chive, For Cod, Dry, Schwartz*	1 Serving/19g	74	388	9.4	64.1	10.4	0.0
Parsley Lemon Caper, New Covent Garden Food Co*	1/4 Carton/65ml	137	211	2.5	8.7	18.6	0.8
Parsley, Dry, Colman's*	1 Sachet/20g	64	320	10.4	66.0	1.7	0.0
Parsley, Fresh, Sainsbury's*	1/2 Pot/150g	183	122	2.5	7.0	9.3	1.3

S

SAUCE

	Measure INFO/WEIGHT	per Measure KCAL	Nutrition Values per 100g / 100ml				
			KCAL	PROT	CARB	FAT	FIBRE
Parsley, Instant, Dry, Asda*	1 Serving/23g	82	355	7.0	66.0	7.0	4.4
Parsley, Made Up, Semi Skim Milk, Sainsbury's*	1/4 Sachet/51ml	34	67	3.5	8.6	2.1	0.1
Pasanda, Almond & Yogurt, Patak's*	1 Jar/420g	634	151	2.2	8.5	12.0	0.5
Pasanda, Patak's*	1 Jar/540g	848	157	2.3	9.2	12.2	0.5
Passata, Basil, Del Monte*	1 Jar/500g	160	32	1.4	5.9	0.2	0.0
Passata, Classic Italian With Onion & Garlic, Sainsbury's*	1oz/28g	10	37	1.4	7.7	0.1	1.3
Passata, Italian, Sainsbury's*	1/4 Jar/175g	51	29	1.1	6.0	0.1	0.8
Passata, Napolina*	1 Bottle/690g	173	25	1.4	4.5	0.1	0.0
Passata, Onion Garlic & Herbs, Safeway*	1 Serving/138g	47	34	1.4	5.7	0.6	1.2
Passata, SmartPrice, Asda*	1 Serving/15g	4	25	1.4	4.5	0.1	0.2
Passata, Valfrutta*	1 Serving/50g	13	25	1.4	4.5	0.1	0.0
Passata, With Fresh Leaf Basil, Waitrose*	1/4 Jar/170g	44	26	1.0	5.2	0.1	0.8
Passata, With Garlic & Herbs, Roughly Chopped, Tesco*	1 Serving/200g	56	28	1.4	5.5	0.0	1.0
Passata, With Garlic & Italian Herbs, Tesco*	1 Serving/165g	53	32	1.2	6.4	0.2	1.1
Peanut, Sainsbury's*	1 Sachet/70g	185	264	1.9	34.7	13.1	1.6
Peking Lemon, Stir Fry, Blue Dragon*	1 Serving/35g	58	166	0.3	36.8	1.9	0.1
Peking, Sizzle & Stir, Chicken Tonight*	1 Jar/510g	617	121	0.8	9.4	8.9	1.6
Pepper & Brandy, Pour Over, Knorr*	1oz/28g	29	104	1.0	4.0	9.0	0.0
Pepper, Creamy, Dry, Colman's*	1 Pack/25g	88	352	13.0	50.0	11.0	0.0
Pepper, Creamy, Dry, Schwartz*	1 Serving/25g	92	368	17.6	61.0	5.9	0.0
Pepper, Creamy, Tesco*	1 Serving/85ml	128	151	1.2	6.4	13.4	0.5
Peppercorn, Creamy, Asda*	1/4 Jar/137g	137	100	1.1	6.0	8.0	0.2
Peppercorn, Creamy, Chicken Tonight*	1/4 Jar/125g	100	80	1.0	3.8	6.7	0.5
Peppercorn, Marks & Spencer*	1oz/28g	38	135	1.8	7.1	10.8	0.2
Peppercorn, Mild, Creamy, Cooked, Schwartz*	1 Serving/125g	133	106	4.7	8.7	5.9	0.8
Perfect Plum Stir-Fry, Amoy*	.5 Pack/75g	191	255	0.2	62.6	0.4	0.0
Peri-Peri, Hot, Nando's*	1oz/28g	18	63	0.1	4.5	2.7	1.4
Peri-Peri, Sweet, Nando's*	1 Tbsp/25g	36	142	0.5	30.7	2.1	0.1
Pesto Rosso, Bertolli*	1/4 Jar/47g	183	389	6.6	8.1	36.7	0.0
Pesto, Basil, Stir In, Waitrose*	1/2 Bottle/85g	394	463	12.8	8.2	42.1	1.4
Pesto, Bertolli*	1 Serving/20g	78	391	5.6	4.4	39.0	1.4
Pesto, Black Olive, Sacla*	1oz/28g	115	409	2.9	4.3	42.2	0.0
Pesto, Chargrilled Aubergine, Sacla*	3 Tbsp/30g	102	339	2.4	3.8	34.9	0.0
Pesto, Classic Green, Sacla*	1oz/28g	142	507	4.1	8.5	50.7	0.0
Pesto, Classsic, Sacla*	1 Serving/45g	209	465	5.5	5.6	46.7	0.0
Pesto, Creamy, Pasta Reale*	1 Pack/200g	302	151	2.1	4.5	13.8	0.2
Pesto, Fresh, Waitrose*	1 Tbsp/26g	120	463	12.8	8.2	42.1	1.4
Pesto, Green, Asda*	1 Tsp/5g	21	429	4.7	3.5	44.0	1.4
Pesto, Green, BGTY, Sainsbury's*	1 Hpd Tsp/20g	60	299	13.0	5.9	24.8	0.1
Pesto, Green, Free From, Sainsbury's*	1/3 Jar/70g	298	425	4.1	5.4	43.0	2.8
Pesto, Green, Fresh, Sainsbury's*	1 Serving/60g	328	546	9.4	8.3	52.8	0.1
Pesto, Green, Fresh, Tesco*	1oz/28g	141	505	6.5	12.2	48.0	0.1
Pesto, Green, Half the Fat, Grandissimo*	1 Serving/48g	85	177	4.4	2.2	16.7	0.0
Pesto, Green, Less Than 60% Fat, BGTY, Sainsbury's*	1/4 Jar/48g	61	128	4.2	2.6	11.2	0.0
Pesto, Green, Morrisons*	1 Serving/50g	255	510	10.7	4.7	49.8	0.0
Pesto, Green, Sainsbury's*	1oz/28g	117	419	5.6	9.5	39.8	1.2
Pesto, Italian, Waitrose*	1 Serving/50g	179	358	3.7	1.1	37.7	2.8
Pesto, Knorr*	1 Serving/100g	216	216	2.7	3.8	21.1	0.0
Pesto, Marks & Spencer*	1oz/28g	115	411	3.2	3.5	43.3	3.9
Pesto, Red Pepper, Barilla*	1 Serving/25g	91	364	2.8	22.9	29.0	0.0
Pesto, Red Pepper, Sainsbury's*	1 Serving/37g	118	320	4.3	5.0	31.4	0.0
Pesto, Red, Fresh, Sainsbury's*	1 Serving/60g	233	389	4.5	8.6	37.4	0.7
Pesto, Red, Marks & Spencer*	1oz/28g	93	331	3.6	6.9	33.2	3.5

S

SAUCE

Measure INFO/WEIGHT	per Measure KCAL	KCAL	PROT	CARB	FAT	FIBRE
Pesto, Red, Sacla*	1 Serving/25g	82	327	4.3	8.9	30.4	0.0
Pesto, Red, Sainsbury's*	1 Serving/60g	209	348	4.8	7.0	33.4	0.0
Pesto, Roasted Pepper, Sacla*	1 Serving/47.6g	115	239	4.5	6.0	23.0	0.0
Pesto, Spinach & Parmesan, Sainsbury's*	1/2 Heap Tsp/16g	63	396	5.6	3.4	40.0	0.0
Pesto, Verde, Bertolli*	1 Serving/47g	270	575	5.7	4.3	59.5	0.0
Piemontese, Sainsbury's*	1 Serving/170g	129	76	1.3	6.0	5.2	0.2
Pineapple & Red Pepper, Kwazulu, New World, Knorr*	1 Pack/500g	260	52	0.2	12.4	0.1	0.5
Pineapple Juice & Sweet Chilli, Stir Fry, Marks & Spencer*	1 Pot/120g	192	160	1.6	36.8	0.5	0.5
Piquant Pepper Coriander & Lime, Sainsbury's*	1/3 Pot/100g	43	43	1.2	8.4	0.5	0.8
Plum & Ginger, Stir Fry, Asda*	1/2 Jar/97g	94	97	0.7	22.0	0.7	0.3
Plum & Sesame, Stir Fry, Marks & Spencer*	1/2 Jar/115g	138	120	0.9	29.0	0.1	1.8
Plum, Sharwood's*	1 Serving/50g	121	241	0.5	59.4	0.2	0.6
Prawn Cocktail, Frank Cooper*	1 Tbsp/15g	47	316	0.8	18.3	26.7	0.1
Primavera, Loyd Grossman*	1/4 Jar/88g	86	98	1.4	6.3	7.4	0.9
Puttanesca, Fresh, Waitrose*	1/2 Pot/176.1g	118	67	1.8	6.2	4.4	1.2
Raspberry, Dessert, Marks & Spencer*	1 Serving/20g	24	120	0.5	28.7	0.3	2.6
Red & Yellow Pepper, Roasted, Sacla*	1 Serving/290g	232	80	1.1	5.5	5.9	0.0
Red Pepper, Fresh, Asda*	1/4 Pot/82g	35	43	1.4	6.8	1.2	1.1
Red Pepper, GFY, Asda*	1 Serving/100g	43	43	1.2	7.0	1.1	0.0
Red Thai, Cooking, Perfectly Balanced, Waitrose*	1 Jar/430g	267	62	1.1	6.2	3.6	1.6
Red Thai, Loyd Grossman*	1oz/28g	35	125	2.8	13.7	6.5	1.5
Red Wine & Herb, Safeway*	1 Jar/680g	347	51	1.1	8.3	1.5	0.5
Red Wine & Herbs, Ragu*	1/4 Jar/130g	81	62	2.1	8.8	2.0	1.1
Red Wine & Onion, Rich, Simply Sausages, Colman's*	1/4 Jar/125g	49	39	0.9	8.5	0.2	1.3
Red Wine Cooking, Homepride*	1 Serving/250ml	115	46	0.4	9.8	0.6	0.0
Red Wine, Cook In, Homepride*	1/4 Can/98g	47	48	0.5	10.1	0.6	0.0
Red Wine, Cooking, BGTY, Sainsbury's*	1 Serving/125g	53	42	0.5	8.8	0.5	0.8
Redcurrant, Colman's*	1 Tsp/12g	44	368	0.7	90.0	0.0	0.0
Risotto, Mushroom & White Wine, Sacla*	1 Serving/95g	151	159	3.7	6.9	13.0	0.0
Roast Vegetable With Basil & Tomato, Marks & Spencer*	1 Serving/100g	85	85	2.0	9.5	4.1	1.2
Roasted Peanut Satay, Stir Fry, Amoy*	1 Serving/75g	221	294	7.9	25.5	17.8	0.0
Roasted Vegetable, Finest, Tesco*	1 Serving/175g	102	58	1.4	7.8	2.4	1.0
Roasted Vegetable, Stir In, Dolmio*	1oz/28g	38	135	1.5	9.1	10.3	0.0
Rogan Josh, 99% Fat Free, Homepride*	1/3 Jar/153g	92	60	1.8	11.6	0.7	2.0
Rogan Josh, Asda*	1/4 Jar/125g	135	108	0.9	8.0	8.0	0.6
Rogan Josh, Loyd Grossman*	1/2 Jar/212.5g	413	194	2.4	10.5	15.8	1.5
Rogan Josh, Medium, Sharwood's*	1/2 Jar/210g	151	72	1.4	8.6	3.6	0.5
Rogan Josh, Patak's*	1 Serving/270g	383	142	2.1	9.2	10.8	2.2
Rogan Josh, Tesco*	1/2 Can/220g	156	71	1.3	5.9	4.7	1.4
Royal Korma, Tilda*	1 Pack/400ml	824	206	1.9	8.4	18.3	0.7
Rum, With Lambs Navy* Rum, Finest, Tesco*	1/4 Pot/125ml	378	302	2.1	13.1	25.1	1.5
Saffron Tikka Masala, Patak's*	1 Serving/140g	147	105	1.3	7.9	7.5	1.0
Salmon, Oriental, Schwartz*	1 Serving/105g	138	131	2.0	27.5	1.5	0.0
Satay, Amoy*	1 Tsp/5ml	10	198	10.2	11.6	12.3	0.0
Satay, Indonesian, Sharwood's*	1oz/28g	45	159	5.4	10.0	10.8	5.1
Satay, Stir Fry & Dipping, Finest, Tesco*	1 Tsp/5g	22	432	9.0	20.7	34.8	2.7
Seafood, 25% Less Fat, Tesco*	1 Tsp/5g	17	344	2.7	18.2	28.5	0.3
Seafood, Asda*	1 Serving/10g	45	448	1.6	16.0	42.0	0.2
Seafood, BGTY, Sainsbury's*	1 Serving/15ml	23	152	1.3	12.1	10.9	0.2
Seafood, Baxters*	1oz/28g	149	533	1.5	9.9	54.2	0.7
Seafood, Colman's*	1 Serving/14ml	47	335	0.9	20.0	28.0	0.0
Seafood, GFY, Asda*	1 Dstp/10ml	31	313	0.6	17.0	27.0	0.0
Seafood, Organic, Simply Delicious*	1 Serving/35g	192	549	2.3	13.6	53.9	0.3

SAUCE

INFO/WEIGHT	Measure	per Measure KCAL	Nutrition Values per 100g / 100ml KCAL	PROT	CARB	FAT	FIBRE
Seafood, Sainsbury's*	1 Tbsp/15g	50	330	0.7	17.6	28.2	0.1
Seafood, Tesco	1 Serving/10g	47	465	1.8	15.6	43.5	0.3
Sichuan, Marks & Spencer*	1 Serving/120g	192	160	1.6	36.8	0.5	0.5
Singapore, Curry, Blue Dragon*	1 Sachet/120g	89	74	1.8	9.0	3.4	3.7
Sizzling Szechuan, Uncle Ben's*	1 Serving/260g	289	111	0.9	10.8	7.1	0.0
Smoked Ham & Cheese, For Pasta, Eat Smart, Safeway*	1 Serving/125g	94	75	5.8	6.1	2.5	0.9
Smoked Paprika & Tomato, Marks & Spencer*	1 Serving/300g	135	45	1.3	6.1	1.7	0.9
Smokey Bacon & Tomato, Stir In, Dolmio*	1 Pot/150g	248	165	5.5	6.9	12.8	0.0
Smokey Texan, Sizzle & Stir, Chicken Tonight*	1 Serving/150g	149	99	1.1	5.8	7.9	1.8
Soy	1 Tsp/5ml	3	64	8.7	8.3	0.0	0.0
Soy Ginger & Garlic, Stir Fry, Asda*	1 Pack/100ml	82	82	0.8	19.0	0.3	0.0
Soy, Dark, Amoy*	1 Tsp/5ml	4	73	1.9	16.3	0.0	0.0
Soy, Kikkoman*	1 Tbsp/15g	11	74	10.3	8.1	0.0	0.0
Soy, Light, Amoy*	1 Tsp/5ml	2	40	2.5	7.5	0.0	0.0
Soy, Light, Sharwood's*	1 Tsp/5ml	2	37	2.7	6.4	0.2	0.0
Soy, Reduced Salt, Amoy*	1 Tsp/5ml	3	56	4.0	10.0	0.0	0.0
Soy, Rich, Sharwood's*	1 Tsp/5ml	2	48	4.6	7.5	0.0	0.3
Soy, Superior Dark, Amoy*	1 Tsp/5ml	3	63	1.9	16.3	0.0	0.0
Soya, Japanese, Waitrose*	1 Tbsp/15ml	11	74	7.7	9.4	0.6	0.8
Spaghetti Bolognese, Dolmio*	1 Serving/100g	39	39	1.6	8.0	0.0	0.0
Spaghetti Bolognese, Dry, Colman's*	1 Pack/45g	135	300	8.8	64.0	1.0	5.3
Spanish Chicken, Chicken Tonight, Knorr*	1 serving/250g	115	46	1.5	7.0	1.4	0.6
Spiced Tomato Tagine, Sainsbury's*	1 Jar/355g	227	64	1.7	10.6	1.6	4.3
Spicy Bolognese, Cooking, Ragu*	1 Jar/510g	326	64	1.6	9.3	2.3	1.2
Spicy Durban, New World, Knorr*	1 Pack/500g	305	61	0.6	8.7	2.7	0.4
Spicy Peanut, Sharwood's*	1oz/28g	29	103	2.5	12.1	5.0	0.6
Spicy Pepper & Tomato, Stir Through, Marks & Spencer*	1/2 Jar/95g	166	175	1.6	7.5	15.4	0.0
Spicy Pepper, Eat Smart, Safeway*	1 Serving/84g	42	50	1.4	7.0	1.7	1.3
Spicy Red Pepper & Roasted Vegetable, For Pasta, Asda*	1 Serving/175g	140	80	1.2	9.0	4.4	1.0
Spicy Red Pepper & Roasted Vegetable, Sainsbury's*	1 Pot/302g	220	73	1.5	8.9	3.4	1.0
Spicy Sweet & Sour, Sharwood's*	1 Serving/138g	142	103	0.7	23.8	0.5	0.4
Spicy Szechuan Tomato, Stir Fry, Sharwood's*	1/3 Jar/140g	73	52	1.1	10.2	0.8	0.9
Spicy Tikka, Cooking, Sharwood's*	1oz/28g	27	95	1.3	9.4	5.9	0.8
Spicy Tomato & Pesto, COU, Marks & Spencer*	1 Serving/100g	60	60	2.2	6.8	2.5	1.3
Spicy Tomato, Fresh, Somerfield*	1/3 Pot/100g	41	41	0.8	6.4	1.3	1.1
Spicy Tomato, Italian, Somerfield*	1/2 Pot/149.1g	79	53	1.2	6.1	2.6	0.8
Spinach & Ricotta, Fresh, Perfectly Balanced, Waitrose*	1/2 Pot/175g	96	55	3.3	5.7	2.1	0.9
Stir Fry, Black Bean, Safeway*	1/2 Sachet/37.5ml	70	185	4.1	17.3	10.8	1.5
Stir Fry, Chow Mein, Safeway*	1 Serving/105g	79	75	1.1	16.2	0.6	1.3
Stir Fry, Fragrant Sichuan, Marks & Spencer*	1 Jar/155g	194	125	0.7	24.4	2.9	0.3
Stroganoff, Asda*	1 Serving/285g	305	107	1.5	5.0	9.0	0.3
Stroganoff, Marks & Spencer*	1oz/28g	30	107	3.8	4.9	8.0	0.6
Stroganoff, Tesco*	1 Serving/100g	89	89	0.7	5.3	7.3	0.4
Sun Dried Tomato & Basil, Free From, Sainsbury's*	1 Serving/175g	126	72	2.9	8.7	2.8	1.5
Sun Dried Tomato & Basil, Seeds Of Change*	1 Serving/100g	169	169	1.8	9.3	13.2	0.0
Sun Dried Tomato For Pasta, Stir & Serve, Homepride*	1 Serving/100g	62	62	1.0	7.6	3.0	0.0
Sun Dried Tomato With Vodka & Chilli, TTD, Sainsbury's*	1/2 Pot/150g	99	66	1.7	6.9	3.5	0.5
Sun Dried Tomato, Heinz*	1 Serving/10ml	7	73	1.5	14.9	0.6	0.9
Sun Dried Tomato, Mozzarella & Basil, Safeway*	1/2 Pot/159.1g	175	110	3.5	8.7	6.7	1.4
Sun Dried Tomato, Stir-In, Dolmio*	1 Serving/75g	124	165	1.5	9.3	14.0	0.0
Swedish Mustard & Dill, Safeway*	1 Serving/20g	32	162	17.1	1.5	9.8	0.2
Sweet & Sour, Chinese, Sainsbury's*	1/2 Jar/150g	222	148	0.2	36.6	0.1	0.1
Sweet & Sour, Cooking, GFY, Asda*	1 Jar/500g	310	62	0.9	14.0	0.3	0.6

SAUCE

INFO/WEIGHT	Measure	per Measure KCAL	KCAL	PROT	CARB	FAT	FIBRE
Sweet & Sour, Cooking, Healthy Choice, Asda*	1 Jar/500g	175	35	0.6	8.0	0.1	0.5
Sweet & Sour, Cooking, Healthy Living, Tesco*	1 Serving/125g	80	64	0.4	15.4	0.1	0.5
Sweet & Sour, Cooking, Organic, Sainsbury's*	1/3 Jar/150g	150	100	0.8	22.1	0.9	0.5
Sweet & Sour, Dry, Colman's*	1 Pack/40g	134	334	3.4	78.0	0.1	0.0
Sweet & Sour, Extra Pineapple, Asda*	1/4 Jar/148.4g	138	93	0.5	22.0	0.3	0.3
Sweet & Sour, Extra Pineapple, Chinatown, Knorr*	1 Jar/525g	441	84	0.4	20.4	0.1	0.6
Sweet & Sour, Extra Pineapple, Uncle Ben's*	1 Serving/165g	144	87	0.3	21.4	0.0	0.0
Sweet & Sour, Fresh Ideas, Tesco*	1 Serving/50ml	77	154	1.1	34.3	1.4	0.5
Sweet & Sour, Fresh, Safeway*	1 Sachet/50g	101	201	0.9	37.8	5.1	0.3
Sweet & Sour, Fresh, Sainsbury's*	1 Sachet/50ml	103	205	0.8	31.2	8.6	0.3
Sweet & Sour, GFY, Asda*	1/2 Jar/163.8g	77	47	0.4	11.0	0.2	0.3
Sweet & Sour, Healthy Living, Tesco*	1 Jar/510g	326	64	0.4	15.4	0.1	0.5
Sweet & Sour, Homepride*	1 Serving/195g	179	92	0.3	22.5	0.1	1.0
Sweet & Sour, Light, Uncle Ben's*	1 Serving/200g	128	64	0.5	15.5	0.0	0.0
Sweet & Sour, Oriental, Chicken Tonight*	1/2 Jar/262g	241	92	0.6	20.9	0.7	0.9
Sweet & Sour, Original, Uncle Ben's*	1 Pack/300g	264	88	0.5	21.7	0.0	0.0
Sweet & Sour, Peking Style, Finest, Tesco*	1 Serving/175g	147	84	0.6	20.1	0.1	0.5
Sweet & Sour, Perfectly Balanced, Waitrose*	1 Serving/175g	140	80	0.6	18.9	0.2	1.1
Sweet & Sour, Seeds Of Change*	1 Serving/200g	174	87	0.3	21.3	0.0	0.7
Sweet & Sour, Sizzle & Stir, Chicken Tonight*	1 Jar/465g	693	149	0.6	19.5	7.7	1.6
Sweet & Sour, Sizzle & Stir, Knorr*	1 Serving/460g	676	147	0.6	15.6	9.0	0.2
Sweet & Sour, Sizzling, Homepride*	1/4 Jar/125g	88	70	0.4	16.8	0.1	0.0
Sweet & Sour, Sizzling, Uncle Ben's*	1/2 Jar/270g	375	139	0.6	19.2	6.7	0.0
Sweet & Sour, Spicy, Stir Fry, Sainsbury's*	1 Jar/500g	430	86	0.7	20.0	0.1	0.7
Sweet & Sour, Spicy, Uncle Ben's*	1 Jar/400g	364	91	0.6	22.1	0.1	0.0
Sweet & Sour, Stir Fry Additions, Tesco*	1 Sachet/50g	84	167	0.8	38.7	1.0	0.5
Sweet & Sour, Stir Fry, Asda*	1 Serving/63g	146	232	0.8	46.0	5.0	0.0
Sweet & Sour, Stir Fry, Blue Dragon*	1 Serving/120g	137	114	0.6	25.6	1.1	0.6
Sweet & Sour, Stir Fry, GFY, Asda*	1/2 Pack/51ml	43	85	0.9	11.0	4.1	3.4
Sweet & Sour, Stir Fry, Marks & Spencer*	1 Serving/165g	215	130	0.6	32.0	0.2	0.7
Sweet & Sour, Stir Fry, Sainsbury's*	1/2 Sachet/50ml	100	200	0.7	36.7	5.6	3.2
Sweet & Sour, Stir Fry, Sharwood's*	1 Jar 160g	160	100	0.8	24.1	0.1	1.0
Sweet & Sour, Stir Fry, Straight To Wok, Amoy*	1 Pack/220g	486	221	0.5	54.6	0.2	0.0
Sweet & Sour, Stir Fry, Tesco*	1/2 Jar/222g	164	74	0.6	17.0	0.2	0.4
Sweet & Sour, Stir Fry, Waitrose*	1 Serving/50ml	94	187	1.2	35.6	4.4	1.8
Sweet & Sour, Straight To Wok*	1oz/28g	52	186	0.3	45.5	0.3	0.0
Sweet & Sour, Take-Away	1oz/28g	44	157	0.2	32.8	3.4	0.0
Sweet & Sour, Two Stage, Uncle Ben's*	1/2 Jar/200g	314	157	1.0	18.1	9.1	0.0
Sweet & Sour, Uncle Ben's*	1 Serving/200g	168	84	0.4	21.7	0.0	0.0
Sweet & Sour, Value, Tesco*	1 serving/100g	83	83	0.3	20.0	0.2	1.0
Sweet & Sour, With Mango, Sharwood's*	1/3 Jar/138g	134	97	0.7	23.3	0.1	1.3
Sweet Barbecue, 97% Fat Free, Homepride*	1 Serving/230g	166	72	1.4	11.7	2.7	2.3
Sweet Barbecue, Deliciously Good, Homepride*	1/3 Jar/149g	110	74	1.4	12.0	2.2	1.2
Sweet Chilli & Coriander, Sharwood's*	1 Pack/370g	407	110	0.3	24.4	1.2	0.1
Sweet Chilli & Coriander, Sizzling, Homepride*	1 Serving/100g	51	51	0.7	11.5	0.2	0.0
Sweet Chilli & Garlic Noodle, Sharwood's*	1oz/28g	30	107	0.9	18.9	3.1	0.4
Sweet Chilli & Garlic, Stir Fry & Dipping, Tesco*	1/2 Jar/95ml	78	82	0.3	20.1	0.0	0.1
Sweet Chilli & Ginger, Stir Fry, Marks & Spencer*	1 Serving/60ml	207	345	0.5	44.9	18.1	0.6
Sweet Chilli & Lemon Grass, Sharwood's*	1 Serving/155g	127	82	0.3	19.7	0.1	0.3
Sweet Chilli & Lime, Chinatown, Knorr*	1 Jar/525g	635	121	0.6	22.0	3.3	0.5
Sweet Chilli & Red Pepper, Sharwood's*	1 Serving/250g	178	71	0.8	16.4	0.2	1.1
Sweet Chilli Dipping, Blue Dragon*	1 Tsp/5ml	12	230	0.0	56.0	0.0	0.0
Sweet Chilli Dipping, Marks & Spencer*	1 Tbsp/15g	37	245	0.2	61.1	0.1	0.5

SAUCE

INFO/WEIGHT	Measure per Measure KCAL	Nutrition Values per 100g / 100ml KCAL	PROT	CARB	FAT	FIBRE
Sweet Chilli, Asda*	1 Tbsp/15ml	18	123	0.4	30.0	0.1	0.8
Sweet Chilli, Sharwood's*	1 Jar/150ml	281	187	0.6	44.4	0.8	1.5
Sweet Chilli, Stir Fry, Additions, Tesco*	1 Serving/50g	106	211	0.3	35.2	7.6	0.6
Sweet Curry, Eazy Squirt, Heinz*	1 Serving/10ml	12	124	0.7	29.0	0.3	0.5
Sweet N Sour, Sauces From Afar, Princes*	1 Jar/475g	485	102	0.1	25.2	0.1	0.0
Sweet Pepper, Stir In, Dolmio*	1/2 Pot/75g	103	137	1.5	9.7	10.3	0.0
Sweet Soy & Sesame, Uncle Ben's*	1 Serving/100g	110	110	0.7	23.0	1.7	0.0
Sweet Soy Chow Mein, Stir Fry, Amoy*	1/2 Pack/75g	146	195	0.3	35.0	6.0	0.0
Szechuan Spicy Tomato, Stir Fry, Blue Dragon*	1 Sachet/120g	151	126	1.3	17.6	5.6	2.0
Szechuan Style, Stir Fry, Fresh Ideas, Tesco*	1 Sachet/50g	114	228	1.9	33.4	9.7	0.1
Szechuan Sweet & Sour, Sainsbury's*	1/2 Jar/100g	151	151	0.5	37.0	0.1	0.1
Szechuan, Cooking, Safeway*	1 Jar/440g	458	104	1.3	13.0	5.0	1.2
Szechuan, Hot n Spicy, Safeway*	1 Jar/225g	281	125	1.2	17.9	5.4	0.9
Szechuan, Stir Fry, Sharwood's*	1 Jar/150g	126	84	3.0	15.5	1.1	0.4
Szechuan, Stir Fry, Tesco*	1/2 Jar/220g	205	93	1.0	14.7	3.2	0.9
Tagine, Cooking, Perfectly Balanced, Waitrose*	1 Jar/430g	258	60	1.0	9.6	2.0	1.5
Tamarind & Lime, Stir Fry, Sainsbury's*	1 Serving/75g	88	117	1.1	11.4	7.4	0.8
Tangine & Spiced Tomato, Sainsbury's*	1 Serving/335g	214	64	1.7	10.6	1.6	4.3
Tartare	1oz/28g	84	299	1.3	17.9	24.6	0.0
Tartare, Baxters*	1oz/28g	144	515	1.0	8.0	53.3	0.3
Tartare, Sainsbury's*	1 Serving/20ml	94	469	0.4	5.8	49.0	1.0
Tartare, Tesco*	1 Tbsp/15g	43	287	1.5	19.6	21.8	0.3
Tartare, With Olives, EPC*	1 Tbsp/15g	64	425	2.2	5.7	43.7	0.7
Teriyaki, Asda*	1 Serving/98g	99	101	2.1	23.0	0.1	0.0
Teriyaki, Blue Dragon*	1/2 Pack/60g	104	173	2.0	41.3	0.0	0.0
Teriyaki, Stir Fry, Fresh Ideas, Tesco*	1 Serving/25g	33	133	1.1	26.9	2.3	0.0
Teriyaki, Stir Fry, Sharwood's*	1 Jar/150g	144	96	0.9	22.5	0.3	0.3
Texan Barbeque, Stir It Up, Chicken Tonight*	1/2 Pot/40g	241	602	4.4	33.8	52.5	5.8
Texan Honey & Hickory, Safeway*	1 Serving/110g	173	157	1.7	17.7	8.8	1.3
Thai Chilli, Dipping, Sainsbury's*	1 Tbsp/15g	30	201	0.2	49.8	0.0	5.0
Thai Chilli, Sharwood's*	1 Serving/10g	16	164	1.8	39.1	0.0	0.3
Thai Fish, Amoy*	1 Tbsp/15ml	12	80	13.4	6.7	0.0	0.0
Thai Green, Barts*	1/2 Pack/150ml	210	140	2.0	6.0	12.0	0.0
Thai Green, Sainsbury's*	1/4 Pack/125g	170	136	1.8	10.8	9.5	2.1
Thai Kaffir Lime, Chilli & Basil, Stir Fry, Sainsbury's*	1/2 Jar/175g	166	95	1.3	9.2	5.9	1.1
Thai Lemongrass, Coconut & Coriander, Covent Garden*	1 Carton/260g	252	97	2.6	6.0	6.9	0.9
Thai Panang, Sainsbury's*	1/3 Pack/166g	229	138	1.4	6.6	11.8	1.4
Thai Satay, Sharwood's*	1oz/28g	160	573	17.2	18.0	48.0	6.3
Thai Sweet Chilli, Dipping, Blue Dragon*	1 Serving/30ml	65	215	0.8	52.3	0.0	0.9
Thai Sweet Chilli, Sizzle & Stir, Chicken Tonight*	1 Jar/510g	694	136	0.6	7.5	11.4	2.9
Thai, Ginger & Lemon Grass, Stir Fry, Sainsbury's*	1/2 Pack/150g	159	106	0.9	9.2	7.3	3.2
Thai, Lemongrass, Lime, & Chili, Stir Fry, Sainsbury's*	1 Serving/50ml	145	290	4.0	10.2	26.5	3.5
Three Pepper, Bottled, Heinz*	1 Tbsp/10g	33	329	1.5	8.7	32.0	0.0
Tikka Bhuna, Sizzle & Stir, Chicken Tonight*	1 Jar/460g	561	122	1.1	7.2	9.9	2.7
Tikka Masala Curry, Loyd Grossman*	1 Serving/150g	309	206	2.6	12.5	16.2	1.0
Tikka Masala For One, Express, Uncle Ben's*	1 Sachet/170g	168	99	1.5	9.0	6.3	0.0
Tikka Masala Lemon & Coriander, Patak's*	1 Jar/270g	265	98	2.6	10.8	4.9	0.0
Tikka Masala, 98% Fat Free, Homepride*	1oz/28g	14	49	1.4	7.9	1.7	0.8
Tikka Masala, COU, Marks & Spencer*	1/2 Pack/100g	80	80	4.5	9.9	2.6	1.7
Tikka Masala, Cooking, BGTY, Sainsbury's*	1 Jar/516g	516	100	1.5	12.1	4.9	1.3
Tikka Masala, Cooking, Eat Smart, Safeway*	1/2 Jar/180g	117	65	1.9	9.9	1.7	1.1
Tikka Masala, Cooking, Healthy Eating, Tesco*	1 Serving/250g	220	88	2.1	8.1	5.1	0.8
Tikka Masala, Cooking, Sharwood's*	1 Tsp/2g	2	122	1.2	11.9	7.8	0.9

SAUCE

INFO/WEIGHT	KCAL	KCAL	PROT	CARB	FAT	FIBRE
Tikka Masala, Cooking, Tesco*	1 Jar/735g	1095	149	2.0	9.6	11.2	0.7
Tikka Masala, Deliciously Good, Homepride*	1/4 Jar/149g	121	81	2.1	10.0	3.6	1.5
Tikka Masala, Fresh, Somerfield*	1 Pack/250g	308	123	3.0	10.0	8.0	0.0
Tikka Masala, GFY, Asda*	1/2 Jar/250g	190	76	2.9	9.0	3.2	0.5
Tikka Masala, Healthy Living, Tesco*	1 Serving/500g	325	65	2.3	3.3	4.7	1.1
Tikka Masala, Jar, Sharwood's*	1 Jar/435g	492	113	1.4	9.6	7.6	1.4
Tikka Masala, Lemon & Coriander, Cooking, Patak's*	1 Serving/70g	119	170	2.8	10.3	13.0	1.6
Tikka Masala, Lemon & Coriander, Original, Patak's*	1 Serving/125g	111	89	1.2	6.2	6.6	0.5
Tikka Masala, Loyd Grossman*	1 Serving/100g	206	206	2.6	12.5	16.2	1.0
Tikka Masala, Organic, Seeds Of Change*	1 Jar/385g	343	89	1.7	9.1	5.5	0.7
Tikka Masala, Organic, Tesco*	1/2 Jar/220g	229	104	1.9	9.4	6.2	0.8
Tikka Masala, Shere Khan*	1 Serving/212.5ml	177	83	1.3	3.9	6.9	0.0
Tikka Masala, Sizzle & Stir, Chicken Tonight*	1/3 Jar/168g	336	200	2.0	8.4	17.3	2.6
Tikka Masala, Sizzle & Stir, Knorr*	1 Jar/455g	851	187	1.2	8.3	16.5	3.9
Tikka Masala, Spicy, Sharwood's*	1 Jar/420g	449	107	1.2	9.6	7.1	0.1
Tikka Masala, Uncle Ben's*	1 Serving/200g	212	106	1.3	8.7	7.3	0.0
Tikka, BFY, Morrisons*	1/2 Jar/237.5g	259	109	2.3	17.2	3.4	1.3
Tikka, Cooking, BGTY, Sainsbury's*	1 Jar/500g	370	74	1.2	12.9	1.9	0.3
Tikka, Creamy, Chicken Tonight*	1oz/28g	36	129	1.7	12.1	8.2	0.7
Tikka, Indian Style, Iceland*	1 Serving/225g	284	126	1.7	12.9	7.5	2.2
Toffee Fudge, Sainsbury's*	1 Serving/40g	134	336	1.9	73.9	3.7	0.4
Toffee, GFY, Asda*	1 Serving/5g	15	306	2.2	68.0	2.8	0.0
Tomato & Basil For Pasta Stir & Serve, Homepride*	1 Jar/480g	278	58	1.2	6.7	2.9	0.0
Tomato & Basil, Cooking, BGTY, Sainsbury's*	1 Jar/500g	335	67	2.6	11.3	1.3	0.7
Tomato & Basil, Cooking, Marks & Spencer*	1 Serving/130g	78	60	1.4	5.7	3.4	1.2
Tomato & Basil, Eat Smart, Safeway*	1 Serving/250g	150	60	1.7	7.4	2.5	1.4
Tomato & Basil, Fresh, Organic, Waitrose*	1/4 Pot/175g	77	44	1.0	6.2	1.7	0.8
Tomato & Basil, Sun-Ripened, Microwaveable, Dolmio*	1 Sachet/170g	95	56	1.4	7.9	2.1	0.0
Tomato & Basil, Tesco*	1/2 Jar/175g	84	48	0.7	3.8	3.3	0.8
Tomato & Chilli, Loyd Grossman*	1/2 Jar/175g	154	88	1.7	7.3	5.7	0.9
Tomato & Chorizo Sausage, Tesco*	1 Serving/175g	131	75	3.4	6.1	4.1	1.0
Tomato & Creme Fraiche, Perfectly Balananced, Waitrose*	1/2 Pot/175g	84	48	1.8	7.1	1.3	2.0
Tomato & Garlic, For Pasta, Asda*	1/4 Jar/125g	80	64	2.7	8.0	2.3	1.1
Tomato & Herb, Fresh, Perfectly Balanced, Waitrose*	1 Pot/353g	173	49	1.2	5.3	2.6	0.9
Tomato & Herb, Perfectly Balanced, Waitrose*	1/2 Pot/176g	65	37	1.3	5.3	1.2	2.3
Tomato & Herbs, Italienne, Stir It Up, Chicken Tonight*	1/3 Pot/26g	164	632	4.8	18.3	60.0	4.4
Tomato & Marscapone, Finest, Tesco*	1 Serving/350g	270	77	2.7	5.4	5.0	0.8
Tomato & Marscapone, Italiano, Tesco*	1 Serving/175g	194	111	2.8	5.4	8.7	0.6
Tomato & Mascarpone, BGTY, Sainsbury's*	1 Pot/300g	150	50	2.0	3.6	3.0	3.6
Tomato & Mascarpone, Fresh, Sainsbury's*	1/3 Pot/100g	91	91	2.1	5.9	6.6	1.2
Tomato & Mascarpone, Fresh, Tesco*	1/2 Pot/175g	207	118	2.8	7.1	8.7	0.6
Tomato & Mozarella, Finest, Tesco*	1 Serving/175g	89	51	1.6	4.1	3.2	0.6
Tomato & Onion, Cook In, Homepride*	1 Can/390g	183	47	0.9	9.8	0.5	0.0
Tomato & Roasted Garlic, Stir In, Dolmio*	1/2 Pack/75g	94	125	1.2	7.7	10.2	0.0
Tomato & Wild Mushroom, Organic, Fresh, Sainsbury's*	1 Serving/152g	102	67	1.9	3.9	4.9	1.7
Tomato & Worcester, Table, Lea & Perrins*	1 Serving/10g	10	102	0.8	23.0	0.5	0.7
Tomato Base For Recipes, Salsina*	1oz/28g	7	24	1.6	4.5	0.0	1.4
Tomato Frito, Heinz*	1oz/28g	20	73	1.3	7.7	4.1	0.8
Tomato, Indian, Sizzling, Homepride*	1 Serving/240g	82	34	0.9	7.0	0.2	0.0
Tomato, Mozarella & Wild Rocket, Bistro, Waitrose*	1/2 Pot/175g	96	55	1.6	7.0	2.9	1.5
Tomato, Olive & Rosemary, Schwartz*	1 Serving/50g	45	90	2.8	6.3	6.0	1.0
Tomato, Organic, Heinz*	1 Tsp/5g	5	105	1.3	24.0	0.1	0.9
Tomato, Parmesan & Dill, Tesco*	1 Serving/70g	81	115	3.1	4.8	9.2	0.7

S

	Measure INFO/WEIGHT	per Measure KCAL	Nutrition Values per 100g / 100ml				
			KCAL	PROT	CARB	FAT	FIBRE
SAUCE							
Tomato, Roasted Garlic & Mushroom, Bertolli*	1/4 Jar/125g	68	54	1.9	6.4	2.0	1.5
Tomato, Value, Tesco*	1 Serving/10g	14	139	2.3	32.2	0.1	1.4
Vegetable & Garlic, For Pasta, Dolmio*	1 Serving/150g	108	72	1.3	7.4	4.1	0.0
Vegetable, Chunky, Tesco*	1 Can/455g	155	34	1.2	7.0	0.2	1.0
Vegetables, Hoi Sin & Plum, Stir Fry, Sharwood's*	1 Pack/360g	367	102	1.1	21.4	1.3	0.2
Vine Ripened Tomato & Mascarpone, Stir Through, Sacla*	1/2 Jar/100g	171	171	1.4	5.9	15.8	0.0
Vodka & Chilli, Finest, Tesco*	1 Serving/350g	343	98	2.2	9.4	5.7	2.1
Vongole, Sainsbury's*	1/2 Pot/150g	107	71	3.1	7.8	3.0	1.9
Watercress, Marks & Spencer*	1oz/28g	32	115	3.4	6.5	8.2	0.7
Watercress, TTD, Sainsbury's*	1 Serving/100g	82	82	2.3	2.7	6.9	4.4
White Granules, Sauce In Seconds, Dry, Asda*	1 Pack/57g	237	415	3.7	73.0	12.0	0.9
White Wine & Cream, Homepride*	1 Jar/500g	405	81	1.1	9.0	4.5	0.0
White Wine & Mushroom, BGTY, Sainsbury's*	1/4 Jar/125g	81	65	2.8	9.0	2.0	0.3
White Wine Mushroom & Herb, 98% Fat Free, Homepride*	1 Jar/450g	180	40	0.8	7.0	1.2	0.5
White Wine, Chardonnay, Marks & Spencer*	1 Serving/160ml	184	115	1.4	4.6	10.0	0.9
White, Savoury, Dry, Colman's*	1 Pack/25g	86	343	12.1	53.3	9.0	6.0
White, Savoury, Made With Semi-Skimmed Milk	1oz/28g	36	128	4.2	11.1	7.8	0.2
White, Savoury, Made With Whole Milk	1oz/28g	42	150	4.1	10.9	10.3	0.2
Wild Mushroom, Finest, Tesco*	1/2 Pack/175g	158	90	1.9	5.2	6.8	0.4
Worcestershire	1 Tsp/5g	3	65	1.4	15.5	0.1	0.0
Worcestershire, Lea & Perrins*	1 Tsp/5ml	4	88	1.1	22.0	0.0	0.0
Yellow Bean & Cashew, Tesco*	1/2 Jar/210g	170	81	1.6	11.9	2.9	0.3
Yellow Bean & Ginger, Stir Fry, Finest, Tesco*	1 Jar/350g	319	91	2.1	18.3	1.0	1.1
Yellow Bean, Sharwood's*	1 Jar/160g	128	80	0.3	19.2	0.2	0.3
Yellow Bean, Stir Fry, Sainsbury's*	1/2 Jar/100g	126	126	1.8	26.7	1.3	0.8
Yellow Bean, Stir Fry, Sharwood's*	1 Jar/195g	156	80	0.3	19.2	0.2	0.3
Yellow Bean, Stir Fry, Straight To Wok, Amoy*	1oz/28g	44	159	1.6	36.9	0.5	0.0
Yellowbean & Cashew Nut, Asda*	1 Serving/50g	60	119	2.7	21.0	2.7	0.9
SAUCE MIX							
Beef Stroganoff, Colman's*	1 Pack/40g	160	399	12.4	48.4	17.3	6.4
Bread, Colman's*	1 Pack/40g	130	325	12.0	66.0	1.3	0.0
Bread, Knorr*	1/2 Pint/40g	177	442	7.9	49.9	23.3	2.1
Cheddar Cheese, Colman's*	1 Serving/40g	158	394	19.7	45.2	14.9	1.5
Cheese, Instant, Made Up, Mrs Carters*	1 Serving/100ml	59	59	1.0	10.7	1.4	0.1
Cheese, Instant, Safeway*	1 Pack/54g	202	374	4.1	62.0	12.2	8.5
Cheese, Knorr*	1 Pack/58g	132	227	7.8	38.0	4.9	1.8
Cheese, Made Up With Skimmed Milk	1 Serving/60g	47	78	5.4	9.5	2.3	0.0
Cheese, Made Up, Crosse & Blackwell*	1 Pack/30g	26	86	5.1	9.2	3.2	0.7
Chicken Chasseur, Casserole, Morrisons*	1 Pack/40g	115	288	9.2	59.8	1.2	0.0
Chicken Chasseur, Colman's*	1 Pack/45g	124	276	12.1	54.1	1.2	4.8
Chicken Chasseur, Schwartz*	1/2 Pack/20g	64	322	9.1	64.5	3.1	0.0
Chicken Korma, Colman's*	1/2 Pack/50g	230	459	6.6	38.8	30.8	13.2
Chicken Supreme, Colman's*	1/2 Pack/20g	72	358	12.0	56.8	9.3	2.5
Chilli Con Carne, Colman's*	1 Serving/13g	41	316	7.7	67.0	1.9	4.9
Chilli Con Carne, Schwartz*	1 Serving/10g	31	308	8.2	64.6	1.9	0.5
Coq Au Vin, Colman's*	1 Pack/50g	141	281	7.5	59.0	1.0	0.0
Creamy Cheese & Bacon, For Pasta, Colman's*	1 Pack/50g	197	394	16.6	44.6	16.6	5.7
Four Cheese, Colman's*	1 Pack/35g	145	414	17.8	40.5	20.1	3.8
Garlic Mushrooms, Creamy, Schwartz*	1 Pack/35g	109	310	7.1	60.1	4.6	0.0
Lamb Hot Pot, Colman's*	1 Serving/13.5g	37	282	7.3	59.8	1.5	2.7
Mediterranean Roasted Vegetables, Schwartz*	1/2 Pack/15g	47	311	7.0	64.3	2.9	0.8
Mustard & Sweet Dill, TTD, Sainsbury's*	1/4 Sachet/10g	25	248	2.8	25.8	14.9	2.6

S

	Measure INFO/WEIGHT	per Measure KCAL	Nutrition Values per 100g / 100ml				
			KCAL	PROT	CARB	FAT	FIBRE
SAUCE MIX							
Parsley, Colman's*	1 Serving/20g	61	307	8.1	65.3	1.5	3.7
Parsley, Knorr*	1 Sachet/48g	210	437	4.2	50.6	24.2	0.8
Pepper, Instant, Safeway*	1 Serving/22g	77	348	3.2	66.3	7.5	4.1
Pork Casserole, Morrisons*	1 Pack/36g	118	327	8.1	70.6	1.4	0.0
Rum Flavour, Kraft*	1oz/28g	116	415	6.1	76.5	9.5	0.0
Satay, Thai Chicken, Schwartz*	1 Serving/9g	29	321	3.8	72.5	1.8	0.8
Spaghetti Bolognese, Schwartz*	1 Serving/40g	122	306	10.0	63.0	1.0	0.0
Spanish Roasted Vegetables, Schwartz*	1 Pack/15g	43	287	8.1	45.8	7.9	9.3
Tuna & Mushroom Pasta Melt, Schwartz*	1 Pack/40g	133	332	9.9	54.8	8.1	0.5
Tuna & Pasta Bake, Colman's*	1 Pack/45g	144	319	10.4	57.1	5.4	5.2
Tuna Napolitana, Schwartz*	1 Sachet/29g	107	368	9.7	53.0	13.0	0.0
White, Instant, Made Up, Sainsbury's*	1 Serving/90ml	65	72	0.8	10.9	2.8	0.1
White, Made Up With Semi-Skimmed Milk	1oz/28g	20	73	4.0	9.6	2.4	0.0
White, Made Up With Skimmed Milk	1oz/28g	17	59	4.0	9.6	0.9	0.0
White, Savoury, Knorr*	1/2 Pint Pack/16g	46	290	7.8	52.2	5.6	5.2
SAUERKRAUT							
Average	1oz/28g	4	13	1.3	1.9	0.1	1.1
SAUSAGE							
Beef, Average	1 Sausage/60g	151	252	14.5	7.0	18.5	0.6
Beef, With Onion & Red Wine, Finest, Tesco*	1 Sausage/63g	117	185	13.2	8.5	10.9	1.2
Billy Bear, Kids, Tesco*	1 Slice/20g	37	185	13.7	7.5	11.2	0.4
Bockwurst, Average	1 Sausage/45g	114	253	10.8	0.8	23.0	0.0
Cambridge Gluten Free, Waitrose*	1 Sausage/121g	258	213	14.6	1.9	16.3	1.3
Cheese & Leek, Tesco*	1 Sausage/55g	135	246	6.9	24.0	13.6	1.7
Chicken & Tarragon, Butchers Choice, Sainsbury's*	1 Sausage/47g	106	225	18.1	5.8	14.4	0.2
Chicken, Manor Farm*	1 Sausage/65g	126	194	13.7	6.6	12.5	1.2
Chilli Beef, Boston Style, Waitrose*	1 Sausage/66.5g	136	203	14.7	3.4	14.6	0.9
Chipolata, Average	1 Sausage/28g	81	291	12.1	8.7	23.1	0.7
Chipolata, Chicken & Sweet Chilli, TTD, Sainsbury's*	4 Chipolatas/150g	309	206	18.4	5.4	13.3	1.2
Chipolata, Cumberland, Average	1 Chipolata/28g	74	264	15.3	7.2	19.3	0.9
Chipolata, Lamb & Rosemary, Tesco*	1 Sausage/31.6g	69	218	11.3	8.3	15.5	0.0
Chipolata, Pork & Tomato, Organic, Tesco*	1 Chipolata/28g	79	283	12.2	4.3	24.1	0.9
Chipolata, Pork, Extra Lean, BGTY, Sainsbury's*	1 Chipolata	46	189	16.9	10.9	8.6	0.5
Chipolata, Premium, Average	1 Serving/80g	187	234	14.9	4.7	17.3	1.2
Chorizo, & Jalapeño, Pizzadella, Tesco*	1 Pizza/600g	1272	212	9.9	27.9	6.8	1.7
Chorizo, Average	1 Serving/80g	250	313	21.1	2.6	24.2	0.2
Chorizo, Lean, Average	1 Sausage/67g	131	195	15.7	2.3	13.7	0.8
Classic Sicilian Style, TTD, Sainsbury's*	1 Sausage/49g	135	275	16.8	0.5	22.5	0.9
Classic Toulouse, TTD, Sainsbury's*	1 Sausage/44.5g	138	310	23.2	2.1	23.3	0.9
Cocktail, Average	1oz/28g	90	323	12.1	8.6	26.7	0.9
Cumberland, Average	1 Sausage/57g	167	293	13.8	8.6	22.7	0.8
Cumberland, Healthy Range, Average	1 Sausage/52.6g	75	142	17.4	9.0	4.1	0.9
Duck & Orange, TTD, Sainsbury's*	1 Sausage/40.9g	123	301	13.8	3.2	25.9	0.9
Free From Wheat & Gulten, Sainsbury's*	1 Serving/22.8g	62	268	15.2	4.5	21.0	1.8
French Saucisson, Tesco*	1 Slice/5g	19	379	26.7	4.1	28.4	0.0
Garlic, Average	1 Slice/11g	25	227	15.7	0.8	18.2	0.0
German Extrawurst, Waitrose*	1 Slice/12.5g	39	303	13.8	0.8	27.2	0.0
German Schinkenwurst, Waitrose*	1 Slice/12.5g	29	224	16.0	0.8	17.6	0.0
German, Bierwurst, Selection, Sainsbury's*	1 Slice/4g	8	224	15.0	1.0	17.8	0.1
German, Extrawurst, Selection, Sainsbury's*	1 Slice/3g	9	279	13.1	0.5	25.0	0.1
German, Schinkenwurst, Selection, Sainsbury's*	1 Slice/3g	8	251	13.1	0.3	21.9	0.1
Glamorgan With Cheese & Leek, TTD, Sainsbury's*	1 Sausage/53g	171	323	18.9	3.3	26.0	0.6
Glamorgan, Organic, Waitrose*	1 Sausage/41.8g	81	194	14.5	11.2	10.1	1.7

SAUSAGE

	Measure INFO/WEIGHT	per Measure KCAL	Nutrition Values per 100g / 100ml				
			KCAL	PROT	CARB	FAT	FIBRE
Hot & Spicy Pork Cocktail, Cooked, Asda*	1 Sausage/10g	31	312	13.0	11.0	24.0	1.3
Hot Mustard Porker, Tesco*	1 Sausage/52g	143	275	16.1	8.1	19.8	3.1
Irish Recipe, Average	1 Sausage/40g	119	298	10.7	17.2	20.7	0.7
Lamb & Mint, Marks & Spencer*	1oz/28g	63	225	13.3	6.6	16.3	1.7
Lincolnshire, Average	1 Sausage/42g	122	291	14.6	9.2	21.8	0.6
Lincolnshire, Healthy Range, Average	1 Sausage/50g	89	177	15.8	9.0	8.6	0.8
Lorne, Average	1 Sausage/25g	78	312	10.8	16.0	23.1	0.6
Mediterranean Style Paprika, Waitrose*	1 Sausage/67g	190	283	12.1	4.6	24.0	1.9
Mediterranean Style, 95% Fat Free, Bowyers*	1 Sausage/50g	60	120	13.9	8.9	3.2	0.0
Mortadella, Sainsbury's*	1 Slice/13g	34	261	17.3	0.1	21.2	0.1
Pancetta, & Parmesan, TTD, Sainsbury's*	1 Sausage/58g	156	269	20.8	4.7	18.6	1.2
Pistachio, Waitrose*	1 Slice/12g	32	267	14.0	1.0	23.0	0.1
Polish Kabanos, Sainsbury's*	1 Sausage/25g	92	366	23.0	0.1	30.4	0.1
Polony Slicing, Asda*	1oz/28g	60	214	11.0	11.0	14.0	0.0
Polony, Slicing, Value, Tesco*	1 Serving/40g	92	229	10.0	10.0	16.5	1.0
Pork & Apple, Average	1 Sausage/57g	146	256	14.5	7.5	18.8	1.9
Pork & Apple, Lean Recipe, Wall's*	1 Sausage/57g	79	139	14.5	9.4	4.5	2.3
Pork & Beef, Average	1 Sausage/45g	133	295	8.7	13.7	22.7	0.5
Pork & Chilli, Tesco*	1 Sausage/67g	124	186	16.4	3.2	12.0	1.1
Pork & Herb, Average	1 Sausage/75g	231	308	13.2	5.5	26.0	0.4
Pork & Herb, Healthy Range, Average	1 Sausage/59g	75	127	16.1	10.8	2.4	1.1
Pork & Leek, Average	1oz/28g	73	262	14.6	6.0	19.9	1.1
Pork & Onion, Gluten Free, Asda*	1 Sausage/40.9g	105	257	20.0	6.0	17.0	1.8
Pork & Smoked Bacon, Finest, Tesco*	1oz/28g	76	271	13.9	4.8	21.8	0.2
Pork & Stilton, Average	1 Sausage/57g	180	317	13.2	5.9	26.7	0.3
Pork & Tomato, Average	1 Sausage/46.5g	126	273	13.9	7.5	20.8	0.4
Pork With Mozzarella, Italian Style, Tesco*	1 Sausage/75.6g	206	271	12.0	10.1	20.3	1.0
Pork, & Sweet Chilli, Waitrose*	1 Sausage/67g	146	219	15.6	4.6	15.3	0.8
Pork, Apricot & Lovage, Waitrose*	1 Sausage/67g	165	246	11.2	12.9	16.6	1.3
Pork, Average	1 Sausage/24g	73	305	12.8	9.8	23.8	0.8
Pork, Bacon & Cheese, Asda*	1/4 Pack/114g	329	289	18.0	7.0	21.0	0.4
Pork, Battered, Thick, Average	1oz/28g	126	448	17.3	21.7	36.3	2.0
Pork, Chilli & Coriander, Grilled, Sainsbury's*	1 Sausage/54g	123	228	18.9	3.5	15.4	1.8
Pork, Extra Lean, Average	1 Sausage/54g	84	155	17.3	6.1	6.9	0.9
Pork, Free From, Tesco*	1 Sausage/57g	124	218	12.1	8.5	15.0	2.2
Pork, Frozen, Fried	1oz/28g	88	316	13.8	10.0	24.8	0.0
Pork, Frozen, Grilled	1oz/28g	81	289	14.8	10.5	21.2	0.0
Pork, Garlic & Herb, Average	1 Sausage/75.6g	204	269	12.0	6.0	21.9	1.2
Pork, Ham & Asparagus, Tesco*	1 Sausage/75.7g	173	228	14.9	3.8	17.0	1.1
Pork, Honey Roast, Westaways*	1 Sausage/75g	183	244	13.1	12.8	15.6	0.0
Pork, Premium, Average	1 Sausage/74g	191	258	14.9	8.3	18.4	1.0
Pork, Reduced Fat, Chilled, Grilled	1oz/28g	64	230	16.2	10.8	13.8	1.5
Pork, Reduced Fat, Healthy Range, Average	1 Sausage/57g	86	151	15.7	9.0	6.0	0.9
Pork, Roasted Pepper & Chilli, COU, Marks & Spencer*	1 Sausage/57g	57	100	15.2	7.1	2.0	2.1
Pork, Skinless, Average	1oz/28g	81	291	11.7	8.2	23.6	0.6
Pork, Smoked Bacon, & Garlic, Finest, Tesco*	1 Sausage/67g	115	173	14.7	0.2	12.6	0.4
Pork, Thick, Average	1 Sausage/38.8g	116	296	13.3	10.0	22.4	1.0
Pork, Thick, Reduced Fat, Healthy Range, Average	1 Sausage/52g	90	173	14.1	12.3	7.4	0.8
Premium, Chilled, Fried	1oz/28g	77	275	15.8	6.7	20.7	0.0
Premium, Chilled, Grilled	1oz/28g	82	292	16.8	6.3	22.4	0.0
Rich Venison & Redcurrant, Grilled, TTD, Sainsbury's*	1 Sausage/46g	138	299	21.2	3.0	22.5	1.8
Round, Breakfast Pack, Healthy Choice, Asda*	1 Sausage/53g	85	160	23.0	6.0	4.9	0.0
Saucisson Montagne, Waitrose*	1 Slice/5g	21	421	20.7	1.9	36.7	0.0

S

SAUSAGE	Measure INFO/WEIGHT	per Measure KCAL	Nutrition Values per 100g / 100ml				
			KCAL	PROT	CARB	FAT	FIBRE
Smoked, Average	1 Sausage/174g	498	286	13.3	2.0	25.6	0.6
Smoky Cajun, TTD, Sainsbury's*	1 Sausage/46.4g	115	250	24.2	1.6	16.3	0.9
Spanish, Wafer Thin, Asda*	1 Slice/4g	12	298	25.4	4.1	20.0	0.0
Spicy Pork & Pepper, Summer Selection, Sainsbury's*	1 Sausage/33g	86	260	20.1	6.0	17.3	1.6
Spicy, Pork, Polenta & Sun Dried Tomato, Waitrose*	1 Sausage/67g	165	247	11.8	9.8	17.8	0.9
Sticky, Marks & Spencer*	1oz/28g	62	220	7.1	18.2	12.8	1.5
Toulouse, Marks & Spencer*	1 Sausage/57g	123	215	12.4	5.8	15.6	1.3
Toulouse, TTD, Sainsbury's*	1 Sausage/67g	186	277	22.0	0.3	20.9	1.2
Tuna & Herb, Sainsbury's*	1 Sausage/47g	109	231	19.6	10.0	12.5	1.5
Tuna & Smoked Salmon, Healthy Living, Tesco*	1 Sausage/67g	90	134	17.9	2.8	5.7	2.0
Tuna, Mediterranean Style, Sainsbury's*	1 Serving/50g	102	204	15.1	14.7	9.5	1.2
Turkey & Chicken, Average	1 Sausage/56.7g	126	222	14.5	8.2	14.6	1.8
Turkey & Ham, Tesco*	1 Sausage/57g	101	178	13.8	8.3	10.0	1.0
Turkey & Pork, Bernard Matthews*	1 Sausage/55g	137	249	10.2	13.1	17.3	0.0
Turkey, Average	1 Sausage/57g	90	157	15.7	6.3	8.0	0.0
Tuscan, Marks & Spencer*	1 Sausage/66g	145	220	14.9	4.6	16.0	0.6
Venison, & Red Wine,TTD, Sainsbury's*	1 Sausage/66g	150	226	19.7	6.8	13.3	1.7
With Baked Beans, Heinz*	1 Serving/70g	135	193	13.3	11.5	10.4	2.5
SAUSAGE & MASH							
BGTY, Sainsbury's*	1 Serving/490g	387	79	4.7	10.1	2.2	1.8
British Classic, Tesco*	1 Pack/450g	675	150	5.1	11.1	9.5	0.9
Eat Smart, Safeway*	1 Pack/400g	340	85	4.6	12.4	1.8	1.3
GFY, Asda*	1 Pack/400g	330	83	4.3	10.8	2.5	1.8
Healthy Living, Tesco*	1 Pack/450g	369	82	4.6	11.3	2.1	1.0
Onion, Marks & Spencer*	1 Pack/300g	315	105	4.1	9.0	5.7	1.5
Safeway*	1 Pack/486.1g	875	180	5.9	9.3	12.9	2.2
Vegetarian, GFY, Asda*	1 Pack/400g	292	73	4.2	9.0	2.2	2.1
Vegetarian, Safeway*	1 Pack/450g	450	100	5.5	8.9	4.7	1.8
Vegetarian, Tesco*	1 Pack/410g	398	97	4.6	11.1	3.8	2.0
With Onion Gravy, Healthy Eating, Tesco*	1 Pack/450g	369	82	4.6	11.3	2.1	1.0
With Onion Gravy, Tesco*	1 Pack/500g	525	105	3.0	11.1	5.4	1.6
SAUSAGE MEAT							
Pork, Average	1oz/28g	96	344	9.9	10.2	29.5	0.7
SAUSAGE MEAT FREE							
Asda*	1 Sausage/43g	81	189	20.0	7.0	9.0	2.9
Glamorgan Leek & Cheese, Sainsbury's*	1 Sausage/50g	108	216	5.6	20.4	12.4	2.6
Premium, Realeat*	1 Sausage/50g	71	142	14.8	3.7	7.5	3.0
SAUSAGE ROLL							
Asda*	1 Roll/64g	216	337	7.0	21.0	25.0	0.8
BGTY, Sainsbury's*	1 Roll/65g	200	308	9.6	27.9	17.6	1.4
Basics, Party Size, Somerfield*	1 Roll/13g	45	343	7.0	29.0	22.0	0.0
Buffet, Healthy Eating, Tesco*	1 Roll/30g	83	278	9.6	31.2	12.8	1.5
Cocktail, Marks & Spencer*	1oz/28g	113	405	9.2	25.2	29.7	1.0
Cocktail, Sainsbury's*	1 Roll/15g	57	381	8.2	26.4	27.0	1.0
Ginsters*	1 Roll/140g	753	538	13.0	33.7	39.1	2.2
Go Large, Asda*	1 Roll/170g	660	388	9.0	25.0	28.0	0.9
Healthy Eating, Tesco*	1 Roll/70g	195	278	9.6	31.2	12.8	1.5
Jumbo, Sainsbury's*	1 Roll/145g	492	339	8.2	23.2	23.7	1.5
Kingsize, Pork Farms*	1/2 Roll/49.9g	242	483	10.5	39.9	31.8	0.0
Large, Sainsbury's*	1 Roll/43g	164	382	7.3	28.1	26.7	1.2
Large, Tesco*	1 Roll/100g	360	360	8.4	27.8	23.8	0.7
Lincolnshire, COU, Marks & Spencer*	1 Roll/175g	280	160	10.0	23.2	2.7	2.6
Lincolnshire, Geo Adams*	1 Serving/130g	475	365	8.3	28.2	24.3	1.1

S

	Measure INFO/WEIGHT	per Measure KCAL	Nutrition Values per 100g / 100ml				
			KCAL	PROT	CARB	FAT	FIBRE
SAUSAGE ROLL							
Marks & Spencer*	1 Roll/32g	122	380	10.5	21.0	28.4	0.9
Mini, Marks & Spencer*	1oz/28g	122	435	9.8	29.6	30.9	1.8
Mini, Tesco*	1 Roll/15g	53	356	9.0	23.9	24.9	1.5
Party Size, Tesco*	1 Roll/12g	39	327	6.2	26.2	21.9	1.3
Party, Sainsbury's*	1 Roll/12g	54	422	8.7	26.7	31.1	1.2
Party, Value, Tesco*	1 Roll/12g	33	274	6.8	35.9	11.5	0.6
Pork Farms*	1 Roll/54g	196	363	7.9	30.0	23.9	0.0
Pork, Large, Marks & Spencer*	1 Roll/63g	236	375	9.0	22.5	27.9	0.7
Pork, Morrisons*	1 Roll/70g	195	278	9.6	31.2	12.8	1.5
Puff Pastry	1oz/28g	107	383	9.9	25.4	27.6	1.0
Puff Pastry, Large, Marks & Spencer*	1 Roll/63g	236	375	9.0	22.5	27.9	0.7
Puff Pastry, Sainsbury's*	1 Roll/65g	250	384	8.3	25.0	27.9	0.9
Reduced Fat, Sainsbury's*	1 Roll/66g	191	289	10.5	29.8	14.2	1.8
Snack Size, Tesco*	1 Roll/32g	118	369	9.1	21.7	27.4	2.3
Snack, GFY, Asda*	1 Roll/34g	112	329	9.4	26.5	20.6	0.9
Snack, Sainsbury's*	1 Roll/33g	125	378	7.5	25.5	27.3	1.0
Somerfield*	1 Roll/35g	149	426	9.0	32.0	29.0	0.0
Tesco*	1 Roll/67g	221	330	9.1	23.8	22.0	2.6
Value, Tesco*	1 Roll/64g	211	330	6.8	29.1	20.7	4.1
Waitrose*	1 Roll/75g	287	383	10.1	27.0	26.1	1.3
SAUSAGE ROLL VEGETARIAN							
Linda McCartney*	1 Roll/51g	133	260	10.9	23.1	14.5	1.6
SAUSAGE VEGETABLE							
Granose*	1oz/28g	63	226	8.5	17.5	13.5	0.0
SAUSAGE VEGETARIAN							
Cumberland, Grilled, Cauldron*	1 Sausage/50g	80	160	12.6	12.3	6.7	2.4
Cumberland, Waitrose*	1 Sausage/50g	80	160	12.6	12.3	6.7	2.4
Garlic & Oregano, Roasted, Cauldron*	1 Sausage/50g	90	179	13.1	9.0	10.1	2.1
Hot Dog, Tesco*	1 sausage/30g	81	271	19.0	6.0	19.0	2.0
Leek & Cheese, Organic, Cauldron*	1 Sausage/41g	80	194	14.4	11.3	10.1	1.7
Lincolnshire, Cauldron*	1 Sausage/50g	85	170	10.0	10.5	9.8	1.8
Lincolnshire, Tesco*	1 Sausage/50g	85	170	10.0	10.5	9.8	1.8
Linda McCartney*	1 Sausage/35g	88	252	23.2	8.6	13.8	1.2
Mushroom & Herb, Waitrose*	1 Sausage/50g	62	123	10.2	8.1	5.4	0.5
Mushroom & Tarragon, Wicken Fen*	1 Sausage/47g	82	175	10.1	17.0	7.4	2.4
Safeway*	2 Sausages/89.7g	149	165	17.2	2.0	9.8	8.1
Smoked Paprika & Chilli, Cauldron*	1 Sausage/50g	76	152	7.8	11.8	8.2	2.6
Spinach, Leek & Cheese, Gourmet, Wicken Fen*	1 Sausage/46g	92	201	10.3	17.0	10.2	1.9
Sun Dried Tomato & Black Olive, Cauldron*	1 Serving/50g	71	142	8.7	9.4	7.7	2.6
Sun Dried Tomato & Herb, Linda McCartney*	1 Sausage/35g	93	266	21.8	10.1	15.4	1.7
SAVOURY EGGS							
Mini, Asda*	1 Egg/19g	58	303	10.3	17.7	21.2	1.5
Mini, Iceland*	1 Egg/20g	66	327	11.0	17.5	23.7	1.1
Mini, New Improved Recipe, Tesco*	1 Egg/20g	65	323	12.5	18.3	22.2	1.3
Mini, Tesco*	1 Egg/20g	68	342	11.2	23.0	22.8	0.9
SCALLOPS							
Breaded, With Plum & Chilli Dipping Sauce, Tesco*	1 Pack/210g	441	210	10.6	25.6	7.2	0.8
Hotbake Shells, Sainsbury's*	1 Serving/140g	241	172	9.5	8.4	11.2	0.8
King, Finest, Tesco*	1 Serving/170g	129	76	16.9	0.1	0.9	0.0
King, Marks & Spencer*	1 Serving/260g	182	70	15.5	1.2	0.1	1.2
King, Trimmed by Hand, Sainsbury's*	1 Pack/200g	142	71	16.0	1.4	0.1	0.2
Lemon & Pepper, TTD, Sainsbury's*	1 Serving/100g	213	213	13.8	20.6	8.4	1.7
Lemon Grass & Ginger, Tesco*	1/2 Pack/112g	90	80	15.2	2.5	1.0	0.6

S

	Measure	per Measure		Nutrition Values per 100g / 100ml				
	INFO/WEIGHT	KCAL		KCAL	PROT	CARB	FAT	FIBRE
SCALLOPS								
Meat, Asda*	1oz/28g	33		118	23.2	1.4	1.4	0.0
Queen, Kintyre*	1 Serving/100g	105		105	23.2	0.1	1.4	0.1
Queen, Scottish, Sainsbury's*	1 Pack/200g	350		175	30.4	0.8	5.5	0.0
Steamed	1oz/28g	33		118	23.2	3.4	1.4	0.0
Thai Style Breaded With Plum Sauce, Finest, Tesco*	1 Serving/210g	401		191	11.5	20.6	7.0	0.8
With Lemon Pepper Butter, Cook, Marks & Spencer*	1 Serving/105g	158		150	13.9	1.6	9.8	0.3
With Roasted Garlic Butter, Finest, Tesco*	1 Serving/100g	201		201	16.2	1.8	14.3	0.4
SCAMPI								
Breaded, Average	1/2 Pack/255g	565		222	10.7	20.5	10.7	1.0
SCAMPI &								
Chips, Tesco*	1 Serving/450g	689		153	5.1	22.4	4.8	1.6
Chips, Young's*	1oz/28g	42		150	5.0	20.3	5.4	1.7
SCHNITZELS								
Vegetarian, Tivall*	1 Schnitzel/100g	172		172	16.0	9.0	8.0	5.0
SCONE								
3% Fat, Marks & Spencer*	1 Scone/65g	179		275	7.2	55.1	2.5	2.3
All Butter, Tesco*	1 Scone/41g	126		308	7.2	52.3	7.8	1.6
Cheese	1 Scone/40g	145		363	10.1	43.2	17.8	1.6
Cheese & Black Pepper, Mini, Marks & Spencer*	1 Scone/18g	67		370	10.2	41.1	18.3	1.7
Cheese, Marks & Spencer*	1 Scone/60g	237		395	10.3	38.9	21.9	1.6
Cheese, Sainsbury's*	1 Scone/70g	250		357	10.6	36.9	18.6	2.0
Cherry, Marks & Spencer*	1 Scone/60g	202		337	6.9	49.7	12.2	1.9
Cream, Sainsbury's*	1 Scone/50g	173		345	4.6	42.5	17.4	3.1
Derby, Asda*	1 Scone/59g	202		342	7.0	56.0	10.0	0.0
Derby, Mothers Pride*	1 Scone/60g	208		347	5.2	49.8	14.0	1.5
Derby, Tesco*	1 Scone/60g	201		335	7.2	53.7	10.2	2.0
Devon, Sainsbury's*	1 Scone/54g	201		372	7.1	51.1	15.5	1.6
Devon, Waitrose*	1 Scone/71.8g	269		373	7.5	56.0	13.2	2.3
Fresh Cream With Strawberry Jam, Tesco*	1 Scone/83g	290		352	4.7	40.7	18.9	1.1
Fresh Cream, Finest, Tesco*	1 Serving/133g	469		354	4.6	44.5	17.5	1.7
Fresh Cream, TTD, Sainsbury's*	1 Serving/110g	379		346	5.8	48.1	14.5	2.6
Fresh Cream, Tesco*	1 Scone/79.5g	244		304	15.8	32.3	12.5	0.9
Fruit	1 Scone/40g	126		316	7.3	52.9	9.8	0.0
Fruit, Economy, Sainsbury's*	1 Scone/34g	111		326	7.9	52.5	9.4	1.7
Fruit, SmartPrice, Asda*	1 Scone/41g	139		338	7.0	55.0	10.0	3.0
Fruit, Somerfield*	1 Scone/35g	116		332	8.0	53.0	10.0	0.0
Fruited, Waitrose*	1 Serving/78g	268		344	4.4	37.2	19.6	0.9
Plain	1 Scone/40g	145		362	7.2	53.8	14.6	1.9
Potato	1 Scone/40g	118		296	5.1	39.1	14.3	1.6
Potato, Mothers Pride*	1 Scone/37g	77		207	4.7	42.0	2.2	4.3
Potato, Warburtons*	1 Scone/48g	123		256	5.6	35.1	10.1	0.0
Strawberry, Fresh Cream, BGTY, Sainsbury's*	1 Scone/50g	155		309	5.1	47.0	11.2	1.1
Strawberry, Marks & Spencer*	1 Scone/55g	132		240	3.2	23.0	14.9	0.7
Sultana, BGTY, Sainsbury's*	1 Scone/63g	178		283	7.7	56.7	2.8	2.4
Sultana, Finest, Tesco*	1 Scone/70g	225		321	8.9	46.7	10.9	2.1
Sultana, Less Than 5% Fat, Asda*	1 Scone/60g	198		330	7.0	62.0	6.0	1.8
Sultana, Low Fat, Marks & Spencer*	1 Scone/65g	179		275	7.2	55.1	2.5	2.3
Sultana, Marks & Spencer*	1 Scone/60g	235		392	7.0	58.7	13.8	2.8
Sultana, Reduced Fat, Waitrose*	1 Scone/65g	187		287	6.6	53.2	5.3	2.6
Sultana, Sainsbury's*	1 Scone/53.8g	177		327	6.9	50.2	11.0	6.5
Sultana, Tesco*	1 Scone/70g	215		307	6.8	53.8	7.2	2.0
Sultana, Value, Tesco*	1 Scone/40g	138		346	7.0	53.8	11.5	2.3
Wholemeal	1 Scone/40g	130		326	8.7	43.1	14.4	5.2

S

	Measure INFO/WEIGHT	per Measure KCAL	Nutrition Values per 100g / 100ml				
			KCAL	PROT	CARB	FAT	FIBRE
SCONE							
Wholemeal, Fruit	1 Scone/40g	130	324	8.1	47.2	12.8	4.9
SCONE MIX							
Fruit, Asda	1 Scone/47.5g	144	301	7.0	57.0	5.0	3.7
SCOTCH EGGS							
Bar, Ginsters*	1 Bar/90g	256	284	11.8	20.1	17.4	1.7
Finest, Tesco*	1 Egg/114g	280	247	11.6	10.4	17.7	1.1
Ginsters*	1 Egg/95g	228	240	15.3	9.7	15.9	0.6
Mini, 40% Less Fat, Sainsbury's*	1 Egg/20g	46	231	12.8	15.3	13.2	1.4
Mini, Sainsbury's*	1 Egg/12.2g	39	329	10.9	18.9	23.3	1.0
Retail	1 Egg/120g	301	251	12.0	13.1	17.1	0.0
Sainsbury's*	1 Egg/116g	319	275	11.1	14.2	19.3	0.9
Tesco*	1 Egg/114g	294	258	10.8	12.7	18.2	1.3
SEAFOOD COCKTAIL							
Asda*	1oz/28g	26	92	14.0	5.7	1.5	0.1
Average	1oz/28g	24	87	15.6	2.9	1.5	0.0
Somerfield*	1oz/28g	23	81	14.0	2.0	2.0	0.0
SEAFOOD COLLECTION							
Premium, Frozen, Tesco*	1 Serving/100g	70	70	12.2	2.4	1.3	0.0
SEAFOOD MEDLEY							
Sainsbury's*	1/2 Pack/175g	158	90	14.3	4.0	1.9	0.5
Steam Cuisine, Marks & Spencer*	1 Pack/400g	320	80	8.5	4.5	3.1	1.3
SEAFOOD SELECTION							
Asda*	1 Pack/213g	211	99	12.0	9.0	1.4	0.0
Frozen, Sainsbury's*	1 Serving/100g	76	76	14.2	2.3	1.1	0.2
Healthy Eating, Tesco*	1 Pack/250g	175	70	12.2	2.4	1.3	0.0
Luxury, Safeway*	1 Pack/250g	215	86	13.8	3.1	2.0	0.0
Marks & Spencer*	1 Serving/200g	170	85	17.4	1.6	1.0	0.5
Ready To Eat, Drained, Sainsbury's*	1 Serving/125g	85	68	14.6	0.8	1.0	2.5
Sainsbury's*	1/2 Pack/125g	125	100	18.6	2.2	1.9	0.1
Tesco*	1 Serving/100g	93	93	17.4	1.7	1.8	0.0
SEAFOOD STICKS							
Average	1 Stick/15g	16	106	8.0	18.4	0.2	0.2
Low Price, Sainsbury's*	1 Stick/16g	16	101	7.3	16.0	0.9	0.6
With Cocktail Dip, Asda*	1 Pot/95g	126	133	6.0	16.0	5.0	0.1
With Garlic & Lemon Dip, Asda*	1 Pot/97.9g	184	188	7.0	13.0	12.0	0.0
SEASONING							
Aromat, Knorr*	1oz/28g	46	164	12.4	20.5	3.6	1.0
Sushi, Mitsukan*	2 Tbsp/30ml	50	167	0.0	36.7	3.3	0.0
SEASONING CUBES							
For Potato, Garlic Parsley, Knorr*	1 Serving/10g	55	550	6.0	22.0	48.0	2.0
For Potato, Mint, Perfect Potato, Knorr*	1 Cube/10g	56	560	5.1	21.2	50.5	1.8
For Rice, Pilau, Knorr*	1 Cube/10g	31	305	11.4	13.9	22.6	1.4
For Rice, Saffron, Knorr*	1 Cube/10g	29	291	13.8	17.5	18.4	2.2
For Stir Fry, Oriental Spices, Knorr*	1 Cube/10g	41	414	9.7	25.0	30.6	1.1
Oriental Spice, Knorr*	1 Cube/10g	41	409	9.5	23.7	30.7	0.0
Perfect Pasta, Knorr*	1 Cube/10g	28	278	10.3	5.2	24.0	0.0
Wild Mushroom, Knorr*	1 Cube/10g	37	365	10.3	21.3	26.5	0.2
SEASONING MIX							
Beef Taco, Colman's*	1 Pack/30g	76	252	9.1	26.9	12.0	14.0
Chilli, Old El Paso*	Packet/39g	117	301	7.0	57.0	5.0	0.0
Fajita, Chicken, Colman's*	1 Pack/40g	149	373	10.8	13.3	30.7	13.8
Fajita, Old El Paso*	1oz/28g	88	313	11.0	56.0	5.0	0.0
Garlic & Herb Potato Wedge, Schwartz*	1/2 Serving/337g	546	162	3.4	26.4	4.7	0.0

S

	Measure INFO/WEIGHT	per Measure KCAL	Nutrition Values per 100g / 100ml				
			KCAL	PROT	CARB	FAT	FIBRE
SEASONING MIX							
Mediterranean Roast Vegetable, Schwartz*	1oz/28g	92	330	7.0	65.6	4.4	0.0
Shepherd's Pie, Colman's*	1 Pack/50g	131	262	14.3	48.6	1.1	4.1
Shepherd's Pie, Schwartz*	1 Pack/38g	110	289	9.3	58.5	2.0	0.0
Taco, Old El Paso*	1/4 Pack/9g	30	334	5.5	69.0	4.0	0.0
Whole Grain Mustard & Herb Potato Mash, Colman's*	1 Pack/30g	153	510	9.7	19.1	44.1	0.0
SEAWEED							
Crispy, Average	1oz/28g	182	651	7.5	15.6	61.9	7.0
Irish Moss, Raw	1oz/28g	2	8	1.5	0.0	0.2	12.3
Kombu, Dried, Raw	1oz/28g	12	43	7.1	0.0	1.6	58.7
Nori, Dried, Raw	1oz/28g	38	136	30.7	0.0	1.5	44.4
Wakame, Dried, Raw	1oz/28g	20	71	12.4	0.0	2.4	47.1
SEEDS							
Melon, Average	1 Tbsp/15g	87	583	28.5	9.9	47.7	0.0
Poppy, Asda*	1 Serving/2g	11	556	21.0	19.0	44.0	0.0
Pumpkin, Average	1 Tbsp/10g	57	568	27.9	13.0	45.9	3.9
Sesame, Tesco*	1 Tsp/4g	24	598	18.2	0.9	58.0	7.9
Sunflower, Average	1 Tbsp/10g	59	585	23.4	15.0	48.7	5.7
SEMOLINA							
Average	1oz/28g	98	348	11.0	75.2	1.8	2.1
Pudding, Creamed, Ambrosia*	1 Can/425g	344	81	3.3	13.1	1.7	0.2
Pudding, Creamed, Co-Op*	1 Can/425g	383	90	4.0	15.0	2.0	0.0
SHAKE							
Chocolate, Nutrition, Myoplex*	1 Serving/76g	279	367	55.0	31.0	2.2	1.1
Chocolate, Ready To Drink, Advantage, Atkins*	1 Carton/330ml	172	52	6.0	0.6	2.8	1.2
Chocolate, Ready To Drink, Myoplex*	1 Shake/330ml	150	45	7.6	1.5	1.1	0.0
Herbalife*	1 Serving/250ml	245	98	10.0	8.8	2.6	1.0
Strawberry, Ready To Drink, Myoplex*	1 Shake/330ml	150	45	7.6	1.5	1.1	0.0
Vanilla, Advant Edge, Ready To Drink, EAS*	1 Serving/250ml	150	60	4.5	7.6	1.3	0.4
Vanilla, Ready To Drink, Advantage, Atkins*	1 Carton/330ml	175	53	6.2	0.6	2.7	0.9
Vanilla, Ready To Drink, Myoplex*	1 Shake/330ml	150	45	7.6	1.5	1.1	0.0
SHAKE MIX							
Chocolate, Advantage, Atkins*	1 Serving/33.5g	123	361	49.0	8.1	12.5	15.5
SHALLOTS							
Pickled, In Hot & Spicy Vinegar, Tesco*	1 Onion/18g	14	77	1.0	18.0	0.1	1.9
Raw	1oz/28g	6	20	1.5	3.3	0.2	1.4
SHANDY							
Bitter, Original, Ben Shaws*	1 Can/330ml	89	27	0.0	6.0	0.0	0.0
Homemade	1 Pint/568ml	148	26	0.2	2.9	0.0	0.0
Lemonade, Schweppes*	1 Can/330ml	76	23	0.0	5.1	0.0	0.0
Lemonade, Traditional Style, Tesco*	1 Can/330ml	63	19	0.0	4.7	0.0	0.0
SHARK							
Raw	1oz/28g	29	102	23.0	0.0	1.1	0.0
SHARON FRUIT							
Average	1oz/28g	20	73	0.8	18.6	0.0	1.6
SHERRY							
Dry	1 Serving/50ml	58	116	0.2	1.4	0.0	0.0
Medium	1 Serving/50ml	58	116	0.1	5.9	0.0	0.0
Sweet	1 Serving/50ml	68	136	0.3	6.9	0.0	0.0
SHORTBREAD							
All Butter, Assorted, Parkwood, Aldi*	1oz/28g	143	511	6.5	61.0	26.8	2.0
All Butter, McVitie's*	Twin Finger/40g	216	541	6.3	62.6	29.5	1.9
All Butter, Petticoat Tails, Gardiners Of Scotland*	1 Wedge/12g	64	514	5.2	62.1	27.2	0.0
All Butter, Scottish, Marks & Spencer*	1 Biscuit/34g	173	510	5.7	58.9	27.8	1.8

S

SHORTBREAD

INFO/WEIGHT	Measure	KCAL	KCAL	PROT	CARB	FAT	FIBRE
All Butter, Thins, Marks & Spencer*	1 Biscuit/10.3g	49	485	5.8	68.4	21.1	3.5
All Butter, Trufree*	1 Biscuit/11g	58	524	2.0	66.0	28.0	0.9
Average	1oz/28g	139	498	5.9	63.9	26.1	1.9
Butter, Extra Special, Asda*	1 Serving/19g	101	531	7.0	56.0	31.0	1.8
Choc Chip, Fair Trade, Co-Op*	1 Biscuit/19g	100	526	5.3	57.9	31.6	2.6
Chocolate & Caramel, TTD, Sainsbury's*	1 Serving/55g	245	446	4.7	45.0	27.7	1.3
Chocolate Caramel, Co-Op*	1 Cake/49g	245	500	4.1	61.2	26.5	1.0
Chocolate Chip, Jacobs*	1 Biscuit/17g	87	513	5.2	61.2	27.5	1.8
Chocolate, Waitrose*	1oz/28g	144	516	5.5	61.2	27.7	1.8
Clotted Cream & Choc Chip, Furniss*	1 Biscuit/8g	43	516	6.2	60.7	27.7	0.0
Clotted Cream, Finest, Tesco*	1 Biscuit/20g	109	543	5.2	58.0	32.2	1.7
Cookie, Choc Chip, Low Carb, Carbolite*	1 Cookie/30g	120	400	13.3	19.0	30.0	13.3
Crawfords*	1 Biscuit/12.5g	64	533	6.6	65.0	27.4	2.0
Double Choc Chip, Petit Four, Scottish, Tesco*	1 Serving/50g	266	531	5.1	60.4	30.0	1.7
Farmhouse, TTD, Sainsbury's*	1 Finger/20g	106	528	5.1	61.6	29.0	1.7
Fingers, All Butter, Tesco*	1 Finger/13g	67	519	5.8	60.3	28.3	1.8
Fingers, All Butter, Traditional, Scottish, Tesco*	1 Finger/17.8g	94	520	6.0	58.5	29.1	1.8
Fingers, Asda*	1 Finger/18g	93	519	5.8	60.3	28.3	18.0
Fingers, Clotted Cream, Furniss*	1 Finger/15g	70	464	5.9	56.9	23.8	0.0
Fingers, Cornish Cookie*	2 Fingers/50g	249	498	6.4	61.0	25.5	0.0
Fingers, Deans*	1 Finger/24g	115	488	5.1	60.1	24.8	1.4
Fingers, Highland, Organic, Sainsbury's*	1 Serving/16g	84	527	5.8	58.7	29.9	1.9
Fingers, Highland, Sainsbury's*	1 Finger/20g	106	528	5.6	57.8	30.5	1.9
Fingers, Light & Buttery, TTD, Sainsbury's*	1 Finger/20g	105	528	5.1	61.6	29.0	0.7
Fingers, Marks & Spencer*	1oz/28g	143	510	5.9	60.8	27.0	1.6
Fingers, Scottish, Finest, Tesco*	1 Pack/165g	822	498	5.1	65.5	23.9	2.0
Fingers, Scottish, Marks & Spencer*	1oz/28g	143	510	5.9	60.8	27.0	1.6
Free From, Sainsbury's*	1 Biscuit/20g	98	490	6.0	58.0	26.0	6.0
Highland Demerara Rounds, Sainsbury's*	1 Biscuit/20g	113	565	5.5	70.5	29.0	2.0
Highland, Organic, Duchy Originals*	1 Biscuit/16g	80	515	5.2	61.8	27.4	1.7
Highland, Petticoat Tails, Sainsbury's*	1 Segment/12.5g	67	518	5.7	60.8	28.0	1.8
Luxury Spices, Extra Special, Asda*	1 Biscuit/20g	97	486	4.9	67.0	22.0	2.1
Mini Bites, Country Table*	1 Biscuit/10g	53	525	7.1	59.3	29.5	1.5
Orange Marmalade & Oatflake, Deans*	1 Biscuit/20g	105	524	6.7	59.3	29.6	3.2
Pecan & Caramel, TTD, Sainsbury's*	1 Slice/52g	259	497	5.1	53.1	29.4	1.6
Pecan All Butter, Sainsbury's*	1 Biscuit/18g	99	548	5.3	49.9	36.3	2.5
Petticoat Tails, Sainsbury's*	1 Segment/13g	68	520	5.4	60.5	28.5	1.8
Pure Butter, Jacobs*	1 Biscuit/20g	105	525	5.7	58.6	29.7	1.8
Raspberry & Oatmeal, Deans*	1 Biscuit/20g	103	514	4.7	63.1	28.6	1.4
Reduced Sugar, Tesco*	1 Biscuit/17g	86	519	6.7	57.1	29.4	2.1
Rounds, TTD, Sainsbury's*	1 Biscuit/20g	108	538	5.0	59.5	31.1	1.6
Scottish, Marks & Spencer*	1oz/28g	143	512	4.4	59.7	27.9	2.6
Shrewsbury, Marks & Spencer*	1oz/28g	128	458	7.5	63.9	23.3	4.5
St. Clements Farmhouse Style, TTD, Sainsbury's*	1 Biscuit/20.2g	105	526	4.8	58.4	30.3	2.0
Stem Ginger, Waitrose*	1 Biscuit/15g	71	487	4.7	66.0	22.7	1.6
The Best, Safeway*	1 Finger/20g	100	500	4.8	65.5	23.9	2.0
Wheat & Gluten Free, Free From Range, Tesco*	1 Biscuit/20g	98	490	6.0	58.0	26.0	6.0

SHRIMPS

INFO/WEIGHT	Measure	KCAL	KCAL	PROT	CARB	FAT	FIBRE
Boiled	1oz/28g	33	117	23.8	0.0	2.4	0.0
Dried	1oz/28g	69	245	55.8	0.0	2.4	0.0
Frozen	1oz/28g	20	73	16.5	0.0	0.8	0.0
In Brine, Canned, Drained	1oz/28g	26	94	20.8	0.0	1.2	0.0

	Measure INFO/WEIGHT	per Measure KCAL	Nutrition Values per 100g / 100ml				
			KCAL	PROT	CARB	FAT	FIBRE
SKATE							
Grilled	1oz/28g	22	79	18.9	0.0	0.5	0.0
In Batter, Fried in Blended Oil	1oz/28g	47	168	14.7	4.9	10.1	0.2
Raw	1oz/28g	18	64	15.1	0.0	0.4	0.0
SKIPS							
Bacon, KP*	1 Pack/17.1g	81	474	6.5	62.1	22.2	2.3
Easy Cheesy, KP*	1 Bag/19g	100	525	3.9	59.5	30.1	0.9
Pickled Onion, KP*	1 Pack/13.1g	67	512	3.4	56.4	30.3	1.4
Prawn Cocktail, KP*	1 Bag/17g	88	517	3.3	59.8	29.4	1.3
Prawn Cocktail, KP*	1 Pack/25g	88	352	2.4	40.8	20.0	0.8
Tangy Tomato, KP*	1 Bag/17g	88	517	3.2	59.6	29.5	1.2
SKITTLES							
Fruits, Mars*	1 Pack/18g	72	399	0.0	90.4	4.2	0.0
Mars*	1 Pack/55g	220	400	0.0	90.5	4.2	0.0
SLICES							
Bacon & Cheese, Savoury, Somerfield*	1 Slice/165.0g	490	297	7.4	21.2	20.3	1.5
Bacon & Cheese, Tesco*	1 Slice/165g	480	291	7.4	21.7	19.4	1.0
Beef, Minced Steak & Onion, Tesco*	1 Slice/150g	425	283	8.7	21.3	18.1	1.6
Beef, Minced With Onion, Sainsbury's*	1 Slice/120g	328	273	6.8	24.5	16.4	1.1
Beef, Minced, Morrisons*	1 Slice/143g	457	320	8.8	24.6	20.7	1.0
Cheddar Cheese & Onion, Ginsters*	1 Slice/180g	583	324	7.1	22.8	22.7	1.0
Cheese & Garlic, Safeway*	1 Slice/31g	123	398	11.4	44.1	19.5	2.2
Cheese & Ham, Sainsbury's*	1 Slice/118g	352	298	7.8	22.5	17.9	1.8
Cheese & Ham, Savoury, Somerfield*	1 Slice/150g	399	266	7.0	23.0	16.0	0.6
Cheese & Onion, Savoury, Somerfield*	1 Slice/165g	518	314	7.4	24.0	20.9	0.6
Cheese & Onion, Tesco*	1 Slice/150g	503	335	8.0	20.1	24.7	1.4
Cheese, Potato & Onion, Taste!*	1 Serving/155.1g	501	323	8.6	28.1	19.6	0.0
Chicken & Ham, Taste!*	1 Slice/154.8g	357	230	10.8	24.2	9.9	0.0
Chicken & Leek, Taste!*	1 Slice/155g	406	262	10.1	27.6	12.3	0.0
Chicken & Mushroom, Asda*	1 Serving/127.8g	355	277	7.0	24.0	17.0	2.1
Chicken & Mushroom, Ginsters*	1 Slice/155g	420	271	6.6	21.8	17.5	1.7
Chicken & Mushroom, Sainsbury's*	1 Slice/164g	427	259	7.3	21.3	16.1	1.0
Chicken & Mushroom, Tesco*	1 Slice/165g	457	277	9.2	20.6	17.5	0.9
Chicken Breast, Bacon & Cheese Food, Tesco*	1 Serving/150g	237	158	20.7	1.2	7.8	0.5
Chicken, Spicy, Deep Fill, Ginsters*	1 Slice/180g	499	277	9.2	21.8	17.0	1.4
Fresh Cream, Tesco*	1 Slice/75g	311	414	3.5	37.4	27.9	1.0
Ham & Cheese, Ginsters*	1 Slice/155g	625	403	9.8	31.9	28.2	4.2
Minced Steak & Onion, Sainsbury's*	1 Slice/165g	475	288	15.2	16.0	18.1	2.5
Peppered Steak, Asda*	1 Serving/164g	483	295	9.0	22.0	19.0	1.2
Pork & Egg, Gala, Tesco*	1 Slice/105g	333	317	10.3	17.2	23.0	3.4
Prawn & Avocado, Plait, Extra Special, Asda*	1 Serving/198g	331	167	11.0	23.0	3.4	1.3
Salmon, & Watercress, Honey Roast, Plait, Asda*	1 Plait/166g	421	254	13.0	28.0	10.0	0.4
Sausage Meat, With Onion Gravy, Lattice, Asda*	1 Serving/278g	595	214	10.0	12.0	14.0	1.7
Smoked Cheese With Ham, Aldi*	1 Slice/21g	66	313	21.0	1.0	25.0	0.1
Spinach & Ricotta, Sainsbury's*	1 Slice/165g	500	303	6.5	21.1	21.4	2.9
Steak & Onion, Aberdeen Angus, Tesco*	1 Slice/165g	444	269	8.7	20.7	16.8	1.3
Steak, Peppered, Deep Fill, Ginsters*	1 Slice/180g	513	285	9.4	16.1	20.1	3.1
Steak, Peppered, Ginsters*	1 Slice/155g	415	268	9.9	21.5	15.8	1.9
Vegetable, Tesco*	1 Slice/165g	452	274	5.6	21.4	18.5	3.3
SLIMFAST*							
Banana Deluxe Meal Replacement Drink	1 Serving/325ml	215	66	4.2	11.3	0.8	1.4
Chocolate Royale, Ready To Drink, Ultra	1 Serving/11floz	220	71	3.2	12.8	0.9	1.6
Chocolate Shake	1 Can/325ml	218	67	4.2	10.6	0.8	1.8
Coffee Mocha, Ready to Drink	1 Shake/325ml	215	66	4.2	10.6	0.8	1.5

	Measure INFO/WEIGHT	per Measure KCAL	Nutrition Values per 100g / 100ml				
			KCAL	PROT	CARB	FAT	FIBRE
SLIMFAST*							
French Vanilla, Ready To Drink	1 Can/325ml	215	66	4.2	10.6	0.8	1.5
Shake, Chocolate, Dry	1 Serving/35g	123	351	13.6	54.3	9.3	17.1
Shake, Peach	1 Can/325ml	215	66	4.2	10.6	0.8	1.5
Shake, Strawberry	1 Can/325ml	215	66	4.2	10.6	0.8	1.5
Shake, Vanilla, Dry	1 Serving/35g	123	351	12.7	57.0	7.5	17.1
Shake, Vanilla, Ready to Drink	1 Can/325ml	215	66	4.2	10.6	0.8	1.5
Strawberry Supreme, Ready To Drink	1 Can/325ml	215	66	4.2	10.6	0.8	1.5
SMARTIES							
Biscuits, Nestle*	1 Biscuit/5g	26	519	7.7	57.6	28.6	0.0
Giants, Nestle*	1 Pack/186g	882	474	4.6	70.4	19.3	0.7
Mini Cones, Nestle*	1 Serving/44g	145	330	4.5	45.0	13.1	0.0
Mini Eggs, Nestle*	1 Lge Bag/112g	535	478	4.8	69.6	20.0	0.7
Minis, Nestle*	1 Serving/14.8g	69	458	4.1	73.5	16.4	0.6
Nestle*	3 Smarties/3g	14	458	4.1	73.5	16.4	0.6
Tree Decoration, Nestle*	1 Chocolate/18.0g	95	529	5.6	58.9	30.1	0.8
SMOOTHIE							
Apple, Grapes & Blackcurrant, P & J*	1 Bottle/250ml	125	50	0.8	11.1	0.3	0.7
Apple, Kiwi & Lime, SunJuice*	1 Serving/250ml	133	53	0.5	13.4	0.1	0.8
Apple, Strawberry, Cherry & Banana, Marks & Spencer*	1 Bottle/250ml	125	50	0.5	11.2	0.3	0.6
Apricot & Peach, COU, Marks & Spencer*	1 Serving/250ml	100	40	0.9	8.3	0.4	0.4
Banana, Dairy, Probiotic, Boots*	1 Bottle/250ml	148	59	1.6	12.0	0.5	1.0
Banana, Dairy, Tesco*	1 Serving/250ml	165	66	1.6	14.0	0.4	0.4
Banana, Marks & Spencer*	1 Bottle/500ml	270	54	1.7	12.2	0.1	0.8
Blackberry & Blueberry, Innocent*	1 Bottle/250ml	120	48	0.6	11.5	0.1	0.0
Blackcurrant & Apple, For Kids, Innocent*	1 Carton/180ml	112	62	0.4	14.5	0.2	0.0
Blackcurrants & Gooseberries, For Autuman, Innocent*	1 Bottle/250ml	118	47	0.5	12.5	0.1	0.0
Boysenberry & Raspberry, Fruit, TTD, Sainsbury's*	1 Bottle/250ml	108	43	0.7	10.0	0.1	1.6
Cherries & Strawberries, Innocent*	1 Bottle/250ml	123	49	0.6	12.6	0.1	0.0
Cranberries & Raspberries, Pure Fruit, Innocent*	1 Bottle/250ml	113	45	0.5	13.1	0.1	0.0
Cranberries & Strawberries, Innocent*	1 Serving/250ml	103	41	0.5	9.5	0.2	0.0
Daily Detox, P & J*	1 Bottle/250ml	143	57	0.8	13.1	0.2	0.0
Ginseng & Ace Vitamins, Marks & Spencer*	1 Bottle/250ml	138	55	0.7	13.0	0.2	0.9
It's Alive, P & J*	1 Bottle/250ml	150	60	0.7	13.6	0.3	0.0
Mango & Orange, Smoothie Smile*	1 Bottle/250ml	130	52	0.4	11.7	0.4	0.0
Mango & Passion Fruit, Innocent*	1 Bottle/250ml	138	55	0.4	12.8	0.2	0.0
Mango & West Indian Cherry, Plus, Tesco*	1 Serving/250ml	133	53	0.6	12.2	0.2	0.5
Mango, Pineapple & Passion Fruit, Eat Smart, Safeway*	1 Bottle/250ml	135	54	0.5	12.6	0.0	1.1
Orange & Mango, Fruit, Morrisons*	1 Serving/250ml	145	58	0.5	14.0	0.0	0.7
Orange & Mango, Safeway*	1 Bottle/250ml	130	52	0.5	12.1	0.2	0.7
Orange, Banana & Pineapple, Innocent*	1 Bottle/250ml	120	48	0.6	10.8	0.4	0.0
Orange, Mango & Apricot, COU, Marks & Spencer*	1 Bottle/250ml	130	52	0.6	11.0	0.6	0.6
Orange, Mango, Banana & Passion Fruit, Asda*	1 Serving/100ml	55	55	0.8	12.0	0.2	1.1
Orange, Strawberry & Guava, Sainsbury's*	1 Serving/300ml	159	53	0.3	12.0	0.2	0.8
Oranges & Mangoes, Get Your Vits, P & J*	1 Bottle/250ml	128	51	0.6	11.6	0.2	0.0
Oranges Mangos & Bananas, P & J*	1 Bottle/330ml	195	59	0.9	13.6	0.2	0.7
Passionfruit Lychee, SunJuice*	1 Sm Bottle/250ml	145	58	0.5	13.5	0.2	0.8
Peach, Mild & Fruity, Campina*	1 Bottle/330ml	211	64	2.7	13.1	0.0	0.0
Peaches & Bananas, P & J*	1 Bottle/330ml	188	57	0.7	13.6	0.3	0.0
Pineapple, Banana & Mango Fruit, Finest, Tesco*	1 Glass/200ml	94	47	0.1	11.2	0.2	0.0
Pineapple, Banana & Pear, Asda*	1 Bottle/250ml	147	59	0.5	13.6	0.1	0.3
Pineapple, Banana & Pear, Princes*	1 Bottle/250ml	153	61	0.5	13.9	0.2	0.5
Pineapple, Mango & Lime, Way To Five, Sainsbury's*	1 Bottle/250g	120	48	0.4	11.3	0.1	0.3
Pineapple, Mango & Passion Fruit, Extra Special, Asda*	1/2 Bottle/250ml	100	40	0.5	9.0	0.2	1.3

INFO/WEIGHT	Measure	per Measure KCAL	Nutrition Values per 100g / 100ml KCAL	PROT	CARB	FAT	FIBRE

SMOOTHIE

	Measure	per Measure	KCAL	PROT	CARB	FAT	FIBRE
Pineapple, Mango & Passionfruit, 100% Fruit, Sainsbury's*	1 Bottle/250ml	163	65	0.7	15.2	0.1	1.0
Pineapple, Strawberries & Passion Fruit, P & J*	1 Bottle/330ml	152	46	0.6	10.8	0.1	1.3
Rasberry & Cranberry, Smoothie Plus, Tesco*	1 Serving/250ml	140	56	0.6	13.0	0.2	3.0
Raspberry & Bio Yogurt, Marks & Spencer*	1 Bottle/500ml	275	55	2.0	10.8	0.3	0.9
Raspberry & Blueberry, Plus, Tesco*	1 Serving/100ml	59	59	2.6	11.6	0.3	0.5
Raspberry, Banana & Peach, Sainsbury's*	1 Bottle/250.9ml	138	55	0.8	12.8	0.1	1.5
Raspberry, Marks & Spencer*	1 Serving/250ml	138	55	1.7	12.2	0.6	1.9
Strawberries & Bananas, Innocent*	1 Bottle/250ml	118	47	0.4	10.7	0.2	0.0
Strawberries & Bananas, P & J*	1 Bottle/330ml	172	52	0.9	11.5	0.3	0.0
Strawberry & Banana, Fruit, Finest, Tesco*	1 Bottle/250ml	135	54	0.3	12.5	0.3	0.5
Strawberry & Banana, Full Of Fruit, Tesco*	1 Bottle/250ml	115	46	0.6	10.1	0.2	0.8
Strawberry & Cherry, Organic, Marks & Spencer*	1 Bottle/250ml	138	55	0.8	12.3	0.3	0.4
Strawberry & Raspberry, COU, Marks & Spencer*	1 Bottle/250ml	113	45	0.6	10.2	0.2	0.9
Strawberry & Raspberry, Shapers, Boots*	1 Bottle/250ml	110	44	0.6	10.0	0.2	0.6
Strawberry & White Chocolate, Marks & Spencer*	1 Serving/250ml	100	40	2.5	5.5	1.0	0.1
Strawberry Dairy, Shapers, Boots*	1 Bottle/250ml	120	48	1.7	9.7	0.3	0.5
Strawberry, Dairy, Finest, Tesco*	1 Bottle/250ml	163	65	2.9	13.2	0.1	0.1
Strawberry, Raspberry & Banana, Waitrose*	1 Serving/250ml	123	49	0.7	10.8	0.1	0.8
Strawberry, Raspberry, Apple & Banana, P & J*	1 Bottle/250ml	133	53	0.8	11.9	0.3	0.7
Strawberry, Raspberry, Bio Yoghurt, Eat Smart, Safeway*	1 Bottle/250ml	163	65	2.0	12.5	0.6	0.6
Summer Fruits, Tesco*	1 Serving/250ml	140	56	0.2	13.8	0.0	0.5
Vanilla & Honey, Sainsbury's*	1 Bottle/250ml	238	95	3.2	14.8	2.4	0.3
Vanilla Bean, Marks & Spencer*	1 Bottle/500ml	450	90	3.3	13.9	2.6	0.0

SNACK EGGS

	Measure	per Measure	KCAL	PROT	CARB	FAT	FIBRE
Tesco*	1 Egg/45g	133	295	9.2	18.5	20.5	1.1

SNACK MIX

	Measure	per Measure	KCAL	PROT	CARB	FAT	FIBRE
Bowl, Bombay, Tesco*	1/4 Bowl/131g	626	477	19.5	40.0	26.6	3.6
Bowl, Oriental Style, Tesco*	1/4 Bowl/80g	298	373	7.2	84.2	0.8	1.0
Roasted, Organic, Clearspring*	1 Bag/60.1g	271	451	37.5	11.1	28.5	14.4

SNACK SALAD

	Measure	per Measure	KCAL	PROT	CARB	FAT	FIBRE
Prawn, Lime & Chilli, Good Intentions, Somerfield*	1 Pack/226g	276	122	4.1	17.3	4.1	1.8

SNACK STOP

	Measure	per Measure	KCAL	PROT	CARB	FAT	FIBRE
Bolognese Style, Big, Made Up, Crosse & Blackwell*	1 Pot/407.1g	403	99	2.8	19.5	1.1	0.0
Chicken & Mushroom Flavour Pasta, Crosse & Blackwell*	1 Pot/60g	251	418	10.3	74.3	8.8	0.0
Creamy Cheese Pasta, Made Up, Crosse & Blackwell*	1 Pot/218.3g	251	115	3.0	19.2	2.9	0.0
Creamy Chicken Pasta, Made Up, Crosse & Blackwell*	1 Pot/247g	210	85	2.7	15.7	1.6	0.0
Macaroni Cheese, Light, Made Up, Crosse & Blackwell*	1 Pack/248g	260	105	3.2	16.4	3.0	0.9
Mushroom Pasta Twirls, Made Up, Crosse & Blackwell*	1 Pot/248g	248	100	3.1	15.9	2.7	0.9
Roast Onion & Potato, Made Up, Crosse & Blackwell*	1 Pot/210g	210	100	1.7	14.4	3.7	0.0
Roast Parsnip & Potato, Made Up, Crosse & Blackwell*	1 Pot/210g	200	95	1.7	13.6	3.6	0.0
Spicy Tomato Pasta, Made Up, Crosse & Blackwell*	1 Pot/412g	358	87	2.4	15.9	1.5	0.0

SNACK-A-JACKS

	Measure	per Measure	KCAL	PROT	CARB	FAT	FIBRE
Apple & Cinnamon Flavour, Jumbo, Quaker*	1 Cake/10g	38	376	6.2	83.1	2.2	3.9
Barbecue Flavour, Quaker*	1 Pack/30g	126	421	6.5	77.0	10.0	1.0
Barbecue, Invidual Bag, Quaker*	1 Bag/30g	125	416	7.0	80.0	7.0	1.0
Caramel, Quaker*	1 Bag/35g	140	401	5.5	86.0	3.5	0.5
Cheddar Cheese Flavour, Quaker*	1 Bag/30g	128	427	8.0	73.0	10.0	1.0
Chocolate Flavour, Quaker*	1 Cake/14g	57	406	5.5	85.0	4.5	1.0
Creamy Lemon Flavour, Quaker*	1 Pack/35g	137	390	5.0	87.0	2.5	1.0
Crispy Caramel, Quaker*	1 Pack/35g	140	400	5.4	86.0	3.4	0.6
Crispy Cheese, Quaker*	1 Bag/30g	123	409	8.0	75.0	8.5	1.0
Crispy Chocolate Flavour, Quaker*	1 Pack/30g	122	407	5.5	85.0	4.5	1.0
Crispy Vanilla Flavour, Quaker*	1 Pack/35g	137	390	5.0	87.0	2.5	1.0

S

	Measure INFO/WEIGHT	per Measure KCAL	Nutrition Values per 100g / 100ml KCAL	PROT	CARB	FAT	FIBRE
SNACK-A-JACKS							
Jumbo, Apple Danish Flavour, Quaker*	1 Serving/13g	51	392	5.4	86.9	2.3	0.8
Jumbo, Barbecue Flavour, Quaker*	1 Serving/10g	38	376	7.0	80.0	2.5	1.0
Jumbo, Caramel Flavour, Quaker*	1 Cake/13g	52	397	5.0	87.0	2.5	1.0
Jumbo, Cheddar Cheese Flavour, Quaker*	1 Cake/10g	38	383	8.0	81.0	3.0	1.0
Jumbo, Chocolate, Quaker*	1 Cake/12g	49	406	5.5	85.0	4.5	1.0
Jumbo, Sour Cream & Chive, Quaker*	1 Cake/10g	38	380	8.0	82.0	3.0	2.0
Mini Bites, Mature Cheddar & Red Onion, Quaker*	1 Bag/28g	116	414	7.5	76.1	8.9	2.1
Mini Bites, Sour Cream & Sweet Chilli, Quaker*	1 Packet/28g	114	408	6.5	77.5	8.0	2.0
Mini Bites, Tangy Tomato & Red Pepper, Quaker*	1 Bag/28g	114	406	6.0	77.5	8.0	2.0
Salt & Vinegar, Quaker*	1 Bag/30g	123	410	6.5	77.0	8.0	1.0
Savoury Salted, Quaker*	1 Bag/30g	124	414	7.5	77.0	8.0	1.0
Sour Cream & Chive, Quaker*	1 Pack/30g	123	410	7.5	77.0	8.0	1.0
Spudz, Oriental Barbecue, Quaker*	1 Bag/20g	79	395	6.0	73.0	8.5	1.5
Spudz, Smoked Bacon & Cheese, Quaker*	1 Bag/20g	80	398	7.5	76.5	10.0	1.5
Spudz, Sour Cream & Sweet Chilli, Quaker*	1/4 Pack/30g	118	394	6.5	75.0	7.5	2.0
Tomato & Herb Flavour, Quaker*	1 Pack/30g	125	415	6.5	78.0	8.5	1.0
Vanilla, Quaker*	1 Pack/35.1g	137	390	5.0	87.0	2.5	1.0
SNACKS							
Bacon Flavour, Carbolite*	1 Bag/20g	110	545	62.0	2.6	32.0	0.3
SNAPPER							
Red, Fried in Blended Oil	1oz/28g	35	126	24.5	0.0	3.1	0.0
Red, Raw	1oz/28g	25	90	19.6	0.0	1.3	0.0
SNAPS							
Spicy Tomato Flavour, Walkers*	1 Bag/17.9g	91	508	1.5	65.5	26.8	0.0
SNICKERS							
Cruncher, Mars*	1 Bar/40g	209	523	9.0	57.0	30.0	2.3
Mars*	1 Standard/64.5g	323	501	9.3	52.9	28.1	0.0
SORBET							
A Really Lemon, The Real Ice Cream Company*	1 Serving/100g	117	117	0.1	29.1	0.1	0.4
Blackcurrant, Del Monte*	1oz/28g	30	106	0.4	27.1	0.1	0.0
Exotic Fruit, Sainsbury's*	1 Serving/75g	90	120	1.2	24.1	2.0	0.0
Kiwi & Papaya, World Fruit, Del Monte*	1 Lolly/90ml	61	68	0.2	16.2	0.3	0.0
Lemon	1 Scoop/60g	79	131	0.9	34.2	0.0	0.0
Lemon Harmony, Haagen-Dazs*	1 Serving/90ml	214	238	1.5	32.5	11.3	0.0
Lemon, Asda*	1 Serving/100g	120	120	0.0	30.0	0.0	0.0
Lemon, Del Monte*	1 Sorbet/500g	570	114	0.1	29.2	0.1	0.0
Lemon, Organic, Evernat*	1oz/28g	27	96	0.1	22.8	0.5	0.0
Lemon, Sainsbury's*	1/4 Pot/89g	100	112	0.0	28.1	0.0	0.1
Lemon, Sticks, Haagen-Dazs*	1oz/28g	67	238	1.5	32.5	11.3	0.0
Lemon, Tesco*	1 Serving/75g	80	106	0.0	26.2	0.0	0.4
Mango Lemon, Fruit Ice, BGTY, Sainsbury's*	1 Lolly/72g	84	116	0.3	28.1	0.3	0.5
Mango, Del Monte*	1 Sorbet/500g	575	115	0.2	29.6	0.1	0.0
Mango, Organic, Marks & Spencer*	1 Serving/100g	99	99	0.3	24.1	0.1	0.9
Mango, Sainsbury's*	1/4 Pot/88.9g	104	117	0.2	28.9	0.1	0.7
Mango, Tesco*	1 Serving/100g	107	107	0.1	26.5	0.0	0.3
Mango, Tropicale, Haagen-Dazs*	1oz/28g	32	116	0.2	28.6	0.1	0.0
Mango, Waitrose*	1 Pot/100g	90	90	0.1	22.1	0.0	0.6
Orange, Del Monte*	1 Sorbet/500g	625	125	0.2	32.1	0.1	0.0
Passion Fruit, Fat Free, Marks & Spencer*	1 Sorbet/125g	129	103	0.4	25.0	0.0	0.4
Peach & Strawberry, Haagen-Dazs*	1oz/28g	30	108	0.0	27.0	0.0	0.0
Peach & Vanilla Fruit Swirl, Healthy Living, Tesco*	1 Pot/73g	93	127	1.1	28.9	0.8	0.5
Pear, Organic, Evernat*	1oz/28g	33	119	0.0	28.3	0.6	0.0
Pineapple, Del Monte*	1 Sorbet/500g	600	120	0.3	30.6	0.1	0.0

S

INFO/WEIGHT	Measure	per Measure KCAL	Nutrition Values per 100g / 100ml				
			KCAL	PROT	CARB	FAT	FIBRE
SORBET							
Raspberry & Blackberry, Fat Free, Marks & Spencer*	1 Sorbet/125g	140	112	0.4	27.5	0.0	0.6
Raspberry, Haagen-Dazs*	1/2 Cup/105g	120	114	0.0	28.6	0.0	1.9
Raspberry, Select, Safeway*	1/2 Cup/105g	100	95	0.0	27.6	0.0	1.0
Raspberry, Sticks, Haagen-Dazs*	1oz/28g	28	99	0.2	24.2	0.1	0.0
Raspberry, Tesco*	1 Serving/70ml	97	138	0.5	34.0	0.0	0.0
Strawberry & Champagne, Sainsbury's*	1/4 Pot/89g	95	107	0.2	25.5	0.0	0.6
Strawberry, Fruit Ice, Starburst, Mars*	1 Stick/93ml	99	106	0.1	26.7	0.1	0.0
Strawberry, Marks & Spencer*	1oz/28g	27	95	0.3	23.4	0.1	0.5
Summer Berry, Swirl, Asda*	1/4 Pack/89g	97	109	3.0	26.0	0.4	0.0
Swirl, Raspberry & Blackcurrant, Safeway*	1 Serving/50g	58	115	0.6	27.0	0.0	1.6
Tropical, Really Fruity, Asda*	1 Scoop/75g	90	120	0.1	30.0	0.0	0.3
Zesty Lemon, Haagen-Dazs*	1 Serving/125ml	120	96	0.0	24.8	0.0	1.0
SORBET CONE							
Raspberry, Yoghurt & Sorbet, BGTY, Sainsbury's*	1 Cone/69g	151	219	2.6	37.5	6.5	1.3
SOSMIX							
Direct Foods*	1oz/28g	124	443	18.5	27.0	29.0	0.0
SOUFFLE							
Cheese	1oz/28g	71	253	11.4	9.3	19.2	0.3
Cheese, Mini, Waitrose*	1 Souffle/14g	32	232	16.0	2.9	17.4	2.4
Chocolate & Toffee, Gu*	1 Pot/95g	353	372	4.6	46.4	16.6	2.5
Chocolate, Gu*	1 Pot/70g	307	439	6.3	24.4	35.6	2.9
Lemon, Finest, Tesco*	1 Pot/80g	270	338	2.9	24.1	25.6	0.2
Plain	1oz/28g	56	201	7.6	10.4	14.7	0.3
Raspberry & Amaretto, Marks & Spencer*	1oz/28g	83	298	2.8	33.1	16.7	0.1
Ricotta & Spinach, Marks & Spencer*	1 Serving/120g	186	155	8.0	6.2	11.1	2.1
Strawberry, Marks & Spencer*	1 Serving/95g	171	180	1.6	19.5	10.6	0.9
SOUP							
Asparagus & Chicken, Waitrose*	1 Can/415g	166	40	2.1	5.3	1.1	0.7
Asparagus With Croutons, In a Cup, Sainsbury's*	1 Serving/200ml	103	52	1.0	6.4	2.5	1.7
Asparagus, Batchelors*	1 Serving/223g	143	64	0.5	9.2	2.8	0.4
Asparagus, Fresh, Marks & Spencer*	1 Serving/300g	135	45	1.1	2.5	3.6	0.9
Asparagus, Fresh, New Covent Garden Food Co*	1 Carton/600g	324	54	2.1	1.8	4.3	0.9
Asparagus, Knorr*	1 Serving/300ml	114	38	0.7	4.8	1.7	0.1
Asparagus, Less Than 60 Cals, Waitrose*	1 Serving/204ml	51	25	0.4	4.3	0.7	0.7
Asparagus, Marks & Spencer*	1 Serving/300g	180	60	1.1	3.3	4.5	0.7
Asparagus, New Covent Garden Food Co*	1/2 Carton/300g	99	33	1.2	3.9	1.4	1.2
Aubergine & Red Pepper, New Covent Garden Food Co*	1/2 Pint/284ml	68	24	0.9	4.8	0.1	0.4
Autumn Vegetable With Mild Spice, Baxters*	1 Can/415g	199	48	2.2	9.2	0.3	1.5
Autumn Vegetable, Baxters*	1 Can/425g	170	40	1.8	8.0	0.2	1.5
Autumn Vegetable, Healthy Choice, Baxters*	1/2 Can/208g	100	48	2.2	9.2	0.3	1.5
Autumn Vegetable, Vie, Knorr*	1 Pack/500ml	190	38	0.7	4.3	2.0	0.7
Bean, Italian Style, Tesco*	1 Can/300g	153	51	2.8	7.3	1.2	1.1
Beef & Tomato, Cup A Soup, Batchelors*	1 Serving/215g	71	33	0.6	7.3	0.2	0.5
Beef & Tomato, In A Cup, Sainsbury's*	1 Serving/210.3ml	61	29	0.6	5.6	0.5	0.2
Beef & Vegetable Big, Heinz*	1/2 Can/200g	90	45	2.4	7.3	0.7	0.9
Beef & Vegetable Broth, Marks & Spencer*	1 Can/415g	166	40	1.9	6.4	0.8	0.6
Beef & Vegetable Mighty, Asda*	1/2 Can/81g	32	40	2.3	6.0	0.8	0.6
Beef & Vegetable, Chunky, Meal, Tesco*	1 Can/400g	344	86	7.0	5.3	4.8	0.6
Beef & Vegetable, Tesco*	1 Serving/410g	312	76	2.0	5.3	4.8	0.6
Beef Broth, Big, Heinz*	1/2 Can/200g	82	41	2.0	6.8	0.6	0.7
Beef Chilli Baked Potato Big, Heinz*	1 Can/400g	232	58	3.4	9.1	0.9	1.3
Beef Consomme, Sainsbury's*	1 Can/415g	46	11	2.0	0.7	0.0	0.0
Beef, Big, Heinz*	1 Can/400g	180	45	2.4	7.2	0.7	0.9

S

SOUP

	Measure INFO/WEIGHT	per Measure KCAL	Nutrition Values per 100g / 100ml				
			KCAL	PROT	CARB	FAT	FIBRE
Beetroot & Rosemary, New Covent Garden Food Co*	1 Pack/600g	138	23	1.3	4.0	0.2	1.2
Big Red Tomato, Heinz*	1/2 Can/210g	63	30	0.5	6.4	0.4	0.0
Blended Autumn Vegetable, Heinz*	1/2 Can/200g	114	57	1.2	6.4	3.0	0.7
Blended Carrot & Coriander, Heinz*	1/2 Can/200g	104	52	0.7	6.2	2.7	0.6
Blended Leek & Bacon, Heinz*	1/2 Can/200g	108	54	1.9	5.0	2.9	0.5
Blended Red Pepper With Tomato, Heinz*	1/2 Can/200g	102	51	0.8	5.2	2.9	0.7
Blended Sweetcorn & Yellow Pepper, Heinz*	1/2 Can/200g	98	49	0.9	6.6	2.1	0.6
Bloody Mary, Sainsbury's*	1fl oz/30ml	7	22	0.4	4.3	0.3	0.9
Boston Bean & Ham, New Covent Garden Food Co*	1/2 Pack/300g	180	60	3.5	6.7	2.1	1.7
Broccoli & Blue Stilton, New Covent Garden Food Co*	1 Carton/600g	378	63	3.5	2.9	4.2	1.2
Broccoli & Cauliflower, Cup, BFY, Morrisons*	1 Sachet/15g	56	376	4.9	57.2	14.2	4.9
Broccoli & Cauliflower, Thick & Creamy, Batchelors*	1 Serving/100g	120	120	1.9	17.2	4.8	0.6
Broccoli & Cheddar, Heinz*	1 Can/430g	340	79	2.6	4.4	5.6	0.6
Broccoli & Cheddar, Snack, Made Up, Weight Watchers*	1 Serving/26g	124	477	11.2	78.1	13.5	1.9
Broccoli & Dolcelatte Cheese, Soupreme, Aldi*	1/2 Carton/250g	60	24	3.3	1.1	1.0	1.0
Broccoli & Melton Mowbray Stilton, Marks & Spencer*	1/2 Pot/300g	240	80	2.8	3.3	6.4	0.9
Broccoli & Potato, Organic, Baxters*	1 Can/425g	162	38	1.5	6.2	0.8	0.7
Broccoli & Stilton, Canned, Sainsbury's*	1/2 Can/207g	126	61	1.7	4.8	3.9	0.4
Broccoli & Stilton, Canned, Tesco*	1 Can/400g	224	56	1.8	4.2	3.5	0.3
Broccoli & Stilton, Fresh, Safeway*	1 Serving/300g	180	60	2.7	3.7	3.6	0.6
Broccoli & Stilton, Fresh, Sainsbury's*	1/2 Bottle/300ml	156	52	2.1	3.9	3.1	0.9
Broccoli & Stilton, Fresh, Tesco*	1/2 Pot/300g	207	69	3.2	3.8	4.5	0.7
Broccoli & Stilton, Somerfield*	1/2 Pack/250g	140	56	1.6	3.5	3.9	1.5
Broccoli & Stilton, Special Recipe, Sainsbury's*	1/2 Can/208g	127	61	1.7	4.8	3.9	0.4
Broccoli & Stilton, Tesco*	1 Pack/600g	564	94	2.9	2.5	8.1	0.7
Broccoli With Mustard, New Covent Garden Food Co*	1 Carton/568g	204	36	1.3	3.3	1.9	1.2
Broccoli With Stilton, New Covent Garden Food Co*	1floz/30ml	17	56	2.3	1.8	4.4	0.7
Broccoli, Baxters*	1 Can/425g	191	45	1.3	5.9	1.8	0.4
Brocoli & Stilton, Fresh, Safeway*	1 Serving/500g	290	58	3.5	4.8	2.8	0.7
Butternut Squash & Red Pepper, Baxters*	1 Can/425g	153	36	0.7	6.1	1.0	0.6
Butternut Squash, Fresh, Waitrose*	1/2 Pot/300g	153	51	0.5	5.8	2.9	0.8
Cantonese Chicken & Sweetcorn, Fresh, Sainsbury's*	1/2 Bottle/300ml	135	45	2.1	7.9	0.5	0.5
Cantonese Hot & Sour Noodle, Baxters*	1 Serving/215g	133	62	1.4	11.1	1.3	0.5
Carrot & Butterbean, Baxters*	1 Can/425g	230	54	1.6	7.7	1.9	1.7
Carrot & Coriander, 'a' Meal, Feeling Great, Findus*	1 Serving/371g	130	35	1.5	5.5	1.0	1.5
Carrot & Coriander, BGTY, Sainsbury's*	1/2 Can/200g	62	31	0.8	4.8	1.0	0.9
Carrot & Coriander, Baxters*	1 Can/425g	174	41	0.8	6.0	1.5	0.8
Carrot & Coriander, COU, Marks & Spencer*	1oz/28g	7	25	0.4	4.3	0.7	0.5
Carrot & Coriander, Can, Marks & Spencer*	1/2 Can/210g	95	45	0.8	6.3	1.9	0.9
Carrot & Coriander, Carton, Campbell's*	1 Serving/250ml	110	44	0.7	5.4	2.2	0.0
Carrot & Coriander, Classic Homestyle, Marks & Spencer*	1 Can/425g	170	40	0.6	5.6	2.0	0.7
Carrot & Coriander, Delicious, Tesco*	1 Serving/300g	105	35	0.9	4.1	1.7	0.9
Carrot & Coriander, Eat Smart, Safeway*	1 Serving/300g	105	35	0.7	4.8	1.4	1.1
Carrot & Coriander, Fresh, Marks & Spencer*	1/2 Pot/300g	90	30	0.4	4.2	1.5	0.5
Carrot & Coriander, Fresh, Organic, Simply Organic*	1 Serving/250g	115	46	0.5	4.5	3.0	1.3
Carrot & Coriander, Fresh, Tesco*	1 Pack/600g	246	41	0.6	4.5	2.3	1.2
Carrot & Coriander, GFY, Asda*	1/2 Pot/251g	88	35	1.2	4.0	1.6	0.4
Carrot & Coriander, Heinz*	1 Can/400g	196	49	0.5	5.6	2.7	1.0
Carrot & Coriander, Less Than 5% Fat, Asda	1 Serving/300g	96	32	1.0	6.0	0.3	0.8
Carrot & Coriander, New Covent Garden Food Co*	1floz/30ml	12	40	0.8	6.2	1.3	0.5
Carrot & Coriander, Packet, Sainsbury's*	1oz/28g	7	24	0.7	3.9	0.6	0.7
Carrot & Coriander, Perfectly Balanced, Waitrose*	1 Can/413ml	68	16	0.5	3.1	0.2	1.0
Carrot & Coriander, Seeds Of Change*	1 Pack/500g	210	42	0.5	5.7	1.9	0.9

SOUP

	Measure INFO/WEIGHT	per Measure KCAL	Nutrition Values per 100g / 100ml KCAL	PROT	CARB	FAT	FIBRE
Carrot & Coriander, Selection, Campbell's*	1 Carton/500ml	185	37	0.6	6.4	1.0	0.6
Carrot & Coriander, Soup In A Cup, Tesco*	1 Serving/21g	80	381	4.8	66.4	10.7	5.1
Carrot & Coriander, Soup-A-Cup, Asda*	1 Serving/26g	102	392	4.6	62.0	14.0	4.5
Carrot & Coriander, Special Recipe, Sainsbury's*	1 Can/415g	170	41	0.7	4.7	2.1	0.7
Carrot & Coriander, Tesco*	1/2 Can/210g	92	44	0.7	5.4	2.2	0.8
Carrot & Coriander, Vie, Knorr*	1 Pack/500ml	190	38	0.6	3.9	2.2	1.0
Carrot & Coriander, Waistline, Crosse & Blackwell*	1 Sachet/300g	111	37	0.7	6.8	0.8	1.0
Carrot & Ginger, Perfectly Balanced, Waitrose*	1/2 Pot/300g	66	22	0.4	3.1	0.9	1.0
Carrot & Lentil, Microwave, Heinz*	1 Can/303.2g	94	31	1.5	6.1	0.1	0.8
Carrot & Lentil, Weight Watchers*	1 Can/295g	91	31	1.4	6.0	0.1	0.7
Carrot & Orange	1oz/28g	6	20	0.4	3.7	0.5	1.0
Carrot & Orange, Baxters*	1 Can/415g	174	42	1.0	8.3	0.5	0.4
Carrot & Orange, Finest, Tesco*	1/2 Tub/300g	150	50	0.7	7.5	1.9	1.1
Carrot & Orange, Sainsbury's*	1/2 Carton/300g	54	18	0.4	4.2	0.1	0.9
Carrot & Parsnip, Marks & Spencer*	1oz/28g	9	32	0.5	4.9	1.2	0.9
Carrot With Creme Fraiche, Baxters*	1 Can/415g	170	41	0.5	5.9	1.7	0.7
Carrot, Eat Smart, Safeway*	1/2 Pot/225g	79	35	0.6	5.5	1.3	0.4
Carrot, Onion & Chick Pea, Healthy Choice, Baxters*	1 Can/425g	174	41	1.8	7.7	0.3	1.0
Carrot, Orange & Coriander, COU, Marks & Spencer*	1 Pack/415g	145	35	0.6	6.9	0.6	1.2
Carrot, Orange & Ginger, Go Organic*	1 Jar/495g	119	24	0.5	3.6	0.8	1.4
Carrot, Parsnip & Nutmeg, Organic, Baxters*	1 Can/425g	145	34	0.7	6.6	0.5	1.1
Carrot, Potato & Coriander, Weight Watchers*	1 Can/295g	74	25	0.5	5.5	0.1	0.6
Cauliflower Cheese, Safeway*	1 Serving/300g	135	45	2.3	3.7	2.3	0.8
Cauliflower Cheese, Somerfield*	1 Pack/500g	345	69	3.0	3.0	5.0	0.0
Celeriac & Bacon, New Covent Garden Food Co*	1 Serving/300g	228	76	1.1	3.0	7.1	1.6
Celeriac & Truffle, New Covent Garden Food Co*	1 Serving/300g	225	75	1.1	4.3	5.9	0.7
Cheese & Bacon, With Pasta, Meal In A Mug, Tesco*	1 Serving/37g	142	383	9.1	69.5	7.6	2.8
Cheese, Leek & Bacon, Somerfield*	1 Carton/300g	441	147	5.0	5.0	12.0	0.0
Chicken Vegetable, Big Soup, Heinz*	1 Can/400g	188	47	2.4	7.2	1.0	0.8
Chicken & Bacon, With Pasta, Meal In A Mug, Tesco*	1 Sachet/37g	142	384	9.2	69.5	7.6	2.7
Chicken & Broccoli, Soup a Cups, GFY, Asda*	1 Cup/226.1ml	52	23	0.5	4.0	0.6	0.4
Chicken & Broccoli, Soup-a-Slim, Asda*	1 Sachet/16g	55	341	7.0	58.0	9.0	6.0
Chicken & Ham, Big, Heinz*	1/2 Can/200g	92	46	2.3	6.9	1.0	0.7
Chicken & King Prawn Noodle, Tesco*	1 Pot/400g	180	45	4.7	5.5	0.4	0.4
Chicken & Leek, Big, Heinz*	1/2 Can/200g	118	59	2.3	7.8	2.0	0.5
Chicken & Leek, Cup A Soup, Batchelors*	1 Serving/213g	77	36	0.6	6.7	0.9	0.3
Chicken & Leek, In A Mug, Slim Choice, Safeway*	1 Sachet/12g	53	439	7.2	55.9	20.7	10.0
Chicken & Leek, In a Cup, Symingtons*	1 Serving/224.5ml	110	49	0.5	6.0	2.5	1.2
Chicken & Leek, Soup In A Cup, Sainsbury's*	1 Serving/200ml	72	36	0.5	4.9	1.6	0.9
Chicken & Leek, TTD, Sainsbury's*	1/2 Bottle/300ml	177	59	4.7	2.1	3.5	0.3
Chicken & Mushroom In A Cup, Sainsbury's*	1 Sachet/223ml	107	48	0.7	7.1	1.9	0.1
Chicken & Mushroom, BFY, Dry, Morrisons*	1 Serving/14g	47	337	16.0	54.8	6.1	2.5
Chicken & Mushroom, Extra, Slim A Soup, Batchelors*	1 Serving/257.1g	90	35	1.4	5.9	0.6	0.3
Chicken & Mushroom, In A Cup, Tesco*	1 Sachet/15g	9	57	1.4	8.5	2.0	0.2
Chicken & Mushroom, Meal In A Mug, Tesco*	1 Sachet/40g	146	366	10.8	65.3	6.8	5.1
Chicken & Mushroom, Tesco*	1 Serving/100g	53	53	0.8	5.7	3.0	0.4
Chicken & Pasta Big, Heinz*	1/2 Can/200g	68	34	1.8	5.9	0.4	0.8
Chicken & Red Pepper Noodle, Fresh, Tesco*	1 Serving/400ml	200	50	3.6	8.5	0.3	0.4
Chicken & Sweetcorn With Croutons, Sainsbury's*	1oz/28g	17	60	1.4	8.2	2.4	0.4
Chicken & Sweetcorn, BGTY, Sainsbury's*	1 Serving/200g	42	21	1.2	3.5	0.2	0.1
Chicken & Sweetcorn, Baxters*	1 Can/425g	166	39	1.6	6.2	0.9	0.6
Chicken & Sweetcorn, Fresh, Asda*	1 Pack/500g	260	52	2.6	6.0	1.9	0.0
Chicken & Sweetcorn, GFY, Asda*	1 Can/400g	108	27	1.5	4.2	0.5	0.2

SOUP

Measure INFO/WEIGHT	per Measure KCAL	Nutrition Values per 100g / 100ml				
		KCAL	PROT	CARB	FAT	FIBRE
Chicken & Sweetcorn, Healthy Eating, Tesco* — 1 Serving/200ml	64	32	1.5	5.3	0.5	0.2
Chicken & Sweetcorn, In A Cup, BGTY, Sainsbury's* — 1 Sachet/200ml	50	25	0.7	3.8	0.8	0.6
Chicken & Sweetcorn, In A Mug, Tesco* — 1 Sachet/28g	122	434	4.8	63.4	17.9	1.1
Chicken & Sweetcorn, New Improved, Sainsbury's* — 1/2 Bottle/300g	138	46	3.1	8.1	0.3	0.7
Chicken & Sweetcorn, Slim A Soup, Batchelors* — 1 Sachet/203g	59	29	0.6	4.5	0.9	0.1
Chicken & Sweetcorn, Soupreme* — 1 Serving/250g	90	36	2.7	5.6	0.3	1.7
Chicken & Sweetcorn, Tesco* — 1 Can/400ml	128	32	1.5	5.3	0.5	0.2
Chicken & Tarragon, Thick & Creamy, Batchelors* — 1 Sachet/281g	118	42	0.8	5.7	2.3	0.3
Chicken & Vegetable Broth, Morrisons* — 1 Serving/200g	50	25	1.2	4.5	0.2	0.5
Chicken & Vegetable With Croutons, Sainsbury's* — 1 Serving/227ml	89	39	0.8	4.9	1.8	1.3
Chicken & Vegetable, Big, Heinz* — 1 Can/400g	188	47	2.9	7.4	0.6	0.9
Chicken & Vegetable, Cup A Soup, Batchelors* — 1 Sachet/30g	131	437	4.8	62.7	18.6	1.1
Chicken & Vegetable, Cup, Tesco* — 1 Sachet/29ml	122	422	5.6	61.3	17.1	0.5
Chicken & Vegetable, Eat Smart, Safeway* — 1 Serving/300g	165	55	4.5	5.2	1.6	0.8
Chicken & Vegetable, Fresh, Somerfield* — 1/2 Pot/300g	177	59	2.9	5.6	2.8	3.0
Chicken & Vegetable, Healthy Choice, Baxters* — 1 Can/426g	153	36	1.7	6.1	0.5	1.2
Chicken & Vegetable, In A Mug, Tesco* — 1 Sachet/22g	86	390	5.0	59.1	14.8	5.8
Chicken & Vegetable, Loyd Grossman* — 1 Pouch/420g	126	30	1.8	2.6	1.4	0.6
Chicken & Vegetable, Marks & Spencer* — 1oz/28g	17	59	5.3	5.7	1.7	1.1
Chicken & Vegetable, Mighty, Asda* — 1 Can/410g	176	43	2.5	6.8	1.3	0.7
Chicken & Vegetable, Perfectly Balanced, Waitrose* — 1 Can/68g	23	34	1.8	5.4	0.6	1.0
Chicken & Vegetable, Simply, Dry, Kwik Save* — 1 Serving/22g	83	379	4.6	56.4	15.0	7.8
Chicken & Vegetable, Soup In A Mug, Value, Tesco* — 1 Serving/19g	75	395	4.4	64.1	13.4	1.6
Chicken & Vegetable, Thick, Heinz* — 1 Can/400g	152	38	1.2	6.2	0.9	0.6
Chicken & White Wine, Campbell's* — 1 Serving/295g	145	49	1.0	4.0	3.3	0.0
Chicken Broth, Fresh, Baxters* — 1 Serving/300g	117	39	4.9	2.1	1.2	0.7
Chicken Broth, Traditional, Baxters* — 1/2 Can/207g	64	31	1.5	5.4	0.4	0.6
Chicken Flavour, Calorie Counter, Dry, Co-Op* — 1 Serving/10g	32	320	6.0	49.0	11.0	7.0
Chicken Fusion, Fresh, New Covent Garden Food Co* — 1/2 Carton/300g	213	71	2.5	5.3	4.4	0.5
Chicken Mulligatawny, Asda* — 1 Serving/300g	150	50	3.8	7.0	0.8	0.8
Chicken Mulligatawny, Perfectly Balanced, Waitrose* — 1 Serving/300g	138	46	1.7	5.3	2.0	0.4
Chicken Mulligatawny, Tesco* — 1 Pack/600g	576	96	3.6	10.0	4.7	0.9
Chicken Noodle & Vegetable, Slim A Soup, Batchelors* — 1 Serving/203g	55	27	0.8	4.8	0.5	0.6
Chicken Noodle, Asda* — 1 Can/400g	80	20	0.8	3.4	0.4	0.1
Chicken Noodle, Batchelors* — 1 Pack/284g	71	25	1.6	4.2	0.2	0.3
Chicken Noodle, Canned, Sainsbury's* — 1/2 Can/216.7g	78	36	1.7	7.4	0.3	0.7
Chicken Noodle, Chinese Style, Meal In A Mug, Tesco* — 1 Sachet/29g	95	326	11.2	67.0	1.5	5.1
Chicken Noodle, Chinese, Soup In A Cup, Tesco* — 1 Serving/13g	41	317	8.9	66.6	1.7	3.2
Chicken Noodle, Cup A Soup, Batchelors* — 1 Serving/217g	89	41	1.7	7.4	0.6	0.2
Chicken Noodle, Cup, Asda* — 1 Sachet/13g	40	305	9.0	63.0	1.9	3.6
Chicken Noodle, Dry, Morrisons* — 1oz/28g	88	314	13.1	56.0	4.0	5.1
Chicken Noodle, Dry, Nissin* — 1 Pack/85g	364	428	9.5	62.0	16.6	3.3
Chicken Noodle, Dry, Symingtons* — 1/2 Pack/15g	48	318	8.6	65.4	2.4	2.4
Chicken Noodle, Healthy Eating, Tesco* — 1 Pack/500g	215	43	1.6	6.6	1.1	0.4
Chicken Noodle, Heinz* — 1oz/28g	8	27	1.1	4.9	0.3	0.2
Chicken Noodle, In a Mug, Safeway* — 1 Sachet/100g	325	325	8.4	69.5	1.5	0.0
Chicken Noodle, Safeway* — 1 Can/425g	111	26	1.4	3.5	0.7	0.3
Chicken Noodle, Simmer & Serve, Sainsbury's* — 1 Pack/600ml	102	17	0.8	2.9	0.2	0.0
Chicken Noodle, Soup In A Cup, Made Up, Sainsbury's* — 1 Serving/200ml	44	22	0.7	4.7	0.1	0.2
Chicken Noodle, Weight Watchers* — 1 Can/295g	49	17	0.7	3.1	0.1	0.2
Chicken, Campbell's* — 1 Can/295g	142	48	1.1	3.5	3.6	0.0
Chicken, Coconut & Lemon Grass, Fresh, Waitrose* — 1/2 Pot/300g	303	101	2.6	4.1	8.3	0.8
Chicken, Condensed, 99% Fat Free, Campbell's* — 1 Can/295g	74	25	0.9	3.7	0.7	0.0

S

SOUP

INFO/WEIGHT	per Measure KCAL	KCAL	PROT	CARB	FAT	FIBRE
Chicken, Cream Of, Canned	1oz/28g	16	58	1.7	4.5	3.8	0.0
Chicken, Cup A Soup, Batchelors*	1 Serving/213g	77	36	0.7	3.5	2.1	0.6
Chicken, Cup A Soup, Original, Batchelors*	1 Pack/213g	98	46	0.7	5.8	2.2	0.3
Chicken, In A Cup, Dry, Symingtons*	1 Serving/22g	93	424	7.0	57.7	18.4	11.7
Chicken, In A Cup, Sainsbury's*	1 Serving/221ml	86	39	0.7	5.3	1.7	0.1
Chicken, Leek & White Wine, Finest, Tesco*	1 Pack/300g	216	72	2.8	5.7	4.2	0.3
Chicken, Marks & Spencer*	1 Pack/213g	196	92	1.6	5.5	7.2	0.2
Chicken, Mushroom & Potato, Big, Heinz*	1/2 Can/200g	132	66	3.4	8.1	2.3	0.4
Chicken, Mushroom & Rice, Chilled, Marks & Spencer*	1/2 Pot/300g	240	80	3.4	8.6	3.8	0.6
Chicken, Our Best, New Covent Garden Food Co*	1 Carton/600ml	804	134	4.7	12.2	7.4	0.9
Chicken, Packet, Knorr*	1 Packet/85g	423	498	7.7	44.3	32.3	0.2
Chicken, Sainsbury's*	1 Serving/300g	126	42	2.3	3.2	2.2	0.7
Chicken, Sweetcorn & Potato, Heinz*	1 Can/400g	204	51	1.2	5.4	2.8	0.3
Chicken, Thai Blend, Baxters*	1/2 Pot/300g	282	94	1.7	5.3	7.3	0.4
Chicken, Thai Style, Thick & Creamy, In A Mug, Tesco*	1 Sachet/28g	107	390	3.7	61.3	14.5	5.1
Chicken, Thick & Creamy, Marks & Spencer*	1oz/28g	31	110	5.8	3.9	8.0	0.5
Chicken, Weight Watchers*	1 Can/295g	89	30	1.2	4.1	1.0	0.1
Chilli Bean, Marks & Spencer*	1/2 Carton/300g	150	50	2.5	4.7	2.5	2.7
Chilli Pumpkin, Sainsbury's*	1 Serving/300g	120	40	0.6	4.0	2.4	1.3
Chilli Tomato & Pasta, COU, Marks & Spencer*	1 Serving/300g	150	50	1.3	7.2	1.9	0.9
Chinese Chicken Noodle, Cup A Soup, Extra, Batchelors*	1 Sachet/281g	101	36	1.3	6.8	0.4	0.7
Chinese Chicken Noodle, Dry, Knorr*	1 Pack/45g	138	307	15.1	51.8	4.4	2.9
Chinese Chicken Noodle, Slim A Soup Extra, Batchelors*	1 Sachet/246.4g	69	28	1.0	5.3	0.3	0.4
Chorizo & Tomato With Vegetables, Sainsbury's*	1 Pack/400g	228	57	2.6	4.9	3.0	0.3
Chowder, Clam, New England, Select, Campbell's*	1 Cup/240ml	221	92	2.5	6.0	6.0	0.8
Chowder, Haddock, Smoked, Asda*	1 Serving/300g	135	45	2.4	6.0	1.3	0.7
Chowder, Prawn, Manhattan, Sainsbury's*	1 Pack/300ml	177	59	1.6	7.9	2.3	0.1
Chowder, Smoked Haddock, Sainsbury's*	1 Serving/100ml	68	68	1.2	5.1	4.7	0.1
Chowder, Spicy Corn, New Covent Garden Food Co*	1/2 Pint/284ml	134	47	1.4	5.9	2.0	0.9
Chowder, Sweetcorn & Chicken, Heinz*	1 Serving/200g	148	74	3.3	9.1	2.8	0.6
Chowder, Sweetcorn, New Covent Garden Food Co*	1/2 Carton/250ml	118	47	1.4	5.9	2.0	0.9
Chowder, Vegetable, New Covent Garden Food Co*	1/2 Carton/300g	159	53	2.9	6.6	1.7	1.1
Chunky Beef & Vegetable, Sainsbury's*	1 Can/400g	176	44	2.7	7.0	0.6	0.0
Chunky Chicken & Vegetable Meal, Tesco*	1 Can/410g	176	43	2.3	7.2	0.5	0.7
Chunky Chicken & Vegetable, Sainsbury's*	1 Can/400g	188	47	3.3	6.9	0.7	0.0
Chunky Chicken Noodle, Campbell's*	1/2 Can/200g	86	43	2.8	6.5	0.6	0.0
Chunky Chicken, Leek & Potato, Heinz*	1 Can/400g	236	59	2.3	7.8	2.0	0.5
Chunky Minestrone Meal, Tesco*	1/2 Can/205g	78	38	1.3	6.8	0.6	0.9
Chunky Roasted Vegetable, Marks & Spencer*	1 Can/400g	140	35	1.3	5.8	0.6	1.1
Chunky Tomato, New Covent Garden Food Co*	1/2 Pack/300g	135	45	1.8	5.3	1.8	1.1
Chunky Tuscan Style Bean & Sausage, Marks & Spencer*	1 Can/415g	249	60	2.4	7.7	2.2	1.0
Chunky Vegetable & Chicken, Safeway*	1 Can/400g	156	39	2.5	6.2	0.5	0.6
Chunky Vegetable, Big, Heinz*	1 Serving/400g	208	52	1.5	8.7	1.3	1.2
Chunky Vegetable, Fresh, Baxters*	1 Serving/300ml	117	39	1.6	7.8	0.2	1.1
Chunky Vegetable, Fresh, Sainsbury's*	1/2 Bottle/296ml	77	26	0.5	4.8	0.5	1.2
Chunky Vegetable, Fresh, Tesco*	1 Serving/300g	123	41	0.6	5.5	1.9	1.0
Chunky Vegetable, Organic, Simply Organic*	1 Pot/500g	255	51	1.9	9.0	1.5	1.4
Chunky Vegetable, Organic, Tesco*	1 Serving/250g	135	54	2.1	7.8	1.7	1.8
Chunky Vegetable, Tesco*	1 Pot/600g	288	48	0.8	5.0	2.9	1.3
Chunky Winter Vegetable, Marks & Spencer*	1 Can/415ml	166	40	1.5	7.5	0.3	0.4
Chunky With Pasta Minestrone, Co-Op*	1 Pack/400g	140	35	1.0	6.0	0.6	0.7
Cock-a-Leekie, Traditional, Baxters*	1 Can/425g	98	23	0.9	4.1	0.3	0.3
Colcannon, Sainsbury's*	1/2 Pack/300g	192	64	0.4	6.7	4.0	1.4

SOUP

INFO/WEIGHT	Measure	per Measure KCAL	KCAL	PROT	CARB	FAT	FIBRE
Country Garden, Baxters*	1 Can/425g	149	35	0.9	6.6	0.6	0.8
Country Mixture, Sainsbury's*	1 Serving/75g	83	110	6.6	20.1	0.4	3.9
Country Mushroom, Baxters*	1 Pot/600g	378	63	0.9	5.5	4.1	0.1
Country Mushroom, Selection, Campbell's*	1 Serving/250ml	80	32	0.6	3.4	1.8	0.5
Country Vegetable, Asda*	1 serving/125g	59	47	0.6	4.5	2.9	0.8
Country Vegetable, Chilled, Marks & Spencer*	1/2 Pot/300g	105	35	0.5	3.2	2.1	1.0
Country Vegetable, Fresh, Asda*	1 Carton/500g	195	39	1.9	7.0	0.4	0.0
Country Vegetable, Fresh, Chilled, Marks & Spencer*	1 Pot/600g	210	35	0.5	3.2	2.1	1.0
Country Vegetable, Fresh, Somerfield*	1/2 Pack/300g	123	41	1.1	4.6	2.0	1.2
Country Vegetable, Heinz*	1oz/28g	14	51	2.3	9.3	0.5	1.1
Country Vegetable, Marks & Spencer*	1oz/28g	14	50	1.8	7.0	1.4	1.0
Country Vegetable, Slim Choice, Dry, Safeway*	1 Serving/16.5g	59	345	6.7	63.6	7.3	9.1
Country Vegetable, Thick, Asda*	1 Pack/410g	176	43	0.9	5.0	2.1	0.8
Country Vegetable, Vie, Knorr*	1 Pack/500ml	160	32	0.9	5.5	0.7	1.2
Country Vegetable, Weight Watchers*	1 Can/295g	103	35	0.7	5.4	1.2	0.6
Courgette & Parmesan, Sainsbury's*	1 Pack/300ml	198	66	1.5	2.5	5.6	0.4
Courgette & Watercress Pesto, TTD, Sainsbury's*	1 Bottle/600g	276	46	0.8	2.7	3.5	0.7
Courgette, Parmesan & Bacon, Somerfield*	1 Pack/500g	255	51	2.0	2.0	4.0	0.0
Cream Of Asparagus, Campbell's*	1/2 Can/150g	68	45	0.5	4.6	2.8	0.0
Cream Of Asparagus, Cup A Soup, Batchelors*	1 Sachet/223g	143	64	0.5	9.2	2.8	0.4
Cream Of Asparagus, Heinz*	1oz/28g	13	46	1.1	4.5	2.6	0.2
Cream Of Celery, Campbell's*	1 Serving/150g	71	47	0.6	3.2	3.4	0.0
Cream Of Chicken & Mushroom, Campbell's*	1 Can/250g	140	56	0.9	3.5	4.4	0.0
Cream Of Chicken & Mushroom, Heinz*	1oz/28g	14	49	1.3	4.6	2.9	0.1
Cream Of Chicken & Mushroom, Sainsbury's*	1 Can/400g	232	58	1.1	5.1	3.7	0.1
Cream Of Chicken, Asda*	1 Can/410g	209	51	1.2	4.0	3.4	0.1
Cream Of Chicken, Batchelors*	1 Pack/289g	165	57	1.1	5.6	3.3	0.3
Cream Of Chicken, Cambell's*	1 Can/590g	283	48	1.1	3.5	3.6	0.0
Cream Of Chicken, Condensed, Made Up, Heinz*	1oz/28g	12	42	1.1	3.1	2.8	0.0
Cream Of Chicken, For One, Heinz*	1 can/290g	148	51	1.3	4.4	3.2	0.1
Cream Of Chicken, Fresh, Tesco*	1 Serving/300g	294	98	3.3	6.3	6.6	0.2
Cream Of Chicken, Fresh, Waitrose*	1 Serving/300g	180	60	2.6	3.7	3.9	0.2
Cream Of Chicken, Heinz*	1oz/28g	14	49	1.6	4.3	2.9	0.1
Cream Of Chicken, Sainsbury's*	1/2 Can/200g	130	65	1.5	6.2	3.8	0.1
Cream Of Chicken, Tesco*	1 Serving/200g	120	60	1.1	5.4	3.8	0.0
Cream Of Mushroom Condensed, Made Up, Heinz*	1oz/28g	12	42	0.9	3.5	2.7	0.1
Cream Of Mushroom In A Bottle, Homepride*	1/4 Bottle/250ml	110	44	0.5	3.5	3.1	0.0
Cream Of Mushroom, Condensed, Campbell's*	1 Can/295ml	204	69	1.7	5.3	4.5	0.0
Cream Of Mushroom, Cup A Soup, Batchelors*	1 Serving/219g	125	57	0.6	7.5	2.8	0.4
Cream Of Mushroom, Fresh, Tesco*	1/2 Pot/250g	108	43	1.0	4.0	2.6	0.2
Cream Of Mushroom, GFY, Asda*	1 Serving/250g	93	37	2.1	6.0	0.5	0.3
Cream Of Mushroom, Heinz*	1oz/28g	14	51	1.4	5.1	2.7	0.1
Cream Of Mushroom, Mug Size, Heinz*	1 Can/290g	145	50	1.5	4.9	2.7	0.1
Cream Of Mushroom, Packet, Knorr*	1 Packet/75g	389	518	5.2	44.8	35.3	0.9
Cream Of Mushroom, Soupreme*	1 Serving/200g	100	50	1.4	4.5	2.9	0.3
Cream Of Mushroom, Tesco*	1 Serving/200g	108	54	0.9	4.6	3.5	0.1
Cream Of Tomato, Asda*	1/2 Can/205g	137	67	1.0	8.0	3.4	0.0
Cream Of Tomato, Campbell's*	1 Can/295g	195	66	0.8	8.5	3.2	0.0
Cream Of Tomato, Condensed, Made Up, Heinz*	1oz/28g	15	55	0.9	7.1	2.6	0.4
Cream Of Tomato, For One, Heinz*	1 Can/300g	189	63	0.8	6.9	3.6	0.4
Cream Of Tomato, Fresh, Waitrose*	1/2 Pot/300g	210	70	1.0	4.9	5.1	0.5
Cream Of Tomato, Heinz*	1oz/28g	16	57	0.9	6.7	3.0	0.4
Cream Of Tomato, Homepride*	1/4 Bottle/250ml	138	55	0.9	7.7	2.6	0.0

SOUP

INFO/WEIGHT	Measure	per Measure KCAL	Nutrition Values per 100g / 100ml KCAL	PROT	CARB	FAT	FIBRE
Cream Of Tomato, Microwave, Heinz*	1 Pack/300g	204	68	0.9	7.5	3.8	0.4
Cream Of Tomato, Microwaveable Cup, Heinz*	1 Cup/275ml	169	61	0.8	6.9	3.4	0.4
Cream Of Tomato, Organic, Heinz*	1 Can/400g	220	55	0.9	7.2	2.5	0.4
Cream Of Tomato, SmartPrice, Asda*	1 Can/408g	290	71	0.7	9.0	3.6	0.0
Cream Of Tomato, Tinned, Tesco*	1/2 Can/200g	142	71	0.9	8.7	3.6	0.5
Cream Of Vegatable, Cup Soup, Soupreme*	1 Serving/27g	110	409	9.2	55.7	16.6	6.2
Cream Of Vegetable, Cup A Soup, Batchelors*	1 Sachet/33g	134	406	5.8	59.8	16.0	6.2
Cream of Asparagus In Seconds, Dry, Knorr*	1 Pack/61g	320	524	6.5	42.2	36.6	1.1
Cream of Asparagus Soup in a Cup, Sainsbury's*	1 Serving/230ml	129	56	0.7	8.2	2.3	0.1
Cream of Asparagus, Baxters*	1 Can/415g	278	67	1.1	6.0	4.3	0.2
Cream of Asparagus, Soup-a-Cup, Asda*	1 Pack/112g	491	438	6.0	54.0	22.0	4.1
Cream of Celery, Asda*	1 Can/410g	189	46	0.6	4.8	2.7	0.2
Cream of Chicken, Baxters*	1/2 Can/209g	144	69	1.8	6.1	4.2	0.1
Cream of Chicken, Homepride*	1/4 Bottle/250ml	113	45	1.3	4.0	2.9	0.0
Cream of Chicken, In Seconds, Dry, Knorr*	1 Pack/58g	300	518	11.2	36.0	36.6	0.3
Cream of Chicken, Simmer, Sainsbury's*	1 Pack/500ml	182	36	0.8	4.9	1.5	0.8
Cream of Chicken, Somerfield*	1 Serving/215g	129	60	1.5	4.4	4.1	0.1
Cream of Leek In Seconds, Dry, Knorr*	1 Pack/64g	326	509	5.9	45.2	33.8	1.4
Cream of Leek, Traditional, Baxters*	1 Can/425g	196	46	0.7	5.2	2.5	0.4
Cream of Mushroom & Garlic, The Best, Safeway*	1oz/28g	19	68	1.6	1.5	6.2	0.7
Cream of Mushroom, Asda*	1 Can/410g	258	63	1.0	6.0	3.9	0.3
Cream of Mushroom, Co-Op*	1 Pack/400g	240	60	1.0	5.0	4.0	0.0
Cream of Mushroom, Dry, Knorr*	1 Serving/25g	125	500	5.2	47.8	31.8	1.0
Cream of Mushroom, Fresh, Waitrose*	1/2 Pot/300g	210	70	1.3	3.7	5.5	0.5
Cream of Mushroom, Sainsbury's*	1 Can/400g	220	55	0.6	1.4	5.2	0.1
Cream of Potato & Leek, Sainsbury's*	1/2 Can/200g	80	40	0.6	6.1	1.5	0.0
Cream of Tomato & Basil, Somerfield*	1 Pack/450g	279	62	1.0	5.0	4.0	0.0
Cream of Tomato, Dry, Knorr*	1 Pack/90g	392	435	4.3	51.3	23.6	3.3
Cream of Tomato, Fresh, Sainsbury's*	1/2 Bottle/300ml	126	42	0.9	7.0	1.2	0.6
Cream of Tomato, Fresh, Tesco*	1/2 Pot/250g	153	61	1.6	8.3	2.4	0.4
Cream of Tomato, Traditional, Baxters*	1 Can/415g	315	76	1.4	11.6	2.7	0.6
Creamed Asparagus, Cup a Soup, Symingtons*	1 Serving/28g	108	384	11.6	34.6	22.1	15.0
Creamed Asparagus, Dry, Asda*	1 Sachet/30g	131	451	6.0	55.0	23.0	1.1
Creamed Tomato, In A Cup, Sainsbury's*	1 Sachet/233ml	112	48	0.7	9.3	0.9	0.1
Creamed Vegetable, In A Mug, Safeway*	1 Sachet/29g	117	405	5.6	57.9	16.8	3.2
Creamy Carrot, In a Mug, Thick, Safeway*	1 Sachet/28g	105	375	2.9	60.7	13.6	5.4
Creamy Chicken & Vegetables, For One, Watties*	1 Can/300g	115	38	0.9	3.8	2.1	0.0
Creamy Leek With Croutons In A Cup, Sainsbury's*	1 Serving/228g	130	57	1.1	7.2	2.6	0.1
Creamy Mushroom, Asda*	1 Pot/500g	228	46	1.1	4.0	2.8	1.3
Creamy Mushroom, Fresh, Asda*	1 Serving/250g	110	44	1.1	3.8	2.7	1.3
Creamy Mushroom, Safeway*	1 Pack/300ml	137	46	1.1	3.8	2.9	0.5
Creamy Mushroom, Somerfield*	1 Pack/450g	225	50	1.0	4.0	3.0	0.0
Creamy Potato & Leek, Cup A Soup, Batchelors*	1 Sachet/280ml	132	47	0.8	7.4	1.5	1.1
Creamy Potato, Bacon & Onion, Cup A Soup, Batchelors*	1 Sachet/280ml	106	38	0.9	7.3	1.0	0.5
Creamy Tomato, Fresh, Asda*	1 Pot/500g	202	40	0.7	4.0	2.4	0.5
Creamy Tomato, Seeds Of Change*	1 Pack/500g	320	64	1.1	10.9	1.8	0.5
Crofter's Thick Vegetable, Dry, Knorr*	1 Pack/66g	240	364	10.8	52.9	12.2	3.3
Cucumber Pea & Mint, New Covent Garden Food Co*	1 Serving/200ml	90	45	1.8	4.7	2.1	0.6
Cullen Skink, Baxters*	1 Can/415g	357	86	6.4	7.7	3.3	0.4
Dutch Curry & Rice Cup A Soup, Continental*	1 Serving/250ml	125	50	0.7	8.8	1.3	0.0
English Asparagus, New Covent Garden Food Co*	1/2 Pack/300g	114	38	0.7	5.5	1.5	0.1
English Broccoli & Stilton, Dry, Knorr*	1 Pack/65g	331	509	11.7	30.3	37.9	1.6
Farmhouse Chicken Leek, Dry, Knorr*	1 Pack/54g	248	459	10.3	39.3	29.0	1.5

S

SOUP

INFO/WEIGHT	Measure	per Measure KCAL	KCAL	PROT	CARB	FAT	FIBRE
Farmhouse Vegetable, BGTY, Sainsbury's*	1 Serving/200ml	52	26	0.5	4.4	0.8	0.9
Farmhouse Vegetable, Fresh, Avonmore*	1/2 Carton/250g	138	55	1.9	7.4	2.0	0.8
Farmhouse Vegetable, Soup-a-Cup, GFY, Asda*	1 Sachet/218.5ml	59	27	0.6	4.9	0.5	0.4
Fire Flamed Tomato & Red Onion, Sainsbury's*	1/2 Bottle/300ml	129	43	0.8	5.0	2.2	1.0
Fire Roasted Tomato & Red Pepper, Asda*	1/2 Tub/265.1g	114	43	0.7	4.1	2.6	1.0
Fish, Frozen, Findus*	1 Serving/85g	128	150	11.0	13.0	5.5	0.0
Flame Roasted Red Pepper & Tomato, Baxters*	1/2 Can/207.1g	116	56	0.9	6.8	2.8	0.6
Florentine Pea, The Best, Safeway*	1/2 Pot/300g	165	55	2.5	4.9	2.5	1.4
Florida Spring Vegetable, Dry, Knorr*	1 Pack/36g	104	290	7.8	52.2	5.6	5.2
Forest Mushroom, Heinz*	1oz/28g	12	43	1.0	4.5	2.3	0.1
Forest Mushroom, Microwaveable Cup, Heinz*	1 Cup/275g	146	53	1.0	4.7	3.3	0.1
Four Mushroom, Loyd Grossman*	1 Pack/420g	202	48	0.8	2.5	3.9	0.2
French Onion	1oz/28g	11	40	0.2	5.7	2.1	1.0
French Onion & Cider, Waitrose*	1 Can/425g	94	22	0.5	4.8	0.1	0.4
French Onion & Croutons, Dry, Tesco*	1 Serving/30g	106	353	7.3	63.7	7.7	2.0
French Onion & Gruyere Cheese, Finest, Tesco*	1/2 Pot/300g	210	70	1.4	4.7	5.1	0.5
French Onion, Baxters*	1 Can/425g	94	22	0.6	4.3	0.2	0.4
French Onion, Chilled, Marks & Spencer*	1/2 Pot/300g	150	50	2.0	7.2	1.5	1.0
French Onion, GFY, Asda*	1/2 Pot/253g	91	36	1.9	6.0	0.5	0.4
French Onion, Heinz*	1 Pack/400g	100	25	0.5	5.7	0.1	0.4
French Onion, Knorr*	1 Pack/40g	118	296	6.0	62.5	2.5	6.6
French Onion, Made Up, Sainsbury's*	1/3 Serving/205g	39	19	0.4	4.0	0.1	0.1
French Onion, Sainsbury's*	1 Serving/300ml	153	51	0.5	5.7	3.0	0.5
French Onion, Simmer & Serve, Sainsbury's*	1/3 sachet/204ml	51	25	0.6	5.3	0.2	0.5
French Onion, Tinned, Marks & Spencer*	1/2 Can/200g	40	20	0.4	3.9	0.2	0.3
Garden Vegetable, Baxters*	1 Serving/200g	70	35	0.9	6.6	0.6	0.8
Garden Vegetable, Dry, SlimFast*	1 Serving/60g	224	373	23.8	45.0	10.3	7.0
Garden Vegetable, Heinz*	1 Can/400g	160	40	0.9	7.2	0.8	0.9
Gazpacho, Fresh, New Covent Garden Food Co*	1 Pack/284g	68	24	0.8	2.6	1.2	0.6
Giant Minestrone, Big, New Recipe, Heinz*	1/2 Can/200g	98	49	1.5	9.3	0.7	1.1
Goats Cheese & Rocket, Sainsbury's*	1 Serving/300g	180	60	2.0	3.2	4.4	0.3
Golden Vegetable With Croutons Cup Soup, Co-Op*	1 Sachet/25g	120	480	4.0	56.0	26.0	2.0
Golden Vegetable With Croutons, Instant, Dry, Morrisons*	1 Sachet/27g	118	438	5.3	60.7	19.3	0.0
Golden Vegetable, Calorie Counter, Cup, Co-Op*	1 Sachet/12g	40	335	7.0	54.0	10.0	5.0
Golden Vegetable, Cup A Soup, Batchelors*	1 Serving/212g	70	33	0.4	5.7	0.9	0.4
Golden Vegetable, Cup, Calorie Counter, Co-Op*	1 Sachet/10.9g	35	320	7.0	50.0	10.0	9.0
Golden Vegetable, Dry, Knorr*	1 Pack/76g	299	394	10.4	45.4	19.0	3.3
Golden Vegetable, Instant, Tesco*	1 Sachet/17g	60	351	8.2	62.0	7.8	3.7
Golden Vegetable, Slim A Soup, Batchelors*	1 Sachet/207g	58	28	0.5	4.7	0.8	0.7
Golden Vegetable, Soup-A-Slim, Asda*	1 Sachet/15g	50	336	6.0	60.0	8.0	1.9
Green Pea & Mint, Fresh, Waitrose*	1oz/28g	27	97	1.8	5.5	7.7	1.2
Green Thai Chicken, Waitrose*	1 Pack/400g	324	81	3.8	5.7	4.8	0.3
Green Vegetables & Lentil, Lima*	1 Serving/300g	96	32	1.6	3.7	1.2	0.5
Haggis Broth, Baxters*	1 Can/425g	221	52	1.8	6.8	1.9	0.7
Harvest Carrot & Lima Bean, Heinz*	1oz/28g	11	40	0.8	6.9	1.0	1.3
Harvest Vegetable, In A Cup With Croutons, Sainsbury's*	1 Sachet/226.3ml	86	38	1.0	5.9	1.2	0.9
Hearty Vegetable, 99% Fat Free, Campbell's*	1 Can/295g	91	31	0.8	6.1	0.4	0.0
Highlanders Broth, Baxters*	1 Can/425g	208	49	1.9	7.0	1.5	0.6
Hot & Sour Mushroom, New Covent Garden Food Co*	1 Carton/600g	72	12	0.7	1.9	0.2	0.4
Italian Bean & Pasta, Healthy Choice, Baxters*	1 Can/415g	174	42	2.0	7.9	0.3	1.1
Italian Chicken & Pasta, Big, Heinz*	1/2 Can/200g	108	54	2.5	9.4	0.7	0.7
Italian Chicken Broth, Healthy Choice, Baxters*	1/2 Can/210g	84	40	1.5	6.6	0.8	0.8
Italian Chunky, New Covent Garden Food Co*	1/2 Carton/300g	111	37	1.5	4.7	1.4	0.9

SOUP

INFO/WEIGHT	Measure per Measure KCAL	Nutrition Values per 100g / 100ml KCAL	PROT	CARB	FAT	FIBRE
Italian Minestrone, Dry, Knorr*	1 Pack/62g	193	311	11.5	57.1	4.1	7.8
Italian Minestrone, Sainsbury's*	1 Can/415g	212	51	2.0	6.6	1.8	1.1
Italian Plum Tomato & Basil, Perfectly Balanced, Waitrose*	1/2 Pot/300g	69	23	0.9	3.8	0.5	0.9
Italian Style Tomato & Basil, Co-Op*	1 Pack/500g	200	40	1.0	4.0	2.0	0.6
Italian Style Tomato & Chicken, BGTY, Sainsbury's*	1 Can/400g	148	37	3.1	5.5	0.3	0.4
Italian Style Tomato, Safeway*	1/2 Pot/248g	134	54	1.3	5.7	2.9	0.9
Italian Tomato & Basil, Go Organic*	Jar/495g	183	37	1.2	3.3	2.1	0.8
Italian Tomato With Basil, Baxters*	1 Can/425g	217	51	2.4	8.4	0.9	0.9
Jamaican Jerk Chicken & Pumpkin, Sainsbury's*	1 Pack/600g	282	47	2.7	5.1	1.7	0.2
Lamb & Cous Cous, Marks & Spencer*	1/2 Can/208g	100	48	2.1	6.2	1.8	0.9
Lamb & Vegetable, Big, Heinz*	1/2 Can/200g	112	56	2.4	9.2	1.0	1.2
Lamb & Vegetable, Mega, Morrisons*	1 Pack/410g	172	42	1.9	6.3	1.0	0.8
Leek & Chicken, Knorr*	1 Serving/300ml	82	27	0.6	2.4	1.7	0.1
Leek & Potato, Chilled, Marks & Spencer*	1 Serving/300g	240	80	0.9	5.2	6.2	0.6
Leek & Potato, Cup A Soup, Batchelors*	1 Sachet/28g	121	432	5.2	63.2	17.6	1.8
Leek & Potato, Eat Smart, Safeway*	1/2 Pot/225g	113	50	1.1	6.0	2.4	0.6
Leek & Potato, Fresh, Sainsbury's*	1 Bowl/300ml	156	52	0.8	5.9	2.8	1.0
Leek & Potato, Fresh, Tesco*	1/2 pack/300g	201	67	1.4	6.3	4.0	0.8
Leek & Potato, Fresh, Waitrose*	1/2 Pot/300g	150	50	1.0	5.9	2.5	1.0
Leek & Potato, GFY, Asda*	1 Sachet/220g	55	25	0.3	5.0	0.4	0.3
Leek & Potato, In A Cup, BGTY, Sainsbury's*	1 Sachet/196ml	55	28	0.3	4.9	0.8	0.8
Leek & Potato, In A Cup, Tesco*	1 Sachet/15g	51	343	5.3	66.4	6.2	3.5
Leek & Potato, New Covent Garden Food Co*	1/2 Carton/284g	148	52	1.3	6.1	2.5	0.5
Leek & Potato, Organic, Sainsbury's*	1/2 Can/200g	84	42	1.6	5.7	1.4	0.9
Leek & Potato, Reduced Calorie Quick, Waitrose*	1 Sachet/190ml	51	27	0.4	5.3	0.5	0.4
Leek & Potato, Slim A Soup, Batchelors*	1 Serving/204g	57	28	0.4	5.0	0.7	0.2
Leek & Potato, Smooth, Vie, Knorr*	1 Pack/500ml	155	31	0.9	4.8	0.9	1.0
Leek & Potato, Soup In A Cup, Made Up, Waitrose*	1 Sachet/204ml	47	23	0.3	4.3	0.5	0.5
Leek & Potato, Soup In A Mug, Healthy Living, Tesco*	1 Serving/16g	54	336	4.3	67.1	5.6	7.4
Leek & Potato, Tastebreaks, Knorr*	1 Pot/225g	162	72	1.1	9.1	3.4	0.5
Leek & Potato, Tesco*	1/2 Can/200g	106	53	0.8	5.7	3.0	0.4
Leek & Potato, Thick & Creamy, Soup In A Mug, Tesco*	1 Serving/25g	95	378	4.2	68.5	9.7	4.9
Leek & Potato, Weight Watchers*	1 Sachet/214.8ml	58	27	0.5	5.1	0.5	0.1
Leek With Croutons In A Cup, Sainsbury's*	1 Sachet/24g	91	379	6.7	42.9	20.0	12.1
Lentil	1 Serving/220g	218	99	4.4	12.7	3.8	1.1
Lentil & Bacon, Baxters*	1 Can/415g	228	55	2.9	7.8	1.3	0.8
Lentil & Bacon, Gluten Free, Baxters*	1 Can/207g	114	55	2.9	7.8	1.3	0.8
Lentil & Bacon, Safeway*	1 Can/400g	160	40	2.7	6.3	0.4	2.9
Lentil & Bacon, Sainsbury's*	1/2 Can/200g	90	45	3.3	7.3	0.3	1.5
Lentil & Bacon, Tesco*	1 Serving/200g	96	48	3.2	7.2	0.7	0.5
Lentil & Chick Pea, Organic, Tesco*	1 Serving/300ml	117	39	1.9	6.1	0.8	0.5
Lentil & Parsley, Organic, Simply Organic*	1 Pot/500g	285	57	4.8	9.1	0.2	1.7
Lentil & Smoked Bacon, Marks & Spencer*	1 Pack/415g	228	55	2.8	8.5	0.9	1.2
Lentil & Tomato, New Covent Garden Food Co*	1/2 Pack/284g	162	57	3.6	8.1	1.1	0.7
Lentil & Vegetable With Bacon, Organic, Baxters*	1/2 Can/211.4g	93	44	1.9	7.6	0.7	1.0
Lentil & Vegetable, Baxters*	1 Can/423g	165	39	2.0	7.1	0.3	0.9
Lentil & Winter, New Covent Garden Food Co*	1 Serving/250ml	133	53	3.1	7.7	1.1	0.9
Lentil, Asda*	1/2 Can/202g	89	44	2.6	8.0	0.2	0.7
Lentil, Bacon & Mixed Bean, Low Fat, Aldi*	1 Meal/400g	260	65	4.7	9.5	0.9	1.6
Lentil, Campbell's*	1 Can/295g	139	47	2.6	7.7	0.6	0.0
Lentil, Canned	1 Serving/220g	86	39	3.1	6.5	0.2	1.2
Lentil, Carrot & Cumin, BGTY, Sainsbury's*	1 Pack/400g	204	51	2.3	8.4	0.9	0.1
Lentil, Heinz*	1 Can/300g	123	41	2.3	7.5	0.2	1.0

SOUP

INFO/WEIGHT	Measure	per Measure KCAL	KCAL	PROT	CARB	FAT	FIBRE
Lobster Bisque, Baxters*	1 Can/415g	187	45	3.0	3.6	2.1	0.2
Lobster Bisque, New Covent Garden Food Co*	1/2 Carton/300g	108	36	3.2	4.4	0.6	0.4
Lobster Bisque, Waitrose*	1/2 Carton/300g	201	67	0.9	5.5	4.6	0.6
Londoner's Pea Souper, New Covent Garden Food Co*	1/2 Carton/300g	153	51	4.3	4.1	2.0	1.1
Luxury Game, Baxters*	1 Can/415g	187	45	3.7	5.9	0.7	0.5
Malaysian Chicken & Sweetcorn, Dry, Knorr*	1 Pack/57g	211	370	10.6	56.3	11.4	1.8
Mediteranean Vegetable, Homepride*	1 Serving/250ml	83	33	0.9	4.3	1.3	0.0
Mediterranean Fish, Waitrose*	1/2 Pot/300g	108	36	3.4	3.5	0.9	0.7
Mediterranean Minestrone, Campbell's*	1/2 Carton/250ml	95	38	0.9	6.1	1.1	0.6
Mediterranean Style Tomato, Healthy Eating, Dry, Tesco*	1 Serving/22g	78	355	9.5	64.1	6.4	3.2
Mediterranean Tomato & Vegetable, Weight Watchers*	1 Can/295g	47	16	0.4	3.0	0.3	0.4
Mediterranean Tomato, Baxters*	1 Can/425g	140	33	1.0	6.8	0.2	0.7
Mediterranean Tomato, COU, Marks & Spencer*	1 Pack/415g	104	25	0.7	4.8	0.5	0.6
Mediterranean Tomato, Campbell's*	1 Can/295g	83	28	0.6	6.4	0.0	0.0
Mediterranean Tomato, Dry, SlimFast*	1 Sachet/62g	213	343	22.6	39.8	9.0	10.7
Mediterranean Tomato, Fresh, Baxters*	1 Can/300g	171	57	2.2	8.1	1.8	1.4
Mediterranean Tomato, Fresh, Organic, Sainsbury's*	1 Serving/250ml	78	31	1.3	3.3	1.4	1.0
Mediterranean Tomato, In A Cup, BGTY, Sainsbury's*	1 Serving/200ml	50	25	0.4	5.2	0.3	0.3
Mediterranean Tomato, In A Cup, Sainsbury's*	1 Serving/214ml	60	28	0.7	5.3	0.4	0.2
Mediterranean Tomato, Instant, Weight Watchers*	1 Serving/200ml	50	25	0.7	5.2	0.1	0.1
Mediterranean Tomato, Slim A Soup, Batchelors*	1 Serving/207g	54	26	0.5	4.7	0.6	0.4
Mediterranean Vegetable, GFY, Asda*	1/2 Pot/250g	80	32	0.5	3.6	1.7	1.6
Mediterranean Vegetable, Tesco*	1/2 Can/200g	76	38	0.6	6.8	0.9	0.5
Melon & Carrot, New Covent Garden Food Co*	1 Serving/300g	60	20	0.6	3.6	0.4	0.6
Mexican Beef Chilli, Mighty, Asda*	1 Can/400g	192	48	3.3	7.0	0.7	0.9
Mexican Black Bean, Extra Special, Asda*	1/2 Pot/262.5g	195	74	2.3	7.0	4.1	1.7
Minestrone	1oz/28g	18	63	1.8	7.6	3.0	0.9
Minestrone With Croutons, Soup in a Cup, Sainsbury's*	1 Sachet/225ml	72	32	0.9	6.3	0.4	0.5
Minestrone With Ribbon Noodles, Extra, Dry, Aldi*	1 Serving/34g	107	315	11.0	62.8	2.2	2.0
Minestrone With Wholemeal Pasta, Baxters*	1 Can/415g	133	32	0.9	6.6	0.2	0.8
Minestrone, Baxters*	1 Can/425g	145	34	1.3	5.9	0.6	0.9
Minestrone, Calorie Counter, Low Calorie Cup, Co-Op*	1 Sachet/13g	40	310	7.0	66.0	2.0	3.0
Minestrone, Canned	1oz/28g	9	32	1.4	5.1	0.8	0.6
Minestrone, Chilled, Marks & Spencer*	1/2 Pot/300g	135	45	2.0	5.8	1.3	1.9
Minestrone, Chunky, Fresh, Baxters*	1 serving/250g	95	38	1.5	6.5	0.7	1.1
Minestrone, Chunky, Sainsbury's*	1/2 Can/200g	80	40	1.5	7.2	0.6	1.2
Minestrone, Chunky, Waitrose*	1 Can/415g	195	47	1.6	8.3	0.8	1.1
Minestrone, Cup A Soup, BGTY, Sainsbury's*	1 Serving/200ml	54	27	0.8	6.0	0.1	0.6
Minestrone, Cup A Soup, Batchelors*	1 Serving/217g	100	46	0.9	8.3	1.1	0.5
Minestrone, Delicious, Tesco*	1 Serving/300g	129	43	1.1	7.2	1.1	0.6
Minestrone, For One, Heinz*	1 Can/300g	96	32	1.4	5.2	0.7	0.7
Minestrone, Fresh, Asda*	1/2 Pot/254.3g	89	35	0.8	6.0	0.9	1.2
Minestrone, Fresh, Baxters*	1 Box/568ml	233	41	1.8	6.2	1.0	0.6
Minestrone, Fresh, Sainsbury's*	1/2 Bottle/300ml	93	31	1.2	4.4	0.9	0.9
Minestrone, Fresh, Waitrose*	1 Pack/600g	240	40	1.1	5.8	1.4	0.8
Minestrone, Healthy Choice, Baxters*	1/2 Can/207.5g	67	32	0.9	6.6	0.2	0.8
Minestrone, Healthy Eating, Tesco*	1 Pack/500g	140	28	1.0	4.4	0.7	0.6
Minestrone, Hearty, 99% Fat Free, Campbell's*	1 Can/295g	77	26	0.7	5.6	0.1	0.0
Minestrone, Heinz*	1 Can/300g	120	40	1.0	5.5	1.6	0.8
Minestrone, In A Mug, Tesco*	1 Sachet/23g	83	359	9.0	62.6	8.1	2.7
Minestrone, In a Cup, BGTY, Sainsbury's*	1 Serving/200ml	54	27	0.8	6.0	0.1	0.6
Minestrone, In a Mug, Healthy Eating, Tesco*	1 Sachet/21g	72	342	3.6	67.7	6.3	3.2
Minestrone, Instant With Croutons, Value, Tesco*	1 Sachet/21g	68	325	6.4	60.2	6.5	1.7

S

SOUP

INFO/WEIGHT		KCAL	KCAL	PROT	CARB	FAT	FIBRE
Minestrone, Instant, Under 60 Calories, Tesco*	1 Sachet/19g	58	307	7.3	63.6	2.6	2.3
Minestrone, Marks & Spencer*	1/2 Pot/300g	120	40	1.3	5.7	1.1	1.2
Minestrone, Mighty, Dry, Asda*	1 Serving/38.2g	130	343	9.0	74.0	1.2	2.4
Minestrone, New Covent Garden Food Co*	1 Serving/250ml	83	33	1.7	5.8	0.4	0.7
Minestrone, Organic, Marks & Spencer*	1 Pack/208g	83	40	1.4	8.9	0.5	1.1
Minestrone, Organic, Seeds Of Change*	1 Sachet/500g	325	65	1.3	7.5	3.2	0.9
Minestrone, Packet, Dry, Knorr*	1 Pack/61g	178	292	9.2	53.9	4.4	6.5
Minestrone, Simmer & Serve, Made Up, Sainsbury's*	1 Pack/600ml	108	18	0.5	3.9	0.0	0.4
Minestrone, Simmer, Dry, Asda*	1 Pack/50g	131	262	6.0	57.0	1.1	15.0
Minestrone, Slim A Soup, Batchelors*	1 Serving/203g	55	27	0.6	4.5	0.6	0.3
Minestrone, Soup In A Cup, Healthy Living, Tesco*	1 Sachet/21g	72	342	3.6	67.7	6.3	3.8
Minestrone, Soup a Slim, Asda*	1 Serving/17g	53	311	6.0	69.0	1.2	4.5
Minestrone, Tesco*	1 Pack/600g	222	37	1.2	7.5	0.3	0.7
Minestrone, Weight Watchers*	1 Can/295g	71	24	0.6	5.1	0.2	0.3
Minestrone, With Croutons, Cup A Soup, Batchelors*	1 Serving	93	37	0.7	7.3	0.5	0.3
Minestrone, With Croutons, Dry, Soupreme*	1 Serving/27g	94	349	7.6	65.3	6.4	4.4
Minestrone, With Pasta, Cup A Soup, Extra, Batchelors*	1 Pack/286g	123	43	1.4	8.5	0.4	0.8
Minestrone, in a Cup, Sainsbury's*	1 Serving/227ml	84	37	1.4	6.3	0.7	0.2
Minted Lamb Hot Pot, Big, Heinz*	1oz/28g	14	51	2.2	8.5	1.0	0.9
Miso, Instant, Blue Dragon*	1 Sachet/18g	25	139	10.0	14.4	3.9	0.0
Miso, Instant, Dry, Sanchi*	1 Sachet/8g	27	336	18.4	48.6	7.6	0.0
Miso, Naga-Negi Instant, Dry, Amano Foods*	1 Serving/7g	25	357	24.3	41.4	10.0	0.0
Mixed Bean & Pepper, Organic, Marks & Spencer*	1 Pack/208g	94	45	2.3	7.7	0.3	1.8
Mixed Vegetable, Dry, Gallina Blanca*	1 Pack/20g	76	378	4.0	68.0	10.0	0.0
Moroccan Chick Pea, Marks & Spencer*	1oz/28g	20	70	3.6	8.8	2.1	2.0
Moroccan Chicken, New Covent Garden Food Co*	1 Serving/300g	108	36	2.1	2.7	1.9	0.4
Moroccan Chicken, Waitrose*	1 Serving/300g	189	63	2.4	8.7	2.1	0.8
Moroccan Lentil, Waitrose*	1/2 Pot/300g	153	51	3.5	8.2	0.5	3.4
Mulligatawny	1 Serving/220g	213	97	1.4	8.2	6.8	0.9
Mulligatawny Beef Curry, Heinz*	1oz/28g	15	54	2.0	7.2	1.9	0.6
Mulligatawny, Asda*	1 Can/400g	172	43	2.2	6.0	1.1	0.3
Mulligatawny, In A Cup, Symingtons*	1 Serving/232ml	95	41	0.7	8.3	0.6	0.5
Mulligatawny, Tesco*	1 Can/400g	144	36	1.2	6.8	0.5	0.3
Mushroom & Chestnut, Finest, Tesco*	1 Serving/250g	130	52	1.1	4.7	3.3	0.7
Mushroom & Chicken, Co-Op*	1 Pack/400g	220	55	0.9	5.0	4.0	0.0
Mushroom & Garlic, Dry, Tesco*	1 Sachet/16g	58	360	5.8	61.1	10.3	3.2
Mushroom & Garlic, Slim Choice, Safeway*	1oz/28g	108	384	8.3	61.4	11.7	6.2
Mushroom & Garlic, Slimming Cup A Soup, Tesco*	1 Serving/16g	58	360	5.8	61.1	10.3	3.2
Mushroom & Madeira Flavour, Soup In A Mug, Safeway*	1 Sachet/28g	114	406	3.2	67.3	13.8	1.0
Mushroom & Mascarpone, TTD, Sainsbury's*	1/2 Bottle/300ml	108	36	0.6	2.8	2.5	0.4
Mushroom & Tarragon, TTD, Sainsbury's*	1 Serving/300ml	201	67	1.4	5.8	4.2	0.7
Mushroom Creme Fraiche, Waistline, Crosse & Blackwell*	1 Carton/300g	69	23	1.2	2.8	0.8	0.3
Mushroom Noodle, Mighty, Dry, Asda*	1 Serving/42g	171	407	8.0	69.0	11.0	1.9
Mushroom Potage, Baxters*	1 Can/415g	320	77	1.5	6.1	5.2	0.3
Mushroom Pottage, Tesco*	1 Can/400g	260	65	1.0	5.0	4.6	0.5
Mushroom, 98% Fat Free, Baxters*	1 Can/425g	170	40	0.9	5.6	1.6	0.3
Mushroom, 99% Fat Free, Campbell's*	1oz/28g	7	24	0.6	3.5	0.9	0.0
Mushroom, Chilled, Marks & Spencer*	1 Pack/300g	135	45	1.9	3.3	2.6	0.5
Mushroom, Condensed, Campbell's*	1 Can/300g	207	69	1.7	5.3	4.5	0.0
Mushroom, Cream of, Canned	1 Serving/220g	101	46	1.1	3.9	3.0	0.1
Mushroom, Delicious, Tesco*	1 Serving/300g	111	37	1.2	3.1	2.2	0.4
Mushroom, Dry, Symingtons*	1 Serving/23g	80	348	17.8	48.4	9.2	6.7
Mushroom, For One, Heinz*	1 Tin/290g	148	51	1.4	5.1	2.7	0.1

SOUP

INFO/WEIGHT	per Measure KCAL	KCAL	PROT	CARB	FAT	FIBRE
Mushroom, Fresh, Sainsbury's*	1 Serving/300g	204	68	1.6	4.7	4.8	0.8
Mushroom, In A Cup, Sainsbury's*	1 Serving/200ml	76	38	0.6	5.0	1.7	0.9
Mushroom, Quick, Knorr*	1 Serving/100g	85	85	2.0	8.5	4.5	0.0
Mushroom, Tesco*	1 serving/250ml	120	48	1.0	5.1	2.6	0.3
Mushroom, Weight Watchers*	1 Can/295g	80	27	1.0	4.4	0.6	0.1
Mushroom, With Croutons, Soup In A Mug, Tesco*	1 Pack/26g	113	435	6.1	63.3	17.5	2.9
Oxtail, Canned	1 Serving/220g	97	44	2.4	5.1	1.7	0.1
Oxtail, Condensed, Classics, Diluted, Campbell's*	1 Can/590g	236	40	1.4	5.3	1.5	0.0
Oxtail, Cup A Soup, Batchelors*	1 Serving/211g	76	36	0.8	6.5	0.8	0.5
Oxtail, Heinz*	1oz/28g	10	37	1.7	6.6	0.5	0.3
Oxtail, Marks & Spencer*	1 Serving/415g	208	50	2.1	6.9	1.4	0.5
Oxtail, Sainsbury's*	1 Can/400g	132	33	2.3	5.1	0.4	0.2
Oxtail, Simmer & Serve, Sainsbury's*	1 Pack/600ml	180	30	0.6	4.9	0.9	0.2
Oxtail, Soup in A Cup, Sainsbury's*	1 Serving/223ml	69	31	1.0	5.7	0.5	0.2
Oxtail, Tesco*	1 Can/400g	152	38	2.0	5.9	0.7	0.3
Paddestoelen, Cup A Soup, Batchelors*	100ml	5	5	0.4	0.6	0.1	0.2
Parsnip & Apple, COU, Marks & Spencer*	1 Can/415g	187	45	0.7	5.4	2.5	1.2
Parsnip & Honey, Sainsbury's*	1/2 Bottle/300g	192	64	1.1	5.4	4.2	1.5
Parsnip, Carrot & Sweet Potato, Baxters*	1 Serving/150g	93	62	0.9	8.5	2.7	1.4
Parsnip, Fresh, Morrisons*	1/2 Pot/250g	100	40	0.9	5.8	1.5	1.4
Parsnip, Honey & Ginger, COU, Marks & Spencer*	1 Can/415g	125	30	0.7	5.3	0.6	0.7
Parsnip, Leek & Ginger, New Covent Garden Food Co*	1 Carton/600g	162	27	1.2	4.9	0.3	1.3
Parsnip, Mr Bean's*	1 Tin/400g	208	52	1.9	6.7	1.9	0.0
Pasta, Tomato & Basil, Bertolli*	1 Serving/100g	47	47	1.5	7.9	1.1	1.6
Pea & Ham	1oz/28g	20	70	4.0	9.2	2.1	1.4
Pea & Ham, Asda*	1/2 Can/205g	94	46	3.2	7.0	0.6	1.6
Pea & Ham, Baxters*	1 Can/425g	234	55	3.0	8.3	1.1	1.2
Pea & Ham, Fresh, Sainsbury's*	1 Serving/400ml	160	40	1.9	7.0	0.5	0.3
Pea & Ham, Tesco*	1 Serving/300g	207	69	3.4	6.6	3.2	1.0
Pea & Ham, Thick, Heinz*	1 Can/400g	204	51	3.2	8.7	0.4	1.0
Pea & Mint, Baxters*	1 Serving/300g	186	62	2.3	6.1	3.2	1.5
Pea & Mint, Fresh, Marks & Spencer*	1 Serving/164g	49	30	1.8	6.3	0.1	1.5
Pea & Mint, Fresh, Tesco*	1 Serving/300g	207	69	2.4	5.1	4.4	0.0
Pea & Mint, Pouch, Tesco*	1/2 Pouch/250g	198	79	2.0	5.6	5.4	1.5
Pea & Mint, Sainsbury's*	1 Serving/200g	86	43	2.1	6.7	0.9	0.5
Pea & Mint, Tinned, Tesco*	1 Can/400g	180	45	2.0	7.8	0.7	1.3
Pea, In a Cup, Symingtons*	1 Sachet/30.5g	97	311	7.2	54.1	7.2	6.9
Peking Shiitake Mushroom Noodle, Baxters*	1 Serving/215g	90	42	1.3	7.5	0.8	0.2
Pepper & Chorizo, Sainsbury's*	1 Bowl/400ml	172	43	7.0	2.0	1.0	0.0
Pork, Chinese Dumpling, New Cultural Revolution*	1 Serving/250ml	156	62	6.4	6.0	1.6	0.4
Potato & Leek	1oz/28g	15	52	1.5	6.2	2.6	0.8
Potato & Leek With Peppers & Chicken, Stockmeyer*	1/2 Can/200g	118	59	2.6	6.7	2.4	0.8
Potato & Leek, Asda*	1/2 Pack/292ml	166	57	0.8	4.4	4.0	0.3
Potato & Leek, Fresh, Asda*	1/2 Pot/250g	98	39	1.2	7.0	0.7	0.0
Potato & Leek, Thick, Heinz*	1 Can/400g	172	43	0.8	6.0	1.8	0.6
Potato, Leek & Chicken, BGTY, Sainsbury's*	1 Can/400g	152	38	2.1	5.4	0.9	0.5
Provencal Vegetable, Marks & Spencer*	1 Serving/300g	150	50	1.0	6.0	2.5	1.1
Pumpkin & Bramley Apple, New Covent Garden Food Co*	1/2 Carton/300g	99	33	1.1	5.9	0.6	0.8
Pumpkin & Ginger, In a Aup, Symingtons*	1 Serving/200ml	66	33	0.4	4.7	1.4	0.4
Pumpkin, New Covent Garden Food Co*	1/2 Pint/284ml	97	34	0.4	5.5	1.1	0.6
Red Lentil & Ham, Waitrose*	1/2 Pot/300g	147	49	3.9	5.8	1.1	2.0
Red Pepper & Tomato, Perfectly Balanced, Waitrose*	1 Can/415g	154	37	0.8	4.5	1.8	0.9
Red Pepper & Tomato, Sainsbury's*	1 Serving/100g	41	41	0.8	4.5	2.2	1.8

SOUP

INFO/WEIGHT	Measure per Measure KCAL	KCAL	PROT	CARB	FAT	FIBRE
Red Pepper & Tomato, Vie, Knorr*	1 Pack/500ml	195	39	0.8	6.4	1.2	1.0
Red Pepper & Tomato, Weight Watchers*	1 Serving/295g	35	12	0.4	2.4	0.1	0.4
Red Pepper, Tomato & Basil, Marks & Spencer*	1 Can/415g	83	20	1.3	2.7	0.3	0.8
Rich Tomato & Basil, Batchelors*	1 Serving/280g	104	37	0.5	6.7	0.9	0.6
Rich Woodland Mushroom, Cup A Soup, Batchelors*	1 Pack/280g	123	44	0.6	5.8	1.9	0.5
Roasted Parsnip, Chunky Carrot & Sweet Potato, Baxters*	1/2 Pot/300g	186	62	0.9	8.5	2.7	1.4
Roasted Pepper, Eat Smart, Safeway*	1/2 Pot/225g	79	35	0.8	3.7	1.8	1.4
Roasted Red Pepper & Tomato, Marks & Spencer*	1 Serving/150g	105	70	1.4	5.0	4.9	0.6
Roasted Red Pepper, Fresh, Waitrose*	1 Pack/600g	172	29	0.8	3.0	1.5	1.0
Roasted Vegetable, Eat Smart, Safeway*	1 Serving/450g	180	40	0.8	4.1	2.2	2.0
Roasted Vegetable, Fresh, Sainsbury's*	1/2 Pot/273ml	71	26	0.5	4.8	0.5	1.2
Roasted Vegetable, TTD, Sainsbury's*	1/2 Pack/297.7g	128	43	0.5	3.4	3.0	1.0
Roasted Winter Vegetable, Sainsbury's*	1 Serving/300ml	129	43	0.5	3.4	3.0	1.0
San Marzano Tomato & Mascarpone, Marks & Spencer*	1 Serving/150g	98	65	1.4	5.7	4.3	2.0
Scotch Broth, Asda*	1/2 Can/205g	82	40	1.1	6.0	1.3	0.4
Scotch Broth, Baxters*	1 Can/415g	195	47	1.9	7.5	1.0	0.9
Scotch Broth, Fresh, Baxters*	1 Serving/300g	108	36	1.6	5.9	0.7	0.6
Scotch Broth, Marks & Spencer*	1 Serving/300g	150	50	2.1	5.1	2.4	1.1
Scotch Broth, New Covent Garden Food Co*	1/2 Pint/284ml	114	40	1.6	2.8	2.5	0.5
Scotch Broth, Sainsbury's*	1/2 Can/200g	100	50	1.7	8.0	1.2	0.7
Scotch Broth, Tesco*	1 Can/400g	152	38	1.5	6.7	0.6	0.8
Scotch Broth, Thick, Heinz*	1/2 Can/200g	70	35	1.2	5.8	0.7	0.6
Scotch Vegetable, Baxters*	1 Can/425g	183	43	1.9	7.4	0.6	1.2
Scottish Vegetable With Lentils & Beef, Heinz*	1 Can/403.8g	210	52	3.4	8.2	0.7	1.2
Seasoned Chicken With Sweetcorn & Croutons, SlimFast*	1 Pack/60g	211	351	23.7	36.8	10.6	9.7
Sicilian Tomato, New Covent Garden Food Co*	1/2 Pint/284ml	114	40	1.6	4.8	1.6	0.8
Smoked Salmon & Dill, Finest, Tesco*	1/2 Carton/300g	240	80	2.2	5.3	5.5	0.6
Snack, Golden Chicken, With Noodles, Weight Watchers*	1 Serving/27g	89	330	6.7	71.9	1.9	1.1
Snack, Mushroom, With Pasta, Weight Watchers*	1 Serving/27g	127	470	10.0	77.0	13.3	1.9
Spiced Chickpea & Fresh Red Pepper, Marks & Spencer*	1 Serving/300g	165	55	2.2	5.8	2.3	2.5
Spiced Spinach & Green Lentil, Asda*	1/2 Pot/250g	123	49	2.7	5.0	2.0	0.0
Spicy Gumbo, Sainsbury's*	1 Carton/600ml	240	40	1.5	4.5	1.8	0.9
Spicy Lentil & Mixed Pepper, Organic, Sainsbury's*	1 Can/400g	204	51	3.0	7.5	1.0	0.8
Spicy Lentil & Tomato, Soup A Slim, Asda*	1 Serving/17g	54	320	12.6	62.9	2.3	5.1
Spicy Lentil & Vegetable, Chilled, Marks & Spencer*	1/2 Serving/600g	300	50	2.7	8.0	0.8	1.1
Spicy Lentil, COU, Marks & Spencer*	1 Pack/415g	187	45	2.6	6.7	0.9	1.2
Spicy Lentil, Seeds Of Change*	1 Pack/500g	345	69	2.8	9.4	2.2	0.8
Spicy Mixed Bean & Vegetable, Eat Smart, Safeway*	1 Can/415g	183	44	2.3	7.5	0.5	3.1
Spicy Parsnip, BGTY, Sainsbury's*	1 Pack/400g	180	45	2.2	7.1	0.9	1.0
Spicy Parsnip, Baxters*	1 Can/425g	217	51	1.1	6.1	2.5	1.5
Spicy Parsnip, Fresh, Tesco*	1 Serving/300g	102	34	0.6	4.5	1.6	1.6
Spicy Parsnip, Perfectly Balanced, Waitrose*	1 Can/415g	125	30	1.0	4.8	0.7	1.1
Spicy Pumpkin, Sainsbury's*	1/2 Bottle/300ml	96	32	0.4	3.8	1.7	0.6
Spicy Red Curry, Blue Dragon*	1 Serving/205g	97	47	0.4	5.8	2.5	0.3
Spicy Red Lentil & Tomato, Marks & Spencer*	1/2 Pack/300g	150	50	2.7	8.0	0.8	1.1
Spicy Sausage & Bean Meal, Tesco*	1 Can/500g	265	53	2.8	6.4	1.4	1.2
Spicy Thai Chicken, Baxters*	1 Can/415g	278	67	1.8	7.1	3.5	0.3
Spicy Tomato & Lentil, BGTY, Sainsbury's*	1 Can/400g	240	60	3.2	10.4	0.7	0.1
Spicy Tomato & Lentil, Tesco*	1 Can/400g	180	45	2.1	8.7	0.2	0.8
Spicy Tomato & Rice With Sweetcorn, Baxters*	1/2 Can/207g	93	45	1.3	9.2	0.3	0.5
Spicy Tomato & Vegetable With Croutons, Sainsbury's*	1 Sachet/23.5g	78	323	5.1	62.1	6.0	6.4
Spicy Tomato & Vegetable, Healthy Living, Co-Op*	1 Can/400g	180	45	2.0	8.0	0.8	2.0
Spicy Tomato, Cup A Soup, Batchelors*	1 Sachet/23g	74	322	7.6	65.8	3.2	3.2

SOUP

INFO/WEIGHT	Measure per Measure KCAL	KCAL	Nutrition Values per 100g / 100ml PROT	CARB	FAT	FIBRE
Spinach & Watercress, New Covent Garden Food Co*	1/2 Carton/298g	60	20	1.3	2.8	0.4	0.8
Spinach With Nutmeg, New Covent Garden Food Co*	1 serving/500ml	245	49	2.5	3.7	2.7	0.6
Split Pea & Ham, Asda*	1 Serving/300g	129	43	3.5	6.9	0.2	0.7
Split Peas, Yellow, Simply Organic*	1 Pot/500g	270	54	3.5	9.7	0.2	2.5
Spring Vegetable, Condensed, Campbell's*	1 Can/295g	62	21	0.5	4.5	0.1	0.0
Spring Vegetable, Heinz*	1 Can/400g	124	31	0.8	6.2	0.4	0.7
Stilton & White Port, Baxters*	1oz/28g	25	88	2.5	5.4	6.3	0.3
Stilton, Celery & Watercress, Morrisons*	1 Serving/250g	273	109	3.9	3.1	9.2	0.3
Sugar Snap Pea & Mint, New Covent Garden Food Co*	1/2 Pack/300g	87	29	1.7	3.0	1.1	1.4
Summer Minestrone, With Basil Pesto, Marks & Spencer*	1/2 Pot/300g	240	80	1.9	5.7	5.4	1.2
Summer Vegetable, With Pasta, Cup A Soup, Batchelors*	1 Serving/33g	17	50	1.4	8.5	1.1	1.0
Sun Dried Tomato & Basil, Heinz*	1 Serving/275ml	124	45	0.6	6.5	1.9	0.1
Sun Dried Tomato & Basil, Microwaveable Cup, Heinz*	1 Cup/275ml	125	45	0.7	6.5	1.9	0.1
Super Chicken Noodle in Seconds, Dry, Knorr*	1 Pack/37g	111	299	17.9	46.1	4.7	0.3
Super Chicken Noodle, Dry, Knorr*	1 Pack/56g	182	325	14.3	56.0	4.9	1.8
Sweet Cherry Tomato, TTD, Sainsbury's*	1 Pack/300g	120	40	0.7	6.0	1.5	1.0
Sweet Potato & Coconut, COU, Marks & Spencer*	1 Can/415g	166	40	0.7	6.7	1.3	0.8
Sweetcorn & Chicken, Cup, Calorie Counter, Co-Op*	1 Sachet/11.1g	35	315	5.0	49.0	11.0	11.0
Sweetcorn & Chilli, COU, Marks & Spencer*	1/2 Can/275g	138	50	0.9	6.1	2.4	0.4
Tangy Tomato, Extra, Slim A Soup, Batchelors*	1 Pack/253.1g	121	48	1.2	9.0	0.8	0.4
Tangy Tomato, Slim A Soup, Batchelors*	1 Serving/230ml	81	35	1.1	6.7	0.4	0.5
Thai Chicken & Coconut, Safeway*	1 Serving/300g	235	78	3.4	4.6	5.2	0.9
Thai Chicken Noodle, Baxters*	1 Serving/430g	202	47	1.7	6.8	1.4	0.3
Thai Chicken, GFY, Asda*	1 Serving/200g	85	43	1.7	5.5	1.5	0.5
Thai Chicken, Safeway*	1 Serving/200g	178	89	4.1	2.5	7.0	1.3
Thai Pumpkin Coconut, New Covent Garden Food Co*	1 Carton/568ml	182	32	1.3	3.5	1.3	1.1
Thai Red Chicken, Fresh, Sainsbury's*	1/2 Pot/300ml	159	53	1.9	5.0	2.8	0.5
Thai Style Chicken, Sainsbury's*	1/2 Can/200g	106	53	2.9	5.5	2.1	0.7
Three Bean, Chunky, Marks & Spencer*	1 Can/415g	208	50	2.3	7.5	1.2	1.8
Three Bean, Organic, Seeds Of Change*	1 Pack/500g	400	80	3.2	13.8	1.3	1.8
Tomato & Basil With Onion, Waistline, Crosse & Blackwell*	1 Serving/300g	87	29	0.9	5.1	0.6	0.3
Tomato & Basil, 1% Fat, Marks & Spencer*	1 Can/400g	152	38	0.6	9.0	0.4	1.4
Tomato & Basil, 99% Fat Free, Baxters*	1/2 Can/207g	75	36	0.7	6.1	1.0	0.6
Tomato & Basil, Campbell's*	1 Pack/500ml	205	41	0.7	6.7	1.3	1.1
Tomato & Basil, Delicious, Tesco*	1 Serving/300ml	150	50	1.0	7.4	1.9	0.7
Tomato & Basil, Finest, Tesco*	1/2 Pot/300g	249	83	1.2	6.5	5.8	0.7
Tomato & Basil, Fresh, Improved, Sainsbury's*	1/2 Bottle/300ml	105	35	1.4	4.1	1.4	0.6
Tomato & Basil, Fresh, Somerfield*	1 Serving/294.7g	112	38	0.7	4.4	1.9	1.4
Tomato & Basil, Fresh, Tesco*	1 Pack/300g	141	47	0.9	7.4	1.6	0.6
Tomato & Basil, Fresh, The Fresh Soup Company*	1/2 Pot/250g	85	34	1.3	5.1	0.9	0.6
Tomato & Basil, GFY, Asda*	1 Serving/250ml	100	40	0.9	6.0	1.4	1.6
Tomato & Basil, Loyd Grossman*	1/2 Pack/210g	88	42	0.8	5.3	2.0	0.3
Tomato & Basil, Marks & Spencer*	1oz/28g	10	35	0.8	5.2	1.2	1.5
Tomato & Basil, New Covent Garden Food Co*	1 Pack/568g	187	33	1.8	5.7	0.4	0.5
Tomato & Basil, Organic, Sainsbury's*	1 Serving/200g	96	48	0.4	7.0	2.0	0.3
Tomato & Basil, Soup-a-Slim, Asda*	1 Sachet/16g	52	326	7.0	70.0	2.0	3.9
Tomato & Basil, Thick & Creamy, Batchelors*	1 Serving/281g	104	37	0.5	6.7	0.9	0.6
Tomato & Basil, Vie, Knorr*	1 Pack/500ml	145	29	0.8	5.5	0.4	0.9
Tomato & Basil, Waitrose*	1 Serving/300ml	84	28	1.0	5.3	0.3	1.0
Tomato & Brown Lentil, Baxters*	1 Can/400g	216	54	2.7	10.4	0.2	1.0
Tomato & Brown Lentil, Healthy Choice, Baxters*	1 Can/415g	191	46	2.6	8.3	0.3	1.3
Tomato & Butterbean, Baxters*	1 Can/425g	225	53	1.9	8.6	1.2	1.8
Tomato & Fresh Basil, Marks & Spencer*	1/2 Pot/300g	105	35	0.8	5.2	1.2	1.5

S

INFO/WEIGHT	Measure	per Measure KCAL	KCAL	PROT	CARB	FAT	FIBRE

SOUP

	Measure INFO/WEIGHT	per Measure KCAL	KCAL	PROT	CARB	FAT	FIBRE
Tomato & Herb, Campbell's*	1 Carton/500ml	180	36	1.0	5.0	1.3	0.0
Tomato & Herb, Marks & Spencer*	1oz/28g	14	50	1.3	7.9	1.6	1.3
Tomato & Lentil, Heinz*	1 Can/400g	216	54	2.7	10.4	0.2	1.0
Tomato & Orange, Baxters*	1 Can/425g	179	42	1.0	8.3	0.5	0.4
Tomato & Orange, Healthy Eating, Tesco*	1 Pack/400g	132	33	0.6	7.1	0.2	0.4
Tomato & Red Pepper, Campbell's*	1 Can/590g	366	62	0.5	7.7	3.3	0.0
Tomato & Red Pepper, Soupreme*	1 Serving/250ml	90	36	1.1	5.7	1.0	1.7
Tomato & Red Pepper, Weight Watchers*	1 Serving/205g	25	12	0.4	2.5	0.1	0.4
Tomato & Roasted Red Pepper, COU, Marks & Spencer*	1 Serving/415g	145	35	1.0	7.6	0.1	0.9
Tomato & Spinach, Organic, Waitrose*	1 Serving/300g	126	42	1.4	4.9	1.9	0.7
Tomato & Three Bean, BGTY, Sainsbury's*	1 Can/400g	216	54	2.9	8.5	0.9	0.8
Tomato & Vegetable, Cup A Soup, Batchelors*	1 Serving/218g	107	49	1.1	8.5	1.2	0.6
Tomato & Vegetable, Cup, Soupreme*	1 Sachet/24g	87	361	6.0	64.6	8.7	1.4
Tomato & Vegetable, In A Mug, Tesco*	1 Sachet/24g	88	366	5.5	62.3	10.5	4.3
Tomato & Vegetable, Organic, Baxters*	1 Can/400g	200	50	1.6	9.2	0.8	0.8
Tomato & Vegetable, Spicy, Meal In A Mug, Tesco*	1 Serving/34g	123	362	8.2	68.2	6.5	5.9
Tomato & Vegetable, With Croutons, Dry, Soupreme*	1 Serving/27g	106	394	7.2	59.9	13.9	4.8
Tomato Rice, Campbell's*	1oz/28g	13	46	0.9	8.3	1.0	0.0
Tomato, 99% Fat Free, Campbell's*	1 Can/295g	130	44	0.7	8.0	1.0	0.0
Tomato, 99% Fat Free, Watties*	1 Serving/105g	32	31	1.0	5.6	0.4	1.1
Tomato, Cannellini & Borlotti Bean, Marks & Spencer*	1/2 Pot/300g	195	65	2.1	6.7	3.3	2.5
Tomato, Cream of, Canned	1oz/28g	15	52	0.8	5.9	3.0	0.7
Tomato, Creme Fraiche & Basil, The Best, Safeway*	1/3 Pot/200g	130	65	1.0	5.0	4.2	1.0
Tomato, Cup A Soup, Batchelors*	1 Serving/212g	85	40	0.3	7.5	1.0	0.3
Tomato, Fresh Country, New Covent Garden Food Co*	1 fl oz/30ml	12	40	1.9	6.4	0.8	0.8
Tomato, Fresh, Tesco*	1 Serving/100g	44	44	0.7	5.2	2.3	0.4
Tomato, In A Cup, Gluten Free, Symingtons*	1 Serving/19.1g	68	356	5.2	45.8	16.9	13.0
Tomato, In A Cup, Tesco*	1 Serving/23g	75	328	6.4	68.5	3.2	0.1
Tomato, In a Cup, Symingtons*	1 Sachet/31.5g	99	308	3.5	62.0	5.0	3.8
Tomato, Mediterranean, Rich, Fresh, Baxters*	1 Carton/600g	318	53	1.8	7.7	1.7	1.1
Tomato, Mixed Bean & Vegetable, Chunky, Sainsbury's*	1 Can/400g	232	58	2.2	11.5	0.3	1.6
Tomato, Mixed Bean & Vegetable, Tesco	1oz/28g	18	64	2.4	9.8	0.3	1.6
Tomato, Onion & Basil, GFY, Asda*	1 Can/400g	96	24	1.0	3.4	0.7	1.7
Tomato, Pasta & Basil Cup, Good Intentions, Somerfield*	1 Serving/26g	92	355	5.4	69.1	6.3	5.1
Tomato, Pepper & Basil, Eat Smart, Safeway*	1 Can/415g	162	39	0.9	4.8	1.7	1.8
Tomato, Pepper & Basil, Safeway*	1 Can/415.4g	162	39	0.9	4.8	1.7	1.8
Tomato, Thick & Creamy, In A Mug, Tesco*	1 Serving/26g	95	365	5.0	66.5	8.8	5.4
Tomato, Weight Watchers*	1 Tin/295g	74	25	0.7	4.6	0.5	0.3
Tuscan Bean, GFY, Asda*	1 Carton/400ml	224	56	2.9	9.0	0.9	0.8
Tuscan Bean, New Covent Garden Food Co*	1/2 Carton/300g	171	57	3.9	8.8	0.7	2.4
Tuscan Bean, Organic, Sainsbury's*	1 Pack/400g	171	43	2.6	6.3	0.8	2.0
Tuscan Bean, Perfectly Balanced, Waitrose*	1/2 Pot/300g	147	49	2.0	6.1	1.8	1.8
Vegetable	1oz/28g	15	52	0.9	3.2	4.0	0.9
Vegetable & Barley Broth, Organic, Sainsbury's*	1/2 Can/200g	48	24	1.4	3.7	0.4	0.9
Vegetable & Beef, Sainsbury's*	1 Can/400g	260	65	2.1	8.5	2.5	1.3
Vegetable & Lentil, Fresh, Somerfield*	1/2 Pack/300g	183	61	2.7	8.4	1.9	1.5
Vegetable & Lentil, Somerfield*	1 Serving/300g	120	40	1.6	4.9	1.5	2.4
Vegetable Broth, Healthy Eating, Tesco*	1 Can/400g	148	37	1.2	7.4	0.2	1.0
Vegetable Broth, Marks & Spencer*	1 Pack/213g	85	40	1.0	6.3	1.4	0.8
Vegetable, & Rosemary, Chunky, Tesco*	1/2 Pot/250g	113	45	1.0	5.8	2.0	1.4
Vegetable, 99% Fat Free, Watties*	1 Serving/105g	30	29	0.8	5.9	0.2	0.8
Vegetable, Asda*	1 Can/400g	144	36	1.1	7.0	0.4	0.8
Vegetable, Bean & Pasta, Organic, Baxters*	1 Can/415g	212	51	2.2	8.7	0.8	1.4

S

INFO/WEIGHT	Measure	per Measure KCAL	KCAL	PROT	CARB	FAT	FIBRE
			Nutrition Values per 100g / 100ml				

SOUP

	Measure INFO/WEIGHT	per Measure KCAL	KCAL	PROT	CARB	FAT	FIBRE
Vegetable, Canned	1oz/28g	13	48	1.4	9.9	0.6	1.5
Vegetable, Chunky, Simply Organic*	1 Pot/500g	270	54	2.1	7.8	1.7	1.8
Vegetable, Condensed, Campbell's*	1 Can/295g	103	35	0.8	6.2	0.8	0.0
Vegetable, Cup, Soupreme*	1 Sachet/26g	111	444	8.1	49.7	23.6	2.3
Vegetable, Extra Thick, Sainsbury's*	1 Can/400g	176	44	1.6	8.0	0.6	1.3
Vegetable, Heinz*	1 Can/400g	188	47	1.4	8.4	0.9	1.1
Vegetable, In A Cup, BGTY, Sainsbury's*	1 Sachet/200g	52	26	0.5	4.4	0.8	0.9
Vegetable, In A Cup, Healthy Living, Tesco*	1 Sachet/18g	66	367	7.2	66.1	7.8	2.8
Vegetable, Instant, Weight Watchers*	1 Sachet/219.2ml	57	26	0.5	4.8	0.5	0.2
Vegetable, New Covent Garden Food Co*	1/2 Pint/284ml	88	31	1.1	5.9	0.4	1.1
Vegetable, Sainsbury's*	1 Can/400g	184	46	1.5	8.3	0.7	1.2
Vegetable, Soup In A Mug, Healthy Living, Tesco*	1 Sachet/18g	66	365	7.0	66.3	8.0	2.6
Vegetable, Soup-a-Cups, Asda*	1 Sachet/200ml	59	30	0.7	5.5	0.6	0.5
Vegetable, Tesco*	1/2 Can/200g	88	44	1.3	9.3	0.2	1.0
Vegetable, Thick & Creamy, Soup In A Mug, Tesco*	1 Serving/26g	104	399	5.2	57.4	16.5	7.5
Vegetable, Vie, Knorr*	1 Pack/500ml	160	32	0.9	5.5	0.7	1.2
Vegetable, Weight Watchers*	1 Serving/295ml	83	28	0.9	5.6	0.2	0.8
Vegetable, With Croutons, Soup In A Mug, Tesco*	1 Pack/23g	90	392	6.2	55.2	16.3	8.0
Watercress & Courgette Pesto Soup, TTD, Sainsbury's*	1/2 pack/300g	138	46	0.8	2.7	3.5	0.7
Watercress & Cream, Soup Chef*	1 Jar/780g	413	53	0.8	5.9	2.9	0.3
Watercress, Marks & Spencer*	1/2 Pot/300g	75	25	1.3	1.5	1.7	0.6
Wild Mushroom & Maderia, Finest, Tesco*	1 Serving/300g	156	52	1.4	5.0	2.9	0.3
Wild Mushroom & Porcini Pieces, BGTY, Sainsbury's*	1 Serving/196.4g	55	28	0.5	4.7	0.8	0.6
Wild Mushroom & Truffle, The Best, Safeway*	1/2 Pot/300g	180	60	1.1	3.5	4.5	0.9
Wild Mushroom Cup, Good Intentions, Somerfield*	1 Serving/20g	74	369	4.1	68.9	8.5	4.5
Wild Mushroom in a Cup, BGTY, Sainsbury's*	1 Serving/200ml	56	28	0.5	4.7	0.8	0.6
Wild Mushroom, Dry, SlimFast*	1 Pack/60g	209	349	23.3	37.5	10.2	10.4
Wild Mushroom, Fresh, Tesco*	1 Serving/300g	159	53	1.3	4.7	3.2	0.3
Wild Mushroom, New Covent Garden Food Co*	1 fl oz/30ml	11	36	1.5	5.0	1.1	0.5
Wild Mushroom, Soupreme*	1 Carton/500g	135	27	1.1	2.9	1.2	0.5
Winter Vegetable & Lentil, New Covent Garden Food Co*	1 Serving/300g	243	81	5.1	12.0	1.4	2.6
Winter Vegetable, Organic, Sainsbury's*	1/2 Can/200g	100	50	2.3	7.9	1.0	1.3
Winter Warmer, New Covent Garden Food Co*	1 Serving/300g	180	60	2.5	10.5	0.9	2.3
Won Ton, Blue Dragon*	1 Can/410g	103	25	1.2	2.0	1.3	0.2

SOUP MIX

	Measure INFO/WEIGHT	per Measure KCAL	KCAL	PROT	CARB	FAT	FIBRE
Leek & Potato, Made Up, Sainsbury's*	1/2 Pack/204g	39	19	0.6	3.6	0.2	0.5
Minestrone, Made Up, Sainsbury's*	1 Serving/200ml	44	22	0.3	6.0	0.0	0.3
Scotch Broth, Made Up, Sainsbury's*	1 Serving/175g	32	18	0.2	3.8	0.2	0.6

SOYA

	Measure INFO/WEIGHT	per Measure KCAL	KCAL	PROT	CARB	FAT	FIBRE
Bolognese Style, Sainsbury's*	1/2 Pack/168g	113	67	3.1	13.9	0.7	2.7
Chunks, Dried, Cooked, Sainsbury's*	1oz/28g	27	98	14.0	9.8	0.3	1.1
Mince, Dried, Cooked, Sainsbury's*	1 Serving/200g	164	82	11.8	8.3	0.2	0.9
Mince, Dry Weight, Sainsbury's*	1 Serving/50g	164	328	47.2	33.2	0.8	3.6
Mince, Granules	1oz/28g	74	263	43.2	11.0	5.4	0.0
Mince, Unflavoured, Nature's Harvest*	1 serving/100g	345	345	50.0	35.0	1.0	4.0
Mince, With Onion, Cooked, Sainsbury's*	1/2 Pack/180g	122	68	5.4	8.0	1.6	1.8
Protein Powder, Holland & Barratt*	1oz/28g	109	390	88.0	0.5	4.0	0.0

SPACE RAIDERS*

	Measure INFO/WEIGHT	per Measure KCAL	KCAL	PROT	CARB	FAT	FIBRE
Beef Flavour	1 Pack/17g	82	482	8.3	61.0	22.7	2.6
Cheese	1 Bag/16g	76	473	7.1	61.6	22.0	3.1
Pickled Onion	1 Bag/16g	77	479	7.4	61.5	22.6	2.4
Salt & Vinegar	1 Bag/16.9g	81	478	6.9	61.7	22.6	2.2

S

	Measure INFO/WEIGHT	per Measure KCAL	Nutrition Values per 100g / 100ml				
			KCAL	PROT	CARB	FAT	FIBRE
SPAGHETTI							
Canned in Tomato Sauce	1oz/28g	18	64	1.9	14.1	0.4	0.7
Chicken, BGTY, Sainsbury's*	1 Serving/300g	281	94	9.8	11.6	0.9	2.3
Cooked, Average	1oz/28g	33	119	4.1	24.8	0.7	1.1
Dry, Average	1oz/28g	98	350	12.1	72.1	1.5	2.4
Dry, Carb Check, Heinz*	1 Serving/75g	219	292	52.7	15.2	2.3	20.8
Durum Wheat, Dry, Average	1oz/28g	97	348	12.4	71.8	0.4	1.5
Fresh, Cooked, Average	1 Serving/125g	182	146	6.1	26.9	1.7	1.8
Fresh, Dry, Average	1 Serving/100g	278	278	10.8	53.0	3.0	2.2
In Rich Tomato Sauce, Asda*	1 Serving/200g	128	64	1.6	14.0	0.2	0.5
In Tomato & Cheese, Sainsbury's*	1 Serving/300g	345	115	4.4	16.8	3.4	1.4
In Tomato Sauce With Parsley, Weight Watchers*	1 Can/400g	196	49	1.8	10.0	0.2	0.6
In Tomato Sauce, HP*	1 Can/410g	247	60	1.5	13.1	0.2	0.4
In Tomato Sauce, Heinz*	1 Can/400g	244	61	1.7	13.0	0.2	0.5
In Tomato Sauce, Organic, Sainsbury's*	1/2 Can/205g	133	65	1.8	13.9	0.2	1.0
In Tomato Sauce, Sainsbury's*	1 Can/410g	262	64	1.9	13.3	0.4	0.5
In Tomato Sauce, Tesco*	1 Can/410g	246	60	1.6	12.9	0.2	0.5
In Tomato Sauce, Value, Tesco*	1/2 Can/205g	131	64	1.9	13.3	0.4	0.5
In Tomato Sauce, Weight Watchers*	1 Serving/200g	98	49	1.8	10.0	0.2	0.6
In Tomato Sauce, Whole Wheat, Sainsbury's*	1 Serving/205g	125	61	2.0	11.9	0.6	1.1
Quick Cook, Dry, Average	1 Serving/50g	176	351	12.8	70.8	1.9	2.7
Weight Watchers*, Cooked	1 Serving/200g	99	50	1.8	10.0	0.2	0.6
Wheat Free, Tesco*	1 Serving/100g	340	340	8.0	72.5	2.0	2.5
Whole Wheat, Dry, Average	1 Serving/100g	326	326	13.5	62.2	2.6	8.0
Wholemeal, Boiled	1oz/28g	32	113	4.7	23.2	0.9	3.5
Wholemeal, Raw	1oz/28g	91	324	13.4	66.2	2.5	8.4
With Cheese & Broccoli, GFY, Asda*	1 Pack/369.8g	477	129	4.3	20.0	3.5	0.8
With Sausages, Heinz*	1 Can/400g	352	88	3.5	10.8	3.4	0.5
With Tomato & Cheese, Tesco*	1/2 Pack/250g	280	112	4.0	18.1	2.6	1.1
With Tomatoes & Mozzerella, GFY, Asda*	1 Pack/120g	542	452	16.0	79.0	8.0	3.0
SPAGHETTI & MEATBALLS							
American, Superbowl, Asda*	1 Pack/453.4g	593	131	11.0	13.0	3.9	1.1
BGTY, Sainsbury's*	1 Pack/300g	249	83	5.9	12.7	0.9	3.1
COU, Marks & Spencer*	1 Pack/360g	360	100	6.8	14.2	1.9	1.9
Chicken in Tomato Sauce, Heinz*	1 Can/400g	352	88	4.1	11.0	3.0	0.5
Italian, Healthy Living, Tesco*	1 Pack/400g	392	98	5.4	13.5	2.5	0.4
Italian, Sainsbury's*	1 Pack/450g	495	110	5.0	11.9	4.7	2.7
Sainsbury's*	1 Pack/400g	497	124	6.5	14.2	4.6	2.8
Somerfield*	1 Pack/900g	1035	115	5.0	15.0	4.0	0.0
Tesco*	1 Serving/475g	641	135	5.1	14.1	6.5	0.9
Vegetarian, Safeway*	1 Pack/350g	382	109	5.0	13.7	3.8	0.5
SPAGHETTI BOLOGNESE							
Al Forno, Sainsbury's*	1 Pack/400g	460	115	7.8	10.0	4.9	1.1
Asda*	1 Pack/400g	432	108	6.0	17.0	1.8	0.9
Average	1 Serving/450g	581	129	7.8	12.5	5.6	0.9
BGTY, Sainsbury's*	1 Pack/450g	396	88	6.0	13.4	1.1	3.0
Basics, Sainsbury's*	1 Pack/300g	207	69	4.2	11.7	0.6	3.6
Bean & Mushroom, Safeway*	1 Pack/435.3g	370	85	3.7	12.8	2.1	3.7
Birds Eye*	1 Pack/362g	404	112	4.8	13.4	4.4	0.9
COU, Marks & Spencer*	1 Pack/360g	378	105	7.3	13.9	2.2	1.0
Canned, Asda*	1/2 Can/205g	174	85	4.2	10.7	2.8	0.6
Eat Smart, Safeway*	1 Pack/393g	350	89	5.9	13.1	1.4	1.3
Finest, Tesco*	1 Pack/400g	548	137	9.5	12.3	5.5	1.2
Flavour, Sainsbury's*	1 Serving/233g	231	99	2.9	19.1	1.2	2.1

	Measure INFO/WEIGHT	per Measure KCAL	Nutrition Values per 100g / 100ml				
			KCAL	PROT	CARB	FAT	FIBRE
SPAGHETTI BOLOGNESE							
Frozen, Tesco*	1 Serving/400g	472	118	4.7	15.9	3.9	0.4
GFY, Asda*	1 Serving/250g	208	83	5.0	12.0	1.7	0.7
Good Intentions, Somerfield*	1 Serving/400g	380	95	6.2	12.4	2.3	1.4
HP*	1 Pack/410g	312	76	3.8	11.3	1.9	0.7
Healthy Living, Tesco*	1 Serving/400g	448	112	5.2	16.9	2.6	0.6
Heinz*	1 Can/400g	296	74	2.7	12.9	1.4	0.5
In Tomato & Beef Sauce, Carlini, Aldi*	1 Can/410g	324	79	3.7	10.2	2.6	1.2
Italia, Marks & Spencer*	1 Pack/400g	600	150	8.8	14.0	6.3	1.1
Italiano, Tesco*	1 Pack/340g	388	114	6.4	12.6	4.2	1.1
Lean Cuisine, Findus*	1 Pack/320g	275	86	4.5	11.5	2.3	1.1
Loved by Kids, Marks & Spencer*	1/2 Pack/200g	250	125	6.6	15.3	4.4	1.9
Meat Free, Canned, Sainsbury's*	1 Can/400g	280	70	3.4	12.0	0.9	1.2
Meat Free, Heinz*	1 Serving/200g	162	81	3.3	13.1	1.7	0.6
Mega Value, Somerfield*	1 Pack/500g	450	90	4.9	15.6	0.9	1.5
Perfectly Balanced, Waitrose*	1 Pack/350g	319	91	4.2	10.0	3.8	1.0
Quick Pasta, Dry, Sainsbury's*	1 Serving/63g	231	367	10.8	71.0	4.4	3.3
Ready Meals, Marks & Spencer*	1 Pack/360g	576	160	8.8	12.7	8.1	1.2
Ross*	1 Serving/320g	288	90	4.2	15.7	1.1	0.9
SmartPrice, Asda*	1/2 Can/205g	215	105	3.2	12.0	4.9	0.8
Somerfield*	1 Pack/300g	339	113	5.3	18.0	2.2	2.0
Spar*	1 Pack/500g	440	88	5.6	8.6	3.5	1.5
Tesco*	1 Pack/257g	339	132	6.5	14.1	5.5	1.2
Value, Tesco*	1 Pack/300g	294	98	5.2	11.8	3.3	0.5
Vegetarian, Tesco*	1 Pack/340g	374	110	5.1	13.7	3.9	1.2
Waitrose*	1 Serving/250g	253	101	7.6	11.7	2.6	1.0
Weight Watchers*	1 Pack/320g	290	91	5.9	12.9	1.6	0.8
With Mushrooms, Colman's*	1 Pack/45g	67	149	4.0	29.9	1.4	2.8
SPAGHETTI CARBONARA							
COU, Marks & Spencer*	1 Pack/330g	347	105	5.7	15.5	2.0	1.8
Cappelletti, Balanced Lifestyle, Carlini, Aldi*	1 Can/400g	328	82	4.1	10.0	2.8	0.6
Chicken & Asparagus, Sainsbury's*	1 Pack/450g	657	146	6.6	16.2	6.1	1.1
Chicken, Mushroom & Ham, Asda*	1 Pack/700g	686	98	10.0	10.0	2.0	1.5
GFY, Asda*	1 Pack/120g	151	126	4.4	20.0	3.2	0.7
Italian Express*	1 Pack/320g	310	97	4.3	11.6	3.7	1.1
Italiano, Tesco*	1 Pack/450g	702	156	6.9	14.8	7.7	1.7
Marks & Spencer*	1 Pack/360g	630	175	7.6	14.3	9.5	0.1
Safeway*	1 Pack/360g	569	158	7.9	15.7	7.1	1.2
Sainsbury's*	1 Pack/450g	558	124	7.3	14.2	4.2	0.9
Tesco*	1 Pack/450g	612	136	5.9	15.2	5.7	1.3
SPAGHETTI HOOPS							
& Sausages, Tesco*	1 Serving/205g	185	90	3.1	11.9	3.3	0.2
'N' Hot Dogs, Heinz*	1 Can/400g	304	76	2.8	11.0	2.4	0.4
In Tomato Sauce, Heinz*	1 Can/400g	224	56	1.9	11.7	0.2	0.6
Tesco*	1/2 Can/205g	123	60	1.6	12.9	0.2	0.5
SPAGHETTI LOOPS							
SmartPrice, Asda*	1 Serving/205g	127	62	1.7	13.0	0.3	0.4
SPAGHETTI MARINARA							
GFY, Asda*	1 Pack/400g	520	130	8.0	15.0	4.2	0.9
SPAGHETTI RINGS							
Sainsbury's*	1 Serving/213g	136	64	1.9	13.3	0.4	0.5
SPAM*							
Pork & Ham, Chopped	1 Serving/100g	296	296	14.5	3.2	24.2	0.0

S

	Measure INFO/WEIGHT	per Measure KCAL	KCAL	PROT	CARB	FAT	FIBRE
SPICE BLEND							
Balti, Sharwood's*	1oz/28g	34	122	1.8	7.1	9.6	1.2
Thai, Sharwood's*	1 Pack 260g	424	163	1.8	12.0	11.9	1.0
Tikka, Sharwood's*	1 Pack/260g	263	101	2.7	10.2	5.4	1.7
SPICE MIX							
Chicken Tikka Masala & Pilau Rice, Colman's*	1 Pack/85g	309	364	11.5	39.9	18.0	11.2
Chili Mix for Chilli, Schwartz*	1oz/28g	96	344	9.6	63.6	5.7	1.0
Chilli & Garlic Seed, The Food Doctor*	1 Serving/15g	88	584	30.5	3.7	49.7	11.0
Chilli Con Carne, Colman's*	1 Pack/50g	154	308	8.6	62.0	1.7	0.0
Chilli Con Carne, Hot, Schwartz*	1 Pack/41g	141	344	10.8	59.0	7.2	0.0
Curry, Green Thai, For Chicken, Schwartz*	1 Pack/41g	137	334	11.3	67.6	3.2	0.3
Fajita, Old El Paso*	1/2 pack/17.5g	55	306	9.0	54.0	6.0	0.0
Smoky BBQ Pork, Seasoning, Shotz, Schwartz*	1oz/28g	64	228	1.0	53.8	1.0	0.0
SPINACH							
& Carrot Pilau, Waitrose*	1oz/28g	44	158	5.8	22.9	5.8	0.0
Baby, Average	1 Serving/90g	23	25	2.8	1.6	0.8	2.1
Boiled Or Steamed, Average	1oz/28g	6	21	2.6	0.9	0.8	2.1
Canned, Average	1oz/28g	6	23	3.1	1.5	0.5	3.0
Chopped, Frozen, Fresh, Somerfield*	1 Serving/90g	22	24	2.8	1.5	0.8	2.7
Leaf In Water, Salt Added, Sainsbury's*	1 Can/265g	53	20	3.3	1.0	0.3	2.8
Leaf, Frozen, Organic, Waitrose*	7 Pieces/90g	23	25	2.8	1.6	0.8	2.1
Raw, Average	1oz/28g	7	24	2.9	1.3	0.8	2.1
SPIRA							
Cadbury*	2 Twists/40g	210	525	7.8	56.8	29.4	0.0
SPIRALI							
Dry, Average	1 Serving/50g	176	352	12.2	72.6	1.7	2.8
SPIRITS							
37.5% Volume	1 Shot/25ml	48	207	0.0	0.0	0.0	0.0
40% Volume	1 Shot/25ml	51	222	0.0	0.0	0.0	0.0
SPLIT PEAS							
Dried, Average	1oz/28g	89	319	22.1	57.4	1.7	3.2
Dried, Boiled, Average	1 Tbsp/35g	40	115	8.3	19.8	0.6	3.9
SPONGE FINGERS							
Boudoir, Sainsbury's*	1 Biscuit/5g	20	396	8.1	82.8	3.6	0.4
Tesco*	1 Finger/5g	19	386	7.6	80.6	3.7	1.0
SPONGE PUDDING							
Average	1 Portion/170g	578	340	5.8	45.3	16.3	1.1
Banoffee, Heinz*	1/4 Can/78g	239	307	2.8	46.6	12.2	0.6
Banoffee, Morrisons*	1 Pudding/109.8g	316	287	3.0	59.6	2.9	0.7
Blackberry & Apple, Healthy Eating, Tesco*	1 Pot/102.5g	159	155	3.1	32.6	1.4	0.7
Blackcurrant, BGTY, Sainsbury's*	1 Serving/110g	155	141	2.5	30.7	0.9	3.2
Blackcurrant, Low Fat, Iceland*	1 Pudding/90g	159	177	2.2	39.5	1.1	1.6
Canned	1 Portion/75g	214	285	3.1	45.4	11.4	0.8
Cherry & Almond Flavour, Sainsbury's*	1/4 Pudding/110g	334	304	3.5	40.3	14.3	0.7
Cherry & Chocolate, Eat Smart, Safeway*	1 Serving/86g	151	175	2.7	35.6	2.4	0.8
Chocolate & Chocolate Sauce, Healthy Eating, Tesco*	1 Pudding/90g	186	207	3.9	38.7	4.1	2.1
Chocolate & Sauce, Co-Op*	1 Pack/225g	608	270	5.0	34.0	13.0	0.6
Chocolate Chip, Healthy Eating, Tesco*	1 Serving/103g	197	191	4.4	34.7	3.8	0.9
Chocolate, GFY, Asda*	1 Pudding/105g	201	191	6.0	37.0	2.1	2.5
Chocolate, Healthy Eating, Tesco*	1 Pudding/90g	184	204	4.2	45.4	0.6	1.3
Chocolate, Healthy Living, Tesco*	1 Pudding/102.5g	197	191	4.4	34.7	3.8	0.9
Chocolate, Heinz*	1 Serving/50g	150	300	4.8	45.0	11.2	1.2
Chocolate, Marks & Spencer*	1/4 Pudding/131g	524	400	6.1	38.6	24.6	1.8
Chocolate, Sainsbury's*	1/4 Pudding/110g	464	422	5.4	42.3	25.7	0.8

S

SPONGE PUDDING

	Measure INFO/WEIGHT	per Measure KCAL	Nutrition Values per 100g / 100ml				
			KCAL	PROT	CARB	FAT	FIBRE
Chocolate, Somerfield*	1/4 Pudding/100g	369	369	5.0	35.0	23.0	0.0
Chocolate, Tesco*	1 Pudding/110g	337	306	4.7	37.7	15.1	1.8
Chocolate, Weight Watchers*	1 Serving/102.5g	202	196	4.5	35.6	3.9	0.9
Chocolate, With Cadbury's Caramel Sticky Sauce, Heinz*	1 Serving/200g	762	381	3.5	52.3	16.9	0.6
Circus, & Custard, Weight Watchers*	1 Serving/140g	239	171	4.2	32.1	2.9	0.9
Citrus, BGTY, Sainsbury's*	1 Pudding/110g	230	209	3.5	39.7	4.0	0.7
Double Chocolate, BGTY, Sainsbury's*	1 Pot/110g	293	266	4.3	51.5	4.7	0.6
Fruit, Co-Op*	1 Can/300g	1110	370	3.0	53.0	16.0	2.0
Fruited With Brandy Sauce, Sainsbury's*	1 Pudding/125g	261	209	3.6	33.6	6.7	0.8
Fruits Of The Forest, Asda*	1 Pudding/115g	323	281	2.8	59.0	3.8	1.3
Ginger, With Plum Sauce, Waitrose*	1 Pudding/120g	424	353	3.1	51.7	14.9	0.7
Golden Syrup, Co-Op*	1 Can/300g	945	315	2.0	47.0	13.0	0.6
Jam & Custard, Co-Op*	1 Pack/244g	598	245	3.0	37.0	9.0	0.3
Jam & Custard, Somerfield*	1/4 Pudding/62g	143	231	3.0	38.0	8.0	0.0
Jam, Marks & Spencer*	1oz/28g	87	311	3.6	51.5	10.1	1.6
Jam, Safeway*	1 Serving/110g	396	360	3.6	55.6	13.7	2.3
Jam, Tesco*	1 Pudding/110g	367	334	3.3	53.3	11.9	0.5
Lemon Curd, Heinz*	1/4 Can/78g	236	302	2.6	46.7	11.7	0.6
Lemon, COU, Marks & Spencer*	1 Pudding/100g	157	157	2.0	32.1	2.3	1.9
Lemon, Healthy Eating, Tesco*	1 Pudding/102g	195	191	3.7	40.1	2.0	0.5
Lemon, Marks & Spencer*	1 Pudding/105g	326	310	4.3	39.4	15.2	2.3
Lemon, Waitrose*	1 Serving/105g	212	202	3.4	41.7	2.4	1.4
Raspberry Jam, Asda*	1/2 Pudding/147.4g	481	327	3.1	54.0	11.0	4.1
St Clements, GFY, Asda*	1 Pudding/116g	332	286	2.6	60.0	3.9	1.2
Sticky Toffee, COU, Marks & Spencer*	1 Pack/150g	278	185	2.5	39.3	1.7	1.8
Sticky Toffee, Heinz*	1/4 Can/77g	235	305	3.1	45.2	12.5	0.7
Sticky Toffee, Mini, Somerfield*	1 Pudding/110g	349	349	3.0	54.0	13.0	0.0
Sticky Toffee, Somerfield*	1 Pudding/440g	1456	364	3.0	56.0	14.0	0.0
Strawberry Jam, Heinz*	1/4 Can/82g	230	281	2.6	50.4	7.6	0.6
Sultana, With Toffee Sauce, Healthy Eating, Tesco*	1 Serving/80g	223	279	3.3	60.3	2.8	1.0
Summer Fruits, BGTY, Sainsbury's*	1 Serving/110g	243	221	2.7	42.9	4.3	1.0
Syrup, & Custard, Marks & Spencer*	1oz/28g	76	271	3.3	44.9	8.7	1.1
Syrup, BGTY, Sainsbury's*	1 Pudding/110g	338	307	2.8	64.6	4.1	0.4
Syrup, Finest, Tesco*	1 Pudding/115g	330	287	3.1	51.2	7.8	0.6
Syrup, GFY, Asda*	1 Sponge/105g	256	244	3.0	50.0	3.6	0.6
Syrup, Marks & Spencer*	1oz/28g	104	370	4.1	65.9	10.2	1.1
Syrup, Sainsbury's*	1/4 Pudding/110g	404	371	2.7	63.5	11.8	0.4
Syrup, Tesco*	1 Pudding/110g	375	341	3.2	55.8	11.7	0.4
Treacle, With Custard, Farmfoods*	1 Serving/145g	539	372	3.2	38.4	22.8	0.8
Very Fruity Cherry, Marks & Spencer*	1 Pot/110g	286	260	3.5	38.6	10.3	1.8
With Dried Fruit	1oz/28g	93	331	5.4	48.1	14.3	1.2
With Jam or Treacle	1oz/28g	93	333	5.1	48.7	14.4	1.0
With Lyles Golden Syrup, Heinz*	1/2 Pudding/95.3g	367	386	3.1	53.3	15.1	0.5

SPOTTED DICK

Average	1oz/28g	92	327	4.2	42.7	16.7	1.0
Pudding, Individual, Sainsbury's*	1 Serving/110g	347	315	3.8	48.7	11.7	2.2
Puddings, 2 Pack, Tesco*	1 Pudding/110g	354	322	3.3	49.2	12.4	1.3

SPRATS

Fried	1oz/28g	116	415	24.9	0.0	35.0	0.0
Raw	1oz/28g	48	172	18.3	0.0	11.0	0.0

SPREAD

63% Fat, Benecol*	1 Serving/12g	69	573	0.6	1.0	63.0	0.0
Beef, Classic, Shippams*	1 Pot/75g	133	177	15.5	2.2	11.8	0.0

SPREAD

INFO/WEIGHT	Measure	per Measure KCAL	KCAL	PROT	CARB	FAT	FIBRE
Blackcurrant, Weight Watchers*	1 Tsp/5.7g	6	106	0.2	26.3	0.0	0.9
Butter & Olive, Olivio, Bertolli*	Thin Spread/7g	38	536	0.2	1.0	59.0	0.0
Butter Me Up, Light, Healthy Living, Tesco*	1 Serving/15g	52	345	0.3	0.5	38.0	0.0
Butterlicious, Sainsbury's*	Thin Spread/7g	44	628	0.6	1.1	69.0	0.0
Buttery Gold, Somerfield*	1 Tbsp/15g	94	627	0.5	1.0	69.0	0.0
Buttery Taste, Benecol*	1 Tsp/7g	40	573	0.6	1.0	63.0	0.0
Chicken, Classic, Shippams*	1 Serving/35g	64	182	15.5	1.8	12.5	0.0
Chocolate Hazelnut, Tesco*	1 Tsp/10g	54	542	7.0	50.8	34.5	3.7
Crab, Classic, Shippams*	1 Jar/35g	48	138	14.1	6.0	6.4	0.0
Diet, Delight*	1oz/28g	64	228	3.6	1.6	23.0	0.0
Diet, Flora*	1 Tbsp/10g	23	227	3.5	1.6	23.0	0.0
Fat, Carapelli, St Ivel*	Thin Spread/7g	38	537	0.6	0.8	59.0	0.0
Flora Buttery, Flora*	Thin Spread/7g	45	637	1.1	0.5	70.0	0.0
Flora Light, Flora*	1 Serving/10g	37	366	0.1	6.0	38.0	0.0
Flora Original, Flora*	1 Serving/10g	53	531	0.1	0.1	59.0	0.0
Flora Pro-Activ, Flora*	1 Serving/10g	33	328	0.1	3.2	35.0	0.3
Flora, Low Salt, Flora*	1oz/28g	176	630	0.1	0.1	70.0	0.0
From Soya, Kallo*	1 Tsp/7g	27	380	7.0	6.0	37.0	0.0
Gold, Low Fat, St Ivel*	Thin Spread/7g	25	359	0.5	3.3	38.0	0.0
Gold, Lowest, Low Fat, St Ivel*	Thin Spread/7g	18	259	0.7	3.3	27.0	0.0
Golden, Light, Healthy Eating, Tesco*	1 Serving/10g	35	354	1.5	1.5	38.0	0.0
Hazelnut & Chocolate, Organic, Green & Black's*	1 Serving/28g	155	553	5.9	53.0	35.0	0.0
Light, Benecol*	2 Tsp/12g	38	318	2.8	0.2	34.0	0.0
Light, Olivio*	Thin Soread/7g	34	486	0.0	0.0	55.0	0.0
Low Fat 32%, Benecol*	1 Serving/12g	36	300	2.8	0.2	32.0	0.0
Low Fat, Better By Far, Morrisons*	1 Serving/10g	63	630	0.0	1.0	69.0	0.0
Low-Fat	Thin Spread/7g	27	390	5.8	0.5	40.5	0.0
Morning Gold, Low Fat, Morrisons*	1 Tbsp/15g	56	372	7.5	0.0	38.0	0.0
Olive Gold, Reduced Fat, Co-Op*	1oz/28g	150	535	0.2	1.0	59.0	0.0
Olive Gold, With Olive Oil, Low Fat, Asda*	1 Serving/10g	54	537	0.2	1.2	59.0	0.0
Olive Light, Low Fat, BGTY, Sainsbury's*	Thin Spread/ 7g	19	265	0.1	0.8	29.0	0.0
Olive Light, Low Fat, Healthy Living, Tesco*	1 Serving/15g	52	348	1.5	0.0	38.0	0.0
Olive Light, Safeway*	1 Tsp/10g	35	346	1.0	0.0	38.0	0.0
Olive Oil, 55% Reduced Fat, Benecol*	Thin Spread/7g	35	498	0.3	0.5	55.0	0.0
Olive Oil, 59% Reduced Fat, Safeway*	Thin Spread/7g	37	532	0.1	0.1	59.0	0.0
Olive Oil, 59% Vegetable Fat, Olivio*	Thin Spread/7g	38	536	0.2	1.0	59.0	0.0
Olive, BGTY, Sainsbury's*	1 Serving/10g	27	265	0.1	0.8	29.0	0.0
Olive, Reduced Fat, Morrisons*	Thin Spread/7g	38	537	0.9	0.0	59.3	0.3
Olive, Reduced Fat, Organic, Sainsbury's*	Thin Spread/7g	37	531	0.0	0.0	59.0	0.0
Olive, Tesco*	1 Serving/28g	150	537	0.2	1.2	59.0	0.0
Olive, Waitrose*	1 Serving/10g	53	534	0.2	0.5	59.0	0.0
Olivio, Van Den Bergh Foods Ltd*	Thin Spread/7g	38	536	0.2	1.0	59.0	0.0
Olivite, Low Fat, Weight Watchers*	Thin Spread/7g	25	351	0.0	0.2	38.9	0.0
Organic, Dairy Free, Marks & Spencer*	1 Serving/5g	27	531	0.0	0.0	59.0	0.0
Pure Gold, GFY, Asda*	1 Serving/10g	35	353	1.7	1.0	38.0	0.0
Pure Gold, Light, 65% Less Fat, Asda*	1 Serving/10g	24	239	2.5	1.0	25.0	0.0
Salmon, Classic, Shippams*	1 Serving/35g	70	200	14.7	4.2	14.1	0.0
Soft, Dairy Free, Free From, Sainsbury's*	1 Serving/30g	89	296	2.5	4.0	30.0	0.0
Soft, Economy, Sainsbury's*	1oz/28g	126	450	0.2	1.0	50.0	0.0
Soft, Reduced Fat, SmartPrice, Asda*	1 Serving/7g	32	455	0.2	1.0	50.0	0.0
Soft, Sainsbury's*	1 Serving/75g	473	630	0.1	0.1	70.0	0.0
Sunflower, Asda*	1 Serving/10g	64	635	0.2	1.0	70.0	0.0
Sunflower, Light, 38% Less Fat, Asda*	Thin Spread/7g	24	342	0.0	0.0	38.0	0.0

S

	Measure INFO/WEIGHT	per Measure KCAL	Nutrition Values per 100g / 100ml				
			KCAL	PROT	CARB	FAT	FIBRE
SPREAD							
Sunflower, Light, BGTY, Sainsbury's*	1 Serving/10g	35	352	1.0	1.5	38.0	0.0
Sunflower, Light, GFY, Asda*	1 Serving/10g	35	351	0.0	0.0	39.0	0.0
Sunflower, Light, Healthy Eating, Tesco*	1 Serving/6g	21	347	0.3	1.0	38.0	0.0
Sunflower, Light, Tesco*	Thin Spread/7g	24	348	1.4	0.0	38.0	0.0
Sunflower, Low Fat, Good Intentions, Somerfield*	1 Serving/10g	35	347	0.0	0.0	38.6	0.0
Sunflower, Low Fat, Marks & Spencer*	1 Serving/14g	48	342	0.0	0.0	38.0	1.0
Sunflower, Low Fat, Somerfield*	1 Serving/10g	34	342	0.0	0.0	38.0	0.0
Sunflower, Lowest, Healthy Eating, Tesco*	Thin Spread/7g	8	109	2.0	14.0	5.0	10.0
Sunflower, Marks & Spencer*	Thin Spread/7g	44	635	0.2	1.0	70.0	0.0
Sunflower, Probiotic, Tesco*	1 Serving/15g	52	347	0.2	1.0	38.0	0.0
Sunflower, Reduced Fat, Asda*	Thin Spread/7g	37	531	0.2	1.0	58.5	0.0
Sunflower, Sainsbury's*	Thin Spread/7g	37	532	0.1	0.2	59.0	0.0
Sunflower, Substitute, Low Fat, Tesco*	1 Tsp/10g	11	109	2.0	14.0	5.0	10.0
Sunflower, Tesco*	1 Serving/15g	80	532	0.0	0.2	59.0	0.0
Sunflower, Value, Tesco*	Thin Spread/7g	31	439	0.1	0.4	48.6	0.0
Sunflower, Waitrose*	1 Serving/5g	32	631	0.0	0.2	70.0	0.0
Tuna & Mayonnaise, Shippams*	1 Pot/75g	189	252	18.3	3.1	18.5	0.0
Vegetable, Dairy Free, Free From, Sainsbury's*	1 Serving/10g	63	630	0.0	0.0	70.0	3.0
Vegetable, Soft, Tesco*	1 Tbsp/15g	99	661	0.1	1.0	73.0	0.0
Vegetable, Soft, Value, Tesco*	1 Serving/10g	43	433	0.0	0.0	48.1	0.0
Vitalite, Lite, St Ivel*	Thin Spread/7g	24	348	1.5	0.0	38.0	0.0
Vitalite, St Ivel*	Thin Spread/7g	40	578	0.4	1.2	63.0	0.0
With Garlic & Herb, Soft, Free From, Sainsbury's*	1 Serving/30g	91	302	2.5	5.5	30.0	0.1
With Pure Olive Oil, Bertolli*	1 Serving/10g	54	536	0.2	1.0	59.0	0.0
With Soya, Dairy Free, Pure*	1 Serving/10g	53	531	0.0	0.0	59.0	0.0
SPRING GREENS							
Boiled, Average	1oz/28g	6	20	1.9	1.6	0.7	2.6
Raw	1oz/28g	9	33	3.0	3.1	1.0	3.4
SPRING ONIONS							
Bulbs Only, Raw	1oz/28g	10	35	0.9	8.5	0.0	1.7
Raw, Average	1oz/28g	7	24	2.0	3.0	0.5	1.5
SPRING ROLLS							
Cantonese Chicken & Chilli, Sainsbury's*	1 Roll/51g	85	166	9.7	19.4	5.5	0.6
Cantonese Selection, Sainsbury's*	1 Serving/35.2g	68	193	4.1	26.9	7.7	1.4
Cantonese Vegetable, Sainsbury's*	1 Roll/36.1g	84	233	3.6	28.1	11.7	1.4
Char Sui Pork & Bacon, Marks & Spencer*	1 Pack/220g	528	240	4.8	33.9	9.4	0.6
Chicken & Chilli, Sainsbury's*	1 Roll/50g	93	185	9.6	15.6	9.3	2.8
Chicken, Asda*	1 Roll/58g	115	199	4.6	25.0	9.0	3.4
Chicken, Finest, Tesco*	1 Roll/60g	118	196	10.1	20.1	8.3	1.0
Chicken, Oriental Snack Selection, Sainsbury's*	1 Roll/15g	38	256	11.5	30.3	9.9	1.7
Chicken, Oriental, Asda*	1 Roll/59.6g	107	178	3.7	25.0	7.0	0.4
Chicken, Tesco*	1 Roll/50g	116	231	8.1	24.5	11.2	1.5
Chinese Takeaway, Tesco*	1 Roll/50g	101	201	4.4	26.4	8.6	1.5
Dim Sum, Sainsbury's*	1 Roll/12g	26	216	4.1	28.2	9.6	2.9
Duck With Sweet Chilli Sauce, Waitrose*	1 Roll/72g	66	92	5.1	14.0	1.9	0.9
Duck, Morrisons*	1 Roll/30g	68	226	6.2	27.2	10.3	1.2
Duck, Party Bites, Sainsbury's*	1 Roll/20g	49	245	10.1	31.4	8.8	1.0
Marks & Spencer*	1 Pack/180g	333	185	3.5	24.2	8.4	2.3
Mini, Asda*	1 Roll/20g	35	175	3.5	33.6	3.0	1.9
Mini, Sainsbury's*	1 Roll/12g	27	221	4.2	28.7	9.9	1.6
Mini, Tesco*	1 Roll/18g	47	263	3.9	24.9	16.5	1.9
Prawn, Cantonese, Sainsbury's*	1 Roll/28g	46	162	6.8	20.3	6.0	2.5
Prawn, Chinese, Sainsbury's*	1 Roll/30g	65	217	9.6	21.8	10.2	1.3

S

	Measure	per Measure		Nutrition Values per 100g / 100ml				
	INFO/WEIGHT	KCAL		KCAL	PROT	CARB	FAT	FIBRE
SPRING ROLLS								
Prawn, Marks & Spencer*	1oz/28g	62		220	9.4	21.4	10.8	1.6
Prawn, Tesco*	3 Rolls/100g	211		211	8.7	22.8	9.4	1.4
Roast Duck, Marks & Spencer*	1 Roll/30.9g	85		275	7.8	26.2	15.7	1.4
Thai Prawn, Waitrose*	1 Roll/50g	110		219	8.0	25.4	9.5	2.4
Thai, Sainsbury's*	1 Roll/30g	69		229	2.9	28.8	11.3	3.5
Vegetable & Chicken, Tesco*	1 Roll/60g	110		183	6.1	22.2	7.7	2.5
Vegetable, Asda*	1 Roll/62g	126		203	3.5	27.0	9.0	2.7
Vegetable, Chinese Takeaway, Sainsbury's*	1Roll/59g	100		170	4.0	24.4	6.3	2.8
Vegetable, Chinese, Sainsbury's*	1 Roll/26g	69		193	4.1	26.9	7.7	1.4
Vegetable, Cocktail, Tiger Tiger*	1 Roll/15g	38		254	6.4	26.7	13.4	2.0
Vegetable, Frozen, Tesco*	1 Roll/60g	107		179	4.1	20.8	8.8	3.5
Vegetable, Marks & Spencer*	1 Roll/29g	62		215	3.2	27.7	10.3	2.4
Vegetable, Mini, Occasions, Sainsbury's*	1 Roll/24g	52		216	4.1	28.2	9.6	2.9
Vegetable, Mini, Oriental Selection, Waitrose*	1 Roll/18.2g	35		192	4.2	28.6	6.8	1.7
Vegetable, Occasions, Sainsbury's*	1 Roll/25g	52		206	3.7	24.4	10.4	2.1
Vegetable, Oriental Style, Party, Tesco*	1 Roll/20.2g	47		235	3.0	29.0	12.0	1.5
Vegetable, Safeway*	1 Serving/117g	242		207	3.5	27.1	9.4	2.7
Vegetable, Tempura, Marks & Spencer*	1 Pack/140g	280		200	2.8	27.9	8.6	1.8
Vegetable, Tesco*	1 Roll/60g	100		166	4.0	21.2	7.2	2.0
Vegetable, Waitrose*	1 Roll/57g	107		187	3.7	22.1	9.3	3.4
SQUARES								
Rice Krispies, Chewy, Marshmellow, Kellogg's*	1 Med Bar/18g	74		410	3.0	78.0	10.0	1.0
Rice Krispies, Chocolate Caramel, Kellogg's*	1 Bar/21g	89		425	4.5	73.0	13.0	2.0
Rice Krispies, Chocolate, Kellogg's*	1 Bar/18g	74		410	4.0	75.0	11.0	1.5
SQUASH								
Acorn, Baked	1oz/28g	16		56	1.1	12.6	0.1	3.2
Acorn, Raw	1oz/28g	11		40	0.8	9.0	0.1	2.3
Apple & Blackcurrant, Special R, Diluted, Robinson's*	1fl oz/30ml	2		8	0.1	1.1	0.1	0.0
Apple & Strawberry High Juice, Sainsbury's*	1 Serving/250ml	83		33	0.1	8.2	0.1	0.1
Apple, Blackcurrant, Low Sugar, Diluted, Sainsbury's*	1 Glass/250ml	5		2	0.1	0.2	0.1	0.1
Apple, Hi Juice, Tesco*	1fl oz/30ml	52		173	0.0	42.5	0.0	0.0
Blackcurrant, High Juice, Marks & Spencer*	1 Glass/250ml	50		20	0.1	5.2	0.0	0.1
Blackcurrant, High Juice, Tesco*	1 Serving/75ml	215		287	0.3	70.0	0.0	0.0
Blackcurrant, Sainsbury's*	1 Serving/250ml	8		3	0.1	0.5	0.1	0.1
Butternut, Baked	1oz/28g	9		32	0.9	7.4	0.1	1.4
Butternut, Courgette & Mange Tout, Marks & Spencer*	1 Pack/80g	24		30	2.0	5.8	0.2	2.3
Butternut, Raw, Average	1oz/28g	11		38	1.1	8.3	0.1	1.6
Dandelion & Burdock, Morrisons*	1 Serving/50ml	2		3	0.0	0.0	0.0	0.0
Forest Fruits, High Juice, Undiluted, Robinson's*	1 Serving/25ml	52		206	0.2	50.0	0.1	0.0
Grape & Passion Fruit, High Juice, Diluted, Sainsbury's*	1 serving/250ml	100		40	0.1	9.8	0.1	0.1
Lemon, High Juice, Diluted, Sainsbury's*	1 Glass /250ml	98		39	0.1	9.1	0.1	0.1
Lemon, High Juice, Tesco*	1 Serving/80ml	141		176	0.3	43.6	0.1	0.0
Lemon, No Sugar, Asda*	1 Serving/200ml	5		3	0.1	0.3	0.1	0.1
Lemon, Whole, Low Sugar, Sainsbury's*	1 Glass/250ml	5		2	0.1	0.2	0.1	0.1
Mixed Fruit, Low Sugar, Sainsbury's*	1 Glass/250ml	5		2	0.1	0.2	0.1	0.1
Mixed Fruit, Tesco*	1 Serving/75ml	13		17	0.0	3.5	0.0	0.0
Orange & Mango, Low Sugar, Sainsbury's*	1 Serving/250ml	5		2	0.1	0.2	0.1	0.1
Orange & Mango, Special R, Diluted, Robinson's	1 Serving/250ml	20		8	0.2	0.9	0.0	0.0
Orange & Pineapple, Original, Undiluted, Robinson's*	1 Serving/250ml	138		55	1.0	13.0	0.0	0.0
Orange, Hi Juice, Tesco*	1 Serving/75ml	140		187	0.3	45.0	0.1	0.0
Orange, High Juice, Undiluted, Robinson's*	1 Serving/200ml	364		182	0.3	44.0	0.1	0.0
Orange, No Added Sugar, High Juice, Sainsbury's*	1 Serving/100ml	6		6	0.1	1.1	0.1	0.1
Orange, No Added Sugar, Undiluted, Pennywise, Crystal*	1 Serving/40ml	3		8	0.1	1.2	0.0	0.0

S

INFO/WEIGHT	Measure	per Measure KCAL	KCAL	PROT	CARB	FAT	FIBRE
SQUASH							
Orange, Sainsbury's*	1 Glass/250ml	8	3	0.1	0.5	0.1	0.1
Orange, Special R, Diluted, Robinson's*	1fl oz/30ml	2	8	0.2	0.7	0.1	0.0
Orange, Undiluted, Pennywise, Crystal*	1 Serving/40ml	7	17	0.1	3.5	0.0	0.0
Peach, High Juice, Undiluted, Robinson's*	1fl oz/30ml	54	181	0.5	43.0	0.1	0.0
Pink Grapefruit, High Juice, Low Sugar, Tesco*	1 Serving/75ml	12	16	0.2	3.7	0.1	0.0
Pink Grapefruit, High Juice, Sainsbury's*	1 Serving/250ml	103	41	0.1	9.9	0.1	0.1
Pink Grapefruit, High Juice, Tesco*	1 Serving/75ml	135	180	0.2	44.6	0.1	0.0
Pink Grapefruit, High Juice, Undiluted, Robinson's*	1 Glass/250ml	455	182	0.2	43.3	0.1	0.0
Spaghetti, Baked	1oz/28g	6	23	0.7	4.3	0.3	2.1
Spaghetti, Raw	1oz/28g	7	26	0.6	4.6	0.6	2.3
Summer Fruits, High Juice, Undiluted, Robinson's*	1fl oz/30ml	61	203	0.1	49.0	0.1	0.0
Summer Fruits, High Juice, Waitrose*	1 Serving/250ml	102	41	0.0	10.0	0.0	0.0
Tropical Fruits, High Juice Sainsbury's*	1 Serving/250ml	95	38	0.1	9.3	0.1	0.1
Tropical, High Juice, Tesco*	1 Glass/75ml	141	188	0.2	46.6	0.1	0.1
Whole Orange, Tesco*	1 Serving/100ml	45	45	0.2	10.1	1.0	1.0
SQUID							
Dried	1oz/28g	88	313	63.3	4.8	4.6	0.0
In Batter, Fried in Blended Oil	1oz/28g	55	195	11.5	15.7	10.0	0.5
Raw, Average	1oz/28g	23	81	15.4	1.2	1.7	0.0
STAR FRUIT							
Average, Tesco*	1oz/28g	9	32	0.5	7.3	0.3	1.3
STARBAR							
Cadbury*	1 Bar/53g	260	491	10.7	49.0	27.9	0.0
STARBURST							
Fruit Chews, Tropical, Mars*	1 Tube/45g	168	373	0.0	76.9	7.3	0.0
Joosters, Mars*	1 Pack/45g	160	356	0.0	88.8	0.1	0.0
Juicy Gums, Mars*	1 Pack/45g	139	309	5.9	71.0	4.1	0.0
Mars*	1 Pack/45g	185	411	0.3	85.3	7.6	0.0
STARS							
Chargrilled Chicken & Herb, Shapers, Boots*	1 Pack/12.0g	46	382	6.4	83.0	2.7	3.3
Chicken Flavour, Healthy Eating, Tesco*	1 Serving/12g	43	357	5.1	81.0	1.4	3.4
Spicy, COU, Marks & Spencer*	1 Bag/20g	69	345	4.2	82.6	1.6	4.0
STEAK							
Au Poivre, Finest, Tesco*	1/2 Packet/225g	405	180	16.3	2.6	11.6	0.9
Diane, Finest, Tesco*	1 Serving/225g	331	147	14.2	3.9	8.3	0.7
STEAK &							
Ale, With Vintage Cheddar Mash, Finest, Tesco*	1 Serving/550g	594	108	8.0	8.6	4.6	0.6
Vegetable Medley, Healthy Eating, Tesco*	1 Pack/400g	264	66	7.6	5.3	1.6	0.8
STEAK & KIDNEY PUDDING							
Fray Bentos*	1 Tin/213g	477	224	7.8	19.8	12.6	0.0
Marks & Spencer*	1 Pudding/100g	215	215	10.5	18.1	11.3	1.0
Sainsbury's*	1 Pudding/435g	1135	261	10.5	22.3	14.4	0.8
Tesco*	1 Serving/190g	437	230	10.0	20.7	11.9	1.2
Waitrose*	1 Pudding/223g	497	223	8.9	20.4	11.7	1.2
STEAK CHASSEUR							
Healthy Eating, Tesco*	1 Pack/450g	347	77	10.0	5.3	1.8	0.5
STEAK IN							
Rich Gravy, Stewed, Extra Lean, Sainsbury's*	1 Sm Can/220g	249	113	20.3	1.6	2.8	1.6
STEAK PEPPERED							
With Garlic Butter, Somerfield*	1 Serving/170g	265	156	24.9	1.7	5.5	0.3
With Potato Gratin, Healthy Living, Tesco*	1 Pack/450g	459	102	9.8	9.7	2.7	1.0
STEAK STEWED							
& Onions With Gravy, John West*	1/2 Can/205g	269	131	14.0	3.0	7.0	0.0

S

	Measure INFO/WEIGHT	per Measure KCAL	Nutrition Values per 100g / 100ml				
			KCAL	PROT	CARB	FAT	FIBRE
STEAK STEWED							
Tesco*	1/2 Can/200g	230	115	17.5	4.5	3.0	0.0
With Gravy, John West*	1oz/28g	30	107	18.0	2.0	3.0	0.2
STEAK WITH							
Red Wine & Shallot Sauce, Rump, Waitrose*	1 Serving/205g	242	118	16.4	0.9	5.6	0.3
STEAMED PUDDING							
Apple & Sultana, BGTY, Sainsbury's*	1 Pudding/110g	294	267	2.9	57.4	2.9	0.8
Apple With Wild Berry Sauce, BGTY, Sainsbury's*	1 Pudding/110g	308	280	2.6	59.7	3.4	1.4
Chocolate Flavour, BGTY, Sainsbury's*	1 Serving/110g	300	273	3.3	58.4	2.5	1.3
Chocolate Fudge, Aunty's*	1 Pudding/110g	314	285	3.0	59.0	4.2	1.8
Chocolate, BGTY, Sainsbury's*	1 Pudding/110g	308	280	3.0	59.0	3.6	1.8
Golden Syrup, Aunty's*	1 Pudding/110g	366	333	2.6	69.0	5.0	2.3
Lemon, BGTY, Sainsbury's*	1 Pudding/110g	307	279	3.0	60.2	2.9	0.7
Lemon, Sainsbury's*	1 Serving/110.0g	307	279	3.0	60.2	2.9	0.7
Toffee & Date, Aunty's*	1 Serving/110g	320	291	2.6	59.1	4.6	1.1
STEW							
Beef & Dumplings, Asda*	1 Pack/400g	392	98	6.0	11.0	3.3	0.8
Beef & Dumplings, Birds Eye*	1 Pack/320g	275	86	6.4	10.2	2.2	0.7
Beef & Dumplings, British Classics, Tesco*	1 Pack/450g	563	125	7.9	8.6	6.6	0.5
Beef & Dumplings, Eat Smart, Safeway*	1 Pack/394g	335	85	8.1	6.8	2.5	1.1
Beef & Dumplings, Frozen, Asda*	1 Pack/400g	392	98	6.0	11.0	3.3	0.8
Beef & Dumplings, Ready Meals, Waitrose*	1oz/28g	38	136	8.0	13.3	5.6	0.8
Beef & Dumplings, Traditional English Meals, Birds Eye*	1 Pack/338g	355	105	6.7	11.5	3.6	0.0
Beef & Dumplings, Weight Watchers*	1 Pack/327g	262	80	5.2	10.0	2.1	0.8
Beef With Dumplings, COU, Marks & Spencer*	1 Pack/454g	431	95	8.9	9.1	2.6	0.8
Beef With Dumplings, Classic British, Sainsbury's*	1 Pack/450g	531	118	7.7	10.2	5.2	0.5
Beef With Dumplings, GFY, Asda*	1 Pack/400g	429	107	11.5	10.3	2.3	0.9
Beef With Dumplings, Sainsbury's*	1 Pack/450g	545	121	7.1	10.9	5.4	0.7
Beef, Asda*	1/2 Can/196g	178	91	10.0	7.0	2.5	1.5
Beef, Meal for One, Marks & Spencer*	1 Pack/440g	350	80	7.0	8.7	1.9	2.0
Chicken & Dumplings, Birds Eye*	1 Pack/320g	282	88	7.0	8.9	2.7	0.5
Chicken & Dumplings, Tesco*	1 Serving/450g	567	126	7.6	9.1	6.6	0.7
Chicken, Morrisons*	1 Pack/400g	492	123	17.6	8.9	1.9	0.5
Irish, Sainsbury's*	1 Pack/450g	275	61	5.7	4.8	2.1	0.5
Irish, SmartPrice, Asda*	1 Can/392g	298	76	3.0	8.0	3.6	0.9
Irish, Tesco*	1 Can/400g	308	77	7.0	5.9	2.8	0.8
Lentil & Winter Vegetable, Organic, Pure & Pronto*	1 Pack/400g	364	91	3.6	14.0	2.4	4.0
Lentil & Winter Vegetable, Simply Organic*	1 Pack/400g	364	91	3.6	14.0	2.4	4.0
Mixed Vegetable Topped With Herb Dumplings, Tesco*	1 Pack/420g	508	121	1.9	14.5	6.2	1.3
STIR FRY							
Baby Leaf, Marks & Spencer*	1 Serving/125g	31	25	1.7	4.6	0.3	1.9
Baby Vegetable & Pak Choi, Two Step, Tesco*	1/2 Pack/95g	29	31	2.1	4.0	0.8	2.3
Bean Sprout & Vegetable, Tesco*	1 Serving/150g	47	31	2.1	4.8	0.4	1.9
Bean Sprout Mix, Safeway*	1 Serving/175g	123	70	2.5	4.6	4.6	1.9
Bean Sprout, Chinese, Sainsbury's*	1 Pack/300g	144	48	1.9	5.1	2.8	1.5
Bean Sprout, Ready To Eat, Washed, Sainsbury's*	1 Serving/150g	83	55	1.5	3.3	3.9	1.8
Bean Sprouts & Vegetables, Asda*	1/2 Pack/173g	107	62	2.0	4.5	4.0	1.8
Bean Sprouts, Asda*	1/2 Pack/175g	56	32	2.9	4.0	0.5	1.5
Beef & Black Bean, Sizzling, Oriental Express*	1 Pack/400g	420	105	7.2	14.0	2.1	2.1
Beef, BGTY, Sainsbury's*	1/2 Pack/125g	156	125	22.0	0.1	4.1	0.0
Beef, Less Than 10% Fat, Asda*	1 Pack/227g	275	121	24.0	0.0	2.8	0.8
Beef, Less Than 3% Fat, BGTY, Sainsbury's*	1/2 Pack/125g	134	107	22.1	0.1	2.1	0.1
Cherry Tomato & Noodle, Waitrose*	1 Pack/400g	304	76	2.1	8.5	3.8	1.5
Chicken Chow Mein, Fresh, Heathly Living, Tesco*	1 Pack/400g	312	78	5.7	11.4	1.2	1.3

STIR FRY

INFO/WEIGHT	Measure	per Measure KCAL	KCAL	PROT	CARB	FAT	FIBRE
Chicken Chow Mein, Orient Express, Oriental Express*	1 Pack/400g	384	96	7.3	10.7	2.7	2.2
Chicken Noodle, GFY, Asda*	1 Pack/330g	403	122	7.0	16.0	3.3	2.4
Chicken, Safeway*	1 Serving/200g	204	102	22.0	0.0	1.6	0.0
Chinese Bean Sprout, Sainsbury's*	1/2 Pack/313g	150	48	1.9	5.1	2.8	1.5
Chinese Chicken, Sizzling, Oriental Express*	1 Pack/400g	400	100	6.6	13.8	2.0	1.7
Chinese Chop Suey Veg, Sharwood's*	1 Pack/310g	223	72	1.5	13.9	1.1	0.6
Chinese Exotic Vegetable, Sainsbury's*	1 Pack/350g	133	38	1.7	2.8	2.2	1.8
Chinese Mixed Vegetable, Sainsbury's*	1 Serving/150g	75	50	1.7	4.7	2.7	0.0
Chinese Mushroom, Sainsbury's*	1 Serving/175g	67	38	1.7	2.4	2.4	1.7
Chinese Noodles, Oriental Express*	1oz/28g	20	70	2.7	14.7	0.5	1.4
Chinese Prawn, Asda*	1 Serving/375g	345	92	3.6	18.0	0.6	1.8
Chinese Prawns, Sizzling, Oriental Express*	1 Pack/400g	384	96	3.9	14.7	2.4	1.6
Chinese Style Chicken, GFY, Asda*	1 Pack/338.3g	362	107	6.0	17.0	1.7	1.5
Chinese Style Prawn, GFY, Asda*	1 Pack/400g	324	81	3.6	13.0	1.6	1.6
Chinese Style Rice With Vegetables, Tesco*	1 Serving/550g	495	90	2.2	14.8	2.5	0.3
Chinese Style, Tesco*	1 Pack/350g	140	40	2.5	6.6	0.4	1.4
Chinese Vegetable & Oyster Sauce, Asda*	1 Serving/150g	93	62	1.9	8.0	2.5	0.0
Chinese Vegetables, Oriental Express*	1/2 Pack/200g	44	22	1.4	3.7	0.2	2.2
Chinese Vegetables, Tesco*	1 Serving/175g	93	53	1.6	10.8	0.4	1.3
Chinese Vegetables, With Oyster Sauce, Tesco*	1 Pack/350g	98	28	2.0	4.6	0.2	1.1
Chinese, Eastern Inspirations*	1/2 Pack/170g	49	29	2.7	3.5	0.5	1.8
Chinese, Family, Sainsbury's*	1 Serving/150g	60	40	2.3	3.3	2.0	3.6
Chinese, With Oriental Sauce, Tesco*	1 Pack/530g	180	34	2.3	5.4	0.4	1.5
Chow Mein, Safeway*	1 Pack/400g	536	134	3.8	15.2	6.4	1.9
Creamy Coconut & Lime, The Best, Safeway*	1/2 Pack/165g	231	140	3.4	14.4	7.2	2.1
Exotic, Tesco*	1 Pack/191g	42	22	1.3	3.8	0.2	1.5
Family, Tesco*	1 Serving/150g	33	22	1.8	2.6	0.4	1.1
Green Vegetable, Marks & Spencer*	1 Pack/220g	165	75	3.1	2.5	5.9	2.2
Mediterranean Style, Eastern Inspirations*	1/2 Pack/153g	41	27	1.6	4.0	0.4	2.2
Mediterranean Style, Waitrose*	1 Pack/305g	82	27	1.6	4.6	0.4	2.2
Mexican Vegetables, Lidl*	1 Serving/100g	97	97	3.4	8.1	5.7	0.0
Mixed Pepper & Sweet Chilli Sauce, Asda*	1 Pack/300g	180	60	1.6	9.0	2.0	2.6
Mixed Pepper & Vegetable, Asda*	1/2 Pack/150g	42	28	1.6	3.2	1.0	2.6
Mixed Pepper, Healthy Living, Tesco*	1 Pack/325g	62	19	1.9	2.6	0.1	1.5
Mixed Pepper, Tesco*	1/2 Pack/170g	114	67	1.8	5.3	4.3	1.8
Mixed Vegetable, Safeway*	1 Serving/150g	105	70	2.1	6.2	3.6	2.5
Mixed Vegetables, Sainsbury's*	1/2 Pack/140g	70	50	1.7	4.7	2.7	3.0
Mushroom, 2 Step, Tesco*	1/2 Pack/180g	34	19	2.3	2.1	0.2	0.7
Mushroom, Mixed, Asda*	1 Pack/283g	113	40	2.5	3.4	1.8	2.5
Mushroom, Sainsbury's*	1/2 Pack/159g	84	53	1.8	3.1	3.7	2.2
Mushroom, Tesco*	1 Pack/350g	102	29	2.4	4.0	0.4	1.7
Noodles & Bean Sprouts, Tesco*	1 Serving/125g	119	95	4.4	14.6	2.1	1.5
Orient Inspired, Marks & Spencer*	1 Serving/250g	50	20	1.6	3.4	0.3	1.6
Oriental Chinese, Waitrose*	1 Serving/150g	41	27	2.2	3.9	0.4	1.4
Oriental Leaf, Marks & Spencer*	1/2 Pack/125g	25	20	1.9	2.5	0.5	2.2
Oriental Style Pak Choi, Marks & Spencer*	1 Pack/220g	165	75	2.2	3.5	5.7	2.4
Oriental Vegetable, Frozen, Asda*	1 Serving/150g	116	77	2.1	7.0	4.5	1.7
Oriental Vegetables, Safeway*	1 Serving/175g	196	112	2.6	15.5	4.4	0.5
Oriental, Marks & Spencer*	1/2 Pack/150g	45	30	3.1	2.5	0.6	1.8
Pineapple, Safeway*	1 Pack/300g	237	79	3.6	4.7	5.1	0.5
Plum Hoisin Noodle, Tesco*	1 Carton/400g	392	98	3.6	17.5	1.5	1.8
Prawns, Chinese Sizzling, Oriental Express*	1 Pack/400g	384	96	3.9	14.7	2.4	1.6
Singaporean Noodle, Sainsbury's*	1/2 Pack/160g	202	126	3.2	11.9	7.3	2.4

	Measure INFO/WEIGHT	per Measure KCAL	Nutrition Values per 100g / 100ml				
			KCAL	PROT	CARB	FAT	FIBRE
STIR FRY							
Spicy Oriental Vegetable, Sainsbury's*	1/2 Pack/175g	112	64	1.3	4.9	4.4	1.7
Spicy Thai Style Noodle, Tesco*	1 Pack/500g	335	67	2.6	8.4	2.6	1.3
Sweet & Crunchy, Waitrose*	1/2 Pack/150g	35	23	1.8	3.6	0.1	1.4
Sweet & Sour Vegetable, Somerfield*	1 Pack/350g	249	71	2.0	14.0	1.0	0.0
Sweet & Sour, Co-Op*	1/2 Pack/187g	103	55	2.0	10.0	0.9	3.0
Sweet & Sour, Tesco*	1 Pack/350g	161	46	1.8	9.1	0.3	1.3
Sweet Pepper, Marks & Spencer*	1 Pack/400g	160	40	2.3	3.5	1.8	0.6
Szechuan Spicy Oriental Vegetable, Sainsbury's*	1 Pack/350g	224	64	1.3	4.9	4.4	1.7
Tatsoi & Sugar Snap Pea, Marks & Spencer*	1/2 Pack/125g	25	20	2.0	3.0	0.3	1.9
Tender Shoot, Sainsbury's*	1/2 Pack/126g	113	90	4.4	2.8	6.6	0.8
Thai Style Vegetables, Amoy*	1 Pack/220g	41	19	0.7	3.5	0.2	0.0
Thai Style, Eastern Inspirations*	1 Pack/330g	92	28	2.9	3.2	0.5	1.3
Thai Style, Marks & Spencer*	1 Serving/150g	75	50	2.3	3.0	3.0	1.2
Thai Style, Tesco*	1 Pack/350g	301	86	3.9	6.2	5.1	1.9
Thai, Vegetable, Safeway*	1 Serving/300g	220	73	2.6	5.6	4.3	2.3
Tomato & Basil, Sundried, Tesco*	1 Pack/325g	205	63	1.6	6.2	3.6	2.2
Turkey, Fresh, Good Intentions, Somerfield*	1/2 Pack/150g	246	164	31.0	0.0	4.5	0.0
Vegetable & Beansprout, With Peanut Sauce, Tesco*	1 Serving/475g	409	86	3.9	6.2	5.0	1.9
Vegetable & Mushroom, Asda*	1/2 Pack/160g	59	37	2.4	3.4	1.5	3.4
Vegetable & Noodle, Tesco*	1 Pack/300g	261	87	3.5	12.3	2.6	1.5
Vegetable & Sprouting Beans, Waitrose*	1 Pack/300g	213	71	4.8	10.4	1.1	2.7
Vegetable Noodles, BGTY, Sainsbury's*	1 Pack/455g	391	86	3.2	14.0	2.0	1.4
Vegetable, Asda*	1 Pack/300g	132	44	1.6	4.2	2.3	3.1
Vegetable, Cantonese, Sainsbury's*	1 Serving/150g	90	60	2.8	4.2	3.5	2.7
Vegetable, Chinese Style, Asda*	1 Pack/300g	81	27	1.6	3.6	0.7	2.8
Vegetable, Crispy, Oriental Inspired, Marks & Spencer*	1 Pack/300g	81	27	3.1	2.5	0.6	1.8
Vegetable, Mixed, Sainsbury's*	1 Pack/600g	240	40	2.3	3.3	2.0	3.6
Vegetable, Premium, Sainsbury's*	1/2 Pack/150g	90	60	2.8	4.2	3.5	2.7
Vegetable, Tesco*	1 Pack/300g	90	30	1.7	4.9	0.4	2.1
Vegetables & Bean Sprout, Marks & Spencer*	1 Pack/350g	105	30	1.8	4.6	0.4	2.0
Vegetables With Oyster Sauce, Asda*	1 Serving/150g	93	62	1.9	8.0	2.5	0.0
Vegetables, Amoy*	1 Can/250g	30	12	1.0	2.1	0.0	2.7
Vegetables, Cantonese Style, Tesco*	1 Serving/125g	40	32	2.0	4.1	0.9	1.4
Vegetables, Fresh, Asda*	1/2 Pack/150g	107	71	1.7	4.9	5.0	1.7
Vegetables, Somerfield*	1 Pack/300g	93	31	2.0	5.0	0.0	0.0
STOCK							
Beef, Fresh, Tesco*	1 Serving/300ml	54	18	2.1	1.6	0.3	0.5
Beef, Slowly Prepared, Sainsbury's*	1 Serving/100g	7	7	0.7	0.3	0.3	0.5
Chicken, Asda*	1/2 Pot/150g	26	17	1.8	0.7	0.9	0.2
Chicken, Concentrated, Marks & Spencer*	1 Serving/5g	16	315	25.6	12.2	18.1	0.8
Chicken, Fresh, Sainsbury's*	1/2 Pot/142ml	23	16	3.7	0.1	0.1	0.3
Chicken, Fresh, Tesco*	1 Serving/300ml	27	9	1.6	0.5	0.1	0.5
Chicken, Homemade, Average	1 fl oz/28ml	5	16	3.7	0.1	0.1	0.3
Chicken, Knorr*	1 Pack/150g	348	232	13.1	36.5	3.7	0.4
Chicken, Prepared, Tesco*	1 Serving/300ml	54	18	2.4	1.8	0.1	0.5
Chicken, Simply, Knorr*	1oz/28g	2	6	1.6	0.1	0.0	0.1
Fish, Fresh, Finest, Tesco*	1 Serving/100g	10	10	0.6	1.8	0.0	0.5
Fresh, Finest, Tesco*	1 Pot/300g	33	11	1.9	0.8	0.0	0.2
Vegetable, Campbell's*	1 Serving/250ml	38	15	0.3	2.0	0.7	0.0
Vegetable, Knorr*	1 Serving/9g	18	199	8.5	39.9	0.6	0.9
Vegetable, Tablets, Sainsbury's*	1 Tablet/11g	1	7	0.4	0.2	0.5	0.1
Vegetable, Waitrose*	1 Serving/50g	3	6	0.4	1.2	0.0	0.0

S

	INFO/WEIGHT	KCAL	KCAL	PROT	CARB	FAT	FIBRE
STOCK CUBES							
Beef, Dry, As Sold, Bovril*	1 Cube/5.9g	12	197	10.8	29.3	4.1	0.0
Beef, Dry, As Sold, Oxo*	1 Cube/5.8	15	265	17.3	38.4	4.7	1.5
Beef, Knorr*	1 Cube/10g	33	326	11.1	21.0	22.0	0.2
Beef, Organic, Kallo*	1 Cube/12g	25	208	16.7	16.7	8.3	0.0
Beef, SmartPrice, Asda*	1 Cube/11g	31	279	10.0	8.0	23.0	0.0
Beef, Tesco*	1 Serving/7g	17	260	9.7	48.9	2.8	1.3
Beef, Value, Tesco*	1 Cube/10g	19	189	11.2	17.0	8.5	0.1
Chicken	1 Cube/6g	14	237	15.4	9.9	15.4	0.0
Chicken, Dry, As Sold, Oxo*	1 Cube/6g	13	224	11.1	37.1	3.5	1.4
Chicken, Just Bouillon, Kallo*	1 Cube/12g	30	247	11.8	26.1	10.6	1.0
Chicken, Knorr*	1 Cube/10g	30	301	10.1	23.6	18.5	0.2
Chicken, Made Up, Sainsbury's*	1 Cube/200ml	16	8	0.3	1.4	0.1	0.1
Chicken, Tesco*	1 Cube/11g	32	290	10.5	11.1	22.6	0.7
Chinese, Dry, As Sold, Oxo*	1 Cube/6g	16	263	11.0	40.9	6.1	3.6
Fish, Knorr*	1 Cube/10g	32	321	18.9	15.9	20.2	0.7
Fish, Sainsbury's*	1 Cube/11g	31	282	19.1	7.3	20.0	0.9
Garlic, Dry, As Sold, Oxo*	1 Cube/6g	18	298	13.4	48.5	5.5	3.6
Ham, Knorr*	1 Cube/10g	31	313	11.8	24.4	18.7	0.0
Indian, Dry, As Sold, Oxo*	1 Cube/6g	17	291	11.5	43.9	7.7	6.7
Lamb, Knorr*	1 Cube/10g	30	301	14.7	12.9	21.2	0.2
Mexican, Dry, As Sold, Oxo*	1 Cube/6g	15	248	11.8	36.8	6.0	3.7
Vegetable	1 Cube/7g	18	253	13.5	11.6	17.3	0.0
Vegetable Bouillon, Yeast Free, Made Up, Marigold*	1 Serving/250ml	19	8	0.0	0.5	0.6	0.0
Vegetable, Dry, As Sold, Oxo*	1 Cube/6g	15	253	11.2	41.9	4.5	1.7
Vegetable, Knorr*	1 Pack/80g	246	308	11.9	21.7	19.3	1.3
Vegetable, Low Salt, Organic, Made Up, Kallo*	1 Serving/100ml	8	8	0.5	0.9	0.3	0.1
Vegetable, Made Up, Organic, Kallo*	2 Cubes/100ml	4	4	0.2	0.4	0.2	0.0
Vegetable, Organic, Evernat*	1oz/28g	2	6	0.3	0.0	0.5	0.0
Vegetable, Premium, Made Up, Kallo*	1 Serving/125ml	7	6	0.4	0.4	0.3	0.1
Vegetable, Tesco*	1/2 Cube/4.8g	10	207	8.0	25.7	8.0	0.3
Vegetable, Yeast Free, Made Up, Kallo*	1oz/28g	1	5	0.4	0.4	0.3	0.1
STORTELLI							
Microwaveable, Dolmio*	1 Serving/220g	299	136	5.3	26.3	1.0	0.0
STRAWBERRIES							
Fresh, Average	1oz/28g	8	28	0.8	6.0	0.1	0.9
In Fruit Juice, Average	1/3 Can/127g	58	46	0.5	11.0	0.0	1.0
In Light Syrup, Canned, Drained, Tesco*	1 Can/149g	100	67	0.5	16.0	0.1	0.7
In Raspberry Sauce, WTF, Sainsbury's*	1 Serving/170g	111	65	0.7	15.3	0.1	2.3
STREAKY STRIPS							
Meat Free, Morningstar Farms*	1 Strip/8g	28	348	11.5	13.4	27.6	3.9
STREUSEL							
Baked Apple & Plum, Healthy Eating, Tesco*	1 Serving/120g	161	134	1.9	29.4	1.0	2.0
STROGANOFF							
Beef, Asda*	1 Serving/120g	276	230	16.0	3.3	17.0	0.6
Beef, BGTY, Sainsbury's*	1 Pack/400g	416	104	5.6	14.6	2.6	0.6
Beef, Eat Smart, Morrisons*	1 Pack/400g	344	86	5.0	11.2	2.3	0.9
Beef, Finest, Tesco*	1 Pack/200g	200	100	13.4	3.9	3.4	0.0
Beef, Large Pack, Finest, Tesco*	1 Serving/500g	625	125	8.9	14.9	3.3	0.9
Beef, Sainsbury's*	1 Can/200g	232	116	12.5	3.0	6.0	0.2
Beef, TTD, Sainsbury's*	1 Pack/300g	491	164	11.9	5.2	10.6	0.4
Beef, With Long Grain & Wild Rice, Somerfield*	1 Pack/400g	485	121	7.3	13.8	4.1	1.6
Beef, With Parsley Rice, Tesco*	1 Serving/460g	561	122	4.6	17.6	3.7	0.6
Beef, With Rice, Tesco*	1 Pack/475g	518	109	5.6	13.7	3.5	3.4

	Measure INFO/WEIGHT	per Measure KCAL	Nutrition Values per 100g / 100ml				
			KCAL	PROT	CARB	FAT	FIBRE
STROGANOFF							
Chicken & Mushroom, COU, Marks & Spencer*	1 Serving/400g	360	90	8.6	9.0	2.0	1.0
Chicken, Healthy Living, Tesco*	1 Pack/450g	491	109	7.7	13.5	2.7	0.6
Mushroom With Rice, Eat Smart, Safeway*	1 Pack/400g	280	70	2.7	11.3	1.3	1.6
Mushroom With Rice, Healthy Eating, Tesco*	1 Pack/450g	396	88	3.8	13.3	2.2	1.2
Mushroom With Rice, Tesco*	1 Pack/450g	486	108	3.6	14.4	4.0	0.6
Mushroom, BGTY, Sainsbury's*	1 Pack/451g	392	87	3.2	17.4	0.5	0.5
Mushroom, GFY, Asda*	1 Pack/450g	351	78	2.8	13.0	1.6	0.3
Mushroom, Vegetarian, Tesco*	1 Serving/460g	460	100	1.8	17.4	2.6	1.3
Pork With Rice, Healthy Eating, Tesco*	1 Pack/450g	482	107	7.0	15.8	1.8	0.5
STRUDEL							
Apple & Mincemeat, Tesco*	1 Serving/100g	322	322	3.3	39.6	16.7	2.0
Apple & Sultana, Tesco*	1/2 Slice/150g	333	222	2.8	23.8	12.8	4.3
Apple, Frozen, Sainsbury's*	1 Serving/100g	283	283	3.2	32.8	15.4	1.9
Apple, Safeway*	1/4 Strudel/150g	414	276	3.1	35.7	14.4	2.4
Apple, Sainsbury's*	1/6 Portion/90g	269	299	3.6	36.4	15.4	1.9
Apple, Tesco*	1 Serving/150g	432	288	3.3	36.4	14.4	2.8
Woodland Fruit, Tesco*	1 Serving/100g	257	257	3.2	31.5	13.1	1.8
Wooland Fruit, Sainsbury's*	1/6 Strudel/95.2g	276	290	3.7	34.0	15.5	2.0
STUFFING							
Apricot & Walnut, Made Up, Celebrations, Paxo*	1 Serving/50g	81	161	4.3	28.0	3.5	2.8
Chestnut & Pork, Marks & Spencer*	1oz/28g	67	240	6.6	16.3	16.7	2.9
Olde English Chestnut, Sainsbury's*	1 Serving/110g	216	196	9.4	13.5	11.6	2.1
Parsley & Thyme, Co-Op*	1 Serving/28g	95	340	10.0	67.0	3.0	6.0
Parsley, Thyme & Lemon Stuffing, Paxo*	1 Serving/45g	68	150	4.3	28.4	2.1	2.4
Pork, Sage & Onion, Marks & Spencer*	1 Serving/85g	183	215	11.2	10.5	14.3	2.4
Sage & Onion, Somerfield*	1oz/28g	100	358	6.0	74.0	5.0	0.0
Sage and Onion, Made Up, Safeway*	1 Serving/60g	90	150	4.5	30.8	0.7	3.2
Sausagemeat & Thyme, Made Up, Celebrations, Paxo*	1 Serving/50g	80	160	6.3	25.8	3.5	4.0
Sausagemeat, Sainsbury's*	1 Serving/100g	175	175	7.0	27.0	4.2	2.3
STUFFING BALLS							
Sage & Onion, Aunt Bessie's*	1 Stuffing Ball/26g	56	214	7.5	29.6	7.3	2.4
Sage & Onion, Meat-Free, Aunt Bessie's*	1 Ball/28g	54	193	5.4	28.0	6.7	1.7
Sage & Onion, Tesco*	1 Serving/20g	64	322	10.0	21.1	22.0	1.9
STUFFING MIX							
Apple & Herb, Special Recipe, Sainsbury's*	1 Serving/41g	68	165	3.8	32.4	2.2	2.2
Apple Mustard & Herb, Paxo*	1 Serving/50g	83	166	4.2	32.8	2.0	4.0
Chestnut & Cranberry, Celebration, Paxo*	1 Serving/25g	35	141	4.0	26.7	2.0	2.4
Chestnut, Morrisons*	1 Serving/20g	33	165	4.6	29.1	3.4	3.7
Date & Walnut, TTD, Sainsbury's*	1 Serving/50g	66	131	4.4	24.2	1.8	3.4
Date, Walnut & Stilton, Special Recipe, Sainsbury's*	1 Serving/25g	49	196	5.2	25.0	8.4	2.0
Parsley, Thyme & Lemon, Sainsbury's*	1 Pack/170g	240	141	4.2	28.2	1.3	1.3
Sage & Onion, Asda*	1 Serving/27g	29	107	3.4	22.0	0.6	1.3
Sage & Onion, Made Up, Paxo*,	1 Serving/60g	74	123	3.6	23.0	1.8	1.7
Sage & Onion, SmartPrice, Asda*	1/4 Pack/75g	262	349	11.0	68.0	3.7	4.7
Sage & Onion, Tesco*	1 Pack/85g	295	347	11.3	71.0	2.0	4.4
Sage, Red Onion & Lemon TTD, Sainsbury's*	1 Serving/50g	53	106	3.8	23.9	1.3	4.2
SUET							
Beef, Tesco*	1 Serving/100g	854	854	0.6	6.2	91.9	0.1
Shredded Vegetable, Atora Light*	1oz/28g	197	704	3.8	28.5	63.9	1.2
Shredded, Original, Atora*	1oz/28g	232	828	1.6	9.4	87.1	0.4
Vegetable	1oz/28g	234	836	1.2	10.1	87.9	0.0
SUET PUDDING							
Average	1oz/28g	94	335	4.4	40.5	18.3	0.9

S

	Measure INFO/WEIGHT	per Measure KCAL	Nutrition Values per 100g / 100ml				
			KCAL	PROT	CARB	FAT	FIBRE
SUGAR							
Brown, Soft, Average	1 Tsp/4g	15	382	0.0	96.5	0.0	0.0
Canem Demerara, Unrefined, Sainsbury's*	1 Tsp/5.1g	20	396	0.0	99.0	0.0	0.0
Caster, Average	1 Tbsp/12g	48	399	0.0	99.8	0.0	0.0
Dark Brown, Muscovado, Average	1 Tsp/7g	27	380	0.3	94.8	0.0	0.0
Dark Brown, Soft, Average	1 Tsp/5g	18	369	0.1	92.0	0.0	0.0
Demerara, Average	1 Tsp/5g	18	368	0.3	99.2	0.0	0.0
For Making Jam, Silver Spoon*	1oz/28g	111	398	0.0	99.5	0.0	0.0
Golden, Unrefined, Average	1 Tsp/4g	16	399	0.0	99.8	0.0	0.0
Granulated, Organic, Average	1 Tsp/4g	16	398	0.2	99.7	0.0	0.0
Icing, Average	1 Tsp/4g	16	395	0.0	102.2	0.0	0.0
Light, Silver Spoon*	1 Tsp/5g	12	240	0.0	60.0	0.0	0.0
White, Granulated, Average	1 Tsp/5g	20	397	0.0	100.7	0.0	0.0
SULTANAS							
Average	1oz/28g	82	292	2.5	69.7	0.4	2.0
SUMMER FRUITS							
Asda*	1 Serving/30g	8	28	0.9	6.0	0.0	2.5
Frozen, Asda*	1 Serving/100g	28	28	0.9	6.0	0.0	2.5
Frozen, Sainsbury's*	1 Serving/80g	26	33	0.9	7.4	0.1	2.4
In Syrup, Sainsbury's*	1 Pudding/289g	188	65	0.5	15.6	0.1	1.2
Mix, Marks & Spencer*	1oz/28g	9	33	1.0	6.7	0.3	2.5
Mix, Sainsbury's*	1 Serving/80g	26	32	0.9	7.4	0.0	2.4
SUNDAE							
Banoffee, Perfectly Balanced, Waitrose*	1 Pot/115g	143	124	3.1	23.6	1.9	0.8
Blackcurrant, Marks & Spencer*	1 Sundae/49g	196	400	4.5	51.7	19.5	1.9
Blackcurrant, Tesco*	1 Cake/48g	183	385	3.4	52.2	18.1	5.1
Butter Toffee, Mini, Eat Smart, Safeway*	1 Pot/62.5g	101	160	2.9	32.5	1.8	3.7
Butterscotch, Perfectly Balanced, Waitrose*	1 Sundae/150ml	135	90	1.9	17.3	1.3	1.0
Chocolate & Vanilla Ice Cream, Tesco*	1 Sundae/70.2g	139	199	2.8	27.5	8.6	0.5
Chocolate & Vanilla, Healthy Living, Tesco*	1 Sundae/120g	193	161	2.8	31.5	2.6	0.6
Chocolate Brownie, Finest, Tesco*	1 Serving/215g	778	362	2.7	28.7	26.3	2.3
Chocolate Mint, COU, Marks & Spencer*	1 Pot/90g	108	120	5.4	17.8	2.6	0.5
Chocolate Nut	1 Portion/70g	195	278	3.0	34.2	15.3	0.1
Chocolate, Healthy Eating, Tesco*	1 Serving/130g	199	153	4.5	24.9	3.9	0.6
Chocolate, Mini, Asda*	1 Pot/86g	199	231	3.1	21.0	15.0	1.7
Chocolate, Sainsbury's*	1 Pot/140g	393	281	2.5	19.3	21.3	0.6
Galaxy Caramel, Eden Vale*	1 Serving/128g	300	234	4.8	26.5	12.4	0.7
Mango & Passionfruit, Tesco*	1 Pot/78g	112	143	1.1	32.7	0.8	0.4
Peach & Apricot, Perfectly Balanced, Waitrose*	1 Pot/175g	142	81	1.7	17.7	0.4	0.0
Raspberry, Eat Smart, Safeway*	1 Serving/97g	150	155	3.0	30.9	2.1	2.8
Raspberry, Perfectly Balanced, Waitrose*	1 Pot/175ml	151	86	1.7	18.9	0.6	0.0
Strawberry & Vanilla Ice Cream, Tesco*	1 Serving/68g	120	177	2.0	29.5	5.7	0.1
Strawberry & Vanilla, Weight Watchers*	1 Pot/105g	148	141	1.2	29.1	2.1	0.3
Strawberry, Marks & Spencer*	1 Sundae/45g	173	385	3.4	53.3	17.8	1.0
Strawberry, Tesco*	1 Sundae/48g	194	408	3.3	57.6	18.3	1.3
Toffee & Vanilla Ice Cream, Tesco*	1 Serving/70g	133	189	2.1	30.7	6.4	0.1
Toffee, Asda*	1 Serving/120g	322	268	2.1	29.0	16.0	0.0
SUNNY DELIGHT*							
Apple & Kiwi Kick	1 Glass/200ml	15	7	0.2	1.3	0.2	0.2
Californian Style, No Added Sugar	1 Serving/200ml	20	10	0.1	1.4	0.2	0.1
Original	1 Glass/200ml	88	44	0.1	10.0	0.2	0.0
SUSHI							
Advent, Medium, Tesco*	1 Serving/210g	307	146	3.8	25.7	3.1	0.9
Aya Set, Waitrose*	1 Pack/110g	200	182	5.4	31.7	3.9	1.5

S

	Measure INFO/WEIGHT	per Measure KCAL	Nutrition Values per 100g / 100ml				
			KCAL	PROT	CARB	FAT	FIBRE
SUSHI							
California Roll Box, Marks & Spencer*	1 Box/230g	391	170	7.0	22.0	5.2	1.1
California, Roll Selection, Tesco*	1 Pack/100g	161	161	7.1	24.7	3.8	2.7
Californian Rolls, Sainsbury's*	1 Pack/237g	363	153	5.9	22.6	4.3	0.9
Californian, Selection, Marks & Spencer*	1 Serving/145g	203	140	4.4	25.9	2.1	2.3
Californian, Yakatori, Marks & Spencer*	1 Serving/200g	340	170	6.4	25.0	4.7	1.0
Fish Medium Box, Marks & Spencer*	1 Serving/100g	285	285	13.3	39.8	8.1	1.4
Fish Nigiri, Adventurous, Tesco*	1 Med Pack/200g	270	135	7.1	21.7	2.2	0.5
Fish Selection Box, Marks & Spencer*	1 Serving/220g	396	180	6.6	27.1	4.5	0.9
Fish Selection, Marks & Spencer*	1 Serving/210g	315	150	6.5	25.8	2.3	1.0
Fish, Large Box, Tesco*	1 Box/290g	423	146	4.9	25.8	2.6	0.8
Fish, Medium Box, Tesco*	1 Box/195g	281	144	5.1	25.7	2.3	0.7
Fish, Small, Tesco*	1 Serving/105g	148	141	5.9	23.9	2.4	0.6
Fish, Tesco*	1 Pack/105g	155	148	6.2	25.1	2.5	0.6
GFY, Asda*	1 Pack/220g	352	160	4.9	32.0	1.4	0.0
Hana Set, Waitrose*	1 Serving/175g	324	185	5.4	35.7	2.3	1.4
Irodori Sushi Set, Waitrose*	1 Serving/281g	486	173	5.2	33.4	3.3	1.4
Komachi Set, Waitrose*	1 Box/235g	425	181	6.1	31.3	3.5	1.4
Large Box, Food To Go, Marks & Spencer*	1oz/28g	41	145	5.1	27.4	1.5	0.5
Large, Boots*	1 Pack/324g	480	148	5.0	28.0	1.8	0.7
Large, Sainsbury's*	1 Serving/228g	372	163	5.9	28.4	2.9	0.7
Maki Rolls Box, Sainsbury's*	1 Box/127g	197	155	4.5	30.5	1.7	0.8
Maki Selection, Shapers, Boots*	1 Pack/158g	225	142	3.5	29.0	1.3	1.1
Medium Box, Marks & Spencer*	1 Serving/215g	366	170	9.7	24.3	2.8	0.9
Medium Selection Pack, Tesco*	1 Pack/195g	312	160	5.6	27.9	2.9	1.4
Mini, Boots*	1 Pack/99g	153	155	5.5	29.0	1.9	0.8
Mixed Box, Somerfield*	1 Pack/220g	339	154	4.6	31.4	1.1	0.0
Nigiri, Marks & Spencer*	1 Serving/190g	285	150	5.2	25.7	2.5	0.9
Nigiri, Sainsbury's*	1 Serving/155.8g	251	161	8.5	27.7	1.8	0.7
Nigiri, Taiko, Set, Waitrose*	1 Serving/165g	252	153	6.3	26.0	2.6	0.6
Nigri, Californian Roll, Maki Roll, Sainsbury's*	1 Pack/195g	283	145	5.3	27.4	1.5	1.9
Oriental Fish Box, Marks & Spencer*	1 Box/205g	318	155	6.1	23.3	4.1	0.9
Pot, Sainsbury's*	1 Pot/79.9g	127	159	5.9	27.7	2.7	0.8
Prawn & Salmon Selection, Marks & Spencer*	1 Serving/175g	255	146	5.5	27.4	1.7	0.6
Prawn Feast, Marks & Spencer*	1 Box/219g	350	160	5.7	25.8	3.7	1.1
Roll Selection, Tesco*	1 Pack/140g	221	158	4.6	30.5	1.9	1.9
Salmon & Roll Set, Small, Sainsbury's*	1 Serving/101g	167	165	4.9	30.4	2.6	0.8
Salmon Feast Box, Marks & Spencer*	1 Pack/200g	330	165	5.6	27.0	2.9	1.0
Salmon, Nigri Crayfish, Red Pepper, Sainsbury's*	1 Serving/150g	233	155	5.5	26.4	3.0	1.0
Selection, Boots*	1 Pack/268g	434	162	5.5	27.0	3.6	1.6
Selection, Shapers, Boots*	1 Pack/189g	301	159	5.2	28.0	3.0	0.7
Taiko Hagi Set, Waitrose*	1 Box/370g	688	186	7.1	33.6	2.6	1.1
Taiko Vegetable Set, Waitrose*	1 Serving/135g	254	188	4.4	37.1	2.4	1.4
Tokyo Set, Marks & Spencer*	1 Pack/150g	240	160	7.3	25.3	3.1	0.6
Trial Pack, Asda*	1 Pack/115g	186	162	4.1	31.0	2.4	0.0
Tuna, To Snack Selection, Food To Go, Marks & Spencer*	1 Serving/150g	225	150	5.2	26.4	2.6	2.3
Vegetarian, Marks & Spencer*	1 Pack/223g	290	130	4.1	25.5	1.5	1.3
Vegetarian, Taiko, Medium, Waitrose*	1 Pack/316g	499	158	4.1	28.8	2.1	1.8
Vegetarian, Tesco*	1 Pack/132g	185	140	3.1	27.2	2.1	0.9
Yo!, Bento Box, Sainsbury's*	1 Pack/208g	530	255	8.4	48.7	3.0	0.9
Yo!, Salmon Lunch Set, Sainsbury's*	1 Pack/150g	242	161	5.9	28.1	2.8	0.8
SWEDE							
Boiled, Average	1oz/28g	3	11	0.3	2.3	0.1	0.7
Mash, COU, Marks & Spencer*	1oz/28g	15	55	1.1	9.5	1.2	2.1

	Measure INFO/WEIGHT	per Measure KCAL	Nutrition Values per 100g / 100ml				
			KCAL	PROT	CARB	FAT	FIBRE
SWEDE							
Raw, Average	1oz/28g	6	21	0.8	4.4	0.3	1.9
SWEET & SOUR							
Beef, Feeling Great, New, Findus*	1 Pack/350g	420	120	4.5	20.0	2.5	1.3
Chicken & Egg Fried Rice, BGTY, Sainsbury's*	1 Pack/450g	477	106	5.4	17.3	1.7	1.0
Chicken & Noodles, BGTY, Sainsbury's*	1 Pack/400g	356	89	7.5	13.3	0.6	0.7
Chicken & Rice, Morrisons*	1 Pack/400g	452	113	3.6	18.8	2.6	0.8
Chicken Cantonese, Sainsbury's*	1 Pack/350g	368	105	10.4	14.6	0.6	0.6
Chicken In Crispy Batter, Cantonese, Sainsbury's*	1 Pack/300g	546	182	9.0	21.4	6.7	1.1
Chicken With Rice, Asda*	1 Pack/400g	440	110	4.7	22.0	0.3	0.6
Chicken With Rice, Eat Smart, Safeway*	1 Pack/390g	312	80	5.4	12.2	0.9	1.2
Chicken With Rice, Iceland*	1 Pack/400g	516	129	5.4	25.7	0.5	0.4
Chicken With Rice, Oriental Express*	1 Pack/340g	350	103	4.4	21.3	0.6	0.7
Chicken With Vegetable Rice, COU, Marks & Spencer*	1 Pack/400g	320	80	6.7	10.7	1.2	1.0
Chicken, & Noodles, Chinese Takeaway, Tesco*	1 Pack/350g	350	100	5.7	18.8	0.2	0.2
Chicken, & Rice, Mega, Value, Tesco*	1 Pack/500g	675	135	4.4	25.0	1.9	1.9
Chicken, Battered, Chinese, Sainsbury's*	1 Pack/350g	532	152	9.1	22.5	2.9	0.7
Chicken, Battered, Healthy Living, Tesco*	1 Pack/350g	434	124	7.6	18.4	2.2	0.5
Chicken, Breasts, Tesco*	1 Serving/185g	172	93	14.6	6.5	1.0	0.1
Chicken, Canned, Tesco*	1 Can/400g	408	102	9.6	12.4	1.6	1.1
Chicken, Cantonese, Sainsbury's*	1/2 Pack/200g	176	88	8.2	11.8	0.9	0.8
Chicken, Chinese Takeaway, Sainsbury's*	1 Pack/264g	515	195	13.1	21.3	6.4	1.0
Chicken, Crispy, Iceland*	1 Serving/125g	221	177	18.3	14.2	5.2	1.2
Chicken, GFY, Asda*	1 Serving/165g	163	99	4.5	19.0	0.5	0.9
Chicken, Healthy Living, Tesco*	1 Serving/350g	315	90	7.2	12.5	1.2	2.0
Chicken, Marks & Spencer*	1 Pack/300g	465	155	6.6	24.4	3.6	0.8
Chicken, Somerfield*	1 Serving/175g	156	89	9.5	12.6	0.1	0.6
Chicken, Take It Away, Marks & Spencer*	1 Pack/200g	200	100	9.4	13.2	0.8	1.2
Chicken, Tesco*	1 Pack/350g	319	91	6.4	12.9	1.5	4.0
Chicken, Tinned, Marks & Spencer*	1 Serving/481g	553	115	11.4	7.8	4.2	1.9
Chicken, Waitrose*	1 Serving/400g	372	93	9.8	11.7	0.8	1.4
Chicken, Weight Watchers*	1 Pack/320g	304	95	5.2	17.4	0.4	0.3
Chicken, With Egg Fried Rice, Healthy Eating, Tesco*	1 Pack/450g	468	104	7.4	15.5	1.4	1.2
Chicken, With Egg Fried Rice, Somerfield*	1 Pack/400g	428	107	8.5	16.7	0.7	2.0
Chicken, With Noodles, Steamed, Healthy Eating, Tesco*	1 Pack/370g	289	78	8.3	10.8	0.2	0.6
Chicken, With Noodles, Tesco*	1 Pack/350g	441	126	5.7	24.4	0.6	1.4
Chicken, With Rice, BGTY, Sainsbury's*	1 Pack/400g	408	102	7.2	17.1	0.5	1.9
Chicken, With Rice, Healthy Eating, Tesco*	1 Pack/450g	450	100	8.0	16.3	0.3	0.8
Chicken, With Rice, Sainsbury's*	1 Pack/400g	448	112	4.1	21.1	1.2	0.3
Chicken, With Rice, Value, Tesco*	1 Pack/300g	348	116	5.9	22.3	0.3	0.7
Pork	1oz/28g	48	172	12.7	11.3	8.8	0.6
Pork, Battered, Sainsbury's*	1/2 Pack/175g	306	175	7.3	25.1	5.0	0.6
Pork, Cantonese, & Egg Fried Rice, Farmfoods*	1 Pack/327g	520	159	4.8	22.0	5.8	0.1
Pork, In Crispy Batter, Sainsbury's*	1/2 Pack/150g	293	195	10.0	20.0	8.3	1.1
Roasted Vegetables, Cantonese, Sainsbury's*	1 Pack/348g	327	94	1.1	19.6	1.2	0.9
Vegetables With Rice, Waitrose*	1 Pack/400g	384	96	1.9	19.5	1.1	1.1
SWEET POTATO							
Baked	1oz/28g	32	115	1.6	27.9	0.4	3.3
Boiled in Salted Water	1oz/28g	24	84	1.1	20.5	0.3	2.3
Raw	1oz/28g	24	87	1.2	21.3	0.3	2.4
Steamed	1oz/28g	24	84	1.1	20.4	0.3	2.3
SWEETBREAD							
Lamb, Fried	1oz/28g	61	217	28.7	0.0	11.4	0.0
Lamb, Raw	1oz/28g	37	131	15.3	0.0	7.8	0.0

	Measure	per Measure	Nutrition Values per 100g / 100ml				
	INFO/WEIGHT	KCAL	KCAL	PROT	CARB	FAT	FIBRE
SWEETCORN							
& Petit Pois, Marks & Spencer*	1oz/28g	20	73	4.6	10.8	1.3	3.6
Baby, & Mangetout, Somerfield*	1 Pack/150g	42	28	3.2	3.0	0.3	1.9
Baby, Canned, Drained	1oz/28g	6	23	2.9	2.0	0.4	1.5
Baby, Frozen, Average	1oz/28g	7	24	2.5	2.7	0.4	1.7
Boiled, Average	1oz/28g	31	111	4.2	19.6	2.3	2.2
Canned, In Water, No Sugar & Salt, Average	1/2 Can/125g	99	79	2.7	14.9	1.1	1.6
Canned, With Sugar & Salt, Average	1/2 Can/71g	79	111	3.2	21.9	1.2	1.9
Carrot Batons & Broccoli Florets, Microsteam, Birds Eye*	1 Serving/113.2g	60	53	2.6	8.5	0.9	2.2
Easy Steam, Sainsbury's*	1 Serving/115g	127	110	4.2	18.0	2.3	2.2
Fritters With Chilli Dip, Sainsbury's*	1 Fritter/40g	60	151	3.0	27.0	3.4	3.0
Frozen, Average	1 Sachet/115g	121	105	3.8	17.9	2.1	1.8
With Peppers, Canned, Average	1 Serving/50g	40	79	2.7	16.5	0.3	0.6
SWEETENER							
Aspartamo, Artificial Sugar, Zen*	1 Tbsp/2g	8	383	1.8	94.0	0.0	0.0
Canderel, Spoonful, Canderel*	2 Tsp/1g	4	384	2.9	93.0	0.0	0.0
Granulated, Asda*	1 Tsp/1g	4	400	3.0	97.0	0.0	0.0
Granulated, Aspartame, Safeway*	1 Tsp/0.5g	4	392	3.0	95.0	0.0	0.0
Granulated, Splenda*	1 Tsp/1g	4	391	0.0	97.7	0.0	0.0
Granulated, Tesco*	1 Tsp/1g	4	400	3.0	97.0	0.0	0.0
Power, Canderel*	1 Tsp/2g	8	380	1.4	93.7	0.0	0.0
Silver Spoon*	1 Tablet/0.05g	0	325	10.0	71.0	0.0	0.0
SlendaSweet, Sainsbury's*	1 Tsp/1g	4	395	1.8	97.0	0.0	0.1
Spoonfull, Low Calorie, SupaSweet*	1 Tsp/1g	4	392	3.0	95.0	0.0	0.0
Sweet N Low*	1 Sachet/1g	3	368	0.0	92.0	0.0	0.0
Tablets, Low Calorie, Canderel*	1 Tablet/0.1g	0	342	13.0	72.4	0.0	0.0
Tablets, Splenda*	1 Tablet/0.1g	0	345	10.0	76.2	0.0	1.6
SWEETS							
Allsorts, Fruit, Bassett's*	1 serving/100g	320	320	1.8	76.9	0.4	0.0
Banana, Baby Foam, Marks & Spencer*	1/3 Pack/34g	131	385	4.1	92.7	0.0	0.0
Black Jacks & Fruit Salad, Bassett's*	1 Serving/190g	760	400	0.7	84.9	6.2	0.0
Body Parts, Rowntree's*	1 Pack/42g	146	348	4.3	82.9	0.0	0.0
Bursting Bugs, Rowntree's*	1 Pack/175g	583	333	4.8	78.1	0.2	0.0
Candy Butter, Werther's Original*	1 Sweet/5g	22	430	1.0	86.0	9.0	0.0
Candy Cane, Average	1oz/28g	100	357	3.6	85.7	0.0	0.0
Chew	1oz/28g	107	381	1.0	87.0	5.6	1.0
Chews, Calcium, Ellactiva*	2 Chews/14g	49	350	1.4	51.4	15.7	0.0
Chews, Fruity, Starburst*	1 serving/100g	401	401	0.0	83.9	7.3	0.0
Chews, Just Fruit, Fruittella	1 serving/42.5g	172	400	0.9	79.5	6.5	0.0
Cola Bottles, Fizzy, Marks & Spencer*	1 Pack/200g	650	325	6.4	75.0	0.0	0.0
Drumstick, Matlow's*	1pack/40g	164	409	0.4	88.3	5.5	0.0
Fizzy Lemon Fish, Asda*	1 Sweet/4.3g	13	325	5.0	76.0	0.1	0.0
Fizzy Mix, Tesco*	1/2 Bag/50g	166	332	5.2	75.2	0.0	0.0
Flipsters, Starburst*	1pack/37g	145	392	0.0	98.1	0.0	0.0
Flumps, Bassett's*	1 Serving/5g	16	325	4.0	77.0	0.0	0.0
Flying Suacers, Asda*	1 Serving/23.1g	82	355	0.1	83.0	2.5	0.8
Fruit Gums & Jellies	1 Tube/33g	107	324	6.5	79.5	0.0	0.0
Fruit Puffs, Allen's*	1 Serving/25g	91	364	2.2	92.4	0.0	0.0
Fruity Mallows, Fizzy, Asda*	1 Pack/400g	1252	313	4.3	74.0	0.0	0.0
Gummy Mix, Tesco*	1 Pack/100g	327	327	5.9	75.7	0.1	0.0
Kisses, Hershey*	1 Kiss/5g	28	561	7.0	59.0	32.0	0.0
Lances, Strawberry & Cream Flavour, Tesco*	1 Bag/75g	276	368	3.2	86.1	1.2	2.1
Lances, Strawberry Flavour, Fizzy, Tesco*	1/2 Pack/50g	177	354	2.8	79.8	2.6	1.8
Lovehearts, Swizzels*	1oz/28g	100	359	0.7	88.2	0.0	0.0

S

	Measure	per Measure	Nutrition Values per 100g / 100ml				
	INFO/WEIGHT	KCAL	KCAL	PROT	CARB	FAT	FIBRE
SWEETS							
Maynards Sours, Trebor*	1 Pack/52g	166	320	3.9	74.9	0.1	0.0
Rhubarb & Custard, Marks & Spencer*	1 Pack/113g	424	375	0.0	93.9	0.0	0.0
Scary Mix, Tesco*	1 Bag/100g	327	327	9.5	71.1	0.5	0.3
Sherbert Cocktails, Sainsbury's*	1 Sweet/9g	36	400	0.0	83.1	7.5	0.0
Sherbert Lemons, Marks & Spencer*	1 Serving/20g	76	380	0.0	93.9	0.0	0.0
Shrimps & Bananas, Sainsbury's*	1/2 Pack/50g	188	376	2.5	91.3	0.1	0.5
Sour Apple Sticks, Fizzy Wizzy, Woolworths*	1 Stick/5g	18	358	2.8	79.8	2.7	0.0
Squidgy Cars, Shannon*	1 Sweet/8g	27	342	5.3	80.0	0.1	0.0
Sugar Free, Sula*	1 sweet/3g	7	231	0.0	96.1	0.0	0.0
Sweetshop Favourites, Bassett's*	1 Sweet/5g	17	340	0.0	84.3	0.0	0.0
Toffo*	1 Tube/43g	194	451	2.2	69.8	22.0	0.0
Wazzly Wobble Drops, Wonka*	1 Bag/42g	186	443	3.0	71.6	16.1	0.2
Wiggly Worms, Sainsbury's*	1 Serving/10g	32	317	5.6	72.7	0.4	0.2
SWORDFISH							
Grilled	1oz/28g	39	139	22.9	0.0	5.2	0.0
Raw, Average	1oz/28g	42	149	21.1	0.0	7.2	0.0
SYRUP							
Coffee, Caramel, Lyle's*	2 Tsps/10ml	33	329	0.0	83.0	0.0	0.0
Corn, Dark	1 Tbsp/20g	56	282	0.0	76.6	0.0	0.0
Golden, Average	1 Tbsp/20g	61	304	0.4	78.3	0.0	0.0
Maple	1 Tbsp/20g	52	262	0.0	67.2	0.2	0.0

S

INFO/WEIGHT	Measure	per Measure KCAL	Nutrition Values per 100g / 100ml				
			KCAL	PROT	CARB	FAT	FIBRE
TABOO*							
Average	1 Serving/30ml	69	230	0.0	33.0	0.0	0.0
TABOULEH							
Average	1oz/28g	33	119	2.6	17.2	4.6	0.0
TACO SHELLS							
Corn, Crunchy, Old El Paso*	1 Taco/10g	51	506	7.0	61.0	26.0	0.0
Old El Paso*	1 Taco/12g	57	478	7.4	60.8	22.8	0.0
Traditional, Discovery*	1 Shell/11g	51	448	6.7	51.0	24.1	6.4
TADKA DAAL							
Sainsbury's*	1/2 Pack/150g	137	91	5.5	12.7	2.0	3.0
TAGINE							
Apricot & Coriander, Al'fez*	1 Serving/175g	224	128	1.4	19.0	5.1	1.2
Vegetable, Filo Topped, Marks & Spencer*	1 Serving/281.8g	310	110	3.3	18.7	2.3	3.9
TAGLIATELLE							
Basil, Marks & Spencer*	1 Serving/100g	365	365	15.1	69.0	2.8	4.0
Bicolore, Asda*	1/4 Pack/125g	203	162	7.0	28.0	2.4	1.4
Carbonara, Frozen, Tesco*	1 Pack/400g	480	120	4.2	12.5	5.9	1.4
Carbonara, Italiano, Tesco*	1 Serving/325g	757	233	8.6	23.8	11.5	1.2
Carbonara, Low Fat, Bertorelli*	1 Pack/350g	301	86	5.3	12.0	2.2	0.9
Carbonara, Naturally Less 5% Fat, Asda*	1 Pack/400g	440	110	4.2	18.0	2.4	0.8
Carbonara, Perfectly Balanced, Waitrose*	1 Pack/350g	357	102	5.3	12.1	3.6	0.7
Carbonara, Reduced Fat, Waitrose*	1 Pack/350g	399	114	5.0	12.1	5.1	0.6
Chicken & Mushroom, GFY, Asda*	1 Pack/400g	359	90	7.3	11.3	1.8	0.7
Chicken & Tomato, Eat Smart, Safeway*	1 Pack/400g	360	90	7.5	10.8	1.4	1.1
Chicken & Tomato, Italiano, Tesco*	1 Pack/400g	416	104	6.6	14.8	2.1	0.8
Chicken, Italia, Marks & Spencer*	1 Pack/360g	342	95	8.1	12.1	1.8	1.2
Chicken, Italian, Sainsbury's*	1 Pack/450g	567	126	6.5	17.0	3.5	2.6
Dry, Average	1 Serving/100g	357	357	12.6	72.4	1.8	1.1
Egg & Spinach, Marks & Spencer*	1 Serving/100g	365	365	15.5	69.6	2.7	3.0
Egg, Dry, Average	1 Serving/75g	272	362	14.3	68.8	3.3	2.3
Egg, Fresh, Dry, Average	1 Serving/125g	345	276	10.6	53.0	2.8	2.1
Fresh, Dry, Average	1 Serving/75g	211	281	11.4	53.3	2.6	2.6
Garlic & Herb, Fresh, Asda*	1/2 Pack/150.7g	202	134	3.5	21.0	4.0	2.1
Garlic & Herb, Fresh, Sainsbury's*	1 Serving/125g	184	147	6.5	26.2	1.8	1.9
Garlic & Herb, Fresh, Tesco*	1 Serving/125g	361	289	12.0	51.8	3.7	1.5
Garlic & Herb, Italiano, Tesco*	1 Serving/85g	236	278	11.4	52.0	2.7	2.4
Garlic & Herb, Safeway*	1 Serving/125g	175	140	5.7	25.5	1.8	1.9
Garlic & Herbs, Cooked, Pasta Reale*	1 Pack/250g	390	156	6.2	30.4	1.1	1.0
Garlic Mushroom, BGTY, Sainsbury's*	1 Pack/400g	416	104	4.7	16.2	2.3	2.0
Garlic Mushroom, Italiano, Tesco*	1 Pack/450g	738	164	5.2	15.2	9.1	0.6
Ham & Mushroom, Asda*	1 Pack/340g	469	138	6.0	20.0	3.8	0.2
Ham & Mushroom, BGTY, Sainsbury's*	1 Pack/450g	486	108	5.3	14.5	3.2	0.8
Ham & Mushroom, COU, Marks & Spencer*	1 Serving/360g	324	90	5.6	10.9	2.6	1.1
Ham & Mushroom, Eat Smart, Safeway*	1 Pack/400g	380	95	5.0	13.0	2.5	1.2
Ham & Mushroom, GFY, Asda*	1 Pack/400g	366	92	4.3	13.0	2.5	0.6
Ham & Mushroom, Good Intentions, Somerfield*	1 Serving/300g	333	111	5.6	15.6	2.9	0.3
Ham & Mushroom, Healthy Eating, Tesco*	1 Meal/340g	306	90	4.3	13.6	2.0	0.9
Ham & Mushroom, Italiano, Tesco*	1 Pack/380g	475	125	5.4	13.3	5.6	0.4
Ham, Ready Meals, Marks & Spencer*	1 Pack/360g	414	115	5.8	10.5	5.7	1.0
Meditarranean Style Chicken, Eat Smart, Safeway*	1 Pack/400g	320	80	5.6	8.7	2.5	1.4
Mushroom & Bacon, BGTY, Sainsbury's*	1 Pack/400g	413	103	6.9	15.3	1.6	2.4
Mushroom & Bacon, Sainsbury's*	1 Pack/450g	585	130	7.1	13.8	5.2	0.5
Mushroom & Tomato, Asda*	1 Pack/340g	211	62	2.5	10.0	1.3	1.2
Nests, Dry, Napolina*	1oz/28g	93	332	11.5	68.0	1.5	3.7

	Measure INFO/WEIGHT	per Measure KCAL	Nutrition Values per 100g / 100ml				
			KCAL	PROT	CARB	FAT	FIBRE
TAGLIATELLE							
Prawn, Eat Smart, Morrisons*	1 Pack/380g	296	78	6.1	9.4	1.8	0.9
Red Pepper, Organic, Sainsbury's*	1/2 Bag/125g	183	146	5.4	27.8	1.5	1.4
Salmon & Prawn, Perfectly Balanced, Waitrose*	1 Pack/401.2g	341	85	6.8	7.1	3.3	1.1
Salmon, Perfectly Balanced, Waitrose*	1 Pack/400g	376	94	5.4	11.7	2.7	0.8
Smoked Salmon, Ready Meals, Marks & Spencer*	1 Pack/360g	612	170	6.2	10.6	11.2	0.9
Sundried Tomato, Fresh, Morrisons*	1 Packet/250g	748	299	11.1	56.4	3.3	3.5
Tomato & Basil Chicken, Weight Watchers*	1 Pack/330g	322	98	7.5	14.1	1.2	0.3
Tricolore, Waitrose*	1/2 Pack/125g	351	281	12.0	51.6	2.9	1.6
Vegetables, Retail	1oz/28g	21	74	1.6	11.0	3.0	0.7
Verdi, Dry, Barilla*	1 Serving/150g	555	370	14.0	70.5	3.5	0.0
Verdi, Fresh, Average	1 Serving/125g	171	137	5.5	25.5	1.5	1.8
With Chicken & Pancetta, Sainsbury's*	1/2 Pack/351g	453	129	9.5	10.4	5.5	0.7
With Chicken, Garlic & Lemon, New, BGTY, Sainsbury's*	1 Pack/300g	324	108	9.2	15.1	1.2	1.7
With Ham & Mushroom, New, BGTY, Sainsbury's*	1 Pack/450g	401	89	5.3	11.8	2.3	1.4
With Roasted Vegetables, Good Intentions, Somerfield*	1 Pack/340g	349	103	3.7	16.6	2.4	1.7
Wth Ham, COU, Marks & Spencer*	1 Pack/357.9g	340	95	5.4	13.1	2.3	1.1
TAHINI PASTE							
Average	1 Heaped Tsp/19g	115	607	18.5	0.9	58.9	8.0
TAMARILLOS							
Average	1oz/28g	8	28	2.0	4.7	0.3	0.0
TAMARIND							
Average	1oz/28g	72	256	2.8	60.5	0.3	0.0
Leaves, Fresh	1oz/28g	32	115	5.8	18.2	2.1	0.0
Pulp	1oz/28g	76	273	3.2	64.5	0.3	0.0
TANGERINES							
Fresh, Raw	1oz/28g	10	35	0.9	8.0	0.1	1.3
Weighed With Peel & Pips	1 Med/70g	18	25	0.7	5.8	0.1	0.9
TANGO*							
Britvic	1 Can/330ml	103	31	0.0	7.7	0.0	0.0
TAPENADE							
Green Olive, Best, Safeway*	1 Tsp/15g	71	470	1.6	10.2	47.0	1.7
Olive With Capers & Anchovy, Safeway*	1 Tbsp/20g	103	513	2.1	1.0	55.6	2.2
Sundried Tomato & Jalapeno Pepper, Finest, Tesco*	1 Jar/90g	392	436	3.4	13.1	41.0	5.0
TAPIOCA							
Creamed, Ambrosia*	1/2 Can/212.5g	160	75	2.6	12.6	1.6	0.2
Raw	1oz/28g	101	359	0.4	95.0	0.1	0.4
TARAMASALATA							
Fresh, Healthy Eating, Tesco*	1 Pot/170g	430	253	4.3	13.5	20.2	0.7
Fresh, Safeway*	1 Pot/170g	797	469	3.4	8.7	46.7	0.0
Marks & Spencer*	1 Serving/100g	480	480	4.9	6.4	48.9	0.7
Reduced Fat, Waitrose*	1 Pot/170g	598	352	4.2	9.6	33.0	0.6
Smoked Salmon, Tesco*	1 Serving/95g	474	499	3.1	7.7	50.7	0.3
Somerfield*	1/2 Pot/85g	434	510	3.4	9.8	50.8	0.7
Supreme, Waitrose*	1 Serving/20g	84	421	7.4	6.3	40.7	2.9
Tesco*	1 Serving/50g	220	440	7.4	8.8	41.7	0.3
TARRAGON							
Dried, Ground	1 Tsp/1.6g	6	295	22.8	42.8	7.2	0.0
Fresh	1oz/28g	14	49	3.4	6.3	1.1	0.0
TART							
Apricot Lattice, Sainsbury's*	1 Slice/125g	321	257	3.4	35.3	11.4	2.6
Assorted, Oakdale*	1 Serving/26.9g	104	386	3.1	62.0	14.0	1.7
Aubergine & Feta, Roast Marinated, Sainsbury's*	1 Serving/105g	227	216	4.8	16.6	14.5	1.7
Bakewell	1oz/28g	128	456	6.3	43.5	29.7	1.9

TART

INFO/WEIGHT	Measure per Measure	KCAL	Nutrition Values per 100g / 100ml KCAL	PROT	CARB	FAT	FIBRE
Bakewell, Free From, Tesco*	1 Cake/50g	170	340	1.6	63.0	9.2	4.8
Bakewell, Large, Tesco*	1 Serving/57g	247	433	4.3	59.5	19.7	1.7
Bakewell, Lemon, Holmefield Bakery*	1 Tart/46.1g	207	449	4.8	52.9	24.6	0.0
Bakewell, Lyons*	1/6 Tart/51.6g	206	397	3.8	56.7	17.2	0.9
Bakewell, Marks & Spencer*	1/4 Tart/75g	345	460	7.5	48.1	26.7	2.1
Bakewell, Weight Watchers*	1 Cake/43.0g	156	363	3.6	65.2	11.7	3.2
Bannoffi, Finest, Tesco*	1/6 Tart/87g	291	334	3.0	37.2	19.3	0.5
Blackcurrant Sundae, Asda*	1 Tart/55g	227	413	3.5	57.0	19.0	2.3
Cherry Tomato & Mascarpone, Asda*	1 Tart/160g	290	181	4.4	15.6	11.3	1.1
Cherry Tomato & Mascarpone, Extra Special, Asda*	1 Tart/153g	290	190	4.6	16.0	12.0	1.1
Chocolate, Co-Op*	1 Tart/22g	102	465	4.0	42.0	31.0	0.7
Chocolate, TTD, Sainsbury's*	1 Tart/93.1g	389	418	4.8	37.6	27.6	3.0
Coconut & Cherry, Asda*	1 Serving/50g	215	430	4.4	58.0	20.0	4.0
Coconut & Raspberry, Waitrose*	1 Tart/48g	204	426	5.0	45.0	24.0	3.9
Coconut, Marks & Spencer*	1 Tart/53g	220	415	5.8	57.8	18.1	3.6
Congress, Morrisons*	1 Tart/38g	149	393	6.0	59.7	14.4	2.4
Custard, Individual	1 Tart/94g	260	277	6.3	32.4	14.5	1.2
Date Pecan & Almond, Sticky, Sainsbury's*	1/8 Pie/75g	298	397	5.0	63.5	13.7	1.7
Egg Custard, Marks & Spencer*	1 Tart/85g	243	286	6.3	34.7	14.5	0.7
Egg Custard, Sainsbury's	1 Tart/85g	230	270	6.1	30.1	14.1	0.7
Egg Custard, Tesco*	1 Cake/82g	214	261	6.2	31.5	12.2	1.1
Feta Cheese & Spinach, Puff Pastry, Tesco*	1 Tart/108g	306	283	7.1	23.5	17.8	0.9
Filo Asparagus Tartlette, Marks & Spencer*	1 Serving/15g	45	300	4.4	25.2	20.4	2.1
Fruit, Safeway*	1 Tart/180g	425	236	2.7	30.6	11.4	0.0
Goats Cheese & Onion, Marks & Spencer*	1 Serving/161g	451	280	5.8	22.4	18.7	1.5
Italian Lemon & Almond, Sainsbury's*	1 Slice/49g	182	371	7.4	31.9	23.7	4.1
Jam	1 Slice/90g	342	380	3.3	62.0	14.9	1.6
Jam, Assorted, Tesco*	1 Tart/35g	123	351	3.4	51.9	14.4	1.2
Jam, Farmfoods*	1 Tart/34g	132	387	3.6	60.5	14.5	2.8
Jam, Real Fruit, Mr Kipling*	1 Tart/35g	136	389	3.5	61.0	14.5	1.3
Jam, Real Fruit, Sainsbury's*	1 Tart/37g	142	383	3.4	60.9	14.0	1.4
Leek & Stilton, Morrisons*	1 Serving/125g	393	314	6.9	23.1	21.5	0.3
Lemon & Raspberry, Finest, Tesco*	1 Tart/120g	360	300	5.2	38.4	14.0	2.9
Lemon Curd, Lyons*	1 Tart/30g	122	406	3.7	59.3	17.0	0.0
Lemon, Marks & Spencer*	1/6 Tart/50g	208	415	5.0	32.7	29.3	0.9
Lutowska Cherry Amaretto Frangipane, Sainsbury's*	1 Serving/66g	264	400	6.0	50.0	19.5	1.3
Manchester, Marks & Spencer*	1oz/28g	104	370	4.1	36.0	23.5	1.1
Mixed Fruit, Waitrose*	1 Tart/146g	318	218	2.3	27.3	11.2	1.0
Normandy Apple & Calvados, Finest, Tesco*	1/6 Tart/100g	256	256	3.2	41.4	7.6	1.9
Pear & Chocolate With Brandy, TTD, Sainsbury's*	1/6 Tart/90g	261	290	3.5	32.0	16.4	1.4
Raspberry & Blueberry, Tesco*	1 Serving/85g	168	198	2.7	27.0	8.8	2.8
Raspberry Flavoured, Value, Tesco*	1 Tart/29.0g	113	389	3.8	56.6	16.4	1.6
Raspberry, Reduced Sugar, Asda*	1 Tart/34g	129	380	4.6	67.5	10.1	1.2
Red Pepper, Serrano Ham & Goats Cheese, Waitrose*	1 Serving/100g	293	293	8.7	21.3	19.2	3.2
Roasted Vegetable, Finest, Tesco*	1 Serving/130g	250	192	3.0	19.6	11.3	1.2
Sao Tome Chocolate, TTD, Sainsbury's*	1 Slice/66g	314	476	5.6	46.1	29.1	1.8
Strawberry & Fresh Cream, Finest, Tesco*	1 Tart/129g	350	271	3.3	31.1	14.8	1.2
Strawberry Custard, Asda*	1 Tart/100g	335	335	3.1	47.0	15.0	0.0
Strawberry Sundae, Asda*	1 Tart/46g	187	407	3.3	58.0	18.0	1.3
Strawberry, Marks & Spencer*	1 Tart/120g	312	260	2.6	26.4	16.0	0.7
Strawberry, Reduced Sugar, Asda*	1 Tart/37g	141	380	4.6	67.5	10.1	1.2
Strawberry, Sainsbury's*	1 Serving/206g	521	253	2.6	32.0	12.7	0.7
Toffee Apple, Co-Op*	1 Tart/20g	69	345	3.0	47.0	16.0	0.7

T

Food	Measure INFO/WEIGHT	per Measure KCAL	Nutrition Values per 100g / 100ml KCAL	PROT	CARB	FAT	FIBRE
TART							
Toffee Bakewell, Sainsbury's*	1 Tart/45.0g	200	444	3.4	64.2	19.3	1.1
Toffee Pecan, Marks & Spencer*	1 Tart/91g	414	455	6.0	48.5	26.5	2.0
Tomato, Mozzarella & Basil Puff, Sainsbury's*	1/3 Tart/120g	318	265	9.2	10.2	20.8	0.9
Treacle	1oz/28g	103	368	3.7	60.4	14.1	1.1
Treacle & Pecan, Mini, TTD, Sainsbury's*	1 Tart/27.1g	107	395	4.4	59.3	15.6	1.7
Treacle Lattice, Mr Kipling*	1/6 Tart/70g	256	365	4.4	59.8	12.1	1.1
Treacle, & Custard, Apetito*	1 Pack/142g	330	232	2.0	39.2	7.2	0.8
Treacle, Large, Tesco*	1/6 Tart/59g	237	402	3.3	74.1	10.3	1.7
Treacle, Lattice, Lyons*	1/6 Tart/70g	255	364	4.4	59.3	12.0	1.1
Treacle, Sainsbury's*	1 Serving/100g	369	369	4.3	60.6	12.1	1.2
TARTE							
Au Chocolat, Finest, Tesco*	1/6 Tarte/85g	421	495	5.1	44.0	33.2	1.6
Au Chocolat, Twin Pack, Finest, Tesco*	1 Serving/110g	477	434	4.8	44.6	26.3	3.3
Au Citron, TTD, Sainsbury's*	1 Tart/105g	360	343	3.7	36.6	20.2	0.6
Au Citron, Tesco*	1 Serving/104g	235	225	3.2	29.8	11.4	0.7
Au Citron, Waitrose*	1 Tart/100g	325	325	4.9	35.7	18.1	1.0
Aux Cerises, Finest, Tesco*	1 Serving/98g	219	225	4.9	35.4	7.2	0.6
Aux Fruits, Finest, Tesco*	1 Tart/147g	345	235	3.0	33.4	9.9	1.1
Aux Pommes, TTD, Sainsbury's*	1/6 Tarte/71g	270	381	6.4	46.0	19.0	1.7
Bacon, Leek & Roquefort, Bistro, Waitrose*	1/6 Tarte/100g	189	189	6.6	10.8	13.2	2.1
Citron, Marks & Spencer*	1oz/28g	98	350	5.7	36.2	20.9	0.4
Goats Cheese & Spinach Flambe, Sainsbury's*	1/3 Tart/76.8g	223	289	7.4	15.9	21.8	0.9
Normande, French Style, Marks & Spencer*	1/6 Tarte/84.5g	244	290	3.3	26.8	19.0	0.7
Tatin, Sainsbury's*	1 Serving/120g	244	203	2.9	32.8	6.7	1.9
TARTLETS							
Caramelised Onion & Gruyere, Sainsbury's*	1 Tart/145g	381	263	5.8	17.3	19.0	1.3
Cheese & Roast Onion, Asda*	1 Tartlet/50g	135	270	6.0	28.0	15.0	1.9
Cherry Tomato & Aubergine, Marks & Spencer*	1 Tartlet/160g	320	200	3.1	17.8	12.6	1.7
Mandarin, Mini, Marks & Spencer*	1 Tartlet/28.6g	81	280	3.4	30.4	16.3	0.6
Mushroom & Watercress, Waitrose*	1 Tartlet/120g	308	257	8.4	19.1	20.5	2.6
Mushroom Medley, BGTY, Sainsbury's*	1 Serving/80g	134	167	4.7	14.5	10.0	3.4
Mushroom, Bacon & Spinach, Safeway*	1 Tartlet/120g	312	260	7.0	13.0	20.0	1.0
Onion, Caramelised, Creamy, Somerfield*	1 Tartlet/105g	310	295	4.0	21.0	22.0	0.0
Raspberry, Mini, Marks & Spencer*	1 Tartlet/27.3g	89	330	4.3	34.4	19.6	0.5
Red Onion & Goats Cheese, Sainsbury's*	1 Tart/112.8g	336	297	7.0	23.7	19.3	1.5
Redcurrant & Blackcurrant, Mini, Marks & Spencer*	1 Tartlet/29.3g	84	290	3.9	30.5	16.8	1.1
Roast Pepper & Mascarpone, Sainsbury's*	1 Tart/100g	232	232	3.5	17.7	16.4	1.5
Roast Vegetable, Filo, Mini, Somerfield*	1oz/28g	71	255	8.0	34.0	10.0	0.0
Roasted Red Pepper, BGTY, Sainsbury's*	1 Tartlet/80g	143	179	3.1	21.0	9.2	3.4
Salmon & Watercress, Hot Smoked, Waitrose*	1 Serving/130g	315	242	8.1	18.0	15.3	3.0
Sausage & Tomato, Sainsbury's*	1 Tartlet/135g	323	239	4.8	19.5	15.8	1.6
Tomato & Goats Cheese, Waitrose*	1 Tartlet/130g	295	227	6.6	17.4	14.6	2.0
TARTLETTE							
Cherry & Almond, Go Ahead, McVitie's*	1 Tartlette/46.0g	165	359	4.1	67.5	9.8	0.7
TEA							
Camomile, Smile, Tetley*	1oz/28g	1	2	0.0	0.5	0.0	0.0
Earl Grey, Infusion With Water, Average	1 Mug/250ml	3	1	0.0	0.2	0.0	0.0
Fruit Or Herbal, Made With Water, Twinings*	1 Mug/200ml	8	4	0.0	1.0	0.0	0.0
Fruit Punch, London Fruit & Herb Company*	1 Mug/200ml	4	2	0.0	0.5	0.0	0.0
Green & Lemon, Twinings*	1 Serving/250ml	65	26	0.0	7.3	0.0	0.0
Green, With Jasmine, Wellbeing Selection, Flavia*	1 Cup/200ml	14	7	0.5	1.2	0.1	0.0
Herbal, Fruit Burst, London Fruit & Herb Company*	1 Serving/200ml	4	2	0.0	0.5	0.0	0.0
Iced, Green & Lemon, Twinings*	1 Serving/250ml	75	30	0.1	7.3	0.1	0.0

TEA

	Measure	per Measure					
Iced, Lemon, San Benedetto*	1 Sm Bottle/500ml	170	34	0.1	8.3	0.0	0.0
Iced, Mango, Lipton*	1fl oz/30ml	10	33	0.0	8.1	0.0	0.0
Iced, Peach, Twinings*	1 Serving/200ml	60	30	0.1	7.3	0.1	0.0
Iced, Pickwick*	1 Serving/250ml	33	13	0.0	3.3	0.0	0.0
Lemon & Limeflower, Infused, Marks & Spencer*	1 Bottle/330ml	99	30	0.0	7.8	0.0	0.0
Lemon, Instant Drink, Reduced Sweetness, Lift*	1 Serving/15g	53	352	0.0	87.0	0.0	0.0
Lemon, Instant, Tesco*	1 Serving/7g	23	326	1.0	80.5	0.0	0.0
Lemon, Original, Instant Drink, Lift*	1 Serving/15g	53	352	0.0	87.0	0.0	0.0
Made With Water	1 Mug/227ml	0	0	0.1	0.0	0.0	0.0
Made With Water With Semi-Skimmed Milk	1 Cup/200ml	14	7	0.5	0.7	0.2	0.0
Made With Water With Skimmed Milk	1 Mug/227ml	14	6	0.5	0.7	0.2	0.0
Made With Water With Whole Milk	1 Cup/200ml	16	8	0.4	0.5	0.4	0.0
Peach Flavour, Lift*	1 Cup/15g	58	384	0.3	95.6	0.0	0.0
Raspberry & Cranberry, T Of Life, Tetley*	1 Serving/100ml	36	36	0.0	9.0	0.0	0.0

TEACAKES

	Measure	per Measure					
Chocolate, Tunnock's*	1 Cake/22g	91	413	5.3	61.0	18.1	0.0
Currant, Sainsbury's*	1 Serving/100g	283	283	7.7	50.9	5.4	3.8
Fresh	1oz/28g	83	296	8.0	52.5	7.5	0.0
Fruit, Lidl*	1 Cake/62g	166	267	10.6	46.3	4.4	2.2
Fruited, Marks & Spencer*	1 Cake/60g	156	260	8.9	53.4	1.0	2.0
Fruited, Warburtons*	1 Cake/62g	162	261	9.7	48.0	3.4	2.7
Fruity, Warburtons*	1 Teacake/63g	166	264	8.8	49.5	3.4	2.7
Jam, Burton's*	1 Cake/10g	45	448	4.2	71.4	16.2	1.6
Large, Sainsbury's*	1 Cake/100g	291	291	8.3	49.1	6.8	3.4
Lees*	1 Cake/19g	81	426	4.2	67.7	15.4	0.0
Mallow, Value, Tesco*	1 Teacake/14g	63	450	4.1	65.4	19.1	1.0
Milk Chocolate, Marks & Spencer*	1 Teacake/17.5g	77	430	5.0	65.4	16.7	1.0
Milk Chocolate, Tunnock's*	1 Serving/22g	91	413	5.3	61.0	18.1	0.0
Reduced Fat, Marks & Spencer*	1 Cake/17g	68	401	5.0	69.1	11.7	0.9
Richly Fruited, Waitrose*	1 Cake/72g	205	285	7.8	55.0	3.7	2.2
Sainsbury's*	1 Cake/70g	171	244	8.0	45.0	3.6	2.6
Somerfield*	1 Teacake/62g	165	267	10.6	46.3	4.4	2.2
Tesco*	1 Cake/61g	163	267	7.8	51.1	3.5	2.4
Toasted	1oz/28g	92	329	8.9	58.3	8.3	0.0
Value, Tesco*	1oz/28g	74	265	7.5	49.1	4.3	2.3
With Fruit, Morning Fresh, Aldi*	1 Cake/65g	155	239	7.4	44.6	3.4	2.3
With Orange Filling, Marks & Spencer*	1 Teacake/20g	80	410	4.5	66.6	14.2	0.9
With Sultanas, Raisins & Currants, Sainsbury's*	1 Teacake/73g	207	284	8.2	53.7	4.0	2.5

TEMPEH

	Measure	per Measure					
Average	1oz/28g	46	166	20.7	6.4	6.4	4.3

TERRINE

	Measure	per Measure					
Chicken, With Pork, Sage & Onion Stuffing, Somerfield*	1oz/28g	32	114	25.0	1.0	1.0	0.0
Lobster & Prawn, Slices, Marks & Spencer*	1 Serving/55g	107	195	18.2	0.7	13.4	0.7
Poached Salmon, Tesco*	1 Pack/113g	349	309	15.5	0.8	27.1	0.0
Prawn, TTD, Sainsbury's*	1 Serving/60g	115	192	9.0	3.7	15.7	0.4
Salmon & Crayfish, Slice, Finest, Tesco*	1 Slice/110g	149	135	21.9	0.1	5.2	0.1
Salmon & King Prawn, Waitrose*	1 Serving/75g	98	130	19.3	1.3	5.3	0.0
Salmon & Lemon, Luxury, Tesco*	1 Segment/50g	98	196	10.6	3.2	15.7	0.8
Salmon, Reduced Fat, Tesco*	1 Serving/56g	100	179	15.5	1.1	12.5	3.5
Salmon, Three, Marks & Spencer*	1 Serving/80g	168	210	17.6	0.8	15.3	0.9
Salmon, With Prawn & Lobster, Marks & Spencer*	1 Serving/55g	107	195	18.2	0.7	13.4	0.7
Scottish Smoked Salmon, Tesco*	1 Slice/25g	56	225	13.9	4.9	16.6	0.5
Trout, TTD, Sainsbury's*	1 Serving/60g	138	230	14.7	2.6	17.9	0.2

T

	Measure INFO/WEIGHT	per Measure KCAL	Nutrition Values per 100g / 100ml				
			KCAL	PROT	CARB	FAT	FIBRE
TEX MEX PLATTER							
Marks & Spencer*	1 Pack/415g	934	225	12.6	10.5	14.6	0.9
THAI BITES							
Lightly Salted, Jacobs*	1 Pack/25g	94	375	6.9	79.7	3.2	0.1
Mild Thai Flavour, Jacobs*	1 Bag/25g	93	373	6.9	79.0	3.3	1.0
Oriental Spice, Jacobs*	1 Pack/25g	93	373	7.1	78.0	3.6	0.2
Red Curry & Coriander, Fusions, Jacobs*	1 Bag/30g	110	367	6.0	72.3	6.0	1.0
Roasted Chilli Flavour, Fusions, Jacobs*	1 Bag/30g	109	363	5.5	72.3	5.8	1.2
Seaweed Flavour, Jacobs*	1 Pack/25g	94	377	7.1	80.0	3.2	0.5
Sesame & Prawn, Fusions, Jacobs*	1 Serving/25g	92	366	6.3	71.2	5.9	1.3
Sweet Herb, Jacobs*	1 Pack/25g	93	372	7.1	78.8	3.2	0.2
THYME							
Dried, Ground	1 Tsp/1.2g	3	276	9.1	45.3	7.4	0.0
Fresh	1 Tsp/0.8g	1	95	3.0	15.1	2.5	0.0
TIA MARIA							
Original	1 Serving/25ml	75	300	0.0	0.0	0.0	0.0
TIC TAC							
Extra Strong Mint, Ferrero*	2 Tic tacs/1g	4	381	0.0	95.2	0.0	0.0
Fresh Mint, Ferrero*	2 Tic Tacs/1g	4	390	0.0	97.5	0.0	0.0
Lime & Orange, Ferrero*	2 Tic Tacs/1g	4	386	0.0	95.5	0.0	0.0
Orange, Ferrero*	2 Tic Tacs/1g	4	385	0.0	95.5	0.0	0.0
Spearmint, Ferrero*	1 Box/16g	62	390	0.0	97.5	0.0	0.0
TIDGY PUDS							
Aunt Bessie's*	4 Puds/16.9g	55	326	9.6	38.4	14.8	2.1
Tryton Foods*	1oz/28g	97	346	11.3	43.5	14.1	2.1
TIDGY TOADS							
Aunt Bessie's*	1 Serving/45g	125	278	14.7	25.3	13.2	1.1
TIKKA MASALA							
Cauliflower & Potato, With Pilau Rice, Safeway*	1 Serving/414.3g	435	105	2.4	13.9	4.1	2.2
Chicken & Basmati Rice, Patak's*	1 Pack/400g	580	145	9.9	15.1	5.0	0.2
Chicken & Pilau Rice, Asda*	1 Pack/400g	548	137	7.0	16.0	5.0	1.6
Chicken & Pilau Rice, GFY, Asda*	1 Pack/400g	440	110	6.0	17.0	2.0	0.8
Chicken & Pilau Rice, Safeway*	1 Pack/399g	654	164	7.5	16.5	7.5	1.4
Chicken & Rice, COU, Marks & Spencer*	1 Pack/400g	420	105	7.8	14.6	1.6	2.1
Chicken & Rice, Healthy Living, Tesco*	1 Serving/450g	495	110	6.9	16.7	1.7	1.1
Chicken & Rice, Takeaway, Tesco*	1 Pack/350g	525	150	4.4	20.3	5.7	1.2
Chicken With Basmati Rice, Eat Smart, Safeway*	1 Pack/363g	290	80	6.4	9.6	1.4	0.7
Chicken With Fruit & Nut Pilau Rice, Sainsbury's*	1 Pack/500g	885	177	7.6	16.1	9.1	2.8
Chicken With Golden Rice, Iceland*	1 Pack/500g	885	177	6.2	19.4	8.3	1.1
Chicken With Pilau Rice, Eat Smart, Safeway*	1 Pack/400g	396	99	5.7	14.3	2.1	1.6
Chicken With Rice, Healthy Eating, Tesco*	1 Pack/400g	472	118	6.1	17.0	2.8	1.8
Chicken With Rice, Healthy Living, Co-Op*	1 Pack/499g	518	104	8.0	15.5	1.2	1.0
Chicken With Rice, Patak's*	1 Carton/350g	571	163	5.1	21.8	6.1	4.4
Chicken With Rice, Sainsbury's*	1 Pack/500g	960	192	8.3	21.2	8.2	0.1
Chicken With Tumeric Rice, BGTY, Sainsbury's*	1 Pack/369g	446	121	6.7	20.5	1.3	0.4
Chicken With White Rice, BGTY, Sainsbury's*	1 Pack/400g	436	109	5.8	16.1	2.4	0.7
Chicken, & Pilau Rice, BGTY, Sainsbury's*	1 Serving/400g	340	85	7.9	11.1	1.0	2.5
Chicken, BGTY, Sainsbury's*	1 Pack/450g	513	114	8.6	17.0	1.3	1.1
Chicken, Boiled Rice & Nan, Meal For One, GFY, Asda*	1 Pack/605g	823	136	6.0	21.0	3.1	0.0
Chicken, Breast, GFY, Asda*	1 Pack/380g	426	112	13.0	6.0	4.0	0.7
Chicken, COU, Marks & Spencer*	1 Pack/300g	300	100	12.1	6.0	2.8	1.3
Chicken, Feeling Great, Findus*	1 Pack/350g	420	120	5.5	17.0	3.5	2.0
Chicken, Good Intentions, Somerfield*	1 Pack/400g	612	153	7.6	26.0	2.1	1.7
Chicken, Healthy Choice, Iceland*	1 Pack/399g	431	108	6.5	18.0	1.1	0.9

	Measure INFO/WEIGHT	per Measure KCAL	Nutrition Values per 100g / 100ml KCAL	PROT	CARB	FAT	FIBRE
TIKKA MASALA							
Chicken, Healthy Living, Tesco*	1 Serving/400g	380	95	4.6	16.0	1.4	1.3
Chicken, Hot, Sainsbury's*	1 Pack/400g	604	151	13.2	3.6	9.3	1.5
Chicken, Indian Meal for One, BGTY, Sainsbury's*	1 Serving/241.0g	200	83	13.9	5.1	0.8	1.0
Chicken, Indian Takeaway, Tesco*	1 Serving/125g	114	91	8.1	3.9	4.8	1.8
Chicken, Indian, Medium, Sainsbury's*	1 Pack/400g	848	212	13.2	5.3	15.3	0.1
Chicken, Large, Sainsbury's*	1 Pack/650g	1105	170	11.7	7.0	10.6	0.3
Chicken, Low Fat, Iceland*	1 Pack/400g	360	90	7.8	12.5	1.0	0.5
Chicken, Marks & Spencer*	1 Pack/300g	495	165	12.3	7.4	9.3	1.2
Chicken, Medium, Tesco*	1 Pack/350g	532	152	11.2	4.9	9.8	0.6
Chicken, Microwave In Two Minutes, Patak's*	1 Pack/300g	354	118	4.3	17.8	3.3	0.4
Chicken, Microwave Meal, Good Choice, Iceland*	1 Pack/400g	488	122	6.6	20.4	1.5	0.6
Chicken, Sainsbury's*	1 Pack/400g	736	184	12.8	4.6	12.7	0.2
Chicken, Sharwood's*	1 Pack/375g	563	150	7.2	15.1	6.7	0.8
Chicken, SmartPrice, Asda*	1 Pack/300g	405	135	7.0	17.0	4.3	0.3
Chicken, Somerfield*	1 Pack/350g	553	158	11.7	3.6	10.8	1.5
Chicken, Take Away Menu, BGTY, Sainsbury's*	1 Pack/251g	226	90	13.4	4.2	2.2	1.3
Chicken, Take Away, Tesco*	1 Pack/350g	613	175	11.3	2.0	13.5	1.1
Chicken, Tesco*	1 Pack/350g	511	146	11.1	4.3	9.4	1.5
Chicken, The Authentic Food Company*	1 Serving/375g	510	136	10.6	5.5	8.4	0.9
Chicken, Tinned, Asda*	1/2 Can/200g	238	119	8.0	6.0	7.0	0.9
Chicken, Waitrose*	1/2 Pack/200g	298	149	12.8	2.6	9.7	1.6
Chicken, With Pilau Rice, Perfectly Balanced, Waitrose*	1 Pack/400g	476	119	8.2	15.8	2.5	1.8
Chicken, With Pilau Rice, Waitrose*	1 Pack/399g	674	169	9.3	14.6	8.1	2.1
Green, Asda*	1 Jar/340g	401	118	1.2	8.0	9.0	0.4
Healthy Eating, Tesco*	1 Serving/220g	191	87	1.0	10.2	4.7	0.5
Vegetable & Rice, Patak's*	1 Pack/370g	503	136	2.5	19.0	6.1	0.9
Vegetable, Asda*	1/2 Can/204g	190	93	2.0	10.0	5.0	2.0
Vegetable, Canned, Waitrose*	1 Can/200g	204	102	2.4	6.4	7.4	0.0
Vegetable, Indian, Tesco*	1 Pack/225g	234	104	2.4	10.4	6.0	2.4
Vegetable, With Rice, Tesco*	1 Pack/450g	500	111	2.6	15.5	4.3	0.9
Vegetarian, With Pilau Rice, Tesco*	1 Serving/440g	519	118	5.0	15.6	3.9	1.5
TIME OUT							
Break Pack, Cadbury*	1 serving/19.8g	106	530	6.2	58.3	30.7	0.0
Cadbury*	2 Fingers/35g	186	530	6.2	58.3	30.7	0.0
Orange, Snack Size, Cadbury*	1 Finger/11g	61	555	5.0	59.4	32.9	0.0
TIP TOP							
Nestle*	1 Serving/40g	45	112	4.8	9.0	6.3	0.0
TIRAMISU							
Asda*	1 Pot/100g	252	252	4.3	34.0	11.0	0.5
BGTY, Sainsbury's*	1 Pot/90g	140	156	4.5	28.3	2.7	0.3
COU, Marks & Spencer*	1 Serving/95g	138	145	3.7	26.9	2.7	0.6
Eat Smart, Safeway*	1 Serving/90g	149	165	5.3	29.4	2.6	1.6
Family Size, Tesco*	1 Serving/125g	356	285	4.3	34.5	14.5	4.3
Healthy Living, Tesco*	1 Pot/90g	172	191	7.8	27.4	4.3	2.0
Italian, Safeway*	1 Serving/125g	353	282	4.4	34.4	14.0	1.6
Raspberry, Marks & Spencer*	1 Serving/84g	197	235	3.8	22.9	14.4	0.2
Sainsbury's*	1 Serving/100g	263	263	4.4	40.2	10.0	0.1
Single Size, Tesco*	1 Pot/100g	290	290	3.8	35.1	12.9	4.5
Somerfield*	1 Pot/100g	286	286	5.0	39.0	11.0	0.0
Trifle, Sainsbury's*	1 Serving/100g	243	243	2.3	23.2	15.7	0.6
TOAD IN THE HOLE							
Asda*	1/4 Pack/100g	251	251	11.0	18.0	15.0	2.5
Average	1oz/28g	78	277	11.9	19.5	17.4	1.1

T

	Measure INFO/WEIGHT	per Measure KCAL	Nutrition Values per 100g / 100ml				
			KCAL	PROT	CARB	FAT	FIBRE
TOAD IN THE HOLE							
Large, Great Value, Asda*	1/4 Pack/81.2g	237	293	10.0	25.0	17.0	2.3
Sainsbury's*	1 Serving/144g	449	312	11.5	23.4	19.2	0.9
Tesco*	1 Serving/188g	461	245	8.5	18.7	15.1	2.6
Vegetarian, Aunt Bessie's*	1 Pack/190g	481	253	13.1	19.9	13.6	1.2
Vegetarian, Linda McCartney*	1 Pack/190g	359	189	13.6	13.9	8.8	1.1
Vegetarian, Meat Free, Asda*	1 Toad/173g	407	235	9.0	25.0	11.0	3.1
Vegetarian, Tesco*	1 Pack/190g	471	248	13.1	26.5	10.0	2.8
Vegetarian, Tryton Foods*	1oz/28g	73	262	14.8	18.6	14.2	1.6
With Three Sausages, Asda*	1 Pack/150g	435	290	10.0	22.0	18.0	1.0
TOAST TOPPERS							
Chicken & Mushroom, Heinz*	1 Serving/56g	31	56	5.1	5.7	1.4	0.2
Ham & Cheese, Heinz*	1oz/28g	27	96	7.4	7.3	4.1	0.1
Mushroom & Bacon, Heinz*	1 Serving/56g	53	94	6.9	6.6	4.4	0.3
TOASTIE							
All Day Breakfast, Marks & Spencer*	1 Serving/174.4g	374	215	11.2	25.0	7.9	1.7
Cheese & Pickle, Marks & Spencer*	1 Toastie/136g	320	235	10.4	33.5	6.7	2.6
Ham & Cheddar, British, Marks & Spencer*	1 Pack/128g	269	210	15.5	22.3	6.7	1.3
Ham & Cheese, Tesco*	1 Serving/138g	388	281	11.5	29.1	13.2	1.0
TOBLERONE							
Milk, Toblerone*	1oz/28g	152	542	5.4	61.2	30.8	2.3
TOFFEE							
Assorted, Bassett's*	1 Toffee/8g	35	434	3.8	73.1	14.0	0.0
Assorted, Sainsbury's*	1 Sweet/8g	37	457	2.2	76.5	15.8	0.2
Butter, SmartPrice, Asda*	1 Toffee/8.4g	35	440	1.3	75.0	15.0	0.0
Chocolate Coated, Thorntons*	1 Bag/100g	521	521	3.5	57.9	30.7	0.3
Dairy, Tesco*	1 Toffee/7g	33	476	2.2	73.3	19.3	0.0
Dairy, Waitrose*	1 Toffee/14g	64	458	2.0	80.2	14.3	0.5
Devon Butter, Thorntons*	1 Sweet/9g	40	444	1.7	72.2	16.7	0.0
Double Devon, Marks & Spencer*	1 Sweet/8g	37	460	1.8	73.1	19.9	0.0
English Butter, Co-Op*	1 Toffee/8g	38	470	2.0	71.0	20.0	0.0
Liquorice, Thorntons*	1 Bag/100g	506	506	1.9	58.8	29.4	0.0
Mixed	1oz/28g	119	426	2.2	66.7	18.6	0.0
No Added Sugar, Boots*	1 Serving/7.1g	23	324	1.3	52.0	14.0	0.0
Original, Thorntons*	1 Bag/100g	514	514	1.8	59.3	30.1	0.0
Squares, No Added Sugar, Russell Stover*	1 Piece/15g	57	380	6.0	49.3	26.0	1.3
TOFFEE CRISP							
Biscuit, Nestle*	1 Biscuit/25g	115	460	4.0	55.2	24.8	0.8
Mini, Nestle*	1 Bar/18g	93	511	4.3	60.6	27.9	0.0
Nestle*	1 Bar/48g	243	507	4.5	61.1	27.9	0.0
Snack Size, Nestle*	1 Bar/30.1g	153	511	4.3	60.6	27.9	0.0
TOFU							
Average	1 Pack/250g	297	119	13.4	1.4	6.6	0.1
Fried, Average	1oz/28g	75	268	28.6	9.3	14.1	0.0
Pieces, Marinated, Golden, Organic, Cauldron*	1oz/28g	64	230	19.3	2.4	15.9	0.7
Savoury Beech, Smoked, Organic, Cauldron*	1/2 Pack/110g	163	148	16.0	1.0	8.9	0.3
Sheets, Dried, H.K. Huizenhou Foods*	10g	5	50	4.0	5.0	4.0	0.0
Smoked, Organic, Evernat*	1oz/28g	36	127	16.3	0.8	6.6	0.0
TOMATO PUREE							
Average	1oz/28g	21	76	4.5	14.1	0.2	2.3
TOMATOES							
Cherry, Average	1 Serving/73g	14	19	0.9	3.3	0.3	1.0
Cherry, On the Vine, Average	1 Serving/50g	9	18	0.7	3.1	0.3	1.0
Chopped, Canned, Average	1 Serving/130g	27	21	1.1	3.8	0.1	0.8

T

	Measure INFO/WEIGHT	per Measure KCAL	Nutrition Values per 100g / 100ml				
			KCAL	PROT	CARB	FAT	FIBRE
TOMATOES							
Chopped, Italian, Average	1/2 Can/200g	47	23	1.3	4.4	0.1	0.9
Chopped, Italian, With Olive Oil & Garlic, Waitrose*	1 Serving/100g	33	33	1.1	3.6	1.6	0.0
Chopped, Italian, With Olives, Waitrose*	1 Can/400g	184	46	1.4	6.0	1.8	0.8
Chopped, Sugocasa, Premium, Sainsbury's*	1/4 Jar/172g	59	34	1.6	6.5	0.2	0.9
Chopped, With Chilli & Peppers, Asda*	1 Pack/400g	92	23	1.0	4.0	0.3	0.0
Chopped, With Chilli, Sainsbury's*	1/2 Can/200g	44	22	1.0	3.5	0.5	0.9
Chopped, With Garlic, Average	1/2 Can/200g	43	21	1.2	3.8	0.1	0.8
Chopped, With Herbs, Average	1/2 Can/200g	42	21	1.1	3.8	0.1	0.8
Chopped, With Olive Oil & Roasted Garlic, Sainsbury's*	1 Pack/390g	187	48	1.3	5.9	2.1	1.0
Chopped, With Onion & Herbs, Napolina*	1 Can/400g	84	21	1.0	4.0	0.1	0.4
Chopped, With Onions, Italian, Tesco*	1/2 Can/200g	58	29	1.1	5.7	0.2	0.7
Chopped, With Peppers & Onions, Sainsbury's*	1/2 Can/200g	40	20	1.2	3.5	0.1	0.9
Chopped, With Sliced Green & Black Olives, Sainsbury's*	1 Pack/390g	183	47	1.3	5.6	2.1	0.7
Creamed, Sainsbury's*	1 Carton/500g	150	30	1.1	6.0	0.1	0.8
Fresh, Raw, Average	1 Med/85g	15	18	0.8	3.2	0.3	1.1
Fried in Blended Oil	1 Av Tomato/85g	77	91	0.7	5.0	7.7	1.3
Grilled	1oz/28g	14	49	2.0	8.9	0.9	2.9
Plum, Baby, Average	1 Serving/50g	9	18	1.5	2.3	0.3	1.0
Plum, In Tomato Juice, Average	1 Can/400g	71	18	1.0	3.3	0.1	0.7
Plum, In Tomato Juice, Premium, Average	1 Can/400g	93	23	1.3	3.8	0.3	0.7
Pomodorino, TTD, Sainsbury's*	1 Serving/50g	9	18	0.8	3.0	0.4	1.0
Ripened On The Vine, Average	1oz/28g	5	18	0.7	3.0	0.3	0.7
Semi Dried, In Olive Oil, TTD, Sainsbury's*	1 Serving/20g	33	167	4.2	19.5	8.0	0.0
Stuffed With Rice	1oz/28g	59	212	2.1	22.2	13.4	1.1
Sun Dried, Average	3 Pieces/20g	43	214	4.7	13.0	15.9	3.3
Sun Dried, In Seasoned Oil, Asda*	1 Serving/25g	51	205	4.3	11.0	16.0	6.0
Sun Dried, Marinated, Waitrose*	1 Serving/100g	126	126	2.4	8.0	9.4	1.2
Sun Dried, Moist, Waitrose*	1 Serving/25g	44	175	11.8	27.4	2.0	7.2
Sundried, With Chianti, TTD, Sainsbury's*	1/2 Pot/150g	108	72	1.8	8.2	3.5	1.0
TONDO'S							
Lightly Salted, Ryvita*	1 Serving/25g	99	397	7.0	86.1	2.7	0.7
Salsa Flavour, Ryvita*	1 Serving/25g	99	395	7.1	84.8	3.0	0.9
Smokey Barbecue Flavour, Ryvita*	1 Bag/25g	98	393	7.0	84.6	3.0	0.7
TONGUE							
Lunch, Average	1oz/28g	51	181	20.1	1.8	10.7	0.0
Slices	1oz/28g	56	201	18.7	0.0	14.0	0.0
TONIC WATER							
Average	1 Glass/250ml	83	33	0.0	8.8	0.0	0.0
Diet, Asda*	1 Glass/200ml	2	1	0.0	0.0	0.0	0.0
Indian, Slimline, Schweppes*	1 Measure/188ml	3	2	0.4	0.1	0.0	0.0
TOOTY FROOTIES							
Rowntree's*	1oz/28g	113	402	0.4	92.1	3.6	0.0
TOPIC							
Mars*	1 Bar/47g	232	493	6.0	58.1	26.3	0.0
TOPPING							
Bruschetta	1serving/115g	30	26	1.2	3.6	0.8	1.1
Bruschetta, Sainsbury's*	1 Sm Tin/230g	60	26	1.2	3.6	0.8	1.1
Bruschetta, Tesco*	1 can/230g	58	25	1.2	3.2	0.8	1.1
Cake Covering, Milk Chocolate Flavoured, Tesco*	1 Pack/300g	1761	587	2.1	57.3	38.8	2.6
For Cappuccino, Creamy, Flavia*	1 Serving/15g	38	253	14.7	33.3	6.7	0.0
Ice Cream, Monster Crackin, Silver Spoon*	1 Tbsp/15g	92	612	0.0	50.8	45.5	0.0
Mediterranean, For Cod, Schwartz*	1/2 Jar/147g	128	87	1.7	9.5	4.7	0.0
Pizza, Italian Tomato & Herb, Sainsbury's*	1/5 Jar/50g	19	38	1.6	7.1	0.4	1.1

T

INFO/WEIGHT	Measure	per Measure KCAL	Nutrition Values per 100g / 100ml				
			KCAL	PROT	CARB	FAT	FIBRE

TOPPING

	Measure INFO/WEIGHT	per Measure KCAL	KCAL	PROT	CARB	FAT	FIBRE
Pizza, Tomato With Cheese & Onion, Napolina*	1 Jar/250g	195	78	2.9	7.0	4.0	0.8
Pizza, Traditional Tomato With Basil, Napolina*	1 Jar/250g	153	61	1.2	7.8	2.6	0.7
Pizza, With Herbs, Napolina*	1 Serving/100g	49	49	0.9	6.3	2.2	0.6

TORCHIETTI

Egg, With Parmesan & Rocket, TTD, Sainsbury's*	1/4 Pot/62.5g	123	195	7.1	21.4	9.0	1.6

TORTE

Chocolate Orange & Almond, Gu*	1 Serving/65g	273	420	5.0	28.2	30.5	2.7
Chocolate Truffle, Waitrose*	1 Serving/116g	359	309	4.6	30.1	17.3	1.4
Chocolate, Safeway*	1/6 Torte/55g	122	221	4.1	27.6	10.5	1.5
Chocolate, Tesco*	1 Serving/50g	126	251	3.6	32.3	11.9	1.0
Lemon & Mango, Waitrose*	1 Serving/80g	142	177	3.9	33.6	3.0	0.6
Lemon, Farmfoods*	1/6 Cake/70g	137	195	4.3	21.9	10.0	0.5
Lemon, Somerfield*	1 Serving/45g	71	157	0.8	32.6	2.6	0.8
Lemon, Tesco*	1 Serving/62g	142	230	2.3	32.9	9.9	0.5
Raspberry, BGTY, Sainsbury's*	1 Serving/100g	154	154	2.6	27.0	3.9	1.2
Raspberry, Safeway*	1/6 Serving/54g	93	172	1.2	25.1	7.4	1.5

TORTELLINI

3 Cheese, Sainsbury's*	1 Serving/50g	196	391	14.4	63.8	8.7	3.0
Aubergine & Pecorino, Sainsbury's*	1/2 Pack/150g	354	236	8.9	40.3	4.3	3.2
Beef & Red Wine, Italian, Asda*	1/2 Pack/150.3g	242	161	9.0	25.0	2.8	0.0
Carbonara, Sainsbury's*	1 Serving/250g	515	206	9.1	23.9	8.2	2.3
Cheese & Ham, Italiano, Tesco*	1/2 Pack/150g	426	284	12.3	37.9	9.2	1.8
Cheese & Tomato, Marks & Spencer*	1 Meal/125g	238	190	10.0	29.1	3.6	1.8
Cheese, Fresh, Sainsbury's*	1/2 Pack/180g	329	183	7.6	26.8	5.0	1.7
Cheese, Healthy Living, Tesco*	1 Serving/400g	368	92	3.2	13.4	2.8	0.6
Cheese, Tomato & Basil, Sainsbury's*	1 Serving/100g	181	181	6.9	27.4	4.9	1.9
Cheese, Weight Watchers*	1 Can/395g	233	59	2.1	8.5	1.8	0.5
Four Cheese & Tomato, Italian, Asda*	1 Serving/150g	249	166	8.0	25.0	3.8	0.0
Four Cheese With Tomato & Basil Sauce, Tesco*	1 Pack/400g	500	125	6.1	16.9	3.7	0.6
Four Cheese, Asda*	1 Serving/150g	201	134	6.0	20.0	3.3	0.0
Four Cheese, Tesco*	1 Serving/125g	314	251	10.8	38.3	6.1	2.4
Garlic & Herb, Fresh, Sainsbury's*	1/2 Pack/150g	365	243	11.1	32.2	7.8	1.8
Garlic, Basil & Ricotta, Asda*	1/2 Pack/175g	319	182	6.0	26.0	6.0	2.6
Ham & Cheese, Asda*	1 Serving/125g	191	153	7.0	20.0	5.0	1.8
Ham & Cheese, Fresh, Asda*	1/2 Pack/150g	198	132	6.0	20.0	3.1	0.0
Ham & Cheese, Tesco*	1 Serving/225g	578	257	13.5	38.1	5.6	1.8
Italian Meat, Tesco*	1 Serving/125g	333	266	10.6	38.9	7.6	2.3
Italiana, Weight Watchers*	1 Can/395g	237	60	2.1	8.5	1.9	0.5
Mozzarella & Tomato, Fresh, Asda*	1oz/28g	46	166	8.0	25.0	3.8	0.0
Mushroom, BGTY, Sainsbury's*	1/2 Can/200g	180	90	2.2	13.2	3.1	0.7
Mushroom, Perfectly Balanced, Waitrose*	1 Pack/250g	573	229	9.4	39.8	3.6	2.4
Pepperoni, Italian, Asda*	1/2 Pack/150g	250	167	6.7	26.0	4.0	0.0
Pesto & Goats Cheese, Sainsbury's*	1/2 Pack/125g	259	207	8.9	24.6	8.1	2.6
Pork & Beef, BGTY, Sainsbury's*	1/2 Can/200g	142	71	2.3	11.9	1.6	1.2
Sausage & Ham, Italiano, Tesco*	1 Pack/300g	816	272	13.1	34.0	9.3	3.7
Smoked Bacon & Tomato, Asda*	1 Pack/300g	591	197	9.0	29.0	5.0	0.0
Smoked Ham & Cheese, Ready Meals, Waitrose*	1oz/28g	73	261	12.9	38.7	6.1	1.3
Smoked, Ham, Bacon & Tomato, Tesco*	1 Serving/100g	254	254	12.1	33.4	8.0	3.2
Spicy Pepperoni, Asda*	1/2 Pack/150g	252	168	7.0	26.0	4.0	0.0
Spicy Pepperoni, Fresh, Asda*	1/2 Pack/150g	249	166	7.0	26.0	4.0	0.0
Spinach & Ricotta, Italian, Asda*	1/2 Pack/150g	189	126	5.0	21.0	2.4	0.6
Spinach & Ricotta, Italiano, Tesco*	1/2 Pack/125g	303	242	11.3	36.8	5.5	2.2
Spinach & Ricotta, Pasta Reale*	1/2 Pack/125g	314	251	10.4	44.5	5.1	3.7

INFO/WEIGHT	per Measure KCAL	Nutrition Values per 100g / 100ml				
		KCAL	PROT	CARB	FAT	FIBRE

TORTELLINI

	INFO/WEIGHT	per Measure KCAL	KCAL	PROT	CARB	FAT	FIBRE
Spinach & Ricotta, Sainsbury's*	1oz/28g	109	388	15.0	62.5	8.7	2.2
Spinach & Ricotta, Tesco*	1 Serving/125g	361	289	11.6	38.5	9.9	3.4
Spinach & Ricotta, Verdi, Asda*	1 Serving/125g	186	149	6.0	21.0	4.5	2.4
Spinach & Ricotta, Waistline, Crosse & Blackwell*	1 Serving/300g	219	73	2.9	10.1	2.4	1.3
Tomato & Mozzarella, Fresh, Asda*	1/2 Pack/150g	236	157	8.0	25.0	2.8	0.0
Tomato & Mozzarella, Sainsbury's*	1 Serving/150g	291	194	7.5	23.0	8.0	3.4
Trio, Fresh, Tesco*	1/2 Pack/125g	323	258	12.8	35.8	7.1	2.0
Walnut & Gorgonzola, Sainsbury's*	1/2 Pack/125g	246	197	8.4	27.8	5.8	4.3
With Tomato, Basil, & Paprika, Easy Cook, Napolina*	1 Pack/120g	481	401	12.4	60.7	12.1	0.0

TORTELLONI

	INFO/WEIGHT	per Measure KCAL	KCAL	PROT	CARB	FAT	FIBRE
Arrabbiata, Sainsbury's*	1/2 Pack/125g	343	274	11.2	36.0	9.5	2.2
Beef, Red Wine, & Mushroom, Asda*	1/2 Pack/150g	242	161	7.0	29.0	1.9	2.8
Carbonara, Sainsbury's*	1 Serving/250g	515	206	9.1	23.9	8.2	2.3
Cheese & Chive, Safeway*	1 Serving/100g	200	200	8.3	26.4	6.3	1.7
Cheese & Ham, Co-Op*	1 Serving/125g	344	275	12.0	42.0	7.0	3.0
Cheese & Pesto, Somerfield*	1 Pack/250g	788	315	12.0	40.0	12.0	0.0
Cheese & Smoked Ham, Waitrose*	1 Serving/250g	625	250	11.5	35.8	6.8	1.8
Cheese & Sun Dried Tomato, Fresh, Safeway*	1/2 Pack/199g	364	183	7.7	24.2	6.2	2.7
Cheese, Garlic & Herb, Co-Op*	1 Serving/125g	331	265	10.0	43.0	6.0	0.0
Cheese, Heinz*	1 Can/395g	233	59	2.1	8.6	1.8	0.5
Cheese, Tomato, & Basil, Sainsbury's*	1/2 Pack/150g	272	181	8.0	22.7	6.5	1.7
Chicken & Ham, Morrisons*	1 Serving/150g	366	244	12.3	38.6	3.9	2.4
Five Cheese, Safeway*	1 Serving/150g	275	183	7.8	24.2	6.2	2.7
Five Cheese, Sainsbury's*	1 Serving/125g	285	228	10.8	25.2	9.3	2.9
Four Cheese, Express, Dolmio*	1 Pack/220g	411	187	7.6	22.1	7.6	0.0
Four Cheese, Waitrose*	1/2 Pack/125g	298	238	10.3	34.2	6.7	1.6
Garlic & Herb, Cooked, Pasta Reale*	1 Pack/300g	546	182	6.7	30.1	3.9	0.9
Garlic Mushroom & Onion, Eat Smart, Safeway*	1 Serving/125g	231	185	9.3	31.4	2.0	1.4
Goats Cheese & Basil, Somerfield*	1 Serving/250g	650	260	11.1	38.7	6.8	1.8
Goats Cheese & Pesto, Sainsbury's*	1/2 Pack/125g	259	207	8.9	23.6	8.1	2.6
Meat & Cheese, Fresh, Sainsbury's*	1/2 Pack/125g	304	243	13.5	28.3	8.4	2.6
Meat, Italian, Asda*	1/2 Pack/150g	266	177	7.0	27.0	4.5	2.4
Mediterranean Vegetable, Perfectly Balanced, Waitrose*	1/2 Pack/125g	286	229	9.1	40.1	3.6	2.5
Mozzarella, Tomato & Basil, Italian, Somerfield*	1/2 Pack/125g	314	251	10.5	43.1	4.1	1.9
Mushroom, Perfectly Balanced, Waitrose*	1/2 Pack/125g	300	240	10.9	41.8	3.2	2.2
Olive & Ricotta, Sainsbury's*	1/2 Pack/175.2g	403	230	8.8	25.1	10.5	2.3
Parma Ham & Parmesan, Safeway*	1 Serving/125g	269	215	9.9	27.8	6.7	1.5
Porcini & Pancetta, TTD, Sainsbury's*	1 Serving/175g	294	168	7.1	20.8	6.3	3.4
Potato & Rosemary, Fresh, Sainsbury's*	1/2 Pack/175g	364	208	5.7	26.6	8.8	2.3
Red Pepper & Mozzarella, Cooked, Somerfield*	1/2 Pack/124g	325	263	10.8	40.1	6.6	1.8
Roasted Vegetable, TTD, Sainsbury's*	1/2 Pack/125g	259	207	8.4	23.3	8.9	4.0
Spinach & Ricotta, Fresh, Safeway*	1/2 Pack/202g	341	169	7.4	24.0	4.8	2.4
Spinach & Ricotta, Fresh, Sainsbury's*	1/2 Pack/125g	294	235	10.3	27.8	9.1	2.9
Spinach & Ricotta, Waitrose*	1/2 Pack/125g	328	262	11.3	38.4	7.0	2.4
Taleggio & Leek, Fresh, Sainsbury's*	1/2 Pack/175g	450	257	9.7	38.8	7.1	2.6
Tomato & Mozzarella, Sainsbury's*	1 Serving/175g	340	194	7.5	23.0	8.0	3.4
Walnut & Gorgonzola, Fresh, Sainsbury's*	1/2 Pack/175g	345	197	8.4	27.8	5.8	2.4

TORTIGLIONI

	INFO/WEIGHT	per Measure KCAL	KCAL	PROT	CARB	FAT	FIBRE
Dry, Average	1 Serving/75g	267	355	12.5	72.2	1.9	2.1

TORTILLA CHIPS

	INFO/WEIGHT	per Measure KCAL	KCAL	PROT	CARB	FAT	FIBRE
Blazing BBQ, Sainsbury's*	1 Serving/50g	237	474	6.8	58.9	23.5	4.6
Blue, Organic, Sainsbury's*	1 Serving/50g	252	504	7.7	65.8	23.4	5.6
Cajun, Organic, Apache*	1 Serving/25g	113	450	6.0	58.0	22.0	0.0

TORTILLA CHIPS

INFO/WEIGHT	Measure	per Measure KCAL	KCAL	PROT	CARB	FAT	FIBRE
Chilli Flavour, Somerfield*	1 Serving/50g	242	484	6.8	60.1	24.1	5.3
Chilli, Organic, Evernat*	1oz/28g	137	490	8.0	65.0	22.0	0.0
Classic Mexican, Phileas Fogg*	1 Serving/35g	162	464	5.9	67.2	19.1	3.8
Cool Flavour, Sainsbury's*	1 Serving/50g	232	463	5.7	68.1	18.7	3.7
Cool, Asda*	1 Serving/26g	118	454	7.0	57.0	22.0	9.0
Cool, Salted, Sainsbury's*	1 Serving/50g	253	506	6.5	58.6	27.3	4.3
Cool, Tesco*	1 Serving/50g	227	453	6.4	57.4	22.0	8.1
Easy Cheesy!, Sainsbury's*	1 Serving/50g	249	498	7.1	58.7	26.1	4.5
Lightly Salted, Marks & Spencer*	1 Serving/20g	99	495	7.0	62.2	25.0	4.0
Lightly Salted, SmartPrice, Asda*	1/4 Bag/50g	251	502	7.0	60.0	26.0	5.0
Lightly Salted, Tesco*	1 Serving/50g	248	495	4.8	56.8	27.6	7.5
Nacho Cheese Flavour, Marks & Spencer*	1 Serving/25g	126	505	8.0	57.5	26.8	3.0
Nacho Cheese Flavour, Mexican Style, Co-Op*	1 Serving/50g	248	495	7.0	58.0	27.0	4.0
Nacho Cheese Flavour, Morrisons*	1 Serving/25g	126	504	7.2	59.4	26.4	3.6
Nachos Kit, Asda*	1 Serving/100g	448	448	7.0	51.0	24.0	0.7
Natural, Evernat*	1oz/28g	137	490	8.0	65.0	22.0	0.0
Salsa Flavour, Somerfield*	1oz/28g	140	499	6.0	62.0	25.0	0.0
Salsa, Asda*	1 Serving/25g	122	488	6.0	62.0	24.0	6.0
Salsa, Marks & Spencer*	1/2 Bag/75g	364	485	5.7	59.1	25.1	6.1
Slightly Salted, Organic, Sainsbury's*	1 Serving/50g	227	453	10.0	73.3	13.3	13.3
Taco, Tesco*	1 Serving/50g	248	495	7.4	59.3	25.4	4.4
Waitrose*	1 Serving/25g	128	510	7.9	65.5	24.0	4.5

TORTILLAS

INFO/WEIGHT	Measure	per Measure KCAL	KCAL	PROT	CARB	FAT	FIBRE
Corn, Discovery*	1 Serving/15g	36	243	5.4	53.8	2.3	3.8
Corn, Soft, Old El Paso*	1 Tortilla/38g	129	343	10.0	60.0	7.0	0.0
Flour, 10 Pack, Asda*	1 Tortilla/30g	95	315	9.0	54.0	7.0	2.5
Flour, American Style, Sainsbury's*	1 Tortilla/34.5g	110	313	8.6	53.9	7.0	2.5
Flour, Bakery, Asda*	1 Tortilla/42.6g	130	303	9.0	51.0	7.0	2.5
Flour, For Soft Tacos & Fajitas, Old El Paso*	1 Tortilla/25g	80	320	6.0	52.0	9.0	0.0
Flour, Mexican Style, Morrisons*	1 Tortilla/33g	103	313	8.6	53.9	7.0	2.5
Flour, Salsa, Old El Paso*	1 tortilla/41g	132	323	9.0	52.0	9.0	0.0
Flour, Soft, Old El Paso*	2 Tortillas/81g	278	343	10.0	60.0	7.0	0.0
Flour, Tex "n" Mex 12, Sainsbury's*	1 Tortilla/26g	85	326	8.6	53.9	9.6	2.5
Made With Wheat Flour	1oz/28g	73	262	7.2	59.7	1.0	2.4
Mexican Cheese, Phileas Fogg*	1 Pack/278g	1404	505	6.5	61.4	26.0	3.0
Mexicana Cheddar, Kettle*	1 Serving/50g	249	498	7.9	56.7	26.6	5.1
Plain Wheat, Waitrose*	1 Tortilla/43g	134	311	8.1	51.5	8.1	3.0
Plain, BGTY, Sainsbury's*	1 Serving/50g	126	251	7.8	50.1	2.2	2.9
Plain, Wheat Flour, Wraps, Sainsbury's*	1 Tortilla/56g	175	313	8.6	53.0	7.0	2.5
Soft Flour, Discovery*	1 Serving/39g	122	313	8.6	53.9	7.0	2.5
Soft Flour, Garlic & Coriander, Discovery*	1 Tortilla/40g	125	313	8.5	54.0	7.0	2.5
Soft Flour, Old El Paso*	1 Tortilla/41g	141	343	10.0	60.0	7.0	0.0
Wheat Flour, Waitrose*	1 Wrap/62g	203	327	8.5	51.5	9.8	0.0
Wrap, Bueno, Aldi*	1 Tortilla/62.9g	171	272	6.9	48.2	5.7	2.0
Wrap, Discovery*	1 Serving/39.9g	125	313	8.6	53.9	7.0	2.5
Wrap, Garlic & Parsley, Sainsbury's*	1 Tortilla/60g	166	277	7.2	48.0	6.2	1.8
Wrap, Healthy Living, Tesco*	1 Wrap/50g	125	249	8.1	50.0	1.9	2.5
Wrap, Low Carb, Tesco*	1 Tortilla/17g	77	453	39.4	53.5	8.8	23.5
Wrap, Low Fat, Marks & Spencer*	1 Serving/180g	225	125	6.3	20.6	2.2	1.9
Wrap, Marks & Spencer*	1 Wrap/40g	106	265	9.0	49.9	3.5	3.4
Wrap, Morrisons*	1 Serving/35g	84	240	6.8	45.8	3.8	1.9
Wrap, Organic, Tesco*	1 Tortilla/173g	529	306	8.1	51.1	7.8	1.9
Wrap, Original, Wrappin Roll, Discovery*	1 Serving/56g	166	296	8.1	50.6	6.8	1.9

INFO/WEIGHT	Measure per Measure KCAL		Nutrition Values per 100g / 100ml				
			KCAL	PROT	CARB	FAT	FIBRE

TORTILLAS

	Measure INFO/WEIGHT	per Measure KCAL	KCAL	PROT	CARB	FAT	FIBRE
Wrap, Plain, Tesco*	1 Wrap/60g	163	272	6.9	48.2	5.7	2.0
Wrap, Spicy Tomato, Tesco*	1 Wrap/63g	175	278	7.8	49.2	5.6	2.4
Wrap, Tomato & Herb, Tesco*	1 Serving/63g	165	262	7.9	45.1	5.5	2.1
Wrap, Tomato & Herbs, Sainsbury's*	1 Tortilla/52g	157	302	7.8	54.1	6.0	2.4
Wraps, 8 Pack, Asda*	1 Wrap/50g	143	286	8.0	50.0	6.0	1.8

TRAIL MIX

Average	1oz/28g	121	432	9.1	37.2	28.5	4.3

TREACLE

Black	1 Tbsp/20g	51	257	1.2	67.2	0.0	0.0

TRIFLE

Average	1oz/28g	45	160	3.6	22.3	6.3	0.5
Banana & Mandarin, Co-Op*	1/4 Trifle/125g	238	190	2.0	21.0	11.0	0.1
Black Forest, Asda*	1 Serving/100g	237	237	3.1	36.0	9.0	0.0
Blackforest, BGTY, Sainsbury's*	1 Pot/125g	171	137	2.1	21.9	4.5	1.6
Caramel, Galaxy, Mars*	1 Pot/100g	255	255	4.5	30.0	13.0	1.0
Cherry & Almond, Somerfield*	1 Trifle/125g	230	184	2.0	23.0	9.0	0.0
Cherry, Finest, Tesco*	1/4 Trifle/163g	340	209	2.6	22.9	11.9	0.3
Chocolate, Asda*	1 Serving/125.3g	271	217	4.1	21.0	13.0	0.5
Chocolate, Healthy Living, Tesco*	1 Serving/150g	189	126	4.0	21.4	2.7	4.6
Chocolate, Light Milk, Cadbury*	1 Pot/90g	171	190	5.6	25.5	7.3	0.0
Chocolate, Tesco*	1 Serving/125g	313	250	4.3	24.0	15.2	0.7
Cream Mandarin, GFY, Asda*	1 Serving/113g	151	134	1.6	27.0	4.4	0.2
Fruit Cocktail, COU, Marks & Spencer*	1 Trifle/140g	175	125	2.8	23.1	2.3	0.5
Fruit Cocktail, Individual, Shape*	1 Trifle/115g	136	118	3.2	19.6	2.7	1.6
Fruit Cocktail, Individual, Tesco*	1 Pot/113g	175	155	1.7	19.6	7.8	0.6
Fruit Cocktail, Low Fat, Danone*	1 Pot/114.8g	140	122	2.2	24.0	1.8	0.4
Fruit Cocktail, Luxury Devonshire, St Ivel*	1 Trifle/125g	211	169	1.9	22.6	7.9	0.2
Fruit Cocktail, Sainsbury's*	1 Trifle/150g	241	161	1.8	24.8	6.0	0.4
Fruit, Sainsbury's*	1 Serving/125g	233	186	2.3	21.7	10.0	0.3
Mango & Passion Fruit, Danone*	1oz/28g	50	177	2.6	30.7	4.9	0.4
Peach & Zabaglione, COU, Marks & Spencer*	1 Glass/130g	150	115	2.8	20.6	2.3	0.8
Raspberry, Asda*	1 Serving/100g	175	175	1.8	24.0	8.0	0.1
Raspberry, Individual, Safeway*	1 Pot/125g	259	207	2.7	26.2	10.2	0.0
Raspberry, Sainsbury's*	1 Pot/125g	204	163	1.7	21.5	7.8	0.6
Raspberry, Somerfield*	1 Trifle/125g	208	166	2.0	22.0	8.0	0.0
Raspberry, Tesco*	1 Pot/150g	210	140	1.7	18.5	6.5	1.0
Raspberry, Waitrose*	1 Serving/150g	207	138	1.9	20.4	5.4	0.8
Sherry, Sainsbury's*	1 Serving/132g	215	162	2.4	20.1	7.5	0.3
Sherry, BGTY, Sainsbury's*	1 Pot/135g	146	108	3.0	20.2	1.7	0.5
Sherry, TTD, Sainsbury's*	1 Serving/125g	219	175	1.7	21.5	9.1	0.5
Strawberry, COU, Marks & Spencer*	1 Pot/140g	168	120	3.0	21.8	2.3	0.3
Strawberry, Healthy Living, Tesco*	1 Pot/150g	161	107	2.3	19.3	2.3	2.7
Strawberry, Individual, Shape*	1 Pot/115g	137	119	3.3	19.8	2.7	1.6
Strawberry, Individual, Somerfield*	1 Trifle/125g	186	149	1.8	20.5	6.6	0.6
Strawberry, Individual, Waitrose*	1 Pot/150g	206	137	1.8	19.7	5.7	1.0
Strawberry, Low Fat Goodies, Danone*	1 Pot/115g	148	129	2.2	26.0	1.8	0.3
Strawberry, Low Fat, Shape*	1oz/28g	38	137	3.8	22.8	3.1	1.8
Strawberry, Luxury Devonshire, St Ivel*	1 Trifle/125g	208	166	2.0	21.7	7.9	0.2
Strawberry, Marks & Spencer*	1 Trifle/50g	81	161	2.0	17.7	9.2	0.6
Strawberry, Sainsbury's*	1/4 Trifle/125g	232	186	2.2	21.7	10.0	0.2
Strawberry, St Ivel*	1 Trifle/113g	194	172	2.4	21.0	8.7	0.2
Strawberry, Tesco*	1 Serving/83g	140	169	1.6	17.7	10.2	0.7
Summerfruit, BGTY, Sainsbury's*	1 Trifle/125g	151	121	1.2	19.2	4.4	0.5

T

	Measure	per Measure		Nutrition Values per 100g / 100ml				
	INFO/WEIGHT	KCAL		KCAL	PROT	CARB	FAT	FIBRE

TRIFLE

Triple Chocolate, Farmfoods*	1/4 Trifle/86.25g	223		259	2.1	21.6	18.2	1.2

TRIFLE MIX

Strawberry Flavour, Bird's*	1oz/28g	119		425	2.7	78.0	10.5	1.2

TRIFLE SPONGES

Safeway*	1 Sponge/23g	73		318	5.3	70.8	1.5	1.1
Sainsbury's*	1 Sponge/24g	77		323	5.3	71.9	1.6	1.1
Somerfield*	1 Sponge/24g	81		339	5.0	76.0	2.0	0.0
Tesco*	1 Sponge/24g	75		311	5.3	66.6	2.6	1.1

TRIPE &

Onions, Stewed	1oz/28g	26		93	8.3	9.5	2.7	0.7

TROFIE

Waitrose*	1 Serving/75g	256		341	12.5	68.8	1.3	3.7

TROMPRETTI

Egg, Somerfield*	1 Serving/75g	265		353	14.0	67.6	3.0	3.5
Fresh, Waitrose*	1 Serving/125g	339		271	11.7	50.6	2.4	2.0
Tricolour, Fresh, Tesco*	1 Pack/250g	675		270	11.2	48.6	3.4	4.0

TROTTOLE

Dry, Sainsbury's*	1 Serving/90g	338		375	12.3	73.1	1.7	2.5
Tricolore, Sainsbury's*	1 Serving/90g	321		357	12.3	73.1	1.7	2.5

TROUT

Fillets, In Lemon & Dill Marinade, Safeway*	1 Fillet/110g	215		195	19.5	0.0	12.7	0.6
Rainbow, Fillets, With Thyme & Lemon Butter, Asda*	1 Serving/147g	210		143	20.0	0.9	7.0	0.5
Rainbow, Grilled	1 Serving/120g	162		135	21.5	0.0	5.4	0.0
Rainbow, Raw, Average	1oz/28g	36		127	20.5	0.0	5.1	0.0
Rainbow, Smoked, Average	1 Pack/135g	190		141	21.7	0.8	5.7	0.0
Raw, Average	1 Serving/120g	159		132	20.6	0.0	5.4	0.0
Roasting, Lemon & Rosemary, TTD, Sainsbury's*	1 Fish/269.9g	475		176	20.2	0.0	10.6	0.5
Rosemary Crusted, Finest, Tesco*	1 Trout/150g	264		176	16.2	12.2	6.9	1.0
Smoked, Average	1oz/28g	39		139	22.7	0.3	5.2	0.1

TUACA*

Alcoholic Beverage	1 Serving/25ml	67		267	0.0	0.0	0.0	0.0

TUNA

Chunks, In Brine, Average, Drained	1 Can /130g	141		108	25.9	0.0	0.5	0.0
Chunks, In Spring Water, Average, Drained	1 Can /130g	140		108	25.4	0.0	0.6	0.1
Chunks, In Sunflower Oil, Average, Drained	1 Can/138g	260		189	26.5	0.0	9.2	0.0
Chunks, Skipjack, In Brine, Average	1 Can/138g	141		102	24.3	0.0	0.6	0.0
Coronation Style, Average	1 Can/80g	122		152	10.2	6.5	9.5	0.6
Coronation, BGTY, Sainsbury's*	1 Can/80g	90		112	16.5	5.7	2.6	1.0
Flakes, In Brine, Average	1oz/28g	29		104	24.8	0.0	0.6	0.0
In A Lime & Black Pepper Dressing, Princes*	1 Can/80g	102		127	16.3	3.5	5.3	0.0
In A Red Chilli & Lime Dressing, Princes*	1 Sachet/85g	102		120	21.5	1.0	3.3	0.0
In A Tikka Dressing, Princes*	1 Sachet/85g	116		137	18.6	5.5	4.5	0.0
In Chilli Sauce, Safeway*	1 Serving/100g	158		158	16.8	4.8	7.9	0.5
In Sweet & Sour Sauce, Safeway*	1 Can/185g	148		80	10.9	5.6	1.6	1.0
In Thousand Island Dressing, John West*	1 Can/185g	287		155	18.0	5.1	7.0	0.2
In Water, Average	1 Serving/120g	126		105	24.0	0.1	0.8	0.0
Steaks, Chargrilled, Italian, Sainsbury's*	1 Serving/125g	199		159	25.1	0.2	6.4	0.5
Steaks, In Brine, Average	1 Sm Can/99g	106		107	25.6	0.0	0.6	0.0
Steaks, In Cajun Marinade, Sainsbury's*	1 Steak/100g	141		141	29.8	0.0	2.4	0.0
Steaks, In Olive Oil, Average	1 Serving/111g	211		190	25.8	0.0	9.6	0.0
Steaks, In Sunflower Oil, Average	1 Can/150g	276		184	26.7	0.0	8.6	0.0
Steaks, In Water, Average	1 Serving/200g	215		107	25.6	0.0	0.4	0.0
Steaks, Lemon & Herb Marinade, Seared, Sainsbury's*	1/2 Pack/118.6g	192		161	23.4	0.1	7.4	0.0

T

	Measure INFO/WEIGHT	per Measure KCAL	Nutrition Values per 100g / 100ml				
			KCAL	PROT	CARB	FAT	FIBRE
TUNA							
Steaks, Raw, Average	1 Serving/140g	185	132	28.5	0.1	2.0	0.2
Steaks, Skipjack, In Brine, Average	1/2 Can/75g	73	98	23.2	0.0	0.6	0.0
Steaks, Thai Style Butter, Tesco*	1 Serving/110g	191	174	24.7	0.0	8.3	0.0
Steaks, With Lime & Coriander Dressing, Tesco*	1 Serving/150g	156	104	21.6	3.6	0.4	0.6
Steaks, With Sweet Red Pepper Glaze, Sainsbury's*	1 Steak/100g	135	135	28.5	5.0	0.1	0.1
With Basil Butter, Microwave Easy Steam, Sainsbury's*	1 Pack/170g	292	172	23.3	0.5	8.5	0.1
With Onion, John West*	1oz/28g	33	118	19.0	6.0	2.0	0.0
With Salsa Verde, Sainsbury's*	1 Serving/125g	310	248	25.5	0.6	16.0	0.0
With a Twist, French Dressing, John West*	1 Pack/85g	135	159	15.2	2.8	9.7	0.1
With a Twist, Lime & Black Pepper Dressing, John West*	1 Pack/85g	133	156	15.6	2.8	9.2	0.0
With a Twist, Oven Dried Tomato & Herb, John West*	1 Pack/85g	129	152	16.1	3.9	8.0	0.1
TUNA LUNCH							
French Style, Light, John West*	1 Pack/250g	208	83	7.8	7.6	2.4	1.0
Indian Style, John West*	1 Pack/240g	401	167	7.7	12.3	9.6	0.6
Mediterranean, Light, John West*	1 Pack/250g	193	77	8.3	6.4	2.0	1.6
Nicoise Style, Light, John West*	1 Pack/250g	241	96	10.4	8.9	2.1	2.8
Tomato Salsa, Light, John West*	1 Serving/250g	180	72	8.0	7.5	1.1	1.1
TUNA MAYONNAISE							
& Sweetcorn, BGTY, Sainsbury's*	1/2 Pack/50g	46	92	13.8	5.9	1.5	1.1
Garlic & Herb, John West*	1/2 Can/92g	243	264	12.0	4.0	22.2	0.2
Lemon, Light, Princes*	1 Can/80g	104	130	22.0	2.8	3.5	0.0
Lemon, Light, Slimming World, Princes*	1 Can/80g	99	124	16.8	3.5	4.8	0.0
Light, Princes*	1 Sachet/100g	112	112	20.5	3.0	2.0	0.0
Light, Slimming World*	1 Serving/80g	96	120	17.3	3.6	4.1	0.0
Style Dressing, With Sweetcorn, Weight Watchers*	1 Can/80g	114	142	11.5	6.2	7.9	0.1
Weight Watchers*	1 Can/80g	111	139	11.3	6.1	7.7	0.1
With Sweetcorn And Green Peppers, GFY, Asda*	1 Pack/100g	103	103	14.0	5.0	3.0	0.8
With Sweetcorn, John West*	1/2 Can/92g	231	251	12.0	4.5	20.6	0.2
TUNA MEAL							
Italian, Light, All Day, John West*	1 Serving/100g	141	141	11.0	13.0	5.0	0.0
TUNA SNACK POT							
Italian, Weight Watchers*	1 Pot/240g	245	102	9.1	8.5	3.6	0.5
Oriental, Weight Watchers*	1 Pot/240g	269	112	9.0	12.6	2.9	0.3
Provencale, Weight Watchers*	1 Pot/240g	266	111	9.8	10.2	3.4	0.5
TURBOT							
Grilled	1oz/28g	34	122	22.7	0.0	3.5	0.0
Raw	1oz/28g	27	95	17.7	0.0	2.7	0.0
TURKEY							
Breast, Butter Basted, Average	1 Serving/75g	110	146	23.7	1.9	4.9	0.4
Breast, Canned, Average	1 Can/200g	194	97	18.3	0.7	2.4	0.1
Breast, Diced, Healthy Range, Average	1oz/28g	30	108	23.9	0.1	1.3	0.1
Breast, Hand Sliced, Butter Roasted, TTD, Sainsbury's*	1 Pack/150g	177	118	24.5	0.3	2.1	0.5
Breast, Honey Roast, Sliced, Average	1 Serving/50g	57	115	24.0	1.6	1.4	0.3
Breast, Joint, Lemon & Pepper Basted, Tesco*	1/4 Pack/132g	238	180	19.7	0.0	11.2	0.0
Breast, Joint, Raw, Average	1 Serving/125g	134	108	21.3	0.7	2.1	0.6
Breast, Joint, With Sage & Onion Stuffing, Waitrose*	1 Serving/325g	377	116	19.2	1.4	4.1	0.1
Breast, Raw, Average	1oz/28g	33	117	24.1	0.5	2.0	0.1
Breast, Roasted, Average	1oz/28g	37	131	24.6	0.7	3.3	0.1
Breast, Roll, Cooked, Average	1 Slice/10g	9	92	17.6	3.5	0.8	0.0
Breast, Slices, Cooked, Average	1 Slice/20g	23	114	24.1	1.2	1.4	0.3
Breast, Smoked, Sliced, Average	1 Slice/20g	23	113	23.4	0.7	2.0	0.0
Breast, Spicy Tikka Flavoured, Safeway*	1 Pack/450g	698	155	28.8	5.4	1.7	1.2
Breast, Steaks, In Crumbs, Average	1 Steak/76g	217	286	13.7	16.4	18.5	0.2

	Measure INFO/WEIGHT	per Measure KCAL	Nutrition Values per 100g / 100ml				
			KCAL	PROT	CARB	FAT	FIBRE
TURKEY							
Breast, Steaks, Raw, Average	1oz/28g	30	107	24.3	0.0	1.1	0.0
Breast, Steaks, Thai, Bernard Matthews*	1 Serving/175g	280	160	29.4	4.6	2.7	0.0
Breast, Strips, Chinese Style, Sainsbury's*	1 Pack/650g	1274	196	26.4	12.5	4.5	0.5
Breast, Strips, For Stir Fry, Average	1 Serving/175g	205	117	25.6	0.1	1.6	0.0
Breast, Wafer Thin, Chinese Style, Bernard Matthews*	1 Pack/100g	110	110	18.0	6.1	1.5	0.0
Butter Roast, TTD, Sainsbury's*	2 Slices/102g	120	118	24.5	0.3	2.1	0.5
Butter Roasted, Finest, Tesco*	1 Serving/40g	60	150	25.2	1.2	4.9	0.3
Dark Meat, Raw	1oz/28g	29	104	20.4	0.0	2.5	0.0
Dark Meat, Roasted	1oz/28g	50	177	29.4	0.0	6.6	0.0
Drummers, Golden, Bernard Matthews*	1 Drummer/57g	146	256	12.2	10.1	18.6	0.9
Drumsticks, Tesco*	1 Serving/200g	272	136	19.9	0.0	6.3	0.0
Escalope, Average	1 Escalope/138g	341	247	13.5	16.7	14.0	0.6
Escalope, Creamy Pepper Topped, Tesco*	1 Escalope/165g	337	204	11.5	15.3	10.7	1.7
Escalope, Lemon & Pepper, Average	1 Escalope/143g	371	260	12.6	16.7	15.8	0.5
Escalope, Spicy Mango, Bernard Matthews*	1 Escalope/136g	354	260	11.6	24.6	12.8	0.0
Fillets, Chinese Marinated, Bernard Matthews*	1 Pack/200g	304	152	23.4	7.2	3.3	0.0
Fillets, Tikka Marinated, Bernard Matthews*	1 Pack/200g	310	155	21.8	5.2	5.2	1.6
Goujons, Bernard Matthews*	1 Goujon/32g	78	245	11.3	18.1	14.1	0.0
Leg, Roast, Bernard Matthews*	1 Leg/567g	777	137	15.4	0.5	5.4	1.2
Leg, Roast, Uncooked, Bernard Matthews*	1 Serving/283g	317	112	15.4	0.5	5.4	0.0
Light Meat, Raw	1oz/28g	29	105	24.4	0.0	0.8	0.0
Mince, Average	1oz/28g	45	161	23.9	0.0	7.2	0.0
Mince, Free From, Sainsbury's*	1 Serving/100g	148	148	23.0	0.1	6.2	0.0
Mince, Lean, Healthy Range, Average	1oz/28g	33	118	20.3	0.0	4.1	0.0
On The Bone, Honey Roast, Somerfield*	1oz/28g	42	149	26.0	0.0	5.0	0.0
Rashers, Average	1 Rasher/26g	26	101	19.1	2.3	1.6	0.0
Rashers, Smoked, Average	1 Serving/75g	76	101	19.8	1.5	1.8	0.0
Roast, Meat & Skin	1oz/28g	48	171	28.0	0.0	6.5	0.0
Roll, Dinosaur, Cooked, Bernard Matthews*	1 Slice/10g	17	170	13.6	6.0	10.2	1.1
Schnitzel, Lidl*	1 Schnitzel/115g	210	183	19.0	11.0	7.0	0.0
Sticks, Honey Roast, Mini, Tesco*	1 Serving/90g	101	112	20.0	3.6	1.9	0.0
Sticks, With Nacho Cheese Dip, Tesco*	1 Serving/35g	161	459	5.5	1.5	47.9	0.0
Strips, Stir-Fried	1oz/28g	46	164	31.0	0.0	4.5	0.0
Thigh, Diced, Average	1oz/28g	33	117	19.7	0.0	4.3	0.0
Thigh, Joint, Cooked, Sainsbury's*	1 Serving/150g	366	244	27.7	2.1	13.9	0.1
Wafer Thin, Cooked, Average	1 Slice/10g	12	122	19.0	3.2	3.7	0.0
Wafer Thin, Honey Roast, Average	1 Slice/10g	11	109	19.2	4.2	1.7	0.2
Wafer Thin, Smoked, Average	1 Slice/10g	12	119	18.1	3.6	3.7	0.0
Whole, Raw, Average	1/2 Joint/254g	389	153	22.6	0.9	6.6	0.1
TURKEY DINNER							
Roast, Birds Eye*	1 Pack/340g	395	116	7.4	13.8	3.5	1.5
TURKEY IN							
BBQ Marinade, Steaks, Asda*	1 Serving/225g	356	158	30.0	4.4	2.3	0.9
Pepper Sauce, Escalope, Bernard Matthews*	1 Escalope/143g	350	245	9.4	18.2	15.0	1.5
TURKEY WITH							
A Cheese & Leek Sauce, Escalope, Bernard Matthews*	1 Portion/134g	340	254	9.2	17.6	16.3	0.0
Cranberry & Orange Glaze, Breast Joint, Sainsbury's*	1 Serving/180g	281	156	29.6	3.0	2.9	1.0
Sage & Onion, Breast Joint, Glazed, GFY, Asda*	1 Serving/100g	101	101	19.0	2.5	1.7	1.0
Sausagemeat, Sage & Onion Stuffing, Breast, Tesco*	1 Serving/300g	417	139	17.9	2.8	6.2	0.8
Stuffing, Breast, Cooked, Somerfield*	1oz/28g	29	104	17.0	6.0	2.0	0.0
TURKISH DELIGHT							
Cadbury*	1 Bar/51g	186	365	2.0	73.3	7.2	0.0
Dark, Thorntons*	1 Chocolate/10g	39	390	2.7	69.0	11.0	2.0

T

	Measure INFO/WEIGHT	per Measure KCAL	Nutrition Values per 100g / 100ml KCAL	PROT	CARB	FAT	FIBRE
TURKISH DELIGHT							
Fry's*	1 Bar/51g	186	365	2.0	73.3	7.2	0.0
Sultan, Delight*	1 Serving/16g	58	360	0.0	90.0	0.0	0.0
With Mixed Nuts, Hazer Baba, Delight*	1 Piece/12g	47	389	1.6	88.5	1.7	0.0
With Rose, Hazer Baba, Delight*	1 Square/18g	70	389	1.6	88.6	1.7	0.0
TURMERIC							
Powder	1 Tsp/3g	11	354	7.8	58.2	9.9	0.0
TURNIP							
Boiled, Average	1oz/28g	3	12	0.6	2.0	0.2	1.9
Raw	1oz/28g	6	23	0.9	4.7	0.3	2.4
TURNOVER							
Apple, Bramley, Tesco*	1 Turnover/88g	304	346	0.0	25.4	25.9	0.9
Apple, Dairy Cream, Safeway*	1 Turnover/91.8g	350	380	3.8	32.9	25.9	0.9
Apple, Dutch, Sainsbury's*	1 Serving/33g	130	393	3.6	56.9	16.8	1.4
Apple, Fresh Cream, Sainsbury's*	1 Turnover/84g	292	347	4.1	26.9	24.8	2.5
Apple, Tesco*	1 Turnover/88g	294	334	3.2	29.8	22.4	0.9
Mincemeat, Fresh Cream, Tesco*	1 Turnover/83g	334	405	3.1	37.5	26.9	1.1
Rasperry, Fresh Cream, Asda*	1 Cake/100g	411	411	6.0	45.0	23.0	2.1
TWIGLETS							
Curry, Jacobs*	1 Bag/30g	134	448	8.0	55.7	21.5	6.0
Original, Jacobs*	1 Bag/30g	117	390	12.0	61.3	10.8	6.8
Tangy, Jacobs*	1 Bag/30g	136	454	8.1	55.9	22.0	5.4
TWIRL							
Cadbury*	1 Finger/22g	116	525	8.1	55.9	30.1	0.0
Snack Size, Cadbury*	1 Finger/21.9g	116	525	7.0	55.3	30.9	0.0
TWIRLS							
Prawn Cocktail, Bobby's*	1 Pack/26g	116	445	3.4	65.9	18.6	0.0
Salt & Vinegar, Co-Op*	1 Bag/40g	170	425	5.0	57.5	20.0	5.0
Salt & Vinegar, Sainsbury's*	1/2 Bag/40g	167	418	3.0	70.1	14.0	3.0
Salt & Vinegar, Tesco*	1 Bag/80g	349	436	3.9	65.8	17.5	2.4
TWISTS							
Apple, Sainsbury's*	1 Serving/10g	38	375	1.7	82.7	3.0	0.1
Black Olive & Basil, Finest, Tesco*	1/4 Pack/31g	151	483	11.3	53.1	25.1	3.9
Strawberry, Sainsbury's*	1 Serving/10g	38	375	1.7	82.7	3.0	0.1
Tomato & Herb, Shapers, Boots*	1 Pack/20g	94	468	3.7	66.0	21.0	3.9
TWIX							
Fingers, Mars*	1 Bar/29g	143	494	4.6	64.8	24.1	0.0
Fun Size, Mars*	1 finger/25g	125	500	4.4	64.8	24.8	0.0
Mars*	1 Single Bar/29g	143	494	4.6	64.8	24.1	0.0
Top, Mars*	1 Bar/28g	143	511	5.2	60.2	27.7	0.0
Twixels, Mars*	1 Finger/6g	31	513	5.0	64.0	26.1	0.0
TZATZIKI							
Average	1oz/28g	18	66	3.7	2.0	4.9	0.2
Fresh, Sainsbury's*	1oz/28g	35	126	4.0	3.7	10.6	0.3
Marks & Spencer*	1oz/28g	41	145	5.6	5.9	10.9	0.4
Safeway*	1 Serving/85g	67	79	7.9	5.6	2.8	0.2
Somerfield*	1/2 Pot/85g	108	127	5.8	4.8	9.4	1.5
Tesco*	1 Serving/85g	112	132	5.1	4.9	10.2	2.2
Total*	1oz/28g	27	98	4.9	4.1	7.0	0.0
Waitrose*	1 Serving/50g	57	113	6.8	5.0	7.3	0.7

T

	Measure INFO/WEIGHT	per Measure KCAL	Nutrition Values per 100g / 100ml				
			KCAL	PROT	CARB	FAT	FIBRE

VANILLA EXTRACT

Pure, Nielsen Massey Vanillas*	1oz/28g	45	160	0.1	39.5	0.2	0.1

VEAL

Cutlet, Breaded, Marks & Spencer*	1 Serving/130g	293	225	13.6	18.7	10.7	0.4
Escalope, Fried	1oz/28g	55	196	33.7	0.0	6.8	0.0
Mince, Raw	1oz/28g	40	144	20.3	0.0	7.0	0.0

VEGEMITE

Australian, Kraft*	1 Tsp/5g	9	173	23.5	19.7	0.0	0.0
Kraft*	Thin Spread/1g	2	180	30.0	14.0	0.0	0.0

VEGETABLE ARRABBIATA

Roast, Healthy Eating, Tesco*	1 Pack/450g	437	97	3.3	18.4	1.1	1.1

VEGETABLE ESCALOPE

Indian Style, Dalepak*	1 Escalope/160g	410	256	4.3	24.3	15.7	1.6
Italian Style, Dalepak*	1 Escalope/163g	355	218	4.3	26.5	11.9	1.0

VEGETABLE FINGERS

Crispy Crunchy, Dalepak*	1 Finger/28g	62	223	4.2	26.7	11.0	15.0
Crispy, Birds Eye*	1 Finger/29g	50	171	3.8	21.0	8.0	1.2
Sweetcorn, Tesco*	1 Finger/28g	66	236	7.7	23.0	12.6	3.0
Tesco*	1 Finger/27g	73	269	4.1	24.8	17.0	2.0

VEGETABLE MEDLEY

& Carrot, Waitrose*	1/2 Pack/100g	28	28	1.5	4.7	0.4	2.2
& New Potato, Asda*	1/2 Pack/175g	102	58	2.5	7.0	2.2	5.0
Asda*	1 Serving/150g	39	26	1.9	3.0	0.7	0.0
Asparagus Tips, Perfectly Balanced, Waitrose*	1 Serving/225g	122	54	1.3	4.6	3.4	1.4
Basil & Oregano Butter, Waitrose*	1 Serving/113g	59	52	1.7	3.7	3.4	1.9
Buttered, Sainsbury's*	1/2 Pack/175g	123	70	1.7	7.0	3.9	1.8
Carrot, Courgette, Fine Bean & Baby Corn, Tesco*	1 Serving/100g	36	36	1.1	2.4	2.4	3.0
Carrots, Broccoli, Baby Corn, Sugar Snap Peas, Co-Op*	1/3 Pack/88.9g	40	45	3.0	7.0	0.8	3.0
Crunchy, Marks & Spencer*	1 Pack/250g	75	30	3.3	2.7	0.8	2.9
Green, Healthy Living, Tesco*	1 Serving/125g	59	47	3.7	4.1	1.8	4.1
Green, Sainsbury's*	1 Pack/220g	178	81	3.0	2.5	6.5	2.9
Green, Tesco*	1 Pack/250g	218	87	3.5	7.4	4.9	1.2
Mediterranean Style, Asda*	1 serving/410g	226	55	1.7	7.9	1.8	1.3
Tesco*	1 Serving/200g	52	26	1.8	3.6	0.5	2.4
Winter, Safeway*	1 Serving/250g	68	27	1.4	3.6	0.8	2.4
With Herby Butter, Marks & Spencer*	1 Pack/300g	180	60	1.4	5.2	3.6	1.5

VEGETABLE SELECTION

Baby, Tesco*	1/2 Pack/100g	25	25	1.6	3.7	0.4	1.0
Casserole, Somerfield*	1 Pack/600g	174	29	1.0	5.7	0.3	1.4
Chefs, Marks & Spencer*	1 Pack/250g	75	30	2.7	3.8	0.6	2.4
Country, Way To Five, Sainsbury's*	1/2 Pack/125g	36	29	2.1	3.7	0.6	2.2
Five, Sainsbury's*	1/2 Pack/125g	43	34	2.6	4.3	0.8	3.1
Fresh, Finest, Tesco*	1 Pack/250g	183	73	1.9	3.2	5.8	2.2
Garden, Tesco*	1 Pack/275g	124	45	1.2	2.7	3.3	1.2
Green, Fresh, Finest, Tesco*	1 Pack/250g	138	55	3.3	4.8	2.5	2.3
Marks & Spencer*	1/2 Pack/150g	105	70	1.6	6.5	4.3	2.7
Ready To Cook, Morrisons*	1 Serving/150g	51	34	2.4	4.8	0.6	2.3
Roast, COU, Marks & Spencer*	1 Serving/250g	95	38	1.2	6.1	0.8	0.6
Sainsbury's*	1oz/28g	7	25	1.9	3.0	0.6	2.2
Winter, Marks & Spencer*	1 Bag/400g	80	20	2.2	3.2	0.0	3.1
Winter, Ready to Roast, Safeway*	1/2 Pack/175g	140	80	0.8	12.4	2.7	3.5
With Chilli & Garlic Dressing, Finest, Tesco*	1 serving/250g	258	103	2.0	12.8	4.9	1.0
With Herb Butter, Waitrose*	1 Pack/300g	270	90	1.9	8.1	5.6	2.1

VEGETABLES

INFO/WEIGHT	Measure per Measure KCAL		KCAL	PROT	CARB	FAT	FIBRE
& Feta Cheese, Roasted, BGTY, Sainsbury's*	1 Pack/200g	264	132	6.4	21.7	2.2	0.0
Baby Mix, Freshly Frozen, Iceland*	1 Serving/100g	26	26	1.8	3.9	0.3	1.9
Baby, Frozen, Asda*	1 Serving/100g	25	25	1.9	3.7	0.3	1.9
Broccoli & Cauliflower, Layered, Marks & Spencer*	1/2 Pack/135g	95	70	1.5	7.6	3.4	1.2
Carrot, Broccoli & Cauliflower, Organic, Sainsbury's*	1 Serving/250g	63	25	1.9	3.0	0.6	2.2
Carrots, Broccoli & Sweetcorn, Steam Veg, Tesco*	1 serving/120g	60	50	1.8	10.6	0.1	2.4
Carrots, Cauliflower & Green Beans, Steam Veg, Tesco*	1 serving/120g	23	19	1.2	2.8	0.3	2.9
Casserole, Frozen, Morrisons*	1 Serving/150g	21	14	0.5	2.8	0.2	1.5
Casserole, Ready To Cook, Sainsbury's*	1/2 Pack/240g	74	31	0.9	6.2	0.3	1.4
Casserole, With Baby Potatoes, Marks & Spencer*	1/2 Pack/350g	140	40	1.2	7.8	0.3	2.1
Chargrilled With Tomato Sauce, GFY, Asda*	1 Serving/260g	164	63	1.4	8.0	2.8	0.0
Chinese Glazed, Tesco*	1 Pack/200g	110	55	1.3	7.7	2.2	1.2
Chinese Inspired, Crisp, Marks & Spencer*	1 Pack/250g	63	25	1.7	4.6	0.3	1.9
Chinese Water, Amoy*	1 Pack/200g	46	23	1.8	3.7	0.3	1.5
Chinese, Stir Fry, Tesco*	1 Serving/175g	49	28	2.0	4.6	0.2	1.1
Chunky, Somerfield*	1 Serving/100g	26	26	0.1	5.8	0.3	0.0
Country Mix, Easy Steam, Sainsbury's*	1 Pack/115g	35	30	1.6	4.4	0.7	3.1
Country, Way To Five, Sainsbury's*	1 Serving/250g	73	29	2.1	3.7	0.6	2.2
Crispy, Ready To Cook, Sainsbury's*	1 Serving/100g	24	24	1.8	3.6	0.3	2.2
Crispy, Tesco*	1 Pack/200g	54	27	1.9	3.9	0.4	2.3
Crudite Selection, Prepared, Marks & Spencer*	1 Serving/250g	75	30	1.4	5.8	0.4	2.0
Diamond Sliced, Ready To Cook, Waitrose*	1/2 Pack/125g	31	25	1.6	3.7	0.5	2.1
Farmhouse Mix, Frozen, Asda*	1 Serving/100g	25	25	2.5	2.2	0.8	0.0
Favourite Five Selection, Marks & Spencer*	1/2 Pack/125g	25	20	1.8	2.4	0.6	2.9
For Casserole, Ready To Cook, Sainsbury's*	1/2 Pack/217g	50	23	0.8	4.2	0.3	1.4
For Honey Chicken Pancakes, Sainsbury's*	1 Pack/92g	12	13	0.8	2.3	0.1	0.5
For Roasting, Marks & Spencer*	1/2 Pack/223.5g	190	85	1.2	7.7	5.6	2.4
Garden, Sainsbury's*	1 bag/250g	60	24	2.1	2.5	0.6	1.9
Garden, Washed, Tesco*	1 Bag/250g	65	26	3.0	1.9	0.7	2.0
Garden, With Asparagus, Way To Five, Sainsbury's*	1 Serving/230g	55	24	2.1	2.5	0.6	1.9
Green, Selection, Finest, Tesco*	1 Pack/250g	220	88	3.0	4.9	6.3	3.4
Italiano Marinated, Roasted, Tesco*	1/2 Tub/100g	121	121	1.7	9.2	8.6	0.8
Julienne, Tesco*	1 serving/100g	30	30	1.1	5.7	0.3	1.9
Layered, GFY, Asda*	1/2 Pack/150g	81	54	1.2	6.0	2.8	2.0
Layered, Marks & Spencer*	1 Serving/100g	85	85	1.6	9.1	4.5	1.8
Layered, Tesco*	1 Serving/280g	202	72	1.6	4.8	5.2	1.6
Layered, With Butter, Waitrose*	1 Pack/280g	207	74	1.7	3.6	5.8	2.4
Mediterranean Roast, Ready To Eat, Waitrose*	1 Serving/200g	128	64	1.3	5.6	4.0	1.6
Mediterranean Roasted, Sainsbury's*	1 Serving/150g	119	79	2.2	9.5	3.6	3.4
Mediterranean Style Roasting, Tesco*	1 serving/200g	72	36	1.1	5.7	1.0	1.3
Mediterranean Style Vegetables, Safeway*	1 Serving/205g	110	54	1.7	7.4	1.9	2.4
Mediterranean Style, Asda*	1/2 Pack/205g	113	55	1.7	7.9	1.8	1.3
Mediterranean Style, Finest, Tesco*	1 Serving/150g	153	102	1.9	7.3	7.2	1.2
Mediterranean Style, Marks & Spencer*	1/2 Pack/200g	170	85	2.0	9.5	4.1	1.2
Mediterranean Style, Ready to Roast, Sainsbury's*	1/2 Pack/200g	138	69	2.3	9.9	2.2	2.2
Mediterranean Style, Roasting, Tesco*	1 Serving/200g	72	36	1.1	5.7	1.0	1.3
Mediterranean Style, Somerfield*	1 Serving/200g	50	25	1.2	4.5	0.3	1.5
Mixed Crunchy, Tesco*	1 Pack/210g	63	30	1.7	5.0	0.4	2.4
Mixed, Farmhouse, Tesco*	1 Serving/100g	40	40	3.6	4.7	0.8	3.0
Moroccan, COU, Marks & Spencer*	1 Pack/300g	165	55	2.4	8.2	1.5	1.7
Oriental Inspired, Marks & Spencer*	1 Pack/260g	78	30	1.9	4.6	0.5	2.7
Oriental Stir Fry, Frozen, Sainsbury's*	1/2 Pack/225g	142	63	1.5	5.4	3.9	1.5
Oven Roasted, Somerfield*	1oz/28g	36	129	1.0	19.0	5.0	0.0

	Measure INFO/WEIGHT	per Measure KCAL	Nutrition Values per 100g / 100ml				
			KCAL	PROT	CARB	FAT	FIBRE
VEGETABLES							
Ready To Roast Mediterranean, Woolworths*	1 Punnet/660g	378	57	1.9	1.6	4.8	3.2
Roast, Marks & Spencer*	1 Pack/420g	273	65	1.4	4.9	4.2	0.4
Roasted Root, Extra Special, Asda*	1/2 Pack/205g	160	78	1.1	15.0	1.5	6.0
Roasted Winter, Healthy Living, Tesco*	1/2 Pack/200g	160	80	1.9	12.7	2.5	3.6
Roasted Winter, Tesco*	1 Serving/200g	170	85	2.2	10.0	4.0	2.0
Roasted, & Olive Sauce, TTD, Sainsbury's*	1 Serving/75g	42	56	1.7	6.9	2.4	2.0
Roasted, Italian, Marks & Spencer*	1 Serving/95g	219	230	1.8	7.1	21.0	1.7
Roasted, Selection, COU, Marks & Spencer*	1 Pack/250g	88	35	1.2	6.1	0.8	0.6
Roasting, Summer, Tesco*	1/4 of Pack/137.5g	68	49	1.3	5.6	2.4	1.6
Roasting, Tesco*	1 Serving/350g	161	46	1.0	9.4	0.5	1.0
Root, Honey Roast, BGTY, Sainsbury's*	1/2 Pack/150g	174	116	2.5	23.1	1.5	5.5
Root, Honey Roast, Sainsbury's*	1 Pack/400g	748	187	0.0	25.8	8.7	5.2
Root, Ready to Roast, Sainsbury's*	1/2 Pack/200g	188	94	1.3	13.0	4.3	2.2
Seasonal, Pack, Sainsbury's*	1 Serving/261g	60	23	0.7	4.6	0.3	2.0
Special Mix, Sainsbury's*	1 Serving/80g	54	68	3.4	9.7	1.7	3.2
Steam Fresh, Birds Eye*	1 Bag/121.2g	40	33	2.0	5.0	0.5	2.2
Steam, Tesco*	1 Serving/120g	23	19	1.1	2.3	0.6	3.6
Stew Pack, Budgens*	1 Serving/80g	32	40	0.9	8.4	0.3	1.2
Sun Dried Tomato, Selection, Finest, Tesco*	1 Pack/340g	303	89	1.8	8.9	5.1	1.1
Sweet & Crunchy, Tesco*	1 Serving/50g	22	43	2.3	7.0	0.6	2.4
Sweet Summer, Safeway*	1 Serving/115g	60	52	3.7	7.8	0.7	3.5
Szechuan Style, Ready Prepared, Waitrose*	1 Pack/300g	132	44	2.3	5.7	1.3	1.9
Vietnamese, Wok, Findus*	1 Serving/100g	25	25	1.5	4.5	0.5	0.0
Winter Crunchy, Marks & Spencer*	1/2 Pack/125g	31	25	2.0	3.1	0.8	2.7
Winter, Ready to Roast, Fresh, Sainsbury's*	1 Pack/272g	226	83	1.2	13.2	2.8	0.0
Winter, Sainsbury's*	1 Serving/125g	38	30	2.0	3.6	0.8	2.2
Winter, Tesco*	1 Pack/250g	73	29	2.0	3.3	0.8	2.6
With Sun Dried Tomato, Roasted, Finest, Tesco*	1/2 Pack/150g	153	102	1.9	7.3	7.2	1.2
Wok Classic, Findus*	1 Serving/500g	150	30	2.0	5.0	0.3	0.0
VEGETABLES IN							
Tomato Sauce, Mediterranean, Marks & Spencer*	1 Pack/300g	105	35	2.5	4.3	0.7	2.2
VEGETARIAN MINCE							
Easy Cook, Linda McCartney*	1oz/28g	35	126	21.4	9.3	0.4	1.7
Meat Free, Asda*	1oz/28g	49	176	27.0	7.0	4.4	4.1
Safeway*	1 Pack/454g	781	172	17.3	4.5	9.5	1.8
Tesco*	1 Serving/76g	116	153	18.0	7.2	5.8	6.0
Vegemince, Realeat*	1 Serving/125g	220	176	15.5	6.0	10.0	2.0
VEGETARIAN SUPREME							
With Leeks & Parsley Rice, Tesco*	1 serving/460g	469	102	3.6	16.7	2.3	0.6
VENISON							
Grill Steak, Average	1 Grillsteak/150g	179	119	19.0	5.0	2.5	1.0
Roasted	1oz/28g	46	165	35.6	0.0	2.5	0.0
Steak, Raw, Average	1oz/28g	30	108	22.8	0.0	1.9	0.0
VENISON IN							
Red Wine & Port, Average	1oz/28g	21	76	9.8	3.5	2.6	0.4
VERMICELLI							
Dry	1oz/28g	99	355	8.7	78.3	0.4	0.0
Egg, Cooked, Average	1 Serving/185g	239	129	5.0	24.0	1.4	1.0
VERMOUTH							
Dry	1 Shot/50ml	55	109	0.1	3.0	0.0	0.0
Sweet	1 Shot/50ml	76	151	0.0	15.9	0.0	0.0
VICE VERSAS							
Nestle*	1 Bag/45.6g	223	485	5.0	69.3	20.9	0.0

	Measure	per Measure	Nutrition Values per 100g / 100ml				
	INFO/WEIGHT	KCAL	KCAL	PROT	CARB	FAT	FIBRE
VIMTO*							
Cordial	1 Serving/10ml	3	30	0.0	7.4	0.0	0.0
Cordial, No Added Sugar, Diluted	1 Glass/250ml	6	2	0.1	0.4	0.1	0.0
Grape Blackcurrant & Raspberry Juice Drink	1 Bottle/500ml	223	45	0.0	11.0	0.0	0.0
VINAIGRETTE							
Balsamic Vinegar & Pistachio, Finest, Tesco*	1 Tbsp/15ml	56	370	0.2	2.8	39.2	0.0
Balsamic, Newman's Own*	1 Serving/20g	67	333	0.5	3.9	35.0	0.0
Blush Wine, Briannas*	2 Tbsp/30ml	100	333	0.0	40.0	20.0	0.0
Finest, Tesco*	1 Serving/50ml	248	495	0.9	13.2	48.7	0.5
Frank Cooper*	1 Pot/28g	46	163	1.0	14.1	11.4	0.3
French Style, Finest, Tesco*	1 Tbsp/15ml	69	461	0.8	5.9	47.4	0.2
French, Real, Briannas*	2 Tbsp/30ml	150	500	0.0	0.0	56.7	0.0
Light, Hellmann's*	1 Serving/15ml	7	49	0.0	12.2	0.0	0.2
Luxury French, Hellmann's*	1 Tsp/5ml	15	305	0.8	16.0	26.1	0.4
Newman's Own*	1/2 Tbsp/5g	17	333	0.5	3.9	35.0	0.0
Olive Oil & Lemon, Amoy*	1/2 Sachet/15ml	38	250	0.3	3.0	24.0	0.0
Perfectly Balanced, Waitrose*	1 Tsp/5ml	4	89	0.4	20.9	0.4	0.5
Portuguese, Nando's*	1 Tbsp/15g	61	409	1.0	2.1	44.0	0.3
Waistline, 99% Fat Free, Crosse & Blackwell*	1 Tbsp/15ml	1	9	1.0	0.7	0.2	0.2
With Mustard, Delhaize*	1 Serving/20g	93	464	0.8	0.7	50.9	0.0
VINE LEAVES							
Preserved in Brine	1oz/28g	4	15	3.6	0.2	0.0	0.0
Stuffed With Rice	1oz/28g	73	262	2.8	23.8	18.0	0.0
Stuffed With Rice & Mixed Herbs, Sainsbury's*	1 Leaf/36.7g	44	120	2.6	16.3	4.9	1.2
Stuffed, Marks & Spencer*	1 Vine Leaf/38.1g	40	105	2.6	14.2	4.1	1.2
VINEGAR							
Balsamic	5ml	0	3	0.3	0.6	0.0	0.0
Balsamic, Dipping Oil, Finest, Tesco*	1 Tsp/5ml	33	668	0.0	4.4	71.7	0.0
Balsamic, Marks & Spencer*	1 Tbsp/20g	24	120	0.9	29.1	0.0	0.3
Balsamic, Of Modena, Monari Federzoni*	1 Serving/5ml	3	69	0.6	16.0	0.0	0.0
Balsamic, Of Modena, TTD, Sainsbury's*	1 Tbsp/15ml	18	120	2.0	25.0	2.0	2.0
Malt	1 Tbsp/15g	1	4	0.4	0.6	0.0	0.0
Rice, White, Amoy*	1 Tsp/5ml	0	4	0.0	1.0	0.0	0.0
VODKA							
37.5% Volume	1 Shot/25ml	52	207	0.0	0.0	0.0	0.0
40% Volume	1 Shot/25ml	56	222	0.0	0.0	0.0	0.0
VOL AU VENTS							
Broccoli, Marks & Spencer*	1oz/28g	105	375	6.8	28.5	26.4	1.0
Chicken & Mushroom, Marks & Spencer*	1oz/28g	98	350	7.7	25.2	24.3	2.1
Garlic Mushroom, Mini, Asda*	1 Vol au Vent/16.7g	59	347	5.0	21.0	27.0	0.0
Ham & Cheese, Marks & Spencer*	1oz/28g	106	380	8.8	25.7	26.7	1.8
Mushroom, Marks & Spencer*	1oz/28g	94	335	6.3	24.2	23.6	1.5
Mushroom, Sainsbury's*	1 Vol Au Vent/14g	49	350	6.9	30.8	22.1	1.4
Party Seafood, Young's*	1 Vol Au Vent/17g	60	354	8.3	26.0	24.8	1.0
Prawn, Marks & Spencer*	1oz/28g	101	360	8.0	26.2	24.7	1.9
Tomato, Marks & Spencer*	1oz/28g	87	310	4.5	26.7	20.4	1.7

	Measure INFO/WEIGHT	per Measure KCAL	Nutrition Values per 100g / 100ml				
			KCAL	PROT	CARB	FAT	FIBRE
WAFERS							
Apricot & Peach, Highlights, Cadbury*	1 Wafer/19g	80	430	5.2	70.6	14.3	1.4
Cafe Curls, Rolled, Askeys*	1 Curl/5g	21	422	5.8	80.3	8.6	0.0
Cannoli, Sainsbury's*	1 Biscuit/9g	45	496	3.5	71.0	22.0	0.0
Caramel, Dark Chocolate, Tunnock's*	1 Wafer/26g	128	492	5.2	60.7	25.4	0.0
Caramel, Marks & Spencer*	1oz/28g	136	486	5.4	63.1	23.5	0.5
Caramel, Milk Chocolate, Marks & Spencer*	1oz/28g	133	475	5.9	61.9	22.8	3.1
Caramel, Tunnock's*	1 Biscuit/26g	118	454	4.6	68.0	20.1	0.0
Caramel, Value, Tesco*	1 Wafer/23.1g	102	443	4.6	64.0	18.7	0.9
Chocolate Curl, Mini, Marks & Spencer*	1 Biscuit/5g	28	550	5.8	56.0	33.6	1.5
Chocolate Mint, Plain, Somerfield*	1oz/28g	151	538	9.0	56.0	31.0	0.0
Chocolate, Cadbury*	1oz/28g	147	526	7.0	61.2	29.8	0.0
Cornets, Askeys*	1 Serving/4g	13	325	10.0	65.0	2.5	2.5
Filled	1oz/28g	150	535	4.7	66.0	29.9	0.0
Ice Cream, Askeys*	2 Wafers/3g	12	388	11.4	79.0	2.9	0.0
Milk Chocolate, Sainsbury's*	1 Biscuit/10g	51	506	6.2	60.5	26.7	1.4
Orange Break, Somerfield*	1oz/28g	149	531	8.0	57.0	30.0	0.0
Orange, Highlights, Cadbury*	1 Wafer/19g	80	430	5.2	70.6	14.3	1.4
Raspberry, Highlights, Cadbury*	1 Wafer/19g	80	430	5.2	70.6	14.3	1.5
WAFFLES							
Bacon Flavour, BFY, Morrisons*	1 Bag/12g	40	333	6.7	80.0	1.7	2.5
Barbecue Flavour, American Style, Shapers, Boots*	1 Pack/20g	95	476	4.5	65.0	22.0	3.7
Caramel, The Big Cereal Company*	1 Serving/23g	84	367	7.5	80.1	1.9	2.8
Cheese & Onion, Marks & Spencer*	1 Pack/50g	253	505	5.1	56.0	28.7	2.6
Ready Salted, Marks & Spencer*	1 Bag/40g	194	485	2.1	65.6	23.6	1.6
Smokey Bacon, BGTY, Sainsbury's*	1 Bag/12g	41	344	5.6	76.3	1.8	1.5
Sweet, American Style, Sainsbury's*	1 Waffle/35.0g	153	437	9.5	51.5	21.4	3.3
Toasting, McVitie's*	1 Waffle/23g	108	469	5.9	53.9	25.6	0.9
WAGON WHEEL							
Burton's*	1 Wheel/36g	159	441	4.9	67.3	16.9	1.3
Chocolate, Burton's*	1 Wheel/39g	164	420	5.4	67.3	14.8	2.2
WALNUT WHIP							
The Classic, Marks & Spencer*	1 Whip/26g	127	490	7.2	54.9	27.4	1.1
Vanilla, Nestle*	1 Whip/34g	160	486	5.7	60.5	24.6	0.0
WALNUTS							
Average	6 Halves/20g	138	691	15.6	3.2	68.5	3.5
Halves, Average	1 Serving/25g	167	669	17.4	6.3	65.0	4.7
WATER							
Blackcurrant Flavour, Still, Danone*	1 Serving/120ml	25	21	0.0	5.0	0.0	0.0
Elderflower Presse, Bottle Green*	1 Serving/250ml	88	35	0.0	8.9	0.0	0.0
Grapefruit Flavoured, Balanced Lifestyle, Aldi*	1 Serving/100ml	2	2	0.1	0.4	0.0	0.1
Mandarin & Cranberry, Still, Marks & Spencer*	1 Bottle/500ml	100	20	0.0	5.0	0.0	0.0
Mineral Or Tap	1 Glass/200ml	0	0	0.0	0.0	0.0	0.0
Mineral, Apple & Elderflower, Hedgerow*	1 Serving/250ml	85	34	0.0	8.2	0.0	0.0
Mineral, Energy, Vittel*	1fl oz/30ml	7	23	0.0	5.5	0.0	0.0
Peach & Lemon, Still, Marks & Spencer*	1 Bottle/500ml	100	20	0.0	5.0	0.0	0.0
Sparkling, Fruit, Aqua Libra*	1 Glass/200ml	54	27	0.0	5.1	0.0	0.0
Spring Peach, Safeway*	1 Bottle/500ml	10	2	0.1	0.2	0.1	0.1
Spring, Apple & Blackcurrant, Hadrian*	1 Bottle/365ml	3	1	0.1	0.1	0.0	0.0
Spring, Apple & Cherry Flavoured, Sparkling, Sainsbury's*	1 Glass/250ml	5	2	0.1	0.2	0.1	0.1
Spring, Apple & Raspberry, Sparkling, Tesco*	1 Tall Glass/330ml	7	2	0.0	0.5	0.0	0.0
Spring, Blackberry & Blueberry Flavoured, Sainsbury's*	1 Serving/1000ml	20	2	0.1	0.2	0.1	0.1
Spring, Elderflower & Pear, Sainsbury's*	1 Glass/250g	5	2	0.1	0.2	0.1	0.1
Spring, Lemon & Lime Flavoured, Sparkling, Sainsbury's*	1 Lge Bottle/1000ml	17	2	0.1	0.1	0.1	0.1

W

	Measure INFO/WEIGHT	per Measure KCAL	Nutrition Values per 100g / 100ml				
			KCAL	PROT	CARB	FAT	FIBRE
WATER							
Spring, Peach Flavoured, Sainsbury's*	1 Glass/250ml	5	2	0.1	0.2	0.1	0.1
Spring, Raspberry & Cranberry, Shapers, Boots*	1 Bottle/500ml	10	2	0.0	0.5	0.0	0.0
Spring, Stawberry & Vanilla, Sainsbury's*	1 Glass/250ml	5	2	0.1	0.2	0.1	0.1
Spring, Strawberry & Aloe Vera, Marks & Spencer*	1 Bottle/500ml	5	1	0.0	0.2	0.0	0.0
Spring, White Grape & Blackberry, Tesco*	1 Glass/200ml	4	2	0.0	0.5	0.0	0.0
Spring, Wild Berries, The Simpsons*	1oz/28g	0	1	0.0	0.0	0.0	0.0
Spring, With Cranberry, Tesco*	1 Glass/250ml	3	1	0.0	0.3	0.0	0.0
WATER CHESTNUTS							
Raw, Average	1oz/28g	10	34	1.0	7.8	0.1	0.1
With Bamboo Shoots, Sainsbury's*	1 Serving/50g	29	58	2.0	12.0	0.2	1.1
WATER ICE							
Fruit, Iceland*	1 Lolly/75ml	74	98	0.2	24.4	0.0	0.2
Orange, Iceland*	1 Ice/75ml	73	98	0.2	24.4	0.0	0.2
Pineapple, Iceland*	1 Ice/75ml	65	86	0.0	21.5	0.0	0.2
Raspberry, Iceland*	1 Ice/75ml	67	89	0.0	22.2	0.0	0.2
WATERCRESS							
& Creme Fraiche Sauce, COU, Marks & Spencer*	1/2 Pack/153.8g	100	65	3.2	9.2	1.8	0.5
Raw, Average	1oz/28g	6	23	3.0	0.4	1.0	1.5
WATERMELON							
Average	1 Serving/250g	75	30	0.4	7.0	0.3	0.4
WHEAT							
Ebly*	1oz/28g	98	351	12.1	71.9	1.7	5.4
WHEAT CRUNCHIES							
Bacon, Crispy, Golden Wonder*	1 Bag/35g	172	492	9.7	56.0	25.5	3.9
Golden Wonder*	1 Pack/35g	172	491	11.1	55.9	24.8	0.0
Salt & Vinegar, Golden Wonder*	1 Bag/34g	165	484	10.5	54.5	24.9	2.8
Spicy Tomato, Golden Wonder*	1 Bag/35g	172	491	9.4	56.0	25.5	3.9
Worcester Sauce, Golden Wonder*	1 Bag/35g	172	492	9.3	56.4	25.5	3.9
WHEATGERM							
Average	1oz/28g	100	357	26.7	44.7	9.2	15.6
WHELKS							
Boiled	1oz/28g	25	89	19.5	0.0	1.2	0.0
WHIPS							
Double Chocolate, Marks & Spencer*	1 Whip/28.9g	141	485	6.6	57.8	25.3	1.0
WHISKEY							
37.5% Volume	1 Shot/25ml	52	207	0.0	0.0	0.0	0.0
40% Volume	1 Shot/25ml	56	222	0.0	0.0	0.0	0.0
Jack Daniels*	1 Shot/25ml	56	222	0.0	0.0	0.0	0.0
Teacher's*	1 Shot/25ml	56	222	0.0	0.0	0.0	0.0
WHISKY							
Scotch, 37.5% Volume	1 Shot/25ml	52	207	0.0	0.0	0.0	0.0
Scotch, 40% Volume	1 Shot/25ml	56	222	0.0	0.0	0.0	0.0
WHITE PUDDING							
Average	1oz/28g	126	450	7.0	36.3	31.8	0.0
WHITEBAIT							
In Flour, Fried	1oz/28g	147	525	19.5	5.3	47.5	0.2
WHITECURRANTS							
Raw	1oz/28g	7	26	1.3	5.6	0.0	3.4
WHITING							
In Crumbs, Fried in Blended Oil	1 Serving/180g	344	191	18.1	7.0	10.3	0.2
Raw	1oz/28g	23	81	18.7	0.0	0.7	0.0
Steamed	1 Serving/85g	78	92	20.9	0.0	0.9	0.0

	Measure INFO/WEIGHT	per Measure KCAL	Nutrition Values per 100g / 100ml				
			KCAL	PROT	CARB	FAT	FIBRE
WIENER SCHNITZEL							
Average	1oz/28g	62	223	20.9	13.1	10.0	0.4
WINDERS							
Real Fruit, Kellogg's*	1 Serving/18g	67	370	0.5	77.0	7.0	3.0
WINE							
Mulled, Homemade	1 Glass/120ml	227	196	0.1	25.2	0.0	0.0
Mulled, Sainsbury's*	1 Serving/125ml	113	90	0.0	8.6	0.0	0.0
Red	1 Glass/120ml	80	68	0.1	0.2	0.0	0.0
Rose, Medium,	1 Glass/120ml	83	71	0.1	2.5	0.0	0.0
Sparkling, Alcohol Free, Sainsbury's*	1 Glass/175ml	35	20	0.0	4.9	0.0	0.0
Strong Ale Barley	1 Can/440ml	290	66	0.7	6.1	0.0	0.0
White, Dry	1 Glass/120ml	77	66	0.1	0.6	0.0	0.0
White, Medium	1 Glass/120ml	87	74	0.1	3.0	0.0	0.0
White, Non Alcoholic, Ame*	1 Glass/120ml	46	38	0.0	9.5	0.0	0.0
White, Sparkling	1 Glass/120ml	87	74	0.3	5.1	0.0	0.0
White, Sweet	1 Glass/120ml	110	94	0.2	5.9	0.0	0.0
WINE GUMS							
Marks & Spencer*	1oz/28g	60	214	2.9	54.3	0.0	0.0
Maynards*	1 Sweet/5g	17	331	6.0	76.6	0.0	0.0
Mini, Co-Op*	1 Sweet/2g	7	330	6.0	76.0	0.1	0.0
Mini, Rowntree's*	1 Sm Bag/36g	125	348	6.7	80.5	0.0	0.0
SmartPrice, Asda*	1 Sweet/6.0g	20	332	4.0	79.0	0.0	0.0
Sour, Bassett's*	1/4 Bag/50g	160	319	3.7	78.0	0.0	0.0
Tesco*	1 Serving/100g	316	316	7.7	70.7	0.2	0.1
WINKLES							
Boiled	1oz/28g	20	72	15.4	0.0	1.2	0.0
WISPA							
Bite, With Biscuit In Caramel, Cadbury*	1 Bar/47g	240	510	6.4	56.9	28.6	0.0
Cadbury*	1 Treatsize/15g	83	550	7.1	53.9	34.2	0.0
Gold, Cadbury*	1 Bar/52g	263	505	5.7	57.0	28.0	0.0
Mint, Cadbury*	1 Bar/50g	275	550	7.0	54.7	33.6	0.0
WOK							
Chinese, Findus*	1 Serving/250g	113	45	1.5	9.5	0.2	0.0
Classic, Findus*	1 Serving/250g	113	45	2.0	7.5	0.5	0.0
Sambal Oelek, Findus*	1 Serving/200g	170	85	3.0	17.0	0.4	0.0
Thai, Findus*	1/2 Pack/250g	88	35	1.5	7.0	0.3	0.0
WONTON							
Chicken, Asda*	1 Wonton/15g	46	306	14.0	18.0	20.0	1.9
Chinese Prawn, Sainsbury's*	1 Wonton/16g	38	252	11.9	16.5	15.4	1.2
Prawn, Dim Sum Selection, Sainsbury's*	1 Wonton/10g	26	259	11.3	26.8	11.8	1.3
Prawn, Oriental Selection, Waitrose*	1 Wonton/17.9g	45	252	9.1	29.2	11.0	1.1
Prawn, Oriental Snack Selection, Sainsbury's*	1 Wonton/20g	53	265	10.6	25.6	13.4	2.0
WOTSITS							
BBQ, Walkers*	1 Bag/21g	109	521	7.2	55.8	29.9	1.2
Cheesy Wafflers, Walkers*	1 Bag/31g	160	515	6.5	50.0	32.0	1.3
Cheesy, Walkers*	1 Pack/19g	101	530	6.0	55.0	32.0	1.0
Flamin' Hot, Walkers*	1 Pack/19g	99	520	5.0	57.0	30.0	1.2
Mild Cheese, Walkers*	1 Serving/19.1g	102	535	6.0	54.0	33.0	1.0
Prawn Cocktail, Walkers*	1 Pack/21g	109	520	5.5	55.0	31.0	1.1
WRAP							
All Day Breakfast, Marks & Spencer*	1 Pack/196g	529	270	10.8	21.2	16.0	1.4
American Deli, Shapers, Boots*	1 Pack/171.7g	249	145	9.5	21.0	2.6	2.0
Aromatic Duck, Safeway*	1 Pack/180g	376	209	9.1	21.3	9.7	1.6
BBQ Chicken, Shapers, Boots*	1 Serving/165.4g	267	162	10.0	25.0	2.3	1.2

W

WRAP

	INFO/WEIGHT	KCAL	KCAL	PROT	CARB	FAT	FIBRE
BBQ Chicken, Tesco*	1 Wrap/215g	389	181	10.4	23.6	5.0	2.6
BBQ Steak, Marks & Spencer*	1 Pack/253g	506	200	10.6	24.8	6.8	1.8
Beef in Black Bean, Marks & Spencer*	1 Pack/150g	338	225	10.2	20.5	11.4	1.6
Brie & Cranberry, Marks & Spencer*	1 Pack/224.5g	549	245	6.1	27.3	12.4	1.7
Cajun Chicken Louisiana Style, Sainsbury's*	1 Pack/190g	395	209	11.1	23.9	7.6	0.0
Cajun Chicken Pizzatilla, Marks & Spencer*	1 Pack/240.4g	564	235	10.0	25.8	10.4	2.2
Cajun Chicken, King- Keele University, Sandwich King*	1 Pack/138.2g	386	279	12.3	25.1	14.4	0.0
Cajun, GFY, Asda*	1 Pack/176.3g	231	131	9.0	21.0	1.2	0.9
Chargrilled Chicken, Perfectly Balanced, Waitrose*	1 Pack/230g	361	157	10.3	22.7	2.9	2.9
Cheese & Bean, Tesco*	1 Pack/105g	235	224	7.0	28.6	9.0	1.0
Cheese, Pickle & Ham, Sainsbury's*	1 Pack/237.9g	614	258	11.8	22.3	13.5	0.0
Cheestring & Ham, Attack-a-Snak, Golden Vale*	1 Pack/109.9g	266	242	13.4	28.0	8.2	1.4
Chicken & Bacon Caesar Salad, Asda*	1 Pack/160g	565	353	18.0	20.8	22.0	0.9
Chicken & Bacon, Simple Solutions, Tesco*	1 Pack/300g	474	158	20.7	1.2	7.8	0.5
Chicken & Cous Cous, BGTY, Sainsbury's*	1 Pack/230g	359	156	8.8	21.5	3.9	0.0
Chicken & Cous Cous, Moroccan Inspired, Sainsbury's*	1 Serving/212g	420	198	8.7	31.0	4.4	2.2
Chicken Caesar, Boots*	1 Pack/160.4g	254	159	13.0	22.0	2.1	2.0
Chicken Caesar, Good Intentions, Somerfield*	1 Pack/184g	357	194	13.0	25.7	4.3	1.1
Chicken Caesar, Healthy Living, Tesco*	1 Pack/200g	296	148	10.2	22.3	2.0	2.2
Chicken Caesar, Marks & Spencer*	1 Pack/225g	575	255	9.5	22.5	14.3	1.5
Chicken Caesar, Menu, Boots*	1 Pack/225.8g	551	244	11.0	23.0	12.0	1.3
Chicken Caesar, Tesco*	1 Wrap/100g	224	224	10.4	24.3	9.4	1.6
Chicken Fajita Red, Yellow Peppers, Weight Watchers*	1 Pack/177g	297	168	9.0	24.7	3.7	1.7
Chicken Fajita, Asda*	1 Pack/180g	369	205	9.4	20.6	9.4	0.4
Chicken Fajita, Finest, Tesco*	1 Pack/213g	422	198	9.0	24.0	7.3	1.9
Chicken Fajita, Perfectly Balanced, Waitrose*	1 Serving/218g	368	169	10.5	26.0	2.6	1.9
Chicken Fajita, Shapers, Boots*	1 Pack/201.3g	302	150	11.0	21.0	2.6	1.8
Chicken Fajita, Tesco*	1 Pack/220g	383	174	9.3	22.3	5.3	1.9
Chicken Fillet With Cheese & Bacon, Asda*	1 Pack/164.1g	366	223	25.0	1.4	13.0	0.0
Chicken Jalfrezi, Boots*	1 Pack/215g	456	212	8.6	28.0	7.3	1.7
Chicken Korma, Patak's*	1 Pack/150g	294	196	7.6	20.0	9.5	0.0
Chicken Louisiana, Benedicts*	1 Pack/250g	410	164	13.4	24.2	2.2	0.0
Chicken Salad, Roast, Sainsbury's*	1 Serving/220g	497	226	10.4	23.2	10.2	1.6
Chicken Salad, Sainsbury's*	1 Pack/211.0g	519	246	10.2	21.6	13.2	0.0
Chicken Salsa, Healthy Living, Tesco*	1 Pack/240g	350	146	8.5	21.4	3.0	1.9
Chicken Salsa, Taste!*	1 Pack/175.3g	298	170	4.8	22.9	6.6	0.0
Chicken Southern Style, Ginsters*	1 Pack/150g	290	193	9.5	25.1	6.4	0.8
Chicken Sweet & Sour, Ginsters*	1 Pack/150g	378	252	13.4	40.8	3.9	2.4
Chicken Thai Style, Boots*	1 Pack/156g	290	186	11.0	21.0	6.4	2.2
Chicken Tikka Masala, Patak's*	1 Pack/150g	252	168	7.8	19.3	6.6	0.0
Chicken Tikka, Finest, Tesco*	1 Wrap/227g	402	177	5.1	24.9	6.3	2.0
Chicken Tikka, French Cuisiniers*	1 Pack/130.0g	185	142	15.4	18.3	1.3	1.5
Chicken Tikka, Ginsters*	1 Pack/150g	278	185	8.9	25.5	5.3	1.6
Chicken Tikka, Healthy Living, Tesco*	1 Pack/206g	317	154	11.3	22.1	2.3	1.3
Chicken Tikka, Mattessons*	1 Pack/150g	284	189	9.8	21.5	7.0	3.2
Chicken With Stilton & Pear, Sainsbury's*	1 Serving/150g	264	176	25.4	2.1	7.3	0.1
Chicken, Cheddar & Peppers, Cajun, Sainsbury's*	1 Pack/242g	535	221	10.4	19.8	11.0	2.1
Chicken, Eat Smart, Safeway*	1 Pack/153g	230	150	12.5	19.7	1.9	2.0
Chicken, Louisiana Style, GFY, Asda*	1 Pack/195g	355	182	11.0	31.0	1.5	2.0
Chicken, Marks & Spencer*	1 Pack/246.5g	531	215	8.2	23.4	10.1	1.6
Chicken, Meditteranean Style, Waitrose*	1 Pack/182.7g	296	162	8.3	18.6	6.0	2.3
Chicken, Mexican Style, Good Intentions, Somerfield*	1 Pack/220g	387	176	8.3	26.0	4.3	1.4
Chicken, Moroccan, BGTY, Sainsbury's*	1 Pack/207.2g	315	152	9.4	25.3	1.5	0.0

WRAP

INFO/WEIGHT	Measure per Measure KCAL	Nutrition Values per 100g / 100ml KCAL	PROT	CARB	FAT	FIBRE
Chicken, Morrocan, Shapers, Boots*	1 Serving/154g	271	176	9.6	26.0	3.7	1.7
Chicken, Southern Fried, Tesco*	1 Serving/225g	590	262	8.0	23.6	15.1	1.7
Chicken, Tandoori Style, Good Intentions, Somerfield*	1 Pack/175g	299	171	10.9	28.8	1.4	1.6
Chicken, Tasties*	1 Pack/148.6g	325	218	11.7	26.5	7.1	0.0
Chilli Beef, COU, Marks & Spencer*	1 Pack/179g	269	150	10.1	23.4	1.6	2.6
Chilli Beef, Co-Op*	1 Pack/163g	310	190	10.0	26.0	6.0	2.0
Chilli Chicken, BGTY, Sainsbury's*	1 Pack/180g	313	174	10.2	28.0	2.4	0.0
Chinese Chicken, Asda*	1 Pack/200g	404	202	9.0	28.0	6.0	0.0
Chinese Chicken, Marks & Spencer*	1 Pack/155g	239	154	14.0	22.3	1.0	2.0
Coronation Chicken, Waitrose*	1 Pack/163.6g	284	173	10.1	21.3	5.1	2.2
Cous Cous, Moroccan Style, Tesco*	1 Serving/240g	370	154	5.3	27.3	2.7	1.3
Dhansak Prawn, Marks & Spencer*	1 Pack/208.1g	385	185	7.1	23.3	7.2	2.4
Duck, Food To Go, Marks & Spencer*	1 Pack/257g	474	185	8.5	25.5	5.4	1.0
Duck, Hoi Sin, Delicious, Boots*	1 Pack/214g	393	184	10.0	25.0	5.1	1.8
Egg & Cress, Sainsbury's*	1 Pack/247g	543	220	8.4	19.3	12.1	0.0
Egg Mayonnaise, Tomato & Cress, Sainsbury's*	1 Pack/255g	592	232	7.3	17.7	15.0	0.0
Feta Cheese Flat Bread, COU, Marks & Spencer*	1 Pack/180g	225	125	6.3	20.6	2.2	1.9
Feta Cheese, GFY, Asda*	1 Pack/165g	256	155	7.0	22.0	4.3	2.1
Fiery Mexican Cheese, Ginsters*	1 Pack/150g	291	194	7.4	25.0	7.3	1.8
Goats Cheese & Tomato, TTD, Sainsbury's*	1 Pack/204g	420	206	7.0	25.6	8.4	0.0
Goats Cheese, & Grilled Pepper, Asda*	1 Wrap/75g	194	259	5.0	26.0	15.0	2.1
Greek Feta Salad, Shapers, Boots*	1 pack/157.5g	242	153	6.4	24.0	3.6	1.2
Greek Feta, Tortilla, Shapers, Boots*	1 Pack/169.4g	270	160	6.7	27.0	2.7	1.6
Greek Salad, COU, Marks & Spencer*	1 Pack/180g	288	160	6.0	27.2	2.7	2.3
Greek Salad, Marks & Spencer*	1 Pack/178.6g	251	140	8.1	21.5	2.5	1.0
Greek Salad, Sainsbury's*	1 Pack/167g	242	145	6.7	21.2	3.7	1.8
Green Thai Chicken, Sainsbury's*	1 Pack/212g	481	227	8.8	24.3	10.5	1.6
Green Thai Chicken, Tortilla, Shapers, Boots*	1 Pack/175.5g	278	159	13.0	21.0	2.6	1.4
Green Thai Prawn, BGTY, Sainsbury's*	1 Pack/200g	237	119	7.0	19.2	1.5	1.5
Gressingham Duck & Hoi Sin Sauce, TTD, Sainsbury's*	1 Pack/199g	354	178	9.3	24.8	4.6	0.0
Ham, Cheese & Pickle Tortilla, Weight Watchers*	1 Pack/170.1g	296	174	10.9	26.4	2.8	1.2
Ham, Cheese & Pickle, Sainsbury's*	1 Pack/195g	503	258	11.9	24.4	12.5	3.6
Hoisin Duck, Marks & Spencer*	1 Serving/236.1g	425	180	7.7	24.6	5.8	1.9
Hoisin Duck, Tesco*	1 Serving/222g	424	191	7.4	24.6	7.0	0.8
Houmous, Taste!*	1 Pack/170.2g	291	171	5.4	26.4	4.9	0.0
Italian Chicken, Just Cook, Sainsbury's*	1 Pack/225g	329	146	16.7	3.5	7.2	0.7
Italian Chicken, Sainsbury's*	1/2 Pack/211g	395	187	15.7	6.2	11.0	0.9
King Prawn, Shapers, Boots*	1 Pack/154.4g	226	147	9.2	24.0	1.4	2.1
Mexican Bean & Potato In Spinach Tortilla, Daily Bread*	1 Pack/195.8g	329	168	4.9	25.0	5.4	0.0
Mexican Bean, BGTY, Sainsbury's*	1 Pack/216g	330	153	9.3	25.1	2.6	2.9
Mexican Bean, GFY, Asda*	1 Pack/173g	303	175	5.0	31.0	3.4	2.3
Mexican Chicken, Marks & Spencer*	1 Serving/218g	447	205	8.6	19.7	10.3	1.3
Mexican Sweet Potato & Three Bean, Marks & Spencer*	1 Pack/222g	522	235	7.6	26.4	11.0	1.4
Mexican Three Bean, Marks & Spencer*	1 Pack/246.8g	580	235	7.6	26.4	11.0	1.4
Mild Chicken Curry, Patak's*	1 Pack/150g	239	159	8.1	21.3	6.0	2.8
Monterey Jack & Ham, Tesco*	1 Pack/200g	522	261	7.9	25.9	14.1	0.2
Nacho Chicken, COU, Marks & Spencer*	1 Pack/181.5g	246	136	9.6	19.7	2.1	1.4
Nacho Chicken, Marks & Spencer*	1 pack/181.5g	244	135	9.6	19.7	2.1	1.4
Peking Duck, Asda*	1 Pack/172g	427	248	9.4	28.5	10.7	1.1
Peking Duck, Boots*	1 Pack/229g	440	192	8.3	30.0	4.3	2.6
Peking Duck, Finest, Tesco*	1 Pack/200g	378	189	8.4	29.5	4.2	0.3
Peking Duck, Shapers, Boots*	1 Pack/161.6g	258	159	9.1	28.0	1.1	1.6
Pepperoni, Tesco*	1 Pack/153g	271	177	6.4	26.9	4.9	1.4

	Measure	per Measure	Nutrition Values per 100g / 100ml				
	INFO/WEIGHT	KCAL	KCAL	PROT	CARB	FAT	FIBRE
WRAP							
Plain Tortilla, Morrisons*	1 Pack/35g	84	240	6.8	45.8	3.8	1.9
Pork Caribbean Spicy, Ginsters*	1 Pack/150g	396	264	11.3	34.1	9.1	2.3
Red Thai Chicken, BGTY, Sainsbury's*	1 Pack/194g	384	198	11.3	29.3	3.9	1.0
Red Thai Chicken, Shapers, Boots*	1 Pack/158g	254	161	12.0	22.0	2.6	1.4
Red Thai Prawns, Somerfield*	1oz/28g	81	288	10.0	20.0	19.0	0.0
Roasted Vegetable & Feta, BGTY, Sainsbury's*	1 Serving/200g	318	159	5.8	25.0	4.0	0.0
Sausage & Bacon, Asda*	1 Pack/21g	52	249	18.0	15.0	13.0	0.5
Smoked Salmon & Prawn, Finest, Tesco*	1 Serving/58.5g	84	143	14.3	1.0	9.1	0.0
Smoked Salmon, Finest, Tesco*	1 Pack/58g	113	194	15.5	0.6	14.4	0.3
Soft Cheese & Spinach, To Go*	1 Serving/250g	278	111	4.5	17.4	2.7	0.0
Sushi Salmon & Cucumber, Waitrose*	1 Pack/180g	299	166	6.3	27.2	3.6	1.6
Sweet & Sour Prawn, Eat Smart, Safeway*	1 Pack/204g	275	135	6.4	24.0	1.2	1.4
Sweet Chili Chicken, Waitrose*	1 Wrap/200g	390	195	10.3	22.0	7.4	2.4
Sweet Chilli Chicken, Shapers, Boots*	1 Serving/178.9g	315	176	12.0	27.0	2.2	2.0
Sweet Chilli Noodle, Sainsbury's*	1 Pack/210g	399	190	10.6	26.1	4.8	2.1
Tandoori Chicken, GFY, Asda*	1 Pack/167g	281	168	10.0	26.0	2.7	1.7
Thai Prawn, COU, Marks & Spencer*	1 Pack/181g	235	130	8.3	20.4	1.6	1.9
Tomato & Chilli, Discovery*	1 Pack/55.9g	161	288	7.9	53.5	5.9	2.5
Tortilla, Chicken, Asda*	1 Pack/125g	253	202	9.6	36.9	1.8	3.3
Tortilla, Vegetable, Asda*	1 Pack/125g	245	196	6.8	37.2	2.2	0.8
Tuna Nicoise, BGTY, Sainsbury's*	1 Pack/181g	273	151	11.0	18.0	3.9	0.0
Tuna Nicoise, Healthy Eating, Tesco*	1 Pack/117g	160	137	8.3	20.6	2.3	0.5
Tuna Salsa, Healthy Eating, Wild Bean Cafe*	1 Pack/159g	245	154	11.3	23.5	1.7	1.5
Tuna, Sweetcorn & Red Pepper, BGTY, Sainsbury's*	1 Pack/178g	306	172	11.5	21.2	4.6	2.1
Turkey, Bacon & Cranberry, COU, Marks & Spencer*	1 Pack/143.8g	230	160	9.6	27.1	1.5	2.3
WRAP KIT							
Chapatis Bread, Tikka Masala, Patak's*	1 Bread/42.2g	121	287	7.5	53.1	6.4	3.2
Moroccan Style, Sainsbury's*	1 Wrap/62g	205	332	8.0	41.1	15.1	3.6

	Measure INFO/WEIGHT	per Measure KCAL	Nutrition Values per 100g / 100ml				
			KCAL	PROT	CARB	FAT	FIBRE
YAM							
Baked	1oz/28g	43	153	2.1	37.5	0.4	1.7
Boiled, Average	1oz/28g	37	133	1.7	33.0	0.3	1.4
Raw	1oz/28g	32	114	1.5	28.2	0.3	1.3
YEAST							
Bakers, Compressed	1oz/28g	15	53	11.4	1.1	0.4	0.0
Dried	1oz/28g	47	169	35.6	3.5	1.5	0.0
Extract	1 Tsp/9g	16	180	40.7	3.5	0.4	0.0
YOGHURT							
0.1%fat, Lidl*	1 Pot/150g	119	79	4.0	15.6	0.1	0.0
Adore Vanilla With Choc Flakes, Ehrmann*	1 Pot/150g	215	143	3.1	17.0	7.0	0.0
Apple & Blackberry, Bio, Sainsbury's*	1 Pot/125g	134	107	4.1	16.6	2.7	0.2
Apple & Blackberry, Custard Style, Co-Op*	1 Pot/150g	195	130	3.7	15.9	5.3	0.1
Apple & Blackberry, Deep Fill Fruit, Ski*	1 Pot/160g	139	87	4.0	14.2	1.6	0.0
Apple & Blackberry, Organic, Yeo Valley*	1 Pot/125g	121	97	4.3	12.5	3.3	0.1
Apple & Cinnamon Crumble, Ski*	1 Pot/125g	151	121	3.8	19.6	3.0	0.0
Apple & Cinnamon, COU, Marks & Spencer*	1 Pot/150g	68	45	4.2	6.1	0.1	0.2
Apple & Cinnamon, Dessert, Low Fat, Sainsbury's*	1 Pot/125g	115	92	4.5	14.7	1.7	0.1
Apple & Cinnamon, Tine Jubileum*	1 Carton/125g	166	133	3.2	18.5	5.2	0.0
Apple & Cranberry, Bio Fruit, Shape*	1 Pot/175g	130	74	4.5	13.8	0.1	0.0
Apple & Cranberry, Fat Free, Bio Fruit, Shape, Danone*	1 Pot/120g	85	71	4.3	13.2	0.1	0.1
Apple & Custard, Low Fat, Sainsbury's*	1 Pot/125g	116	93	4.3	15.5	1.5	0.2
Apple & Pear, Low Fat, Sainsbury's*	1 Pot/125g	115	92	4.3	15.2	1.5	0.2
Apple & Prune, Fat Free, Yeo Valley*	1 Pot/125g	98	78	5.1	14.1	0.1	0.2
Apple & Spice Bio, Virtually Fat Free, Shape*	1 Pot/120g	67	56	5.6	7.3	0.1	0.2
Apple Custard & Crumble, Muller*	1 Pot/190g	287	151	11.6	17.7	3.7	0.0
Apple Danish Fruit Pudding Style, Healthy Eating, Tesco*	1 Pot/125g	99	79	4.1	14.1	0.7	0.2
Apple Strude, Custard Style, Shape, St Ivel*	1 Pot/100g	58	58	4.1	7.9	0.8	0.2
Apple, Light, Muller*	1 Pot/200g	108	54	4.4	9.0	0.1	0.0
Apricot & Mango Tropical Fruit, Ski*	1 Pot/125g	124	99	4.9	15.7	1.9	0.2
Apricot & Mango, 25% Extra Fruit, Low Fat, Asda*	1 Pot/125g	120	96	4.6	17.0	1.1	0.0
Apricot & Mango, Best There Is, Yoplait*	1 Pot/125g	130	104	4.7	17.4	1.6	0.0
Apricot & Mango, Low Fat, Tesco*	1 Pot/125g	126	101	4.9	16.3	1.8	0.0
Apricot & Mango, Thick & Creamy, Sainsbury's*	1 Pot/150g	179	119	4.3	17.3	3.6	0.2
Apricot & Nectarine, Healthy Eating, Tesco*	1 Pot/175g	79	45	2.1	8.9	0.1	0.3
Apricot & Nectarine, Sunshine Selection, Sainsbury's*	1 Pot/125g	115	92	4.4	15.3	1.5	0.1
Apricot & Passion Fruit, Fat Free, Yeo Valley*	1 Pot/125g	95	76	5.2	13.6	0.1	0.1
Apricot & Peach, Healthy Living, Tesco*	1 Pot/200g	82	41	3.9	6.2	0.1	1.0
Apricot Bio, Healthy Eating, Tesco*	1 Pot/125g	58	46	4.2	7.1	0.1	0.0
Apricot Tart Style, Sveltesse, Nestle*	1 Pot/125g	98	78	4.8	14.2	0.2	0.1
Apricot, Custard Style, Shapers, Boots*	1 Pot/146g	82	56	3.9	8.3	0.8	0.2
Apricot, Fat Free, Bio Live, Rachel's Organic*	1 Pot/142g	81	57	3.5	10.5	0.1	0.0
Apricot, French Style Smooth, Tesco*	1 Pot/125g	123	98	3.6	14.1	3.0	0.0
Apricot, Healthy Living, Tesco*	1 Pot/125g	68	54	5.1	7.9	0.3	1.1
Apricot, Jubileum, Tine*	1 Pot/135g	146	108	3.1	13.3	4.8	0.0
Apricot, Layered Fruit, Thick & Creamy, Sainsbury's*	1 Pot/125g	141	113	4.1	18.0	2.7	0.2
Apricot, Light, Healthy Living, Tesco*	1 Pot/125g	54	43	4.1	6.3	0.2	0.9
Apricot, Low Fat, Benecol*	1 Pot/150g	119	79	3.7	14.6	0.6	0.0
Apricot, Low Fat, Sainsbury's*	1 Pot/125g	115	92	4.3	15.2	1.5	0.1
Apricot, Low Fat, Tesco*	1 Pot/125g	113	90	4.3	14.1	1.8	0.0
Apricot, Organic, Low Fat, Tesco*	1 Pot/125g	111	89	5.3	14.6	1.0	0.2
Apricot, Organic, Yeo Valley*	1 Pot/150g	152	101	4.1	12.4	3.9	0.1
Apricot, Smooth Set French, Sainsbury's*	1 Pot/125g	100	80	3.5	13.6	1.2	0.0
Apricot, Vitality, Muller*	1 Pot/175g	172	98	4.7	15.8	1.8	0.0

YOGHURT

INFO/WEIGHT	KCAL	KCAL	PROT	CARB	FAT	FIBRE
Banana & Orange, Low Fat, 25% Extra Fruit, Asda*	1 Pot/125g	125	100	4.6	18.0	1.1	0.0
Banana Choco Flakes Corner, Muller*	1 Pot/150g	218	145	4.1	22.5	4.3	0.0
Banana Smooth, Marks & Spencer	1 Pot/150g	165	110	4.8	19.3	1.7	0.2
Banana Toffee, Low Fat, Somerfield*	1 Pot/125g	123	98	4.1	18.0	1.1	0.0
Banana, Bio & Cereal Clusters, Rumblers*	1 Pot/167g	261	156	4.2	21.9	5.6	1.1
Banana, Childrens, Co-Op*	1 Pot/125g	124	99	3.7	15.1	2.6	0.2
Banana, Custard Style, Asda*	1 Pot/150g	224	149	3.7	20.0	6.0	0.2
Banana, Light, Muller*	1 Pot/200g	106	53	4.4	8.7	0.1	0.0
Banana, Low Fat, Sainsbury's*	1 Pot/125g	116	93	4.4	15.4	1.5	0.1
Banoffee, Dessert, Low Fat, Sainsbury's*	1 Pot/125g	123	98	4.5	16.1	1.7	0.2
Banoffee, Fat Free, Bio, Eat Smart, Safeway*	1 Pot/125g	69	55	4.7	8.5	0.1	0.2
Banoffee, Low Fat, Asda*	1 Pot/125g	126	101	4.6	18.2	1.2	1.0
Banoffee, Thick & Creamy, Safeway*	1 Pot/150g	189	126	4.3	18.2	4.0	0.1
Berry Sunshine Grove, Shape*	1 Pot/100g	63	63	4.7	8.3	1.0	0.2
Bio Activia, With Cereals, Danone*	1 Pot/125g	123	98	4.1	15.6	2.1	0.0
Bio Activia, With Prunes, Danone*	1 Pot/125g	124	99	3.3	15.2	2.8	0.0
Bio Activia, With Raspberry, Danone*	1 Pot/125g	113	90	3.5	12.8	2.8	2.0
Bio Activia, With Strawberry, Danone*	1 Pot/125g	124	99	3.7	14.0	3.2	1.6
Bio Fruits With Cherries, 0% Fat, Danone*	1 Pot/125g	65	52	3.6	9.1	0.1	0.0
Bio, Low Fat, Spelga*	1 Pot/125g	125	100	3.9	17.0	1.7	0.0
Black Cherry Live Bio, Perfeclty Balanced, Waitrose*	1 Pot/125g	115	92	4.6	18.3	0.1	0.1
Black Cherry, BGTY, Sainsbury's*	1 Pot/125g	68	54	4.4	8.8	0.1	1.1
Black Cherry, Best There Is, Yoplait*	1 Pot/125g	134	107	4.2	17.8	1.6	0.0
Black Cherry, Bodyline*	1 Pot/113g	50	44	3.0	7.7	0.1	0.3
Black Cherry, Economy, Tesco*	1 Pot/125g	85	68	3.0	11.9	1.0	0.1
Black Cherry, Extra Fruit, Low Fat, Ski*	1 Pot/125g	120	96	3.4	17.2	1.5	0.1
Black Cherry, Extra Fruity, Low Fat, Safeway*	1 Pot/150g	143	95	3.9	17.7	0.9	0.5
Black Cherry, Extremely Fruity, Bio, Marks & Spencer*	1 Pot/150g	165	110	4.9	18.4	1.5	0.2
Black Cherry, Extremely Fruity, Marks & Spencer*	1 Pot/200g	220	110	4.9	18.4	1.5	0.2
Black Cherry, Fat Free, Safeway*	1 Pot/125g	75	60	5.2	9.2	0.0	0.1
Black Cherry, Frozen, Marks & Spencer*	1 Pot/125g	164	131	3.1	27.1	1.1	0.5
Black Cherry, Fruit Corner, Low Fat, Muller*	1 Pot/95g	78	82	4.5	12.5	1.5	0.0
Black Cherry, Healthy Balance, Corner, Muller*	1 Pot/160g	142	89	3.8	15.2	1.5	1.0
Black Cherry, Healthy Living, Tesco*	1 Pot/200g	90	45	3.9	7.0	0.1	1.0
Black Cherry, Live, Turner's Dairies*	1 Pot/125g	86	69	4.9	11.9	0.3	0.0
Black Cherry, Low Fat, Asda*	1 Pot/150g	143	95	4.6	17.4	1.0	0.2
Black Cherry, Low Fat, Sainsbury's*	1 Pot/125g	123	98	4.6	17.3	1.1	0.2
Black Cherry, Low Fat, Tesco*	1 Pot/150g	137	91	4.3	14.3	1.8	0.0
Black Cherry, Low Fat, Value, Tesco*	1 Pot/125g	100	80	2.3	16.0	0.7	0.1
Black Cherry, Marks & Spencer*	1 Pot/150g	149	99	4.8	16.5	1.6	0.2
Black Cherry, Perfectly Balanced, Waitrose*	1 Pot/150g	120	80	4.2	15.6	0.1	0.3
Black Cherry, So-Good*	1 Pot/120g	92	77	2.1	16.6	1.3	0.0
Black Cherry, Swiss, Finest, Tesco*	1 Pot/150g	210	140	3.4	16.0	6.9	0.5
Black Cherry, Thick & Creamy, Waitrose*	1 Pot/125g	139	111	3.7	18.3	2.5	0.4
Black Cherry, Thick & Fruity, Weight Watchers*	1 Pot/120.8g	58	48	4.2	7.5	0.1	0.1
Black Cherry, Variety Selection, Ski*	1 Pot/125g	128	102	4.8	16.7	1.8	0.2
Black Cherry, Virtually Fat Free, Shapers, Boots*	1 Pot/125g	71	57	5.3	8.8	0.1	0.1
Blackberry & Apple, BGTY, Sainsbury's*	1 Pot/122g	61	50	4.7	7.2	0.2	0.3
Blackberry & Apple, Best There Is, Yoplait	1 Pot/124g	133	107	4.7	18.0	1.6	0.0
Blackberry & Apple, Healthy Living, Tesco*	1 Serving/176g	86	49	2.1	10.0	0.1	1.5
Blackberry & Apple, Low Fat, Sainsbury's*	1 Pot/125g	116	93	4.3	15.5	1.5	0.2
Blackberry & Raspberry Flip, Morrisons*	1 Pot/175g	207	118	3.4	15.8	4.6	0.5
Blackberry & Raspberry, Fruit Corner, Muller*	1 Pot/175g	193	110	3.7	15.0	3.9	0.0

Y

YOGHURT

INFO/WEIGHT	per Measure KCAL	KCAL	PROT	CARB	FAT	FIBRE
	Measure		Nutrition Values per 100g / 100ml			

	Measure INFO/WEIGHT	per Measure KCAL	KCAL	PROT	CARB	FAT	FIBRE
Blackberry & Raspberry, Low Fat, Ski*	1 Pot/126g	67	53	5.7	7.2	0.0	2.0
Blackberry & Raspberry, Simply Berries, Shape, Danone*	1 Pot/120g	61	51	4.4	8.1	0.1	1.2
Blackberry, BGTY, Sainsbury's*	1 Pot/150g	107	71	3.4	13.5	0.4	1.6
Blackberry, Boysenberry & William Pear, Marks & Spencer*	1 Pot/150g	188	125	4.0	13.6	6.5	2.4
Blackberry, Elderberry & Lavender, Biowild, Onken*	1 Pot/175g	159	91	4.4	14.7	1.6	0.4
Blackberry, Farmhouse, BGTY, Sainsbury's*	1 Pot/150g	107	71	3.4	13.5	0.4	1.6
Blackberry, Fat Free, BGTY, Sainsbury's*	1 Pot/150g	101	67	3.4	13.6	0.1	1.6
Blackberry, Sveltesse 0%, Nestle*	1 Pot/125g	69	55	4.7	8.8	0.1	0.3
Blackberry, Weight Watchers*	1 Pot/120g	49	41	4.2	5.8	0.1	0.3
Blackcherry, Everyday, Low Fat, Co-Op*	1 Pot/125g	88	70	3.0	13.0	0.7	0.0
Blackcurrant & Vanilla, TTD, Sainsbury's*	1 Pot/143g	136	95	3.6	13.6	2.9	1.0
Blackcurrant Smooth, Ski*	1 Pot/125g	125	100	4.9	15.9	1.9	0.5
Blackcurrant With Liquorice, Tesco*	1 Pot/150g	138	92	4.6	15.8	1.1	0.4
Blackcurrant, BGTY, Sainsbury's*	1 Pot/200g	100	50	4.8	7.3	0.2	0.1
Blackcurrant, Bio Live, Organic, Yeo Valley*	1 Pot/150g	152	101	4.1	12.4	3.9	0.2
Blackcurrant, Extra Special, Asda*	1 Pot/100g	163	163	2.6	18.0	9.0	0.0
Blackcurrant, Light, Muller*	1 Pot/200g	108	54	4.4	8.8	0.1	0.6
Blackcurrant, Limited Edition, Light, Muller*	1 Serving/200g	110	55	4.7	8.9	0.1	0.0
Blackcurrant, Low Fat, Sainsbury's*	1 Pot/125g	116	93	4.2	15.9	1.4	0.6
Blackcurrant, Low Fat, Tesco*	1 Pot/125g	110	88	4.9	13.2	1.7	0.4
Blackcurrant, Marks & Spencer*	1 Pot/150g	147	98	4.8	16.1	1.6	0.8
Blackcurrant, Munch Bunch, Nestle*	1 Pot/100g	107	107	4.4	15.3	3.1	0.5
Blackcurrant, Thick & Creamy, Sainsbury's*	1 Pot/150g	171	114	4.3	15.9	3.6	0.4
Blueberry & Elderberry, Optifit, Aldi*	1 Pot/250g	153	61	4.9	7.0	1.5	1.4
Blueberry Bio, Co-Op*	1 Pot/125g	141	113	4.5	16.5	2.8	0.4
Blueberry Flip, Morrisons*	1 Pot/175g	201	115	3.1	15.1	4.6	0.5
Blueberry Loganberry, Layered, Bio, Sainsbury's*	1 Serving/125g	134	107	4.0	16.6	2.7	0.2
Blueberry Muffin, Fat Free, Eat Smart, Safeway*	1 Pot/125g	66	53	4.7	8.2	0.1	0.3
Blueberry, Fruit Corner, Muller*	1 Pot/175g	196	112	3.7	15.5	3.9	0.0
Blueberry, Light, Muller*	1 Pot/200g	98	49	4.4	7.7	0.1	0.0
Blueberry, Low Lactose, Valio*	2 Servings/200g	160	80	3.2	13.0	2.1	0.0
Blueberry, Marks & Spencer*	1 Pot/150g	141	94	4.7	15.8	1.6	0.4
Blueberry, Wholemilk, Organic, Sainsbury's*	1 Pot/150g	123	82	3.5	9.2	3.5	0.1
Boysenberry, Low Fat, Yoplait*	1 Pot/100g	49	49	5.3	6.7	0.1	0.0
Cappuccino, Thick & Creamy, Safeway*	1 Pot/150g	228	152	4.5	20.8	5.6	0.0
Caramel & Praline, Indulgent Greek Style, Somerfield*	1 Pot/125g	245	196	4.0	28.0	8.0	0.0
Caramel, Organic, Onken*	1 Serving/50g	56	111	4.6	15.6	3.3	0.0
Caramelised Orange, COU, Marks & Spencer*	1 Pot/145g	65	45	4.2	6.1	0.1	0.2
Champagne Rhubarb & Vanilla, Marks & Spencer*	1 Pot/150g	195	130	3.8	15.7	5.8	0.8
Champagne Rhubarb, Finest, Tesco*	1 Pot/150g	213	142	3.3	16.8	6.9	0.2
Cherry & Vanilla Flavour, Light, Brooklea*	1 Pot/200g	138	69	5.5	11.4	0.1	0.6
Cherry Flip, BFY, Morrisons*	1 Pot/175g	93	53	3.9	8.7	0.3	0.4
Cherry Morello Bio, Tesco*	1 Pot/124g	51	41	4.4	5.4	0.2	0.9
Cherry Pie Layered, Custard Style, Healthy Eating, Tesco*	1 Pot/125g	99	79	4.1	13.9	0.8	0.2
Cherry, 0% Fat, Yoplait*	1 Pot/125g	70	56	3.8	9.8	0.1	0.0
Cherry, Fat Free, Bio, Shape*	1 Pot/120g	90	75	4.5	14.0	0.1	0.0
Cherry, Fruit Corner, Muller*	1 Pot/175g	193	110	3.7	15.0	3.9	0.0
Cherry, Greek Style, Shape*	1 Pot/125.4g	143	114	6.0	16.4	2.7	0.0
Cherry, Healthy Eating, Tesco*	1 Pot/200g	96	48	4.2	7.5	0.1	0.0
Cherry, Light, Muller*	1 Pot/200g	100	50	4.4	7.9	0.1	0.0
Cherry, Low Fat, Benecol*	1 Pot/150g	122	81	3.8	15.2	0.6	0.0
Cherry, Muller*	1 Pot/150g	177	118	3.3	17.0	3.7	0.0
Cherry, Probiotic, Vitality, Muller*	1 Pot/150g	155	103	4.7	17.0	1.8	0.0

Y

YOGHURT

INFO/WEIGHT	Measure	per Measure KCAL	KCAL	PROT	CARB	FAT	FIBRE
			Nutrition Values per 100g / 100ml				
Cherry, Virtually Fat Free Bio, Morrisons*	1 Pot/200g	120	60	5.4	9.2	0.2	0.0
Chocolate & Toffee Selection, Shape*	1 Pot/100g	99	99	4.6	15.4	1.8	0.0
Chocolate Chip, Dessert Recipes, Ski*	1 Pot/125g	163	130	3.8	19.3	4.2	0.0
Chocolate, GFY, Asda*	1 Pot/200g	110	55	4.7	8.0	0.5	0.1
Chocolate, Light, Muller*	1 Pot/200g	108	54	4.8	8.1	0.3	0.0
Chocolate, Seriously Smooth, Waitrose*	1 Pot/125g	158	126	6.0	20.1	2.4	0.1
Chocolate, Shape*	1 Pot/100g	111	111	4.9	17.4	2.0	0.2
Chocolate, Village Dairy*	1 Pot/125g	181	145	6.3	23.5	3.0	0.0
Chocolate, Vitaline*	1 Pot/125g	103	82	3.5	15.8	0.5	0.0
Citrus Fruit, Fat Free, Weight Watchers*	1 Pot/120g	52	43	4.1	6.3	0.1	0.2
Citrus Fruit, Tesco*	1 Serving/117g	53	45	4.2	6.5	0.1	0.1
Coconut, Greek Style, Bio Live, Rachel's Organic*	1 Pot/450g	702	156	3.6	10.5	11.0	0.0
Coconut, Muller*	1 Pot/150g	156	104	3.4	13.0	3.9	0.0
Coconut, Ski*	1 Pot/125g	126	101	4.9	15.8	2.0	0.0
Country Berries, Virtually Fat Free, Light, Muller*	1 Pot/200g	104	52	4.4	8.3	0.1	0.0
Cranberry & Blackcurrant, Fat Free, Bio, Shape*	1 Pot/120g	54	45	4.6	5.7	0.1	0.3
Cranberry & Blackcurrant, Low Fat Bio, Ocean Spray*	1 Pot/150g	147	98	4.6	17.4	1.1	0.0
Cranberry & Blackcurrant, Shape, Danone*	1 Pot/120g	62	52	4.4	8.4	0.1	1.0
Cranberry & Pink Grapefruit, Low Fat Bio, Ocean Spray*	1 Pot/125g	118	94	4.6	16.5	1.1	0.0
Cranberry & Raspberry, Fat Free Bio, Eat Smart, Safeway*	1 Pot/125g	69	55	4.7	8.2	0.1	0.5
Cranberry & Raspberry, Low Fat Bio, Ocean Spray*	1 Pot/150g	144	96	4.6	17.0	1.1	0.0
Cranberry & Raspberry, Perfectly Balanced, Waitrose*	1 Pot/150g	135	90	4.5	17.8	0.1	0.6
Cranberry Classic, Low Fat Bio, Ocean Spray*	1 Pot/150g	144	96	4.6	17.0	1.1	0.0
Cranberry, Blueberry & Guarana, Probiotic, Ocean Spray*	1 Pot/170g	162	95	4.7	16.6	1.1	0.0
Creamy Cranberry & Raspberry, Shapers, Boots*	1 Pot/150g	86	57	4.0	7.0	1.1	1.1
Dairy Toffee, Shape*	1 Pot/100g	99	99	4.6	15.4	1.8	0.0
Dessert With Honey, Perfectly Balanced, Waitrose*	1 Pot/125ml	128	102	3.5	19.4	1.2	0.1
Devon Toffee, Low Fat, Sainsbury's*	1 Pot/126g	137	109	4.3	19.6	1.5	0.0
Devon Toffee, Shape, Danone*	1 Pot/125g	129	103	4.9	16.2	2.0	1.0
Diet, Yoplait*	1 Pot/125g	100	80	4.0	16.0	0.0	0.0
Double Caramel, Frozen, Dream*	1 Serving/50g	88	175	4.0	28.0	5.0	0.0
English Plum, The Best, Safeway*	1 Pot/175g	245	140	3.2	17.4	6.4	0.3
Exotic Fruits French Set Wholemilk, Asda*	1 Pot/125g	125	100	3.6	14.1	3.2	0.0
Farmhouse Strawberry & Redcurrant, Ann Forshaw's*	1 Pot/150g	194	129	3.8	17.4	4.9	0.2
Forest Fruits, French Set Wholemilk, Asda*	1 Pot/125g	125	100	3.6	14.1	3.2	0.0
Forest Fruits, Layered Greek Style, Shapers, Boots*	1 Pot/150g	86	57	3.2	7.9	1.4	2.2
Forest Fruits, Marks & Spencer*	1 Pot/150g	149	99	4.7	16.8	1.6	0.5
French Set, Waitrose*	1 Pot/125g	120	96	3.5	13.4	3.1	0.0
French Style, Whole Milk, Smooth Set, Tesco*	1 Pot/125g	123	98	3.6	14.1	3.0	0.0
Fruit & Nut Layer, Indulgent Greek Style, Somerfield*	1 Pot/125g	214	171	3.0	24.0	7.0	0.0
Fruit Bio, Low Fat, Sainsbury's*	1 Pot/150g	156	104	4.6	18.9	1.1	0.3
Fruit Halo Strawberry & Vanilla, Light, Muller*	1 Pot/145g	116	80	3.6	15.8	0.3	0.0
Fruit Halo, Raspberry, Light, Muller*	1 Pot/144.0g	121	84	3.7	16.5	0.3	0.0
Fruit Whole Milk	1 Pot/150g	158	105	5.1	15.7	2.8	0.0
Fruit, Brooklea, Aldi*	1 Pot/120g	97	81	2.7	17.0	0.2	0.0
Fruit, Deep Fill, Ski*	1 Pot/160g	138	86	4.0	13.8	1.6	0.0
Fruit, Low Fat	1 Pot/120g	108	90	4.1	17.9	0.7	0.0
Fruit, Low Fat, Safeway*	1 Pot/125ml	88	70	2.1	13.7	0.8	0.0
Fruits Of The Forest, Smooth Set, Co-Op*	1 Pot/125g	95	76	3.7	12.5	0.9	0.0
Fruits of the Forest, Lite, Yoplait*	1 Pot/200g	184	92	5.0	15.9	0.9	0.0
Fruits of the Forest, Nestle*	1 Pot/125g	123	98	3.4	16.7	1.6	0.0
Fruity Favourites, Organic, Yeo Valley*	1 Pot/125g	126	101	4.1	12.4	3.9	0.2
Fudge Layer, Indulgent Greek Style, Somerfield*	1 Pot/125g	226	181	3.0	26.0	7.0	0.0

YOGHURT

INFO/WEIGHT	Measure	per Measure KCAL	Nutrition Values per 100g / 100ml KCAL	PROT	CARB	FAT	FIBRE
Fudge, Devonshire Style, Finest, Tesco*	1 Pot/150g	281	187	3.7	22.4	9.2	0.0
Fudge, Thick & Creamy, Co-Op*	1 Pot/150g	197	131	3.8	17.6	5.0	0.0
Fudge, Thick & Creamy, Marks & Spencer*	1 Pot/150g	195	130	4.4	17.3	5.0	0.7
Fudge, Thick & Creamy, Waitrose*	1 Pot/150g	197	131	4.4	21.5	3.0	0.0
Garden Fruit, Wholemilk, Bio Live, Rachel's Organic*	1 Pot/125g	109	87	3.5	10.5	3.4	0.0
Goats Whole Milk	1 Carton/150g	95	63	3.5	3.9	3.8	0.0
Gooseberry & Vanilla, TTD, Sainsbury's*	1 Pot/150g	143	95	3.7	13.6	2.9	0.4
Gooseberry, Custard Style, Somerfield*	1 Pot/125g	151	121	3.0	17.0	5.0	0.0
Gooseberry, Low Fat, Sainsbury's*	1 Pot/125g	113	90	4.4	14.6	1.5	0.2
Gooseberry, Low Fat, Tesco*	1 Pot/125g	114	91	4.3	14.5	1.8	0.0
Greek Style With Honey, Asda*	1 Pot/150g	225	150	4.0	13.9	8.7	0.0
Greek Style With Strawberries, Asda*	1 Pot/125g	159	127	3.2	13.6	6.6	0.2
Greek Style With Toffee & Hazelnuts, Asda*	1 Pot/125g	230	184	3.7	23.1	8.6	0.1
Greek Style With Tropical Fruits, Asda*	1 Pot/125g	164	131	3.3	14.5	6.6	0.3
Greek Style, Healthy Living, Tesco*	1 Pot/150g	152	101	5.6	8.1	5.1	0.0
Greek Style, Honey Topped, Tesco*	1 Pot/140g	203	145	3.6	13.4	8.6	0.0
Greek Style, Honey, Selection Pack, Organic, Tesco*	1 Pot/100g	156	156	4.1	15.3	8.7	0.0
Greek Style, Layered, Honey, Shapers, Boots*	1 Serving/150g	137	91	4.2	14.0	2.0	0.0
Greek Style, Lemon, Low Fat, Bio, Shape*	1 Pot/125g	141	113	6.0	16.2	2.7	0.0
Greek Style, Luxury, Loseley*	1 Pot/175g	226	129	4.8	4.5	10.2	0.0
Greek Style, Natural, Tesco*	1 Serving/125g	179	143	4.5	6.6	11.0	0.0
Greek Style, Orange, Low Fat, Bio, Shape*	1 Pot/125g	143	114	6.0	16.3	2.7	0.0
Greek Style, Sainsbury's*	1 Serving/200g	258	129	4.6	4.8	10.2	0.0
Greek, 0% Fat, Total*	1 Pot/150g	84	56	10.0	4.0	0.0	0.0
Greek, Light, Total*	1 Pot/150g	120	80	6.0	3.0	5.0	0.0
Greek, Original, Total*	1oz/28g	36	130	6.0	4.0	10.0	0.0
Greek, With Honey & Nuts, Duettino*	1 Pot/185g	278	150	3.6	15.9	8.0	0.0
Greek, With Strawberry, Total*	1 Pot/150g	189	126	4.7	8.7	8.0	0.0
Guava & Orange, Fat Free, Organic, Yeo Valley*	1 Pot/125g	93	74	5.1	13.2	0.1	0.3
Guava & Passion Fruit, Virtually Fat Free, Tesco*	1 Pot/125g	56	45	4.2	6.7	0.2	1.2
Hazelnut Crunchy, Jordans*	1oz/28g	43	154	5.2	22.2	4.0	1.1
Hazelnut, Low Fat, Sainsbury's*	1 Pot/125g	135	108	4.5	16.4	2.7	0.2
Hazelnut, Low Fat, Tesco*	1 Pot/150g	159	106	4.5	16.0	2.7	0.0
Hazelnut, Sainsbury's*	1 Serving/150g	183	122	5.0	20.3	2.3	0.2
Hazelnut, Yoplait*	1 Pot/125g	166	133	4.6	19.6	4.0	0.0
Hazelnut, Longley Farm*	1 Pot/150g	206	137	5.5	16.0	5.7	0.0
Hazelnut, Low Fat, Somerfield*	1 Pot/150g	126	84	4.0	15.0	1.0	0.0
Hint Of Coconut, Bio Activia, Danone*	1 Pot/125g	119	95	3.6	13.2	3.1	0.0
Honey & Ginger, Tesco*	1 Pot/150g	150	100	4.6	18.0	1.1	0.0
Honey & Greek, Total*	1 Pot/150g	245	163	4.8	19.2	8.0	0.0
Honey & Muesli, Breakfast Break, Tesco*	1 Pot/170g	207	122	3.9	20.5	2.7	0.6
Honey & Multigrain, Breakfast Selection, Sainsbury's*	1 Pot/125g	126	101	4.4	17.4	1.5	0.2
Honey, Greek Style, Boots*	1 Pot/140g	204	146	3.1	18.0	6.8	0.0
Honey, Greek Style, Organic, Sainsbury's*	1 Pot/100g	156	156	4.1	15.3	8.7	0.1
Honey, Low Fat, Asda*	1 Pot/125g	130	104	4.6	19.0	1.1	0.0
Italian Lemon, Muller*	1 Pot/150g	210	140	2.3	15.0	7.9	0.0
Jaffa Cakes Corner, McVitie's, Muller*	1 Pot/150g	237	158	4.0	24.6	4.8	0.0
Jaffa Orange, Low Fat, Co-Op*	1 Pot/150g	126	84	3.9	15.0	0.9	0.4
Jaffa Orange, Morrisons*	1 Pot/150g	134	89	3.6	16.2	1.1	0.0
Jubileum Kiwi, Tine*	1 Pot/135g	149	110	3.2	13.5	4.9	0.0
Jubileum Raspberry, Tine*	1 Pot/135g	163	121	3.2	16.1	4.8	0.0
Kellogg's Coco Pops Corner, Muller*	1 Pot/150g	180	120	4.0	19.0	3.1	0.0
Kellogg's Frosties Crunch Corner, Muller*	1 Pot/150g	185	123	4.0	20.1	2.9	0.0

YOGHURT

INFO/WEIGHT	Measure	per Measure KCAL	KCAL	PROT	CARB	FAT	FIBRE
Kellogg's With Rice Krispies, Muller*	1 Pot/150g	185	123	4.1	19.9	3.0	0.0
Kiwi, BGTY, Sainsbury's*	1 Pot/125g	61	49	4.6	7.5	0.1	0.2
Layered, Eat Smart, Safeway*	1 Pot/125g	81	65	4.1	11.3	0.1	0.4
Lemon & Lime, BGTY, Sainsbury's*	1 Pot/125g	66	53	4.6	8.3	0.1	1.1
Lemon & Lime, Bio, Shape*	1 Pot/120g	54	45	5.7	5.7	0.1	0.1
Lemon & Lime, Fat Free, Shape*	1 Pot/120g	61	51	4.5	7.3	0.1	0.1
Lemon & Lime, Light, Muller*	1 Pot/200g	106	53	4.7	8.2	0.1	0.0
Lemon & Lime, Weight Watchers*	1 Pot/119ml	50	42	4.1	5.9	0.1	0.0
Lemon Cheesecake, Corner, Muller*	1 Pot/150g	224	149	3.7	23.9	4.3	0.0
Lemon Cheesecake, Dessert Recipes, Ski*	1 Pot/125g	154	123	3.8	19.0	3.5	0.0
Lemon Cheesecake, Sveltesse, Nestle*	1 Pot/125g	101	81	4.8	13.8	0.7	0.1
Lemon Curd, Dessert, Waitrose*	1 Pot/150g	278	185	4.1	21.5	9.2	0.0
Lemon Curd, Farmhouse, TTD, Sainsbury's*	1 Pot/149.6g	182	121	4.1	17.7	3.7	0.2
Lemon Curd, Farmhouse, Waitrose*	1 Pot/150g	245	163	4.3	18.7	7.9	0.2
Lemon Lime Mousse, Shapers, Boots*	1 Pot/90g	89	99	4.2	11.0	4.2	0.1
Lemon Meringue, Eat Smart, Safeway*	1 Pot/125g	68	54	4.7	8.6	0.1	0.0
Lemon Meringue, Sveltesse 0%, Nestle*	1 Pot/125g	60	48	4.1	7.7	0.1	0.0
Lemon Smooth Set, Co-Op*	1 Pot/125g	95	76	3.7	12.5	0.9	0.0
Lemon Sunshine Grove, Low Fat, Shape*	1 Pot/100g	64	64	4.6	8.5	1.0	0.0
Lemon, Amore Luxury, Muller*	1 Pot/150g	210	140	2.3	15.0	7.9	0.0
Lemon, COU, Marks & Spencer*	1 Pot/200g	90	45	4.2	6.6	0.1	0.4
Lemon, Fat Free, Weight Watchers*	1 Pot/120g	49	41	4.0	5.8	0.1	0.0
Lemon, Greek Style, GFY, Asda*	1 Pot/150g	125	83	4.1	10.0	2.9	0.1
Lemon, Low Fat, Asda*	1 Pot/125g	130	104	4.6	19.0	1.1	0.0
Lemon, Low Fat, Organic, Sainsbury's*	1 Pot/125g	121	97	5.1	17.0	1.0	0.1
Lemon, Smooth Set French, Low Fat, Sainsbury's*	1 Pot/125g	100	80	3.5	13.6	1.2	0.0
Lemon, Summer, Biopot, Onken*	1 Pot/150g	155	103	3.9	15.9	2.6	0.1
Lemon, Virtually Fat Free, Morrisons*	1 Pot/200g	118	59	5.4	8.9	0.2	0.0
Light, Muller*	1 Serving/200g	110	55	4.3	9.2	0.1	0.0
Loganberry, Low Fat, Sainsbury's*	1 Pot/125g	111	89	4.2	14.5	1.5	0.2
Loganberry, Sainsbury's*	1 Pot/150g	194	129	3.9	14.2	6.2	0.6
Low Calorie	1 Pot/120g	49	41	4.3	6.0	0.2	0.0
Mandarin, Light, Muller*	1 Pot/200g	108	54	4.3	9.0	0.1	0.0
Mandarin, Longley Farm*	1 Pot/150g	161	107	4.9	13.3	3.8	0.0
Mandarin, Low Fat, Safeway*	1 Pot/150g	141	94	4.6	16.4	1.1	0.2
Mango & Guava, Fat Free, Weight Watchers*	1 Pot/120g	55	46	4.1	6.8	0.1	0.3
Mango & Guava, Sunshine Selection, Sainsbury's*	1 Pot/125g	145	116	5.4	19.3	1.9	0.3
Mango & Passionfruit, Biopot, Onken*	1 Serving/100g	101	101	3.9	15.6	2.6	0.2
Mango & Pineapple, BGTY, Sainsbury's*	1 Pot/124g	63	51	4.6	7.6	0.2	0.2
Mango Bio, Healthy Eating, Tesco*	1 Pot/125g	59	47	4.7	6.8	0.1	0.2
Mango Bio, Virtually Fat Free, Shape*	1 Pot/120g	60	50	4.7	6.8	0.1	0.2
Mango Passion, D'lite, Ski*	1 Pot/200g	186	93	5.1	14.9	0.9	0.0
Mango Passionfruit, D'lite 0.2 Ski, Nestle*	1 Pot/125g	103	82	4.6	15.7	0.1	0.1
Mango Smooth, Marks & Spencer*	1 Pot/150g	158	105	4.7	18.0	1.6	0.5
Mango, BGTY, Sainsbury's*	1 Pot/125g	66	53	4.8	8.3	0.1	1.2
Mango, Light, Healthy Living, Tesco*	1 Serving/125g	56	45	4.1	6.6	0.2	0.9
Mango, Light, Muller*	1 Pot/200g	110	55	4.3	9.2	0.1	0.0
Mango, Papaya & Passion Fruit, Onken*	1 Serving/100g	101	101	3.9	15.6	2.6	0.2
Mango, Ski*	1 Pot/125g	125	100	4.9	15.8	1.9	0.1
Mango, Weight Watchers*	1 Pot/120g	54	45	3.9	7.1	0.1	1.1
Melon & Passion Fruit, Weight Watchers*	1 Pot/120g	54	45	4.0	7.0	0.1	0.0
Milchcafe, Onken*	1 Serving/200g	222	111	4.1	15.9	3.4	0.0
Mississippi Mud Pie Corner, Muller*	1 Pot/150g	254	169	4.1	26.3	5.3	0.0

YOGHURT

INFO/WEIGHT	Measure	per Measure KCAL	KCAL	PROT	CARB	FAT	FIBRE
Mississippi Mud Pie, Shape, St Ivel*	1 Pot/120g	166	138	3.8	24.5	2.8	0.8
Mixed Berry, Fat Free, Shape*	1 Pot/120g	62	52	4.4	8.2	0.1	1.0
Morello Cherry, Healthy Living, Tesco*	1 Pot/125g	56	45	4.1	6.6	0.2	0.9
Morello Cherry, Seriously Fruity, Low Fat, Waitrose*	1 Pot/150g	146	97	4.4	17.5	1.0	0.3
Muesli Nut, Low Fat	1 Pot/120g	134	112	5.0	19.2	2.2	0.0
Multifruits, Yop Petit Déjeuner, Yoplait*	1 Bottle/180g	155	86	2.7	16.0	1.2	0.0
Natural With Honey, Greek Style, Sainsbury's*	1 Sm Pot/150g	243	162	4.0	15.4	9.4	0.0
Natural With Prunes, Bio Activia, Danone*	1 Pot/125g	124	99	3.3	15.2	2.8	0.0
Natural, Bio Activia, Danone*	1 Pot/125g	89	71	4.2	5.8	3.4	0.0
Natural, Bio Activia, Low Fat, Danone*	1 Pot/125g	68	54	4.1	9.2	0.1	1.0
Natural, Bio Life, Easiyo*	1 Pot/150g	95	63	5.0	6.7	1.8	0.0
Natural, Bio Live, Organic, Yeo Valley*	1 Pot/100g	82	82	4.5	6.6	4.2	0.0
Natural, Bio Set, Low Fat, Sainsbury's*	1 Pot/150g	78	52	3.9	5.7	1.5	0.0
Natural, Bio Wholemilk, Waitrose*	1 Pot/125g	100	80	4.8	6.9	3.7	0.0
Natural, Bio, Ann Forshaw's*	1 Pot/125g	53	42	5.0	5.5	0.1	0.0
Natural, Bio, Fat Free, Waitrose*	1 Pot/150g	90	60	6.1	8.6	0.1	0.0
Natural, Bio, Healthy Living, Tesco*	1 Serving/100g	53	53	5.4	7.6	0.1	0.0
Natural, Bio, Low Fat, Sainsbury's*	1 Serving/100g	48	48	4.0	4.6	1.5	0.0
Natural, Bio, Unsweetened, Marks & Spencer*	1 Serving/100g	80	80	6.7	8.5	1.8	0.0
Natural, Bio, Very Low Fat, Somerfield*	1 Pot/150g	98	65	7.0	9.0	0.0	0.0
Natural, Bio, Virtually Fat Free, Healthy Living, Tesco*	1 Serving/100g	47	47	5.5	5.8	0.2	0.1
Natural, Biopot, Set, Onken*	1 Pot/150g	101	67	3.9	4.8	3.6	0.0
Natural, Biopot, Stirred, Onken*	1 Bowl/200g	118	59	5.9	5.0	1.5	0.0
Natural, Danone*	1 Pot/125g	71	57	3.2	3.8	2.9	0.0
Natural, Farmhouse, Virtually Fat Free, TTD, Sainsbury's*	1 Serving/100g	44	44	4.5	6.6	0.2	0.0
Natural, Fat Free, Organic, Yeo Valley*	1 Serving/100g	58	58	5.9	8.4	0.1	0.0
Natural, Fat Free, Rachel's Organic*	1 Pot/500g	180	36	3.9	4.8	0.4	0.0
Natural, Greek Style, Asda*	1oz/28g	36	129	4.6	4.8	10.8	0.0
Natural, Greek Style, BGTY, Sainsbury's*	1 Serving/50g	48	95	6.2	6.4	5.0	0.0
Natural, Greek Style, GFY, Asda*	1 Pot/100g	101	101	6.0	8.0	4.8	0.0
Natural, Greek Style, Healthy Eating, Tesco*	1oz/28g	22	79	6.5	4.0	4.1	0.0
Natural, Greek Style, Organic, Tesco*	1oz/28g	37	133	4.5	6.2	10.0	0.0
Natural, Greek Style, Sainsbury's*	1 Serving/100g	78	78	5.5	7.9	2.7	0.0
Natural, Greek Style, Unsweetened, Marks & Spencer*	1 Pot/100g	130	130	5.5	4.6	10.1	0.1
Natural, Greek Style, Waitrose*	1 Pot/150g	210	140	4.8	6.9	10.3	0.0
Natural, Greek Style, With Honey Sauce, Sainsbury's*	1 Pot/140g	206	147	3.3	15.7	7.9	0.0
Natural, Greek, Half Fat, Safeway*	1 Serving/100g	101	101	5.7	8.1	5.1	0.0
Natural, Low Fat, Bio, Safeway*	1 Serving/100g	72	72	6.6	8.8	1.1	0.0
Natural, Low Fat, Bio, Sainsbury's*	1 Pot/125g	85	68	5.6	7.9	1.5	0.0
Natural, Low Fat, Live, Waitrose*	1 Pot/175g	114	65	5.8	8.2	1.0	0.0
Natural, Low Fat, Onken*	1 Pot/75g	36	48	5.3	6.4	0.1	0.0
Natural, Low Fat, Organic, Sainsbury's*	1 Pot/150g	107	71	6.2	8.8	1.2	0.0
Natural, Low Fat, Organic, Yeo Valley*	1 Serving/100g	68	68	5.9	8.5	1.2	0.0
Natural, Low Fat, Safeway*	1 Serving/100g	52	52	4.6	5.9	1.1	0.0
Natural, Low Fat, Somerfield*	1 Pot/150g	78	52	4.5	5.9	1.1	0.0
Natural, Low Fat, Stirred, Sainsbury's*	1 Serving/124g	83	67	5.5	7.8	1.5	0.0
Natural, Low Fat, TTD, Sainsbury's*	1 Pot/125g	80	64	6.7	4.6	1.8	0.0
Natural, Low Fat, Tesco*	1 Pot/200g	134	67	5.5	7.8	1.5	0.0
Natural, Low Fat, Ubley*	1 Serving/100g	67	67	5.5	7.8	1.5	0.0
Natural, Organic, Evernat*	1oz/28g	29	104	3.9	12.9	4.1	0.0
Natural, Organic, Low Fat, Sainsbury's*	1oz/28g	20	71	6.2	8.8	1.2	0.0
Natural, Organic, Yeo Valley*	1 Pot/150g	120	80	4.7	6.9	3.7	0.0
Natural, Set, Asda*	1oz/28g	16	57	5.1	6.8	1.0	0.0

YOGHURT

	Measure INFO/WEIGHT	per Measure KCAL	KCAL	PROT	CARB	FAT	FIBRE
Natural, Set, Low Fat, Waitrose*	1 Pot/150g	99	66	5.7	8.1	1.2	0.0
Natural, Sojasun*	1 Serving/100g	51	51	4.6	2.0	2.7	0.0
Natural, Unsweetened, Bio, Marks & Spencer*	1 Pot/225g	135	60	5.6	5.5	1.8	0.0
Natural, Very Low Fat, Good Intentions, Somerfield*	1 Serving/125g	66	53	5.4	7.6	0.1	0.0
Natural, Very Low Fat, Longley Farm*	1 Serving/80g	46	57	6.5	7.5	0.1	0.0
Natural, Virtually Fat Free, Bio, Safeway*	1 Pot/100g	65	65	6.4	9.4	0.2	0.0
Natural, Vitality Probiotic, Low Fat, Muller*	1 Serving/100g	67	67	5.5	6.9	1.9	0.0
Natural, Weight Watchers*	1 Serving/100g	42	42	4.9	5.3	0.1	0.2
Natural, Wholemilk, Organic, Sainsbury's*	1 Pot/125g	86	69	3.7	5.0	3.8	0.1
Natural, With Cow's Milk, Greek Style, Sainsbury's*	1/2 Pot/100g	143	143	4.5	6.6	10.9	0.1
Nectarine & Apricot Bio, Virtually Fat Free, Shape*	1 Pot/120g	53	44	4.8	5.3	0.1	0.1
Nectarine & Orange, Best There Is, Yoplait	1 Pot/122g	131	107	4.7	18.0	1.6	0.0
Nectarine & Orange, Channel Island, Marks & Spencer*	1 Pot/150g	158	105	4.5	14.7	3.3	0.3
Nectarine & Orange, Fat Free, BFY, Morrisons*	1 Serving/200g	128	64	5.9	9.5	0.3	0.1
Nectarine & Orange, Marks & Spencer*	1 Pot/150g	147	98	4.9	16.0	1.6	0.3
Nectarine & Orange, Virtually Fat Free, Shape*	1 Pot/120g	55	46	4.7	5.8	0.1	0.1
Nectarine & Orange, Virtually Fat Free, Tesco*	1 Pot/125g	58	46	4.1	7.2	0.1	0.0
Nectarine & Passion Fruit, BGTY, Sainsbury's*	1 Pot/151g	122	81	3.2	16.3	0.4	0.6
Nectarine & Passion Fruit, Fat Free, Weight Watchers	1 Pot/120g	54	45	4.2	6.6	0.1	0.1
Nectarine & Raspberry, Low Fat, Somerfield*	1 Pot/150g	134	89	4.0	17.0	1.0	0.0
Nectarine & Raspberry, Very Low Fat, Somerfield*	1 Pot/125g	60	48	5.0	7.0	0.0	0.0
Nectarines & Greek Style, Food To Go, Marks & Spencer*	1 Pack/200g	100	50	2.9	6.3	2.1	1.0
Orange & Guava Tropical Fruit, Ski*	1 Pot/125g	123	98	4.9	15.5	1.9	0.2
Orange & Lemon, BGTY, Sainsbury's*	1 Pot/125g	63	50	4.7	7.3	0.2	0.2
Orange & Mango, COU, Marks & Spencer*	1 Serving/145g	65	45	4.3	6.0	0.1	0.2
Orange & Nectarine, Light, Spelga*	1 Pot/175g	79	45	4.4	7.1	0.2	0.0
Orange & Nectarine, Weight Watchers*	1 Pot/120g	54	45	4.2	6.5	0.1	0.1
Orange Blossom Honey, Finest, Tesco*	1 Pot/150g	237	158	3.5	20.1	7.1	0.0
Orange With Chocolate Flakes, Shape*	1 Pot/150g	140	93	4.6	11.8	2.8	0.2
Orange With Grains, Good Intentions, Somerfield*	1 Pot/125g	91	73	5.9	11.6	0.3	0.1
Orange, BGTY, Sainsbury's*	1 Pot/125g	63	50	4.5	7.7	0.1	1.1
Orange, Fat Free, Shape*	1 Pot/120g	61	51	4.5	8.7	0.2	0.1
Orange, Greek Style, Shape*	1 Pot/100g	105	105	7.7	9.4	3.6	0.1
Orange, Low Fat, Tesco*	1 Pot/125g	114	91	4.3	14.5	1.8	0.0
Orange, Shape, Fat Free, Danone*	1 Pot/119.4g	86	72	4.3	13.5	0.1	0.0
Passion Fruit & Peach, Fruit Corner, Muller*	1 Pot/175g	186	106	3.7	14.1	3.9	0.0
Passion Fruit With Elderflower Extract, Tesco*	1 Pot/150g	147	98	4.7	17.3	1.1	0.2
Peach & Apricot, Bio Fruit, Fat Free, Shape, Danone*	1 Pot/119.7g	85	71	4.3	13.1	0.1	0.0
Peach & Apricot, Extremely Fruity, Marks & Spencer*	1 Pot/200g	194	97	4.8	15.8	1.6	0.4
Peach & Apricot, Fat Free, Bio, Shape*	1 Serving/120g	89	74	4.5	13.6	0.1	0.0
Peach & Apricot, Fruit Corner, Muller*	1 Pot/175g	193	110	3.7	15.0	3.9	0.0
Peach & Apricot, Healthy Living, Tesco*	1 Pot/92g	40	44	4.1	6.4	0.2	0.9
Peach & Apricot, Large, Healthy Living, Tesco*	1 Pot/200g	82	41	3.9	6.2	0.1	1.0
Peach & Apricot, Shape*	1 Pot/120g	54	45	4.6	5.8	0.1	0.1
Peach & Apricot, Smooth, Bio, Fat Free, Shape, Danone*	1 Pot/120g	86	72	4.3	13.7	0.1	0.0
Peach & Apricot, Virtually Fat Free, Bio, Shape*	1 Pot/120g	95	79	4.0	13.7	0.9	0.0
Peach & Lemon Balm, Biowild, Onken*	1 Pot/175g	158	90	4.3	14.9	1.5	0.1
Peach & Mango, Juicy, Shapers, Boots*	1 Pot/150g	89	59	4.0	8.3	1.1	0.5
Peach & Mango, Thick & Creamy, Waitrose*	1 Pot/125g	136	109	3.7	17.8	2.5	0.3
Peach & Maracuya, Light, Muller*	1 Pot/200g	102	51	4.5	8.1	0.1	0.0
Peach & Papaya, Fat Free, Yeo Valley*	1 Pot/125g	95	76	5.1	13.6	0.1	0.1
Peach & Papaya, Waitrose*	1 Pot/150g	129	86	4.2	17.1	0.1	0.2
Peach & Passion Fruit Flip, Morrisons*	1 Pot/175g	89	51	3.9	8.2	0.3	0.6

Y

YOGHURT

INFO/WEIGHT	Measure	per Measure KCAL	Nutrition Values per 100g / 100ml KCAL	PROT	CARB	FAT	FIBRE
Peach & Passion Fruit, Fruit Layered, Bio, GFY, Asda*	1 Pot/126.2g	77	61	4.0	11.0	0.1	0.5
Peach & Passion Fruit, Lite Biopot, Onken*	1 Serving/100g	45	45	4.6	6.0	0.2	0.2
Peach & Passion Fruit, Low Fat, Ski*	1 Pot/125g	124	99	4.9	15.7	1.9	0.2
Peach & Passion Fruit, Organic, Muller*	1 Pot/150g	147	98	3.9	16.6	1.8	0.0
Peach & Passion Fruit, Very Low Fat, Somerfield*	1 Pot/125g	61	49	5.0	7.0	0.0	0.0
Peach & Passionfruit, BGTY, Sainsbury's*	1 Pot/125g	69	55	4.9	8.6	0.1	0.1
Peach & Pear, Seriously Fruity, Low Fat, Waitrose*	1 Pot/125g	110	88	4.5	15.3	1.0	0.3
Peach & Pineapple, Fat Free, Weight Watchers*	1 Pot/120g	53	44	4.1	6.5	0.1	0.1
Peach & Pineapple, Light, Ski*	1 Pot/125g	68	54	5.7	7.5	0.1	2.0
Peach & Raspberry, Custard Style, Fat Free, Shape*	1 Pot/170g	77	45	4.1	6.3	0.1	0.2
Peach & Raspberry, Marks & Spencer*	1 Pot/150g	144	96	4.8	15.7	1.6	0.4
Peach & Vanilla Flip, Morrisons*	1 Pot/175g	212	121	3.4	16.5	4.6	0.6
Peach & Vanilla, Healthy Living, Tesco*	1 Pot/125g	54	43	4.1	6.3	0.2	1.0
Peach & Vanilla, Thick & Creamy, Co-Op*	1 Pot/150g	180	120	3.6	16.0	4.6	0.1
Peach 'n' Mango, D'lite, Ski*	1 Pot/200g	182	91	5.1	14.5	0.9	0.0
Peach Melba, Everyday Low Fat, Co-Op*	1 Pot/125g	88	70	3.0	13.0	0.7	0.0
Peach Melba, Low Fat, Tesco*	1 Pot/125g	100	80	2.3	16.0	0.7	0.1
Peach Melba, Sveltesse 0%, Nestle*	1 Pot/125.5g	70	56	4.7	9.1	0.1	0.2
Peach, BGTY, Sainsbury's*	1 Pot/125g	61	49	4.7	7.2	0.2	0.2
Peach, Bio Activia 0%, Danone*	1 Pot/125g	64	51	3.7	8.9	0.0	0.0
Peach, Bio, Virtually Fat Free, Shape*	1 Pot/120g	55	46	4.7	5.8	0.1	0.1
Peach, Corner Squeezer, Muller*	1 Serving/64g	65	101	3.2	15.2	3.0	0.0
Peach, Custard Style, Low Fat, Sainsbury's*	1 Pot/125g	110	88	4.4	14.2	1.5	0.1
Peach, D'lite, Ski*	1 Pot/125g	100	80	4.6	15.2	0.1	0.2
Peach, Economy, Sainsbury's*	1 Pot/125g	93	74	2.8	14.7	0.4	0.0
Peach, Extra Fruit, Low Fat, Ski*	1 Pot/125g	114	91	3.5	15.7	1.5	0.1
Peach, Fat Free, Skips*	1 Pot/125g	100	80	4.6	15.2	0.1	0.2
Peach, Fat Free, Weight Watchers*	1 Pot/118g	53	45	4.2	6.7	0.1	0.2
Peach, Honey & Grain, Eat Smart, Safeway*	1 Serving/200g	120	60	4.7	9.4	0.2	0.3
Peach, Light, Ski*	1 Pot/125g	100	80	4.6	15.2	0.1	0.2
Peach, Low Fat, Asda*	1 Pot/125g	118	95	4.7	16.7	1.1	0.2
Peach, Low Fat, Basics, Sainsbury's*	1 Pot/125g	84	67	4.0	10.4	1.0	0.1
Peach, Low Fat, Muller*	1 Pot/150g	152	101	4.8	16.1	1.9	0.0
Peach, Low Fat, Probiotic, Tesco*	1 Pot/125g	106	85	3.9	14.3	1.4	0.3
Peach, Low Fat, Sainsbury's*	1 Pot/125g	114	91	4.3	15.0	1.5	0.1
Peach, Low Fat, Ski*	1 Pot/125g	123	98	4.9	15.5	1.8	0.2
Peach, Low Fat, Yeo Valley*	1 Pot/125g	113	90	4.6	15.3	1.1	0.1
Peach, Optimel, Campina*	1 Serving/200ml	70	35	4.0	4.5	0.0	0.0
Peach, Organic, Alpro Soya*	1 Serving/125g	109	87	3.8	12.4	2.2	0.3
Peach, Pineapple Passion Fruit, Very Low Fat, Loseley*	1 Pot/140g	99	71	3.3	14.3	0.0	0.0
Peach, Shape*	1 Pot/120g	55	46	4.7	5.8	0.1	0.1
Peach, Smooth, Ski*	1 Pot/125g	128	102	4.9	16.3	1.9	0.0
Peach, Thick & Fruity, Weight Watchers*	1 Pot/120g	55	46	4.2	7.1	0.1	0.2
Peach, Vitality Probiotic, Muller*	1 Pot/150g	113	75	2.6	13.0	1.4	0.0
Peach, Whole Grain, Biopot, Onken*	1 Serving/200g	226	113	4.2	17.9	2.7	0.3
Peaches, Farmhouse, BGTY, Sainsbury's*	1 Pot/150g	134	89	3.2	17.8	0.4	0.3
Peanut Toffee, Low Fat, Somerfield*	1 Pot/150g	131	87	4.0	15.0	1.0	0.0
Pear & Butterscotch, Finest, Tesco*	1 Pot/150g	413	275	5.0	32.3	14.0	0.5
Pear, Rosehip & Marigold, Biowild, Onken*	1 Pot/175g	161	92	4.4	15.1	1.5	0.3
Pear, Tine Jubileum*	1 Carton/125g	168	134	3.2	18.6	5.2	0.0
Pianola, Lidl*	1 Serving/125g	108	86	4.3	16.1	0.1	0.0
Pineapple & Coconut, Weight Watchers*	1 Pot/120g	56	47	3.9	7.4	0.1	0.1
Pineapple & Grapefruit, BGTY, Sainsbury's*	1 Pot/125g	68	54	4.4	8.8	0.1	0.1

YOGHURT

	Measure INFO/WEIGHT	per Measure KCAL	KCAL	PROT	CARB	FAT	FIBRE
Pineapple & Papaya, Ski*	1 Pot/125g	123	98	4.8	15.5	1.8	0.1
Pineapple & Peach, Virtually Fat Free, Light, Muller*	1 Pot/200g	106	53	4.4	8.7	0.1	0.0
Pineapple Or Peach, Low Fat, Organic, Tesco*	1 Serving/125g	108	86	5.1	14.1	1.0	0.1
Pineapple, BGTY, Sainsbury's*	1 Pot/125g	66	53	4.8	8.3	0.1	1.1
Pineapple, Channel Island, Marks & Spencer*	1 Pot/150g	165	110	4.3	15.9	3.3	0.3
Pineapple, D'Lite 0.2, Ski, Nestle*	1 Pot/125g	100	80	4.4	15.3	0.1	0.1
Pineapple, Eat Smart, Safeway*	1 Pot/125g	66	53	4.5	8.4	0.1	0.1
Pineapple, Extremely Fruity, Marks & Spencer*	1 Pot/200g	200	100	4.3	17.6	1.4	0.2
Pineapple, Finest, Tesco*	1 Pot/200g	220	110	3.5	17.5	2.9	0.2
Pineapple, Healthy Living, Tesco*	1 Pot/125g	69	55	5.1	8.1	0.3	1.1
Pineapple, Low Fat, Bio, Asda*	1 Pot/150g	144	96	4.6	17.0	1.1	0.1
Pineapple, Low Fat, Tesco*	1 Pot/125g	111	89	4.6	13.4	1.7	0.0
Pineapple, Thick & Creamy, Waitrose*	1 Pot/125g	136	109	3.6	17.9	2.5	0.2
Pineapple, Truly Fruity, Shape*	1 Pot/120g	61	51	4.5	7.3	0.1	0.1
Pineapple, Virtually Fat Free, Tesco*	1 Pot/125g	55	44	4.1	6.5	0.2	0.9
Pineapple, Weight Watchers*	1 Pot/120g	56	47	3.9	7.7	0.1	0.9
Pink Grapefruit Fruit Corner, Muller*	1 Pot/175g	189	108	4.1	13.9	4.0	0.0
Pink Grapefruit With Grains, Good Intentions, Somerfield*	1 Pot/125g	87	70	6.0	10.8	0.3	0.1
Pink Grapefruit, Breakfast Selection, Sainsbury's*	1 Pot/117g	109	93	4.2	15.9	1.4	0.1
Pink Grapefruit, Low Fat, Sainsbury's*	1 Pot/125g	116	93	4.2	15.9	1.4	0.1
Pink Grapefruit, Weight Watchers*	1 Pot/120g	52	43	4.1	6.3	0.1	0.2
Plain, Low Fat	1 Pot/120g	67	56	5.1	7.5	0.8	0.0
Plum & Hop, Biowild, Onken*	1 Pot/175g	158	90	4.3	14.9	1.5	0.3
Plum, BGTY, Sainsbury's*	1 Pot/125g	69	55	4.8	8.8	0.1	0.1
Plum, Bio Live, Summer Selection, Yeo Valley*	1 Pot/125g	126	101	4.1	12.4	3.9	0.1
Plum, Low Fat, Orchard Grove, Shape*	1 Pot/100g	63	63	4.7	8.3	1.0	0.2
Plum, Low Fat, Ski*	1 Pot/125g	119	95	4.9	14.9	1.8	0.1
Probiotic, Low Fat, Organic, Glenisk*	1 Serving/150g	92	61	4.5	6.4	1.9	0.0
Prune, Breakfast Selection, Sainsbury's*	1 Pot/125g	119	95	4.2	16.3	1.4	0.2
Prune, Probiotic, Tesco*	1 Serving/170g	145	85	3.9	14.3	1.4	1.0
Rapsberry & White Chocolate, Low Fat, Shape*	1 Pot/100g	101	101	4.7	15.6	1.8	0.1
Rasberry, Orange & Grain, Eat Smart, Safeway*	1 Pot/200g	120	60	4.7	9.1	0.2	0.6
Rashaka, Plain, Danone*	1 Serving/180ml	88	49	5.5	6.5	0.0	0.0
Raspberry & Blackberry, Thick & Creamy, Co-Op*	1 Pot/150g	188	125	3.6	17.3	4.6	0.1
Raspberry & Blackcurrant, Ski*	1 Pot/125g	129	103	4.4	14.6	3.0	0.0
Raspberry & Cranberry, BGTY, Sainsbury's*	1 Pot/125g	65	52	4.4	8.4	0.1	0.5
Raspberry & Cranberry, Light, Healthy Living, Tesco*	1 Pot/125g	55	44	4.2	6.3	0.2	1.1
Raspberry & Cranberry, Light, Muller*	1 Pot/200g	106	53	4.5	8.6	0.1	0.5
Raspberry & Elderberry, Organic, Onken*	1 Serving/50g	53	106	3.8	15.0	3.1	0.0
Raspberry & Orange, Fat Free, Organic, Yeo Valley*	1 Serving/100g	77	77	5.1	13.7	0.1	0.1
Raspberry & Redcurrant, Low Fat, Sainsbury's*	1 Pot/125g	109	87	4.2	14.5	1.4	0.5
Raspberry, 0.1% Fat, Shape, Danone*	1 Pot/120g	55	46	4.6	6.7	0.1	2.2
Raspberry, BGTY, Sainsbury's*	1 Pot/125g	64	51	4.4	7.9	0.2	2.0
Raspberry, Bio Pot, Onken*	1 Pot/150g	153	102	4.4	15.1	2.7	0.0
Raspberry, Bio, Virtually Fat Free, Shape*	1 Pot/120g	56	47	4.7	6.1	0.1	0.2
Raspberry, COU, Marks & Spencer*	1 Pot/150g	68	45	4.2	6.9	0.1	0.6
Raspberry, D'lite 0.2%, Ski*	1 Pot/125g	99	79	4.6	14.9	0.1	0.6
Raspberry, Economy, Sainsbury's*	1 Pot/125g	85	68	3.0	11.9	1.0	0.0
Raspberry, Everyday, Low Fat, Co-Op*	1 Pot/125g	88	70	3.0	13.0	0.7	0.0
Raspberry, Extremely Fruity, Marks & Spencer*	1 Pot/200g	190	95	5.0	15.6	1.5	0.5
Raspberry, Farmhouse, TTD, Sainsbury's*	1 Pot/150g	149	99	3.6	15.0	2.8	1.6
Raspberry, Fat Free, BGTY, Sainsbury's*	1 Pot/125g	64	51	4.8	7.7	0.1	1.7
Raspberry, Fat Free, Bio Live, Organic, Yeo Valley*	1 Pot/125g	98	78	5.2	14.0	0.1	0.4

Y

YOGHURT

INFO/WEIGHT	per Measure KCAL	KCAL	PROT	CARB	FAT	FIBRE
Raspberry, Fat Free, Bio, Shape, Danone*	1 Pot/120g	84	70	4.3	12.9	0.1	0.4
Raspberry, Fat Free, Farmhouse, BGTY, Sainsbury's*	1 Pot/150g	101	67	3.4	13.7	0.1	2.0
Raspberry, Fat Free, Weight Watchers*	1 Pot/120g	49	41	4.2	5.7	0.1	0.3
Raspberry, Fimbles, Marks & Spencer*	1 Pot/87.5g	70	80	3.6	11.1	2.6	0.6
Raspberry, French Set Wholemilk, Asda*	1 Pot/125g	125	100	3.6	14.1	3.2	0.0
Raspberry, French Set, Waitrose*	1 Pot/125g	120	96	3.5	13.4	3.1	2.0
Raspberry, Frozen, Handmade Farmhouse, Sainsbury's*	1 Serving/100g	132	132	2.7	21.8	3.8	2.2
Raspberry, Frozen, Orchard Maid*	1 Serving/80ml	89	111	2.8	19.9	2.1	0.0
Raspberry, Frozen, TTD, Sainsbury's*	1/4 Pot/90g	119	132	2.7	21.8	3.8	2.2
Raspberry, Fruit Corner, Muller*	1 Pot/175g	200	114	4.2	15.3	4.0	0.0
Raspberry, Fruit Halo, Muller Light, Muller*	1 Pot/144.0g	121	84	3.7	16.5	0.3	0.0
Raspberry, Fruit Layer, Activa, Danone*	1 Serving/125g	113	90	3.5	12.8	2.8	2.0
Raspberry, Greek Style, Layered, GFY, Asda*	1 Pot/150g	123	82	4.3	10.0	2.7	1.3
Raspberry, Healthy Living, Tesco*	1 Serving/175g	88	50	4.2	8.1	0.1	0.0
Raspberry, Light, Healthy Living, Tesco*	1 Pot/200g	84	42	3.9	6.4	0.1	1.0
Raspberry, Low Fat, Asda*	1 Pot/125g	121	97	4.7	17.0	1.1	0.7
Raspberry, Low Fat, Benecol*	1 Pot/125ml	100	80	3.8	14.5	0.7	0.0
Raspberry, Low Fat, Bio, Sainsbury's*	1 Pot/150g	146	97	4.7	17.0	1.1	0.7
Raspberry, Low Fat, Muller*	1 Pot/150g	152	101	4.8	16.1	1.9	0.0
Raspberry, Low Fat, Organic, Sainsbury's*	1 Serving/125g	106	85	5.1	14.0	1.0	0.2
Raspberry, Low Fat, Probiotic, Tesco*	1 Pot/170g	145	85	3.9	14.3	1.4	0.3
Raspberry, Low Fat, Sainsbury's*	1 Pot/125g	115	92	4.4	15.2	1.5	0.2
Raspberry, Low Fat, Ski*	1 Pot/125g	121	97	4.9	15.2	1.9	0.6
Raspberry, Low Fat, Tesco*	1 Pot/125g	116	93	4.3	14.9	1.8	0.0
Raspberry, Marks & Spencer*	1 Pot/150g	144	96	4.9	15.4	1.6	0.6
Raspberry, Meadow Fresh*	1 Sm Pot/125g	130	104	4.5	18.9	1.0	0.0
Raspberry, Organic, Fat Free, Rachel's Organic*	1 Serving/142g	78	55	3.6	10.0	0.1	0.0
Raspberry, Organic, Low Fat, Tesco*	1 Pot/125g	109	87	5.3	14.1	1.0	0.1
Raspberry, Organic, Yeo Valley*	1 Pot/150g	144	96	4.4	12.3	3.3	0.1
Raspberry, Pavlova, Corner, Muller*	1 Pot/150g	230	153	3.4	24.4	4.7	0.0
Raspberry, Probiotic, Vitality, Low Fat, Muller*	1 Bottle/100g	97	97	4.8	15.4	1.8	0.0
Raspberry, Really, Solo, Shape, Danone*	1 Pot/175g	75	43	4.6	5.9	0.1	2.2
Raspberry, Scottish, Finest, Tesco*	1 Pot/150g	227	151	3.4	18.9	6.9	0.5
Raspberry, Seriously Fruity, Low Fat, Waitrose*	1 Pot/150g	149	99	4.8	16.2	1.7	0.3
Raspberry, Shape, Danone*	1 Serving/120g	55	46	4.6	6.7	0.1	2.2
Raspberry, Smooth, Marks & Spencer*	1 Pot/150g	150	100	4.9	16.2	1.6	0.5
Raspberry, Thick & Creamy, Sainsbury's*	1 Pot/150g	179	119	4.4	17.2	3.7	0.2
Raspberry, Value, Tesco*	1 Serving/125g	100	80	2.3	16.0	0.7	0.1
Raspberry, Virtually Fat Free, Tesco*	1 Pot/125g	51	41	4.1	5.8	0.2	1.1
Raspberry, Vitality, Muller*	1oz/28g	27	97	4.8	15.4	1.8	0.0
Raspberry, Way To Five, Sainsbury's*	1 Pot/151g	104	69	3.3	13.6	0.1	2.1
Red Cherries, Bio Activia 0%, Danone*	1 Pot/125g	65	52	3.6	9.1	0.0	0.0
Red Cherry, Bio, Shape*	1 Pot/120g	58	48	4.6	6.4	0.1	0.1
Red Cherry, D'lite, Ski*	1 Pot/125g	101	81	4.5	15.4	0.1	0.1
Red Cherry, Fruit Layered, GFY, Asda*	1 Pot/125g	75	60	3.7	11.0	0.1	0.0
Red Cherry, Light, 99.9% Fat Free, Ski*	1 Pot/125g	73	58	4.9	9.2	0.1	1.2
Red Cherry, Light, Ski*	1 Pot/125g	101	81	4.5	15.4	0.1	0.1
Red Cherry, Organic, Onken*	1 Serving/28g	29	102	3.6	14.8	3.1	0.0
Red Cherry, Simply Berries, Shape, Danone*	1 Pot/120g	64	53	4.4	8.7	0.1	7.4
Red Cherry, Virtually Fat Free, Ski*	1 Pot/125g	64	51	4.5	7.7	0.2	2.0
Red Fruits, Crumble Style, Sveltesse 0%, Nestle*	1 Pot/125g	69	55	4.3	9.0	0.2	0.2
Rhubarb & Orange, Perfectly Balanced, Waitrose*	1/2 Pot/250ml	218	87	1.9	18.4	0.6	0.2
Rhubarb & Orange, Tesco*	1 Pot/150g	146	97	4.6	17.1	1.1	0.5

YOGHURT

INFO/WEIGHT	Measure	per Measure KCAL	Nutrition Values per 100g / 100ml KCAL	PROT	CARB	FAT	FIBRE
Rhubarb & Vanilla, Onken*	1 Serving/100g	106	106	3.8	16.9	2.6	0.3
Rhubarb Crumble Corner, Muller*	1 Pot/150g	222	148	3.3	21.7	5.3	0.0
Rhubarb Crumble, Layered Style, Healthy Eating, Tesco*	1 Pot/125g	93	74	4.1	12.9	0.7	0.2
Rhubarb, Bio, Activia, Danone*	1 Pot/125g	129	103	3.5	15.0	3.2	1.6
Rhubarb, Custard Style, Somerfield*	1 Pot/125g	149	119	3.0	16.0	5.0	0.0
Rhubarb, Eat Smart, Safeway*	1 Pot/125g	69	55	5.1	7.8	0.1	0.2
Rhubarb, Extremely Fruity, Bio, Marks & Spencer*	1 Pot/150g	158	105	4.5	18.2	1.4	0.4
Rhubarb, Extremely Fruity, Marks & Spencer*	1 Pot/150g	158	105	4.5	18.2	1.4	0.4
Rhubarb, Farmhouse, TTD, Sainsbury's*	1 Pot/150g	149	99	4.3	13.4	3.1	0.3
Rhubarb, Live Bio, Perfectly Balanced, Waitrose*	1 Pot/151g	131	87	4.6	17.0	0.1	0.2
Rhubarb, Low Fat, Bio Live, Rachel's Organic*	1 Pot/100g	73	73	3.5	11.0	1.7	0.0
Rhubarb, Low Fat, Organic, Marks & Spencer*	1 Pot/170g	145	85	4.1	14.7	1.2	0.2
Rhubarb, Low Fat, Organic, Sainsbury's*	1 Pot/125g	99	79	5.1	12.3	1.0	0.2
Rhubarb, Low Fat, Sainsbury's*	1 Pot/125g	114	91	4.5	14.5	1.7	0.2
Rhubarb, Low Fat, Ski*	1 Pot/125g	123	98	4.8	15.7	1.8	0.1
Rhubarb, Low Fat, Tesco*	1 Pot/125g	106	85	4.9	12.4	1.7	0.1
Rhubarb, Marks & Spencer*	1 Pot/150g	149	99	4.4	17.4	1.4	0.3
Rhubarb, Perfectly Balanced, Waitrose*	1 Pot/150g	114	76	4.2	14.5	0.1	0.2
Rhubarb, Very Low Fat, Somerfield*	1 Pot/125g	58	46	5.0	6.0	0.0	0.0
Rich & Creamy, Spelga*	1 Serving/150g	188	125	3.7	17.2	4.7	0.1
Rum Raisin Crunch Corner, Muller*	1 Pot/150g	219	146	4.2	22.0	4.6	0.0
Sheep's Milk, Total*	1oz/28g	25	90	4.8	4.3	6.0	0.0
Simply Strawberry, Low Fat, Ubley*	1 Pot/125g	113	90	4.4	15.7	1.0	0.4
Smooth Toffee & Apple, Low Fat, Co-Op*	1 Pot/125g	150	120	6.0	22.0	1.0	0.1
Smooth Toffee & Orange, Co-Op*	1 Pot/125g	181	145	6.0	27.0	1.0	0.0
Smooth Toffee, Eat Smart, Safeway*	1 Pot/125g	69	55	5.1	8.7	0.1	0.0
Smooth Vanilla, Eat Smart, Safeway*	1 Pot/125g	69	55	5.0	8.3	0.1	0.0
Somerset With Vanilla, TTD, Sainsbury's*	1 Pot/150g	222	148	4.0	18.1	6.6	0.0
Soya	1oz/28g	20	72	5.0	3.9	4.2	0.0
Spanish Lemon, Onken*	1 Serving/100g	100	100	3.9	15.1	2.7	0.0
Spanish Orange, Amore Luxury, Muller*	1 Pot/175g	254	145	2.3	16.3	7.8	0.0
Spiced Orange, Dessert, Low Fat, Sainsbury's*	1 Pot/125g	121	97	4.5	16.0	1.7	0.1
Sticky Toffee Pudding Corner, Muller*	1 Pot/150g	239	159	3.6	24.7	5.1	0.0
Strawberries & Cream, Finest, Tesco*	1 Pot/150g	206	137	3.4	15.4	6.9	0.5
Strawberries & Cream, TTD, Sainsbury's*	1 Serving/150g	194	129	3.6	15.8	5.7	0.5
Strawberry & Cornish Clotted Cream, Marks & Spencer*	1 Pot/150g	218	145	3.2	15.4	7.7	0.5
Strawberry & Orange Crunch Corner, Muller*	1 Pot/150g	218	145	4.1	22.5	4.3	0.0
Strawberry & Raspberry, Bio Live, Organic, Yeo Valley*	1 Pot/125g	125	100	4.2	12.0	3.9	0.1
Strawberry & Raspberry, Bio, GFY, Asda*	1 Pot/125g	75	60	3.8	11.0	0.1	0.0
Strawberry & Raspberry, Healthy Eating, Tesco*	1 Pot/125g	58	46	4.2	7.0	0.1	0.0
Strawberry & Raspberry, Layered, Bio, GFY, Asda*	1 Pot/72g	43	60	3.8	11.0	0.1	0.4
Strawberry & Raspberry, Low Fat, Sainsbury's*	1 Pot/125g	109	87	4.2	14.3	1.4	0.2
Strawberry & Rhubarb, Channel Island, Marks & Spencer*	1 Pot/150g	158	105	3.9	15.4	3.0	0.0
Strawberry & Rhubarb, Low Fat, Sainsbury's*	1 Pot/125g	108	86	4.2	14.1	1.4	0.2
Strawberry & Rhubarb, Onken*	1 Serving/100g	85	85	4.6	16.2	0.1	0.4
Strawberry & Vanilla, Low Fat, Somerfield*	1 Pot/125g	109	87	4.0	15.9	0.8	0.1
Strawberry & Vanilla, Weight Watchers*	1 Pot/120g	54	45	4.2	6.8	0.1	0.1
Strawberry & Wild Strawberry, Sveltesse 0%, Nestle*	1 Pot/125g	58	46	4.3	7.0	0.1	0.0
Strawberry & Wild Strawberry, Weight Watchers*	1 Pot/120g	49	41	4.2	5.8	0.1	0.1
Strawberry Cheescake Corner, Muller*	1 Pot/150g	233	155	3.7	25.3	4.3	0.0
Strawberry Cheesecake, Eat Smart, Safeway*	1 Pot/125g	64	51	4.7	7.7	0.1	0.3
Strawberry Fruit, Deep Fill, Low Fat, Ski*	1 Pot/159g	137	86	4.0	13.8	1.6	0.0
Strawberry Mousse, Shapers, Boots*	1 Pot/90g	88	97	4.1	11.0	4.1	0.1

YOGHURT

INFO/WEIGHT	Measure per Measure KCAL	KCAL	PROT	CARB	FAT	FIBRE
			Nutrition Values per 100g / 100ml			
Strawberry With Grains, Good Intentions, Somerfield*	1 Pot/125g	86	69	6.0	10.6	0.3	0.2
Strawberry With Real Fruit Chunks, Low Fat, Muller*	1 Pot/150g	149	99	4.8	15.7	1.9	0.0
Strawberry, & Muesli, Breakfast, Tesco*	1 Pot/170g	192	113	4.1	17.9	2.8	0.5
Strawberry, & Whole Grain, Bio Break, Tesco*	1 Pot/175g	175	100	4.7	17.8	1.1	0.2
Strawberry, & Wild Strawberry, 0.1% Fat, Shape, Danone*	1 Pot/120g	55	46	4.6	6.7	0.1	2.1
Strawberry, 0.1% Fat, Solo, Shape, Danone*	1 Serving/175g	75	43	4.5	5.9	0.1	2.1
Strawberry, BGTY, Sainsbury's*	1 Pot/125g	64	51	4.8	7.7	0.1	1.2
Strawberry, Balanced Lifestyle, Aldi*	1 Pot/150g	72	48	4.1	7.1	0.3	0.5
Strawberry, Bettabuy, Morrisons*	1 Pot/115g	91	79	4.4	12.8	1.3	0.3
Strawberry, Bio & Cereal Clusters, Rumblers*	1 Pot/168g	267	159	4.3	22.4	5.8	1.1
Strawberry, Bio Activia 0% Fat, Danone*	1 Pot/125g	63	50	3.8	8.4	0.0	0.0
Strawberry, Bio Live, Fat Free, Rachel's Organic*	1 Pot/142g	81	57	3.5	10.5	0.1	0.0
Strawberry, Bio Live, Organic, Yeo Valley*	1 Pot/150g	152	101	4.1	12.3	3.9	0.1
Strawberry, Bio Virtually Fat Free, Tesco*	1 Pot/125g	50	40	4.4	5.3	0.2	0.9
Strawberry, Bio, Healthy Eating, Tesco*	1 Pot/125g	61	49	4.7	7.0	0.2	0.2
Strawberry, Biopot, Onken*	1 Serving/100g	100	100	3.1	15.9	2.7	0.0
Strawberry, COU, Marks & Spencer*	1 Pot/125g	56	45	4.1	7.3	0.1	0.4
Strawberry, Carb Control, Tesco*	1 Pot/125g	61	49	3.7	6.3	1.0	0.2
Strawberry, Crisp, Jordans*	1oz/28g	38	137	4.8	22.8	3.3	1.1
Strawberry, Crumble Corner, Muller*	1 Pot/150g	222	148	3.3	21.7	5.3	0.0
Strawberry, Custard Style, Somerfield*	1 Pot/125g	153	122	3.0	17.0	5.0	0.0
Strawberry, D'lite, Ski*	1 Pot/125g	99	79	4.5	14.7	0.1	0.2
Strawberry, Dessert, Frozen, Tesco*	1 Pot/60g	82	136	2.6	26.5	2.2	0.8
Strawberry, Duo, Co-Op*	1 Pot/175g	219	125	3.0	17.0	5.0	0.7
Strawberry, Everyday Low Fat, Co-Op*	1 Pot/125g	88	70	3.0	13.0	0.7	0.0
Strawberry, Extra Light, 0.1% Fat, Muller*	1 Pot/200g	118	59	5.0	8.8	0.1	0.0
Strawberry, Extremely Fruity, Marks & Spencer*	1 Pot/200g	190	95	4.8	15.4	1.6	0.2
Strawberry, Farmhouse, BGTY, Sainsbury's*	1 Pot/150g	107	71	3.2	13.7	0.4	0.5
Strawberry, Fat Free, Bio Live, Organic, Yeo Valley*	1 Pot/125g	108	86	5.1	14.1	1.0	0.1
Strawberry, Fat Free, Bio, Shape, Danone*	1 Pot/120g	86	72	4.3	13.6	0.1	0.1
Strawberry, Fat Free, Rachel's Organic*	1 Pot/125g	121	97	4.7	15.4	1.8	0.0
Strawberry, Fat Free, Weight Watchers*	1 Pot/120g	52	43	4.1	6.2	0.1	0.1
Strawberry, Fimbles, Marks & Spencer*	1 Pot/88.2g	75	85	3.8	11.1	2.8	0.8
Strawberry, Frozen, Organic, Yeo Valley*	1 Serving/100g	139	139	4.7	23.9	2.7	0.3
Strawberry, Fruit Corner, Muller*	1 Pot/175g	207	118	3.7	17.1	3.9	0.0
Strawberry, Fruit'n'Creamy, Ubley*	1 Pot/150.5g	167	111	4.3	16.9	2.9	0.3
Strawberry, Granose*	1oz/28g	25	90	4.5	15.5	1.6	0.0
Strawberry, Healthy Living, Tesco*	1 Pot/175g	74	42	4.1	6.0	0.2	1.0
Strawberry, Light & Refreshing, Campina*	1 Pot/125g	110	88	2.5	16.9	1.1	0.0
Strawberry, Light, 99.9% Fat Free, Ski*	1 Pot/125g	60	48	4.7	7.7	0.1	1.0
Strawberry, Light, Healthy Living, Tesco*	1 Pot/200g	100	50	4.2	8.1	0.1	0.0
Strawberry, Light, Muller*	1 Pot/200g	108	54	4.5	8.7	0.1	0.0
Strawberry, Lite, Onken*	1 Serving/100g	46	46	4.6	6.5	0.2	0.2
Strawberry, Little Town Dairy*	1 Pot/125g	82	66	2.9	9.9	1.6	0.0
Strawberry, Live, Turner's Dairies*	1 Pot/125g	86	69	4.9	11.9	0.3	0.0
Strawberry, Low Fat, Asda*	1 Pot/125g	114	91	4.4	16.0	1.0	0.0
Strawberry, Low Fat, Basics, Sainsbury's*	1 Pot/125g	74	59	4.0	8.4	1.0	0.1
Strawberry, Low Fat, Benecol*	1 Pot/150g	119	79	3.7	14.8	0.6	0.0
Strawberry, Low Fat, Lakeland*	1 Pot/125g	98	78	4.3	13.4	0.8	0.1
Strawberry, Low Fat, Organic, Muller*	1 Pot/150g	147	98	3.9	16.6	1.8	0.0
Strawberry, Low Fat, Organic, Sainsbury's*	1 Pot/125g	100	80	5.3	12.6	1.0	0.1
Strawberry, Low Fat, Sainsbury's*	1 Pot/125g	115	92	4.3	15.2	1.5	0.1
Strawberry, Low Fat, Ski*	1 Pot/125g	124	99	4.8	15.8	1.8	0.0

YOGHURT

INFO/WEIGHT	per Measure KCAL	KCAL	PROT	CARB	FAT	FIBRE
Strawberry, Low Fat, SmartPrice, Asda*	1 Pot/125g	85	68	2.2	13.0	0.8	0.0
Strawberry, Low Fat, Spelga*	1 Pot/125g	129	103	4.5	18.0	1.8	0.0
Strawberry, Low Fat, Tesco*	1 Pot/125g	113	90	4.2	14.4	1.7	0.0
Strawberry, Low Fat, Value, Tesco*	1 Pot/125g	81	65	2.7	11.8	0.7	0.1
Strawberry, Low Fat, Vitality Probiotic, Muller*	1 Pot/150g	146	97	4.7	15.6	1.8	0.0
Strawberry, Luscious, Shapers, Boots*	1 Pot/150g	83	55	4.0	7.3	1.1	0.6
Strawberry, Marks & Spencer*	1 Pot/150g	143	95	4.8	15.4	1.6	0.2
Strawberry, Organic, Alpro Soya*	1 Serving/125g	104	83	3.8	11.5	2.2	0.3
Strawberry, Organic, Low Fat, Tesco*	1 Pot/125g	104	83	5.3	13.2	1.0	0.1
Strawberry, Organic, Yeo Valley*	1 Pot/150g	144	96	4.3	12.4	3.3	0.1
Strawberry, Perfectly Balanced, Waitrose*	1 Pot/150g	136	91	4.6	17.8	0.1	0.1
Strawberry, Probiotic, Tesco*	1 Pot/170g	145	85	3.9	14.3	1.4	0.3
Strawberry, Redcurrant, Bio Layered, Sainsbury's*	1 Serving/125g	134	107	4.1	16.5	2.7	0.2
Strawberry, Seriously Fruity, Low Fat, Waitrose*	1 Pot/150g	131	87	4.5	15.0	1.0	0.3
Strawberry, Ski*	1 Pot/125g	111	89	3.4	15.3	1.5	0.9
Strawberry, Smooth Set French, Low Fat, Sainsbury's*	1 Pot/125g	100	80	3.5	13.6	1.2	0.0
Strawberry, Smooth, Fat Free, Shape*	1 Pot/120g	85	71	4.3	13.2	0.1	0.1
Strawberry, Smooth, Marks & Spencer*	1 Pot/150g	150	100	4.8	16.1	1.6	0.2
Strawberry, Smooth, Ski*	1 Pot/125g	126	101	4.9	16.1	1.9	0.0
Strawberry, Soyage, GranoVita*	1 Pot/145g	112	77	1.8	16.5	0.4	0.0
Strawberry, Sundae Style, Sveltesse %, Nestle*	1 Pot/124.5g	66	53	4.3	8.7	0.1	0.0
Strawberry, Sveltesse*	1 Pot/125g	70	56	4.7	9.1	0.1	0.2
Strawberry, Thick & Creamy, Co-Op*	1 Pot/150g	182	121	3.6	16.4	4.6	0.1
Strawberry, Thick & Fruity, Weight Watchers*	1 Pot/121g	52	43	4.1	6.2	0.1	0.1
Strawberry, Variety Selection, Nestle*	1 Pot/125g	119	95	4.7	15.1	1.8	0.2
Strawberry, Very Low Fat, Loseley*	1 Pot/140g	92	66	3.3	13.0	0.1	0.0
Strawberry, Virtually Fat Free, Organic, Yeo Valley*	1 Pot/125g	98	78	5.1	14.3	0.1	0.1
Strawberry, Virtually Fat Free, Shapers, Boots*	1 Pot/125g	67	54	5.2	8.1	0.1	0.1
Strawberry, Virtually Fat Free, Ski*	1 Pot/127g	61	48	4.5	7.1	0.2	2.0
Strawberry, Virtually Fat Free, Tesco*	1 Pot/125g	53	42	4.1	6.0	0.2	1.0
Strawberry, Vitality Probiotic, Muller*	1 Pot/175g	138	79	2.6	14.1	1.4	0.0
Strawberry, Whole Grain, Biopot, Onken*	1 Serving/100g	109	109	4.2	16.9	2.7	0.3
Strawberry, Wholemilk, Organic, Sainsbury's*	1 Pot/150g	123	82	3.5	9.2	3.5	0.1
Strawberry, Yoplait*	1 Pot/125g	61	49	4.2	7.6	0.2	0.9
Summer Berries, Fat Free, Shape*	1 Pot/120g	55	46	4.6	6.0	0.1	0.2
Summer Berries, Whole Grain, Lite, Biopot, Onken*	1 Serving/240g	199	83	4.6	15.8	0.2	1.4
Summer Fruits, Cool Country*	1 Serving/150g	137	91	3.0	16.3	1.5	0.0
Summer Fruits, Light, Spelga*	1 Pot/175g	79	45	4.4	7.1	0.2	0.0
Summer Fruits, Strawberry, Light, Healthy Living, Tesco*	1 Pot/125g	53	42	4.1	6.0	0.2	1.0
Summer Selection, Fat Free, Organic, Yeo Valley*	1 Pot/125g	89	71	5.2	12.3	0.1	0.2
Summerfruits Bio, Boots*	1 Pot/150g	140	93	4.1	13.0	2.7	0.4
Summerfruits, Fat Free, Bio Live, Rachel's Organic*	1 Pot/125g	120	96	4.7	15.3	1.8	0.0
Timperley Rhubarb, Seriously Fruity, Waitrose*	1 Pot/125g	111	89	4.4	15.5	1.0	0.2
Toffee Apple, COU, Marks & Spencer*	1 Pot/200g	90	45	4.2	6.3	0.2	0.2
Toffee Apple, Indulgent Greek Style, Somerfield*	1 Pot/125g	225	180	3.0	27.0	7.0	0.0
Toffee Caramel, D'lite, Ski*	1 Pot/180g	153	85	4.8	16.3	0.1	0.0
Toffee Fudge, Low Fat, Sainsbury's*	1 Pot/125g	146	117	4.3	20.4	2.0	0.0
Toffee Hoops, Crunch Corner, Muller*	1 Pot/150g	242	161	4.7	22.3	5.9	0.0
Toffee, Benecol*	1 Pot/125g	124	99	3.8	19.3	0.7	0.0
Toffee, COU, Marks & Spencer*	1 Pot/145g	65	45	4.2	7.7	0.2	0.0
Toffee, Childrens, Co-Op*	1 Pot/125g	143	114	3.6	18.6	2.8	0.0
Toffee, Economy, Sainsbury's*	1 Pot/126g	91	72	3.0	12.8	1.0	0.0
Toffee, Fat Free, Eat Smart, Safeway*	1 Pot/200g	100	50	4.6	7.7	0.1	0.0

YOGHURT

INFO/WEIGHT	Measure	per Measure KCAL	KCAL	PROT	CARB	FAT	FIBRE
Toffee, Light, Healthy Living, Tesco*	1 Pot/200g	80	40	3.9	5.9	0.1	1.0
Toffee, Light, Muller*	1 Pot/200g	108	54	4.3	8.9	0.1	0.0
Toffee, Light, Ski*	1 Pot/120g	60	50	4.6	7.7	0.2	0.6
Toffee, Live Bio, Perfectly Balanced, Waitrose*	1 Pot/150g	156	104	4.2	21.1	0.3	0.0
Toffee, Low Fat, Asda*	1 Pot/150g	174	116	4.6	22.0	1.1	0.0
Toffee, Low Fat, Marks & Spencer*	1 Pot/150g	180	120	4.9	21.6	1.7	0.0
Toffee, Low Fat, SmartPrice, Asda*	1 Pot/125g	96	77	2.2	15.0	0.9	0.0
Toffee, Low Fat, Tesco*	1 Pot/125g	130	104	4.2	17.4	1.9	0.0
Toffee, Seriously Smooth, Low Fat, Waitrose*	1 Pot/150g	156	104	4.7	16.5	2.1	0.1
Toffee, Smooth & Creamy, Fat Free, Weight Watchers*	1 Pot/120g	48	40	3.9	5.9	0.1	0.8
Toffee, Very Low Fat Bio, Somerfield*	1 Pot/200g	100	50	5.0	7.0	0.0	0.0
Toffee, Virtually Fat Free, Boots*	1 Pot/125g	69	55	5.1	8.3	0.1	0.0
Toffee, Weight Watchers*	1 Pot/120g	52	43	4.2	6.2	0.1	0.0
Treacle Toffee, Dessert, Low Fat, Sainsbury's*	1 Pot/125g	149	119	4.3	21.2	1.9	0.0
Tropical Crunch, Healthy Balance, Fruit Corner, Muller*	1 Pot/150g	188	125	5.3	19.7	2.8	1.4
Tropical Fruit, Greek Style, Asda*	1 Pot/125g	170	136	3.3	15.0	7.0	0.0
Tropical Fruit, Greek Style, Shapers, Boots*	1 Pot/150g	101	67	3.6	9.8	1.5	0.8
Tropical Fruit, Healthy Living, Tesco*	1 Serving/125g	56	45	4.1	6.6	0.2	0.9
Tropical, Fat Free, Rachel's Organic*	1 Pot/125g	123	98	4.7	15.7	1.8	0.0
Tropical, Smooth, Ski*	1 Pot/125g	126	101	4.9	16.1	1.9	0.1
Valencia Orange, Layered, Bio, GFY, Asda*	1 Pot/125g	80	64	3.7	12.0	0.1	0.0
Valencia Orange, Seriously Fruity, Low Fat, Waitrose*	1 Pot/150g	147	98	4.3	18.0	1.0	0.3
Vanilla & Chocolate Flakes, Low Fat Bio, Shape*	1 Pot/150g	140	93	4.5	12.0	2.7	0.0
Vanilla & Pineapple, Nestle*	1 Pot/125g	120	96	4.2	16.7	1.5	0.0
Vanilla Choco Balls, Crunch Corner, Muller*	1 Pot/150g	218	145	4.1	22.5	4.3	0.0
Vanilla Creme, D'lite, Ski*	1 Pot/200g	192	96	5.1	15.8	0.8	0.0
Vanilla Flavour, Healthy Living, Light, Tesco*	1 Pot/200g	90	45	4.1	7.0	0.1	0.0
Vanilla Flavour, Organic, Low Fat, Tesco*	1 Pot/125g	114	91	5.3	15.3	1.0	0.0
Vanilla Toffee, Low Fat, Sainsbury's*	1 Pot/125g	145	116	4.3	20.6	1.8	0.0
Vanilla, BGTY, Sainsbury's*	1 Pot/200g	98	49	4.5	7.5	0.1	0.0
Vanilla, Benecol*	1 Serving/125g	99	79	3.7	14.6	0.6	0.0
Vanilla, Bio Live, Low Fat, Rachel's Organic*	1 Pot/142g	104	73	3.7	10.5	1.8	0.0
Vanilla, Breakfast, Tesco*	1 Pot/150g	108	72	2.9	13.9	0.5	0.0
Vanilla, COU, Marks & Spencer*	1 Pot/200g	90	45	4.5	6.3	0.1	0.0
Vanilla, Channel Island, Marks & Spencer*	1 Pot/150g	173	115	4.5	16.5	3.5	0.0
Vanilla, French Set Wholemilk, Asda*	1 Pot/125g	125	100	3.6	14.1	3.2	0.0
Vanilla, Frozen, Less Than 5% Fat, Tesco*	1 Pot/120g	179	149	8.1	23.8	2.4	0.7
Vanilla, Light, Muller*	1 Pot/200g	108	54	4.7	8.5	0.1	0.0
Vanilla, Live Bio, Waitrose*	1 Pot/150g	132	88	4.6	17.3	0.1	0.0
Vanilla, Low Fat, Bio, Sainsbury's*	1 Pot/150g	147	98	4.8	17.2	1.1	0.0
Vanilla, Low Fat, Ski*	1 Pot/125g	123	98	5.0	15.5	1.9	0.0
Vanilla, Low Fat, Tesco*	1 Pot/125g	125	100	4.9	16.3	1.7	0.0
Vanilla, Onken*	1 Serving/25g	25	100	3.1	15.9	2.7	0.0
Vanilla, Organic, Low Fat, Sainsbury's*	1 Pot/125g	114	91	5.3	15.3	1.0	0.0
Vanilla, Perfectly Balanced, Waitrose*	1 Pot/150g	132	88	4.6	17.3	0.1	0.0
Vanilla, Seriously Smooth, Low Fat, Waitrose	1 Pot/150g	149	99	4.7	16.3	1.7	0.0
Vanilla, Smooth Set, Co-Op*	1 Pot/125g	95	76	3.7	12.5	0.9	0.0
Vanilla, Thick & Creamy, Waitrose*	1 Pot/150g	188	125	4.2	20.6	2.9	0.0
Vanilla, Thickie, Innocent*	1 Bottle/250ml	200	80	2.4	12.2	2.0	0.0
Vanilla, Very Low Fat Bio, Somerfield*	1 Pot/200g	98	49	5.0	7.0	0.0	0.0
Vanilla, Virtually Fat Free, Shapers, Boots*	1 Pot/125g	66	53	5.0	7.9	0.1	0.0
Vanilla, Virtually Fat Free, Ski*	1 Pot/120g	59	49	4.7	7.2	0.2	0.6
Vanilla, Virtually Fat Free, Yeo Valley*	1 Pot/150g	122	81	5.1	15.0	0.1	0.0

	Measure INFO/WEIGHT	per Measure KCAL	Nutrition Values per 100g / 100ml				
			KCAL	PROT	CARB	FAT	FIBRE
YOGHURT							
Vanilla, Weight Watchers*	1 Pot/120g	49	41	4.2	5.7	0.1	0.0
Walnut & Honey, Amore Luxury, Muller*	1 Pot/150g	227	151	2.3	16.1	8.6	0.0
Whisp, Marks & Spencer*	1 Pot/100g	115	115	4.5	13.9	4.1	0.1
White Peach, Seriously Fruity, Waitrose*	1 Pot/150g	152	101	4.8	16.5	1.7	0.2
Whole Milk, Plain	1oz/28g	22	79	5.7	7.8	3.0	0.0
Wholemilk, Organic, Marks & Spencer*	1fl oz/30ml	27	90	6.1	7.4	3.6	0.0
Wholemilk, With Maple Syrup, Bio Live, Rachel's Organic*	1 Pot/142g	139	98	3.5	13.0	3.5	0.0
Wicked Wholemilk Vanilla, Bio Live, Rachel's Organic*	1 Pot/125g	125	100	5.2	12.1	3.5	0.0
Wild Berries, Shape, Danone*	1 Pot/120g	55	46	4.6	6.7	0.1	2.1
Wild Blackberry, Seriously Fruity, Waitrose*	1 Pot/125g	120	96	4.4	17.2	1.0	0.4
Wild Blueberry, Finest, Tesco*	1 Pot/150g	212	141	3.4	16.6	6.8	0.5
Wild Blueberry, Sveltesse 0%, Nestle*	1 Pot/125g	59	47	4.3	7.0	0.2	0.0
Winter Medley, COU, Marks & Spencer*	1 Pot/150g	68	45	4.2	6.2	0.1	0.1
With Hazelnut, Low Fat, Safeway*	1 Serving/150g	182	121	4.9	20.1	2.3	0.2
With Large Fruit Chunks, Bio, Waitrose*	1 Serving/170g	170	100	3.7	15.8	2.4	0.4
With Vanilla, Bio-Live, Low Fat, Rachel's Organic*	1/4 Pot/115g	98	85	4.4	12.8	1.8	0.0
With Wild Blueberries, Somerset, TTD, Sainsbury's*	1 Serving/150g	209	139	3.8	16.4	6.2	0.4
Yellow Fruit, Yoplait*	1 Pot/125g	139	111	3.3	18.0	2.9	0.0
Zingy Lemon, D'lite, Ski*	1 Pot/178.5g	141	79	4.5	14.3	0.1	0.0
YOGHURT DRINK							
Actimel, Mixed Fruit, Danone*	1 Serving/100ml	88	88	2.7	16.0	1.5	0.0
Actimel, Orange, Danone*	1fl oz/30ml	26	88	2.7	16.0	1.5	0.0
Actimel, Original, 0% Fat, Danone*	1 Bottle/100g	33	33	2.9	5.1	0.1	2.0
Actimel, Original, Danone*	1fl oz/30ml	25	83	2.8	14.3	1.6	0.0
Actimel, Pineapple, 0.1% Fat, Danone*	1 Bottle/100g	33	33	2.7	5.5	0.0	1.8
Actimel, Strawberry, Danone*	1 Bottle/100g	88	88	2.7	15.9	1.5	0.0
Average	1floz/30ml	19	62	3.1	13.1	0.0	0.0
Benecol*	1 Serving/70g	62	88	2.6	14.2	2.3	0.0
BioActive, Yagua*	1 Bottle/200ml	84	42	0.4	9.9	0.0	0.0
Blueberry & Blackcurrant, Orchard Maid*	1 Carton/250ml	148	59	1.6	13.6	0.0	0.0
Danacol, Original, Danone*	1 Bottle/100ml	64	64	3.2	10.0	1.0	0.0
Danacol, Strawberry, Danone*	1 Bottle/100g	68	68	3.2	11.2	1.2	0.0
Emmi*	1 Serving/500ml	245	49	3.0	7.5	0.8	0.0
Fristi*	1 Carton/330g	191	58	2.6	13.6	0.1	0.0
Light, Yakult*	1 Pot/66ml	31	47	1.3	12.2	0.0	1.8
Orchard Maid*	1 Serving/250g	148	59	1.6	13.0	0.0	0.0
Peach & Mango, Fristi*	1 Carton/330g	191	58	2.6	13.6	0.1	0.0
Peach, Low Fat, Vitality Probiotic, Muller*	1 Bottle/100ml	75	75	2.6	13.0	1.4	0.0
Raspberry & Passion Fruit, Everybody, Yoplait*	1 Bottle/90g	60	67	2.6	12.2	0.9	0.0
Raspberry, Low Fat, Vitality, Probiotic, Muller*	1 Bottle/100g	74	74	2.6	12.8	1.4	0.0
Ski Smooth, Nestle*	1 Bottle/200g	144	72	2.8	13.1	0.9	0.0
Strawberry, Bio, The Best, Safeway*	1 Bottle/250ml	215	86	2.7	13.6	1.9	0.6
Strawberry, Fristi*	1 Carton/250g	165	66	2.6	13.6	0.1	0.0
Strawberry, Froop, Muller*	1 Carton/191ml	183	96	2.7	14.0	2.9	0.0
Strawberry, Low Fat, Vitality Probotic, Muller*	1 Bottle/100g	79	79	2.6	14.1	1.4	0.0
Strawberry, Yop, Yoplait*	1 Bottle/330g	261	79	2.8	14.0	1.3	0.0
Tropical, Vitality, Muller*	1oz/28g	12	42	3.5	6.8	0.1	0.0
Vanilla, Activate, Probiotic, Little Town Dairy*	1 Bottle/265.1g	167	63	2.7	10.0	1.4	0.2
Yakult*	1 Pot/65ml	51	78	1.4	17.8	0.1	0.0
YORK FRUITS							
Terry's*	1 Sweet/9g	30	328	0.0	81.4	0.0	1.0
YORKIE							
Honeycomb, Nestle*	1 Bar/65g	331	509	5.7	63.6	25.8	0.0

	Measure INFO/WEIGHT	per Measure KCAL	Nutrition Values per 100g / 100ml				
			KCAL	PROT	CARB	FAT	FIBRE
YORKIE							
Nestle*	1 Bar/24g	121	504	6.8	60.4	26.1	1.2
Original, Nestle*	1 Bar/68g	357	525	6.5	58.6	29.4	0.0
Raisin & Biscuit, Nestle	1 Bar/63g	307	487	5.9	60.5	24.6	0.0
YORKSHIRE PUDDING							
3", Baked, Aunt Bessie's*	1 Pudding/36g	91	252	9.0	36.4	7.9	1.7
4 Minute, Aunt Bessie's*	1 Pudding/18g	59	326	9.6	38.4	14.8	2.1
7", Baked, Aunt Bessie's*	1 Pudding/110g	290	264	8.5	37.4	9.0	2.0
Average	1oz/28g	58	208	6.6	24.7	9.9	0.9
Baked Sage & Onion, Morrisons*	1 Pudding/19.3g	53	280	8.0	35.0	12.0	2.6
Batters, In Foils, Aunt Bessie's*	1 Pudding/17g	47	276	9.1	32.6	10.8	1.4
Beef Dripping, Marks & Spencer*	1 Pudding/24.7g	106	425	9.2	25.1	32.0	1.2
Chicken & Vegetable, COU, Marks & Spencer*	1 Pudding/150g	195	130	12.2	14.3	2.2	1.3
Filled With Beef & Vegetable, Safeway*	1 Pack/300g	396	132	8.6	15.2	4.1	1.3
Filled With Beef, Tesco*	1 Pudding/300g	408	136	6.1	16.2	5.2	1.1
Filled With Chicken, GFY, Asda*	1 Pack/380.9g	438	115	9.0	14.0	2.6	1.5
Filled With Chicken, Tesco*	1 Pack/300g	366	122	6.5	17.4	2.9	1.3
Filled With Cumberland Sausage, Tesco*	1/2 Pack/350g	536	153	6.8	6.4	11.3	0.5
Filled With Sausage, Tesco*	1 Pack/300g	417	139	5.1	15.2	6.4	1.1
Filled, Chicken Casserole, Farmfoods*	1 Pack/280g	347	124	6.5	19.3	2.3	1.3
Filled, Roast Chicken, COU, Marks & Spencer*	1 Pudding/150g	210	140	12.6	15.7	2.7	0.9
Filled, With Beef, Morrisons*	1 Serving/350g	515	147	7.4	15.7	6.0	0.5
Filled, With Sausage, Sainsbury's*	1 Pack/300g	576	192	6.9	17.5	10.4	0.9
Four Minute, Aunt Bessie's*	1 Pudding/18g	59	326	9.6	38.4	14.8	2.1
Frozen, Ovenbaked, Iceland*	1 Pudding/12.4g	35	290	9.7	45.1	7.9	4.1
Fully Prepared, Marks & Spencer*	1 Pudding/22g	63	285	9.4	31.6	13.2	1.2
Giant, Aunt Bessie's*	1 Pudding/110g	290	264	8.5	37.4	9.0	2.0
Individual, Aunt Bessie's*	1 Pudding/18g	50	276	9.1	32.6	10.8	1.4
Large, Aunt Bessie's*	1 Pudding/39g	104	267	8.8	32.3	11.4	1.4
Large, Safeway*	1 Pudding/45g	123	273	8.5	41.1	8.3	2.5
Large, The Real Yorkshire Pudding Co*	1 Pudding/34g	103	304	11.5	37.3	12.1	2.5
Made From Batter Mix, Sainsbury's*	1 Pudding/100g	248	248	9.9	40.1	5.3	4.0
Minced Beef Filled, Waitrose*	1 Serving/350g	525	150	7.5	14.1	7.1	1.0
Mini, Asda*	1 Pudding/13g	34	260	10.0	37.0	8.0	2.8
Potato & Sausage, Marks & Spencer*	1 Serving/100g	200	200	6.4	14.6	12.9	0.9
Premium, Bisto*	1 Pudding/30g	74	248	7.3	30.3	10.9	2.1
Ready Baked, SmartPrice, Asda*	1 Pudding/12g	36	297	10.0	44.0	9.0	2.8
Ready To Bake, Aunt Bessie's*	1 Pudding/17g	42	246	8.5	35.1	8.0	1.7
Ready To Bake, Sainsbury's*	1 Pudding/18g	48	263	9.9	35.9	8.9	1.3
Riding Lodge*	1 Pudding/16g	44	276	10.0	41.5	7.8	0.0
Sage & Onion, Tesco*	1 Pudding/19g	53	280	8.0	35.0	12.0	2.6
Sausage & Onion Gravy Filled, Safeway*	1 Pudding/300g	540	180	6.2	18.0	9.2	1.2
Steak & Vegetable, COU, Marks & Spencer*	1 Pudding/150g	188	125	9.6	14.9	2.7	0.9
Traditional Style, Asda*	1 Pudding/35.7g	116	322	10.0	39.0	14.0	0.5
Traditional Style, Small, Asda*	1 Pudding/19g	49	259	10.0	39.0	7.0	2.1
YORKSHIRE PUDDING							
Value, Tesco*	1 Pudding/16g	45	282	9.7	34.3	11.8	1.6
YORKSHIRE PUDDING							
With Beef in Gravy, Asda*	1 Serving/290g	406	140	7.0	20.0	3.5	0.7
YULE LOG							
Chocolate, Sainsbury's*	1/8 Log/48g	186	382	5.1	46.5	19.6	0.7
Christmas Range, Tesco*	1 Serving/30g	131	442	4.9	56.8	21.7	2.8
Mini, Marks & Spencer*	1 Cake/35.9g	166	460	5.7	56.9	23.3	1.1

	Measure	per Measure		Nutrition Values per 100g / 100ml			
	INFO/WEIGHT	KCAL	KCAL	PROT	CARB	FAT	FIBRE

BAXTER & PLATTS
SANDWICH
Cheese, & Ham, Baxter & Platts*	1 Pack/168g	408	243	11.3	20.5	13.0	1.7
Chicken, & Salad, Baxter & Platts*	1 Pack/165g	254	154	11.4	17.8	4.2	2.8

BENJYS
BAGEL
Bacon, & Cream Chesse, Benjys*	1 Bagel/149g	386	259	13.6	36.0	6.6	0.0
Buttered With Marmite, Benjys*	1 Bagel/109g	315	289	12.2	49.5	4.8	0.0
Cheese, & Ham, Benjys*	1 Bagel/169g	477	282	13.0	33.3	10.8	0.0
Cheese, Benjys*	1 Bagel/134g	427	319	14.1	39.6	11.5	0.0
Cinnamon, Benjys*	1 Bagel/104g	278	267	7.8	49.2	4.3	0.0
Cinnamon, Buttered With Jam, Benjys*	1 Bagel/119g	317	266	6.8	51.3	3.7	0.0
Cinnamon, With Peanut Butter, Benjys*	1 Bagel/119g	370	311	9.7	44.7	10.5	0.0
Cream Cheese, & Crispy Bacon, Benjys*	1 Bagel/149g	329	221	7.1	35.1	5.9	0.0
Peanut Butter, Benjys*	1 Bagel/119	397	334	12.4	46.2	11.1	0.0
Plain, Buttered With Jam, Benjys*	1 Bagel/119g	343	288	9.6	52.8	4.4	0.0
Plain, Buttered, Benjys*	1 Bagel/104g	304	292	11.0	51.0	5.0	0.0
Smoked Salmon, & Cream Cheese, Benjys*	1 Bagel/154g	373	242	12.7	36.1	5.1	0.0

BAGUETTE
Brie, With Bacon, Benjys*	1 Baguette/250g	695	278	12.5	24.0	15.3	0.0
Chicken Ceaser Salad, Benjys*	1 Serving/232g	657	283	9.4	25.7	16.4	0.0
Chicken, & Salad, Benjys*	1 Baguette/266g	512	192	7.3	22.9	10.0	0.0
Chicken, Red Thai, Benjys*	1 Baguette/251g	353	141	9.2	24.5	1.1	0.0
Ham, & Cheddar, With Branston Pickle, Benjys*	1 Baguette/270g	715	265	12.6	25.6	12.6	0.0
Mozzarella, Tomato, & Basil, Benjys*	1 Baguette/224g	500	223	11.2	26.7	7.7	0.0
Tuna Mayonnaise, & Tomato, Benjys*	1 Baguette/260g	644	248	8.3	24.4	12.2	0.0

BARS
Chocolate Crunch, Benjys*	1 Bar/90g	458	509	5.0	50.0	32.0	0.0

BHAJI
Onion, Benjys*	1 Pack/110g	232	211	4.8	19.7	8.8	0.0

BISCUITS
Clot Cream Fingers, Mini, Benjys*	1 Pack/2.9g	15	517	6.9	58.6	31.0	0.0
Golden Crunch, Five Pack, Benjys*	1 Pack/15g	71	473	5.3	62.7	22.7	0.0
Shortcake, Four Pack, Benjys*	1 Pack/18.8g	94	500	5.9	60.6	27.1	0.0
Shrewsbury, Fruit, Four Pack, Benjys*	1 Pack/18.8g	91	484	4.8	64.9	22.9	0.0
Viennese, Four Pack, Benjys*	1 Pack/18.8g	100	532	5.9	57.5	31.4	0.0

BREAD
Toast, & Butter, Benjys*	1 Serving/140g	395	282	7.5	47.0	7.0	0.0
Toast, & Jam, Benjys*	1 serving	446	279	6.5	49.3	6.1	0.0
Toast, & Marmite, Benjys*	1 Serving/150g	416	277	9.5	45.1	6.5	0.0
Toast, & Peanut Butter, Benjys*	1 Serving/160g	446	279	6.5	49.3	6.1	0.0

BREAKFAST
Full English, Cooked, Benjys*	1 Breakfast/359g	815	227	10.9	24.5	9.7	0.0
Pot, Banana, Benjys*	1 Pot/110g	99	90	5.0	13.4	1.7	0.0

BREAKFAST CEREAL
Alpen, Benjys*	1 Serving/50g	183	366	10.0	66.0	6.8	0.0
Coco Pops, Benjys*	1 Serving/45g	171	380	4.4	85.1	2.4	0.0
Cornflakes, Benjys*	1 Serving/30g	111	370	7.0	84.0	0.7	0.0
Cornflakes, Crunchy Nut, Benjys*	1 Serving/40g	156	390	6.0	83.0	3.5	0.0
Frosties, Benjys*	1 Serving/40g	148	370	4.5	87.0	0.5	0.0
Fruit N Fibre, Benjys*	1 Serving/50g	180	360	8.0	70.0	5.0	0.0
Porridge, Plain, Benjys*	1 Serving/383g	318	83	3.3	10.4	3.1	0.0
Porridge, With Cinnamon, Benjys*	1 Serving/384g	319	83	3.3	10.4	3.1	0.0
Porridge, With Syrup, Benjys*	1 Serving/423g	442	104	3.0	16.7	2.8	0.0

BENJYS

INFO/WEIGHT	Measure per Measure KCAL	Nutrition Values per 100g / 100ml KCAL	PROT	CARB	FAT	FIBRE

BREAKFAST CEREAL

Special K, Benjys*	1 Serving/35g	130	371	15.1	75.1	1.1	0.0
Sugar Puffs, Benjys*	1 Serving/25g	97	388	6.4	86.4	1.2	0.0
Weetabix, Benjys*	1 Serving/37.5g	126	336	11.7	67.2	1.9	0.0

BROWNIE

Benjys*	1 Brownie/65g	274	422	5.1	48.0	23.1	0.0

BUNS

Chelsea, Benjys*	1 Bun/95g	237	249	5.0	55.8	2.2	0.0
Hot Cross, Benjys*	1 Bun/127.5g	402	315	4.1	42.8	15.3	0.0
Iced, Belgian, Benjys*	1 Bun/115g	279	243	5.0	55.2	1.7	0.0

BURRITO

Bean, Vegtable & Chesse, Benjys*	1 Burrito/298g	472	158	7.7	14.7	7.7	0.0
Chicken, Benjys*	1 Burrito/288g	536	186	11.5	15.1	8.9	0.0
Chili Beef, Benjys*	1 Burrito/298g	513	172	8.6	15.7	8.4	0.0

CAKE

Banana, Square, Benjys*	1 Cake/100g	421	421	5.0	43.0	25.0	0.0
Carrot, Square, Benjys*	1 Cake/95g	334	352	5.1	38.0	20.0	0.0
Chocolate, Square, Benjys*	1 Cake/105g	375	357	5.1	41.1	19.1	0.0
Eccles, Benjys*	1 Cake/185g	751	406	4.5	61.6	15.7	0.0
Passion, Wedge, Benjys*	1 Cake/105g	384	366	4.4	36.0	22.7	0.0

CHICKEN

Bites, Italian, Benjys*	1 Pack/150g	84	56	9.2	2.8	1.1	0.0
Drumstick, Roast, Benjys*	1 Pack/210g	304	145	20.8	2.7	5.6	0.0

CIABATTA

Bacon & Chesse, Benjys*	1 Ciabatta/223g	782	351	16.7	31.1	17.7	0.0
Cheese, Tomato & Onion, Benjys*	1 Ciabatta/233g	684	294	11.9	30.3	14.0	0.0
Chicken, & Baby Spinach Leaves, Benjys*	1 Ciabatta/233g	599	257	11.5	30.6	9.9	0.0
Chicken, Bacon, Cheese & BBQ Sauce, Benjys*	1 Ciabatta/275g	838	305	16.4	24.0	15.7	0.0
Ham, Cheddar, & Pesto Mayonnaise, Benjys*	1 Ciabatta/260g	772	297	13.2	27.4	14.3	0.0
Ham, Cheese & Tomato, Benjys*	1 Ciabatta/273g	722	264	12.8	25.6	12.4	0.0
Italian Chicken & Tomato, Benjys*	1 Ciabatta/190g	386	203	11.7	31.5	3.4	0.0
Mozzarella, Tomato, Oregano & Olives, Benjys*	1 Pack/247g	676	274	11.3	29.1	12.1	0.0
Tuna & Cheese Melt, Benjys*	1 Ciabatta/239g	828	346	12.7	30.0	19.8	0.0
Turkey, Bacon, & Gruyere, Benjys*	1 Ciabatta/261g	720	276	14.4	29.1	11.0	0.0

COOKIES

Choc Chip, Benjys*	1 Cookie/60g	298	497	5.8	60.2	25.7	0.0
Oat, Giant, Benjys*	1 Cookie/60g	305	508	5.8	58.7	27.8	0.0
Pecan Maple, Mini, Benjys*	1 Pack/5.6g	29	518	5.4	60.7	26.8	0.0
Shrewsbury, Fruit, Giant, Benjys*	1 Cookies/60g	301	502	4.8	62.3	25.8	0.0

COUS COUS

Moroccan, Benjys*	1 Pack/181g	266	147	2.8	19.2	6.7	0.0

CROISSANT

Almond, Benjys*	1 Croissant/150g	587	391	7.7	34.3	24.8	0.0
Cheese, & Ham, Benjys*	1 Croissant/161g	459	285	12.1	16.8	18.9	0.0
Cheese, Cheddar, Benjys*	1 Croissant/111g	418	377	11.0	24.1	26.4	0.0

CURRY

Chicken, Green Thai, Benjys*	1 Pack/450g	817	182	8.1	16.5	9.2	0.0

DANISH PASTRY

Cinnamon, Benjys*	1 Danish/116g	333	287	4.4	31.0	16.2	0.0
Custard, Benjys*	1 Danish/100g	303	303	5.0	14.1	25.1	0.0

DESSERT

Banana, & Custard, Benjys*	1 Dessert/240g	258	108	2.0	18.6	2.5	0.0
Fruit Cocktail Jelly, & Custard, Benjys*	1 Dessert/351g	300	85	1.6	14.9	1.5	0.0

BENJYS

INFO/WEIGHT	KCAL	KCAL	PROT	CARB	FAT	FIBRE

DESSERT

	INFO/WEIGHT	KCAL	KCAL	PROT	CARB	FAT	FIBRE
Greek Yoghurt, With Mango, & Blueberry, Benjys*	1 Dessert/140g	67	48	4.4	5.3	1.1	0.0
DOUGHNUTS							
Chocolate Chip, Benjys*	1 Doughnut/120g	532	443	6.1	75.4	15.9	0.0
Chocolate, & Nut, Benjys*	1 Doughnut/120g	436	363	7.0	59.8	13.2	0.0
Jam, Single, Benjys*	1 Doughnut/108g	288	267	5.7	53.5	4.4	0.0
White Chocolate Chip, Benjys*	1 Doughnut/120g	532	443	6.0	75.0	16.1	0.0
FLAPJACK							
Fruit, Benjys*	1 Flapjack/70g	287	410	4.6	53.1	19.9	0.0
FRUIT SALAD							
Tropical, Benjys*	1 Serving/200g	76	38	0.6	8.3	0.2	0.0
KORMA							
Chicken, Benjys*	1 Pack/450g	889	198	9.4	15.9	10.7	0.0
MEATBALLS							
Spicy, Benjys*	1 Pack/120g	294	245	14.8	13.0	15.0	0.0
MUFFIN							
Bacon & Egg, With Chesse, Benjys*	1 Muffin/140g	307	219	13.9	22.5	8.1	0.0
Bacon, & Chesse, Toasted, Benjys*	1 Muffin/120g	295	246	16.7	26.3	8.2	0.0
Blueberry, Benjys*	1 Muffin/120g	412	343	4.8	44.0	20.7	0.0
Chocolate Chunk, Benjys*	1 Muffin/125g	525	420	6.3	49.1	25.2	0.0
Cranberry, & Orange, Benjys*	1 Muffin/120g	428	357	5.1	45.1	20.0	0.0
Egg, & Chesse, Toasted, Benjys*	1 Muffin/122.5g	265	216	11.6	25.8	7.3	0.0
Sausage & Egg, With Chesse, Toasted, Benjys*	1 Muffin/172g	420	244	11.4	22.4	12.1	0.0
Sausage, & Chesse, Toasted, Benjys*	1 Muffin/159g	440	277	11.1	26.4	14.3	0.0
PAIN AU CHOCOLATE							
Benjys*	1 Serving/73g	167	229	3.6	23.7	13.3	0.0
PAIN AU RAISIN							
Benjys*	1 Serving/145g	399	275	3.9	36.3	12.8	0.0
PANINI							
Chicken, Cheese & Jalepenos, Benjys*	1 Panini/240g	624	260	14.6	28.6	9.6	0.0
Ham, Chesse & BBQ Sauce, Benjys*	1 Panini/250g	635	254	12.5	30.2	9.1	0.0
Mozzarella & Roasted Mediterranean Vegtables, Benjys*	1 Panini/245g	569	232	8.7	30.4	8.1	0.0
Smoked Turkey, With Mozzarella & Cranberry Jam, Benjys*	1 Panini/243g	572	235	12.0	31.0	6.7	0.0
Tuna & Cheese Melt, Benjys*	1 Panini/268g	864	322	12.0	26.5	18.7	0.0
PASTA SALAD							
Chicken & Bacon Herb, Benjys*	1 Salad/295g	334	113	4.7	14.6	4.2	0.0
Chicken & Bacon, Benjys*	1 Salad/201g	180	90	6.1	8.7	3.4	0.0
Chicken, Tomato & Red Cheddar, Benjys*	1 Salad/226g	294	130	5.7	17.6	5.5	0.0
Prawn Cocktail, Benjys*	1 Salad/256g	111	43	1.2	5.9	1.8	0.0
Spring Vegetable, Benjys*	1 Salad/242g	197	81	3.3	14.4	1.2	0.0
Tuna, Benjys*	1 Salad/250g	150	60	3.8	7.1	2.0	0.0
With Basil, Benjys*	1 Salad/177g	320	181	5.8	31.4	4.6	0.0
PASTY							
Cheese & Onion, Benjys*	1 Pasty/177g	504	285	4.4	29.2	16.6	0.0
Cornish, Benjys*	1 Pasty/215g	542	252	6.8	28.1	12.6	0.0
PIE							
Apple, Benjys*	1 Pie/150g	450	300	4.1	41.3	13.2	0.0
Cherry, Benjys*	1 Pie/135g	474	351	4.3	51.8	14.1	0.0
Chicken & Mushroom, Benjys*	1 Pie/172g	487	283	6.8	23.5	18.0	0.0
Meat & Cheese Feast	1 Pie/250g	489	196	18.3	1.2	13.1	0.0
Mince, Benjys*	1 Pie/170g	663	390	3.9	66.7	11.9	0.0
Steak & Kidney, Benjys*	1 Pie/183g	476	260	8.9	22.5	18.1	0.0

	Measure INFO/WEIGHT	per Measure KCAL	Nutrition Values per 100g / 100ml KCAL	PROT	CARB	FAT	FIBRE
ROLL							
Cheddar, & Spring Onion Mayonnaise, Twill, Benjys*	1 Roll/175g	628	359	12.4	31.0	20.1	0.0
Cheese & Tomato, Benjys*	1 Pack/263g	683	260	11.5	39.2	9.8	0.0
Cheese, & Tomato, Morning, Benjys*	1 Roll/132g	343	260	11.5	39.2	9.8	0.0
Chesse, & Pickle, Morning, Benjys*	1 Roll/122g	366	300	12.5	39.0	10.5	0.0
Chicken Mayonnaise, & Tomato, Twill, Benjys*	1 Roll/170g	482	284	9.7	31.7	14.7	0.0
Egg Mayonnaise, Twill, Benjys*	1 Roll/175g	511	292	10.0	30.2	14.6	0.0
Ham, & Coleslaw, Morning, Benjys*	1 Roll/132g	326	247	8.2	34.7	7.8	0.0
Ham, & Salad, With Heinz Salad Cream, Twill, Benjys*	1 Roll/178g	436	245	8.7	31.1	9.5	0.0
Ham, & Tomato, Morning, Benjys*	1 Roll/137g	270	197	7.8	32.9	3.9	0.0
Ham, Just, Benjys*	1 Serving/210g	418	199	10.1	32.1	3.4	0.0
Tuna Mayonnaise, & Sweetcorn, Twill, Benjys*	1 Roll/194g	562	290	8.7	29.9	15.0	0.0
Turkey, & Stuffing, Twill, Benjys*	1 Roll/178g	433	243	9.4	32.1	8.7	0.0
SALAD							
Baby Plum Tomato, Mozzarella Balls & Spinach, Benjys*	1 Salad/182g	145	80	3.1	5.0	5.4	0.0
Cheese, Layered, Benjys*	1 Salad/255g	184	72	3.3	8.4	3.1	0.0
Chefs, Benjys*	1 Salad/243g	163	67	4.5	1.4	4.6	0.0
Chicken & Mexican Bean, Benjys*	1 Salad/230g	135	59	3.1	3.8	3.5	0.0
Chicken Breast, Orange & Chili Jam, Benjys*	1 Salad/281g	762	271	10.0	41.5	9.0	0.0
Chicken Noodle, Red Thai, Benjys*	1 Salad/296g	670	226	11.8	43.0	0.9	0.0
Chicken, Bacon & Spinach	1 Salad/330g	1064	322	12.1	46.1	12.0	0.0
Coleslaw, Layered, Benjys*	1 Salad/380g	352	93	1.7	9.3	5.6	0.0
Dry Cured Wiltshire Ham, Benjys*	1 Salad/379g	526	139	4.3	7.5	10.4	0.0
Egg Mayonnaise, Layered, Benjys*	1 Salad/381g	406	107	4.5	7.7	6.8	0.0
Goats Cheese & Roasted Pepper, Gourmet, Benjys*	1 Pack/400g	412	103	3.4	12.4	3.8	0.0
Lentil & Rice	1 Salad/251g	233	93	4.3	13.6	2.4	0.0
Mixed, Including Dressing, Benjys*	1 Pack/315g	151	48	0.8	3.5	3.4	1.2
Prawn Noodle, Red Thai, Benjys*	1 Salad/311g	676	217	10.3	42.5	0.7	0.0
Three Bean, Benjys*	1 Salad/251g	185	74	1.6	4.0	5.8	0.0
Tuna Fish & Leaf, Benjys*	1 Salad/145g	65	45	6.0	1.5	0.3	0.0
SAMOSAS							
Chicken, Benjys*	1 Pack/110	263	239	8.3	22.6	12.9	0.0
Lamb, Benjys*	1 Pack/110g	316	287	9.2	29.6	14.7	0.0
SANDWICH							
All Day Breakfast, Brown, Benjys*	1 Sandwich/296g	746	252	12.5	23.7	11.2	0.0
BLT, Brown, Benjys*	1 Sandwich/200g	469	235	10.1	26.4	9.9	0.0
Bacon, & Chesse, Toasted, Benjys*	1 Sandwich/216g	629	291	15.1	30.2	12.2	0.0
Bacon, & Egg Mayonnaise, With Rocket, Brown, Benjys*	1 Sandwich/199g	513	258	10.8	25.6	12.6	0.0
Bacon, & Egg, & Mayonnaise, With Rocket, Benjys*	1 Serving/199g	513	258	10.8	25.6	12.6	0.0
Bacon, & Egg, & Sausage, Torpedo, Benjys*	1 Sandwich/382g	928	243	11.3	24.4	11.3	0.0
Bacon, & Egg, Toasted, Benjys*	1 Sandwich/224g	508	227	11.7	29.9	6.8	0.0
Bacon, & Egg, Torpedo	1 Sandwich/282g	618	219	11.5	28.0	6.9	0.0
Bacon, & Sausage, Toasted, Benjys*	1 Sandwich/236g	609	258	11.4	31.4	9.8	0.0
Bacon, & Sausage, Torpedo, Benjys*	1 Sandwich/306g	814	266	11.1	30.0	11.4	0.0
Bacon, Sausage, & Egg, Toasted, Benjys*	1 Sandwich/324g	820	253	11.5	25.0	12.1	0.0
Bacon, Toasted, Benjys*	1 Sandwich/204g	496	243	13.2	32.9	6.6	0.0
Bacon, Torpedo, Benjys*	1 Sandwich/278g	681	245	15.9	28.5	7.6	0.0
Breakfast, White, Benjys*	1 Sandwich/254g	571	225	8.7	23.4	10.9	0.0
Cheddar, & Branston Pickle, Torpedo, Benjys*	1 Torpedo/235g	699	297	12.6	32.1	13.2	0.0
Cheddar, & Onion, Torpedo, Benjys*	1 Torpedo/235g	613	261	11.1	29.7	11.1	0.0
Cheddar, & Tomato, Torpedo, Benjys*	1 Torpedo/285g	716	251	12.0	24.2	12.0	0.0
Cheddar, Bloomer, Mini, Benjys*	1 Sandwich/175g	528	302	14.5	29.9	14.0	0.0
Cheese, & Coleslaw, White, Benjys*	1 Sandwich/175g	498	285	9.2	30.3	13.3	0.0

BENJYS

SANDWICH

INFO/WEIGHT	Measure per Measure KCAL	Nutrition Values per 100g / 100ml KCAL	PROT	CARB	FAT	FIBRE
Cheese, & Ham, Brown, Benjys*	1 Sandwich/245g 652	266	15.6	22.0	13.0	0.0
Cheese, & Ham, Toasted, Benjys*	1 Sandwich/250g 803	321	11.5	27.4	18.3	0.0
Cheese, & Ham, White, Benjys*	1 Sandwich/185g 442	239	12.4	27.3	8.9	0.0
Cheese, & Onion, Bloomer, Mini, Benjys*	1 Sandwich/155g 415	268	11.4	34.2	9.6	0.0
Cheese, & Onion,Toasted, Benjys*	1 Sandwich/200g 548	274	11.1	33.4	10.7	0.0
Cheese, & Pickle, White, Benjys*	1 Sandwich/195g 594	305	13.3	30.0	14.1	0.0
Cheese, & Tomato, Toasted, Benjys*	1 Sandwich/220g 543	247	10.1	30.2	9.7	0.0
Cheese, Toasted, Benjys*	1 Sandwich/215g 753	350	12.0	30.3	19.9	0.0
Chicken, & Bacon, Brown, Benjys*	1 Sandwich/230g 553	240	16.0	23.0	9.5	0.0
Chicken, & Cheddar, With Tomato Salsa, Torpedo, Benjys*	1 Torpedo/270g 691	256	14.3	25.9	10.4	0.0
Chicken, & Mayonnaise, Brown, Benjys*	1 Sandwich/165g 455	276	11.2	31.3	14.2	0.0
Chicken, & Mozzarella, With Pesto, Brown, Benjys*	1 Sandwich/302g 656	217	14.8	18.5	8.8	0.0
Chicken, & Salad, Brown, Benjys*	1 Sandwich/256g 521	204	11.1	20.7	8.4	0.0
Chicken, & Salad, Torpedo, Benjys*	1 Torpedo/266g 580	218	8.4	26.1	11.0	0.0
Chicken, & Stuffing, White, Benjys*	1 Sandwich/260g 513	197	12.9	24.2	5.5	0.0
Chicken, Tikka, & Mint Sauce, Bloomer, Mini, Benjys*	1 Sandwich/185g 403	218	7.9	30.4	7.1	0.0
Club, Brown, Benjys*	1 Sandwich/233g 566	243	12.2	22.4	13.4	0.0
Cream Cheese, & Roasted Vegetable, Low Fat, Benjys*	1 Pack/190g 333	175	8.2	29.8	2.6	0.0
Egg Mayonnaise, & Bacon, Torpedo, Benjys*	1 Torpedo/325g 781	240	10.5	21.0	12.8	0.0
Egg Mayonnaise, & Smoked Salmon, Brown, Benjys*	1 Sandwich/212g 535	252	11.5	25.4	11.8	0.0
Egg Mayonnaise, & Tomato, Brown, Benjys*	1 Sandwich/205g 443	216	8.1	25.3	9.3	0.0
Egg Mayonnaise, White, Benjys*	1 Sandwich/205g 503	245	9.1	24.7	12.3	0.0
Egg, & Tomato, Benjys*	1 Pack/223g 415	186	9.0	22.0	7.0	0.0
Egg, Toasted, Benjys*	1 Sandwich/226g 477	211	9.0	29.7	6.3	0.0
Egg, Torpedo, Benjys*	1 Sandwich/284g 585	206	9.3	27.8	6.5	0.0
Focaccia, Greek Salad, With Tzatziki, Benjys*	1 Focaccia/240g 487	203	6.5	21.1	10.3	0.0
Ham, & Brie, & Tomato, Brown, Benjys*	1 Sandwich/281g 612	218	11.9	18.9	10.8	0.0
Ham, & Coleslaw, White, Benjys*	1 Sandwich/170g 396	233	7.2	31.2	8.0	0.0
Ham, & Mustard, Bloomer, Mini, Benjys*	1 Sandwich/180g 362	201	10.0	30.9	5.0	0.0
Ham, & Salad, With Mustard Mayonnaise, Brown, Benjys*	1 Sandwich/305g 459	150	9.3	22.7	5.8	0.0
Ham, Benjys*	1 Serving/155g 288	186	9.1	30.5	3.1	0.0
Ham, Torpedo, Benjys*	1 Torpedo/210g 417	199	10.1	32.1	3.4	0.0
Houmous, & Mixed Peppers, Brown, Benjys*	1 Sandwich/201g 513	255	8.0	30.3	11.2	0.0
Ploughman's, Cheddar, Brown, Benjys*	1 Sandwich/277g 578	209	9.4	21.7	9.6	0.0
Prawn Mayonnaise, Brown, Benjys*	1 Sandwich/200g 434	217	10.4	25.7	8.2	0.0
Prawn Mayonnaise, Triple Pack, Benjys*	1 Sandwich/299g 645	216	10.4	25.8	7.9	0.0
Salmon Mayonnaie, & Cucumber, Bloomer, Mini, Benjys*	1 Sandwich/213g 447	210	8.6	25.1	8.5	0.0
Sausage, & Egg, Toasted, Benjys*	1 Sandwich/288g 732	254	9.0	28.1	11.8	0.0
Sausage, & Egg, Torpedo, Benjys*	1 Sandwich/346g 841	243	9.4	26.9	11.1	0.0
Sausage, Toasted, Benjys	1 Sandwich/200g 520	260	8.2	37.0	9.0	0.0
Sausage, Torpedo, Benjys*	1 Sandwich/320g 886	277	9.0	31.3	13.2	0.0
Tuna Mayonnaise, & Cucumber, Torpedo, Benjys*	1 Torpedo/269g 644	239	7.8	26.3	10.5	0.0
Tuna Mayonnaise, & Salad, Torpedo, Benjys*	1 Torpedo/296g 773	261	9.0	29.1	10.9	0.0
Tuna Mayonnaise, & Sweetcorn, White, Benjys*	1 Sandwich/181g 448	248	9.2	29.9	10.2	0.0
Tuna Mayonnaise, With Cucumber, Brown, Benjys*	1 Sandwich/223g 579	260	9.2	24.3	12.7	0.0
Turkey, & Cream Chesse, & Cranberry, Brown, Benjys*	1 Sandwich/229g 426	186	9.4	25.3	5.3	0.0
Wedge, Brie, & Salad, Benjys*	1 Wedge/205g 466	227	9.0	22.9	11.1	0.0
Wedge, Chicken Mayonnaise, Bacon, & Cheddar, Benjys*	1 Wedge/223g 538	241	12.5	21.3	12.8	0.0
Wedge, Tuna, & Heinz Salad Cream, Benjys*	1 Sandwich/207g 384	186	8.7	24.3	6.0	0.0

SAUSAGE

INFO/WEIGHT	Measure per Measure KCAL	KCAL	PROT	CARB	FAT	FIBRE
Mini, Benjys*	1 Pack/150g 468	312	11.0	14.0	24.0	0.0

	INFO/WEIGHT	KCAL	KCAL	PROT	CARB	FAT	FIBRE
BENJYS							
SCONE							
Jam, Benjys*	1 Scone/160g	461	288	5.1	48.3	9.6	0.0
SOUP							
Carrot & Coriander, Benjys*	1 Serving/300g	162	54	0.4	5.4	3.5	0.0
SPRING ROLLS							
Vegetable, Benjys*	1 Pack/140g	267	191	3.7	18.1	11.6	0.0
TART							
Bakewell, Benjys*	1 Tart/130g	553	425	4.7	64.4	16.5	0.0
TIKKA MASALA							
Chicken, Benjys*	1 Pack/450g	783	174	8.3	17.8	7.7	0.0
WRAP							
Light Cream Cheese With Roasted Red Pepper, Benjys*	1 Pack/200g	316	158	7.0	19.1	5.7	0.0
Tuna, & Sweet Chilli Mayonnaise, Benjys*	1 Wrap/208g	473	227	5.8	32.1	8.2	0.0
BURGER KING							
BAGUETTE							
Chicken, Piri Piri, Burger King*	1 Serving/539g	343	64	4.5	9.5	0.7	0.0
BURGERS							
Bacon Double Cheeseburger, Bunless, Burger King*	1 Burger/138g	607	440	30.0	4.0	31.0	0.0
Cheeseburger, Bacon Double, Burger King*	1 Burger/172g	494	287	1.7	39.0	15.1	1.2
Cheeseburger, Burger King*	1 Burger/141g	379	269	15.6	30.0	13.4	1.4
Chicken Flamer, Burger King*	1 Sandwich/162g	308	190	12.6	18.6	7.3	1.9
Chicken Royale, Burger King*	1 Sandwich/204g	560	275	12.3	25.5	13.7	1.5
Chicken Sandwich, Burger King*	1 Sandwich/224g	659	294	11.2	23.6	17.4	1.3
Chicken Whopper, Lite, Burger King*	1 Whopper/159g	339	213	15.3	18.4	8.7	0.0
Double Whopper With Cheese, Burger King*	1 Pack/378g	934	247	14.0	13.0	16.0	1.0
Double Whopper, Burger King*	1 Sandwich/353g	918	260	13.5	15.0	16.1	1.1
Hamburger, Burger King*	1 Burger/128g	339	265	14.8	23.4	12.5	1.5
Spicy Bean, Burger King*	1 Burger/239g	504	211	7.9	26.2	8.3	3.9
Whopper Junior With Cheese, Burger King*	1 Burger/167g	421	252	12.0	18.0	14.0	1.0
Whopper With Cheese, Burger King*	1 Pack/299g	724	242	11.0	16.0	15.0	1.0
Whopper With Mayo, Burger King*	1 Whopper/278g	678	244	10.4	19.0	14.0	1.4
Whopper, Burger King*	1 Whopper/274g	641	234	11.0	17.0	14.0	1.0
BURGERS VEGGIE							
Burger King*	1 Burger/223g	433	194	6.6	24.9	7.6	3.4
CHICKEN							
Fillets, Burger King*	1 Serving/72g	101	140	27.9	0.4	3.1	0.0
COLA							
Coke, Burger King*	1 Med/400g	172	43	0.0	10.6	0.0	0.0
DIP							
Barbeque Sauce, Pot, Burger King*	1 Serving/25g	31	125	0.6	28.7	0.3	0.4
DRESSING							
Honey & Mustard, Burger King*	1 Sachet/40g	32	80	1.5	14.5	2.0	0.8
FRENCH FRIES							
King Size, Salted, Burger King*	1 Bag/170g	539	317	3.5	42.3	14.7	2.9
Medium, Salted, Burger King*	1 Bag/116g	369	318	3.4	42.2	14.6	3.4
Small, Salted, Burger King*	1 Bag/74g	229	310	2.7	41.8	14.8	2.7
FRIES							
Regular, Burger King*	1 Serving/150g	498	332	3.0	43.0	16.0	0.0
HASH BROWNS							
Burger King*	1 Hash/102g	318	312	7.2	32.3	19.4	3.8
KETCHUP							
Dip Pot, Burger King*	1 Pot/25g	27	107	1.0	24.7	0.1	0.6
Sachet, Burger King*	1 Sachet/15g	16	107	1.0	24.7	0.1	0.6

INFO/WEIGHT	Measure	per Measure KCAL	Nutrition Values per 100g / 100ml				
			KCAL	PROT	CARB	FAT	FIBRE

BURGER KING

MILK SHAKE
Chocolate, Burger King*	1 Serving/336ml	291	87	1.5	12.2	3.9	0.0

ONION RINGS
Large, Burger King*	1 Serving/120g	348	290	4.8	36.4	13.9	3.8
Regular, Burger King*	1 Serving/90g	261	290	4.8	36.4	13.9	3.8

PIE
Dutch Apple, Burger King*	1 Pie/113g	339	300	1.7	46.0	12.3	0.8

SALAD
Burger King*	1 Serving/165g	34	21	1.2	3.5	0.2	2.6
Chicken, Burger King*	1 Salad/237g	135	57	9.3	2.6	1.1	1.8

SANDWICH
Bacon, & Egg, Burger King*	1 Pack/139g	296	213	11.1	21.7	9.1	1.9
Chicken, Burger King*	1 Pack/224g	659	294	11.2	23.6	17.4	1.3
Chicken, Club, Burger King*	1 Pack/242g	620	256	12.3	22.3	13.2	1.6
Sausage, Bacon & Egg, Burger King*	1 Pack/182g	430	236	13.2	17.5	12.7	1.7

CAFFE NERO

BARS
Granola, Caffe Nero*	1 Bar/64g	259	404	5.9	55.3	21.7	0.0
Shortbread, Caffe Nero*	1 Pack/50g	243	485	4.8	54.6	27.6	0.0

BREAD
Panettone, Classic, Mini, Caffe Nero*	1 Panettone/100g	362	362	6.1	46.9	16.6	0.0

BROWNIE
Chocolate, Double, Organic, Caffe Nero*	1 Brownie/65g	273	420	6.0	61.2	16.8	0.0

CAKE
Banana & Caramel, Slice, Caffe Nero*	1 Slice/82g	342	417	4.6	45.5	24.1	0.0
Banana & Sultana, Slice, Caffe Nero*	1 Slice/81g	221	276	4.7	53.6	4.8	0.0
Carrot & Raisin, Slice, Organic, Caffe Nero*	1 Slice/70g	309	442	9.5	44.7	25.0	0.0
Chocolate & Orange, Slice, Caffe Nero*	1 Serving/70g	258	369	5.0	43.9	19.3	0.0
Chocolate & Pecan Fudge Brownie, Caffe Nero*	1 Serving/113g	426	377	3.6	47.7	19.1	0.0
Chocolate Fudge, Caffe Nero*	1 Serving/143g	488	341	3.4	36.6	20.1	0.0
Coffee & Pecan, Slice, Caffe Nero*	1 Slice/87g	389	447	5.1	46.2	26.9	0.0
Cranberry & Orange, Slice, Caffe Nero*	1 Slice/60g	196	326	5.1	49.8	11.9	0.0
Lemon Drizzle, Slice, Organic, Caffe Nero*	1 Slice/76g	264	348	4.6	53.6	12.8	0.0
Mocha, Slice, Caffe Nero*	1 Slice/89g	333	375	4.8	43.4	20.2	0.0
Passion, Caffe Nero*	1 Serving/143g	598	418	3.7	42.3	23.8	0.0
White Chocolate & Orange Ganache, Caffe Nero*	1 Serving/135g	558	413	4.0	29.0	31.3	0.0

CHEESE TWISTS
Caffe Nero*	1 Twist/100g	356	356	10.2	27.7	22.7	0.0

CHEESECAKE
Apple & Cinnamon, Baked, Caffe Nero*	1 Serving/138g	406	294	4.1	30.6	17.9	0.0
Chocolate, Simply, Caffe Nero*	1 Serving/125g	475	380	4.4	45.6	20.0	0.0
Chocolate, White & Dark, Caffe Nero*	1 Serving/172g	716	416	5.7	30.8	30.8	0.0
Rhubarb & Vanilla, Caffe Nero*	1 Serving/135g	424	314	5.4	26.9	22.0	0.0
Summer Fruit, Caffe Nero*	1 Serving/157g	388	247	3.4	29.5	13.2	0.0
Toffee Swirl, Caffe Nero*	1 Serving/133g	410	308	6.3	30.0	18.1	0.0

COFFEE BEANS
Cioccafe, Caffe Nero*	1 Serving/25g	117	468	8.5	50.0	26.0	0.0

COOKIES
Belgian Chocolate, Organic, Caffe Nero*	1 Cookie/50g	244	488	6.4	64.8	22.6	0.0
Raisin & Oat, Organic, Caffe Nero*	1 Cookie/50g	223	445	6.3	62.9	18.7	0.0

CRISPS
Sea Salt & Balsamic Vinegar, Caffe Nero*	1 Pack/50g	241	482	7.0	54.1	26.4	0.0
Sea Salt, Caffe Nero*	1 Pack/50g	247	493	7.0	54.0	27.1	0.0

CAFFE NERO

	Measure INFO/WEIGHT	per Measure KCAL	Nutrition Values per 100g / 100ml				
			KCAL	PROT	CARB	FAT	FIBRE
CROISSANT							
Almond, Caffe Nero*	1 Croissant/100g	329	329	5.2	45.4	14.0	0.0
Apricot, Caffe Nero*	1 Croissant/100g	260	260	5.6	37.1	9.9	0.0
Butter, Caffe Nero*	1 Croissant/50g	208	416	8.9	43.1	23.3	0.0
DANISH PASTRY							
Apple, Caffe Nero*	1 Pastry/75g	191	255	4.5	37.0	10.9	0.0
Pear & Chocolate, Caffe Nero*	1 Pastry/90g	238	264	4.7	36.9	12.8	0.0
DESSERT							
Panna Cotta, Raspberry, Caffe Nero*	1 Pot/130g	384	295	1.2	17.2	24.6	0.0
FRUIT SALAD							
Spring, Caffe Nero*	1 Salad/174g	47	27	0.6	6.2	0.1	0.0
LASAGNE							
Beef, Caffe Nero*	1 Serving/370g	485	131	6.1	13.8	6.2	0.0
Vegetable, Caffe Nero*	1 Serving/371g	482	130	5.1	13.9	6.5	0.0
MOUSSE							
Chocolate, Dessert Pot, Caffe Nero*	1 Pot/95g	377	397	3.7	31.1	28.6	0.0
MUFFIN							
Blueberry, Caffe Nero*	1 Muffin/120g	432	360	5.5	40.2	19.7	0.0
Blueberry, Reduced Fat, Caffe Nero*	1 Muffin/120g	353	294	4.2	42.0	12.2	0.0
Carrot & Sultana, Low Fat, Caffe Nero*	1 Muffin/119g	271	227	5.0	44.8	3.0	0.0
Chocolate, White & Dark, Caffe Nero*	1 Muffin/120g	476	396	5.9	45.7	21.1	0.0
Lemon Poppy Seed, Caffe Nero*	1 Muffin/120g	468	390	6.2	42.3	21.8	0.0
White Chocolate & Raspberry, Caffe Nero*	1 Muffin/120g	453	378	6.0	41.0	21.1	0.0
PAIN AU CHOCOLAT							
Almond, Caffe Nero*	1 Pain/120g	624	520	10.4	52.2	31.1	0.0
Caffe Nero*	1 Pain/60g	262	437	8.9	46.4	24.3	0.0
PAIN AU RAISIN							
Caffe Nero*	1 Pain/100g	339	339	6.6	47.3	13.4	0.0
PANINI							
All Day Breakfast, Caffe Nero*	1 Panini/251g	515	205	10.2	24.0	7.6	0.0
Chicken BLT, Caffe Nero*	1 Panini/249g	613	246	9.0	25.6	12.0	0.0
Chicken Caesar, Caffe Nero*	1 Panini/237g	582	246	10.0	25.9	11.3	0.0
Club, Caffe Nero*	1 Panini/224g	498	222	8.8	27.5	8.6	0.0
Club, Italian, Caffe Nero*	1 Panini/212g	581	274	13.2	28.4	11.9	0.0
Herbed Ham, & Smoked Mozzarella, Caffe Nero*	1 Panini/193g	512	265	13.4	31.5	9.5	0.0
Lemon Chicken, Caffe Nero*	1 Panini/212g	478	225	9.1	28.8	8.2	0.0
Meatball, With Tomato Sauce, Italian, Caffe Nero*	1 Panini/245g	533	218	11.1	28.2	6.7	0.0
Mozzarella, & Plum Tomato, Caffe Nero*	1 Panini/217g	535	247	9.2	28.2	10.8	0.0
Parma Ham, & Mascarpone, Caffe Nero*	1 Panini/195g	536	275	11.3	30.6	11.9	0.0
Tricolore, Caffe Nero*	1 Panini/239g	540	226	8.3	25.7	10.0	0.0
PASTA SALAD							
Basil Pesto, Caffe Nero*	1 Serving/200g	510	255	5.9	24.1	15.1	0.4
Sunkissed Tomato, Caffe Nero*	1 Salad/285g	755	265	6.7	24.6	15.5	0.0
PASTRY							
Almond Torta, Caffe Nero*	1 Pastry/150g	522	348	2.7	51.1	14.8	0.0
Creamed Spinach, Savoury, Caffe Nero*	1 Pastry/120g	372	310	5.7	27.8	19.5	0.0
Ham & Cheese, Puff Pastry, Savoury, Caffe Nero*	1 Pastry/110g	394	358	11.5	26.9	22.7	0.0
PENNE							
With Roasted Red Pepper Sauce, Caffe Nero*	1 Serving/321g	507	158	5.1	23.6	4.8	0.0
RAVIOLI							
Mushroom, With Chestnut Mushroom Sauce, Caffe Nero*	1 Serving/310g	565	182	6.9	15.3	10.3	0.0
SALAD							
Crayfish, Caffe Nero*	1 Salad/205g	279	136	5.2	17.0	5.4	0.0

	INFO/WEIGHT	KCAL	KCAL	PROT	CARB	FAT	FIBRE
CAFFE NERO							
SALAD							
Tuna Nicoise, Caffe Nero*	1 Salad/232g	260	112	5.5	5.0	7.8	0.0
SANDWICH							
Cheddar, & Ham, Mature, Caffe Nero*	1 Serving/168g	457	272	15.7	20.7	14.0	0.0
Cheese, Simply, Caffe Nero*	1 Serving/161g	516	320	16.1	26.1	16.8	0.0
Chicken, Italian, Caffe Nero*	1 Serving/174g	361	207	9.6	21.0	9.4	0.0
Crayfish, With Lemon Mayonnaise, Caffe Nero*	1 Serving/156g	370	237	8.3	22.4	12.7	0.0
Egg Mayonnaise, & Cress, Caffe Nero*	1 Serving/168g	351	209	10.4	20.6	9.4	0.0
Foccacia, Mozzarella, Mushroom, & Spinach, Caffe Nero*	1 Serving/215g	480	223	9.0	28.0	8.3	0.0
Foccacia, Parma Ham, & Parmesan, Caffe Nero*	1 Serving/218g	569	261	14.9	25.4	11.1	0.0
Foccacia, Salami, Provolone, & Spinach, Caffe Nero*	1 Serving/242g	591	244	9.9	22.7	12.6	0.0
Salmon, Smoked, & Lemon Mayonnaise, Caffe Nero*	1 Serving/159g	497	313	10.6	21.8	20.3	0.0
SLICE							
Caramel Shortcake, Caffe Nero*	1 Slice/98g	514	524	2.7	49.6	31.1	0.0
SOUP							
Broccoli & Blue Cheese, Less Than 5% Fat, Caffe Nero*	1 Serving/331g	205	62	1.8	3.0	4.8	0.0
Cream Of Tomato & Basil, Caffe Nero*	1 Serving/330g	234	71	1.0	5.8	5.1	0.0
Creamy Mushroom, Caffe Nero*	1 Serving/331g	185	56	1.0	4.1	4.1	0.0
Roast Vegetable, Caffe Nero*	1 Serving/332g	73	22	0.6	2.2	1.3	0.0
Roasted Tomato, Caffe Nero*	1 Serving/329g	112	34	0.8	5.1	1.1	0.0
TART							
Blueberry, Caffe Nero*	1 Serving/111g	414	373	6.0	43.3	20.0	0.0
Winter Fruit, Caffe Nero*	1 Serving/145g	434	299	2.9	46.6	11.2	0.0
TIRAMISU							
Caffe Nero*	1 Serving/96g	302	315	4.1	22.0	23.4	0.0
WRAP							
Chicken, Spicy, Hot, Caffe Nero*	1 Serving/176g	296	168	11.1	23.5	3.3	0.0
Cream Cheese, Grilled Vegetable, & Tomato, Caffe Nero*	1 Serving/216g	344	159	4.8	22.9	5.3	0.0
Ham, Mushroom, & Mozzarella, Hot, Caffe Nero*	1 Serving/166g	355	214	12.0	21.7	8.7	0.0
COFFEE REPUBLIC							
FLAPJACK							
Chewy Nutty, Coffee Republic*	1 Flapjack/33g	145	440	7.1	50.9	23.2	2.0
PANINI							
Ham & Swiss Cheese, Coffee Republic*	1 Panini/223g	558	250	15.7	20.5	11.7	0.0
Mozzarella & Tomato, Coffee Republic*	1 Panini/255g	566	222	11.1	23.6	10.0	0.0
SANDWICH							
Cheese, & Ham, Toasted, Coffee Republic*	1 Pack/160g	429	268	15.7	24.4	12.7	0.0
Ham, & Salad, Coffee Republic*	1 Pack/224g	309	138	8.6	19.9	2.7	0.0
Mozzarella, & Salad, Coffee Republic*	1 Pack/242g	477	197	8.6	14.4	11.8	0.0
Turkey, & Sun Dried Tomato, Coffee Republic*	1 Pack/215g	445	207	11.8	25.3	6.5	0.0
TOASTIES							
Cheese & Ham, Coffee Republic*	1 Serving/164g	436	266	13.7	30.1	10.1	0.0
COSTA							
CIABATTA							
Ham, With Plum Tomato & Rocket, Italian, Costa*	1 Serving/50g	115	231	23.1	24.9	4.4	0.0
PANINI							
Chicken & Baby Spinach, Costa*	1 Serving/440g	832	189	9.8	32.5	2.5	0.0
Chicken Arrabiata, Costa*	1 Serving/194g	410	211	10.8	30.2	6.1	0.0
Mozzarella, Tomato & Pesto, Costa*	1 Panini/209g	487	233	9.6	35.1	7.2	5.0
SANDWICH							
Brie, Apple & Grape, Costa*	1 Serving/225g	536	238	8.3	28.7	10.9	0.0
Houmous, Costa*	1 Pack/165g	263	160	6.4	25.9	2.8	0.0
Salmon, & Salad, Poached, On Oatmeal, Costa*	1 Pack/151g	224	148	7.7	22.9	2.8	0.0

	Measure	per Measure	Nutrition Values per 100g / 100ml				
	INFO/WEIGHT	KCAL	KCAL	PROT	CARB	FAT	FIBRE

COSTA
SANDWICH
| Sausage, Chorizo, & Vine Ripened Tomato, Costa* | 1 Pack/181.0g | 315 | 174 | 15.5 | 26.1 | 2.1 | 0.0 |

SOUP
| Fish, Bouillabaisse, Costa* | 1 Serving/400g | 180 | 45 | 5.8 | 2.2 | 1.4 | 0.0 |

TEA
| Iced, Lemon, Costa* | 1 Bottle/275ml | 91 | 33 | 0.0 | 8.0 | 0.0 | 0.0 |

CUISINE DE FRANCE
BREAD
| Baguette, Demi, Cuisine De France* | 1 Serving/140g | 360 | 257 | 6.7 | 56.0 | 1.4 | 1.7 |
| Bap, Brown, Soft, Cuisine De France* | 1 Bap/99g | 236 | 238 | 11.5 | 46.0 | 0.9 | 7.3 |

MUFFIN
| Carrot Cake, Cuisine De France* | 1 Muffin/105g | 373 | 355 | 4.7 | 56.9 | 12.0 | 0.0 |

DOMINO'S PIZZA
BREAD
| Garlic, Pizza, Domino's Pizza* | 1 Slice/40g | 115 | 295 | 12.0 | 41.4 | 9.0 | 2.3 |

CHEESECAKE
| Domino's Pizza* | 1 Serving/132g | 396 | 300 | 5.0 | 28.5 | 18.6 | 0.5 |

CHICKEN
| Dunkers, Domino's Pizza* | 1oz/28g | 62 | 220 | 23.5 | 1.5 | 13.3 | 0.5 |
| Strippers, Domino's Pizza* | 1oz/28g | 61 | 219 | 23.3 | 13.4 | 8.0 | 1.0 |

DIP
| Garlic & Herb, Domino's Pizza* | 1 Pot/28g | 194 | 693 | 1.4 | 2.5 | 75.4 | 0.4 |

PIZZA
Cheese Steak Melt, Dominoes*	1 Slice Sm/64g	153	241	15.0	29.8	6.9	1.5
Deluxe, 9.5", Domino's Pizza*	1 Slice/66g	171	259	12.8	29.1	10.1	2.4
Full House, Extravaganza, 9.5", Domino's Pizza*	1 Slice/74g	183	247	12.5	25.5	10.5	1.8
Hawaiian, Domino's Pizza*	1 Slice/68g	148	215	13.5	31.4	3.9	2.5
Hot & Spicy, 9.5", Domino's Pizza*	1 Slice/79g	178	225	12.7	28.7	6.6	2.5
Mighty Meaty, 9.5", Domino's Pizza*	1/6 Pizza/71g	177	249	13.9	25.5	10.2	2.8
Mixed Grill, 9.5", Domino's Pizza*	1 Slice/75g	178	237	12.0	26.2	9.3	2.3
Pepperoni Passion, 11.5", Domino's Pizza*	1 Slice/71g	204	286	13.8	31.5	11.6	2.2
Pepperoni Passion, 9.5", Domino's Pizza*	1 Slice/65g	186	286	13.6	31.5	11.6	1.4
Tandoori Hot, 9.5", Domino's Pizza*	1 Slice/67g	137	205	12.2	27.8	5.2	2.8
Texas BBQ, Domino's Pizza*	1 Slice Sm/67g	152	227	12.1	34.1	4.7	2.8
Veg-a-Roma Without Cheese, Domino's Pizza*	1 Sm Pizza/354g	712	201	8.4	33.4	3.8	2.7
Vegetarian, Supreme, 14", Domino's Pizza*	1 Slice/133g	263	198	8.3	29.3	6.0	1.5
Vegetarian, Supreme, 9.5", Domino's Pizza*	1 Slice/71g	137	193	10.8	27.0	4.6	2.4

POTATO WEDGES
| Domino's Pizza* | 1 Serving/198g | 428 | 216 | 4.1 | 30.3 | 8.7 | 0.0 |

EAT
COFFEE
| Cappuccino, Skimmed Milk, EAT* | 1 Tall/355ml | 85 | 24 | 2.6 | 3.1 | 0.1 | 0.0 |

HOT CHOCOLATE
| Soya Milk, EAT* | 1 Tall/278ml | 115 | 42 | 3.5 | 2.1 | 2.2 | 0.0 |

SALAD
Chef's, EAT*	1 Serving/200g	414	207	8.5	1.8	18.4	0.9
Chicken Caesar, EAT*	1oz/28g	105	374	17.8	11.6	28.6	1.8
Crayfish & Avocado, EAT*	1oz/28g	108	387	12.1	2.7	36.7	2.8

SANDWICH
Chicken, & Salad, EAT*	1 Pack/250g	436	174	9.3	19.3	6.6	2.1
Club, EAT*	1 Pack/200g	861	431	23.1	37.1	21.2	1.7
Crayfish, & Rocket, EAT*	1 Sandwich/200g	519	260	11.3	21.9	14.1	2.6
Crayfish, & Rocket, Low Calorie, EAT*	1 Serving/200g	399	200	11.2	22.4	7.2	2.6

	Measure INFO/WEIGHT	per Measure KCAL	Nutrition Values per 100g / 100ml				
			KCAL	PROT	CARB	FAT	FIBRE

EAT
SANDWICH
	Measure INFO/WEIGHT	per Measure KCAL	KCAL	PROT	CARB	FAT	FIBRE
Egg, & Cress, EAT*	1 Pack/200g	530	265	11.0	23.2	14.3	2.9

SOUP
Black Bean Chilli Con Carne, EAT*	1 Serving/450ml	358	80	7.1	7.1	2.6	1.3
Butternut Squash, With Parmesan, EAT*	1 Can/400ml	127	32	1.9	1.7	2.0	0.5
Carrot & Coriander, EAT*	1 Serving/82.7ml	141	169	2.2	11.5	13.0	3.0
Carrot, Honey & Ginger, EAT*	1 Serving/474ml	255	54	0.7	5.6	3.3	1.2
Chicken Laksa, EAT*	1 Serving/30ml	3	115	5.2	8.2	6.8	0.8
Chicken Noodle, Old Fashioned, EAT*	1 Can/400ml	240	60	6.0	5.5	1.6	0.6
Chicken Pot Pie, EAT*	1 Serving/343g	298	87	5.4	7.8	3.9	1.3
Chicken, Coconut & Sweet Potato, EAT*	1 Pack/343g	235	69	2.0	7.0	3.8	1.1
Chowder, Clam, Manhattan, EAT*	1 Can/400ml	262	66	5.2	5.5	2.6	1.0
Cream Of Corn, EAT*	1 Pack/343g	316	92	1.7	8.4	5.8	0.8
Cream Of Tomato, EAT*	1 Can/400ml	247	62	1.5	3.9	4.3	0.9
French Onion, Eat*	1 Serving/360ml	255	71	1.8	7.0	3.8	0.5
Leek & Potato, EAT*	1 Serving/355ml	156	44	0.8	4.4	2.6	0.6
Minestrone, With Pesto, EAT*	1 Pack/400ml	276	69	2.8	9.2	2.4	2.2
Roast Pumpkin, EAT*	1 Can/400ml	224	56	1.0	5.3	3.5	0.7
Spicy Tomato, EAT*	1 Can/400ml	137	34	0.7	3.6	1.8	0.8
Spinach & Ricotta, EAT*	1 Pack/400ml	224	56	2.1	3.0	4.0	0.7
Sweet Pepper & Tomato, EAT*	1 Serving/473ml	107	23	0.7	4.3	0.3	0.8
Thai Chicken, With Ginger & Coconut, EAT*	1 Serving/340g	244	72	3.4	4.4	4.6	0.6
Tomato & Basil, EAT*	1 Serving/455g	123	27	1.0	4.1	0.7	0.9
Vegetarian Chilli, Eat*	1 Serving/450ml	205	46	2.5	7.3	0.7	2.8
Wild Mushroom, EAT*	1 Serving/500ml	192	38	1.5	2.2	2.7	0.6

YOGHURT
Greek, Fruits Of The Forest, EAT*	1 Pot/125g	94	75	5.0	12.3	0.8	0.2
Greek, With Muesli & Mixed Berries, Low Fat, EAT*	1oz/28g	45	161	8.1	27.5	2.2	2.7

GIA
GARLIC PUREE
In Vegetable Oil, Gia*	1 Tsp/5g	20	391	3.3	1.6	41.3	0.0

SAUCE
Green Pesto, Gia*	1 serving/5g	19	383	3.9	0.5	40.8	0.0

TOMATO PUREE
Sun Dried, & Olive Oil, Gia*	1 Serving/20g	41	204	2.6	0.5	21.6	0.0

TOMATOES
Sundried, In Oil, Gia*	1 Serving/10g	15	153	1.9	7.5	13.9	0.0

GREGGS
BAKE
Steak, Greggs*	1 Bake/80g	200	250	10.0	20.0	15.0	1.0

PASTY
Cheese & Onion, Greggs*	1 Pasty/143g	507	355	6.9	27.9	23.1	1.4
Vegetable, Geggs*	1 Pasty/170g	580	341	3.6	27.9	23.9	0.8

HOT STUFF
PIZZA
Garden Style, Hot Stuff*	1 Slice/188g	370	197	0.0	21.3	11.2	1.6

IXXY'S
BAGEL
Chicken & Bacon, Ixxy's*	1 Serving/215g	589	274	12.8	29.3	12.5	0.0
Chicken, Caesar, Ixxy's*	1 Serving/213.8g	404	189	9.6	25.8	5.3	0.0
Salt Beef & Dill Pickle, Ixxy's*	1 Bagel/213g	403	189	11.1	25.5	4.7	1.8
Soft Cheese & Tomato, Low Fat, Ixxy's*	1 Serving/191g	332	174	7.3	33.1	1.4	0.0
Tuna & Cucumber, Ixxy's*	1 Bagel/260g	390	150	11.3	23.1	1.4	0.0

INFO/WEIGHT	Measure	per Measure KCAL	Nutrition Values per 100g / 100ml KCAL	PROT	CARB	FAT	FIBRE

IXXY'S

BAGEL

Tuna Mayonnaise, Ixxy's*	1 Serving/220g	462	210	11.1	26.1	6.8	1.4

JD WETHERSPOON

BALTI

Chicken, Meal, JDW*	1 Serving/720g	1062	148	7.3	19.4	4.5	1.7

BHAJI

Onion, JDW*	1 Bhaji/30g	43	144	5.3	18.7	7.0	5.7

BREAD

Garlic, Ciabatta, JDW*	1 Serving/120g	320	267	6.0	37.6	10.3	1.7
Naan, JDW*	1 Serving/50g	189	378	8.2	47.4	17.2	2.0

BURGERS

Beef, Double, With Cheese, & Chips, JDW*	1 Serving/654g	1586	243	17.7	9.6	15.2	0.4
Beef, Double, With Chips, JDW*	1 Serving/598g	1356	227	17.0	10.5	13.4	0.4
Beef, With Bacon, Cheese & Chips, JDW*	1 Serving/531g	1202	226	17.2	11.6	12.7	0.4
Beef, With Chips, JDW*	1 Serving/428g	851	199	13.0	14.7	9.0	0.5
Chicken, Fillet, With Chips, JDW*	1 Serving/404g	710	176	6.4	18.9	9.0	0.7
Lamb, Double, Minted, With Chips, JDW*	1 Serving/598g	1077	180	14.6	14.1	7.9	0.9
Lamb, Minted, With Chips, JDW*	1 Serving/428g	712	166	11.3	17.2	6.5	0.9

BURGERS VEGETABLE

With Chips, JDW*	1 Serving/393g	571	145	3.6	22.6	5.0	1.2

BUTTY

Bacon & Egg, Brown Bloomer, JDW*	1 Serving/269g	702	261	18.3	21.0	11.6	1.4
Bacon & Egg, White Bloomer, JDW*	1 Serving/269g	689	256	16.7	20.9	12.2	1.2
Bacon, Brown Bloomer, JDW*	1 Serving/309g	869	281	23.3	18.3	12.8	1.2
Chip & Cheese, Brown Bloomer, JDW*	1 Serving/232g	593	256	9.7	31.4	10.5	1.6
Chip & Cheese, White Bloomer, JDW*	1 Serving/232g	580	250	7.9	31.3	11.2	1.4
Chip, Brown Bloomer, JDW*	1 Serving/204g	478	234	7.6	35.7	7.2	1.9
Chip, White Bloomer, JDW*	1 Serving/204g	465	228	5.6	35.6	8.0	1.6
Sausage & Egg, Brown Bloomer, JDW*	1 Serving/331g	885	267	16.8	20.8	14.8	1.3
Sausage & Egg, White Bloomer, JDW*	1 Serving/331g	872	263	11.4	20.7	15.3	1.1

CAKE

Chocolate Fudge, & Ice Cream, JDW*	1 Serving/239g	822	344	4.0	37.6	19.8	0.4

CHEESECAKE

White Chocolate & Raspberry, JDW*	1 Serving/175g	656	375	5.6	40.8	21.1	0.9

CHICKEN ALFREDO

Pasta, JDW*	1 Serving/420g	1003	239	13.6	27.4	9.5	1.5
Pasta, With Garlic Ciabatta, JDW*	1 Serving/540g	1323	245	11.9	29.7	9.7	1.6

CHICKEN PHAAL

Meal, JDW*	1 Serving/720g	1234	171	7.5	21.0	6.4	1.6

CHICKEN ROAST

With Chips & Salad, JDW*	1 Meal/695g	983	141	13.1	5.9	7.5	0.6
With Chips, Peas, Tomatoes, Mushrooms, JDW*	1 Meal/742g	904	122	13.0	5.6	5.2	1.2
With Jacket Potato, Salad, & Salsa, JDW*	1 Meal/785g	1193	152	12.2	10.2	7.3	1.3

CHICKN FORESTIERRE

JDW*	1 Serving/684g	626	92	7.7	8.7	3.8	1.0

CHILLI

Con Carne, With Rice, & Tortilla Chips, JDW*	1 Serving/585g	733	125	6.3	17.7	3.3	1.3

CHIPS

Bowl, JDW*	1 Serving/300g	363	121	2.6	21.7	3.8	0.0
With Cheese, JDW*	1 Serving/356g	593	167	6.1	18.3	8.6	0.0
With Roast Gravy, JDW*	1 Serving/400g	395	99	2.5	17.6	3.1	0.0

CHUTNEY

Mango, JDW*	1 Serving/25g	47	188	0.4	44.8	0.8	0.4

JD WETHERSPOON

	Measure / INFO/WEIGHT	per Measure / KCAL	KCAL	PROT	CARB	FAT	FIBRE
DHANSAK							
Lamb, Meal, JDW*	1 Serving/720g	1110	154	7.2	21.0	5.0	0.8
FISH & CHIPS							
Haddock, JDW*	1 Serving/495g	804	162	7.2	14.4	8.2	2.4
Plaice, Breaded, & Peas, JDW*	1 Serving/460g	550	120	6.8	15.0	3.4	1.7
Traditional, JDW*	1 Serving/495g	804	162	7.2	14.4	8.2	2.4
GAMMON &							
Chips, Peas, Tomato, & Egg, JDW*	1 Meal/564g	844	150	15.0	6.7	7.3	1.3
Chips, Peas, Tomato, & Pineapple, JDW*	1 Meal/575g	799	139	13.6	7.8	6.3	1.4
HAGGIS							
With Neeps & Tatties, JDW*	1 Serving/684g	982	144	4.6	15.0	7.7	1.9
HAM							
& Eggs, JDW*	1 Serving/396g	253	64	4.9	3.5	3.2	0.0
JALFREZI							
Chicken, Meal, JDW*	1 Serving/720g	1170	163	8.5	20.2	5.3	1.7
KORMA							
Chicken, Meal, JDW*	1 Serving/720g	1223	170	7.7	19.8	6.6	1.7
LASAGNE							
Al Forno, With Dressed Side Salad, JDW*	1 Serving/673g	897	133	5.2	14.8	5.9	1.1
MASALA							
Vegetable, Tandoori, Meal, JDW*	1 Serving/720g	1020	142	3.4	20.7	5.0	2.3
MELT							
BBQ Chicken, & Chips, & Dressed Salad, JDW*	1 Serving/643g	849	132	10.4	8.2	6.6	0.4
MIXED GRILL							
With Chips, & Dressed Side Salad, JDW*	1 Serving/784g	1324	169	12.0	5.6	11.1	0.3
MOUSSAKA							
Vegetarian, JDW*	1 Serving/555g	582	105	2.7	7.6	7.0	2.7
NACHOS							
JDW*	1 Serving/366g	1139	311	7.0	29.2	18.4	3.2
With Chilli Con Carne, JDW*	1 Serving/531g	1276	240	7.5	22.6	13.4	2.8
With Fajita Chicken, JDW*	1 Serving/486g	1225	252	5.7	24.7	14.5	2.9
With Five Bean Chilli, JDW*	1 Serving/531g	1174	221	6.0	24.4	12.7	3.4
PANINI							
Cheese & Tomato, JDW*	1 Panini/216g	509	236	10.6	26.1	10.2	0.9
Cheese & Tuna, JDW*	1 Panini/221g	551	249	15.5	24.9	10.1	0.7
Cheese, Tomato, & Bacon, JDW*	1 Panini/261g	630	241	14.3	21.6	11.1	0.8
Club, JDW*	1 Panini/273g	560	205	14.9	20.8	7.2	0.8
Fajita Chicken, JDW*	1 Panini/235g	359	153	4.4	28.8	2.6	1.7
Pepperoni & Mozzarella, JDW*	1 Panini/205g	617	301	11.6	27.5	16.3	1.0
PASTA BAKE							
Mediterranean, JDW*	1 Serving/450g	527	117	4.0	14.4	4.8	0.9
PIE							
Aberdeen Angus, With Chips, & Vegetables, JDW*	1 Serving/780g	1356	174	5.5	15.7	11.1	0.9
Cottage, Meal, JDW*	1 Serving/618g	654	106	4.2	11.2	4.7	2.6
Fish, With Carrot & Broccoli, In Light Herb Butter, JDW*	1 Serving/550g	612	111	4.6	9.7	6.9	2.4
Ice Cream, Toffee & Chocolate, JDW*	1 Serving/140g	542	387	5.2	51.2	21.1	2.3
Scotch, With Chips & Beans, JDW*	1 Serving/435g	603	139	6.8	14.9	5.1	1.5
PLATTER							
Italian Style, JDW*	1 Platter/1020g	1985	195	10.4	22.9	7.4	0.6
Mexican, With Chilli Con Carne, & Sour Cream, JDW*	1 Platter/1062g	2560	241	7.5	22.6	13.3	2.8
Mexican, With Five Bean Chilli, JDW*	1 Platter/1002g	2358	235	6.2	25.6	12.3	3.6
Western, JDW*	1 Platter/1454g	2973	205	16.9	9.1	11.6	0.4

JD WETHERSPOON

INFO/WEIGHT	Measure per Measure KCAL	KCAL	PROT	CARB	FAT	FIBRE
POPPADOMS						
JDW*	1 Poppadom/10g 28	280	21.0	45.0	2.0	10.0
POTATO JACKET						
With Baked Beans, & Dressed Side Salad, JDW*	1 Serving/570g 650	114	3.0	17.2	4.1	2.3
With Cheddar Cheese, & Dressed Side Salad, JDW*	1 Serving/486g 761	157	5.0	15.8	8.6	1.6
With Chilli Con Carne, & Dressed Side Salad, JDW*	1 Serving/595g 668	112	4.2	15.0	4.4	1.8
With Fajita Chicken, & Dressed Side Salad, JDW*	1 Serving/550g 617	112	2.3	16.3	4.7	1.8
With Salmon, Mayonnaise, & Salad, JDW*	1 Serving/471g 800	170	4.8	16.2	10.0	1.5
With Prawn Mayonnaise, & Side Salad, JDW*	1 Serving/486g 682	140	2.2	15.7	8.1	1.5
With Tuna, & Dressed Side Salad, JDW*	1 Serving/640g 977	153	6.9	12.5	8.8	1.2
POTATO SKINS						
Loaded, Chilli Con Carne, JDW*	1 Serving/503g 735	146	5.0	15.7	7.1	1.9
POTATO WEDGES						
Spicy, JDW*	1 Serving/270g 434	161	2.2	27.7	5.8	1.8
Spicy, With Sour Cream, JDW*	1 Serving/330g 558	169	2.3	23.4	8.3	1.5
POTATOES						
Diced, Garlic & Herb, With Dip, JDW*	1 Serving/320g 586	183	2.0	19.9	10.6	2.9
RIBS						
Double, JDW*	1 Serving/350g 767	219	16.7	11.9	11.7	0.4
Double, With Chips, JDW*	1 Serving/500g 949	190	12.5	14.9	9.3	0.3
Double, With Jacket Potato, JDW*	1 Serving/590g 1159	196	11.4	19.2	8.6	1.3
RICE						
JDW*	1 Serving/200g 274	137	2.9	30.9	0.2	0.2
ROGAN JOSH						
Lamb, Meal, JDW*	1 Serving/720g 1245	173	9.8	19.5	6.2	1.2
SALAD						
Breaded Tiger Prawn, With Dressing & Chilli Jam, JDW*	1 Portion/340g 500	147	4.7	10.1	9.7	0.9
Caesar, Chicken, JDW*	1 Serving/150g 634	423	12.1	9.4	37.3	0.7
Caesar, JDW*	1 Salad/192g 634	330	9.5	7.3	29.2	0.6
Chicken & Bacon, Warm, JDW*	1 Salad/427g 688	161	16.2	6.4	7.8	0.5
Chicken, BBQ, With Croutons & BBQ Dressing, JDW*	1 Portion/350g 315	90	9.4	7.5	2.4	0.8
Side, No Dressing, JDW*	1 Salad/195g 125	64	2.0	8.9	2.3	1.1
Side, With Dressing, JDW*	1 Salad/215g 263	122	2.2	8.1	9.1	1.0
Tuna, With Eggs, Olives, & Croutons, JDW*	1 Portion/395g 679	172	10.3	3.2	13.1	0.7
SAMOSAS						
Vegetable, JDW*	1 Samosa/50g 92	184	5.4	28.4	6.2	2.2
SANDWICH						
BLT, Brown Bloomer, JDW*	1 Sandwich/404g 885	219	18.0	14.6	9.8	1.2
BLT, White Bloomer, JDW*	1 Sandwich/404g 872	216	17.0	14.6	8.1	1.0
Beef, Hot, Brown Bloomer, JDW*	1 Sandwich/299g 618	207	11.4	19.9	9.1	1.3
Beef, Hot, White Poppy Seed Bloomer, JD Wetherpoon*	1 Sandwich/299g 605	202	10.0	19.8	9.6	1.1
Cheddar, & Pickle, Brown Bloomer, JDW*	1 Sandwich/260g 651	250	10.8	24.7	12.0	1.7
Cheddar, & Pickle, White Bloomer, JDW*	1 Sandwich/260g 638	245	9.2	24.6	12.6	1.5
Chicken, Cheese, & Bacon, With Mayo, Brown, JDW*	1 Sandwich/312g 763	245	14.8	18.9	12.2	1.4
Chicken, Cheese, & Bacon, With Mayo, White, JDW*	1 Sandwich/312g 710	228	13.5	18.8	12.7	1.2
Chicken, With Half Fat Mayo, Brown Bloomer, Hot, JDW*	1 Sandwich/289g 628	217	11.8	20.7	9.8	1.7
Chicken, With Half Fat Mayo, White Bloomer, Hot, JDW*	1 Sandwich/289g 615	213	11.3	20.6	10.3	1.5
Egg Mayonnaise, Brown Bloomer, JDW*	1 Sandwich/295g 704	239	10.1	19.7	13.4	1.3
Egg Mayonnaise, White Bloomer, JDW*	1 Sandwich/295g 692	235	8.7	19.6	13.9	1.1
Ham, & Tomato, Brown Bloomer, JDW*	1 Sandwich/239g 514	215	11.4	24.4	7.2	1.8
Ham, & Tomato, White Bloomer, JDW*	1 Sandwich/239g 501	210	9.7	24.4	7.8	1.5
Prawn Mayonnaise, Brown Bloomer, JDW*	1 Sandwich/244g 579	237	11.0	23.8	10.9	1.6
Prawn Mayonnaise, White Bloomer, JDW*	1 Sandwich/244g 567	232	9.3	23.7	11.6	1.4

JD WETHERSPOON

	Measure INFO/WEIGHT	per Measure KCAL	Nutrition Values per 100g / 100ml KCAL	PROT	CARB	FAT	FIBRE
SANDWICH							
Salmon, & Lemon Mayo, Poached, Brown Bloomer, JDW*	1 Sandwich/229g	637	278	11.4	25.4	14.7	1.7
Salmon, & Lemon Mayo, Poached, White Bloomer, JDW*	1 Sandwich/229g	625	273	9.6	25.2	15.4	1.4
Tuna Mayonnaise, Half Fat Mayo, Brown Bloomer, JDW*	1 Sandwich/389g	841	216	12.3	15.7	11.7	1.1
Tuna Mayonnaise, Half Fat Mayo, White Bloomer, JDW*	1 Serving/389g	828	213	11.2	15.6	12.1	1.0
SAUSAGE & MASH							
JDW*	1 Serving/712g	1045	147	6.5	10.1	8.7	1.2
SAUSAGES WITH							
Bacon & Egg, JDW*	1 Serving/582g	1040	179	11.7	11.3	9.9	1.0
Beans & Chips, JDW*	1 Serving/518g	937	181	8.4	13.9	10.5	1.2
Champ, JDW*	1 Serving/678g	974	144	6.4	8.3	9.2	1.4
SCAMPI							
Breaded, With Chips, Peas, & Tartare Sauce, JDW*	1 Serving/490g	793	162	5.7	18.2	7.0	1.8
SOUP							
Mushroom, No Bread, JDW*	1 Serving/305g	500	83	2.8	5.5	5.4	0.4
Mushroom, With Brown Bloomer, JDW*	1 Serving/429g	610	142	5.1	17.1	5.9	1.2
Mushroom, With White Bloomer, JDW*	1 Serving/429g	597	139	4.1	17.0	6.2	1.0
Tomato, No Bread, JDW*	1 Serving/305g	393	65	0.9	3.9	4.6	0.6
Tomato, With Brown Bloomer, JDW*	1 Serving/429g	556	130	3.8	15.9	5.2	1.3
Tomato, With White Bloomer, JDW*	1 Serving/429g	543	127	2.8	15.9	5.6	1.2
STEAK &							
Breaded Scampi, Chips, & Peas, JDW*	1 Serving/816g	1369	168	10.1	11.3	8.9	1.2
STEAK WITH							
Chips, & Dressed Side Salad, Rump, JDW*	1 Meal/634g	922	145	9.5	6.3	9.5	0.3
Chips, & Dressed Side Salad, Sirloin, JDW*	1 Meal/577g	979	170	7.6	6.9	12.7	0.3
Chips, Peas, Tomatoes, & Mushrooms, Rump, JDW*	1 Meal/627g	833	133	10.4	6.1	7.3	1.1
Chips, Peas, Tomatoes, & Mushrooms, Sirloin, JDW*	1 Meal/570g	891	156	8.6	6.8	10.4	1.2
Jacket Potato, Butter, Salad, & Salsa, Rump, JDW*	1 Meal/724g	1132	156	9.0	10.9	8.9	1.1
Jacket Potato, Butter, Salad, & Salsa, Sirloin, JDW*	1 Meal/667g	1189	178	7.3	11.8	11.6	1.2
STEW							
Irish, JDW*	1 Serving/600g	516	86	7.3	5.6	3.9	0.9
TART							
Apple, With Ice Cream, JDW*	1 Serving/235g	464	197	1.6	29.8	8.5	0.4
TIKKA MASALA							
Chicken, Hot, Meal, JDW*	1 Serving/720g	1257	175	8.2	21.2	6.3	1.2
WAFFLES							
Belgian, With Vanilla Ice Cream & Maple Syrup, JDW*	1 Serving/395g	934	237	13.8	28.4	8.5	0.8
WRAP							
Caesar Wetherwrap, JDW*	1 Wrap/159g	478	301	7.0	23.1	20.5	1.5
Caesar Wetherwrap, With Potato Wedges, JDW*	1 Serving/289g	687	238	5.0	25.2	13.9	1.6
Caesar Wetherwrap, With Tortilla Chips & Salsa, JDW*	1 Serving/244g	624	256	5.7	23.4	15.9	1.6
Chicken & Cheese, & Potato Wedges, JDW*	1 Serving/401g	762	190	8.0	22.2	8.5	1.5
Chicken & Cheese, & Tortilla Chips With Salsa, JDW*	1 Serving/356g	699	196	8.8	20.6	9.1	1.5
Chicken & Cheese, JDW*	1 Wrap/271g	553	204	10.7	19.6	9.7	1.4
Chicken & Guacamole, With Potato Wedges, JDW*	1 Serving/318g	537	169	7.2	23.7	5.8	2.0
Chicken & Guacamole, With Tortilla Chips & Salsa, JDW*	1 Serving/273g	474	174	8.2	21.9	6.2	2.0
Chicken, JDW*	1 Wrap/243g	438	180	9.1	21.8	6.9	1.6
Chicken, With Potato Wedges, JDW*	1 Serving/373g	647	174	6.7	23.9	6.5	1.7
Chicken, With Tortilla Chips & Salsa, JDW*	1 Serving/328g	584	178	7.5	22.3	7.0	1.6
Club Wetherwrap, JDW*	1 Wrap/251g	613	244	15.3	14.9	14.2	1.0
Club Wetherwrap, With Potato Wedges, JDW*	1 Serving/381g	822	216	10.9	19.2	11.3	1.2
Club Wetherwrap, With Tortilla Chips & Salsa, JDW*	1 Serving/336g	759	226	12.2	17.1	12.5	1.1
Fajita Chicken, JDW*	1 Wrap/228g	345	151	3.8	21.2	6.2	1.9

JD WETHERSPOON

	INFO/WEIGHT	KCAL	KCAL	PROT	CARB	FAT	FIBRE
WRAP							
Fajita Chicken, With Potato Wedges, JDW*	1 Serving/358g	554	155	3.2	23.5	6.1	1.9
Fajita Chicken, With Tortilla Chips & Salsa, JDW*	1 Serving/313g	491	157	3.5	21.9	6.5	1.9
Poached Salmon & Prawn Salad, JDW*	1 Wrap/355g	512	144	9.8	4.5	9.6	0.5
Poached Salmon, With Potato Wedges, JDW*	1 Serving/298g	656	220	7.1	24.2	11.5	1.5
Poached Salmon, With Tortilla Chips & Salsa, JDW*	1 Serving/203g	573	282	9.9	25.8	16.2	1.6

KENTUCKY FRIED CHICKEN

	INFO/WEIGHT	KCAL	KCAL	PROT	CARB	FAT	FIBRE
BURGERS							
Chicken Fillet, KFC*	1 Burger/213g	469	220	15.0	19.0	9.2	1.6
Fillet Towermeal, KFC*	1 Pack/283g	656	232	13.0	19.8	11.2	1.5
Zinger Fillet, KFC*	1 Serving/185g	445	241	13.9	22.4	10.6	1.4
Zinger Tower, KFC*	1 Serving/256g	620	242	12.4	20.2	12.5	1.3
Zinger, Meal, KFC*	1 Meal/305g	735	241	22.4	10.6	14.0	1.4
CHEESECAKE							
Boysenberry, Chateau, KFC*	1 Cheescake/85g	196	230	4.0	30.0	11.0	0.0
CHICKEN							
Breast, Original Recipe, KFC*	1 Breast/161g	596	370	40.0	11.0	19.0	0.0
Breast, Original, KFC*	1 Breast/161g	370	230	24.8	6.8	11.8	0.0
Popcorn, Large, KFC*	1 Serving/170g	1054	620	30.0	36.0	40.0	0.0
Popcorn, Small, KFC*	1 Serving Sm/99g	358	362	17.0	21.0	23.0	0.2
Strips, Crispy, KFC*	1 Strip/50g	134	268	18.6	14.5	15.1	1.5
Thigh, Original Recipe, Kentucky Fried, KFC*	1 Serving/126g	360	286	17.5	9.5	19.8	0.0
COLESLAW							
KFC*	1 Portion/142g	231	163	1.4	18.3	9.5	2.1
FRIES							
Medium, KFC*	1 Serving/100g	294	294	3.8	36.4	14.8	3.1
GRAVY							
Chicken, KFC*	1oz/28g	39	138	5.2	7.0	9.8	0.0
PIE							
Apple Slice, Colonels Pies, KFC*	1 Slice/113g	310	274	1.7	38.9	12.3	0.0
Strawberry Creme, Slice, KFC*	1 Slice/78g	279	358	5.4	41.0	19.2	2.5
SALAD							
Potato, KFC*	1 Portion/160g	229	143	2.5	14.3	8.7	1.8
Warm Chicken, No Dressing, KFC*	1 Salad/100g	302	302	28.4	22.0	11.1	1.9
TWISTER							
KFC*	1 Twister/240g	600	250	9.1	21.6	14.1	1.6
WRAP							
Twister, KFC*	1 Twister/252g	670	266	10.7	21.8	15.1	1.2

KRISPY KREME

	INFO/WEIGHT	KCAL	KCAL	PROT	CARB	FAT	FIBRE
CAKE							
Chocolate, Glazed, Krispy Kreme*	1 Doughnut/80g	340	425	4.0	53.0	23.0	1.0
DOUGHNUTS							
Blueberry, Powdered, Filled, Krispy Kreme*	1 Doughnut/86g	290	337	3.0	41.0	19.0	1.0
Chocolate Iced, Custard Filled, Krispy Kreme*	1 Doughnut/87g	300	345	3.0	40.0	20.0	1.0
Chocolate Iced, Glazed, Krispy Kreme*	1 Serving/66g	250	379	5.0	50.0	18.0	1.0
Chocolate Iced, With Creme Filling, Krispy Kreme*	1 Doughnut/87g	350	402	3.0	42.0	24.0	1.0
Chocolate Iced, With Sprinkles, Krispy Kreme*	1 Doughnut/71g	260	366	4.0	54.0	17.0	1.0
Cinnamon Apple, Filled, Krispy Kreme*	1 Doughnut/81g	290	358	4.0	40.0	20.0	1.0
Cruller, Glazed, Krispy Kreme*	1 Doughnut/54g	240	444	4.0	48.0	26.0	1.0
Glazed, With A Creme Filling, Krispy Kreme*	1 Doughnut/86g	340	395	3.0	45.0	23.0	1.0
Lemon Filled, Glazed, Krispy Kreme*	1 Doughnut/85g	290	341	4.0	40.0	19.0	1.0
Maple Iced, Krispy Kreme*	1 Doughnut/66g	240	364	3.0	48.0	18.0	1.0
Original Glazed, Krispy Kreme*	1 Doughnut/52g	200	385	4.0	42.0	23.0	1.0

	Measure INFO/WEIGHT	per Measure KCAL	Nutrition Values per 100g / 100ml KCAL	PROT	CARB	FAT	FIBRE
KRISPY KREME							
DOUGHNUTS							
Raspberry, Glazed, Krispy Kreme*	1 Doughnut/86g	300	349	3.0	45.0	19.0	1.0
Sour Cream, Krispy Kreme*	1 Doughnut/80g	340	425	4.0	53.0	23.0	1.0
Strawberry, Powdered, Filled, Krispy Kreme*	1 Doughnut/74g	260	351	4.0	35.0	22.0	1.0
MCDONALD'S							
APPLES							
McDonald's*	1 Apple/140g	59	42	0.3	10.0	0.0	2.2
BREAKFAST							
Big Breakfast Bun, McDonald's*	1 Bun/242g	571	236	13.0	15.1	13.3	0.9
Big Breakfast, McDonald's*	1 Breakfast/256g	591	231	10.2	15.6	14.2	1.6
BROWNIE							
Chocolate Chip, McMini, McDonald's*	1 Brownie/18.9g	68	360	4.9	58.8	12.7	1.9
BURGERS							
Bacon McDouble, With Cheese, McDonald's*	1 Burger/141g	372	264	16.1	19.6	13.5	2.2
Big Mac, McDonald's*	1 Big Mac/215g	492	229	12.4	20.5	10.7	2.7
Big Tasty, McDonald's*	1 Burger/348g	804	231	11.7	14.6	14.5	1.6
Cheeseburger, Double, McDonalds*	1 Burger/171g	438	256	15.5	19.4	11.7	1.8
Cheeseburger, McDonald's*	1 Burger/122g	300	246	13.0	27.2	9.5	2.1
Double Cheeseburger, McDonald's*	1 Burger/171g	438	256	15.5	19.4	12.9	1.8
Filet-O-Fish, McDonald's*	1 Burger/161g	386	240	9.9	25.2	11.1	1.2
Grilled Chicken Caprese, McDonald's*	1 Burger/275g	470	171	12.5	15.0	7.7	2.1
Hamburger, McDonald's*	1 Burger/108g	254	235	12.2	30.6	7.1	2.3
McChicken Grill With BBQ Sauce, McDonald's*	1 Pack/215g	309	144	12.1	18.1	2.6	2.2
McChicken Premiere, McDonald's*	1 Burger/244g	537	220	12.1	21.4	9.5	1.6
McChicken Sandwich, McDonald's*	1 Burger/167g	376	225	9.9	23.2	10.3	2.3
Quarter Pounder, Deluxe, McDonald's*	1 Burger/253g	521	206	11.4	16.1	10.6	1.7
Quarter Pounder, McDonald's*	1 Burger/178g	424	238	14.5	20.9	10.7	2.1
Quarter Pounder, With Cheese, McDonald's*	1 Burger/206g	515	250	15.1	18.2	13.0	1.8
Steak Premiere, McDonald's*	1 Burger/229g	453	198	14.9	19.4	6.2	1.6
BURGERS VEGETABLE							
Deluxe, McDonald's*	1 Burger/210g	475	226	5.1	28.8	10.0	4.9
CADBURY BYTE							
McMini, McDonald*	1 Byte/14.0g	67	478	6.5	64.7	20.7	1.7
CAKE							
Birthday, McDonald's*	1 Portion/158g	640	405	2.7	65.4	14.3	1.0
CAPPUCCINO							
McDonald's*	1 Reg Cup/25ml	92	365	22.4	20.6	14.4	0.0
CHICKEN							
Selects, McDonald's*	2 Selects/82.1g	184	224	13.7	14.8	11.7	1.3
COFFEE							
Latte, McDonald's*	1 Reg Cup/16.2ml	59	364	22.3	20.3	14.3	0.0
UHT Creamer, McDonald's*	1 Cup/14ml	17	123	4.2	4.2	10.0	0.0
COLA							
Coke, Diet, McDonald's*	1 Med/400ml	2	0	0.0	0.0	0.0	0.0
Coke, McDonald's*	1 Med/400ml	172	43	0.0	10.5	0.0	0.0
CROUTONS							
McDonald's*	1 Sachet/14g	58	414	14.6	70.8	8.0	3.0
DOUGHNUTS							
Chocolate Donut, McMini, McDonald's*	1 Donut/17.1g	64	375	6.8	46.9	17.8	1.6
Cinnamon Donut, McDonald's*	1 Donut/72g	302	419	5.1	43.1	25.1	3.8
Sugared Donut, McDonald's*	1 Donut/72g	303	421	5.0	42.6	25.6	3.7
DRESSING							
Balsamic, McDonalds*	1 Sachet/31ml	30	95	0.3	11.9	5.1	0.8

MCDONALD'S

INFO/WEIGHT	Measure per Measure KCAL	Nutrition Values per 100g / 100ml KCAL	PROT	CARB	FAT	FIBRE
DRESSING						
Caesar, Salad, McDonalds*	1 Sachet/75ml	145	188	2.6	10.0	15.3	0.5
Ranch, Salad, McDonalds*	1 Sachet/78ml	107	136	3.1	12.3	8.3	0.8
FANTA						
Orange, McDonald's*	1 Reg/250ml	108	43	0.0	10.4	0.0	0.0
FISH FINGERS						
McDonald's*	3 Fingers/74g	164	221	13.5	20.2	9.6	3.1
FLATBREAD						
Chicken Salsa, McDonald's*	1 Serving/100g	480	480	27.3	57.6	15.5	0.0
Greek, McDonald's*	1 Flatbread/100g	433	433	21.2	47.3	20.7	3.8
FRIES						
McDonald's *	1 Regular/78g	207	265	3.8	36.3	11.5	3.6
FRUIT						
& Yoghurt, McDonald's*	1 Serving/144g	138	96	2.8	15.9	1.9	1.1
A Croquer, McDonald's*	1 Serving/80g	47	59	0.4	13.5	0.4	2.3
Bag, Happy Meal, McDonald's*	1 Bag/80g	43	54	0.3	13.0	0.1	2.3
HASH BROWNS						
McDonald's*	1 Portion/56g	138	247	2.5	28.3	13.8	3.1
HOT CHOCOLATE						
McDonald's*	1 Cup/32.4ml	122	380	7.0	79.0	4.0	0.0
HOT DOG						
& Ketchup, McDonald's*	1 Serving/116g	296	255	9.6	25.8	12.6	1.3
ICE CREAM CONE						
McDonald's*	1 Cone/98g	157	160	4.5	24.4	5.0	0.0
With Flake, McDonald's*	1 Cone/107g	204	191	4.8	27.0	7.2	0.0
LEMONADE						
Sprite, McDonald's*	1 Regular/251ml	108	43	0.0	10.5	0.0	0.0
MCFLURRY						
Creme Egg, Cadbury's, McDonald's*	1 McFlurry/203g	390	192	4.1	29.9	6.5	0.0
Crunchie, McDonald's*	1 McFlurry/183g	319	174	4.1	26.4	6.0	0.0
Dairy Milk, McDonalds's*	1 McFlurry/181g	324	178	4.5	24.3	7.2	0.0
Jammie Dodger, McDonald's*	1 Serving/128g	256	200	3.9	33.6	6.4	0.3
Rolo, McDonald's*	1 McFlurry/205g	390	190	4.0	29.2	6.5	0.1
Smarties, McDonald's*	1 McFlurry/185g	327	177	4.2	26.2	6.2	0.2
MCMUFFIN						
Bacon & Egg, Double, McDonald's*	1 McMuffin/226g	600	265	15.8	16.9	14.9	1.2
Bacon & Egg, McDonald's*	1 McMuffin/141g	345	245	14.2	18.5	12.8	1.3
Egg, McDonald's*	1 McMuffin/127g	281	221	12.2	20.4	10.1	3.2
Sausage & Egg, Double, McDonald's*	1 McMuffin/226.5g	572	253	14.7	11.4	16.4	0.8
Sausage & Egg, Double, No Muffin, McDonald's*	1 Serving/100g	416	416	27.6	0.2	33.5	0.0
Sausage & Egg, McDonald's*	1 McMuffin/176g	426	242	13.8	14.7	14.1	1.0
Scrambled Egg, McDonald's*	1 McMuffin/147g	294	200	10.9	17.5	9.6	1.3
MELT						
Toasted Ham & Cheese, McDonald's*	1 Serving/100g	239	239	11.2	30.6	8.0	1.8
MILK SHAKE						
Banana, McDonald's*	1 Regular/336g	396	118	3.2	20.2	3.0	0.0
Chocolate, McDonald's*	1 Regular/336g	403	120	3.4	19.9	3.0	0.0
Strawberry, McDonald's*	1 Regular/336g	396	118	3.2	20.0	3.0	0.0
Vanilla, McDonald's*	1 Regular/336g	383	114	3.2	18.8	3.0	0.0
MUFFIN						
Buttered, McDonald's*	1 Muffin/63g	158	250	8.6	40.7	5.9	2.9
Buttered, With Preserve, McDonald's*	1 Muffin/93g	234	252	5.9	48.1	4.0	2.0

	Measure	per Measure	Nutrition Values per 100g / 100ml				
	INFO/WEIGHT	KCAL	KCAL	PROT	CARB	FAT	FIBRE

MCDONALD'S

PANCAKE

	Measure	per Measure KCAL	KCAL	PROT	CARB	FAT	FIBRE
& Sausage, McDonald's*	1 Portion/262g	686	262	5.4	33.8	10.8	0.5
& Syrup, McDonald's*	1 Pack/209.4g	531	254	2.4	41.9	7.6	0.6

PIE

Apple, McDonald's*	1 Pie/78g	225	289	2.8	33.2	16.1	1.4

POTATO SKINS

Loaded, Cheese & Bacon, JDW*	1 Serving/439g	949	216	8.9	15.2	13.3	1.5

POTATO WEDGES

McDonald's	1 Portion/176g	368	208	3.3	26.1	10.1	2.2

QUORN*

Burger, Premiere, McDonald's*	1 Burger/210g	311	148	9.1	24.2	2.9	2.7

ROLL

Bacon With Brown Sauce, McDonald's*	1 Roll/118g	289	245	12.8	31.2	8.4	1.4
Bacon, McBacon, McDonald's*	1 Roll/122g	349	286	13.5	30.5	11.5	1.7

SALAD

Caesar, Crispy Chicken With Croutons, McDonalds*	1 Salad/295g	385	131	9.4	8.8	6.2	1.3
Caesar, Crispy Chicken, With Dressing, McDonalds	1 Salad/316g	472	149	8.8	7.5	9.2	1.2
Caesar, Grilled Chicken, With Croutons, McDonalds	1 Salad/294g	280	95	11.5	4.2	3.3	1.3
Caesar, Grilled Chicken, With Dressing, McDonalds*	1 Salad/305g	367	120	11.1	3.3	6.7	1.2
Garden, Side, Without Dressing, McDonald's*	1 Salad/93g	13	14	0.8	2.2	0.3	1.4
Ranch, Crispy Chicken, With Dressing, McDonald's*	1 Salad/401g	501	125	8.3	6.6	7.2	1.1
Ranch, Crispy Chicken, Without Dressing, McDonalds*	1 Salad/320g	394	123	9.5	5.1	6.9	1.1
Ranch, Grilled Chicken, With Dressing, McDonald's*	1 Salad/400g	396	99	9.8	3.1	5.0	1.1
Ranch, Grilled Chicken, Without Dressing, McDonald's*	1 Salad/298g	268	90	11.4	1.4	4.2	1.0

SANDWICH

McChicken Sandwich, New, McDonald's*	1 Sandwich/100g	375	375	16.5	38.6	17.2	3.8

SAUCE

Barbeque, McDonald's*	1 Portion/32g	55	173	2.2	38.3	1.2	0.0
Curry, Sweet, McDonald's*	1 Portion/32g	61	192	1.2	41.1	2.5	0.0
Mustard, Mild, McDonald's*	1 Portion/30g	64	212	1.0	24.8	12.1	0.0
Sweet & Sour, McDonald's*	1 Portion/32g	59	183	0.4	43.5	0.8	0.0

SUNDAE

Hot Caramel, McDonald's*	1 Sundae/189g	357	189	3.8	33.9	4.4	0.0
Hot Fudge, McDonald's*	1 Sundae/187g	352	188	4.5	30.0	5.7	0.0
No Topping, McDonald's*	1 Sundae/149g	219	147	4.2	21.6	5.1	0.0
Strawberry, McDonald's*	1 Sundae/186g	296	159	3.4	27.5	4.1	0.0

TEA

UHT Skimmed Milk, McDonald's*	1 Cup/14ml	10	74	3.7	5.4	4.1	0.0

YOGHURT

Burst, Strawberry, McDoanld's*	1 Yoghurt/40g	21	52	2.9	11.0	0.0	0.9

PIZZA HUT

BREAD

Garlic, Pizza Hut*	1 Slice/24g	101	419	8.7	48.1	21.3	2.7

CHICKEN WITH

Sour Cream & Chive Dip, Wings, Pizza Hut*	1 Pack/178g	680	382	22.8	1.9	31.5	1.3

ICE CREAM

Dairy, Pizza Hut*	1 Portion/141.7g	273	192	4.6	23.3	8.9	0.2

LASAGNE

Pizza Hut*	1 Serving/350g	669	191	11.3	17.8	8.3	2.7

MUSHROOMS

Garlic, With BBQ Dip, Pizza Hut*	1 Pack/112.2g	264	234	6.2	30.5	10.0	3.4
Garlic, With Sour Cream & Chive Dip, Pizza Hut*	1 Pack/112.2g	429	380	6.4	20.0	30.8	3.4

	Measure INFO/WEIGHT	per Measure KCAL	Nutrition Values per 100g / 100ml KCAL	PROT	CARB	FAT	FIBRE
PIZZA HUT							
PIZZA							
Cheese Feast, Grand Pan, Pizza Hut*	1 Serving/97g	270	278	11.3	27.8	13.4	1.0
Chicken Supreme, Medium Pan, Pizza Hut*	1/2 Pizza/300g	810	270	13.0	29.0	12.0	2.0
Farmhouse, Hi Light, Large, Pizza Hut*	1 Slice/83g	191	230	12.2	30.3	6.7	0.0
Farmhouse, Hi Light, Medium, Pizza Hut*	1 Slice/82g	184	225	12.1	29.1	6.7	0.0
Ham & Mushroom, The Italian, Medium 12", Pizza Hut*	1 Slice/96g	270	281	13.6	35.4	10.6	2.6
Ham, Hi Light, Large, Pizza Hut*	1 Slice/83g	191	230	12.2	30.3	6.7	0.0
Ham, Hi Light, Medium, Pizza Hut	1 Slice/82g	184	225	12.1	29.1	6.7	0.0
Hawaiian, Medium Pan, Pizza Hut*	1 Slice/96g	201	210	9.5	29.5	5.7	1.0
Margherita, Medium Pan, Pizza Hut*	1 Slice/85g	239	281	12.7	31.1	11.8	2.1
Margherita, Stuffed Crust Original, Pizza Hut*	1 Slice/125.3g	330	262	14.9	28.5	9.8	1.0
Margherita, The Italian, Medium, Pizza Hut*	1 Slice/95g	292	307	15.2	39.5	10.8	2.3
Meat Feast, Medium Pan, Pizza Hut*	1 Slice/114g	324	284	14.6	24.4	14.2	0.9
Meat Feast, The Italian, 12", Pizza Hut*	1 Slice/113g	341	302	15.4	30.3	14.3	2.3
Meaty, The Edge, Pizza Hut*	1 Slice/64g	207	323	16.6	23.3	18.2	0.0
Pepperoni, The Insider, Pizza Hut*	1 Slice/137g	360	263	12.4	25.5	12.4	1.5
Supreme, Medium Pan, Pizza Hut*	1 Slice/105.7g	292	275	12.6	25.1	13.8	1.2
Supreme, The Italian, Medium, Pizza Hut*	1 Slice/106g	297	280	13.0	33.4	11.4	2.1
Supreme, Vegetable, Italian Pan, Pizza Hut*	1 Slice/112g	180	161	7.1	21.4	5.4	1.8
The Works, The Edge, Pizza Hut*	1 Slice/64g	161	252	12.9	22.0	12.5	0.0
Vegetarian, Original Medium, Pizza Hut*	1 Slice/93.5g	227	241	11.2	28.0	9.4	1.9
Veggie, The Edge, Pizza Hut*	1 Slice/60g	137	228	11.4	24.6	9.3	0.0
POTATO SKINS							
Jacket, Pizza Hut*	1 Portion/ 223.5g	571	255	3.4	23.0	16.6	2.1
Jacket, With Sour Cream & Chive Dip, Pizza Hut*	1 Portion/223.5g	311	139	1.4	9.3	10.8	0.8
Loaded, Cheese & Red Onion, JDW*	1 Serving/414g	835	202	6.0	16.5	12.4	1.6
PRET A MANGER							
BAGUETTE							
Brie, Tomato & Basil, Pret A Manger*	1 Baguette/200g	407	203	9.3	23.9	7.8	0.3
Cheddar & Baby Plum Tomato, Pret A Manger*	1 Baguette/300g	625	208	6.7	18.5	11.9	1.0
Egg & Tomato, Breakfast, Pret A Manger*	1 Av Pack/230g	426	185	8.1	22.8	6.8	0.7
Ham & Greve, Pret A Manger*	1 Av Pack/350g	844	241	12.3	21.9	10.9	0.3
Ham, Kids, Pret A Manger*	1 Baguette/118g	308	261	12.4	26.8	11.6	0.0
New Tuna Salad, Pret A Manger*	1 Baguette/227g	506	223	10.0	21.7	10.7	0.9
Salmon & Egg, Pret A Manger*	1 Av Pack/230g	527	229	10.9	23.0	10.4	2.2
Tuna Mayo, Pret A Manger*	1 Av Pack/230g	535	233	10.8	25.0	10.0	1.7
BARS							
Power, Pret A Manger*	1 Bar/65g	265	408	6.8	41.4	24.0	6.2
BROWNIE							
Pret A Manger*	1 Av Pack/50g	204	408	4.8	53.2	19.8	2.5
CAKE							
Apple, Card Box, Pret A Manger*	1 Cake/116g	356	307	3.9	39.6	14.7	1.8
Apple, Pret A Manger*	1 Av Pack/120g	432	360	5.3	38.8	21.9	2.1
Banana Slice, In A Box, Pret A Manger*	1 Slice/100g	335	335	4.6	39.0	17.8	1.9
Banana, Card Box, Pret A Manger*	1 Cake/103g	345	335	4.6	39.0	17.8	1.9
Carrot, Card Box, Pret A Manger*	1 Cake/112g	402	359	4.0	41.0	19.9	2.3
Carrot, Pret A Manger*	1 Av Pack/120g	288	240	2.9	41.6	6.9	0.2
Fudge, Pret A Manger*	1 Av Pack/140g	537	384	4.1	46.1	20.3	1.3
Lemon, Card Cake, Pret A Manger*	1 Cake/97g	318	328	5.0	42.8	15.2	0.9
Lemon, Pret A Manger*	1 Serving/100g	328	328	5.0	42.8	15.2	0.9
Nut Munch, Pret A Manger*	1 Av Pack/100g	497	497	8.0	38.5	34.6	7.9
Oat & Fruit Slice, Pret a Manger*	1 Slice/100g	427	427	5.3	56.0	20.3	5.1
Pecan Pie, Pret A Manger*	1 Av Pack/70g	344	492	6.3	43.7	32.5	0.8

PRET A MANGER	INFO/WEIGHT	KCAL	KCAL	PROT	CARB	FAT	FIBRE
CHEESECAKE							
Caramel Crunch, Pret A Manger*	1 Serving/150g	564	376	5.3	21.1	30.1	1.2
Lemon, Pret A Manger*	1 Pot/150g	594	396	4.3	26.4	30.3	0.6
CHOCOLATE							
Milk, Organic, Pret A Manger*	1 Bar/40g	216	540	9.5	54.0	32.0	0.0
Plain, Organic, Pret A Manger*	1 Bar/40g	230	575	7.5	45.5	40.5	0.0
White, Organic, Pret A Manger*	1 Bar/40g	230	575	7.5	52.5	37.5	0.0
COFFEE							
Cappuccino, Chocolate, Pret A Manger*	1 Serving/340g	106	31	1.7	2.2	1.7	0.0
Cappuccino, Chocolate, Tall, Pret A Manger*	1 Serving/355ml	106	30	1.7	2.1	1.6	0.0
Cappuccino, Full-Fat Milk, No Chocolate, Pret A Manger*	1 Serving/355ml	102	29	1.7	1.9	1.6	0.0
Latte, Pret A Manger*	1 Serving/336g	192	57	3.1	3.9	3.3	0.0
Mocha, Pret A Manger*	1 Serving/340g	243	72	2.8	7.6	3.4	0.0
Mocha, Skimmed Milk, Pret a Manger*	1 Serving/340ml	91	27	2.6	3.6	0.2	0.0
CRISPS							
Cheddar & Chive, Pret A Manger	1 Bag/40g	187	468	7.0	53.8	24.8	6.0
Lightly Salted, Pret A Manger*	1 Bag/40g	198	495	5.8	58.0	28.5	4.3
Mature Cheddar, & Red Onion, Pret A Manger*	1 Pack/40g	196	490	6.0	60.0	25.0	5.0
Pickled Onion, Pret A Manger*	1 Bag/40g	177	443	7.5	52.0	22.8	7.3
Salt & Vinegar, Pret A Manger*	1 Bag/40g	186	465	6.8	55.0	25.3	6.0
Sea Salt & Black Pepper, Pret A Manger*	1 Bag/40g	180	450	5.8	55.0	23.0	5.3
Sweet Chilli, Pret A Manger*	1 Pack/40g	190	475	5.5	60.5	23.5	6.3
Vegetable Chips, Pret A Manger*	1 Bag/25g	126	504	5.6	37.2	36.8	10.0
CROISSANT							
Almond, Pret A Manger*	1 Croissant/50g	183	365	8.8	34.9	21.1	1.1
Cheese & Tomato, Pret A Manger*	1 Croissant/111g	376	339	11.4	22.5	22.6	0.0
Chocolate, Pret A Manger*	1 Croissant/70g	268	383	5.4	42.3	21.5	0.8
Ham & Cheese, Pret A Manger*	1 Croissant/134g	441	329	13.3	21.4	20.0	2.2
CRUMBLE							
Mincemeat Crumble, Pret A Manger*	1 Serving/70g	275	393	3.9	53.0	17.9	2.1
DESSERT							
Brownie, Pret Pot, Pret A Manger*	1 Pot/121g	201	166	5.7	17.7	8.3	0.7
DOUGHNUTS							
Mixed Berry, Baked, Pret A Manger*	1 Doughnut/100g	337	337	7.6	51.8	11.2	1.5
DRIED FRUIT							
Nuts & Bolts, Pret A Manger*	1 Pack/120g	571	476	15.5	35.7	32.5	4.4
FOOL							
Raspberry, Pret A Manger*	1 Pot/140g	188	134	1.7	12.4	8.9	0.4
FRUIT SALAD							
Fresh, Pret A Manger*	1 Pack/150g	55	37	0.5	8.5	0.1	0.7
Large, Pret A Manger*	1 Pack/315g	120	38	0.5	8.8	0.2	1.1
Pret a Manger*	1 Av Pack/300g	120	40	0.5	9.2	0.2	1.2
GOULASH							
Hungarian, Pret a Manger*	1 Serving/455g	240	53	3.2	6.7	1.7	1.2
GRAPES							
Pret A Manger*	1 Pack/130g	78	60	0.4	15.4	0.1	0.7
ICE CREAM							
Chocolate, Organic, Pret A Manger*	1 Serving/110ml	192	192	3.9	19.5	10.8	0.9
Vanilla, Organic, Pret A Manger*	1 Serving/100ml	156	156	3.3	14.3	9.5	0.1
White Chocolate & Caramel, Organic, Pret A Manger*	1 Serving/100ml	223	100	1.4	10.0	6.1	0.0
JUICE							
Blue Bionic, Pret A Manger*	1 Serving/250g	170	68	2.9	11.3	1.4	1.8
Carrot, Freshly Pressed, Pret a Manger*	1 Serving/250ml	60	24	0.5	5.7	0.1	0.0

PRET A MANGER

	Measure INFO/WEIGHT	per Measure KCAL	Nutrition Values per 100g / 100ml				
			KCAL	PROT	CARB	FAT	FIBRE
JUICE							
Orange, & Raspberry, Pret A Manger*	1 Serving/250g	110	44	0.7	10.0	0.0	0.0
Orange, Large, Pret A Manger*	1 Serving/500ml	229	46	0.6	11.4	0.0	0.1
Orange, Pret A Manger*	1 Serving/260g	114	44	0.6	11.0	0.0	0.1
MILK							
Kids, Pret A Manger*	1 Serving/250g	170	68	3.4	4.7	4.0	0.0
MOUSSE							
Chocolate, Pret A Manger*	1 Pot/110g	314	285	2.7	16.9	22.9	1.3
MUFFIN							
Morning Glory, Pret A Manger*	1 Muffin/140g	521	372	7.4	35.2	22.6	3.2
Orange, & Lemon, Pret A Manger*	1 Muffin/160g	603	377	4.9	38.1	17.6	1.1
POPCORN							
Honey, Organic, Pret A Manger*	1 Bag/35g	157	449	4.0	75.7	17.4	6.3
Sea Salt, Organic, Pret A Manger*	1 Bag/35g	138	394	11.1	52.0	15.7	13.1
PRETZELS							
Pret A Manger*	1 Serving/175g	541	309	10.9	51.6	6.5	2.5
SALAD							
Chicken, Al Fresco, Pret A Manger*	1 Pack/287g	439	153	6.9	4.8	12.0	1.6
Crayfish, Pret a Manger*	1 Av Pack/320g	200	63	3.0	0.8	5.2	0.3
Houmous & Pitta Bread, Pot, Pret a Manger*	1 Pot/200g	393	197	4.8	12.0	14.4	3.4
Pesto Pasta, Pret a Manger*	1 Pot/320g	425	133	2.7	6.9	10.7	0.9
Super Club, Pret a Manger*	1 Av Pack/200g	213	107	10.8	1.6	6.3	0.6
Tuna Nicoise, Pret a Manger*	1 Av Pack/300g	381	127	7.9	3.7	9.1	1.2
Tuna, Pret a Manger*	1 Serving/150g	276	184	11.5	5.4	13.2	1.8
SALAD BOWL							
Crayfish, Pret A Manger*	1 Pack/243.50g	149	61	4.8	4.6	2.6	0.5
Houmous & Feta, Pret A Manger*	1 serving/200g	421	210	5.8	9.1	16.9	1.5
New Tuna Salad, Pret A Manager*	1 Pack/289.20g	368	127	7.9	3.7	9.1	1.2
Pasta, Basil, Pret A Manager*	1 Pack/334.20g	629	188	4.4	17.7	11.0	0.8
SALAD BOWL							
Crayfish, & Smoked Salmon, Pret A Manger*	1 Pack/230.40g	194	84	8.2	4.6	3.7	0.7
SANDWICH							
All Day Breakfast, Pret A Manger*	1 Pack/300g	612	204	8.6	15.5	12.0	1.4
All Day Breakfast, Slim Pret, Pret A Manger*	1 Pack/148.9g	306	206	8.6	15.7	12.0	1.5
Avocado, & Alfalfa Sprout, Pret A Manger*	1 Av Pack/250g	329	132	3.4	11.6	8.0	2.4
BLT, Big, Pret A Manger*	1 Serving/200g	398	199	8.5	15.4	11.6	1.6
BLT, Slim Pret, Pret A Manger*	1 Sandwich/123.9g	248	200	8.5	15.4	11.6	1.7
Beef, & Horseradish, Pret A Manger*	1 Av Pack/250g	382	153	11.2	17.7	4.4	2.5
Big Prawn, Pret A Manger*	1 Pack/208.6g	445	213	10.6	16.5	11.9	1.5
Cheddar, Christmas, Pret A Manger*	1 Av Pack/270g	671	249	8.8	18.3	15.5	2.0
Cheese, Three, & Roasted Tomato, Pret A Manger*	1 Pack/350g	417	119	3.8	11.5	6.2	1.5
Chicken & Pepper Sauce, Special, Pret A Manger*	1 Sandwich/215.4g	397	184	10.1	17.5	8.3	1.9
Chicken Caesar, Slim Pret, Pret A Manger*	1 Sandwich/135.4g	239	177	8.4	14.2	9.3	1.7
Chicken, & Avocado, Pret A Manger*	1 Av Pack/250g	513	205	8.4	14.7	12.6	2.9
Chicken, & Coriander, On Rye, Pret A Manger*	1 Sandwich/200g	500	250	10.8	22.1	13.9	2.0
Chicken, Black Pepper, Bloomer, Pret A Manger*	1 Av Pack/250g	642	257	13.0	29.5	9.7	1.8
Chicken, Caesar, Pret A Manger*	1 Serving/400g	481	120	5.6	10.2	6.1	1.4
Chicken, Coronation, Pret A Manger*	1 Av Pack/250g	415	166	7.9	21.2	5.4	0.2
Christmas Lunch, 2003, Pret A Manger*	1 Av Pack/270g	599	222	11.3	19.0	11.2	2.3
Club, Pret A Manger*	1 Av Pack/250g	542	217	12.8	18.7	10.1	2.3
Club, Super, Pret A Manger*	1 Av Pack/200g	404	202	10.3	13.5	12.0	1.5
Club, Super, Slim Pret, Pret A Manger*	1 Pack/143.40g	290	202	10.3	13.6	12.1	1.6
Crayfish & Rocket, Slim Pret, Pret A Manger*	1 Pack/97.90g	184	188	8.3	18.3	9.0	1.6

PRET A MANGER

INFO/WEIGHT	Measure	per Measure KCAL	KCAL	PROT	CARB	FAT	FIBRE
SANDWICH							
Crayfish, & Rocket, Pret A Manger	1 Av Pack/195.9	341	174	9.4	16.7	7.8	1.5
Crayfish, & White Crab, Pret A Manger*	1 Pack/250g	391	156	5.0	16.8	7.7	2.2
Egg Mayonnaise, Pret A Manger*	1 Av Pack/250g	508	203	9.6	21.0	8.9	1.9
Egg, & Tomato, On Rye, Pret A Manger*	1 Pack/350g	626	179	8.3	17.2	8.5	2.1
Egg, Florentine, No Bread, Pret A Manger*	1 Pack/232g	263	113	5.7	4.9	7.9	0.7
Ham, Cheese, & Pickle, Pret A Manger*	1 Av Pack/250g	592	237	11.9	25.0	11.0	2.4
Houmous Salad, Slim Pret, Pret A Manger*	1 Pack/128.30g	201	157	5.1	18.4	7.1	2.6
Houmous, & Oven Roasted Tomato, Pret A Manger*	1 Pack/350g	404	115	3.5	13.6	5.2	3.1
Lamb, Pea & Mint Relish, Roast, Pret A Manger*	1 Sandwich/250g	938	375	21.8	44.1	12.7	7.4
Mozzarella, More Than, No Bread, Pret A Manger*	1 Pack/311g	413	133	6.0	2.8	10.9	1.7
Pastrami, On Rye, Pret A Manger*	1 Sandwich/200g	391	196	10.3	22.6	7.7	1.9
Prawn, & Rocket, Pret A Manger*	1 Pack/280g	435	155	8.4	14.9	6.9	1.3
Prawn, Gourmet, Pret A Manger*	1 Av Pack/250g	454	182	7.8	15.2	10.2	1.8
Salmon, & Egg, Smoked, No Bread, Pret A Manger*	1 Pack/233g	223	96	6.9	4.0	5.9	0.7
Salmon, & Horseradish, Pret A Manger*	1 Pack/300g	462	154	9.0	14.2	6.7	1.8
Salmon, Salmon, Pret A Manger*	1 Av Pack/250g	370	148	3.8	20.3	5.8	1.8
Soft Cheese, & Spicy Aubergine, Pret A Manger*	1 Av Pack/250g	319	128	4.6	21.2	2.7	2.8
Tuna Mayonnaise, No Bread, Pret A Manger*	1 Pack/233g	193	83	10.8	1.9	3.8	0.5
Tuna Mayonnaise, Pret A Manger*	1 Av Pack/250g	505	202	9.5	16.2	10.9	2.2
Tuna, St Tropez, Pret a Manger*	1 Serving/250g	387	155	7.4	14.7	7.6	2.0
Turkey Club, Pret a Manger*	1 Pack/295.7g	593	200	10.0	15.1	10.6	1.8
SHORTBREAD							
Fingers, Pret A Manger*	1 Pack/28.40g	148	521	5.6	58.5	35.2	2.8
SMOOTHIE							
Mango, Pret A Manger*	1 Serving/250g	130	52	0.6	12.4	0.2	1.2
Strawberry, Pret A Manger*	1 Serving/250g	105	42	0.3	9.6	0.1	0.9
Vitamin Volcano, Pret A Manger*	1 Serving/250ml	103	41	0.4	10.1	0.1	0.9
SOUP							
Celeriac & Mash, Pret A Manger*	1 Container/297g	125	42	0.8	2.2	3.4	1.0
Classic Tomato, Pret A Manger*	1 Serving/336g	179	53	0.9	7.5	2.1	0.7
Fresh Tomato, & Herb, Pret A Manger*	1 Serving/307g	123	40	0.6	3.3	2.2	0.9
Minestrone, Pret A Manger*	1 Serving/455g	187	41	1.7	5.6	1.4	1.5
Porcini Musroom, Pret A Manger*	1 Serving/455g	210	46	1.4	5.6	1.8	0.9
Roasted Red Pepper, & Goats Chesse, Pret A Manger*	1 Serving/282g	175	62	1.8	2.9	4.8	0.9
Smoked Bacon, Pea & Mint, Pret A Manger*	1 Serving/282g	215	76	2.7	5.3	4.9	1.4
Tomato & Basil, Pret A Manger*	1 Serving/453.6g	147	32	0.6	4.7	1.4	0.7
Tomato & Mountain Wheat, Pret A Manger*	1 Serving/455g	220	48	1.3	8.1	1.3	0.7
Tuscan Bean & Sausage, Pret A Manger*	1 Serving/340g	267	79	4.8	8.1	3.3	3.8
SUSHI							
Deluxe, Pret A Manger*	1 Pack/350g	494	141	6.0	25.1	1.4	1.2
Salmon Nigiri, Pret A Manger*	1 Serving/175g	245	140	4.7	24.6	2.1	1.1
WATER							
Blackcurrant, Pure Still, Pret A Manger*	1 Serving/500ml	80	16	0.0	3.6	0.0	0.0
Cranberry, Pure Pret, Pret A Manger*	1 Can/330ml	119	36	0.0	8.6	0.0	0.0
Ginger Beer, Pure Pret, Pret A Manger*	1 Can/330ml	152	46	0.0	11.4	0.0	0.0
Grape & Elderflower, Pure Pret, Pret A Manger*	1 Can/330ml	146	44	0.0	10.6	0.0	0.0
Lemon Barley, Pure Pret, Pret A Manger*	1 Serving/500ml	80	16	0.0	3.7	0.0	0.0
Lemon, Pure Pret, Pret A Manger*	1 Can/330ml	175	53	0.0	12.6	0.0	0.0
Orange, Pure Pret, Pret A Manger*	1 Can/330ml	158	48	0.0	11.3	0.0	0.0
Orange, Still, Pure Pret, Pret A Manger*	1 Serving/500ml	85	17	0.0	3.8	0.0	0.0
WRAP							
Avocado & Salad, Pret A Manger*	1 Serving/200g	416	208	4.6	13.9	15.0	2.8

PRET A MANGER

	INFO/WEIGHT	KCAL	KCAL	PROT	CARB	FAT	FIBRE
WRAP							
Chicken Salad, Pret A Manger*	1 Av Pack/230g	378	164	8.3	15.6	7.7	1.3
Houmous Salad, Pret A Manger*	1 Av Pack/230g	351	153	5.0	17.9	6.8	3.4
Tuna Nicoise, Pret A Manger*	1 Pack/200g	338	169	7.0	15.1	9.1	2.1
YOGHURT							
Red Berry, Blender, Pret A Manger*	1 Av Pack/125g	175	140	5.6	23.0	3.0	2.4
Vanilla, Blender, Pret A Manger*	1 Pot/250ml	230	92	4.5	12.8	2.7	0.0
YOGHURT DRINK							
Blueberry Blender, Pret A Manger*	1 Drink/250g	170	68	2.9	11.3	1.4	1.8
Mango's & Minerals, Pret A Manger*	1 Drink/250g	203	81	2.6	14.4	1.4	0.1

STARBUCKS

	INFO/WEIGHT	KCAL	KCAL	PROT	CARB	FAT	FIBRE
BAGEL							
Cheese, & Jalapeno, Starbucks*	1 Bagel/115g	292	254	10.8	45.8	3.1	1.5
BARS							
Cereal, Granola, Starbucks*	1 Bar/90g	324	360	8.0	38.6	21.3	4.8
BISCUITS							
Biscotti, Starbucks*	1 Biscuit/27g	100	370	7.4	55.6	14.8	0.0
Ginger Snap, Starbucks*	1 Biscuit/21g	89	426	7.9	73.1	11.3	0.0
BREAD							
Bagel, Cinamon & Raisin, Starbucks*	1 Bagel/83g	190	229	44.8	9.4	1.4	1.3
CAKE							
Banana & Date Loaf, Starbucks*	1 Slice/105g	292	278	5.9	57.1	2.9	2.7
Carrot Loaf, Starbucks*	1 Slice/100g	352	352	4.7	38.4	19.9	2.3
Yoghurt & Berry Loaf, Low Fat, Starbucks*	1 Cake/94g	254	270	5.3	50.8	5.1	1.7
CHEESECAKE							
Chocolate, Starbucks*	1 Serving/185g	723	391	6.9	30.5	26.8	0.8
COFFEE							
Brewed, Grande, Starbucks*	1 Grande/473ml	9	2	0.1	0.4	0.0	0.0
Brewed, Tall, Starbucks*	1 Tall/354ml	7	2	0.1	0.3	0.0	0.0
Brewed, Venti, Starbucks*	1 Venti/591ml	14	2	0.1	0.5	0.0	0.0
Caffe Americano, Grande, Starbucks*	1 Grande/473ml	17	4	0.2	0.6	0.0	0.0
Caffe Americano, Tall, Starbucks*	1 Tall/354ml	11	3	0.2	0.6	0.0	0.0
Caffe Americano, Venti, Starbucks*	1 Venti/591ml	23	4	0.3	0.5	0.0	0.0
Caffe Latte, Skimmed Milk, & Syrup, Grande, Starbucks*	1 Grande/473ml	218	46	2.8	8.5	0.0	0.0
Caffe Latte, Skimmed Milk, Grande, Starbucks*	1 Grande/473ml	163	34	3.4	5.1	0.0	0.0
Caffe Latte, Skimmed Milk, Tall, Starbucks*	1 Tall/354ml	122	34	3.4	5.1	0.0	0.0
Caffe Latte, Skimmed Milk, Venti, Starbucks*	1 Venti/591ml	208	35	3.5	5.1	0.0	0.0
Caffe Latte, Skimmed Milk, With Syrup, Tall, Starbucks*	1 Tall/354ml	169	48	3.0	8.8	0.0	0.0
Caffe Latte, Skimmed Milk, With Syrup, Venti, Starbucks*	1 Venti/591ml	274	46	2.9	8.5	0.0	0.0
Caffe Latte, Whole Milk, Grande, Starbucks*	1 Grande/473ml	265	56	3.0	4.4	2.9	0.0
Caffe Latte, Whole Milk, Tall, Starbucks*	1 Tall/354ml	200	57	3.1	4.5	3.0	0.0
Caffe Latte, Whole Milk, Venti, Starbucks*	1 Venti/591ml	341	58	3.1	4.6	3.0	0.0
Caffe Latte, Whole Milk, With Syrup, Grande, Starbucks*	1 Grande/473ml	301	64	2.5	8.0	2.4	0.0
Caffe Latte, Whole Milk, With Syrup, Tall, Starbucks*	1 Tall/354ml	237	67	2.7	8.2	2.6	0.0
Caffe Latte, Whole Milk, With Syrup, Venti, Starbucks*	1 Venti/591ml	380	64	2.6	8.0	2.5	0.0
Caffe Misto, Skimmed Milk, Grande, Starbucks*	1 Grande/473ml	88	19	1.8	2.8	0.0	0.0
Caffe Misto, Skimmed Milk, Tall, Starbucks*	1 Tall/354ml	64	18	1.8	2.5	0.0	0.0
Caffe Misto, Skimmed Milk, Venti, Starbucks*	1 Venti/591ml	109	18	1.8	2.7	0.0	0.0
Caffe Misto, Whole Milk, Grande, Starbucks*	1 Grande/473ml	143	30	1.6	2.3	1.6	0.0
Caffe Misto, Whole Milk, Tall, Starbucks*	1 Tall/354ml	106	30	1.6	2.3	1.6	0.0
Caffe Misto, Whole Milk, Venti, Starbucks*	1 Venti/591ml	179	30	1.6	2.4	1.6	0.0
Caffe Mocha, Skimmed Milk, & Whip, Grande, Starbucks*	1 Grande/473ml	324	69	3.0	9.3	2.5	0.4
Caffe Mocha, Skimmed Milk, Grande, Starbucks*	1 Grande/473ml	223	47	3.0	8.9	0.5	0.4

STARBUCKS
COFFEE

	Measure INFO/WEIGHT	per Measure KCAL	KCAL	PROT	CARB	FAT	FIBRE
			Nutrition Values per 100g / 100ml				
Caffe Mocha, Skimmed Milk, Tall, Starbucks*	1 Tall/354ml	175	49	0.3	9.3	0.4	0.4
Caffe Mocha, Skimmed Milk, Venti, Starbucks*	1 Venti/591ml	287	49	3.1	9.1	0.5	0.4
Caffe Mocha, Skimmed Milk, With Whip, Tall, Starbucks*	1 Tall/354ml	255	72	3.1	9.6	2.6	0.4
Caffe Mocha, Skimmed Milk, With Whip, Venti, Starbucks*	1 Venti/591ml	388	66	3.1	9.5	2.1	0.4
Caffe Mocha, Whole Milk, Grande, Starbucks*	1 Grande/473ml	295	62	2.7	8.5	2.5	0.4
Caffe Mocha, Whole Milk, Tall, Starbucks*	1 Tall/354ml	233	66	2.9	8.8	2.6	0.4
Caffe Mocha, Whole Milk, Venti, Starbucks*	1 Venti/591ml	383	65	2.8	8.6	2.7	0.4
Caffe Mocha, Whole Milk, With Whip, Grande, Starbucks*	1 Grande/473ml	396	84	2.7	8.9	4.5	0.4
Caffe Mocha, Whole Milk, With Whip, Tall, Starbucks*	1 Tall/354ml	313	88	2.9	9.0	4.9	0.4
Caffe Mocha, Whole Milk, With Whip, Venti, Starbucks*	1 Venti/591ml	484	82	2.8	9.0	4.3	0.4
Cappuccino, Skimmed Milk, Grande, Starbucks*	1 Grande/473ml	96	20	2.0	3.0	0.0	0.0
Cappuccino, Skimmed Milk, Tall, Starbucks*	1 Tall/354ml	76	21	2.1	3.1	0.0	0.0
Cappuccino, Skimmed Milk, Venti, Starbucks*	1 Venti/591ml	129	22	2.1	3.2	0.0	0.0
Cappuccino, Whole Milk, Grande, Starbucks*	1 Grande/473ml	153	32	1.8	2.8	1.6	0.0
Cappuccino, Whole Milk, Tall, Starbucks*	1 Tall/354ml	122	34	1.9	2.8	1.8	0.0
Cappuccino, Whole Milk, Venti, Starbucks*	1 Venti/591ml	207	35	1.9	2.9	1.8	0.0
Caramel Macchiato, Skimmed Milk, Grande, Starbucks*	1 Grande/473ml	234	49	2.9	8.5	0.4	0.0
Caramel Macchiato, Skimmed Milk, Tall, Starbucks*	1 Tall/354ml	173	49	3.1	8.5	0.2	0.0
Caramel Macchiato, Skimmed Milk, Venti, Starbucks*	1 Venti/591ml	277	47	3.0	7.8	0.4	0.0
Caramel Macchiato, Whole Milk, Grande, Starbucks*	1 Grande/473ml	319	67	2.6	7.8	2.9	0.0
Caramel Macchiato, Whole Milk, Tall, Starbucks*	1 Tall/354ml	244	69	2.8	7.9	2.9	0.0
Caramel Macchiato, Whole Milk, Venti, Starbucks*	1 Venti/591ml	390	66	2.7	7.3	2.9	0.0
Espresso, Con Panna, Doppio, Starbucks*	1 Doppio/60ml	111	185	1.2	6.7	15.5	0.0
Espresso, Con Panna, Solo, Starbucks*	1 Solo/30ml	105	350	1.3	10.0	31.0	0.0
Espresso, Doppio, Starbucks*	1 Doppio/60ml	11	18	1.2	3.3	0.0	0.0
Espresso, Macchiato, Skimmed Milk, Doppio, Starbucks*	1 Doppio/60ml	14	23	1.7	3.3	0.0	0.0
Espresso, Macchiato, Skimmed Milk, Solo, Starbucks*	1 Solo/30ml	9	30	1.7	3.3	0.0	0.0
Espresso, Macchiato, Whole Milk, Doppio, Starbucks*	1 Doppio/60ml	15	25	1.5	3.3	0.3	0.0
Espresso, Macchiato, Whole Milk, Solo, Starbucks*	1 Solo/30ml	9	30	1.7	3.3	0.7	0.0
Espresso, Solo, Starbucks*	1 Solo/30ml	6	20	1.3	3.3	0.0	0.0
Iced, Americano, Grande, Starbucks*	1 Grande/473ml	18	4	0.2	0.6	0.0	0.0
Iced, Americano, Tall, Starbucks*	1 Tall/354ml	12	3	0.2	0.6	0.0	0.0
Iced, Americano, Venti, Starbucks*	1 Venti/591ml	24	4	0.3	0.7	0.0	0.0
Iced, Caffe Latte, Whole Milk, Venti, Starbucks*	1 Venti/591ml	166	28	1.5	2.4	1.4	0.0
Iced, Caramel Macchiato, Skimmed, Grande, Starbucks*	1 Grande/473ml	197	42	2.3	7.6	0.2	0.0
Iced, Caramel Macchiato, Skimmed, Tall, Starbucks*	1 Tall/354ml	141	40	2.2	7.1	0.2	0.0
Iced, Caramel Macchiato, Skimmed, Venti, Starbucks*	1 Venti/591ml	222	38	1.9	6.9	0.2	0.0
Iced, Caramel Macchiato, Whole, Grande, Starbucks*	1 Grande/473ml	262	55	2.0	7.2	2.1	0.0
Iced, Caramel Macchiato, Whole, Tall, Starbucks*	1 Tall/354ml	189	53	2.0	6.8	2.1	0.0
Iced, Caramel Macchiato, Whole, Venti, Starbucks*	1 Venti/591ml	291	49	1.7	6.6	1.8	0.0
Iced, Grande, Starbucks*	1 Grande/473ml	6	1	0.1	0.2	0.0	0.0
Iced, Latte, Skimmed Milk, & Syrup, Tall, Starbucks*	1 Tall/354ml	122	34	1.8	6.8	0.0	0.0
Iced, Latte, Skimmed Milk, & Syrup, Venti, Starbucks*	1 Venti/591ml	192	32	1.5	6.6	0.0	0.0
Iced, Latte, Skimmed Milk, Grande, Starbucks*	1 Grande/473ml	98	21	2.0	3.0	0.0	0.0
Iced, Latte, Skimmed Milk, Syrup, Grande, Starbucks*	1 Grande/473ml	163	34	1.7	6.8	0.0	0.0
Iced, Latte, Skimmed Milk, Tall, Starbucks*	1 Tall/354ml	73	21	2.0	3.1	0.0	0.0
Iced, Latte, Skimmed Milk, Venti, Starbucks*	1 Venti/591ml	105	18	1.7	2.5	0.0	0.0
Iced, Latte, Whole Milk, & Syrup, Venti, Starbucks*	1 Venti/591ml	244	41	1.3	6.3	1.2	0.0
Iced, Latte, Whole Milk, Grande, Starbucks*	1 Grande/473ml	155	33	1.8	2.8	1.6	0.0
Iced, Latte, Whole Milk, Syrup, Grande, Starbucks*	1 Grande/473ml	212	45	1.5	6.6	1.4	0.0
Iced, Latte, Whole Milk, Tall, Starbucks*	1 Tall/354ml	119	34	1.8	2.8	1.7	0.0
Iced, Latte, Whole Milk, With Syrup, Tall, Starbucks*	1 Tall/354ml	160	45	1.6	6.5	1.5	0.0

STARBUCKS
COFFEE

	INFO/WEIGHT	KCAL	KCAL	PROT	CARB	FAT	FIBRE
Iced, Mocha, Skimmed Milk, Grande, Starbucks*	1 Grande/473ml	178	38	2.0	7.6	0.5	0.0
Iced, Mocha, Skimmed Milk, Tall, Starbucks*	1 Tall/354ml	133	38	2.0	7.3	0.5	0.0
Iced, Mocha, Skimmed Milk, Venti, Starbucks*	1 Venti/591ml	227	38	2.1	7.8	0.5	0.0
Iced, Mocha, Skimmed Milk, Whip & Syrup, Starbucks*	1 Tall/354ml	237	67	1.7	8.8	2.6	0.1
Iced, Mocha, Skimmed Milk, Whip & Syrup, Starbucks*	1 Venti/591ml	363	61	1.5	8.8	2.3	0.2
Iced, Mocha, Skimmed Milk, Whip, Grande, Starbucks*	1 Grande/473ml	309	65	2.0	8.0	3.0	0.4
Iced, Mocha, Skimmed Milk, Whip, Syrup, Starbucks*	1 Grande/473ml	335	71	1.7	9.5	2.8	0.2
Iced, Mocha, Skimmed Milk, Whip, Tall, Starbucks*	1 Tall/354ml	227	64	2.0	7.9	2.9	0.4
Iced, Mocha, Skimmed Milk, Whip, Venti, Starbucks*	1 Venti/591ml	358	61	2.1	8.1	2.5	0.4
Iced, Mocha, Whole Milk, Grande, Starbucks*	1 Grande/473ml	220	47	1.9	7.4	1.7	0.0
Iced, Mocha, Whole Milk, Tall, Starbucks*	1 Tall/354ml	166	47	1.9	7.1	1.8	0.0
Iced, Mocha, Whole Milk, Venti, Starbucks*	1 Venti/591ml	281	48	1.9	7.5	1.7	0.0
Iced, Mocha, Whole Milk, Whip & Syrup, Starbucks*	1 Grande/473ml	374	79	1.5	9.3	4.0	0.2
Iced, Mocha, Whole Milk, Whip & Syrup, Tall, Starbucks*	1 Tall/354ml	270	76	1.6	8.5	3.9	0.1
Iced, Mocha, Whole Milk, Whip & Syrup, Venti, Starbucks*	1 Venti/591ml	408	69	1.4	8.5	3.3	0.2
Iced, Mocha, Whole Milk, Whip, Grande, Starbucks*	1 Grande/473ml	351	74	1.9	7.8	4.3	0.4
Iced, Mocha, Whole Milk, Whip, Tall, Starbucks*	1 Tall/354ml	260	73	1.9	7.6	4.2	0.4
Iced, Mocha, Whole Milk, Whip, Venti, Starbucks*	1 Venti/591ml	412	70	1.9	7.8	3.8	0.4
Iced, Tall, Starbucks*	1 Tall/354ml	4	1	0.1	0.3	0.0	0.0
Iced, Venti, Starbucks*	1 Venti/591ml	7	1	0.1	0.2	0.0	0.0
Mocha, Peppermint, Skimmed, Grande, Starbucks*	1 Grande/473ml	304	64	2.9	13.3	0.5	0.4
Mocha, Peppermint, Skimmed, Tall, Starbucks*	1 Tall/354ml	237	67	3.1	13.6	0.4	0.4
Mocha, Peppermint, Skimmed, Venti, Starbucks*	1 Venti/591ml	385	65	3.0	13.4	0.5	0.4
Mocha, Peppermint, Skimmed, Whip, Grande, Starbucks*	1 Grande/473ml	405	86	2.9	13.7	4.4	0.4
Mocha, Peppermint, Skimmed, Whip, Tall, Starbucks*	1 Tall/354ml	317	90	3.1	13.8	2.7	0.4
Mocha, Peppermint, Skimmed, Whip, Venti, Starbucks*	1 Venti/591ml	486	82	3.0	13.7	2.1	0.4
Mocha, Peppermint, Whole, Grande, Starbucks*	1 Grande/473ml	372	79	2.7	12.9	2.4	0.4
Mocha, Peppermint, Whole, Tall, Starbucks*	1 Tall/354ml	293	83	2.9	13.3	2.5	0.4
Mocha, Peppermint, Whole, Venti, Starbucks*	1 Venti/591ml	475	80	2.8	12.9	2.6	0.4
Mocha, Peppermint, Whole, Whip, Grande, Starbucks*	1 Grande/473ml	473	100	2.7	13.3	4.4	0.4
Mocha, Peppermint, Whole, Whip, Tall, Starbucks*	1 Tall/354ml	373	105	2.9	13.6	4.8	0.4
Mocha, Peppermint, Whole, Whip, Venti, Starbucks*	1 Venti/591ml	576	97	2.8	13.2	4.2	0.4
Mocha, White Chocolate, Skimmed, Grande, Starbucks*	1 Grande/473ml	340	72	3.3	12.3	1.1	0.0
Mocha, White Chocolate, Skimmed, Tall, Starbucks*	1 Tall/354ml	264	75	3.5	12.7	1.0	0.0
Mocha, White Chocolate, Skimmed, Venti, Starbucks*	1 Venti/591ml	429	73	3.4	12.4	1.1	0.0
Mocha, White Chocolate, Skimmed, Whip, Starbucks*	1 Grande/473ml	441	93	3.3	12.7	3.0	0.0
Mocha, White Chocolate, Skimmed, Whip, Starbucks*	1 Tall/354ml	344	97	3.5	13.0	3.2	0.0
Mocha, White Chocolate, Skimmed, Whip, Starbucks*	1 Venti/591ml	530	90	3.4	12.7	2.7	0.0
Mocha, White Chocolate, Whole, Grande, Starbucks*	1 Grande/473ml	414	88	3.0	11.8	3.2	0.0
Mocha, White Chocolate, Whole, Tall, Starbucks*	1 Tall/354ml	326	92	3.3	12.2	3.4	0.0
Mocha, White Chocolate, Whole, Venti, Starbucks*	1 Venti/591ml	527	89	3.1	12.0	3.3	0.0
Mocha, White Chocolate, Whole, Whip, Starbucks*	1 Grande/473ml	515	109	3.0	12.3	5.2	0.0
Mocha, White Chocolate, Whole, Whip, Tall, Starbucks*	1 Tall/354ml	406	115	3.3	12.4	5.6	0.0
Mocha, White Chocolate, Whole, Whip, Venti, Starbucks*	1 Venti/591ml	628	106	3.1	12.4	4.9	0.0

COOKIES

	INFO/WEIGHT	KCAL	KCAL	PROT	CARB	FAT	FIBRE
Fruit & Oat, Starbucks*	1 Cookie/80g	359	449	7.8	72.3	14.4	0.0

CRISPS

	INFO/WEIGHT	KCAL	KCAL	PROT	CARB	FAT	FIBRE
Strong Cheese & Onion, Starbucks*	1 Bag/50g	228	455	7.1	56.2	22.6	4.0

CROISSANT

	INFO/WEIGHT	KCAL	KCAL	PROT	CARB	FAT	FIBRE
Almond Filled, Starbucks*	1 Croissant/92g	330	359	0.0	42.4	19.6	2.2
Butter, Starbucks*	1 Croissant/82g	289	352	5.9	34.9	21.1	0.0

STARBUCKS

FLATBREAD

Falafel & Houmous, Starbucks*	1 Pack/232.8g	405	174	5.9	28.8	3.9	2.5

FRAPPUCCINO

Caramel Cream, Grande, Starbucks*	1 Grande/473ml	339	72	2.8	12.7	1.1	0.0
Caramel Cream, Tall, Starbucks*	1 Tall/354ml	261	74	2.8	13.0	1.1	0.0
Caramel Cream, Venti, Starbucks*	1 Venti/591ml	409	69	2.6	12.4	1.0	0.0
Caramel Cream, With Whip, Grande, Starbucks*	1 Grande/473ml	470	99	2.8	13.1	3.7	0.0
Caramel Cream, With Whip, Tall, Starbucks*	1 Tall/354ml	355	100	2.8	13.6	3.6	0.0
Caramel Cream, With Whip, Venti, Starbucks*	1 Venti/591ml	540	91	2.6	12.7	3.1	0.0
Caramel, Grande, Starbucks*	1 Grande/473ml	294	62	0.0	12.5	0.8	0.0
Caramel, Light, Grande, Starbucks*	1 Grande/473ml	196	41	1.7	8.0	0.4	0.7
Caramel, Light, Tall, Starbucks*	1 Tall/354ml	152	43	1.6	8.5	0.4	0.7
Caramel, Light, Venti, Starbucks*	1 Venti/591ml	271	46	1.8	9.0	0.4	0.7
Caramel, Tall, Starbucks*	1 Tall/354ml	228	64	0.0	12.7	0.9	0.0
Caramel, Venti, Starbucks*	1 Venti/591ml	370	63	0.0	12.7	0.8	0.0
Caramel, With Whip, Grande, Starbucks*	1 Grande/473ml	425	90	1.2	12.9	3.4	0.0
Caramel, With Whip, Tall, Starbucks*	1 Tall/354ml	322	91	1.1	13.3	3.3	0.0
Caramel, With Whip, Venti, Starbucks*	1 Venti/591ml	501	85	1.1	13.0	2.9	0.0
Chocolate, Grande, Starbucks*	1 Grande/473ml	338	71	3.0	12.7	1.2	0.0
Chocolate, Tall, Starbucks*	1 Tall/354ml	260	73	3.0	13.0	1.3	0.0
Chocolate, Venti, Starbucks*	1 Venti/591ml	413	70	2.8	12.7	1.2	0.0
Chocolate, With Whip, Grande, Starbucks*	1 Grande/473ml	469	99	3.0	13.1	3.8	0.1
Chocolate, With Whip, Tall, Starbucks*	1 Tall/354ml	354	100	3.0	13.6	3.7	0.2
Chocolate, With Whip, Venti, Starbucks*	1 Venti/591ml	544	92	2.8	13.0	3.3	0.2
Coffee, Grande, Starbucks*	1 Grande/473ml	261	55	1.2	11.0	2.0	0.0
Coffee, Light, Grande, Starbucks*	1 Grande/473ml	164	35	1.7	6.6	0.3	0.7
Coffee, Light, Tall, Starbucks*	1 Tall/354ml	119	34	1.6	6.5	0.3	0.7
Coffee, Light, Venti, Starbucks*	1 Venti/591ml	216	37	1.8	6.9	0.3	0.7
Coffee, Tall, Starbucks*	1 Tall/354ml	190	54	1.1	10.7	0.7	0.0
Coffee, Venti, Starbucks*	1 Venti/591ml	291	49	1.0	9.8	1.7	0.0
Coffee, With Whip & Syrup, Grande, Starbucks*	1 Grande/473ml	422	89	1.2	13.1	3.3	0.0
Coffee, With Whip & Syrup, Tall, Starbucks*	1 Tall/354ml	313	88	1.1	13.3	3.2	0.0
Coffee, With Whip & Syrup, Venti, Starbucks*	1 Venti/591ml	484	82	1.1	12.7	2.8	0.0
Espresso, Grande, Starbucks*	1 Grande/473ml	233	49	1.1	9.7	0.9	0.0
Espresso, Tall, Starbucks*	1 Tall/354ml	165	47	2.7	9.3	0.6	0.0
Espresso, Venti, Starbucks*	1 Venti/591ml	315	53	1.2	10.7	0.7	0.0
Mocha, Grande, Starbucks*	1 Grande/473ml	287	61	1.3	12.3	0.9	0.1
Mocha, Light, Grande, Starbucks*	1 Grande/473ml	189	40	1.8	8.0	0.4	0.7
Mocha, Light, Tall, Starbucks*	1 Tall/354ml	145	41	1.8	8.2	0.4	0.8
Mocha, Light, Venti, Starbucks*	1 Venti/591ml	268	45	2.0	9.1	0.5	0.9
Mocha, Tall, Starbucks*	1 Tall/354ml	216	61	1.3	12.4	2.5	0.1
Mocha, Venti, Starbucks*	1 Venti/591ml	364	62	1.3	12.7	0.9	0.2
Mocha, With Whip & Syrup, Grande, Starbucks*	1 Grande/473ml	440	93	1.3	14.0	3.5	0.1
Mocha, With Whip & Syrup, Tall, Starbucks*	1 Tall/354ml	331	94	1.3	14.4	5.0	0.1
Mocha, With Whip & Syrup, Venti, Starbucks*	1 Venti/591ml	534	90	1.3	14.7	3.0	0.2
Raspberry Tea, Grande, Starbucks*	1 Grande/473ml	200	42	0.1	11.0	0.0	0.2
Raspberry Tea, Tall, Starbucks*	1 Tall/354ml	144	41	0.1	10.5	0.0	0.2
Raspberry Tea, Venti, Starbucks*	1 Venti/591ml	261	44	0.1	11.3	0.0	0.2
Strawberries & Cream, Grande, Starbucks*	1 Grande/473ml	424	90	2.9	17.3	1.1	0.0
Strawberries & Cream, Tall, Starbucks*	1 Tall/354ml	299	84	2.7	16.4	1.0	0.0
Strawberries & Cream, Venti, Starbucks*	1 Venti/591ml	543	92	3.0	17.6	1.1	0.0
Strawberries & Cream, With Whip, Grande, Starbucks*	1 Grande/473ml	555	117	2.9	17.8	3.7	0.1
Strawberries & Cream, With Whip, Tall, Starbucks*	1 Tall/354ml	393	111	2.7	17.0	3.5	0.1

STARBUCKS

INFO/WEIGHT	Measure	per Measure KCAL	KCAL	PROT	CARB	FAT	FIBRE
FRAPPUCCINO							
Strawberries & Cream, With Whip, Venti, Starbucks*	1 Venti/591ml	674	114	3.0	17.9	3.2	0.1
Tazo Chai, Grande, Starbucks*	1 Grande/473ml	405	86	2.9	16.5	1.1	0.0
Tazo Chai, Tall, Starbucks*	1 Tall/354ml	294	83	2.9	15.8	1.1	0.0
Tazo Chai, Venti, Starbucks*	1 Venti/591ml	487	82	2.7	16.1	1.0	0.0
Tazo Chai, With Whip, Grande, Starbucks*	1 Grande/473ml	536	113	2.9	16.9	3.7	0.0
Tazo Chai, With Whip, Tall, Starbucks*	1 Tall/354ml	388	110	2.9	16.4	3.5	0.0
Tazo Chai, With Whip, Venti, Starbucks*	1 Venti/591ml	618	105	2.7	16.4	3.1	0.0
Tropical Citrus Tea, Grande, Starbucks*	1 Grande/473ml	178	38	0.3	9.3	0.1	0.3
Tropical Citrus Tea, Tall, Starbucks*	1 Tall/354ml	128	36	0.3	9.0	0.1	0.3
Tropical Citrus Tea, Venti, Starbucks*	1 Venti/591ml	232	39	0.3	9.8	0.1	0.3
Vanilla, Grande, Starbucks*	1 Grande/473ml	329	70	2.8	12.3	1.1	0.0
Vanilla, Tall, Starbucks*	1 Tall/354ml	250	71	2.8	12.4	1.1	0.0
Vanilla, Venti, Starbucks*	1 Venti/591ml	459	78	2.6	12.0	1.0	0.0
Vanilla, With Whip, Grande, Starbucks*	1 Grande/473ml	460	97	2.8	12.7	3.6	0.0
Vanilla, With Whip, Tall, Starbucks*	1 Tall/354ml	344	97	2.8	13.0	3.5	0.0
Vanilla, With Whip, Venti, Starbucks*	1 Venti/591ml	530	90	2.6	12.4	3.1	0.0
FRUIT SALAD							
Starbucks*	1 Salad/300g	126	42	0.5	9.7	0.2	1.0
HOT CHOCOLATE							
Skimmed Milk, Grande, Starbucks*	1 Grande/473ml	261	55	3.3	10.6	0.5	0.4
Skimmed Milk, Tall, Starbucks*	1 Tall/354ml	209	59	3.5	11.3	0.4	0.4
Skimmed Milk, Venti, Starbucks*	1 Venti/591ml	340	58	3.3	11.2	0.5	0.4
Skimmed Milk, With Whip, Grande, Starbucks*	1 Grande/473ml	362	77	3.3	11.0	2.5	0.4
Skimmed Milk, With Whip, Tall, Starbucks*	1 Tall/354ml	289	82	3.5	11.6	2.7	0.4
Skimmed Milk, With Whip, Venti, Starbucks*	1 Venti/591ml	441	75	3.3	11.5	2.1	0.4
White, Skimmed Milk, Grande, Starbucks*	1 Grande/473ml	386	82	3.9	14.0	3.8	0.0
White, Skimmed Milk, Tall, Starbucks*	1 Tall/354ml	301	85	4.1	14.4	1.1	0.0
White, Skimmed Milk, Venti, Starbucks*	1 Venti/591ml	493	83	4.0	14.2	1.2	0.0
White, Skimmed Milk, With Whip, Grande, Starbucks*	1 Grande/473ml	487	103	3.9	14.4	3.2	0.0
White, Skimmed Milk, With Whip, Tall, Starbucks*	1 Tall/354ml	381	108	4.1	14.7	3.4	0.0
White, Skimmed Milk, With Whip, Venti, Starbucks*	1 Venti/591ml	594	101	4.0	14.6	2.8	0.0
White, Whole Milk, Grande, Starbucks*	1 Grande/473ml	479	101	3.6	13.3	3.8	0.0
White, Whole Milk, Tall, Starbucks*	1 Tall/354ml	377	107	3.8	13.8	4.0	0.0
White, Whole Milk, Venti, Starbucks*	1 Venti/591ml	618	105	3.7	13.5	4.1	0.0
White, Whole Milk, With Whip, Grande, Starbucks*	1 Grande/473ml	580	123	3.6	13.7	5.8	0.0
White, Whole Milk, With Whip, Tall, Starbucks*	1 Tall/354ml	457	129	3.8	14.1	6.3	0.0
White, Whole Milk, With Whip, Venti, Starbucks*	1 Venti/591ml	719	122	3.7	13.9	5.7	0.0
Whole Milk, Grande, Starbucks*	1 Grande4/473ml	347	73	3.0	9.9	3.0	0.4
Whole Milk, Tall, Starbucks*	1 Tall/354ml	277	78	3.1	10.7	3.0	0.4
Whole Milk, Venti, Starbucks*	1 Venti/591ml	448	76	3.0	10.7	3.0	0.4
Whole Milk, With Whip, Grande, Starbucks*	1 Grande/473ml	448	95	3.0	10.4	5.0	0.4
Whole Milk, With Whip, Tall, Starbucks*	1 Tall/354ml	357	101	3.1	11.0	5.3	0.4
Whole Milk, With Whip, Venti, Starbucks*	1 Venti/591ml	549	93	3.0	11.0	4.6	0.4
HOUMOUS							
With Crunchy Vegetables, Starbucks*	1 Pot/219g	359	164	4.7	26.4	4.4	2.9
MUFFIN							
Bran, Honey Raisin, Starbucks*	1 Muffin/100g	315	315	5.9	38.9	15.2	4.5
Classic Blueberry, Starbucks*	1 Muffin/129g	438	337	4.4	39.7	17.7	1.4
Skinny Blueberry, Starbucks*	1 Muffin/129g	306	236	3.7	47.2	3.2	1.7
Skinny Peach & Raspberry, Starbucks*	1 Muffin/120.2g	286	238	5.1	46.5	3.7	1.4
Skinny Sunrise, Starbucks*	1 Muffin/130g	255	194	4.6	36.7	3.0	1.3
Sunrise, Starbucks*	1 Muffin/150g	592	395	5.5	40.8	23.1	1.9

STARBUCKS

INFO/WEIGHT	Measure	per Measure KCAL	KCAL	PROT	CARB	FAT	FIBRE
MUFFIN							
White Chocolate & Strawberry, Starbucks*	1 Muffin/142g	583	411	5.7	49.0	23.6	2.3
PANINI							
Cheese & Marmite, Breakfast, Starbucks*	1 Serving/100g	441	441	20.0	47.7	18.9	1.3
Egg & Bacon, Starbucks*	1 Panini/210g	458	218	11.1	22.0	9.5	0.0
Grilled Chicken Salsa, Lightly Spiced, Starbucks*	1 Pack/237.7g	386	162	7.9	25.0	3.4	2.0
Grilled Chicken Salsa, With Creme Fraiche, Starbucks*	1 Panini/180g	385	214	10.4	32.9	4.5	0.0
Mozzarella With Sun Dried Tomatoes & Olives, Starbucks*	1 Serving/255g	903	354	6.6	21.6	26.8	0.0
Pastrami, Starbucks*	1 Serving/200g	630	315	15.0	28.5	18.0	0.0
Roasted Vegetables & Cheese, Starbucks*	1 Pack/215g	542	252	8.7	20.6	15.1	0.0
Sausage, Egg & Baked Bean, Starbucks*	1 Panini/100g	395	395	16.9	59.8	9.8	1.5
SALAD							
Chicken Caesar, Starbucks*	1 Serving/233g	403	173	8.7	18.0	7.9	1.2
Salmon Nicoise, Starbucks*	1 Pack/260g	291	112	6.9	7.2	7.0	1.0
SANDWICH							
BLT, Starbucks*	1 Pack/190g	437	230	7.7	28.3	9.6	0.0
Beef, & Horseradish, Roast, Starbucks*	1 Pack/200g	546	273	18.7	23.1	11.1	1.0
Cheddar, & Italian Style Roasted Vegetables, Starbucks*	1 Pack/223g	553	248	5.3	25.8	13.7	0.0
Cheese, & Tomato, & Apple Chutney, Half Fat, Starbucks*	1 Pack/200g	318	159	8.8	21.3	4.2	0.0
Chicken, & Bacon, Club, Starbucks	1 Pack/252g	590	234	11.5	12.8	15.3	0.0
Chicken, Lightly Spiced, Starbucks*	1 Pack/200g	286	143	11.2	18.2	2.4	0.0
Egg Mayonnaise, & Cress, Starbucks*	1 Pack/202g	450	223	9.5	18.5	12.3	0.0
Ham, & Tomato, Smoked, Starbucks*	1 Pack/206g	297	144	5.2	22.0	3.9	0.0
Ham, York, Starbucks*	1 Pack/208g	341	164	10.4	21.2	4.2	2.9
Houmous, With Crunchy Vegetables, Starbucks*	1 Pack/218.9g	359	164	4.7	26.4	4.4	2.9
Soft Cheese, & Tomato, Extra Light, Starbucks*	1 Pack/186g	283	152	8.0	24.0	2.7	3.1
Tuna Mayonnaise, & Spring Onions, Starbucks*	1 Pack/209g	318	152	9.0	19.9	4.0	1.5
Turkey, & Salad, Smoked, Starbucks*	1 Pack/198g	303	153	10.8	22.3	2.4	1.5
Turkey, Pork & Herb, Starbucks*	1 Pack/198g	465	235	11.7	22.6	10.8	2.1
SCONE							
Blueberry, Starbucks*	1 Serving/128g	460	359	3.9	53.1	14.1	2.3
SYRUP							
Hazelnut Flavoured, Starbucks*	1 Pump/10g	20	200	0.0	50.0	0.0	0.0
TEA							
Brewed, Starbucks*	1 Tall/354ml	0	0	0.0	0.0	0.0	0.0
Chai, Latte, Skimmed Milk, Grande, Tazo, Starbucks*	1 Grande/473ml	234	49	1.8	10.8	0.0	0.0
Chai, Latte, Skimmed Milk, Tall, Tazo, Starbucks*	1 Tall/354ml	171	48	1.8	10.5	0.0	0.1
Chai, Latte, Skimmed Milk, Venti, Tazo, Starbucks*	1 Venti/591ml	295	50	1.8	10.8	0.0	0.1
Chai, Latte, Whole Milk, Grande, Tazo, Starbucks*	1 Grande/473ml	286	60	1.6	10.6	1.5	0.0
Chai, Latte, Whole Milk, Tall, Tazo, Starbucks*	1 Tall/354ml	210	59	1.6	10.2	1.5	0.1
Chai, Latte, Whole Milk, Venti, Tazo, Starbucks*	1 Venti/591ml	362	61	1.7	10.5	1.6	0.1
Iced, Chai, Latte, Skimmed Milk, Grande, Tazo,Starbucks*	1 Grande/473ml	225	48	1.6	10.6	0.0	0.0
Iced, Chai, Latte, Skimmed Milk, Tall, Tazo, Starbucks*	1 Tall/354ml	165	47	1.6	10.2	0.0	0.0
Iced, Chai, Latte, Skimmed Milk, Venti, Tazo, Starbucks*	1 Venti/591ml	244	41	1.4	9.0	0.0	0.0
Iced, Chai, Latte, Whole Milk, Grande, Tazo, Starbucks*	1 Grande/473ml	271	57	1.5	10.2	1.4	0.0
Iced, Chai, Latte, Whole Milk, Tall, Tazo, Starbucks*	1 Tall/354ml	199	56	1.4	9.9	1.3	0.0
Iced, Chai, Latte, Whole Milk, Venti, Tazo, Starbucks*	1 Venti/591ml	295	50	1.3	8.8	1.2	0.0
Iced, Starbucks*	1 Tall/354ml	0	0	0.0	0.0	0.0	0.0
WAFFLES							
Caramel, Starbucks*	1 Waffle/30g	140	467	4.3	66.7	20.3	1.3
WRAP							
Houmous & Falafel, Starbucks*	1 Pack/232g	404	174	5.4	28.8	3.9	2.5
Prawn Caesar, Starbucks*	1 Pack/173.1g	464	268	11.4	20.2	15.7	1.1

	Measure INFO/WEIGHT	per Measure KCAL	Nutrition Values per 100g / 100ml				
			KCAL	PROT	CARB	FAT	FIBRE

STARBUCKS

YOGHURT

	Measure INFO/WEIGHT	per Measure KCAL	KCAL	PROT	CARB	FAT	FIBRE
Blueberry, Starbucks*	1 Pot/130g	116	89	4.4	17.8	0.0	0.0

SUBWAY

BACON

Subway*	2 Strips/9g	34	378	22.2	16.7	26.7	0.0

BREAD

Rolls, Deli Style, Subway*	1 Roll/75g	187	249	8.0	49.3	2.8	1.3
Rolls, Honey Oat, Submarine, 6", Subway*	1 Roll/101g	223	221	7.9	40.6	2.9	2.9
Rolls, Monterey Cheddar, Submarine, 6", Subway*	1 Roll/95g	226	238	10.5	36.8	5.4	2.1
Rolls, White, Submarine, 6", Subway*	1 Roll/85g	185	218	8.2	41.2	2.1	2.3

CHEESE

Cheddar, Processed, Subway*	1 Serving/12g	44	367	19.2	2.5	30.0	0.0

COOKIES

Chocolate Chip, Double, Subway*	1 Cookie/47g	213	453	5.1	57.5	23.4	2.3
M & M, Subway*	1 Cookie/47g	206	438	5.1	59.6	19.8	3.2
Oatmeal Raisin, Subway*	1 Cookie/47g	193	411	4.9	59.6	16.6	1.1

DRESSING

Salad, Honey Mustard, Subway*	1 Serving/50g	200	400	0.8	16.0	38.0	0.0
Salad, Ranch, Subway*	1 Serving/50g	98	196	0.0	2.0	20.0	0.0

MAYONNAISE

Subway*	1 Serving/15g	110	733	0.0	0.0	80.0	0.0

OIL

Olive, Blend, Subway*	1 Serving/5g	44	880	0.0	0.0	100.0	0.0

SALAD

Chicken, Grilled, No Dressing, Subway*	1 Salad/385g	146	38	5.2	2.1	0.8	1.0
Club, No Dressing, Subway*	1 Salad/404g	157	39	5.5	2.2	0.7	1.0
Tuna, No Dressing, Subway*	1 Salad/397g	363	91	4.0	2.3	7.3	1.0

SANDWICH

Beef, & Cheese, Roast, Subway*	6" Pack/222g	291	131	8.6	20.3	2.3	1.8
Beef, Roast, Deli Style, Subway*	1 Sandwich/170g	248	146	9.4	22.9	1.8	1.2
Beef, Roast, On White, Plain, Subway*	1 Pack/222g	289	130	8.5	20.0	2.3	1.8
Chicken, & Salad, Subway*	1 serving/236g	330	140	10.2	19.9	2.1	2.1
Chicken, Teriyaki, Subway*	6" Sub/269g	370	138	9.7	21.9	1.9	1.5
Ham, & Salad, Subway*	1 serving/222g	290	131	8.1	20.7	2.3	1.8
Ham, Deli Style, Subway*	1 Sandwich/160g	225	141	6.9	24.4	1.8	1.2
Sub, Beef, Roast, 6", Subway*	1 Sandwich/235g	283	120	8.9	17.0	1.7	1.6
Sub, Chicken, Roasted, 6", Subway*	1 Sandwich/249g	304	122	10.0	15.3	2.1	1.6
Sub, Chicken, Teriyaki, & Sweet Onion, 6", Subway*	1 Sandwich/283g	364	129	8.8	19.1	1.8	0.5
Sub, Ham, & Turkey, Subway*	1 Pack/235g	294	125	8.5	19.6	2.1	1.7
Sub, Ham, 6", Subway*	1 Sandwich/235g	261	111	6.8	16.6	1.7	1.6
Sub, Ham, Honey Mustard, 6", Subway*	1 Sandwich/230g	281	122	7.4	19.1	1.7	1.7
Sub, Italian BMT, 6", Subway*	1 Sandwich/254g	446	176	8.3	15.4	9.1	1.6
Sub, Meatball Marinara, Hot Melt, 6", Subway*	1 Sandwich	441	151	7.9	15.7	6.1	1.4
Sub, Meatballs, With Cheese & Salad, Subway*	1 Pack/286g	526	184	8.4	18.5	9.1	2.1
Sub, Seafood Sensation, 6", Subway*	1 Sandwich/261g	437	167	5.4	17.2	8.4	1.5
Sub, Tuna, 6", Subway*	1 Sandwich/261g	514	197	7.7	14.9	11.9	1.5
Sub, Turkey, & Ham, 6", Subway*	1 Sandwich/244g	271	111	7.8	16.0	1.6	1.6
Sub, Turkey, Ham & Bacon, Hot Melt, 6", Subway*	1 Sandwich/266g	350	132	8.7	15.4	3.8	1.5
Tuna Mayonnaise, Subway*	1 Serving/255g	430	169	7.8	18.0	7.5	2.0
Tuna, & Chesse, Deli Style, Subway*	1 Sandwich/180g	370	206	7.8	21.7	10.0	1.1
Turkey, Deli Style, Subway*	1 Sandwich/170g	236	139	8.2	22.9	1.7	1.2
Veggie Delite, 6", Subway*	1 Sandwich/178g	210	118	3.9	21.4	1.5	2.2

INFO/WEIGHT	Measure	per Measure KCAL	Nutrition Values per 100g / 100ml KCAL	PROT	CARB	FAT	FIBRE

SUBWAY

SAUCE

	Measure INFO/WEIGHT	per Measure KCAL	KCAL	PROT	CARB	FAT	FIBRE
Chipotle, Southwest, Subway*	1 Serving/21g	85	405	1.4	9.5	41.4	0.0
TORTILLA							
Wrap, Plain, Subway*	1 Wrap/70g	109	156	15.7	8.6	5.0	17.1
WRAP							
Chicken, & Bacon Ranch, With Chesse, Subway*	1 Wrap/256g	374	146	13.3	3.9	7.8	5.0
Tuna, & Cheese, Subway*	1 Wrap/210g	406	193	10.0	3.8	14.8	6.1
Turkey & Bacon, With Chipotle Sauce, Melt, Subway*	1 Wrap/242g	386	160	12.0	5.0	9.5	5.3
Turkey, Subway*	1 Wrap/184g	157	85	10.9	4.4	1.9	7.1
WIMPY							
BREAKFAST							
All Day, Wimpy*	1 Breakfast/300g	715	238	10.1	15.3	15.3	0.0
BURGERS							
Cheeseburger, Bacon, Wimpy*	1 Burger/145g	345	238	13.2	22.3	10.6	0.0
Cheeseburger, Wimpy*	1 Burger/125g	315	252	13.4	25.8	10.5	0.0
Hamburger, Wimpy*	1 Burger/105g	270	257	13.1	30.8	9.1	0.0
Quarter Pounders, Wimpy*	1 Burger/170g	918	540	28.1	42.3	29.9	6.7
Quater Pounder, With Chesse, Wimpy*	1 Burger/190g	585	308	16.4	22.3	17.6	0.0
Quorn, In A Bun, Wimpy*	1 Burger/170g	380	224	9.8	22.1	10.7	0.0
Spicy Bean, Wimpy*	1 Burger/205g	520	254	7.9	33.5	10.7	0.0
The Classic, Kingsize, Wimpy*	1 Burger/240g	550	229	10.9	13.9	12.6	0.0
The Classic, Wimpy*	1 Burger/160g	340	213	12.2	20.8	9.1	0.0
The Classic, With Cheese & Bacon, Wimpy*	1 Burger/195g	415	213	12.8	17.1	10.4	0.0
The Classic, With Cheese, Wimpy*	1 Burger/180g	385	214	12.5	18.5	10.0	0.0
CHICKEN &							
Chips, Chunks, Wimpy*	1 Serving/290g	770	266	9.4	27.6	13.1	0.0
CHIPS							
Wimpy*	1 Serving/80g	295	369	4.6	53.0	15.1	0.0
FISH & CHIPS							
Wimpy*	1 Burger/255g	490	192	10.9	18.6	8.3	0.0
FRANKFURTERS							
Wimpy*	1 Frank/150g	405	270	12.4	21.8	14.9	0.0
With Cheese, Wimpy*	1 Frank/170g	450	265	12.7	19.2	17.0	0.0
FRIES							
Wimpy*	1 Serving/100g	369	369	4.6	53.0	15.1	4.4
GRILL							
Bacon, Classic, Wimpy*	1 Grill/310g	740	239	11.8	15.0	15.8	0.0
Classic, Wimpy*	1 Grill/320g	820	256	12.3	14.4	16.7	0.0
Frankfurter, Wimpy*	1 Grill/315g	750	238	10.8	13.6	15.8	0.0
Quaterpounder, Wimpy*	1 Grill/395g	955	242	12.8	11.8	16.1	0.0
RIBS							
Pork, BBQ, In A Bun, Wimpy*	1 Rib/170g	555	326	17.7	20.2	11.4	0.0
ROLL							
Bacon & Egg, In A Bun, Wimpy*	1 Roll/165g	345	209	11.4	19.6	9.3	0.0
Bacon, In A Bun, Wimpy*	1 Roll/105g	230	219	9.8	30.8	6.4	0.0

Useful Resources

Diabetes Advice
Diabetes UK is the leading charity working for people with diabetes. Their mission is to improve the lives of people with diabetes and to work towards a future without diabetes.
Contact: 020 7424 1000
Website: www.diabetes.org.uk

Eating Disorders
The Eating Disorders Association provides information, help and support for people affected by eating disorders, particularly anorexia and bulimia.
Contact 0870 770 3256
Website: www.edauk.com

Exercise Equipment for Home
Diet and Fitness Resources has a range of equipment for exercise at home, along with diet tools such as food diaries and a weight loss kit. at home.
Contact: 01733 345592
Website: www.dietandfitnessresources.co.uk

Healthy Eating
The British Nutrition Foundation has lots of in depth information on healthy eating The Foundation aims to promote the nutritional wellbeing of society through the impartial interpretation and dissemination of scientifically based nutritional knowledge and advice.
Contact: 020 7404 6747
Website: www.nutrition.org.uk

Keep Fit
The Keep Fit Association organises fitness classes throughout the UK.
Contact: 020 8692 9566
Website: www.keepfit.org.uk

Salt and Health
CASH (Consensus Action on Salt and Health) is working to reach a consensus with the food industry and Government to bring about a reduction in the amount of salt in processed foods and in the diet generally.
Contact: 0208 266 6498
Website: www.actiononsalt.org.uk

Safety and Standards
The Food Standards Agency is an independent watchdog, set up to protect the public's health and consumer interests in relation to food.
Contact: 020 7276 8000
Website: www.foodstandards.gov.uk

Vegetarian Diet Advice
The Vegetarian Society is an educational charity promoting understanding and respect for vegetarian lifestyles
They offer advice on nutritional issues and provide free information to individuals, companies and organisations.
Contact: 0161 925 2000
Website: www.vegsoc.org

Weight Loss
Weight Loss Resources is home to the UK's biggest calorie and nutrition database along with diaries and tools for weight loss.
Contact: 01733 345592
Website: www.weightlossresources.co.uk

Feedback

If you have any comments or suggestions about the Calorie, Carb & Fat Bible, or would like further information on Weight Loss Resources, please call, email, or write to them:

Email: helpteam@weightlossresources.co.uk
Tel: 01733 345592
Address: Weight Loss Resources,
            Remus House,
            Peterborough,
            PE2 9JX

Reviews for The Calorie Carb & Fat Bible

WOMAN nutritionist Angela Dowden says: "There are so many faddy diet books around, but what it boils down to is the amount of calories you actually take into your body compared with the amount you expend in exercise and activity. This book gives you all that basic information so you can work out your daily needs, plus the calorie counts of a vast range of supermarket foods."

WOMAN Magazine: 9 Books You Shouldn't Be Without

"To help you make low-cal choices everyday, invest in a copy."

ZEST Magazine

"There's only one way to lose the lard... and that's to eat less. Nobody pretends losing the pounds you so enthusiastically piled on in the first place will be easy. But a good guide to exactly what you're putting in your mouth is the one thing your average slimmer cannot do without.

"So, with two stones down and a fair few still to go, my joy knew no bounds when this weighty tome landed on my desk.

"Jam-packed with info on dieting, and full to bursting point with the calorie, carbohydrate and fat values of thousands of different foods, including branded ones, it's the perfect weight-loss tool for those of us needing to keep an eye on our daily intake."

Evening Express City Edition (Aberdeen)

"What a brilliant book, I know I'll be sinking my teeth into it regularly!"

Amanda Ursell

"As a fitness fanatic and keen sportsman, I constantly monitor weight, and was quite happy with my eleven stone frame. That was, until I looked up my body mass index, in the chart on page 14, of the 2002 edition of 'The Calorie, Carb and Fat Bible'.

"Imagine my surprise, when I found I was nearly in the 'Overweight' category!

"I decided to lose half a stone, which would put me well within the 'Normal weight' range.

"The book contains tables, according to age and activity level, for males and females, of the number of calories required to maintain weight. In order to lose weight, I have to consume less than the figure for my age and activity level.

"Three weeks later, with the help of the book, which gives nutrition values (calories, carbohydrate, protein, fat, fibre and alcohol) of over 15,000 basic and branded foods, I have already lost three pounds.

"I may achieve my goal before Christmas, but there could be a few extra pounds to shed by the New Year!"

South Yorkshire Times

"I felt quite moved by the firm but compassionate tone adopted and the (thank God) no-nonsense fact-based approach... The authors really seem to understand the problem of slimming. Most people (myself included) are very depressed at being overweight and I think the encouraging but not hectoring tone is excellent."

Dr John Campion

"I recently bought your book called the Calorie, Carb & Fat Bible and would love to tell you what a brilliant book it is. I have recently started a weight management programme and I honestly don't know where I'd be without your book. It has helped me a lot and given me some really good advice."

Rachel Mitchell

About Weight Loss Resources

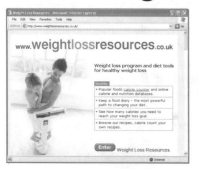

"What this does is put you in control with no guilt, no awful groups and no negativity! Fill in your food diary, get support on the boards and watch it fall off!"

LINDAB, Weight Loss Resources Member

How Does It Work?

Weight Loss Resources is home to the UK's biggest online calorie and nutrition database. You simply tap in your height, weight, age and basic activity level - set a weight loss goal, and the programme does all the necessary calculations.

What Does It Do?

The site enables you to keep a food diary which keeps running totals of calories, fat, fibre, carbs, proteins and portions of fruit and veg. You can also keep an exercise diary which adds the calories you use during exercise. At the end of a week, you update your weight and get reports and graphs on your progress.

How Will It Help?

You'll learn a great deal about how your eating and drinking habits affect your weight and how healthy they are. Using the diaries and other tools you'll be able to make changes that suit your tastes and your lifestyle. The result is weight loss totally tailored to your needs and preferences. A method you can stick with that will help you learn how to eat well for life!

Try It Free!

Go to **www.weightlossresources.co.uk** and take a completely free, no obligation, 3 day trial. If you like what you see you can sign up for membership from £7 per month.